CASES
in Clinical Medicine

Pamela Moyers Scott, PA-C, MPAS, DFAAPA

Center for Graduate Studies
West Coast University
Los Angeles, CA

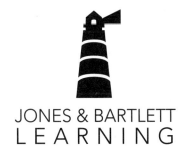

JONES & BARTLETT
LEARNING

World Headquarters

Jones & Bartlett Learning
40 Tall Pine Drive
Sudbury, MA 01776
978-443-5000
info@jblearning.com
www.jblearning.com

Jones & Bartlett Learning
Canada
6339 Ormindale Way
Mississauga, Ontario L5V 1J2
Canada

Jones & Bartlett Learning
International
Barb House, Barb Mews
London W6 7PA
United Kingdom

Jones & Bartlett Learning books and products are available through most bookstores and online booksellers. To contact Jones & Bartlett Learning directly, call 800-832-0034, fax 978-443-8000, or visit our website, www.jblearning.com.

Substantial discounts on bulk quantities of Jones & Bartlett Learning publications are available to corporations, professional associations, and other qualified organizations. For details and specific discount information, contact the special sales department at Jones & Bartlett Learning via the above contact information or send an email to specialsales@jblearning.com.

The author, editor, and publisher have made every effort to provide accurate information. However, they are not responsible for errors, omissions, or for any outcomes related to the use of the contents of this book and take no responsibility for the use of the products and procedures described. Treatments and side effects described in this book may not be applicable to all people; likewise, some people may require a dose or experience a side effect that is not described herein. Drugs and medical devices are discussed that may have limited availability controlled by the Food and Drug Administration (FDA) for use only in a research study or clinical trial. Research, clinical practice, and government regulations often change the accepted standard in this field. When consideration is being given to use of any drug in the clinical setting, the healthcare provider or reader is responsible for determining FDA status of the drug, reading the package insert, and reviewing prescribing information for the most up-to-date recommendations on dose, precautions, and contraindications, and determining the appropriate usage for the product. This is especially important in the case of drugs that are new or seldom used.

Production Credits

Publisher: David Cella
Acquisitions Editor: Katey Birtcher
Associate Editor: Maro Gartside
Production Director: Amy Rose
Senior Production Editor: Renée Sekerak
Marketing Manager: Grace Richards
Manufacturing and Inventory Control Supervisor: Amy Bacus
Composition: Glyph International
Cover Design: Kristin E. Parker

Photo Research and Permissions Supervisor: Christine Myaskovsky
Assistant Photo Researcher: Rebecca Ritter
Cover Images: Nurse assists with egg retrieval © Monkey Business Images/Dreamstime.com; Doctors reviewing a chart © Redbaron/Dreamstime.com; Doctor checking glands © Forestpath/Dreamstime.com; Detail of stethoscope © Olivier Le Queinec/Dreamstime.com
Printing and Binding: Courier Stoughton
Cover Printing: Courier Stoughton

Library of Congress Cataloging-in-Publication Data

Scott, Pamela Moyers.
Cases in clinical medicine / Pamela Moyers Scott.
        p. cm.
    ISBN 978-0-7637-7180-5 (alk. paper)
    1. Clinical medicine—Case studies. 2. Clinical medicine—Problems, exercises, etc. I. Title.
    RC66.S36 2011
    616—dc22

                                                                        2010046759

6048

Printed in the United States of America
15 14 13 12 11   10 9 8 7 6 5 4 3 2 1

This book is dedicated to my father with love.
Thanks for always being there for me.

Contents

Contents

Contents

Introduction

Welcome to one of the most rewarding, challenging, exciting, and fastest-growing careers in the world—the physician assistant (PA) profession!

Cases in Clinical Medicine has been specially developed to assist PA students' transition from the didactic to the clinical portion of their medical training by utilizing case-based learning (CBL). However, it would be appropriate for use by allopathic and osteopathic medical students, nurse practitioner students, and other health professions' students.

Until now, most of your education has been provided in the form of lecture-based learning. This is an appropriate method to obtain a solid core of medical knowledge. By contrast, CBL teaches you by providing a brief case scenario in which you must assimilate your analytical skills with this medical knowledge to appropriately manage this fictitious patient's case as opposed to the traditional method of memorizing and regurgitating facts. Thus, CBL more closely simulates the actual practice of medicine.

Additionally, to this point in your training, most of your history and physical examination skills have been limited to the performance of a complete history and physical (H&P). This too provides you with a sound basis in, and understanding of, the techniques involved. However, unfortunately, in the actual practice of medicine there is insufficient time to perform an entire history and physical examination during every patient encounter. Therefore, in a problem-focused visit, you will be called upon to utilize your clinical skills and knowledge of evidence-based medicine to limit the components of the patient's history, portions of the physical examination, and diagnostic studies to those that are most likely to yield useful clinical information on which to formulate the patient's differential diagnosis list, correct diagnosis, and treatment plan with respect to the patient's chief complaint.

Many guidelines have been developed by reputable organized specialty medical societies and government agencies as a tool to assist you in your evaluation and treatment of the patients with certain medical conditions. However, it is important to remember that these are just what they say they are—guidelines. Therefore, sound medical knowledge and good clinical skills are required to use them appropriately.

Cases in Clinical Medicine has been created to assist you in developing the aforementioned skills. In the first half of each chapter in this book, you will be provided basic histories on fictitious patients. This information will be followed by a series of approximately five options in five different categories; the first three are additional historical data, physical examination components, and diagnostic tests. Utilizing your

medical knowledge, clinical expertise, and analytical skills, you will be asked to determine which of the given choice(s) is/are essential, or pertinent, in working to achieve the correct diagnosis and what is extraneous for each patient complaint. Additionally, you should be able to provide justification for your decisions. Unless stated otherwise, for each question, *none* to *all* of the options can be correct.

Regardless of whether an item in the history, physical examination, and diagnostic study sections is determined to be essential or nonessential, you will be provided with a response for it. For example, if one of the components of a physical examination is a heart examination, you will be provided with the findings of the heart examination in the subsequent physical examination section, regardless of whether a heart examination is essential or nonessential to the patient's complaint. Therefore, you should not let the appearance of this information influence your decisions.

You will note that some of the questions, especially in the history section, have more than one component. The reasoning behind this approach is that in the clinical setting, if you get a positive response to a question, you would follow it up with other ones pertaining to that topic. Or, you might ask a series of questions along the same lines to rule in or eliminate a potential differential diagnosis. Therefore, in order to provide as much information on the topic as possible, these "cluster" questions have been combined into a single option instead of being asked separately. In general, anytime a positive response is elicited from the patient, additional questioning is required for further clarification of the symptom.

Occasionally, you will see terminology stating a certain component of the physical examination is unremarkable. Although this is useful in medical writing to minimize the size of the case presentation, it is never appropriate in the charting of an actual patient encounter. The use of the abbreviation "wnl" for "within normal limits" is likewise not an acceptable charting term. In fact, it is frequently the basis of medical jokes where it is stated to mean "we never looked." In correct charting, you must always list what components were performed along with their findings.

Essentially, by the time you have completed your history and physical examination, you should have a fairly good idea of the patient's diagnosis (or at least a limited differential diagnosis list). Diagnostic studies are utilized to confirm your suspicions. Their only other purpose is to monitor the patient's progress in chronic conditions. They should never be ordered at random in hopes that they will provide a clue to the patient's diagnosis. Therefore, any diagnostic test that is ordered should provide information that assists directly in appropriately evaluating and treating the patient's chief complaint.

Furthermore, it is essential for the healthcare provider (HCP) to realize that the "normal" values established for diagnostic tests are derived from the value that is found in 95% of the adult population (although some do contain age-specific ranges). Therefore, it is possible for a patient to have a result that is slightly lower or slightly higher than the stated "normal" value and still be "normal" for that patient. It goes back to the old axiom, "Treat the patient, not the test."

After you complete these three sections, you will be asked a question regarding the fictitious patient's most likely diagnosis; unless otherwise stated, there will only be a single response for this question. This will be followed by a question regarding the treatment plan for the patient.

Every available option is often *not* going to be included for each case discussed. For example, all treatment plans, regardless of the purpose of the patient's visit, *must* include the following information: patient education regarding his or her current medical condition; nonprescription treatments (if any) and instructions for usage; medication(s) (if any) prescribed, including usage, mechanism of action, and possible adverse effects; when the patient's next appointment is going to be scheduled, why it is being scheduled, and the importance of keeping it; what to do if symptoms increase, adverse effects of the medication occur, or some other question or problem occurs in the interim; and recommended age-appropriate health maintenance visits, including appropriate diagnostic testing and immunizations, if due, past due, or not previously done. Obviously, making each of these an option in all the cases would severely limit the amount of other information that could be included and discussed.

Similarly, problem-focused histories and physical examinations do not contain all the information as a complete H&P does. However, there are some components that are essential to every encounter. In addition to a chief complaint and history of the present illness (HPI), a pertinent review of systems (ROS) is required. Furthermore, the following data need to be reviewed with the patient at every visit: past medical history, past surgical history, past hospitalization history, medications (including prescription, over-the-counter, vitamins, supplements, herbal preparation, and contraceptive methods), medication allergies, smoking history (including number of cigarettes per day, how long patient has smoked, when the patient plans to quit smoking, and when patient quit if a past smoker), alcohol history (including number and type of drinks at setting and frequency), illicit drug use, date and normalcy of last menses in reproductive-aged females, and status of last health maintenance educational examination (including diagnostic testing and immunization). The only requirement for a physical examination is a complete set of vital signs including height, weight, pulse, blood pressure, respirations, and temperature. The only exception would be height on an adult; it is only necessary to perform it once a year.

The usage of electronic medical records (EMRs), summarizing forms, flow charts, and printed patient educational materials can assist in expediting this process. Furthermore, much of this information can be obtained by a trusted nurse, nursing assistant, or medical assistant and reviewed by the HCP to further streamline the process.

Although the majority of the cases in this book follow the typical, structured, nonurgent pattern of medical care—obtaining an appropriate history, performing a focused physical examination, ordering relevant diagnostic studies, establishing a diagnosis, and instituting an appropriate treatment plan—in the real-world practice of medicine many of these steps are going on simultaneously based on the severity of the patient's condition and type of illness.

The second half of each chapter provides you with the correct responses and the reasoning behind why the given response is essential or nonessential (or correct or incorrect) plus additional clinical knowledge and epidemiologic data regarding the case. Those options identified as "nonessential" are designated as such primarily because the information obtained by that selection is extremely unlikely to provide any useful clinical information on which to base the patient's diagnosis and/or treatment plan; hence, they do not need to be performed as part of a problem-focused evaluation. Therefore, in some of these cases, there will be no further explanation regarding their exclusion from the patient's evaluation.

Because the practice of medicine is an art utilizing science, there is not a "one size fits all" or "cookbook" approach that can be used to evaluate patients with similar complaints. As stated previously, the options listed in these cases are *not* the only potential historical questions, physical examination components, diagnostic tests, or treatment options that might be required or considered in an actual clinical situation. Additionally, this book is not meant to be a thorough clinical review of the topics presented in the cases. Therefore, this textbook is not designed and should not be utilized as a reference for the diagnosing and treating of patients in the clinical setting. The names and cases are fictitious; any resemblance to an actual patient is purely coincidental. *Cases in Clinical Medicine* can also be a helpful adjunct to assist you as you prepare for the initial Physician Assistant National Certification Examination (PANCE) sponsored by the National Commission on the Certification of Physician Assistants (NCCPA). The chapters and topics are based on the blueprint provided by the NCCPA regarding the exam content. It can also serve as an appropriate component of review materials for the generalist component of the recertification examination (Physician Assistant National Recertifying Examination [PANRE]).

Best of luck as you begin your career as a physician assistant!

How to Utilize This Textbook

RECOMMENDED

- Read the case presentation.
- From the choices provided, determine which additional components of a medical history are essential to obtain from the case patient in order to formulate an appropriate differential diagnosis list. Remember that none to all of the responses can be correct.
- Review the information provided by the patient and/or his or her legal guardian/accompanying individual. Remember, some type of additional data is going to be supplied for each choice, even if it is a nonessential selection.
- From the choices provided, determine which components of a physical examination are essential in establishing (following) the patient's working diagnosis from the list of differential diagnoses. Remember that none to all of the responses can be correct.
- Review the information obtained from the physical examination, keeping in mind that some type of finding is going to be supplied for each choice, even if it is a nonessential selection.
- From the choices provided, determine which diagnostic studies are essential to confirm the working diagnosis, should be performed as a baseline study, to follow-up on chronic medical condtitions. Again, remember that none to all of the responses could be correct.
- Review the information obtained by the diagnostic studies, keeping in mind that some type of result is going to be supplied for each choice, even if it is a nonessential selection. Laboratory reference ranges are provided.
- Based on this information, select the most likely diagnosis (unless the text specifically instructs you to select more than one) from the choices provided for the patient.
- From the list provided, select the most appropriate components of a treatment plan for the patient, remembering that none to all of the responses could be correct.
- Compare your responses with those provided in the second half of the chapter and review the rationales explaining why the selections were essential versus nonessential (or correct vs incorrect) for all items.
- Remember, you should be able to provide justification to explain why you made your particular selections.

- For additional information on a particular topic, obtain and review the accompanying reference/additional reading materials found at the end of each chapter.

ALTERNATIVE

- Read the case presentation.
- From the choices provided, determine which additional components of a medical history are essential to obtain from the case patient in order to formulate an appropriate differential diagnosis list. Remember that none to all of the responses could be correct.
- Compare responses with those provided in the second half of the chapter and review the rational for each of the selections causing them to be essential versus nonessential.
- Review the information provided in the patient response section in the first part of the chapter. Remember that regardless of whether the item was essential or nonessential, some type of additional data is going to be supplied for each choice.
- From the choices provided, determine which components of a physical examination are essential in establishing the patient's working diagnosis from the list of differential diagnoses. Remember that none to all of the responses could be correct.
- Compare responses with those provided in the second portion of the chapter and review the reasons selections were essential versus nonessential for each item.
- Review the information obtained by the physical examination in the first part of the chapter, keeping in mind that some type of finding is going to be supplied for each choice, even if it is a nonessential selection.
- From the choices provided, determine which diagnostic components are essential to confirm the working diagnosis. Remember that none to all of the responses could be correct.
- Compare responses with those provided in the second half of the chapter and review the rationale for each item regardless if essential or nonessential.
- Review the diagnostic results provided in the first portion of the chapter, keeping in mind that a result is going to appear for each choice, regardless of whether it was determined to be essential or not.

- Based on this information, select the most likely diagnosis (unless the text specifically instructs you to select more than one) from the choices provided for the patient.
- Compare the diagnosis with those provided in the second half of the chapter and review the reasons each selection was correct or incorrect.
- From the list provided in the first part of the chapter, select the most appropriate components of a treatment plan for the patient and explain why. Remember that none to all of the responses could be correct.

- Compare responses with those provided in the second part of the book and review the reasons the selection was correct or incorrect.
- Remember, you should be able to provide justification for why you made your particular selections.
- For additional information on a particular topic, obtain and review the accompanying reference/additional reading materials contained at the end of each chapter.

Reviewers

The author would like to acknowledge and thank the following for their valuable input and assistance in reviewing sections of this book. Without their guidance, this book would not be what it is today. Thank you!

Theresa A. Berry, MD, MEd
Assistant Professor
School of Medicine
Emory University

Kim Cavanagh, MPAS, PA-C
Assistant Professor/Clinical Coordinator
Physician Assistant Department
Gannon University

Jean Covino, DHSc, MPA, PA-C
Associate Clinical Professor
Physician Assistant Studies
Coordinator
Physician Assistant Graduate Education
Physician Assistant Program
PACE University-Lenox Hill Hospital

Jennifer D. Freer, MSPAS, PA-C
Assistant Professor/Clinical Coordinator
Physician Assistant Department
Morosky College of Health Professions and Sciences
Gannon University

Virginia H. Joslin, PA-C, MPH
Assistant Professor and Chief
Physician Assistant Program Division
Department of Family and Preventive Medicine
School of Medicine
Emory University

Jackie Kazik, MA, PA-C
Waukesha Memorial Hospital
Emergency Department
Adjunct Faculty
Marquette University

Mary Ann Laxen, PA-C, MAB
Program Director
School of Medicine and Health Sciences
Department of Family and Community Medicine
Physician Assistant Program
University of North Dakota

Daniela Livingston, MD, PA-C
Instructor
Physician Assistant Program
College of Nursing and Health Professions
Drexel University

Angela Mesa-Taylor, MPAS, PA-C
Assistant Professor
Nova Southeastern University

Karen A. Newell, PA-C, MMSc
Academic Coordinator
School of Medicine
Emory University

Allan Platt, PA-C, MMSc
Faculty
Physician Assistant Program
School of Medicine
Emory University

Evan E. Wolf, MMSc, RPA-C
NCCPA, ACC Cardiac Care Associate
Cardiology Associates of Schenectady

CASES IN CARDIOVASCULAR MEDICINE*

CASE 1-1

Alice Blankenship

Mrs. Blankenship is an 69-year-old African American female who presents for follow-up on her blood pressure (BP). At her regular visit 1 month ago, it was slightly elevated at 138/88 mm Hg. Her only other known medical problem is type 2 diabetes mellitus of 3 years' duration. It is currently well controlled with metformin and lifestyle modifications. However, she admits to not following her diet "as close as I could" and not exercising regularly.

She did have her daughter, who is a nurse, check her BP at home in the interim. The first reading, approximately 3 weeks ago, was 134/80 mm Hg. The second reading roughly 1 week later was 138/82 mm Hg. Her daughter rechecked it last week and it was 136/84 mm Hg.

She has regular health maintenance check-ups with screening diagnostic testing and immunizations as well as regular disease-specific visits and diagnostic evaluations. She has only been hospitalized for childbirth and has never had surgery. Mrs. Blankenship is not taking any other prescription medications. She is not allergic to any medications.

1. Based on this information, which of the following questions are essential to ask Mrs. Blankenship and why?

   A. Has she been experiencing vertigo, presyncope, syncope, palpitations, unusual fatigue, or headaches?
   B. Has she been experiencing weakness in one or more of her extremities, weakness of her facial muscles, difficulty talking, dysphagia, or transient monocular blindness?
   C. Has she noticed any tachycardia, bradycardia, palpitations, changes in her hair or nails, skin rashes or discoloration, diaphoresis, tremor, snoring, or excessive sleepiness?
   D. Is she taking any over-the-counter (OTC) medications, vitamins, supplements, or herbal products?
   E. Does she have a family history of diabetes mellitus?

Patient Responses

She denies vertigo, presyncope, syncope, palpitations, fatigue, headaches, weakness in her extremities, weakness of her facial muscles, difficulty talking, dysphagia, transient monocular blindness, tachycardia, bradycardia, palpitations, changes in her hair or nails, skin rashes or discoloration, diaphoresis, tremor, snoring, or excessive sleepiness.

Mrs. Blankenship admits to daily usage of OTC ibuprofen 100 mg one pill twice a day for "arthritis" in her knees. She states that it controls her pain and stiffness. She denies taking other OTC medications, vitamins, supplements, or herbal products. Her mother and her older sister have hypertension; otherwise, her family history is negative.

2. Based on this information, which of the following components of a physical examination are essential to perform on Mrs. Blankenship and why?

   A. BP and pulse measurements in both arms in lying, sitting, and standing positions as well as BP measurement in both legs with Doppler
   B. Funduscopic examination
   C. Heart and lung examination
   D. Evaluation of all pulses
   E. Rectal examination

Physical Examination Findings

Mrs. Blankenship is 5'3" tall and weighs 165 lb (body mass index [BMI] = 29). Other vital signs are pulse, 86 beats per minute (BPM) and regular; respiratory rate, 12/min and regular; and oral temperature, 98.2°F. Her blood pressure is 134/84 mm Hg in her right arm and 136/82 mm Hg in her left arm lying supine; sitting, it is 134/86 mm Hg in her right arm and 134/88 mm Hg in her left arm; and standing, it is 130/88 mm Hg in her right arm and 134/90 mm Hg in her left arm. The BP is 144/86 mm Hg in

---

*Remember, for each question, none to all of the answers could be correct/essential or incorrect/nonessential. See page 14 for Chapter 1 answers.

her right leg and 144/84 mm Hg in her left leg. Her pulse is 82 BPM lying, 86 BPM sitting, and 90 BPM standing.

Her bilateral funduscopic examination does not reveal any opacities of her lenses. Her discs have distinct margins and a normal cup:disc ratio. There is no evidence of papilledema. Her arteries, veins, and arteriovenous crossings appear normal. Her macular area and retina are normal in color and without any abnormal lesions.

Mrs. Blankenship's heart is regular in rate and rhythm and without any murmurs, gallops, or rubs. Her apical impulse is nondisplaced and without any thrills. Her lungs are clear.

Her knees do not demonstrate any decreased range of motion, deformities, effusions, crepitus, warmth, discoloration, or tenderness.

Her carotid, subclavian, renal, and femoral pulses are normal and equal bilaterally and without bruits. Her brachial, ulnar, radial, popiteal, dorsalis pedis, and posterior tibial pulses are normal and equal bilaterally. Her abdominal aorta is normal in size and pulsation and without bruits.

Her rectal examination is normal.

3. Based on this information, which of the following diagnostic studies are essential to conduct on Mrs. Blankenship and why?

    A. Bilateral magnetic resonance imaging (MRI) of her knees
    B. Urinalysis
    C. Fasting lipid profile
    D. Electrocardiogram (ECG)
    E. Ambulatory BP monitoring

Diagnostic Results

Mrs. Blankenship's MRI, lipid panel, and ambulatory BP monitoring are pending. Her urinalysis was normal except for 1+ glucose. Her hematocrit was 42% (normal for women: 37–47). Her ECG revealed normal sinus rhythm with a rate of 80 BPM, normal axis, and no waveform or segmental changes.

4. Based on this information, in addition to her type 2 diabetes mellitus and obesity, which one of the following is Mrs. Blankenship's most likely diagnosis and why?

    A. White coat syndrome producing pseudo-hypertension
    B. Prehypertension
    C. Hypertension, stage 1
    D. Hypertension, stage 2
    E. Diabetic nephropathy-induced hypertension

5. Based on this diagnosis, which of the following are appropriate components of a treatment plan for Mrs. Blankenship and why?

    A. Dietary modification including low-sodium, low-fat, Dietary Approaches to Stop Hypertension (DASH) eating plan
    B. Start a regular aerobic exercise program, with a goal of 30 minutes daily
    C. Start triamterene 37.5 mg with hydrochlorothiazide 50 mg once every morning
    D. Start valsartan 80 mg once a day
    E. Substitute ibuprofen with acetaminophen 500 mg two pills twice a day

CASE 1-2
Betty Crane

Betty is a 15-year-old white female who presents for a preparticipation sports physical for basketball. Her permission slip has been signed by her mother; however, neither of her parents accompanies her today. She has played for the previous 2 years without difficulty. She denies having any complaints, symptoms, or concerns.

Her only known medical problem is myopia, which is corrected to 20/20 with glasses. She denies any hospitalizations or surgeries. She is not taking any prescription or over-the-counter medications, vitamins, supplements, or herbal preparations. She does not have regular health maintenance examinations; however, her immunizations are up to date. Her menarche began at the age of 13 years. She has been having regular monthly menses since, and her last one was 3 weeks ago. She is not sexually active.

1. Based on this information, which of the following questions are essential to ask Betty and why?

    A. Has she ever experienced chest pain, pressure, or discomfort; presyncope or syncope; dyspnea; or fatigue with exercise?
    B. Has she ever been diagnosed with hypertension or a heart murmur?
    C. Is there a family history of cardiac death or cardiac disability before the age of 50 years?
    D. Is there any known heart disease in the family?
    E. When does she plan on becoming sexually active?

Patient Responses

Betty denies chest pain, pressure, or discomfort; presyncope or syncope; dyspnea; fatigue with exercise; a history of hypertension or a heart murmur; a family history of cardiac death or cardiac disability before the age of 50 years; or heart disease in the family. She does not know when she plans on becoming sexually active.

2. Based on this information, which of the following components of a physical examination are essential to perform on Betty and why?

    A. Funduscopic examination (or preferably slit-lamp examination if available)
    B. Ear and hearing examination
    C. Heart evaluation
    D. Examination of femoral pulse and abdominal aorta
    E. Measurement of arm span from tip of left middle finger to tip of right middle finger and evaluation for arachnodactyly, joint hyperextensibility, joint laxity, and scoliosis

Physical Examination Findings

Betty is 5'11" tall and weighs 120 lb. Other vital signs are BP, 106/56 mm Hg in her right arm and 102/52 mm Hg in her left arm; pulse, 80 BPM and regular; respirations, 10/min and regular; and oral temperature, 97.9°F.

Her bilateral funduscopic examination does not reveal any opacities. Her discs have distinct margins and her cup:disc ratio is normal. There is no evidence of papilledema. Her arteries, veins, and arteriovenous crossings appear normal. Her macular area and retina are normal in color and without any abnormal lesions. Her lenses do not appear to be displaced. However, she does have an incidental finding of a bilaterally elongated ocular globe.

Her ear canals are normal in color and without lesions or abnormal discharge. Her tympanic membranes are normal in color, without any gross lesions; intact; and freely mobile. Her hearing is grossly normal to whisper and watch ticking at appropriate lengths.

Betty's heart is regular in rate and rhythm with a grade 3/6 systolic ejection murmur in her mitral area that radiates to her left axilla and that increases with expiration, standing up, and performing a Valsalva maneuver; however, it softens when she squats or performs isometric exercises. It is unchanged by lying in the left lateral decubitus position. She also has a grade 2/6 diastolic murmur with a click in her aortic area that increases with expiration, squatting, and isometric exercise; however, it decreases with standing upright and with performing a Valsalva maneuver. She does not have any gallops or rubs. Her apical impulse is nondisplaced and not associated with a thrill. Incidentally, pectus excavatum is noted.

Her femoral pulses are normal bilaterally. Her aortic pulse is somewhat bounding, but her aorta is normal in size. There is no bruit.

Her arm span is 6' and she has arachnodactyly as well as hyperextensible, lax joints. Her spinal examination reveals a 15° thoracic scoliosis with curvature to the right as well as a compensatory 10° lumbar scoliosis to the left and mild thoracic kyphosis.

3. Based on this information, which of the following diagnostic studies are essential to conduct on Betty and why?

A. Electrocardiogram (ECG)
B. Echocardiogram
C. Chest x-ray (CXR)
D. Abdominal ultrasound
E. Cardiac-specific troponin T and I

Diagnostic Results

Her ECG revealed normal sinus rhythm (NSR) with a rate of 80 BPM. Her echocardiogram is pending. Her CXR revealed pectus excavatum and confirmed the scoliosis and kyphosis. No other abnormalities were noted. Abdominal ultrasound revealed a normal-sized aorta without abnormal calcifications and/or aneurysms of the walls. Her cardiac troponin T was 0 ng/ml (normal: < 0.2) and her cardiac troponin I was 0 ng/ml (normal: < 0.03).

4. Based on this information, which one of the following is Betty's most likely diagnosis and why?

A. Loeys-Dietz aneurysm syndrome (LDAS)
B. Klinefelter syndrome
C. Marfan syndrome (MFS)
D. Ehlers-Danlos syndrome (EDS)
E. Congenital contractural arachnodactyly (CCA)

5. Based on this diagnosis, which of the following are appropriate components of a treatment plan for Betty and why?

A. Annual echocardiogram
B. Annual eye examination, including a slit lamp, by an ophthalmologist
C. Subacute bacterial endocarditis (SBE) prophylaxis for dental procedures
D. Annual orthopedic evaluation
E. Propranolol 10 to 20 mg twice a day initially; then, titrate every 1 to 2 weeks (to a maximum daily dose of 240 mg) to maintain exercise heart rate below 100 BPM

CASE 1-3
Carl Diaz

Carl is a 15-year-old Hispanic male who presents with his mother for follow-up on an elevated cholesterol level obtained at a free community screening approximately 1 month ago. Carl's level was 237 and his father's was 240. According to Carl's mother, the nurse who performed the test told her Carl's cholesterol was "nothing to worry about because he is still a child"; however, the nurse recommended that Carl's father have a full lipid panel as soon as possible.

His father saw his regular health care provider (HCP) last week for the lipid panel. When the HCP diagnosed her husband with "dangerously high cholesterol," she asked about Carl's test. According to her, the HCP stated, "You might want to get it rechecked," hence prompting this visit.

Carl states (and his mother confirmed) that he has no known medical problems and has never had surgery nor been hospitalized. He is not taking any prescription or over-the-counter medications, vitamins, supplements, or herbal preparations. He is not allergic to any medications. He states that he does not smoke, drink alcohol, or do illicit drugs. He has regular health maintenance check-ups with his pediatrician and his immunizations are up to date.

Carl denies headaches, dizziness, vertigo, presyncope, syncope, palpations, tachycardia, bradycardia, chest pain/pressure, heartburn, gastrointestinal upset, arm or shoulder pain, problems with gait, difficulties with walking, problems using his hands or feet, difficulties talking, problems swallowing, fatigue, diaphoresis, changes in his skin, differences in the texture of his hair and nails, polyuria, polydipsia, and recent weight change.

1. Based on this information, which of the following questions are essential to ask Carl and/or his mother and why?

A. Has Carl ever had his BP checked?
B. Was Carl's cholesterol test done while he was fasting or nonfasting?
C. What is Carl's mother's cholesterol level?
D. Has either of Carl's parents and/or grandparents been diagnosed with a myocardial infarction (MI), coronary artery disease (CAD), sudden cardiac death (SCD), a cerebral vascular accident (CVA), or peripheral vessel disease (PVD) prior to the age of 55 years?
E. Have his parents and/or grandparents been diagnosed with diabetes mellitus (including gestational diabetes) or any other serious medical condition(s)?

Patient Responses

According to Carl's mother, he had his BP checked at his last well-child visit with his pediatrician and was told it was "a little high" and "to lose some weight and get some exercise and it would not be a problem." He has done neither and has not had his BP checked since. When Carl had his cholesterol checked, he was nonfasting. However, he is fasting today.

His father's repeat total cholesterol was 245 mg/dl and he was started on medication. Carl's mother knows he had a lipoprotein panel in addition to the total cholesterol level but cannot remember the exact values. She has never had her cholesterol checked.

Carl's paternal grandfather had a nonfatal MI at the age of 62 years. His maternal grandfather was diagnosed with angina and PVD when he was 58 years old. His paternal grandmother had a CVA at the age of 70 years. All four of his grandparents and both of his parents are obese and hypertensive. His maternal grandfather has type 2 diabetes mellitus.

2. Based on this information, which of the following components of a physical examination are essential to perform on Carl and why?

  A. Ears, nose, and throat (ENT) examination
  B. Thyroid palpation
  C. Heart examination
  D. Abdominal examination
  E. Assessment of pulses

Physical Examination Findings

Carl is 5'5" tall and weighs 225 lb. His BP is 138/86 mm Hg in his right arm and 138/88 mm Hg in his left arm while seated; repeat BP in 5 minutes is 136/86 mm Hg in his right arm and 138/86 mm Hg in his left arm. Other vital signs are pulse, 96 BPM and regular; respirations, 12/min and regular; and oral temperature, 98.7°F.

His ENT and thyroid examinations are normal.

His heart is regular in rate (98 BPM) and rhythm with no murmurs, gallops, or rubs. His apical impulse is nondisplaced and without a thrill.

His abdomen reveals normoactive and equal bowel sounds in all four quadrants. There is no tenderness, masses, or organomegaly. His renal and aortic pulses are normal and without bruits.

His carotid pulses are normal bilaterally and without bruit. His brachial, ulnar, radial, femoral, popiteal, dorsalis pedis, and posterior tibial pulses are normal bilaterally. His feet are normal in color and temperature. His capillary refill is good.

3. Based on this information, which of the following diagnostic studies are essential to conduct on Carl and why?

  A. Fasting blood lipoprotein analysis
  B. Total cholesterol only
  C. Fasting plasma glucose (FPG)
  D. C-reactive protein (CRP)
  E. Glycosylated hemoglobin (Hgb A1C)

Diagnostic Results

Carl's total cholesterol was 222 mg/dl (normal child: 120–200); his low-density lipoproteins (LDLs) were 160 mg/dl (normal: 60–180); his high-density lipoproteins (HDLs) were 30 mg/dl (normal male: > 45); his very low-density lipoproteins (VLDLs) were 32 mg/dl (normal: 7–32); and his triglycerides were 250 mg/dl (normal male, 12–15 years old: 36–138). His FBS was 94 mg/dl (normal child older than 2 years of age to adult: 70–110) and his CRP was 2 mg/dl (normal: < 1.0). His Hgb A1C was 5.0% (nondiabetics and children: < 4).

4. Based on this information, which one of the following is Carl's most likely diagnosis and why?

  A. Hyperlipidemia, hypertension, and type 1 diabetes mellitus
  B. Hyperlipidemia, hypertension, and type 2 diabetes mellitus
  C. Hyperlipidemia, hypertension, obesity, and type 2 diabetes mellitus
  D. Hyperlipidemia, hypotension, and obesity
  E. Hyperlipidemia, hypertension, and overweight for age

5. Based on this diagnosis, which of the following are appropriate components of a treatment plan for Carl and why?

  A. Repeat total lipoprotein analysis in 1 month to obtain LDL average to utilize for monitoring and treatment
  B. Initiate a program of lifestyle modification with a low-fat, low-cholesterol, low-sodium diet; decreased caloric diet; and regular exercise program with goal of 30 minutes of aerobic exercise on most days of the week
  C. Start niacin 500 mg once a day for 2 weeks; then increase to 500 mg twice a day
  D. Thyroid stimulation test (TSH), liver function studies (LFTs), creatinine, and urine protein
  E. Start triamterene 37.5 mg with hydrochlorothiazide 50 mg once every morning

CASE 1-4
Dale Elliott

Mr. Elliott is a 22-year-old white male who presents with the chief complaint, "I've got to get something for this flu—it is killing me." Further questioning reveals that he has been experiencing a moderate-grade fever, chills, malaise, widespread myalgias, generalized arthralgias, cough, and chest pain for approximately 1.5 weeks. The arthralgias involve "all my joints." He feels that all his symptoms are progressively getting worse.

The cough was nonproductive until last night, when he experienced his first episode of hemoptysis, described as a small amount of blood-streaked, clear, thick sputum. Since then, he has had three or four more episodes that are preceded by "coughing hard" and are followed by dyspnea. He has not noticed any stridor, "barking" sounds, wheezing, or rhonchi at any time. He does not have orthopnea. He has also experienced anorexia and has lost 5 or 6 lb since the onset of his illness.

He denies rhinorrhea; sore throat; ear pain; sinus pressure; headache; stiff neck; nausea; vomiting; diarrhea; other changes in his bowel movements; abdominal pain; penile discharge;

dysuria; urinary urgency; urinary frequency; hematuria; confusion; problems using his arms, legs, or facial muscles; dysphagia; difficulty talking; drooling; or abnormalities of gait.

His medical history is negative for any medical conditions, previous surgeries, or hospitalizations. He does not take any prescription or over-the-counter medications, vitamins, supplements, or herbal preparations. He is allergic to penicillin and experienced urticaria, angioedema, dyspnea, and wheezing with last exposure. He has smoked half a pack of cigarettes a day for 6 years. He drinks three beers on Friday and Saturday evenings every week. He denies illicit drug usage. His family history is negative.

1. Based on this information, which of the following questions are essential to ask Mr. Elliott and why?

   A. Where is the chest pain located, does it radiate, what is its nature, what is its intensity, is it constant or intermittent, is it worsening, and are there any known aggravating or alleviating factors?
   B. Has he checked his temperature with a thermometer?
   C. Has he noticed any skin lesions or rash?
   D. Has he experienced any visual abnormalities?
   E. Does he have any pet rabbits at home?

Patient Responses

The chest pain is left anterior in location without radiation. It is sharp in nature and worsens with inspiration. It also appears to be somewhat worse when he lies down. He describes it as 8 out of 10 on the pain scale. He gets moderate relief from the pain when he takes oxycodone that one of his friends gave to him.

He has not checked his temperature with a thermometer. He denies any problem with his vision. He does not own rabbits.

He has noticed some painful, especially if touched or bumped, raised purplish-red lesions on the dorsal surface of some of his fingers; some nontender "red spots" on his palms and soles; and some "red dots" under his nails and in his eyes. He is uncertain how long they have been present. However, they have not changed since he first noticed them.

2. Based on this information, which of the following components of a physical examination are essential to perform on Mr. Elliott and why?

   A. General appearance
   B. Heart examination
   C. Lung auscultation
   D. Digital rectal examination (DRE)
   E. Skin and nail examination

Physical Examination Results

Mr. Elliott is 5'11" tall and weighs 150 lb (BMI = 21). Other vital signs are oral temperature, 100.8°F; BP, 92/62 mm Hg; pulse, 108 BPM and slightly irregular; respirations, 28/min and regular. He looks very ill, and toxic appearing.

His heart is slightly irregular in rhythm and rate (110 BPM) with a grade 1/6 systolic ejection murmur over the tricuspid area, which is unchanged with a Valsalva maneuver. He does

not have any gallops or rubs. His apical impulse is not displaced and he does not have a thrill.

His lungs have occasional inspiratory rhonchi in the bases bilaterally which do not resolve when Mr. Elliott coughs. His lungs are normal to percussion.

His rectal examination reveals good tone and no internal or external lesions.

He has nontender, 1 to 2 mm in diameter, petechial lesions on his conjunctiva surfaces and underneath all of his fingernails. With the exception of his right thumbnail, all his other nails reveal between three and five longitudinal, dark purplish-red to black-colored, enlongated triangular-shaped (tapering proximally), subungual lesions of approximately 2 to 5 mm in length, near the distal ends of his nails (splinter hemorrhages).

His skin reveals irregular, painless, erythematous macular lesions on his palms and fingertips (Janeway lesions) and painful, purplish papules on the dorsal aspect of his fingers (Osler nodes). He refuses to remove his socks to permit visualization of his feet because "my feet get too cold and I've already gotten the chills." He states that his "feet look just like his hands."

3. Based on this information, which of the following diagnostic studies are essential to conduct on Mr. Elliott and why?

   A. Complete blood count with differential (CBC w/diff)
   B. Chest x-ray (CXR)
   C. A minimum of 2 blood cultures with sensitivities and Gram stains drawn at least 1 hour apart
   D. Electrocardiogram (ECG)
   E. Transesophageal echocardiography (TEE)
   F. Urinary drug screen for illicit substances and narcotics

Diagnostic Results

His CBC revealed a red blood cell (RBC) count of 4.8×10^6/μl (normal male: 4.7–6.1) with a mean corpuscular volume (MCV) of 82.3 μm³ (normal adult: 80–95), a mean corpuscular hemoglobin (MCH) of 26.7 pg (normal adult: 27–31), a mean corpuscular hemoglobin concentration (MCHC) of 32.2 g/dl (normal adult: 32–36), and a red blood cell distribution width (RDW) of 12.5% (normal adult: 11–14.5). His white blood cell (WBC) count was 25,500/mm³ (normal adult: 5000–10,000) with 82% neutrophils (normal: 55–70), 10% lymphocytes (normal: 20–40), 4% monocytes (normal: 2–8), 3% eosinophils (normal: 1–4), and 1% basophils (normal: 0.5–1). His hemoglobin (Hgb) was 12.8 g/dl (normal adult male: 14–18) and his hematocrit (HCT) was 39.5% (normal male: 42–52). His platelet (thrombocyte) count was 150,000/mm³ (normal adult: 150,000–400,000) and his mean platelet volume (MPV) was 7.9 fl (normal: 7.4–10.4). His smear was consistent with the aforementioned and revealed no cellular abnormalities except multiple bands.

His CXR revealed no abnormalities.

His blood cultures are pending; however, both of the specimens' Gram stains revealed gram-positive cocci in clusters.

His ECG revealed a sinus tachycardia of 110 BPM with rare unifocal premature ventricular contractions (PVCs). There were no other waveform abnormalities, arrhythmias, or segmental changes present.

His TEE was normal except for a small vegetation on his tricuspid valve with mild to moderate regurgitation.

His urinary drug screen is pending.

4. Based on this information, which one of the following is Mr. Elliott's most likely diagnosis and why?

- **A.** Lymphocytic leukemia
- **B.** Rocky Mountain spotted fever
- **C.** Acute influenza and tricuspid regurgitation
- **D.** Infective endocarditis (IE)
- **E.** Disseminated gonococcal infection (DGI)

5. Based on this diagnosis, which of the following are appropriate components of a treatment plan for Mr. Elliott and why?

- **A.** Cefazolin 2 g IV every 8 hours and gentamicin 70 mg IV every 8 hours until blood cultures and sensitivities are available
- **B.** Vancomycin 1 g IV every 12 hours and gentamicin 70 mg IV every 8 hours until blood cultures and sensitivities are available
- **C.** Hospitalize and observe closely for additional complications
- **D.** Refer for substance abuse treatment
- **E.** Bone marrow biopsy

CASE 1-5
Eric Floyd

Mr. Floyd is a 53-year-old African American male who presents with the chief complaint of chest pain that began when he crashed his all terrain vehicle (ATV) "head-on" into a tree approximately 3 to 4 hours ago. He states that he hit his chest "really hard" against the area between the ATV's handle bars, causing it to dent on the vehicle on the left side.

Currently, he describes his chest pain as a 6 out of 10 on the pain scale, sharp in nature, and located over the left anterior chest wall. It radiates to his left arm and shoulder but does not involve his neck. It is aggravated by breathing, coughing, and lying flat on his back. It feels best when he is sitting up and bending forward. The pain started immediately after impact as an ache that he would have rated as a 3 out of 10 on the pain scale. He assumed it was just "a bad bruise"; however, as it progressively worsened to its current state, he became concerned.

He has been experiencing some exertional fatigue, exertion dyspnea, and orthopnea for approximately the last hour. He denies lightheadedness, vertigo, presyncope, syncope, headache, confusion, chest pressure/tightness, neck pain, nausea, vomiting, hemoptysis, cough, wheezing, stridor, rales, fever, pedal edema, and palpitations.

His only known medical problem is hypertension, which is controlled with triamterene 37.5 mg/hydrochlorothiazide 25 mg every morning, nadolol 40 mg twice a day, and controlled-release dihydropyridine 10 mg every night. He does not take any other prescription or over-the-counter medications, vitamins, supplements, or herbal preparations. He is not allergic to any medications. He has never had any surgery nor been hospitalized. He has regular health maintenance visits and age-appropriate diagnostic testing, and his immunizations are up to date.

He quit smoking 2 years ago after smoking approximately one pack per day since he was 15 years old. He denies drinking alcohol.

1. Based on this information, which of the following questions are essential to ask Mr. Floyd and why?

- **A.** Did he sustain a head injury or loss of consciousness?
- **B.** Is his helmet intact?
- **C.** Did he injure or is he experiencing pain elsewhere in his body?
- **D.** What is his "usual" BP?
- **E.** Does he have a family history of coronary artery disease (CAD)?

Patient Responses

He did not sustain a head injury or loss of consciousness. His helmet was intact after the incident. He denies pain anywhere else in his body or any other type of injury. His "usual" BP is "around" 140/90 mm Hg. His father had a fatal MI at the age of 52 years.

2. Based on this information, which of the following components of a physical examination are essential to perform on Mr. Floyd and why?

- **A.** Heart examination
- **B.** Evaluate for the presence of an elevated jugular venous pressure (JVP), jugular venous distension (JVD), Kussmaul sign, pulsus alternans, pulsus bigeminus, and pulsus paradoxicum
- **C.** Lung evaluation
- **D.** Chest wall examination
- **E.** Cranial nerve evaluation

Physical Examination Findings

Mr. Floyd is 5'8" tall and weighs 250 lb (BMI = 41.6). Other vital signs are pulse, 120 BPM and regular; respirations, 28/min and regular; BP, 96/62 mm Hg, decreases to 80/58 mm Hg with inspiration; and oral temperature, 99.2°F.

At a 30° angle, his right internal jugular vein reveals an estimated central venous pressure of 10 cm. It also shows a prominent x descent but no detectable y descent. It does not change with inspiration (negative Kussmaul sign). Compression of the lower portion of his right external jugular vein results in distension, or JVD.

His carotid pulses are normal bilaterally and without bruits. However, checking his carotid pulse for a full 2 minutes reveals a regular tachycardic rhythm that is unchanged with inspiration. No abnormal beats or PVCs are noted.

His heart reveals distant heart sounds throughout and a regular tachycardia at 120 BPM. He has no murmurs or gallops; however, he has a pericardial friction rub by his left sternal border. It is most pronounced when he sits up and bends forward. His apical impulse is displaced inferiorly and laterally to the seventh intercostal space midway between the midclavicular line and the anterior axillary line. It is slightly increased in size, duration, and amplitude.

His lung sounds are slightly decreased and dull sounding in his left base; tactile fremitus, vocal fremitus, and egophony are detected below the angle of the left scapula (positive Ewart sign). The remainder of the left lung and his right lung are clear to auscultation. His chest wall is tender to palpation from ribs 2 to 8 in an area approximately 2.5 inches wide that centered over his midclavicular line with no flailing or laxity.

His cranial nerves are grossly intact.

3. Based on this information, which of the following diagnostic studies are essential to conduct on Mr. Floyd and why?

A. Chest x-ray (CXR) with rib enhancement
B. Serial cardiac troponin I and T
C. Electrocardiogram (ECG) and cardiac monitoring
D. Echocardiography
E. Tuberculosis skin test (TST)

Diagnostic Results

Mr. Floyd's CXR revealed an enlarged "water bottle shaped" cardiac silhouette and a small pleural effusion in the left base; no other abnormalities were noted.

His cardiac troponin I was slightly elevated at 0.05 ng/ml (normal: < 0.03 ng/ml) and his troponin T was 0.25 ng/ml (normal: < 0.2).

His ECG revealed a sinus tachycardia (rate 110 BPM); diffuse ST-segment elevation of 2 mm in leads I, II, aVF, and V_2 to V_6; PR-segment depression in III, aVR, aVL, and V_1; upright P waves; overall low voltage; and a change in the height of the P, QRS, and/or T waves that occurred at regular intervals (electrical alternans). No Q waves were seen.

His echocardiogram revealed a large pericardial effusion (estimated size ~800 ml) with a moderate decrease of the size of his right ventricle and associated diastolic and right atrial collapse. No myocardial or pericardial thickening or calcifications were observed. His tuberculosis skin test is pending.

4. Based on this information, in addition to his underlying hypertension and his class 3 (extreme) obesity, which one of the following is Mr. Floyd's most likely diagnosis and why?

A. Constrictive pericarditis
B. Cardiac tamponade secondary to a pericardial effusion
C. Tension pneumothorax
D. Restrictive cardiomyopathy
E. Right ventricular myocardial infarction (RVMI)

5. Based on this diagnosis, which of the following are appropriate components of a treatment plan for Mr. Floyd and why?

A. Hospitalize for arterial pressure, venous pressure, and cardiac monitoring; IV fluids; oxygen; further testing; and treatment
B. Pericardiocentesis via subxiphoid approach under echocardiography guidance
C. Evaluation of fluid from tap for cytology, microscopy, bacterial culture and sensitivity, and polymerase chain reaction (PCR) test of DNA of *Mycobacterium tuberculosis*
D. Consultation with a cardiac surgeon
E. Continue his current blood pressure medicines at half strength

CASE 1-6
Frank Gee

Mr. Gee is a 79-year-old Asian American male who presents with the chief complaint of chest pain of 2 hours' duration. He rates it as a 5 out of 10 on the pain scale. He describes it as a substernal ache, but not a true heaviness or pressure. It radiates to both his shoulders and his intrascapular area. It is associated with nausea (without vomiting), weakness, lightheadedness (but no true vertigo), mild diaphoresis, and dyspnea on exertion. It is alleviated some, but does not completely resolve, if he "sits down and rests." It is aggravated by most any form of exertion, including walking. He knows of no other aggravating or alleviating factors.

He states that the sensation feels identical to the pain he was experiencing with his gallstones; however, he knows they cannot be causing the problem because his gallbladder was removed 2 weeks ago. Nevertheless, as with the previous episodes, his chest pain began while he was eating breakfast. Unlike previous episodes, this one did not resolve within a maximum of half an hour. His daughter convinced him to come and have it evaluated because it is not only persisting but also appearing to be worsening.

He has a history of hypertension and hyperlipidemia, which is being treated with herbal therapy by a traditional Chinese physician. He does not know the name of the medication being prescribed; he just makes it into a tea and drinks it four times a day. He has no other known medical problems. His only surgery has been a laparoscopic cholecystectomy. That was his only hospitalization as well. He doesn't take any prescription or over-the-counter medications, vitamins, or supplements. He has no known drug allergies. He is a widower of 20 years and lives with his father. He does the cooking for the two of them and feels it is "healthy."

His father is 102 years old and does not have any medical problems. His family history is positive for cardiac disease. His mother is deceased as a result of a myocardial infarction at the age of 53 years. One of his brothers had a nonfatal MI at the age of 54 years. To his knowledge, there is no other family history of cardiac disease or serious illnesses.

1. Based on this information, which of the following questions are essential to ask Mr. Gee and why?

A. Has he ever tried any Western (i.e., nitroglycerine) or traditional Chinese medications for his chest pain? If yes, what were the treatments and results?
B. Does he smoke, and if so, what is his smoking history?
C. When was his cholesterol last checked and what were the results?
D. What is his "usual" BP?
E. Does he use sildenafil, vardenafil, or tadalafil for his erectile dysfunction (ED)?

Patient Responses

He has not tried any medicines, Western or traditional Chinese, for his chest pain.

He is a smoker and has been smoking one pack of cigarettes per day for the last 65 years.

He had his cholesterol checked before his surgery (~3 weeks ago). According to Mr. Gee, his total cholesterol was 180, his "good" (HDL) cholesterol was 40, his "bad" (LDL) cholesterol was 130, and his triglycerides were 150. His BP generally runs from 130/70 to 140/80.

He denies having ED and being sexually active since his wife died 20 years ago.

2. Based on this information, which of the following components of a physical examination are essential to perform on Mr. Gee and why?

    A. General appearance
    B. Oral examination
    C. Heart auscultation
    D. Lung auscultation
    E. All his pulses

Physical Examination Findings

Mr. Gee is 5'3" tall and weighs 175 lb (BMI = 31). Other vital signs are BP, 164/96 mm Hg in his right arm and 162/98 mm Hg in his left arm; pulse, 112 BPM and regular; respirations, 20/min and regular; and oral temperature, 99.1°F. He appears to be in moderate distress and is slightly diaphoretic. Otherwise, his general appearance is normal.

His oral examination is unremarkable.

His heart is tachycardic at a rate of 112 BPM but regular. He has a faint systolic ejection murmur of his mitral valve that can be heard best in the left lateral decubitus position. Otherwise, no murmurs, rubs, or gallops are heard. His point of maximum intensity is stronger and larger than normal but not displaced. There is not a thrill.

His breath sounds are slightly harsh throughout but clear to auscultation except for bilateral rales in his bases. They are unchanged by coughing or position. Percussion, fremitus, and egophony are normal.

His carotid, renal, and aortic pulses are normal and without bruit. His aorta is not dilated. His brachial, ulnar, radial, femoral, popiteal, dorsalis pedis, and posterior tibial pulses are normal and equal bilaterally. His feet are normal in color and temperature. His capillary refill is good. He has no pedal edema.

3. Based on this information, which of the following diagnostic studies are essential to conduct on Mr. Gee and why?

    A. Cardiac telemetry followed by 12-lead electrocardiogram (ECG)
    B. Oxygen saturation followed by oxygen at 2 L/min via nasal cannula (NC)
    C. Echocardiogram
    D. Gallbladder ultrasound
    E. Cardiac troponin I and T (cTn-I and cTn-T) stat; then repeat in 4 and 8 hours

Diagnostic Results

His cardiac telemetry revealed a sinus tachycardia with a slight downward convexity to his ST segment and an elevation of approximately 2 mm above baseline. His 12-lead ECG also revealed a sinus tachycardia and the same type of ST-segment convexity in all of the peripheral leads but in none of the chest leads; however, the elevation of the ST segment was only apparent in II, III, and aVF. It was approximately 2 mm in all three leads. These three leads also revealed what appeared to be the formation of early Q waves.

His O_2 saturation was 94% on room air but increased to 98% on oxygen at 2 L/min via NC.

His echocardiogram revealed a small area of inferior wall immobility as well as sinus tachycardia. His valves appeared normal. His estimated ejection fraction was greater than 40%.

His gallbladder ultrasound was normal.

His cTn-I was 0.075 ng/ml (normal: < 0.03) and his cTn-T was 0.19 ng/ml (normal: < 0.2).

4. Based on this information, in addition to hypertension, hyperlipidemia, obesity, and current smoker, which one of the following is Mr. Gee's most likely diagnosis and why?

    A. Unstable angina
    B. Old anterior myocardial infarction
    C. Acute anteroseptal myocardial infarction
    D. Choledocholithiasis
    E. Acute inferior myocardial infarction

5. Based on this diagnosis, which of the following are appropriate components of a treatment plan for Mr. Gee and why?

    A. Admit to intensive care unit (ICU), continue telemetry, vital sign monitoring, IV fluids, and oxygen
    B. IV nitroglycerine 2 to 200 μg/min at a dose sufficient enough to alleviate the patient's pain but not so high as to cause adverse effects. If this titration cannot be achieved or maximum dosage fails to alleviate the patient's pain, then give morphine sulfate at 2 to 8 mg IV every 15 minutes as needed, provided no signs of respiratory depression are present
    C. Aspirin 160 to 325 mg stat; then 81 mg enteric-coated aspirin daily with food
    D. Acebutolol 200 mg once a day orally
    E. Fibrinolysis with tissue plasma activator (tPA)
    F. Percutaneous transluminal coronary angiography (PTCA) with stent placement if indicated

CASE 1-7
George Harris

Mr. Harris is a 58-year-old Asian American male who presents with the chief complaint of "coughing up blood" for approximately 2 to 3 weeks. He estimates it to be "less than a teaspoon" and to occur no more frequently than every 3 or 4 hours; however, it does occur "around the clock." It is bright red in color and not associated with sputum, mucus, stomach acid/contents, or "coffee grounds"-looking material. It is unchanged since its onset.

He has been experiencing a nonproductive cough for approximately the last 5 or 6 years. It does not appear to be any different now than it was at its onset. His cough had been nonproductive until the hemoptysis began. He sleeps on three pillows and has paroxysmal nocturnal dyspnea (PND) less than once a week. He admits to occasionally feeling his heart rate increase with exertion; however, he denies noting any other irregularities regarding his heart's rate/beat.

He denies chest pain or pressure, vertigo, lightheadedness, presyncope, syncope, tinnitus, fever, chills, wheezing, stridor, rhonchi, rales, nausea, or vomiting.

He has no known medical problems. He was hospitalized at the age of 16 years for rheumatic fever; however, he denies cardiac involvement and/or long-term antibiotics following the episode. He has never had any surgery. He does not take any OTC or prescription medications, vitamins, supplements, or herbal preparations. He smokes two packs of cigarettes per day and has done so for the past 30 years. He drinks two glasses of red wine every evening. He denies any other alcohol intake. His family history is noncontributory.

1. Based on this information, which of the following questions are essential to ask Mr. Harris and why?

    A. Has he experienced any epistaxis, nasal or oral lesions, or gingival or dental problems recently?
    B. Has he experienced any abdominal pain or change in his bowel movements?
    C. Has he experienced any fatigue, malaise, weight loss, hoarseness, or night sweats?
    D. Has he experienced any dyspnea?
    E. Has he experienced any hallucinations?

Patient Responses

Mr. Harris denies any epistaxis, nasal or oral lesions, gingival or dental problems, abdominal pain, change in bowel movements, nausea, vomiting, heartburn, fatigue, malaise, weight loss, hoarseness, night sweats, or hallucinations.

He has had some dyspnea on exertion daily for several months but denies it worsening. He can climb a flight of steps at a normal pace without having any problems; however, if he tries to do it "too fast," he experiences the dyspnea and occasionally the tachycardia. He can walk more than two blocks, without symptoms, if the ground is level.

2. Based on this information, which of the following components of a physical examination are essential to perform on Mr. Harris and why?

    A. Skin examination
    B. Heart examination
    C. Lung auscultation
    D. Evaluation of jugular venous pressure (JVP), of pulses, and for pedal edema
    E. Joint evaluation

Physical Examination Findings

Mr. Harris is 5'8" tall and weighs 195 lb (BMI = 29.6). Other vital signs are BP, 120/76 mm Hg; pulse, 92 BPM and regular; respiratory rate, 24/min and regular; and oral temperature, 97.9°F. He is overweight and in moderate respiratory distress, bending forward with his hands on his thighs to breathe. He has a bluish discoloration to his face with a malar flushing on his cheeks.

His heart is regular in rate and rhythm. He has a loud opening snap that is more prominent in expiration and with a significant time lapse from the closure of the aortic valve. He has a grade II/VI diastolic murmur and rumble at his apex that is best heard when he is lying on his left side. He has no

gallops or rubs. He does not have a thrill but does have a "tapping" sensation over his apical impulse, which is located in the fifth intercostal margin approximately 8 cm from his midsternal line. He also has a grade I/VI diastolic murmur in his tricuspid area that increases with inspiration.

His breath sounds are harsh throughout but symmetric. He does not have any wheezing, rales, rhonchi, or stridor. Percussion, fremitus, and egophony are normal.

At 30° of head elevation, his JVP is 8.5 cm and he has an elevated α wave.

His carotid and renal pulses are normal, equal bilaterally, and without bruits. His aortic pulsation is normal and does not reveal any evidence of enlargement or a bruit. His brachial, ulnar, femoral, popiteal, dorsalis pedis, and posterior tibial pulses are normal and equal bilaterally. His feet are normal in color and temperature and equal bilaterally. His capillary refill is good. He does not have any pedal edema.

3. Based on this information, which of the following diagnostic studies are essential to conduct on Mr. Harris and why?

    A. Oxygen saturation (O_2 sat) and chest x-ray (CXR)
    B. Electrocardiogram (ECG) and echocardiogram with Doppler
    C. D-dimer
    D. First morning sputum for cytology × 3
    E. Antinuclear antibodies (ANAs); erythrocyte sedimentation rate (ESR); antinative DNA; anticardiolipin antibodies, including lupus anticoagulant; C_3 and C_4 complement assay; systemic lupus erythematosus preparation (SLE prep); and CBC w/diff

Diagnostic Results

Mr. Harris's O_2 sat was 88% (normal adult: ≥ 95). His CXR did not reveal any effusions, lesions, consolidations, or infiltrates. However, it did reveal a cardiac silhouette with a straight left heart border, a large left atrial appendage, and a calcified mitral valve.

His ECG revealed normal sinus rhythm, with large P waves throughout. They were tall and peaked in II and upright in V_1. No other abnormalities were noted.

His echocardiogram confirmed a thickened, immobile, calcified, stenotic mitral valve with left atrial enlargement. His mitral valvular diameter was 0.8 cm² (normal: 4–6 cm²). His tricuspid valve was also slightly stenotic but with a normal valvular diameter. Ejection fraction was estimated to be approximately 35%.

His D-dimer, ANA, ESR, antinative DNA, anticardiolipin antibodies, lupus anticoagulant, C_3 and C_4 complement assay, SLE prep, and CBC w/diff were negative. His sputum cytologies are pending.

4. Based on this information, in addition to his being overweight and a current smoker, which one of the following is Mr. Harris's most likely diagnosis and why?

    A. Lung cancer
    B. Pulmonary embolism
    C. Atypical verrucous endocarditis of Libman-Sacks secondary to systemic lupus erythematous
    D. Left atrial myxoma
    E. Mitral stenosis with associated tricuspid stenosis

5. Based on this diagnosis, which of the following are appropriate components of a treatment plan for Mr. Harris and why?

    A. Hospitalization with oxygen therapy starting at 2 L/min after arterial blood gases and then adjusted accordingly, cardiac monitoring, and IV line to keep vein open (KVO)

    B. Refer to thoracic surgeon and oncologist for evaluation and treatment of lung cancer

    C. Refer to cardiac surgeon for possible cardiac catheterization, possible balloon valvuloplasty, or other interventions

    D. Start on warfarin therapy

    E. Encourage smoking cessation

CASE 1-8

Harriet Issac

Mrs. Issac is a 54-year-old white female who presents with the chief complaint of chest pain and shortness of breath. She describes the chest pain as a "swollen, pressure-like" sensation that is substernal in location and radiates to her left shoulder and arm. It is minimally alleviated by rest and markedly aggravated by activity. She rates it as a 9 out of 10 on the pain scale. It started abruptly approximately 4 hours ago and appears to be getting progressively worse. Her dyspnea started shortly after the chest pain and has been constant since.

She has some mild nausea without vomiting. She has not had any bowel changes, fever, malaise, arthralgias, cough, wheezing, stridor, rhonchi, rales, headache, vertigo, presyncope, syncope, loss of consciousness, visual changes, or edema.

She saw her family physician approximately 1 hour after her pain began and he assured her it was caused by "stress" because she had been involved in a motor vehicle accident (MVA) the previous night. The car she was driving was "T-boned" by a large truck on the passenger side when she drove through an intersection. The accident resulted in the death of her husband and grandson. At this point, she became tearful and stated the police at the scene "said it was all my fault." She admits to being "upset," "crying a lot," and unable to sleep since the incident ~14 hours ago. She feels guilty over her family members' deaths, but she denies thoughts of suicide.

Her only known medical problems are a history of chronic anxiety and depression dating back to her adolescence and problems related to the previous day's MVA consisting of contusions to her left arm, ribs, and thigh; a few minor abrasions and a small laceration to the right side of her face, which was repaired in the emergency department last night; and some mild ecchymosis under both her eyes from the airbag's deployment. None of these symptoms have changed since their onset. She denies any surgery. Her only hospitalizations were for childbirth.

She is taking fluoxetine 40 mg once a day and acetaminophen 500 mg two tablets every 6 to 8 hours as needed for pain. The acetaminophen alleviates all her pain except her chest pain.

She is not taking any other prescription or over-the-counter medications, vitamins, supplements, or herbal preparations. She is allergic to meperidine (it causes generalized hives but no dyspnea). She has never smoked cigarettes or drank alcohol. She has a family history of coronary artery disease (mother: nonfatal myocardial infarction at the age of 70 years).

1. Based on this information, which of the following questions are essential to ask Mrs. Issac and why?

    A. Has she ever experienced similar symptoms in the past?

    B. Is she aware of any other aggravating or alleviating factors?

    C. What type of evaluation and diagnostic tests were performed on her in the emergency department following her MVA, and what were the results?

    D. Has she been experiencing any diaphoresis, palpitations, tachycardia, anxiety, or shakiness?

    E. Does she have any other grandchildren to replace the one she lost?

Patient Responses

Mrs. Issac has never experienced any chest pain or shortness of breath in the past. Her only other known aggravating factor is breathing deeply; and, her only other known alleviating factor is shallow breathing. According to the patient, she had a comprehensive physical examination; radiographs of her neck, back, chest, and left hip; an MRI of her head; an electrocardiogram; and a urinalysis in the ED following her MVA last night. She states she was informed that all the tests were negative and she was "just bruised badly." She denies diaphoresis. She has had some intermittent anxiety, palpations, and shakiness "mostly when I think about my husband and grandson" since the MVA. She has not had any increased stress except for the MVA. She does not have any other grandchildren.

2. Based on this information, which of the following components of a physical examination are essential to perform on Mrs. Issac and why?

    A. Heart examination

    B. Lung auscultation

    C. Palpation of ribs

    D. Evaluation of jugular venous pressure (JVP) and ankles/feet for edema

    E. Visual acuity

Physical Examination Findings

Mrs. Issac is 5'1" tall and weighs 150 lb (BMI = 29.2). Other vital signs are BP, 162/98 mm Hg in her right arm and 166/100 mm Hg in her left arm; pulse, 96 BPM and regular; respirations, 20/min and regular; and oral temperature, 99.2°F.

Her heart is regular in rate and rhythm. There is a midsystolic click followed by a grade 1/6 late systolic murmur in her mitral area that increases in intensity and length with a Valsalva maneuver and standing, and decreases with squatting. She also has an S4 gallop, but no rub. Point of maximal impulse (PMI) is located 15 cm from the left sternal border, in the 8th to 10th intercostal spaces (ICSs), and is 4.5 cm in size.

Her lungs are clear to auscultation and breath sounds are present in all fields. She does not have any chest wall tenderness except from her anterior-axillary line to her midaxillary line over ribs 8 to 10. There is some minor ecchymosis developing on the skin in this area.

Her JVP is not visualized, even with her lying as high as 90° and after performing the abdominojugular reflux test. Her carotid and renal pulses are normal and equal bilaterally; they did not reveal any bruits. Her aorta pulsation is normal, nonenlarged, and without a bruit. Her brachial, ulnar, femoral, popiteal, dorsalis pedis, and posterior tibial pulses are normal and equal bilaterally. Her feet are normal in color and temperature. Her capillary refill is good. She does not have any pedal edema.

Distance vision is 20/25 wearing her corrective lenses.

3. Based on this information, which of the following diagnostic studies are essential to conduct on Mrs. Issac and why?

    A. Brain natriuretic peptide (BNP)
    B. Serial cardiac troponin levels (cTn-I and cTn-T)
    C. Electrocardiogram (ECG) and echocardiogram
    D. Chest x-ray (CXR)
    E. 24-Hour urine vanillylmandelic acid (VMA) and catecholamine levels

Diagnostic Results

Mrs. Issac's BNP was 125 pg/ml (normal: < 100). Her cTn-I was slightly elevated at 0.035 ng/ml (normal: < 0.03), as was her cTn-I at 0.205 ng/ml (normal: < 0.2).

Her ECG revealed ST-segment elevations of 1 mm and deep T-wave inversion in leads V_1 through V_5. Her echocardiogram revealed left ventricular apical ballooning that had a round ampulla shape similar to an "octopus pot" with dyskinesia and mild mitral valve prolapse with mild regurgitation.

Her CXR showed a cardiac silhouette revealing a rounded ampulla of the left ventricle similar to an "octopus pot."

Her VMA level was 8.0 mg/24 hr (normal: < 6.8). Her free catecholamine level was 142 μg/24 hr (normal: < 100) with a dopamine level of 350 μg/24 hr (normal: 65–400), an epinephrine level of 50 μg/24 hr (normal: < 20), a metanephrine level of 1.0 mg/24 hr (normal: < 1.3), a norepinephrine level of 145 μg/24 hr (normal: < 100), and a normetanephrine level of 100 μg/24 hr (normal: 15–80).

4. Based on this information, in addition to her being overweight, which one of the following is Mrs. Issac's most likely diagnosis and why?

    A. Pheochromocytoma
    B. Acute inferior myocardial infarction (AIMI)
    C. Heart failure
    D. Takotsubo cardiomyopathy
    E. Chest pain secondary to stress reaction

5. Based on this diagnosis, which of the following are appropriate components of a treatment plan for Mrs. Issac and why?

    A. Hospitalize with telemetry and close monitoring of vital signs
    B. Repeat cTn-I and cTn-T in 4 and 8 hours

    C. Cardiac catheterization
    D. Meperidine 50 mg IM every 3 to 4 hours as needed
    E. Nebivolol 10 mg orally once a day

CASE 1-9
Ira Jackson

Mr. Jackson is a 78-year-old white male who presents with the chief complaint of "not being able to keep my blood level in the right range, so I keep getting those irregular heartbeats." Upon further questioning, he is referring to his international normalized ratio (INR) for his warfarin, which he started taking approximately 5 years ago when he was diagnosed with atrial fibrillation (AF). His heart rate had been regular and his INR within the desired range since the time of diagnosis until approximately 2 months ago, when he began experiencing palpitations of his heart and fluctuations of his INR.

He states that the palpitations begin without provocation, occur two or three times a day, last for approximately 10 to 15 minutes, and then resolve spontaneously. He is unaware of any aggravating or alleviating factors. They are not associated with weakness, fatigue, tiredness, lightheadedness, vertigo, presyncope, syncope, tinnitus, chest pains, chest pressure, nausea, dyspnea, problems with gait, other difficulties using extremities, abnormalities of speech, lack of coordination, confusion, loss of consciousness, seizures, tremors, anxiety, hunger, or eating.

He has not had any episodes of epistaxis, gingival bleeding with brushing his teeth, vomiting blood or "coffee grounds"-appearing substances, gross hematuria, rectal bleeding, passing dark tarry-appearing stools, or bruising more easily.

According to Mr. Jackson, his INR can be high, low, or, rarely, normal without him doing anything different. He claims his regular physician has not adjusted his warfarin dosage but has just been checking it every week and encouraging him "to take his medication regularly." However, he is unequivocally certain that he takes the same dose of his medication at the same time every day, never missing a dose or taking an extra dose.

His only known medical problems are atrial fibrillation (AF) and hypertension (HTN). His HTN was diagnosed approximately 25 years ago and has always been well controlled with propranolol. His current medications include warfarin 2.5 mg/day and long-acting propranolol 120 mg/day. He is not allergic to any medications. He does not take any other prescription or over-the-counter medications, vitamins, supplements, or herbal preparations. He has never had surgery. His only hospitalization occurred when the AF was first diagnosed. He has never smoked or drank alcohol. His family history is positive for his father and two brothers having AF.

1. Based on this information, which of the following questions are important to ask Mr. Jackson and why?

    A. Were there any changes in his medical condition, medication list (including medications used on an as-needed basis), or life when he began reexperiencing palpitations and having fluctuations of his INR?
    B. Do his medications look different since he started experiencing problems?

C. Does he consume caffeine?

D. Does he alter the amounts of "greens" that he consumes daily?

E. Does he alter the amount of orange juice that he drinks daily?

Patient Responses

Mr. Jackson did not experience any changes in his life/stress level, medical conditions, medications (including over-the-counter drugs, vitamins, supplements, herbal preparations, short-term-usage medications, or as-needed medications), or appearance of his pill. He does not drink caffeine regularly; however, he will have a couple of glasses of iced tea when eating out. This could vary from every day for a couple of days to every couple of weeks. He has never noticed any relationship between the occurrence of the palpitations and the tea consumption; however, he cannot be certain it does not exist. He does vary the amount of "greens" in his diet from no servings a day to four or five servings per day when "fresh" ones are available. He drinks one glass of orange juice each morning for breakfast.

2. Based on this information, which of the following components of a physical examination are essential to perform on Mr. Jackson and why?

A. Nasal and pharyngeal examination

B. Heart examination

C. Lung auscultation

D. Evaluation of jugular venous pulse (JVP)

E. Check for pedal edema

Physical Examination Findings

Mr. Jackson is 5'11" tall and weighs 165 lb (BMI = 23). Other vital signs are pulse, 80 BPM and irregularly irregular; respirations, 10/min and regular; BP, 118/76 mm Hg lying, 124/76 mm Hg sitting, and 128/74 mm Hg standing; and oral temperature, 98.8°F.

His nose and throat examination is unremarkable.

His heart is irregularly irregular in rhythm and its ventricular rate is 78 BPM. There are no murmurs, gallops, or rubs; however, his first heart sound appears to be louder than normal and his fourth heart sound cannot be identified. His apical impulse is located in the third intracostal space approximately 7 cm from his left sternal border. There are no thrills.

His lungs are clear to auscultation. His JVP is also irregularly irregular. He does not have any pedal edema.

3. Based on this information, which of the following diagnostic studies are essential to conduct on Mr. Jackson and why?

A. International normalized ratio (INR)

B. Hematocrit (HCT) and hemoglobin (Hgb), or H&H

C. Electrocardiogram (ECG) and echocardiogram, preferably transesophageal (TEE)

D. Thyroid panel, hepatic function, and renal function

E. Holter monitor (outpatient telemetry)

Diagnostic Results

His INR was 1.6 (patient's goal: 2–3), his HCT was 48% (normal adult male: 42–52), and his Hgb was 16 g/dl (normal adult male: 14–18). His ECG revealed AF with an average ventricular response rate of 72 BPM (see **Figure 1-1**). No other abnormalities were noted. His TEE revealed no areas of myocardial dyskinesis, cardiomegaly, hypertrophy, abnormal chamber sizes, valvular abnormalities, or emboli. His ejection fraction was normal.

His thyroid-stimulating hormone was 5.0 µU/ml (normal adult: 2–10), free thyroxine (FT_4) was 1.3 ng/dl (normal adult: 0.8–2.8), and triiodothyronine by radioimmunoassay (T_3 by RIA) was 60 ng/dl (normal adult older than 50 years: 40–180).

His alkaline phosphatase (ALP) was 50 units/L (normal adult: 30–120), aspartate aminotransferase (AST) was 20 units/L (normal adult: 0–35), alanine aminotransferase (ALT) was 7.5 units/L (normal adult: 4–36), and γ-glutamyl transferase (GTT) was 9.5 units/L (normal adult male: 8–38).

His blood urea nitrogen (BUN) was 12.0 mg/dl (normal adult: 10–20) and his creatinine was 0.8 mg/dl (normal male: 0.6–1.2).

His Holter monitor revealed intermittent bursts of AF lasting 10 to 15 minutes occurring on average three times per day with an average resting ventricular heart rate of 72 BPM and an average ventricular heart rate with exertion of 88 BPM.

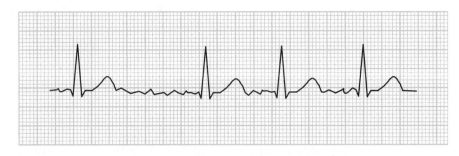

Figure 1-1 ECG strip (lead II) revealing atrial fibrillation.
Source: From Garcia, T.B., and Holtz, N.E. 2003. *Introduction to 12-Lead ECG.* Boston: Jones & Bartlett Learning.

4. Based on this information, which one of the following is Mr. Jackson's most likely diagnosis and why?

    A. Recurrent paroxysmal atrial fibrillation with fluctuations in INR as a result of inconsistent dietary vitamin K intake

    B. Atrial fibrillation with poor medical compliance

    C. Familial atrial fibrillation with fluctuations in INR as a result of inadequate vitamin C in diet

    D. Atrial fibrillation with normal INR

    E. Atrial flutter with excessive propranolol dosage responsible for palpitations and INR fluctuations

5. Based on this diagnosis, which of the following are appropriate components of a treatment plan for Mr. Jackson and why?

    A. Add digoxin 0.125 mg once a day

    B. Schedule for nodal ablation

    C. Schedule for pacemaker implantation

    D. Schedule for cardioversion

    E. Advise patient to consume the same amount of "greens" daily and adjust warfarin dose accordingly

CASE 1-1

Alice Blankenship

1. History

A. Has she been experiencing vertigo, presyncope, syncope, palpitations, unusual fatigue, or headaches?   ESSENTIAL

Hypertension is known as the "silent killer" because the majority of individuals afflicted with the condition are asymptomatic. However, some individuals do have symptoms associated with their hypertension. The most common ones include vertigo, presyncope, syncope, palpitations, unusual fatigue, or headaches. Therefore, it is essential to inquire whether Mrs. Blankenship has been experiencing any of these symptoms. However, it is theorized that these symptoms are not caused by the hypertension itself but reflect symptomatology that is associated with hypertensive cardiovascular disease or, in some cases, a secondary hypertension.

Cardiovascular disease (CVD), including coronary artery disease (CAD), peripheral arterial disease (PAD), renovascular disease (RVD), and heart failure, is seen at twice the rate in individuals who have hypertension compared to those who do not. Some experts estimate the risk of CVD to be doubled with every 20-mm Hg increase in systolic blood pressure (BP) and/or every 10-mm Hg increase in diastolic BP starting with a BP of 115/75. This is significant for Mrs. Blankenship because both diabetes mellitus and obesity can also increase the incidence of these conditions as well. Furthermore, the risks of these three conditions are cumulative.

B. Has she been experiencing weakness in one or more of her extremities, weakness of her facial muscles, difficulty talking, dysphagia, or transient monocular blindness?   ESSENTIAL

These are major signs that are associated with a cerebral vascular accident (CVA) or transient ischemic attack (TIA). Having hypertension doubles a patient's risk of a CVA. Obesity and diabetes mellitus are also associated with an increased risk of CVA. These risks are cumulative.

The length of time the patient experiences these symptoms assists in determining whether they are a TIA or CVA. The current definition of a TIA includes that focal neurologic defects be completely resolved within 24 hours (the majority are resolved in 1–2 hours). However, because approximately 30 to 50% of all individuals with these symptoms have a positive neuroimaging study for a CVA within 24 hours, the American Heart Association and the American Stroke Association Collaborative Guidelines Committee recommends decreasing the length of time that the symptoms could represent a TIA (instead of a CVA) to 1 hour.

A TIA increases a patient's risk of having a CVA within the next 3 months by approximately 10 to 15%. This risk is greatest in the first 48 hours following the TIA. The first month following the TIA is associated with a greater risk than in the subsequent 2 months. Therefore, it is important to inquire whether individuals who are at risk for a CVA are experiencing symptoms suspicious for a TIA and evaluate and treat them promptly, if present.

Transient monocular blindness, or amaurosis fugax, is a TIA symptom that requires immediate evaluation because it is caused by an embolus to the central retinal artery of the ipsilateral eye. This could be from carotid stenosis or local ophthalmic artery disease.

C. Has she noticed any tachycardia, bradycardia, palpitations, changes in her hair or nails, skin rashes or discoloration, diaphoresis, tremor, snoring, or excessive sleepiness?   ESSENTIAL

It is estimated that anywhere from 80 to 95% of all cases of hypertension are essential hypertension, otherwise known as idiopathic or primary hypertension (no identifiable cause). An estimated 5 to 20% of all cases of hypertension are secondary, meaning that they are caused by some other medical condition. Some of the more common of these conditions include fever, aortic regurgitation, aortic insufficiency, calcified arteriosclerosis, arteriolovenous shunt, hyperkinetic heart syndrome, coarctation of the aorta, renovascular disease, hypothyroidism, hyperthyroidism, parathyroid disease, hypercalcemia, acromegaly, primary aldosteronism, pheochromocytoma, Cushing syndrome, Gordon syndrome, obstructive sleep apnea, familial dysautonomia, certain types of polyneuritis, increased intracranial pressure, eclampsia, preeclampsia, excessive alcohol intake, and certain medications.

D. Is she taking any over-the-counter (OTC) medications, vitamins, supplements, or herbal products?   ESSENTIAL

It is essential to specifically inquire about nonprescription products because many patients do not consider these medications and won't list them when asked. Some medications can cause secondary hypertension. The primary ones include oral contraceptives, estrogens, corticosteroids, nasal decongestants, tricyclic antidepressants (TCAs), monamine oxidase inhibitors (MAOIs), and nonsteroidal anti-inflammatory drugs (NSAIDs).

E. Does she have a family history of diabetes mellitus? NONESSENTIAL

Although a family history of type 1 diabetes mellitus is associated with an increased risk of acquiring type 1 diabetes mellitus, the risk is not as defined when it comes to type 2 diabetes mellitus. Regardless, because Mrs. Blankenship has already been diagnosed with diabetes mellitus, the question of risk factors for the disease is moot.

2. Physical Examination

A. BP and pulse measurements in both arms in lying, sitting, and standing positions as well as BP measurement in both legs with Doppler   ESSENTIAL

In evaluating a patient who has an elevated BP, it is essential to evaluate the BP in the contralateral arm as well to determine if there is a significant difference (defined as ≥ 10 mm Hg of the systolic and/or the diastolic BP) in the readings. The most serious cause of this degree of discrepancy is aortic dissection. It could also be representative of an arterial obstruction or compression on the ipsilateral side of the lower BP.

Although the seventh report of the Joint National Committee on Prevention, Detection, Evaluation, and Treatment of High Blood Pressure (JNC 7) utilizes the sitting BP as the reading to determine the presence of an elevated blood pressure and its category, if the BP is elevated, the JNC 7 report recommends that measurements be done in both arms lying, standing, and sitting to ensure that there are no signs of orthostatic hypotension (defined as a ≥ 20-mm Hg drop in systolic blood pressure [SBP] or a ≥ 10-mm Hg drop in diastolic blood pressure [DBP] when measured within 3 minutes of going from supine to standing). If orthostasis is present, then the pulse should be utilized to determine if it is more likely a neurologic or peripheral process causing the condition. If the pulse increased more than 15 beats per minute (BPM), the cause is more likely to be peripheral (e.g., dehydration and/or anemia). However, if it does not increase more than 15 BPM, the cause is more likely to be neurologic (e.g., Shy-Drager syndrome or familial dysautonomia).

Furthermore, the JNC 7 report recommends the measurement of blood pressure in at least one, but preferably both, lower extremities. The systolic values of ankle BP and the sitting BP are useful in determining the ankle-brachial index (ABI). The ABI is the SBP divided by the higher systolic arm value while sitting. Therefore, Mrs. Blankenship's ABI would be 1.1 (144 [her ankle SBP] / 136 [her highest sitting arm SBP]). Any value below 0.9 is considered abnormal and significant

for PAD; if below 0.3, it generally indicates the presence of ischemia secondary to severe PAD. Essentially, the lower the ABI is, the more severe the disease.

B. Funduscopic examination   ESSENTIAL

The fundus of the eye is the only place on the body where direct visualization of the arteries and veins is possible. The arterioles on funduscopic examination can reveal changes that are often associated with the length of time the patient has had hypertension. For example, early in the course of hypertension, the arterioles could reveal either focal or complete spasms resulting in segmental or generalized narrowing of the vessel, respectively. As the disease progresses, the arterial walls begin to thicken and the column of blood that is normally visible in the center of the arterioles changes to a narrow yellowish-red discoloration. This condition is known as "copper wiring." As the disease continues to worsen, the thickening of the walls becomes so severe that the blood column cannot be visualized; this change is referred to as "silver wiring." Arteriovenous (A-V) nicking, AV concealment, and small infarcts of the distal arteriole (called soft exudates or "cotton wool" patches because of their white, fluffy appearance) are other vascular changes from hypertension that can be visualized funduscopically. Retinal changes seen with hypertension include small hemorrhages, flame-shaped hemorrhages, and hard exudates (which are well-demarked creamy to yellowish-colored lesions).

Changes from diabetes mellitus can also be visualized in the fundus; they include deep hemorrhages, microaneurysms of the macular area, and preretinal hemorrhages.

C. Heart and lung examination   ESSENTIAL

The heart examination is important in the evaluation of hypertension to identify signs that could be associated with secondary hypertension (e.g., cardiomegaly, splitting of the heart sounds, cardiac murmurs, an opening snap, or fourth heart sounds). The lungs need to be auscultated for signs suspicious of heart failure.

D. Evaluation of all pulses   ESSENTIAL

Evaluation of the pulses can reveal secondary causes of hypertension. For example, decreased or absent peripheral pulses could indicate PAD or calcified arteriosclerosis. A renal bruit could indicate that a renovascular abnormality is the cause of the secondary hypertension. And a widened pulse pressure could be from aortic regurgitation, aortic insufficiency, fever, arteriovenous shunts, thyrotoxicosis, or hyperkinetic heart syndrome.

E. Rectal examination   NONESSENTIAL

3. Diagnostic Studies

A. Bilateral magnetic resonance imaging (MRI) of her knees NONESSENTIAL

Mrs. Blankenship's knee pain is currently controlled with an OTC agent. Therefore, she does not require further evaluation for this condition at this time. Furthermore, an MRI is not the initial imaging study of choice; it is a knee radiograph.

B. Urinalysis   ESSENTIAL

A urinalysis is indicated to assist in ruling out any renal disease that could be responsible for Mrs. Blankenship's hypertension. This is especially important because her diabetes places her at a greater risk for a nephropathy. A microalbumin on Mrs. Blankenship's urine should also be considered; it has not been done in the past year because of her diabetes.

C. Fasting lipid profile ESSENTIAL

A lipid profile is indicated not only because of her BP level but also for her other risk factors for CVD (e.g., diabetes, obesity, and age). Elevated lipids can further contribute to her risk of CVD. If they are elevated, they also need to be treated promptly and to appropriate levels.

D. Electrocardiogram (ECG) ESSENTIAL

An ECG is indicated to look for signs that are suspicious for ventricular hypertrophy, which is associated with hypertension; silent ischemia caused by her risk factors; or other findings associated with CVD and hypertension (e.g., arrhythmias, hyperkalemia, or hypokalemia).

The JNC 7 also recommends that the initial evaluation of a hypertensive patient include hematocrit, fasting blood glucose, serum potassium, sodium, calcium, blood urea nitrogen and/or creatinine. Additionally, they recommend a urinary albumin:creatinine ratio and a thyroid-stimulating hormone (TSH) as optional tests.

E. Ambulatory BP monitoring NONESSENTIAL

Currently, the primary indication for ambulatory BP monitoring is when it is suspected that the patient is experiencing "white coat syndrome" (the patient's BP is elevated while in the clinical setting but is normal in all other situations). Because Mrs. Blankenship's daughter checked it at home and it was essentially the same as it was during her clinical visits, this condition is unlikely.

The JNC 7 recommends the use of ambulatory monitoring in other situations as well (e.g., treatment-resistant hypertension, symptomatic hypotension, orthostatic hypotension, autonomic failure, and episodic hypertension). Because it does not appear that Mrs. Blankenship is afflicted by any of these conditions at this time, ambulatory BP monitoring is not currently indicated for her.

4. Diagnosis

Mrs. Blankenship's type 2 diabetes mellitus was diagnosed via her history and her mild glucosuria. Her obesity was diagnosed on the basis of her body mass index (BMI). Gender-specific tables are available that can quickly provide the patient's BMI by plotting height against weight. However, these tables generally represent the height in centimeters and the weight in kilograms. Because in the United States patients are generally measured in inches and weighed in pounds, conversions to metric measurements must be completed before one can utilize the table. Even when these tables are in inches and pounds, these tables must be readily accessible if they are going to be used to determine the patient's BMI. Therefore, utilizing the following formula might be the quickest method to calculate the patient's BMI when using weight in pounds and height in inches:

$$\frac{\text{Patient's weight (in pounds)} \times 703}{\text{Patient's height (in inches)}^2}$$

An even quicker method to make this calculation in the clinical setting is:

[(Patient's weight in pounds × 703) ÷ Patient's height in inches] ÷ Patient's height in inches

For example, Mrs. Blankenship is 5'3" (63") tall and weighs 165 lb. Her BMI would be:

[(165 × 703) ÷ 63] ÷ 63 = 29

This would place her BMI in the upper end of the obese category as defined by the National Institutes of Health (NIH). The NIH classification system for obesity according to BMI can be found in **Table 1-1**.

A. White coat syndrome producing pseudo-hypertension INCORRECT

This condition was essentially ruled out because her at-home blood pressure measurements are fundamentally equivalent to her measurements taken in the clinic.

B. Prehypertension CORRECT

According to the JNC 7, the BP readings listed in **Table 1-2** correspond to the diagnostic category for BP. Because all of Mrs. Blankenship's sitting brachial SBPs and DBPs were in the prehypertension range, this is her most likely diagnosis. If the SBP and the DBP values are found in different categories, the higher level is utilized. For example, a BP of 122/90 would be considered hypertension, stage 1.

C. Hypertension, stage 1 INCORRECT

According to the JNC 7 classification scheme, Mrs. Blankenship does not meet the diagnostic criteria for hypertension, stage 1, as defined in Table 1-2.

D. Hypertension, stage 2 INCORRECT

According to the JNC 7 classification scheme, Mrs. Blankenship does not meet the diagnostic criteria for hypertension, stage 2, as defined in Table 1-2.

E. Diabetic nephropathy–induced hypertension INCORRECT

She does have type 2 diabetes mellitus and, as outlined earlier, prehypertension because her BP has consistently been between 120 and 139 mm Hg systolic and/or 80 and 89 mm Hg diastolic. However, it is unlikely that it has a renovascular cause because her physical examination does not reveal a renal bruit and her urinalysis is negative for protein.

Table 1-1 National Institutes of Health Classification System for Obesity According to Body Mass Index

Body Mass Index	Classification
18.5–24.9	Normal
25.0–29.9	Overweight
30.0–34.9	Class 1 obesity
35.0–39.9	Class 2 obesity
≥ 40	Class 3 (extreme) obesity

Table 1-2 Blood Pressure (BP) Readings and Diagnostic Categories

Category	Systolic BP (mm Hg)		Diastolic BP (mm Hg)
Normal	< 120	and	< 80
Prehypertension	120–139	or	80–89
Hypertension, stage 1	140–159	or	90–99
Hypertension, stage 2	≥ 160	or	≥ 100

5. Treatment Plan

A. Dietary modification including low-sodium, low-fat, Dietary Approaches to Stop Hypertension (DASH) eating plan CORRECT

With a history of either diabetes mellitus or chronic kidney disease, the JNC 7 recommends treating patients with prehypertension as well as hypertension. The goal of treatment is BP less than 140/90 mm Hg, unless the aforementioned conditions are present—then the goal is BP less than 130/80 mm Hg. The first step in the treatment of a patient with prehypertension and stage 1 hypertension is lifestyle modification, including dietary restrictions such as following the DASH diet, restricting sodium, restricting caffeine, and limiting or eliminating alcohol. Furthermore, dietary modification is essential in addition to exercise and pharmacological interventions in stage 2 hypertension and other treatments of secondary causes of hypertension. Finally, dietary modification should be continued if a patient who has prehypertension or stage 1 hypertension requires medication therapy.

B. Start a regular aerobic exercise program, with a goal of 30 minutes daily   CORRECT

This recommendation comes from the JNC 7 for the initial treatment of and as an adjunct to medication in all patients being treated for prehypertension and hypertension.

C. Start triamterene 37.5 mg with hydrochlorothiazide 50 mg once every morning   INCORRECT

A diuretic is recommended as a first-line agent for the medical management of hypertension. However, the hydrochlorothiazide dose should never exceed 25 mg/day.

D. Start valsartan 80 mg once a day   INCORRECT

If Mrs. Blankenship required medication at this time for her BP, this would be an excellent choice. Angiotensin receptor blockers (ARBs) and angiotensin-converting enzyme (ACE) inhibitors are good first-line choices, especially in patients with diabetes because they offer some degree of renal protection (however, this indication is not approved by the US Food and Drug Administration [FDA]). ARBs tend to be a better choice than ACE inhibitors because there is a lower incidence of angioedema and cough.

Regardless, with prehypertension, a trial of 1 to 3 months of lifestyle modifications via diet/exercise and frequent at-home and in-office BP measurements are the most appropriate treatment and are approved by the JNC 7. However, if this is not effective or her BP is elevating despite these lifestyle changes, then a medication should be instituted. According to the JNC 7, appropriate first-line agents for patients with diabetes and hypertension include thiazide diuretics, ACE inhibitors, ARBs, calcium channel blockers (CCBs), and beta-blockers.

E. Substitute ibuprofen with acetaminophen 500 mg two pills twice a day   CORRECT

Although she is on a very small dose of ibuprofen, it could be enough to adversely affect her BP. Furthermore, this is a nonselective NSAID. If continuation of this medication is indicated, she should probably be on a proton pump inhibitor (PPI) for gastrointestinal protection because she is likely to require long-term usage. Treating hypertension to goal results in a decreased risk of CVA of 35 to 40%, MI of 20 to 24%, and heart failure of 50%. Most patients require at least two medications to reach goal.

Epidemiologic and Other Data

Estimates of the number of individuals with hypertension in the United States (defined as a systolic BP of ≥ 140 and/or a diastolic BP of ≥ 90) range from approximately 55.4 million to 66 million. The overall incidence is increasing in the United States; experts attribute this to the increasing number of obese individuals and the advancing age of our population, which are well-known risk factors for hypertension. It is estimated that normotensive individuals at the age of 55 years have a 90% lifetime risk for the development of hypertension. It appears that the acquisition of hypertension is a combination of genetic and lifestyle factors. By race, non-Hispanic blacks have the highest incidence, followed by non-Hispanic whites, and then Mexican Americans.

CASE 1-2
Betty Crane
1. History

A. Has she ever experienced chest pain, pressure, or discomfort; presyncope or syncope; dyspnea; or fatigue with exercise?   ESSENTIAL

The American Heart Association (AHA) has developed a consensus statement regarding the preparticipation cardiovascular screening for competitive athletes because of the increasing number of sudden cardiac death in athletes. Its purpose is to screen for individuals who might be at risk for sudden cardiac death and perform additional cardiac testing before making the recommendation that the patient should be able to compete or not. This 12-component screening tool consists of four questions regarding potential symptoms, two questions regarding the patient's personal medical history, and two questions regarding the patient's family history, and defines four essential components required on the physical examination. Additionally, the AHA recommends that for middle and high school students the history be verified with a parent. All positive responses would need to be discussed in detail. This choice asks about these four symptoms.

B. Has she ever been diagnosed with hypertension or a heart murmur?   ESSENTIAL

These are the two personal medical history questions on the AHA screening guideline.

C. Is there a family history of cardiac death or cardiac disability before the age of 50 years?   ESSENTIAL

This is one of the two questions pertaining to family history recommended by the AHA consensus statement.

D. Is there any known heart disease in the family?   ESSENTIAL

This is the second question recommended by the AHA consensus statement regarding the patient's family history. Additionally, it would probably be useful to inquire not only about cardiac disease in the family but also about specific conditions (e.g., hypertrophic or dilated cardiomyopathy, prolonged QT syndromes, other ion channelopathies, significant arrhythmias, sudden cardiac death, and Marfan syndrome).

E. When does she plan on becoming sexually active? NONESSENTIAL

This question does not have anything to do with the patient's ability to participate in sports and is inappropriate as it implies she should be sexually active.

2. Physical Examination

A. Funduscopic examination (or preferably slit-lamp examination if available)   ESSENTIAL

The four essential components of the physical examination, as recommended in the AHA consensus statement regarding the cardiovascular preparticipation evaluation for competitive athletes, include seated blood pressure in both arms; auscultation of the heart supine, standing, and with vagal maneuver; bilateral femoral pulse evaluation; and observation for any signs or symptoms suspicious of Marfan syndrome (MFS).

Therefore, a funduscopic (or the better procedure, a slit-lamp) examination is indicated to look for optical signs that could be consistent with MFS. The most common finding is ectopia lentis (the downward displacement of the lens of the eye). Although generally not progressive, it is associated with the development of cataracts. Other ophthalmologic findings could include retinal detachment, retinal tears, lattice degeneration, optical globe elongation, and myopia.

B. Ear and hearing examination   NONESSENTIAL

C. Heart evaluation   ESSENTIAL

This is one of the areas that the AHA recommends be very carefully evaluated. During the cardiac examination, attention must be focused not only in trying to hear cardiac murmurs but also in attempting to identify other signs suggestive of valvular disease, cardiomegaly, cardiac arrhythmias, extra heart sounds, abnormal splitting of heart sounds, clicks, thrills, parasternal lifts, and changes in heart sounds and/or murmurs (if present). The AHA recommends that the patient's heart be examined supine, standing, squatting, and with a Valsalva maneuver (which increases the intrathoracic pressure). The heart should also be auscultated during respiration and in the left lateral decubitus position (if an abnormal mitral sound is heard or mitral stenosis is suspected). These different maneuvers will enhance or decrease certain heart sounds and cardiac murmurs.

For example, when the patient stands upright or performs a Valsalva maneuver, murmurs tend to lessen in intensity and duration, except for those caused by mitral valve prolapse (it generally becomes louder and longer) and hypertrophic cardiomyopathy (it generally becomes louder).

However, when the patient squats or raises his or her legs while supine, the majority of cardiac murmurs become louder, except for those caused by mitral valve prolapse and hypertrophic cardiomyopathy (these become much softer and can even disappear completely). Isotonic and isometric exercise tends to cause murmurs associated with valvular stenosis (especially mitral and pulmonic) to worsen; however, isometric exercise will only cause regurgitation murmurs to worsen (especially mitral and aortic). A murmur caused by hypertrophic cardiomyopathy will only worsen with hand-grip exercise when maximum exertion is nearly achieved.

Inspiration often intensifies the sound and duration of systolic murmurs caused by tricuspid regurgitation and pulmonary stenosis and diastolic murmurs caused by tricuspid stenosis and pulmonary regurgitation. Expiration often intensifies the sound and duration of systolic murmurs caused by mitral regurgitation and aortic stenosis and diastolic murmurs caused by mitral stenosis and aortic regurgitation.

Bilateral BP measurements are required to determine if they are equivalent. If they are greater than 10 mm Hg, either systolic or diastolic, between the arms, the patient requires additional evaluation to determine the cause (e.g., aortic dissection, arterial obstruction, or arterial compression on the ipsilateral side of the lower BP).

D. Examination of femoral pulse and abdominal aorta   ESSENTIAL

Evaluation of the femoral pulse is also indicated by the AHA guidelines. Decreased pulses could indicate peripheral artery disease and occlusions or obstructions to the arteries in the legs. Comparison of the radial pulse with the ipsilateral femoral pulse evaluates primarily for possible coarctation of the aorta. Femoral pulses are weaker than the radials in this condition.

The aorta needs to be evaluated if the patient has abnormal aortic valvular sounds or is suspected of having Marfan syndrome.

E. Measurement of arm span from tip of left middle finger to tip of right middle finger and evaluation for arachnodactyly, joint hyperextensibility, joint laxity, and scoliosis   ESSENTIAL

Since Betty's physical appearance is suspicious for Marfan syndrome, these additional components should be performed. An arm span greater than the patient's height, arachnodactyly, joint hypermobility, and scoliosis are all signs that could indicate the presence of Marfan syndrome.

Other findings that could be associated with MFS include skin laxity, striae atrophicae (especially on the buttocks and shoulders), pes planus or high pedal arches, high-arched palate, kyphosis, anterior chest asymmetry (such as pectus excavatum or pectus carinatum), spontaneous pneumothorax, dural ectasis, inguinal hernias, incisional hernias, abnormal mitral and/or aortic heart valve leaflets, elongated chordae tendineae, aortic root dilation with dissection and/or rupture, and ocular abnormalities as described earlier.

3. Diagnostic Studies

A. Electrocardiogram (ECG)   ESSENTIAL

An ECG provides information regarding the presence of an arrhythmia, left ventricle hypertrophy, atrial hypertrophy, electrolyte abnormalities, conductive system defects, ischemia, acute infarction, and old infarction(s), with the latter three being extremely rare in adolescents.

B. Echocardiogram   ESSENTIAL

The echocardiogram provides greater detail regarding the valvular components, the aortic root, and wall thickness. It is indicated by Betty's mitral and aortic murmurs.

C. Chest x-ray (CXR)   ESSENTIAL

A CXR is indicated because Betty had findings on her physical examination suspicious for MFS. It will provide information regarding the presence of cardiomegaly, pectus excavatum, pectus carinatum, kyphosis, and thoracic scoliosis, which can be features of the disease.

D. Abdominal ultrasound   ESSENTIAL

The abdominal ultrasound is indicated because Betty has an aortic murmur. Its primary purpose is to evaluate her abdominal aorta for calcification, aneurysm, and/or early dissection.

E. Cardiac-specific troponin T and I   NONESSENTIAL

Cardiac-specific troponin T and I are biochemical markers that are utilized to detect cardiac ischemia. Because Betty does not have any signs or symptoms suspicious for angina or MI, these tests are not indicated.

4. Diagnosis

A. Loeys-Dietz aneurysm syndrome (LDAS)   INCORRECT

This syndrome is considered to be one of the heritable disorders of connective tissue. Like Marfan syndrome, LDAS is associated with a mutation of chromosome 15, but instead of it involving a mutation of the fibrillin-1 (FBN1) gene, it affects the transforming growth factor-β receptor 1 (TGFB1) and the transforming growth factor-β receptor 2 (TGFB2) genes. Although it is associated with the formation of abdominal aneurysms, it affects the ascending aorta more than the descending aorta, as seen in MFS. Additionally, it can be associated with tortuous arteries, hypertelorism, and a cleft palate. Hence, it can be eliminated as Betty's most likely diagnosis.

B. Klinefelter syndrome   INCORRECT

Klinefelter syndrome occurs exclusively in males and is also known as "the extra X-chromosome disease" because its karyotype is typically 47,XXY. Boys with Klinefelter syndrome appear to be typical males until puberty. At that time, they start to grow very long arms and legs, giving them an appearance similar to individuals with MFS. However, they do not exhibit the characteristic cardiovascular and ocular abnormalities.

They do tend to have gynecomastia, a feminine pattern of hair distribution, hypogonadism, small testes, and infertility. Because Klinefelter syndrome only affects males, this is not Betty's most likely diagnosis.

C. Marfan syndrome (MFS)   CORRECT

Marfan syndrome is a connective tissue disease. It is characterized by abnormalities of the cardiovascular, musculoskeletal, and ocular systems. Traditionally, if there is a known family history of Marfan syndrome, the diagnosis can be made when an individual has at least two of the three systems involved with typical signs and symptoms as described earlier. However, if there is no family history, then the patient must have characteristic signs and symptoms of musculoskeletal involvement plus ocular and cardiovascular symptoms, with one of the following major criteria: aortic root dilation, aortic dissection, or ectopia lentis. Thus, this is Betty's most likely diagnosis.

Because specific mutations in the FBN1 gene on chromosome 15 are not always present and the symptomatology of other heritable disorders of connective tissue syndromes/diseases can meet these limited criteria, there is an international movement recommending only the Ghent criteria be utilized to diagnose MFS. It emphasizes the major criteria—the presence of a minimum of four skeletal abnormalities, ectopia lentis, dilation of the ascending aorta, dural ectasia, and a blood relative who also has these abnormalities; however, it is balanced with a combination of minor criteria as well to establish the diagnosis of MFS. Still, other experts in the field feel that if the FBN1 gene abnormality is not present, the patient has another condition (e.g., type II Marfan or Loeys-Dietz aneurysm syndrome).

D. Ehlers-Danlos syndrome (EDS)   INCORRECT

EDS is another heritable disorder of connective tissue. It is characterized by hyperelasticity of the skin and hypermobility of the joints, both of which can be seen with MFS. Additionally, mitral valve prolapse, aortic aneurysms, kyphosis, scoliosis, and hernias are frequently seen. However, unlike MFS, the predominate ocular defect is dependent upon the form of disease the patient has—for example, patients with ocular-scoliotic EDS can have complete eye rupture with very little trauma, and individuals with EDS associated with respiratory impairment can have blue-colored sclerae. Additionally, patients with EDS tend to have bleeding abnormalities. Therefore, this can be eliminated as Betty's most likely diagnosis.

E. Congenital contractural arachnodactyly (CCA)   INCORRECT

CCA is another heritable disorder of connective tissue. It has symptoms that are partially consistent with MFS and partially consistent with osteogenesis imperfecta (OI) but does not completely fulfill the criteria for either. It can be ruled out as Betty's most likely diagnosis because she does not have any joint contractures, which are always associated with CCA.

5. Treatment Plan

A. Annual echocardiogram   CORRECT

An annual echocardiogram is important to monitor the progression of Betty's mitral and/or aortic regurgitation as well as the diameter of her aortic root. In some cases, more frequent echocardiograms may be required.

B. Annual eye examination, including a slit lamp, by an ophthalmologist   CORRECT

An annual eye examination by an ophthalmologist primarily monitors for ectopic lentis, retinal detachment, retinal hemorrhages, amblyopia, and other ocular abnormalities caused by MFS.

C. Subacute bacterial endocarditis (SBE) prophylaxis for dental procedures   INCORRECT

Unless something unusual appears on Betty's subsequent echocardiogram or she requires a valve replacement, she will not require antibiotic prophylaxis for dental procedures.

When the latest American Heart Association's guidelines for SBE prophylaxis were released in 2007, the indications for dental procedures included: history of infective endocarditis, presence of a prosthetic heart valve or a prosthetic material utilized to repair a heart valve, cardiac transplant patients who develop a valvulopathy, and the following congenital heart diseases (CHDs): unrepaired CHD with cyanosis, including palliative shunts and conduits; 6 months following completely repaired CHD when a prosthetic material or device is utilized regardless of procedure used for the intervention; and repaired CHD with residual defects at the site or adjacent to the site inhibiting endothelialization.

These guidelines have subsequently been modified, but not re-written, to state that the only requirement for SBE prophylaxis for dental procedures is for those that could involve manipulation and/or perforation of the gingiva, oral mucosa, and/or periapical areas of the teeth in individuals whose underlying cardiac abnormality places him or her at the highest risk of developing adverse outcomes if infectious endocarditis occurred.

D. Annual orthopedic evaluation   CORRECT

The annual orthopedic examination provides for the monitoring of scoliosis and permits appropriate interventions to prevent deformities. In general, bracing and physical therapy are begun if the degree of scoliosis reaches 20°; surgery is generally required if it reaches 45°.

E. Propranolol 10 to 20 mg twice a day initially; then, titrate every 1 to 2 weeks (to a maximum daily dose of 240 mg) to maintain exercise heart rate below 100 BPM   CORRECT

A beta-blocker, like propranolol, should be given to Betty as it appears to slow the progression of the aortic dilation and hence the need for cardiac surgery.

Epidemiologic and Other Data

Type I Marfan syndrome is a genetic disorder that is generally associated with a mutation of the FBN1 gene on chromosome 15. Approximately 75% of the cases are inherited via autosomal dominant traits. The remainder of the cases consist of new sporadic mutations. The incidence is estimated to be approximately 1 per 3000 to 5000 individuals in the United States. There does not appear to be an increased incidence in any particular race.

CASE 1-3
Carl Diaz
1. History

A. Has Carl ever had his BP checked?   ESSENTIAL

It is important to inquire about Carl's previous BP readings because of his elevated value today. An elevated BP on two occasions is considered to be diagnostic for hypertension.

This is important because having hypertension doubles the patient's risk for CAD, CVA, PAD, heart failure, and renal failure. Multiple clinical trials have proven that normalizing the BP level reduces the risk of developing these complications.

Although it is the standard of care to check the BP of all children at every visit after the age of 3 years, the only organization that makes that recommendation is the National Heart, Lung and Blood Institute (NHLBI). The American Academy of Family Physicians (AAFP) believes that there is insufficient evidence available to make a recommendation for or against routine BP measurements in children to screen for hypertension. However, they recommend checking BP every other year if normal, annually if prehypertensive, and as required if hypertensive. The U.S. Preventative Services Task Force (USPSTF) recommends screening for hypertension beginning at the age of 18 years; however, they do not make a recommendation for frequency.

B. Was Carl's cholesterol test done while he was fasting or nonfasting?   NONESSENTIAL

Total cholesterol levels do not vary significantly regardless of whether they are done in the fasting or nonfasting state. However, it is generally recommended that the patient fast for 8 to 12 hours before having a "cholesterol test" because that term (although technically incorrect) generally involves obtaining an entire lipid panel, which measures not only total cholesterol but also its various components (i.e., high-density lipoproteins [HDLs], low-density lipoproteins [LDLs], very low-density lipoproteins [VLDLs], and non-HDL cholesterol), plus the triglycerides. For an accurate triglyceride measurement, the test must be performed in the fasting state because triglyceride levels can fluctuate significantly during the day.

C. What is Carl's mother's cholesterol level?   NONESSENTIAL

The AHA expanded upon the Third Report of the National Cholesterol Education Program (NCEP) Expert Panel on Detection, Evaluation, and Treatment of High Blood Cholesterol in Adults and developed recommendations for screening children and adolescents (ages 2–18) for hyperlipidemia based on personal and family history. One of the criteria is either parent having a total serum cholesterol measurement of greater than or equal to 240 mg/dl. Because Carl requires screening based on his father's level, his mother's findings are not relevant at this time.

The other criteria are a positive family history of CAD and a personal risk for CAD without any parental risks, defined as one having one or more of the following: hypertension, obesity, diseases known to be associated with hyperlipidemia (e.g., pancreatitis, hepatitis, diabetes mellitus, or Cushing syndrome), medications known to produce hyperlipidemia (e.g., carbamazepine, beta-blockers, glucocorticoids, growth hormone, or iso-tretinoin), or detrimental lifestyle habits (e.g., smoking cigarettes, drinking alcohol, or sedentary lifestyle).

The USPSTF believes that there is not sufficient evidence to recommend for or against routine screening of children and adolescents, regardless of risk factors. However, they do support the screening of high-risk men who are 20 and 35 years old and high-risk women who are 20 to 45 years old; they do not make any recommendations regarding screening frequency if normal. After 35 years of age in men and 45 years of age in women, they recommend "periodic" screening depending on risk factors.

The NCEP III recommends routine screening every 5 years, if normal, beginning at the age of 20 years for both men and women. The AAFP recommends screening at undetermined intervals beginning at the age of 35 years for men and 45 years for women.

D. Has either of Carl's parents and/or grandparents been diagnosed with a myocardial infarction (MI), coronary artery disease (CAD), sudden cardiac death (SCD), a cerebral vascular accident (CVA), or peripheral vessel disease (PVD) prior to the age of 55 years? ESSENTIAL

According to the AHA, a child or adolescent should have a fasting blood lipoprotein analysis if his or her parents and/or grandparents have had a premature MI, CAD, SCD, CVA, and/or PVD (defined as occurring before the age of 55 years).

Furthermore, even if they are not premature, the presence of any of these conditions in a blood relative increases the later risk of these diseases and should be noted.

E. Have his parents and/or grandparents been diagnosed with diabetes mellitus (including gestational diabetes) or any other serious medical condition(s)? ESSENTIAL

This is important because the American Diabetes Association recommends routine screening for diabetes mellitus every other year for children starting at the age of 10 years (or the onset of puberty if before the age of 10 years) if overweight (defined as a BMI > 85th percentile for either age and gender or weight for height OR weight > 120% of ideal height) PLUS the presence of two additional risk factors: type 1 or type 2 diabetes mellitus in any first- or second-degree blood relative (genetic risk is greatest with type 1 diabetes mellitus), maternal gestational diabetes mellitus (GDM), high-risk race (Native American, African American, Hispanic American, Asian American, or Pacific Islander), or any signs, symptoms, or conditions associated with insulin resistance (e.g., hypertension, hyperlipidemia, significantly elevated triglyceride levels, polycystic ovarian disease, and visceral distribution obesity).

No other organization makes a recommendation to routinely screen children or adults. However, the AAFP and the USPSTF do make the recommendation to screen all adults with hypertension with fasting plasma glucose (FPG) measurements for type 2 diabetes mellitus.

2. Physical Examination

A. Ears, nose, and throat (ENT) examination NONESSENTIAL

B. Thyroid palpation ESSENTIAL

Even though a child or adolescent does not require an evaluation for a secondary cause of hyperlipidemia unless he

or she has failed 6 to 12 months of lifestyle modification or is symptomatic, Carl still needs his thyroid palpated because of the association of thyroid disease and hypertension.

C. Heart examination ESSENTIAL

A careful heart examination looking for the abnormalities outlined in Case 1-2 is indicated for Carl because of his weight, BP, cholesterol level, and family history.

D. Abdominal examination ESSENTIAL

Carl should have an abdominal examination primarily because of his elevated BP. In addition to the routine abdominal examination, particular attention should be directed to the aorta (to ensure normal pulsation and size), the renal arteries (to assess for bruits, which could indicate renovascular disease), the kidney and adrenal area (to assess for abnormal sizes and/or masses, which could indicate renal failure, adrenal tumors/masses, or pheochromocytoma), and the bladder (to assess for enlargement, as would be seen with an obstructive uropathy) because these are just a few of the potential causes of secondary hypertension.

E. Assessment of pulses ESSENTIAL

Assessment of the pulses would help ensure Carl is getting good and equal blood flow to all parts of his body. However, it is important to remember that bruits generally disappear when the degree of vascular occlusion becomes greater than 70%; hence, the lack of this abnormality does not necessarily equate with the lack of disease.

Additionally, the strength of the femoral pulses needs to be compared to that of the ipsilateral radial pulse to evaluate for coarctation of the aorta, as discussed in the previous case.

3. Diagnostic Studies

A. Fasting blood lipoprotein analysis ESSENTIAL

The American Heart Association Guidelines recommends that if the initial total cholesterol is greater than 200 mg/dl, then a lipoprotein analysis should be conducted.

B. Total cholesterol only NONESSENTIAL

According to the AHA guidelines, a high-risk adolescent should be screened with a total cholesterol level. However, because Carl already had an elevated screening total cholesterol, an additional one is not indicated (he requires a fasting lipoprotein analysis which includes a total cholesterol).

C. Fasting plasma glucose (FPG) ESSENTIAL

Because Carl is older than the age of 10 years, his weight is greater than 120% for his ideal height and above the 85th percentile of BMI for height (however, the use of BMI in individuals younger than 18 years of age is discouraged by the Centers for Disease Control and Prevention [CDC] to prevent "labeling" a child as "obese"), and his maternal grandfather has diabetes, he meets the criteria set forth by the American Diabetes Association to be screened with an FPG.

D. C-reactive protein (CRP) NONESSENTIAL

CRP is a nonspecific measurement of inflammation in the body, including that associated with endothelium dysfunction. Therefore, it can be utilized in conjunction with the patient's cholesterol and cardiovascular risk factors to provide additional information of a patient's future potential of a cardiovascular event. However, the ideal test is the high-sensitivity CRP (hs-CRP), not just a CRP, because it can detect much smaller levels of inflammation. Nevertheless, neither is indicated as a part of the cardiovascular risk determination in the assessment of children and/or adolescents.

E. Glycosylated hemoglobin (Hgb A1C)   NONESSENTIAL

The Hgb A1C test is a diabetes treatment management tool that is used to monitor the patient's blood sugar level, and hence control, over the past 3 months. It is not indicated as a screening tool at this time; however, there is an ongoing discussion for its potential use as such.

4. Diagnosis

A. Hyperlipidemia, hypertension, and type 1 diabetes mellitus INCORRECT

Carl's total cholesterol was 222 mg/dl, his LDL 160 mg/dl; his HDL 30 mg/dl, his VLDL 32 mg/dl, and his triglycerides 250 mg/dl. Because this was his second total cholesterol measurement, he can be considered to be hyperlipidemic by adult and more appropriately adolescent standards. The AHA and NCEP developed the levels listed in **Table 1-3** regarding hyperlipidemia in children and adolescents (ages 2–18 years).

In adolescents, hypertension is defined as a BP being greater than the 95th percentile for height on at least two occasions. Carl's maximum BP at the 95th percentile would be 135/85 mm Hg; therefore, he can be considered hypertensive.

Prehypertension is defined in adolescents as being between the 90th and 95th percentile for height OR greater than 120/80 mm Hg on two or more occasions for Carl.

Carl's FPG was normal; therefore, he cannot be considered to be diabetic. Hence, this choice is not his most likely diagnosis.

B. Hyperlipidemia, hypertension, and type 2 diabetes mellitus INCORRECT

Carl does meet the diagnostic criteria for hyperlipidemia and hypertension in an adolescent. However, his FPG is not of a sufficient level to diagnose him as having diabetes mellitus. In addition, with his other coexisting medical conditions and a lack of a family history of type 1 diabetes mellitus, if he did have diabetes, he would more than likely have premature type 2. Nevertheless, per the aforementioned definitions, this is also not Carl's most likely diagnosis.

C. Hyperlipidemia, hypertension, obesity, and type 2 diabetes mellitus   INCORRECT

Carl's diagnoses consist of hyperlipidemia and hypertension as defined earlier.

Table 1-3 Hyperlipidemia in Children and Adolescents (Ages 2 to 18 Years)

	Total Cholesterol	Low-Density Lipoprotein Cholesterol
Acceptable	< 170	< 110
Borderline	170–199	110–129
High	≥ 200	≥ 130

Regarding the diagnosis of obesity, many organizations now consider obesity in adolescents to be a BMI for age and gender that is greater than or equal to the 95th percentile. Carl's BMI of 37.4 falls significantly above his projected 95th percentile of BMI for age of 26.5; therefore, it would be appropriate to diagnose him as obese. Additionally, he meets the criteria of obesity defined in individuals younger than the age of 18 years as being greater than 120% of weight for ideal height.

Overweight is classified by most as a BMI for age and gender that is greater than or equal to the 85th percentile but less than the 95th percentile. However, as stated previously, the CDC prefers utilizing the terminology in individuals younger than the age of 20 years as "overweight" if their BMI for age and gender is greater than or equal to the 95th percentile and "at risk of overweight" if their BMI for age and gender is greater than or equal to the 85th percentile but less than the 95th percentile. Currently the Expert Committee on the Assessment, Prevention, and Treatment of Childhood and Adolescent Overweight and Obesity is working with the CDC to develop consistent terminology. Therefore, the more appropriate diagnosis would be overweight for age.

Regardless, he has a normal FPG; hence, he does not meet the diagnostic criteria for diabetes mellitus. Therefore, this is not his most likely diagnosis.

D. Hyperlipidemia, hypotension, and obesity   INCORRECT

For the aforementioned reasons regarding obesity, and Carl's BP being high, not low, this is not his most likely diagnosis.

E. Hyperlipidemia, hypertension, and overweight for age CORRECT

By the aforementioned definitions, this is Carl's most likely diagnosis.

5. Treatment Plan

A. Repeat total lipoprotein analysis in 1 month to obtain LDL average to utilize for monitoring and treatment   CORRECT

According to the AHA guidelines, if the total cholesterol is greater than 200 on the initial screening, then a lipoprotein analysis should be conducted. That analysis should then be repeated in approximately 1 month to obtain the patient's average LDL value. The average LDL value from these two measurements is what his treatment will be based on. His current LDL goal is less than 110 mg/dl or a minimum of less than 130 mg/dl.

B. Initiate a program of lifestyle modification with a low-fat, low-cholesterol, low-sodium diet; decreased caloric diet; and regular exercise program with goal of 30 minutes of aerobic exercise on most days of the week   CORRECT

Lifestyle modification is the cornerstone of treatment for all of Carl's current conditions: overweight for height, hyperlipidemia, and hypertension. Even if lifestyle modifications alone fail to meet his treatment goals, they are still going to be an essential component of any treatment plan for any of these conditions.

C. Start niacin 500 mg once a day for 2 weeks; then increase to 500 mg twice a day   INCORRECT

Medication management for children and adolescents with hyperlipidemia is not indicated until a minimum of

6 to 12 months of dietary modification has failed to be effective. Then, it is only indicated if the LDL is greater than or equal to 190 mg/dl OR the LDL is greater than or equal to 160 mg/dl AND there is a positive family history of premature CAD AND the patient has at least two other risk factors present (hypertension, smoking, diabetes, male gender, sedentary lifestyle, or the suspicion of familial hyperlipidemia). The ideal treatment goal would be an LDL of less than 110 mg/dl; however, less than 130 mg/dl would be acceptable. Statins are currently considered to be the first-line drug and should never be used unless the child is older than 10 years. Other appropriate choices include niacin and bile acid sequestrants. One of these latter two options might soon be the drug of choice as more and more adverse effects are being linked to the statins. However, most would be considered "off-label" usage as few are FDA approved for use in individuals younger than the ages of 18 to 21 years. Those with current FDA approval to be used in children 10 years of age or older include atorvastatin, lovastatin, pravastatin (indication starting at 8 years old), cholestyramine, ezetimibe, and simvastatin.

D. Thyroid stimulation test (TSH), liver function studies (LFTs), creatinine, and urine protein   INCORRECT

These tests are indicated in adults to determine if there is a coexisting medical condition that could be responsible for or contributing to the elevated cholesterol level. The TSH is to screen for hypothyroidism. The LFT will evaluate for hepatic conditions (e.g., hepatitis and cholestasis). The serum creatinine and the urine protein will assist in determining whether chronic renal failure or nephrotic syndrome is present. If the triglycerides are elevated, then an FPG is also indicated to rule out type 2 diabetes mellitus.

However, according to the AHA guidelines, children do not need to be screened for any secondary cause of hyperlipidemia unless they have failed to respond to 6 to 12 months of lifestyle modifications or were symptomatic. Therefore, these tests are not currently indicated for Carl.

E. Start triamterene 37.5 mg with hydrochlorothiazide 50 mg once every morning   INCORRECT

Medical management of hypertension in adolescents (and children) is only indicated if lifestyle modifications fail to decrease the BP to acceptable levels, the adolescent has coexisting type 1 or type 2 diabetes mellitus, the hypertension is caused by another condition (secondary hypertension), the patient has evidence of end-organ damage, or the patient is symptomatic. Because Carl does not fall into any of these groups, he does not require medication at this time.

Additionally, the dosage of hydrochlorothiazide should not exceed 25 mg, because studies indicate that beyond that dosage the BP-lowering effects are negated or reversed. Therefore, instead of increasing hydrochlorothiazide to 50 mg, starting a second agent with an alternative pathway of action is preferable.

Epidemiologic and Other Data

Lipoprotein levels, especially triglycerides, do not remain constant over time. This partially explains the discrepancies between the recommendations of the various organizations as to the optimal time to initiate screening and the appropriate screening interval in adults who have normal levels. Furthermore, it is the justification that some organizations use to never screen a child or adolescent, regardless of levels.

The exact incidence of hypertension in children and adolescents is unknown. Even though the majority of the cases are caused by secondary hypertension, the incidence of essential (or primary) hypertension is increasing in children and adolescents in the United States. This is believed to be associated with the increased rates of overweight and obesity in these groups. African American children, as well as adults, are the racial group with the greatest incidence in the United States.

As with hypertension, the exact incidence of type 2 diabetes mellitus in adolescents is unknown. However, it is also increasing, and it is theorized that that increase is related to the increased rate of overweight and obesity among US teens.

It is estimated that approximately 17% of children and adolescents are overweight in the United States. This equates to approximately 4.2 million children between the ages of 6 and 11 years (with 1.9 million of these being girls) and 5.7 million adolescents (of which 2.6 million are female).

In the last 40 years, the incidence in grade school–aged children being overweight has increased nearly 350%. In the past 35 years, the incidence of overweight adolescents has increased nearly 300%. It is estimated that if these trends continue, by the year 2015, one out of every four children in the United States will be overweight.

CASE 1-4
Dale Elliott
1. History

A. Where is the chest pain located, does it radiate, what is its nature, what is its intensity, is it constant or intermittent, is it worsening, and are there any known aggravating or alleviating factors?   ESSENTIAL

Chest pain can occur with a vast array of cardiac, pulmonary, gastrointestinal, musculoskeletal, dermatologic, metabolic, neurologic, and psychological conditions. They can range from mild problems (e.g., Tietze syndrome or flatulence) to potentially fatal conditions (e.g., myocardial infarction, pneumothorax, or pulmonary embolism). Although certain symptoms are suspicious for some conditions, they are generally not specific (e.g., crushing substernal chest pain alleviated with nitroglycerine could be an esophageal spasm or an acute myocardial infarction, and lateral chest pain aggravated by inspiration could range from a muscle strain to pneumonia). Therefore, the more details that can be obtained regarding Mr. Elliott's chest pain, the more likely an accurate differential diagnosis list will be established to narrow this wide array of possibilities.

B. Has he checked his temperature with a thermometer? ESSENTIAL

Many patients (and parents) base the presence of a fever on whether the skin, especially over the forehead, feels warm or hot. The hotter it feels, the higher they assume the fever. This is not an accurate method of determining core body temperature.

In fact, when the core body temperature is significantly elevated, the patient's skin can feel cool secondary to the vasoconstriction mechanism of the body to dissipate the excessive heat. All patients who feel febrile should have their temperature checked with a thermometer that the user knows how to correctly operate.

C. Has he noticed any skin lesions or rash?   ESSENTIAL

The presence of a rash narrows the list of potential diagnoses for many complaints, especially chest pain. Although it will likely eliminate the possibility of an acute myocardial infarction, it still does not limit the potential diagnoses to benign conditions only. For example, a contusion to the chest wall could cause pain from local tissue trauma or it could represent a serious underlying condition such as cardiac tamponade, ventricular aneurysm, constrictive pericarditis, hemothorax, or diaphragm rupture. Other rashes associated with chest pain are characteristic for specific conditions (e.g., herpes zoster has a dermatomal distribution).

D. Has he experienced any visual abnormalities?   ESSENTIAL

Several viral syndromes (e.g., influenza, herpes zoster, measles, and mumps) can be associated with the visual disturbances of Devic disease (neuromyelitis optica). In view of Mr. Elliott's flulike symptoms, this is an appropriate question to ask. Additionally, chest pain–associated visual abnormality and the presence of Roth spots (exudative lesions of the retina) are frequently associated with acute infectious endocarditis (IE) or SBE.

E. Does he have any pet rabbits at home?   NONESSENTIAL

The concern with constitutional symptoms and rabbits is tularemia. However, Mr. Elliott's other symptoms are not consistent with this diagnosis. Tularemia generally consists of a sudden-onset headache associated with fever, nausea, and a papule at the site of inoculation. This papule quickly ulcerates and is associated with marked regional lymphadenopathy. Additionally, it is rare to acquire the infection by having a rabbit for a pet; generally it takes direct inoculation of the infected tissue (e.g., cutting oneself with the knife while skinning a wild rabbit).

2. Physical Examination

A. General appearance   ESSENTIAL

The patient's general appearance and demeanor is an essential component of the physical examination of each and every patient encounter. It provides a gross assessment of both the patient's physical and psychological condition. However, unless something is grossly abnormal, these finding are rarely recorded in the patient's chart.

The most common elements that should be observed include the patient's overall physical condition (e.g., malnourished, obese, or disheveled), appearance of being seriously ill (e.g., signs of toxicity, acute distress, or altered consciousness), general mental state (e.g., depressed, euphoric, apathetic, or indifferent), other signs of a mental disorder (e.g., poor hygiene, inappropriate dress, or inappropriate affect), incongruency between appearance and chief complaint, and discordance of verbal and body languages. It is important for the HCP not to permit his or her own biases, beliefs, values, and personality to taint this assessment.

B. Heart examination   ESSENTIAL

A careful heart examination looking for the abnormalities outlined in Case 1-2 is indicated because of Mr. Elliott's complaint of left-sided anterior chest pain.

C. Lung auscultation   ESSENTIAL

Auscultation of Mr. Elliott's lung is important to assess that his breath sounds are present and symmetric throughout his lungs, to determine the presence of abnormal breath sounds (e.g., wheezing, rhonchi, rales, and/or stridor), and to evaluate depth and length of inspiration and expiration and their relationship to his pain since he has been experiencing respiratory symptoms.

D. Digital rectal examination (DRE)   NONESSENTIAL

E. Skin and nail examination   ESSENTIAL

Skin and nail changes can be associated with a wide variety of medical conditions. For example, the splinter hemorrhages noted on Mr. Elliott's nails can result from something as simple as trauma to something as severe as SBE. They can also occur without being associated with any specific medical condition in 10 to 20% of all hospitalized patients. Regardless, because Mr. Elliott has dermatologic and nail complaints, these areas need to be evaluated.

3. Diagnostic Studies

A. Complete blood count with differential (CBC w/diff) ESSENTIAL

A CBC w/diff is essential to perform on Mr. Elliott because it provides a lot of information regarding the patient. The primary function of white blood cells (WBCs) is to fight infection and foreign bodies. When they are elevated (leukocytosis), they are associated with infection, inflammation, severe stress (both physical and psychological), severe trauma, tissue necrosis, and some forms of leukemia. A low WBC count (leukopenia) is seen with conditions such as viral infections, some autoimmune diseases, and poor nutrition. The total WBC count is composed of five different types of cells, each one having its own significance: neutrophils, lymphocytes, eosinophils, basocytes, and monocytes. Because the total always has to equal 100%, if one or more types are elevated, then one or more types have to be decreased to compensate. Some of the more common causes for these differential counts to be either elevated or decreased are as follows:

Neutrophil elevations are generally associated with acute bacterial processes, severe inflammation, trauma, metabolic abnormalities, and stress (both physical and psychological). Additionally, if immature neutrophils (bands or stabs) are seen, it is usually indicative of a significant stimulation of the neutrophils and hence a more severe infection or inflammatory process. Neutropenia can be seen with dietary deficiencies, viral infections, overwhelming bacterial infections, and aplastic anemia.

Monocytes are generally elevated in acute viral infections, in inflammatory conditions, and with nongastrointestinal parasites. Monocytopenia is rare and frequently found in patients taking chronic oral corticosteroids and/or chemotherapy.

Eosinophilia is frequently associated with allergic conditions, parasitic infections (primarily gastrointestinal), and autoimmune diseases. They tend to only be decreased when there is abnormal adrenocorticosteroid production.

Basophils tend to be elevated in myeloproliferative diseases and leukemia; basopenia can be found in acute physical or emotional stress or an acute allergic reaction.

Lymphocytosis is generally affiliated with acute viral infections, chronic bacterial infections, and some carcinomas; they are decreased in sepsis, leukemia, immunodeficiency syndromes, and some autoimmune diseases.

The red blood cell (RBC) count, its indices, the hemoglobin, and the hematocrit provide information regarding possible anemia. A patient is considered anemic when his or her hemoglobin and/or hematocrit are decreased. However, early in acute hemorrhage, these values could be normal and the patient could still have significant blood loss.

Anemias are further classified based on the size and hemoglobin concentrations obtained from the RBC indices to assist in determining the most likely type of anemia the patient has. The mean corpuscular volume (MCV) is the average size of a single RBC; from this, an anemia is classified as normocytic, macrocytic, or microcytic. The mean corpuscular hemoglobin (MCH) is a measurement of the average amount of hemoglobin found in a single RBC. It is not a major determinant of the type of anemia the patient is experiencing; however, it tends to match the mean corpuscular hemoglobin concentration (MCHC), which is a measurement of the average percentage of hemoglobin in an RBC. It is this latter value that determines whether the patient's anemia is hypochromic, normochromic, or hyperchromic.

Platelets are necessary for blood to clot properly. The lower the platelet count (thrombocytopenia) is, the more severe the bleeding diathesis tends to be.

B. Chest x-ray (CXR)   ESSENTIAL

Because of the minimal findings on his physical examination, a CXR would not have been generally indicated for Mr. Elliott. However, because he is experiencing hemoptysis, it is recommended to attempt to identify any potential abnormalities that might reveal the cause (e.g., a mass with lung cancer, nodular infiltrates with septic pulmonary infarcts, infiltrates with pneumonia, nodules with tuberculosis [especially in the upper lobes], and left ventricular failure with an enlargement of the ventricular portion of the cardiac shadow).

It is assumed that Mr. Elliott's hemoptysis is secondary to breaking superficial blood vessels in the trachea or bronchi as a result of his severe coughing. However, it could also represent early septic pulmonary infarcts or a malignancy. In theory, his hemoptysis should resolve when his infection resolves. If not, he will probably require a bronchoscopy and/or computed tomography (CT) scan to identify the cause, especially because he is a smoker.

C. A minimum of 2 blood cultures with sensitivities and Gram stains drawn at least 1 hour apart   ESSENTIAL

These are definitely indicated because Mr. Elliott is toxic appearing. It is important to remember to collect the blood for the blood culture BEFORE instituting the empiric antibiotic therapy.

Blood cultures and sensitivities often take up to 72 hours for growth, identification, and sensitivity testing of the organism. Therefore, the Gram stain performed on the specimen to determine whether the sputum is adequate for culture can be utilized to attempt to determine the most likely pathogen (and its empiric treatment) based on its characteristics.

D. Electrocardiogram (ECG)   ESSENTIAL

An ECG is indicated because he has tachycardia, an irregular pulse, and chest pain.

E. Transesophageal echocardiography (TEE)   ESSENTIAL

Because Mr. Elliott's symptoms could represent a heart valve infection, a TEE is indicated. TEE is superior to transthoracic echocardiography (TTE) in attempting to find evidence to diagnose IE because TTE is limited by obesity, large breasts, and/or chronic lung disease. Furthermore, it is less accurate in determining the overall structure and function of the valves. The sensitivity of TTE in determining findings consistent with IE is estimated to be approximately 65% vs approximately 90% with TEE.

F. Urinary drug screen for illicit substances and narcotics ESSENTIAL

Considering that several of the potential conditions on Mr. Elliott's list of differential diagnoses could be associated with or caused by illicit drug use, his admitting to taking oxycodone that was not prescribed for him, and his refusing a foot examination (possibly due to "track marks" being seen) raise suspicions enough to warrant a drug screen. If he has a substance abuse problem that caused, or in addition to, his current condition, it also needs to be addressed and treated.

4. Diagnosis

A. Lymphocytic leukemia   INCORRECT

Mr. Elliott's positive Gram stains for bacteria and his CBC abnormalities of mild leukocytosis with neutrophilia and lymphopenia make lymphocytic leukemia very unlikely to be his most likely diagnosis because the hallmark of lymphocytic leukemia is noninfectious lymphocytosis.

B. Rocky Mountain spotted fever   INCORRECT

Rocky Mountain spotted fever is a serious systemic infection that includes, among other symptoms, a rash on the palms of the hands and the soles of the feet. However, it is a rickettsial infection (hence, it should not be associated with a positive Gram stain) transmitted by ticks (*Dermacentor andersoni* and *variabilis*). Because this is inconsistent with his findings, this is not Mr. Elliott's most likely diagnosis.

C. Acute influenza and tricuspid regurgitation   INCORRECT

Although some of Mr. Elliott's symptoms are consistent with influenza, many of them are not. Uncomplicated acute influenza should be improving, not worsening, after 1.5 weeks of illness. His WBC count and Gram stain indicate a bacterial, not a viral, pathogen is responsible for his illness. And, although his echocardiogram does reveal tricuspid regurgitation, it also reveals vegetation on the tricuspid valve which is inconsistent with uncomplicated tricuspid regurgitation. Hence, this is not his most likely diagnosis.

D. Infective endocarditis (IE)   CORRECT

The Duke criteria have been established to assist in making the clinical diagnosis of IE. It is composed of two major and five minor criteria. The diagnosis of IE can be made by having both major criteria OR one major and three minor criteria OR all five minor criteria.

The major criteria are two separate positive blood cultures for organisms that typically cause IE and echocardiographic evidence of IE. The minor criteria consist of (1) fever of greater than or equal to 38° C (Temperature conversion equations to and from Fahrenheit can be found in **Table 1-4**.), (2) predisposing cardiac condition or IV drug use/abuse, (3) vascular phenomena (e.g., major arterial emboli, septic pulmonary infarctions, intracranial hemorrhage, conjunctival hemorrhages, and/or Janeway lesions), (4) immunologic phenomena (e.g., Osler nodes, Roth spots, or positive rheumatoid factor), and (5) a positive blood culture that did not meet the major criteria's standard OR serologic evidence of an organism associated with IE.

Because Mr. Elliott has one major criterion (perhaps two, if his cultures are positive) and three minor criteria (perhaps four, if he abuses IV drugs), he can be diagnosed with IE. Thus, from the list provided, IE is his most likely diagnosis.

E. Disseminated gonococcal infection (DGI)   INCORRECT

DGI, or gonococcal bacteremia, has some symptoms that are consistent with Mr. Elliott's presentation; however, DGI has other characteristic symptoms that he is not experiencing (i.e., monoarticular arthritis [or occasionally two or three joints maximum] and a sparse macular-papular, pustular, or hemorrhagic rash that is peripherally located). Finally, gonorrhea is a gram-negative intracellular diplococcus. Because of these inconsistencies, this is not his most likely diagnosis.

5. Treatment Plan

A. Cefazolin 2 g IV every 8 hours and gentamicin 70 mg IV every 8 hours until blood cultures and sensitivities are available   INCORRECT

Considering Mr. Elliott's Gram stain reveals gram-positive cocci in clusters; the organisms that most commonly cause infective endocarditis are *Streptococcus viridans, Staphylococcus aureus,* and *Enterococcus*; his tricuspid valve is affected (60% incidence of being due to *S. aureus*); and the suspicion that he uses/abuses IV drugs (which increases the incidence of *S. aureus* even higher), his most likely pathogen is *S. aureus*. However, the offending organism cannot be positively identified until the culture results are available.

Cefazolin would be an acceptable empiric antibiotic treatment regimen for IE caused by *S. aureus* if there were no concerns regarding methicillin-resistant *S. aureus* (MRSA). However, because of the increasing incidence of MRSA in most areas of the United States and the serious nature of his infection, this is not an acceptable empiric choice.

Table 1-4 Temperature Conversions

From Fahrenheit to Celsius:
[(Degrees in Fahrenheit − 32) × 5] ÷ 9 = Degrees in Celsius
From Celsius to Fahrenheit:
[(Degrees in Celsius × 9) ÷ 5] + 32 = Degrees in Fahrenheit

Furthermore, cephalosporins have been known to have a cross-sensitivity to the penicillins; hence, Mr. Elliott could experience a similar (or worse) allergic reaction from the cephalosporins than he did with the penicillin. Thus, this is not an appropriate treatment option for him.

B. Vancomycin 1g IV every 12 hours and gentamicin 70 mg IV every 8 hours until blood cultures and sensitivities are available   CORRECT

Vancomycin alone should cover *S. aureus*, even if it is methicillin resistant. However, until the culture results are available to confirm this suspected pathogen, gentamicin should be added to cover other possible pathogens. Once the cultures' and sensitivities' results are available, his antibiotics can be adjusted accordingly.

C. Hospitalize and observe closely for additional complications   CORRECT

Based on Mr. Elliott's appearance, vital signs, and diagnostic tests, he is considered to be septic. Therefore, hospitalization is indicated for IV fluids, IV antibiotics, additional diagnostic procedures, vital sign monitoring, cardiac monitoring, and close observation.

D. Refer for substance abuse treatment   CORRECT

When the tricuspid valve is involved in IE, it is estimated that 80 to 95% of the cases are secondary to IV drug use/abuse. This combined with the aforementioned reasons for ordering a drug screen is concerning. However, a referral for treatment is not indicated unless his drug screen returns positive, he goes into withdrawal, or he admits to a problem.

E. Bone marrow biopsy   INCORRECT

This painful procedure is not currently indicated for Mr. Elliott. His CBC changes are consistent with his diagnosis; therefore, they should normalize after his IE has responded to therapy. If not, an evaluation is indicated, which may or may not include a bone marrow biopsy.

Epidemiologic and Other Data

It is estimated that there are anywhere from 2 to 7 cases per 100,000 persons of IE in the United States annually. The incidence caused by rheumatic heart disease has been decreasing in recent years; however, the incidence from degenerative valvular disease, prosthetic valves, other implanted intracardiac devices, intra- or post-operative contamination, invasive cardiac procedures, and IV drug use/abuse has been increasing. It is currently estimated that 10 to 30% of all cases of infective endocarditis occur in patients with prosthetic heart valves, with the greatest incidence during the first six months post-operatively. The majority of infections that occur within two months of the surgery is more than likely due to an intra- or post-operative complication. Despite the revised prophylaxis guidelines by the AHA, an estimated 55 to 75% of all cases of IE are associated with an underlying cardiac valvular abnormality (this number includes prosthetic heart valves).

Increased incidence is seen in patients who are male, are immunocompromised (e.g., human immunodeficiency virus [HIV] infection, diabetes, or renal dialysis), are IV drug users/abusers, have a history of rheumatic heart disease (even when SBE prophylaxis is employed), have a history of congenital heart disease (regardless of repair status), have mitral valve prolapse syndrome, or have poor dental hygiene.

CASE 1-5
Eric Floyd
1. History

A. Did he sustain a head injury or loss of consciousness? ESSENTIAL

From the description of his injury, it is apparent that his body was propelled forward, forcing his head over/between the handlebars of the ATV. Because the front of the vehicle directly impacted with the tree, there is a question of whether his head did also. Furthermore, following any type of an impact injury, it is imperative to inquire regarding whether a head injury and/or a loss of consciousness occurred.

B. Is his helmet intact?   ESSENTIAL

If a head injury occurred, a helmet that is relatively unscathed is generally associated with a low incidence of a serious head injury. However, a significantly damaged helmet is not as predictive because this could represent protection of the head or the impact being so severe, both were significantly damaged. Even without a head injury, this question is important because it provides an opportunity to discuss helmet safety.

C. Did he injure, or is he experiencing pain elsewhere in his body?   ESSENTIAL

Inquiring about pain elsewhere in the body enables the full spectrum of potential injuries to be identified instead of focusing on the most obvious symptom. For example, abdominal pain in this patient's case could be the result of a splenic injury and his hypotension could be secondary to acute internal hemorrhage. Obviously, disastrous outcomes could occur if this type of injury was overlooked.

D. What is his "usual" BP?   ESSENTIAL

As discussed in Case 1-1, "normal" BP is essentially defined as less than 120/80 mm Hg. Currently, studies indicate that the better the BP control is, the less the likelihood of developing complications from the disease. Furthermore, some experts believe that BP cannot be decreased "too low" unless the patient becomes symptomatic from the treatment. Although Mr Floyd's current measurement is unlikely to represent his current targeted treatment goal or his "typical" BP, it is therefore essential to obtain his "usual" (or general range) to compare with today's slightly hypotensive reading as part of the assessment of his hemodyanamic stability. This is especially important because Mr. Floyd has a history of hypertension that requires three medications to control.

E. Does he have a family history of coronary artery disease (CAD)   ESSENTIAL

Because he is experiencing chest pain and has several risk factors for CAD (male gender, older age, obesity, previous smoker, and hypertensive), inquiring about additional risk factors for CAD (i.e., family history) is appropriate. If his family history is positive for blood relative(s) with premature CAD (i.e., before the age of 55 years) or for a first-degree relative (i.e., mother, father, or children) with CAD regardless of age, Mr. Floyd's risk of CAD further increases.

2. Physical Examination

A. Heart examination   ESSENTIAL

Because Mr. Floyd is experiencing chest pain, it is important to do a complete heart evaluation looking for the findings as outlined in Case 1-2.

The pericardial friction rub found on his examination can be distinguished from a pleural friction rub because the pleural rub is absent when the patient is not breathing (e.g., between breaths or with breath holding). However, a pericardial rub is present in all stages of the respiratory cycle.

B. Evaluate for the presence of an elevated jugular venous pressure (JVP), jugular venous distension (JVD), Kussmaul sign, pulsus alternans, pulsus bigeminus, and pulsus paradoxicum   ESSENTIAL

The primary purpose of evaluating the internal JVP is to obtain a noninvasive estimate of the patient's central venous pressure (CVP). Less than or equal to 8 cm of blood is considered to be normal. Elevation of the right ventricular diastolic pressure is the main cause of an elevated JVP.

If the JVP is normal but there is still concern regarding the possibility of right ventricular failure, then an abdomino-jugular (or hepatojugular) reflex test is often helpful. The test is considered to be positive if 10 or more seconds of pressure applied to the midabdomen results in an elevation of the CVP AND a 4-cm or greater quick decrease of the pressure.

Another sign of right ventricular failure is the Kussmaul sign. It is an observable increase in the CVP during inspiration (CVP should normally decrease with inspiration).

Pulsus alternans (PA) is a decrease in the intensity or strength of the pulse associated with inspiration, despite an underlying regular cardiac rhythm. It is seen primarily following an episode of paroxysmal supraventricular tachycardia (PSVT) or premature ventricular contraction (PVC). Pulsus bigeminus (PB) is the same type of alterations in the pulse amplitude as seen with PA, except it is observed following a PVC after a regular beat (bigeminy).

Pulsus paradoxicum is a decrease of greater than or equal to 10 to 15 mm Hg in the SBP during inspiration while at the same time, the peripheral pulses decrease or disappear completely. It is associated with pericardial tamponade, airway obstruction, and superior vena cava obstruction.

C. Lung evaluation   ESSENTIAL

Careful lung auscultation is required to identify any increases or decreases in breath sounds that are either localized or generalized through all the lung fields—posteriorly, anteriorly, and laterally. Decreased breath sounds are generally associated with an air-, fluid-, or blood-filled sac compressing normal lung tissue or consolidation of the lungs, as would be the case with severe pneumonia. The presence of wheezing, stridor, rhonchi, and rales indicates that there is an obstruction to airflow in the phase of respiration during which the abnormality is heard. All of these findings can indicate a pulmonary and/or a cardiac disease process. Pleural friction rubs are created when opposing pulmonary serous surfaces are "roughened" acutely by inflammation or chronically by fibrosis.

The presence of intracostal retractions or bulging tends to be associated with severe respiratory distress. Evaluation for symmetry of chest wall movement is essential as it can represent a chest wall abnormality (e.g., rib fracture or severe contusion) or an internal pulmonary process (e.g., pneumothorax or hemithorax). Percussion is sometimes required to distinguish between fluid-/tissue-/air-filled areas. Additionally, vocal and/or tactile fremitus, egophony, bronchophony, and/or whispered pectoriloquy can also be utilized to make this determination.

D. Chest wall examination   ESSENTIAL

Visualization of his chest wall is to evaluate for potential injuries (e.g., contusions, gross deformities or compound rib fractures, lacerations, puncture wounds, and abrasions). His ribs need to be palpated for laxity and tenderness, indicating potential fractured rib(s).

E. Cranial nerve evaluation   NONESSENTIAL

A cranial nerve evaluation is not indicated because Mr. Floyd did not experience a head injury or loss of consciousness with his accident. Furthermore, he has not had nor currently does he have any signs or symptoms suspicious of a neurologic abnormality. However, if his symptoms change or his condition deteriorates, one might be necessary at that time.

3. Diagnostic Studies

A. Chest x-ray (CXR) with rib enhancement   ESSENTIAL

Because Mr. Floyd is experiencing chest wall tenderness, rib pain, and other signs and symptoms that are consistent with musculoskeletal, cardiac and pulmonary disorders, a CXR with rib enhancement is indicated. It can assist in identifying abnormalities such as rib fractures; pleural effusions, contusions, and/or pneumothoraxes; and cardiac conditions such as heart failure, cardiomegaly, and other conditions that could result in abnormal cardiac shadows.

B. Serial cardiac troponin I and T   ESSENTIAL

Serial cardiac troponin levels are biochemical markers that assist in the identification of the presence (or absence) of myocardial ischemia or infarction. Because the cardiac troponins (I and T) can be separated from the troponin found in skeletal muscle by monoclonal antibodies or enzyme-linked immunosorbent assay techniques, they are able to identify myocardial damage with a much higher specificity and sensitivity than even the fractionated creatinine phosphokinase (CPK) levels. Minor elevations of the cardiac troponins can occasionally occur with musculoskeletal trauma; however, the levels tend to be much lower.

Troponin I levels begin to rise in approximately 3 hours from the onset of chest pain and they persist for 7 to 10 days post-MI. Troponin T can actually be elevated for 10 to 14 days post-MI. This is important in attempting to evaluate individuals who delay seeking treatment following an episode of chest pain. Additionally, it appears that the cardiac troponin levels also have prognostic properties in assisting with determining the likelihood of the event being fatal.

C. Electrocardiogram (ECG) and cardiac monitoring   ESSENTIAL

Because the patient is experiencing chest pain, it is important that an ECG be performed. Abnormal ST segments and Q waves are suspicious for cardiac ischemia and/or infarction (especially in conjunction with elevated cardiac troponin levels). Cardiomegaly, atrioventricular (AV), bundle branch blocks, chamber enlargements, arrhythmias, and some electrolyte abnormalities can also be identified based on ECG findings.

D. Echocardiography   ESSENTIAL

Echocardiography is considered to be the "gold standard" for evaluating cardiac structures and identifying areas of ischemia and/infarction. Furthermore, it permits evaluation for any signs of valvular abnormalities, chamber sizes, thickness of the myocardium, thickness of the pericardium, presence of effusions, and other structural blood flow abnormalities. Additionally, it can provide an estimate of the patient's ejection fraction.

E. Tuberculosis skin test (TST)   NONESSENTIAL

Even though TB is a leading cause of cardiac tamponade secondary to a pericardial effusion, with Mr. Floyd's history of trauma, makes an infectious process unlikely. Therefore, this test is not indicated at this time to evaluate his complaint.

4. Diagnosis

A. Constrictive pericarditis   INCORRECT

Constrictive pericarditis is an inflammatory process that is almost always associated with a thickened and frequently scarred pericardium with or without calcifications that produces the "constriction" on the heart. On evaluation, the JVP has both a prominent x and y descent and a positive Kussmaul sign. Because of the absence of a thickened scarred pericardium and a prominent x descent (but no y) constrictive pericarditis is not Mr. Floyd's most likely diagnosis.

B. Cardiac tamponade secondary to a pericardial effusion   CORRECT

Cardiac tamponade's primary diagnostic criteria are known as "Beck's triad." It is a combination of (1) hypotension, (2) diminished or absent heart sounds on auscultation, and (3) JVD with an elevated JVP exhibiting a prominent x descent but an absent y descent.

The presence of a pericardial effusion is confirmed echographically. Additionally, Mr. Floyd's ECG monitoring revealed what is known as electrical alternans. When present, it is considered pathognomonic for a pericardial effusion. It results from the movement of the heart back and forth within a large effusion. Hence, this fulfills the second half of this diagnosis, making cardiac tamponade secondary to a pericardial effusion Mr. Floyd's most likely diagnosis.

Small, slow bleeds are better tolerated than large, massive bleeds because a slow bleed can gradually stretch the pericardial sac, whereas a large bleed cannot be accommodated. Hence, large, fast bleeds are associated with a much greater morbidity and mortality.

C. Tension pneumothorax   INCORRECT

A tension pneumothorax is air (or other gases) trapped between the pleural layers lining the lungs that causes "tension" or pressure on the remaining lung tissue, causing it not to be able to expand and ventilate the body efficiently. Although common with blunt chest trauma, this can be eliminated as Mr. Floyd's most likely diagnosis because there was no evidence of a loss of lung parenchymal tissue markings or a mediastinal shift on his CXR or physical examination.

D. Restrictive cardiomyopathy   INCORRECT

The most striking difference between restrictive cardiomyopathy and cardiac tamponade is the presence of fluid accumulation in the pericardial sac and the small right ventricular size seen with tamponade. Furthermore, restrictive cardiomyopathy is also associated with myocardial thickness; in view of Mr. Floyd's diagnostic studies, this is not his most likely diagnosis.

E. Right ventricular myocardial infarction (RVMI)   INCORRECT

An RVMI is generally associated with an enlarged right ventricle and evidence of infarction on ECG and echocardiography. These findings would be associated with elevated cardiac troponin levels consistent with a myocardial infarction because it has been longer than 3 hours since Mr. Floyd's injury and pain onset. Furthermore, with an RVMI there is no evidence of right atrial collapse, a large pericardial effusion, an *x* descent with JVP measurement, and pulsus paradoxicum. Therefore, RVMI is not Mr. Floyd's most likely diagnosis.

5. Treatment Plan

A. Hospitalize for arterial pressure, venous pressure, and cardiac monitoring; IV fluids; oxygen; further testing; and treatment   CORRECT

With the size of his effusion and the presence of shock (or at least impending shock), Mr. Floyd definitely needs to be hospitalized for more definitive evaluation, monitoring, and treatment.

B. Pericardiocentesis via subxiphoid approach under echocardiography guidance   CORRECT

Because of the rapid accumulation of his effusion and the development of symptoms suggesting an inadequate pumping ability of the heart, he definitely requires pericardiocentesis to alleviate the pressure the effusion is placing on his heart. Because the subxiphoid approach is the easiest method, it is the technique of choice, especially for noncardiac providers.

C. Evaluation of fluid from tap for cytology, microscopy, bacterial culture and sensitivity, polymerase chain reaction (PCR) test of DNA of *Mycobacterium tuberculosis*   CORRECT

A bloody tap is the typical finding with a traumatic pericardial tamponade; however, accepted treatment guidelines include having the fluid analyzed cytologically for malignancy and microscopically for WBC and bacteria counts (which if positive, indicates an infectious process); bacterial cultures and sensitivities to identify the offending agent if a bacterial infection is present; and PCR testing for *M. tuberculosis* (as it is the number one cause of infectious cardiac tamponade). Hence, these tests should be done despite Mr. Floyd's history of trauma and his tap being bloody.

D. Consultation with a cardiac surgeon   CORRECT

In the case of trauma, the pericardiocentesis is highly unlikely to be definitive treatment for this condition because there is a very high likelihood that it will reaccumulate until the underlying pathology is corrected. A cardiac surgeon will

likely order either an MRI or a CT scan to determine the exact cause; then, treat it appropriately and hopefully permanently.

E. Continue his current blood pressure medicines at half strength   INCORRECT

CCBs, such as dihydropyridine, and beta-blockers (BBs), such as nadolol, are contraindicated in patients with cardiac tamponade because they can alter the reflex tachycardia, which compensates for the decreased cardiac output. Furthermore, Mr. Floyd is already hypotensive and the medications are likely to drop his blood pressure even further.

Epidemiologic and Other Data

Over 50% of all cases of cardiac tamponade are secondary to a malignancy. The next most common causes, each accounting for approximately 14% of the cases, are idiopathic pericarditis and renal failure–induced cardiac effusion. Other conditions that can be seen with cardiac tamponade include acute myocardial infarctions (especially if the patient is anticoagulated), adverse events resulting from cardiac surgery or invasive procedures, purulent pericarditis, TB pericarditis, dissected aortic aneurysms, myxedema, and trauma.

CASE 1-6
Frank Gee
1. History

A. Has he ever tried any Western (i.e., nitroglycerine) or traditional Chinese medications for his chest pain? If yes, what were the treatments and results?   ESSENTIAL

From his symptoms description, until proven otherwise, ischemic heart disease has to be his current working diagnosis. Therefore, it is important to know the response of his pain to nitroglycerine. However, it is essential to remember that even though chest pain that resolves with nitroglycerine does not confirm a cardiac cause for the pain. Other conditions, most notably esophageal spasms, are also alleviated by the vasodilatory effects of nitroglycerine.

Additionally, because he is treating his hypertension and hyperlipidemia with a traditional Chinese herbal therapy, it is important to know if he has been utilizing any alternative medications for his chest pain, and if so, what results, if any, occurred.

Attempting to make an accurate diagnosis for his past episodes of chest pain is also important because if he has a history of angina, he already has some degree of CAD. Furthermore, it is estimated that approximately 50% of all patients who develop acute myocardial infarctions (AMIs) have a history of stable angina. The AMI rates among patients with unstable angina are even greater.

B. Does he smoke, and if so, what is his smoking history?   ESSENTIAL

There are many risk factors associated with CAD. Because these tend to be cumulative, the greater number of risk factors a patient possesses, the greater risk he or she has of acquiring CAD. Because Mr. Gee already has several risk factors (hypertension, hyperlipidemia, and obesity), it is important to identify how many of the other ones he possesses. Because smoking is a common (and potentially correctable) risk factor as well as a "significant" comorbid conditions, it is essential to inquire about. In fact, a better question is, "What is your smoking history?"

Studies have found that the significant risk factors for CAD include the presence of the following comorbid conditions: diabetes mellitus, hypertension, hyperlipidemia, prior CAD, obesity, and current smoker. Not as significant, but still important, are the additional risk factors of a positive family history, especially in a first-degree relative or any blood relative who was experienced a fatal MI younger than the age of 55 years; advancing age; male gender until approximately 50 years old, then female gender; sedentary lifestyle; former smokes (especially if recent) poor nutritional habits, especially a diet that is high in saturated fats, salts, and excessive alcohol; elevated homocysteine levels; and elevated levels of highly sensitive C-reactive protein.

It is estimated that as many as 80% of individuals with unstable angina and 87 to 100% of individuals with fatal coronary events have at least one or more risk factors present.

C. When was his cholesterol last checked and what were the results?   ESSENTIAL

In general, the higher the lipoprotein levels are, the greater is the risk of CAD. The exception to this is HDL cholesterol as they appear to be cardioprotective; therefore, higher HDL levels are associated with lower CAD risk. Knowing what Mr. Gee's levels were (and how long ago they were tested) provides additional information regarding his current risk of CAD and its likelihood of being responsible for his current episode of chest pain.

D. What is his "usual" BP?   ESSENTIAL

This is important information to obtain from Mr. Gee because his BP is elevated at this visit. It is important to know if this represents his "usual" BP or if it is resulting from pain or another underlying cause. The associated tachycardia makes pain the more likely culprit.

Furthermore, by knowing the exact numbers for his "usual" BP (and his lipid values from the previous response), his estimated 10-year cardiac risk can be calculated. A high value would provide additional support that his chest pain might be cardiovascular in nature.

The most commonly used 10-year estimation scale is based on data from the Framingham Study and was established by the U.S. Department of Health and Human Services (USDHHS), Public Health Service (PHS), NIH, and NHLBI. There are two separate scales, one for men and one for women. The factors it evaluates are age, total cholesterol level for age, smoking status for age, HDL, systolic BP, and whether or not the patient is on antihypertensive medications. Numerical values are assigned to each of these areas. The total sum of these values is then placed on a scale to determine the individual patient's risk of having a coronary event within the next 10 years. Utilizing this scale, Mr. Gee's 10-year cardiac risk is greater than or equal to 30%.

Higher points are assigned for greater risk; for example, men who are between the ages of 20 and 34 years receive –9 points for age and men between the ages of 75 and 79 receive +13 points. However, with other risk factors such as smoking

and elevated total cholesterol, the younger the patient is, the higher the score assigned. For example, if a man is 20 years old and had a total cholesterol above 280, he would be given +11 points; however, if a man 79 years old had the same cholesterol level, he would only be assigned +1 point. HDL and systolic blood pressure values are assigned without an age status. However, an elevated BP under treatment receives a higher score than the same BP level not being treated for hypertension (the complete tool can be found online at http://hp2010.nhlbihin.net/atpiii/calculator.asp?usertype=pub).

E. Does he use sildenafil, vardenafil, or tadalafil for his erectile dysfunction (ED)?   NONESSENTIAL

This question as stated does not provide much useful information because it is based on two assumptions (both of which are incorrect in Mr. Gee's case): first is that he is sexually active and second that he suffers from ED. Furthermore, it could be considered "insulting" to the patient and could have an adverse impact on the patient–provider relationship.

The information that this question is attempting to ascertain is whether the patient is taking a phosphodiesterase type 5 inhibitor because they can produce tachyarrhythmias and inhibit autonomic regulation of BP. A better approach to obtain this information is to specifically ask about these agents when obtaining his medication list.

2. Physical Examination

A. General appearance   ESSENTIAL

When the patient is presenting with a painful condition, his or her general appearance is useful because it provides an overall impression of the relationship between the complaint and its severity by how the patient looks and acts. Additionally, it provides clues that could support a diagnosis (e.g., diaphoresis is frequently associated with chest pain caused by ischemia).

B. Oral examination   NONESSENTIAL

C. Heart auscultation   ESSENTIAL

Because Mr. Gee is complaining of chest pain, it is essential to conduct a comprehensive heart examination, paying particular attention to the areas outlined in Case 1-2.

D. Lung auscultation   ESSENTIAL

Because Mr. Gee is complaining of chest pain, it is essential to perform a comprehensive lung examination as outlined in Case 1-5.

E. All his pulses   ESSENTIAL

Reduced pulses or a bruit in an artery generally indicates the presence of atherosclerotic vessel disease. Additionally, skin color, skin temperature, and capillary refill are essential components in the evaluation of the patient's pulses; if abnormal, they can indicate reduced circulation even in the presence of a normal pulse. The presence of atherosclerosis would increase the likelihood that Mr. Gee's chest pain is caused by CAD.

However, it is essential to remember than when a blood vessel is more than ~70% occluded, the bruit generally disappears, so significant vessel disease can occur without a bruit. Likewise, up to 30% of bruits are found in normal blood vessels with normal blood flow.

3. Diagnostic Studies

A. Cardiac telemetry followed by 12-lead electrocardiogram (ECG)   ESSENTIAL

Telemetry provides a continuous view of the patient's heart rate and underlying rhythm. Additionally, it permits evaluation of the wave formations, the segment lengths, and their relationship. Furthermore, it is beneficial because any changes in rate and rhythm can be identified quickly; then, any required treatments can be instituted and monitored immediately.

However, it does not provide a complete view of the heart because it is generally conducted in just one lead (usually lead II). Hence, a full 12-lead ECG also needs to be performed. It will provide an overall "snapshot" of the electrical activity of the heart to identify patterns of ischemia, infarction, conduction defects, and other conditions that take more than one lead to correctly diagnose.

B. Oxygen saturation followed by oxygen at 2 L/min via nasal cannula (NC)   ESSENTIAL

Because Mr. Gee has dyspnea (and a strong smoking history), an oxygen saturation (O_2 sat) is required to provide an estimate of the patient's oxygenation status. Regardless of the oxygenation status, any patient with suspected myocardial ischemia should receive oxygen therapy starting at 2 L/min to assist with myocardial perfusion. The amount of oxygen can be increased based on the patient' symptoms, O_2 sat, and arterial blood gases (when indicated).

C. Echocardiogram   ESSENTIAL

If the ECG looks suspicious for ischemia, an echocardiogram (echo) can assist in further determining the area and extent of involvement because it will reveal abnormal motion of the affected area of the myocardium. Furthermore, it can provide a gross estimation of the function of the left ventricle, or the ejection fraction. This additional information can be useful in determining the most appropriate intervention for that individual patient.

However, it is important to remember that segmental wall dysfunction does not necessarily mean that the patient is having an AMI. It can also be seen with scarring from a previous MI, a resolved or mild constrictive pericarditis, or severe ischemia without infarction.

D. Gallbladder ultrasound   NONESSENTIAL

Because the patient had a cholecystectomy, he does not have a gallbladder on which to perform an ultrasound. Therefore, this is not an appropriate diagnostic option for Mr. Gee. However, evaluation of his common bile duct for the presence of a retained gallstone would be appropriate, once more urgent and life-threatening conditions were eliminated, because this would explain why his pain felt like the pain he experienced that was caused by cholelithiasis, and the postoperative window is appropriate for this complication to become symptomatic.

E. Cardiac troponin I and T (cTn-I and cTn-T) stat; then repeat in 4 and 8 hours   ESSENTIAL

Serum cardiac troponin I and T have essentially replaced CPK and/or CPK fractionation as the method of choice for determining myocardial injury because they are more cardiac specific and produce fewer false-positives caused by skeletal muscle damage. They are estimated to be 84 to 96% sensitive and 80 to 95% specific. (For further discussion, please see Case 1-5.)

It is important to remember that a single elevated troponin level is not diagnostic of an AMI, just as a single normal value does not rule out an AMI. Cardiac troponins also elevate in response to any damage to the myocardial muscle; however, the elevation is not nearly as extreme and the increase over time not nearly as significant as is seen with infarction.

Furthermore, if the patient presents early in the course of an AMI, the cardiac troponin levels can still be negative because cardiac troponin levels do not begin to elevate until approximately 3 hours postinjury. Therefore, repeat testing of the levels in 4 hours should reveal a rise in the levels if the chest pain is truly from myocardial ischemia and/or infarction.

Once cardiac troponins are elevated, the cardiac troponin I can still be detected in the serum of the patient for 7 to 10 days and the cardiac troponin T for up to 10 to 14 days.

If the patient is at low risk for an AMI, some experts feel that only two, not three, sets of troponins are adequate to determine chest pain as nonmyocardial in origin (provided the second set is also negative). However, there is a caveat that a minimum of 8 hours must have elapsed since the patient last experienced any chest pain for this to be accurate. Therefore, most HCPs opt for continued monitoring and performing a third set of troponin levels.

4. Diagnosis

A. Unstable angina   INCORRECT

Unstable angina is characterized by ischemic chest discomfort (or equivalent symptoms) with at least one of the following three characteristics: (1) occurs at rest and generally lasts for more than 10 minutes, (2) is described as severe and never experienced before 6 weeks previous, and (3) is a worsening of previous angina (e.g., occurring at more frequent intervals, lasting longer, or increasing in severity of pain [and/or other symptoms]). Although it is considered to be an acute coronary syndrome and associated with myocardial ischemia, infarction is not part of the picture. If tissue death does occur, then the diagnosis is changed to myocardia infarction.

In unstable angina, the typical ST-T-segment change is depression, not elevation, and there are no Q-wave formations as are evident on Mr. Gee's ECG; therefore, despite his first set of cardiac troponin levels being negative, unstable angina is not his most likely diagnosis.

B. Old anterior myocardial infarction   INCORRECT

ST-segment elevation and the beginning of Q waves are characteristic of an AMI. Q waves with resolving ST-segment changes are seen in recent or subacute MIs. Q waves without any ST-segment changes are associated with old or indeterminate-age MIs. Because Mr. Gee's ECG reveals the former, this is not his most likely diagnosis. Furthermore, anterior MIs affect ECG leads V_1 through V_5; Mr. Gee's involvement is currently in II, III, and aVF.

C. Acute anteroseptal myocardial infarction   INCORRECT

This answer would be consistent with Mr. Gee's Q-wave and ST-segment elevations; however, anteroseptal MIs have the affected ST segments in leads V_1 through V_3, not II, III, and aVF as Mr. Gee does. Therefore, this is also not his most likely diagnosis.

D. Choledocholithiasis   INCORRECT

Choledocholithiasis is the presence of a cholelith in the common bile duct. His symptoms and ECG findings prevent this from being his most likely diagnosis.

If there is a high index of suspicion that this is Mr. Gee's diagnosis, then an endoscopic ultrasonography or an endoscopic retrograde cholangiography is indicated.

E. Acute inferior myocardial infarction   CORRECT

As previously stated, Mr. Gee's ECG findings of evolving Q waves and ST-segment elevations are consistent with an AMI. The ST-segmental abnormalities occurring in II, III, and aVF are consistent with an acute inferior myocardial infarction. Despite the negative cardiac troponin levels (which are probably resulting from his early presentation as discussed previously), this is his most likely diagnosis.

It would be appropriate at this time to consider performing some type of assessment to further determine the patient's risk of death from ST-segment elevation MI with negative troponin antibodies (although his are likely to be elevated upon repeat testing).

One such tool developed by **T**hrombolysis **I**n **M**yocardial **I**nfarction (TIMI) is the **U**nstable **A**ngina and **ST**-segment **E**levated **MI** (UA/STEMI). It provides a numerical score ranging from 0 (lowest risk) to 6 (highest risk) that estimates the likelihood of cardiac death cause by either unstable angina or an ST-segment-elevated MI. The scores are divided as follows: 0 to 2, low risk; 3 to 4, moderate risk; and 5 to 6, high risk. It is based on assigning 1 point each to the following six factors: age 65 years or older, history of previous stenosis of 50% or greater, two or more episodes of angina in the past 24 hours, three or more risk factors for CAD, current elevation of cardiac biomarkers, and current ST segment deviations of more than 0.5 mm. CAD risk factors were defined as hypertension, hyperlipidemia, diabetes, current smoke, and positive family history. Mr. Gee's UA/STEMI score is 4, or moderate risk.

The TIMI group has developed 12 different clinical tools for the evaluation of possible cardiac death based on various factors/medications that are available to clinicians to use in appropriate situations. They are based on over 50 clinical trials (all the tools [and trials] can be found at http://timi.org).

5. Treatment Plan

A. Admit to intensive care unit (ICU), continue telemetry, vital sign monitoring, IV fluids, and oxygen   CORRECT

With his symptoms and most likely diagnosis, Mr. Gee needs to be hospitalized for continued telemetry, vital sign monitoring, observation, IV fluids, oxygen, and evaluation.

B. IV nitroglycerine 2 to 200 µg/min at a dose sufficient enough to alleviate the patient's pain but not so high as to cause adverse effects. If this titration cannot be achieved or maximum dosage fails to alleviate the patient's pain, then give morphine sulfate at 2 to 8 mg IV every 15 minutes as needed, provided no signs of respiratory depression are present CORRECT

IV nitroglycerine is generally very effective in alleviating myocardial pain. Nevertheless, regardless of the patient's response to it, it is not diagnostic in either ruling in or ruling out an AMI. If nitroglycerine is ineffective in alleviating the pain, then morphine sulfate IV should be utilized next. In theory, the only ceiling to the maximum dosage is respiratory depression.

C. Aspirin 160 to 325 mg stat; then 81 mg enteric-coated aspirin daily with food   CORRECT

Mr. Gee needs to be given a full-strength aspirin now because he is a candidate for thrombolysis, it will already be "on board." Furthermore, he will need to take low-dose aspirin daily for the rest of his life in hopes of preventing platelet aggravation and clot formation.

D. Acebutolol 200 mg once a day orally   CORRECT

Beta-blockers are indicated immediately in a post-MI patient and also to be continued indefinitely because they are associated with a lower first-year mortality rate from AMIs.

Ideally, the chosen beta-blocker should be one that is β_1 selective because there is less chance of pulmonary complications. With Mr. Gee's smoking history, it would not be unreasonable for him to have chronic bronchitis that could be adversely affected by a beta-blocker. Because he is hospitalized, this complication could be quickly identified and treated.

Furthermore, the beta-blocker should have good membrane-stabilizing activity. Some studies have found it to be advantageous in assisting with the prevention of cardiac arrhythmias. Additionally, it would be preferable for it to possess intrinsic sympathomimetic activity because recent studies indicate this might partially reduce cardiac depression.

Additionally, his herbal products need to be identified and evaluated for efficacy and safety. If that is not possible, then they should be tapered off and replaced with appropriate medications to ensure the best possible outcome and to avoid possible drug–herb interactions.

E. Fibrinolysis with tissue plasma activator (tPA)   INCORRECT

Fibrinolysis therapy, regardless of agent (tPA, streptokinase, tenecteplase [TNK], and reteplase [rPA]) employed, is theoretically contraindicated in Mr. Gee because of his age. In patients between the ages of 76 and 86, studies have failed to reveal any benefit in providing the therapy. However, elderly patients without any other contraindications to fibrinolysis who have a significant amount of myocardium in danger from the AMI need to be individually evaluated as the benefits of fibrinolysis might outweigh the risks.

Regardless, Mr. Gee would not be an acceptable candidate for fibrinolysis therapy because he has a relative contraindication to the treatment—a cholecystectomy 2 weeks ago (relative contraindication is major surgery in the last 3 weeks). Additionally, because the exact details of his surgery are unknown, it is possible that he has another relative contraindication (internal bleeding within the past 2 to 4 weeks) secondary to the surgery. Other relative contraindications include traumatic cardiopulmonary resuscitation (CPR) or CPR that lasted for longer than 10 minutes; bleeding that does not respond appropriately to pressure; ischemic stroke more than 3 months ago; active stomach or duodenal peptic ulcer disease; hypertension, defined a SBP that is greater than 180 and/or as DBP that is greater than 100 at presentation; pregnancy; and currently on anticoagulant therapy.

Absolute contraindications include ischemic CVA longer than 3 hours ago but less than 3 months ago (some experts recommend 1 year), previous intracranial hemorrhage, known structural cerebral vascular lesion (e.g., aneurysm or AV malformation), significant head injury/trauma (including closed) within the past 3 months, brain tumor, known or suspected aortic dissection, or any active internal bleeding. Some experts consider the aforementioned BP criteria as an absolute, not relative, contraindication.

Fibrinolysis therapy is indicated in patients who have ST-segment elevation of greater than 1 mm in two or more contiguous leads, have been symptomatic for less than 12 hours (with an ideal goal of within the first 30 minutes of presentation or within 3 hours of symptom onset), have a true posterior MI, or have appeared to experience an AMI but a bundle branch block (BBB) makes it impossible to determine because of the secondary ST-segment changes from the BBB.

F. Percutaneous transluminal coronary angiography (PTCA) with stent placement if indicated   CORRECT

PTCA with stent placement is a possible option for Mr. Gee. However, he must be at a facility where it and a qualified HCP is available to perform the procedure within 12 hours from the onset of his symptoms. It is indicated in patients who have contraindications to fibrinolysis but have heart failure, recurrent ischemia, a previous MI, and cardiogenic shock.

Interestingly, a meta-analysis was performed on 23 trials with almost 8000 patients and the authors concluded that PTCA for AMI was superior to fibrinolysis therapy. Furthermore, a retrospective analysis of patients who failed to reperfuse with fibrinolysis therapy indicated rescue PTCA to be just as safe and effective as primary PTCA.

Epidemiologic and Other Data

In the United States, there are over 1,000,000 AMIs occurring annually. Approximately 650,000 individuals experience their first AMI annually, and 350,000 AMIs occur in individuals who have had at least one previous AMI.

There appears to be a seasonal relationship to fatal myocardial infarctions. The two months of December and January have 33% more fatal myocardial infarctions than are seen in the 4-month time span from June to September.

In the 30 days after an AMI, the death rate is approximately 30%. Unfortunately, over 50% of this number includes patients who never make it to an emergency department before they die from an AMI. One in every 25 patients who are discharged from the hospital following an AMI is dead at the end of 1 year. In patients older than the age of 75 years, the risk of dying from an AMI is 400% greater compared to individuals experiencing an AMI before the age of 75 years.

CASE 1-7
George Harris
1. History

A. Has he experienced any epistaxis, nasal or oral lesions, or gingival or dental problems recently?   ESSENTIAL

Inquiring about bleeding elsewhere in the body is important because if it is present, it could indicate a bleeding disorder,

thrombocytopenia, vitamin K deficiency, disseminated intravascular coagulation, or unknown ingestion of anticoagulants.

However, if he is experiencing a true hemoptysis, then the major causes include pulmonary infections; carcinomas; abnormalities of the pulmonary vasculature; pulmonary venous hypertension; AV malformations; pulmonary embolism; gastroesophageal reflux disease (GERD), especially with Barrett esophagitis; and some autoimmune diseases.

In the past it was believed that if the hemoptysis was associated with sputum or some other fluid production, it was less serious than if it was just blood alone. However, this has not been proven in any evidenced-based fashion.

B. Has he experienced any abdominal pain or change in his bowel movements?   ESSENTIAL

Knowing if he is experiencing any gastrointestinal bleeding is important to evaluate not only for potential sources for the hemoptysis (e.g., esophageal varices caused by portal hypertension, Barrett esophagitis, and GERD can cause blood to be expelled with coughing as well as dark tarry stools) but also for other sources of bleeding (e.g., bleeding peptic ulcers and inflammatory bowel disease can cause both bleeding and abdominal pain, whereas colon cancer and polyps tend to cause painless bleeding).

C. Has he experienced any fatigue, malaise, weight loss, hoarseness, or night sweats?   ESSENTIAL

The presence of these symptoms is suspicious for a carcinoma. With the hemoptysis, the most likely possibilities would be a lung carcinoma, lung metastasis, or esophageal cancer. However, an acute or chronic pulmonary infection can also present as hemoptysis with these symptoms. In view of the lack of fever and sputum production, an acute lung infection is less likely; however, it certainly cannot be completely ruled out.

D. Has he experienced any dyspnea?   ESSENTIAL

The presence of dyspnea makes a pulmonary abnormality the most likely cause for Mr. Harris's hemoptysis. However, if dyspnea occurs in conjunction with constitutional symptoms, a carcinoma becomes a very likely probability. Poor physical conditioning, medical fragility, psychiatric disorders (e.g., panic attacks, somatization disorders, and malingering), cardiac conditions (e.g., heart failure, arrhythmias, myocardial ischemia, aortic stenosis, and constrictive pericarditis), neurologic conditions (e.g., Guillain-Barré syndrome, amyotrophic lateral sclerosis, and muscular dystrophy), musculoskeletal disorders (kyphoscoliosis or rib fractures), or other conditions (e.g., anemia, hyperthyroidism, and metabolic acidosis) can cause dyspnea, which may be unrelated to his chief complaint.

E. Has he experienced any hallucinations?   NONESSENTIAL

This question would only be relative if he was experiencing neurologic or psychological symptoms, was acting bizarrely, or suddenly ceased drinking alcohol.

2. Physical Examination

A. Skin examination   ESSENTIAL

The skin is important to examine in patients who are experiencing dyspnea to observe for evidence of cyanosis, erythema, and/or pallor. Furthermore, if an infection is suspected, the presence of associated skin lesions can be very helpful in establishing the correct diagnosis. Finally, in patients where there is a suspicion of a metastatic process without an obvious cause, the skin should be examined thoroughly for the presence of a malignant melanoma.

As a general rule, central cyanosis has a pulmonary cause, whereas peripheral cyanosis is related to a cardiovascular condition. Obviously, these are not absolutes and frequently cardiac and pulmonary conditions coexist. For example, congenital cardiac conditions that result in right-to-left shunts can produce central cyanosis. Methemoglobinemia produces central cyanosis without either a cardiovascular or pulmonary cause; conditions like these are generally recognized by the patient's cyanosis failing to improve with oxygen therapy.

B. Heart examination   ESSENTIAL

A careful heart examination following the criteria outlined in Case 1-2 is essential to determine whether Mr. Harris has any cardiac abnormalities that could account for his symptoms.

C. Lung auscultation   ESSENTIAL

Because of Mr. Harris's hemoptysis and dyspnea, a thorough lung examination as outlined in Case 1-5 is essential.

D. Evaluation of jugular venous pressure (JVP), of pulses, and for pedal edema   ESSENTIAL

As stated previously, the primary purpose of evaluating the JVP is to obtain a noninvasive estimate of the patient's CVP. An elevated *a* wave is generally caused by a very forceful right atrial systole.

Normal pulses provide some reassurance that the patient has adequate circulation and perfusion. Bilaterally decreased pulses are generally associated with decreased perfusion or atherosclerosis, whereas a unilaterally decreased pulse is most frequently caused by an obstruction.

The most common cause of bilateral pedal edema is heart failure. However, other conditions can also cause the problem (e.g., hepatic problems, azotemia and/or renal failure, ascites, pleural effusions, and malignancies).

Pedal edema is more accurately dependent edema. Therefore, it is important to remember that when evaluating a patient, the edema is located in the most dependent part of the body. Patients who are bedridden often have presacral edema instead of ankle and foot edema.

E. Joint evaluation   NONESSENTIAL

3. Diagnostic Studies

A. Oxygen saturation (O_2 sat) and chest x-ray (CXR) ESSENTIAL

Because Mr. Harris is experiencing dyspnea, orthopnea, cyanosis, harsh breath sounds, and abnormal cardiac sounds and has a long-standing history of smoking, both an O_2 sat and a CXR are indicated. Although a normal O_2 sat is considered to be 95% or higher, "critical values" are not defined until the level has fallen to 75% or less. However, it is generally accepted to recommend arterial blood gases (ABGs) and oxygen therapy when the O_2 sat falls below 90%, when there is a compelling reason to suspect the reading is incorrect (e.g., poor peripheral circulation, Raynaud disease and/or phenomenon, or dark-colored fingernail polish that cannot be removed), or

when other values identified by the ABGs would provide useful information for managing the case.

B. Electrocardiogram (ECG) and echocardiogram with Doppler   ESSENTIAL

Because two different cardiac murmurs, an abnormal opening snap, and an elevated JVP were discovered during Mr. Harris's physical examination, both an ECG and an echocardiogram with Doppler ultrasound are indicated as part of his evaluation.

An ECG can provide confirmation of the patient's pulse rate; determine his or her current heart rhythm; confirm conduction defects; and provide signs suggestive of ischemia, infarction, chamber enlargement, cardiomegaly, and electrolyte abnormalities.

The echocardiogram is an ultrasound of the heart. It can determine the presence of abnormalities in the motion and/or structure of the heart's chambers, valves, septum, walls, and other components. Furthermore, it can evaluate the valves of the heart for prolapse, regurgitation, stenosis, calcification, vegetation, and other abnormalities; it can also identify cardiomegaly, aneurysms, effusions, tumors, lesions, and emboli. The Doppler component can better visualize the flow and/or turbulence of the blood through the valves and chambers of the heart; hence, it makes it much easier to identify regurgitation and shunts.

C. D-dimer   NONESSENTIAL

D-dimer results from the breakdown of cross-linked fibrin; therefore, values below the established "cut-off" are unlikely to occur in patients with a thromboembolic phenomenon (e.g., deep vein thrombosis or pulmonary embolism). Although some of Mr. Harris's symptoms can be found in patients with a pulmonary embolism, the duration alone of his nonprogressive symptoms essentially rules out this condition. Thus, a D-dimer is not indicated.

D. First morning sputum for cytology × 3   ESSENTIAL

This test is indicated because of Mr. Harris's history of hemoptysis and dyspnea in conjunction with his long-standing smoker status to rule out a primary lung malignancy as the cause of his hemoptysis. Despite the fact that the majority of the other findings of his history and physical examination are not very consistent with this diagnosis, these three symptoms alone justify the testing.

E. Antinuclear antibodies (ANA); erythrocyte sedimentation rate (ESR); antinative DNA; anticardiolipin antibodies, including lupus anticoagulant; C_3 and C_4 complement assay; systemic lupus erythematosus preparation (SLE prep); and CBC w/diff   NONESSENTIAL

Although an autoimmune inflammatory disease could be responsible for Mr. Harris's condition, he lacks sufficient symptomatology to justify an evaluation at this time.

4. Diagnosis

A. Lung cancer   INCORRECT

Even though his sputum cytologies are pending, Mr. Harris's lack of identifiable masses/lesions on CXR, no significant constitutional symptoms, and identified cardiac abnormalities make other diagnoses more likely than lung cancer at this time.

B. Pulmonary embolism   INCORRECT

Even though a pulmonary embolism shares some of the symptoms that Mr. Harris is complaining about, it can be ruled out because of the length of time he has been experiencing his symptoms without progression. Furthermore, he lacks history of unilateral leg edema, leg or pelvic trauma (including surgery), recent immobilization, recent air travel, or other signs, symptoms, and risks consistent with a deep vein thrombosis (DVT), which is nearly universally responsible for a PE.

C. Atypical verrucous endocarditis of Libman-Sacks secondary to systemic lupus erythematous   INCORRECT

Regardless of the cause, the verrucous endocardial growths associated with Libman-Sacks syndrome are almost always apparent on echocardiogram. Furthermore, the other common cardiac manifestations of this condition (e.g., left atrial emboli and mitral regurgitation) are also generally apparent on an echocardiogram. Because Mr. Harris's echocardiogram did not reveal any of these findings (and in fact revealed mitral stenosis), this is not his most likely diagnosis.

D. Left atrial myxoma   INCORRECT

A left atrial myxoma is a benign growth arising from connective tissue of the myocardium that intrudes into the cavity of the left atrium and obstructs the proper emptying of the chamber, producing a diastolic murmur, dyspnea, and several of the hemodynamic findings similar to what Mr. Harris is experiencing. However, a left atrial myxoma is generally associated with systemic symptoms that he denied (e.g., fatigue, weight loss, and fever) as well as some that were not evaluated for (i.e., anemia). Normally they are visible as a mass in the left atrium on echocardiography. In view of this information, a left atrial myxoma is not Mr. Harris's most likely diagnosis.

E. Mitral stenosis with associated tricuspid stenosis   CORRECT

The murmurs identified on Mr. Harris's physical examination and confirmed by echocardiography are typical for both mitral stenosis with regurgitation and tricuspid stenosis with regurgitation.

Furthermore, the opening snap from the mitral valve is normally heard almost immediately following the sound created by the closure of the aortic valve. However, in conditions such as mitral stenosis, these two sounds become more separate and distinct. In fact, the severity of the mitral stenosis is proportional to the length of time between the two sounds. The size of the mitral valve opening on his echocardiogram further confirms the consistency of this finding.

Normal orifice size for the mitral valve is 4 to 6 cm^2. The opening can get as small as 1 to 1.5 cm^2 and still produce a relatively normal cardiac output; however, with exercise, it tends to have a subnormal rise. This degree of stenosis is referred to as moderate. Severe mitral stenosis is associated with a valvular orifice of less than 1 cm^2. If the pulmonary vascular resistance is significantly increased when the orifice is this small, the cardiac output is subnormal at rest and often does not increase but declines further during activity.

His hemoptysis is most likely caused by an elevated pulmonary vascular resistance from rupture of pulmonary–bronchial venous communications and/or a secondary pulmonary venous hypertension. Therefore, from the information that has been gathered thus far, this is his most likely diagnosis.

Additional support is provided for this diagnosis per his ECG findings, facial discoloration, and rash. The large P waves identified are most likely caused by an atrial enlargement. When these are also accompanied by tall, peaked P waves in II and upright P waves in V_1, they are generally caused by a combination of mitral stenosis and tricuspid stenosis and/or pulmonary hypertension. A blue face and malar rash like Mr. Harris has can be attributed to cardiopulmonary conditions (e.g., mitral stenosis associated with tricuspid stenosis and mitral stenosis associated with pulmonary hypertension) or cardiac medications (e.g., amiodarone).

5. Treatment Plan

A. Hospitalization with oxygen therapy starting at 2 L/min after arterial blood gases and then adjusted accordingly, cardiac monitoring, and IV line to keep vein open (KVO)   CORRECT

The seriousness of Mr. Harris's condition, his hypoxia and dyspnea, and the fact that he will require additional cardiac monitoring and interventions support him being hospitalized.

B. Refer to thoracic surgeon and oncologist for evaluation and treatment of lung cancer   INCORRECT

Because there is no current evidence to suggest that Mr. Harris has either a primary or secondary lung cancer, there is no need for these consultations at this time.

If his sputum cytologies come back positive, then this would be appropriate after obtaining a chest CT, with and without contrast, to evaluate for lesions and hilar lymphadenopathy that were too small or "hidden" on his CXR. Ideally, the CT should be performed even if his cytology is negative.

C. Refer to cardiac surgeon for possible cardiac catheterization, possible balloon valvuloplasty, or other interventions CORRECT

Mr. Harris is going to require cardiac catheterization to assess for any evidence of mitral regurgitation that was not identified on the echocardiogram and to provide more accurate and direct measurements of his pulmonary artery, left atrium, and left ventricle. These findings along with his history, physical, and diagnostic studies thus far obtained will permit the cardiac surgeon to determine the most appropriate intervention/treatment for his condition.

Cardiac catheterizations are also indicated if there is discordance between echocardiographic findings and the patient's symptoms, especially if the patient is symptomatic or the pulmonary arteries and the left atrium pressures during exercise don't correlate.

For symptomatic patients with significant disease (in mitral stenosis defined as a valve area of less than 1.5 cm^2 and in tricuspid stenosis defined as a effective orifice of less than 1.5 to 2.0 cm^2 and a diastolic pressure gradient of greater than 4 mm Hg), unless contraindicated, the treatment of choice is valvotomy. This can be accomplished by balloon valvuloplasty or "open" surgical repair for the mitral valve and by surgical correction alone for the tricuspid valve. In asymptomatic patients who meet the aforementioned mitral valvular area criteria PLUS have severe pulmonary hypertension or recurrent embolization (systemic), a valvotomy is also indicated.

In patients who have contraindications to a valvotomy or had a failed valvotomy, valvular replacement is indicated.

Valvotomy patients must be a New York Heart Association (NYHA) II, III, or IV. Valvular replacement patients must be a NYHA III or IV. A class I patient has no impairment and can perform normal activities. A class II patient has some mild limitations in performing activities of daily living (e.g., cannot walk up a flight of steps rapidly, in the cold, after a meal, or carrying objects of minimal weight). Class III individuals have marked physical limitation (e.g., cannot walk one to two blocks on level ground and cannot ascend steps rapidly); however, they are comfortable at rest. Class IV patients have significant difficulty in carrying out activities of daily living and become symptomatic from mild exertion; they often experience symptoms at rest.

D. Start on warfarin therapy   INCORRECT

The primary reason to start patients with tricuspid and mitral regurgitation on warfarin therapy is a coexisting atrial fibrillation, endocarditis, or thromboembolus (which he does not have). However, if he requires a valvular replacement, he will be required to initiate warfarin at that time.

E. Encourage smoking cessation   CORRECT

Mr. Harris needs to be encouraged to quit smoking. Although the number one reason people stop smoking is because their HCP told them to do so, he is not going to be successful until he decides it is a priority. Therefore, utilizing the five A's developed by the Agency for Health Care Policy and Research—**A**sk, **A**dvise, **A**ttempt, **A**ssist, and **A**rrange—is an appropriate plan. Furthermore, smoking cessation should be discussed during each visit with patients who smoke.

Epidemiologic and Other Data

Rheumatic fever is the main cause of both mitral (approximately 40%) and tricuspid stenosis. Typically, the symptoms do not occur until approximately 15 to 20 years after the episode of rheumatic fever beginning with the mitral valve: Then, they tend to be gradual in onset and worse over a 3- to 4-year period. Approximately 66% of all cases occur in women.

The majority of cases (60 to 70%) of hemoptysis that present in the outpatient setting are caused by some type of pulmonary infection (e.g., bronchitis, pneumonia, or tuberculosis).

CASE 1-8
Harriett Issac
1. History

A. Has she ever experienced similar symptoms in the past? ESSENTIAL

This is an excellent question to ask virtually all patients, especially if they are complaining of acute pain. If positive, it provides information regarding prior circumstances, recurrence, progression, and previous diagnosis and suggests a chronic condition.

B. Is she aware of any other aggravating or alleviating factors? ESSENTIAL

Although important with any complaint, knowledge of aggravating and alleviating factors is even more significant when the patient is experiencing pain because the more infor-

mation that is available regarding the condition, the more likely it is that the correct diagnosis will be established.

C. What type of evaluation and diagnostic tests were performed on her in the emergency department following her MVA, and what were the results?   ESSENTIAL

Knowing which components of a physical exam and which diagnostic studies were previously performed and their findings are important when evaluating a patient for continuation of a problem. This provides a baseline assessment from which to work and to compare results while attempting to diagnose the multitude of conditions that could be responsible for Mrs. Issac's chest pain and dyspnea, especially because it is compounded by trauma, depression, and anxiety.

The most common serious conditions that must be included on Mrs. Issac's differential diagnosis list include aortic dissection, aortic root dissection, cardiac contusion, cardiac effusion and/or tamponade, myocardial ischemia, myocardial infarction, cardiomyopathy, ruptured papillary muscles, pneumothorax, and hemithorax.

D. Has she been experiencing any diaphoresis, palpitations, tachycardia, anxiety, or shakiness?   ESSENTIAL

Although virtually any of the aforementioned conditions could be associated with these symptoms, they could also be caused by an excess catecholamine release and/or anxiety. Nevertheless, knowing if she is experiencing them can assist in determining her correct diagnosis.

E. Does she have any other grandchildren to replace the one she lost?   NONESSENTIAL

In attempting to establish good rapport with a patient, especially in nonemergent situations, it is appropriate to inquire about one's family. However, it is inappropriate to even suggest that you can replace a recently deceased person with another. This is especially distasteful given the circumstances surrounding her grandson's death.

2. Physical Examination

A. Heart examination   ESSENTIAL

Because Mrs. Issac is complaining of chest pain, it is essential to perform a careful heart examination as outlined in Case 1-2.

B. Lung auscultation   ESSENTIAL

Because she is experiencing dyspnea, it is essential to perform a comprehensive lung examination as outlined in Case 1-5. In dealing with the combination of chest pain, dyspnea, and trauma, it is important to remember when performing the physical examination and reviewing the CXRs that the apexes of the lungs extend above the clavicles. A small pneumothorax in that area can easily be missed if it is not being diligently sought.

C. Palpation of ribs   ESSENTIAL

Even though Mrs. Issac had rib radiographs the previous evening that were reported as normal, it is still good medical practice to palpate the ribs for tenderness, crepitus, flailness, dislocations, and other signs of rib fracture because rib fractures are notoriously difficult to identify on CXR, especially if rib enhancement films were not performed. The sharp point of a progressing dislocated rib fracture could result in a pneumothorax or a hemothorax, which would produce symptoms very similar to Mrs. Issac's.

Complete rib fractures have also been known to rupture spleens, perforate stomachs, and cause other intra-abdominal trauma resulting in peritoneal hemorrhage. However, if that were the case, Mrs. Issac should be complaining of abdominal pain, experiencing hypotensive and tachycardic episodes, and suffering from lightheadedness, vertigo, presyncope, or syncope. Furthermore, all of these symptoms should be getting progressively worse since their onset.

D. Evaluation of jugular venous pressure (JVP) and ankles/feet for edema   ESSENTIAL

Because cardiomegaly is suggested by her heart examination, it is important to also evaluate her JVP to obtain a quick estimation of her CVP and evidence of right atrium involvement as well as evaluate her feet/ankles for edema, which could suggest the presence of heart failure.

E. Visual acuity   NONESSENTIAL

Because Mrs. Issac did not lose consciousness and has not experienced a headache, visual disturbances, and/or signs or symptoms of an intracranial or cranial nerve injury during or since her accident, checking her visual acuity is not necessary at this time.

3. Diagnostic Studies

A. Brain natriuretic peptide (BNP)   ESSENTIAL

Because Mrs. Issac has abnormal heart sounds, a murmur, and cardiomegaly evident on her physical examination, a BNP is indicated to rule out heart failure. Although it is rare for this condition to exist without the presence of pedal edema, she might regularly wear support/compression stockings and/or sit with her feet supported, which would minimize pedal edema, or she could be spending more time supine and would have presacral edema instead.

Although trauma is not a significant cause of heart failure, traumatic pericardial effusions, hemopericardium, and cardiac tamponade can produce it. Still, it is unlikely to develop this quickly after injury. Nevertheless, there is no guarantee that Mrs. Issac's complaint is related to her accident, so heart failure must be ruled out.

B. Serial cardiac troponin levels (cTn-I and cTn-T)   ESSENTIAL

Any patient who presents with severe, pressurelike chest pain with radiation into their left shoulder and arm (especially if associated with dyspnea) is considered to be having a myocardial infarction until proven otherwise. Hence, it is essential to do serial cardiac troponin levels on Mrs. Issac.

Even though cardiac troponins are very sensitive for myocardial damage, it is not impossible to get a small elevation from myocardial injury without infarction and/or severe or extensive skeletal muscle injury. Furthermore, cardiac troponins can elevate in response to cardiac ischemia as well. However, the rise due to myocardial and skeletal muscle ischemia and contusions is generally not going to be nearly as significant or as predictive as that with myocardial infarction.

C. Electrocardiogram (ECG) and echocardiogram   ESSENTIAL

The presence of pressure-like chest pain, left shoulder and arm pain, dyspnea, trauma, cardiomegaly, and abnormal heart sounds, justifies the performance of both of these tests to further assess Mrs. Issac's cardiac status. The ECG will provide, among other things, information regarding her heart rate, rhythm, conduction, and myocardial oxygenation status.

The echocardiogram can further evaluate for the presence of myocardial dyskinesis, papillary muscle and/or valvular rupture, other valvular abnormalities, the presence of emboli, pericardial effusions, and pericardial and myocardial tissue trauma/damage, as well as provide better estimates of chamber size and volume, overall cardiac size and shape, and an estimation of her ejection fraction.

D. Chest x-ray (CXR)   ESSENTIAL

A CXR is indicated not only to obtain a view of the cardiac shadow but also to look for signs of heart failure that are not yet evident on physical examination, hemothoraxes, pneumothoraxes, and other pulmonary complications or problems.

E. 24-Hour urine vanillylmandelic acid (VMA) and catecholamine levels   ESSENTIAL

Although these tests would likely not be ordered until Mrs. Issac's CXR is viewed, 24-hour urine VMA and catecholamine levels are essential in determining her most likely diagnosis. They are indicated to evaluate for a severe stress reaction with catecholamine release causing the abnormal ballooning pattern of her left ventricle evident on CXR.

The most common indications for these tests is to assist in the diagnosis of pheochromocytoma, a rare cause of secondary hypertension. They are also helpful in diagnosing neuroblastomas and rare adrenal tumors. However, the values can also be elevated with a ganglioneuroma, a ganglioneuroblastoma, some forms of cardiomegaly, strenuous exercise, and acute anxiety.

There is the potential for both false-positives and false-negatives as the levels are affected by strenuous exercise, stress, starvation, some foods (e.g., caffeine, chocolate, and vanilla), and some medications (e.g., aminophylline, clonidine, erythromycin, imipramine, levodopa, lithium, methyldopa, nicotinic acid, nitroglycerine, phenelzine, quinidine, reserpine, salicylates, tetracycline, and tranylcypromine). Hence, multiple factors must be taken into account and caution utilized in interpreting the results of these tests.

4. Diagnosis

A. Pheochromocytoma   INCORRECT

A pheochromocytoma is a functional chromaffinoma that is most commonly derived from adrenal medullary tissue that secretes catecholamines, which results in hypertension and distinct episodes of headaches, nausea (generally without vomiting), palpitations, dyspnea, severe perspiration, and other signs of autonomic dysfunction. Even though Mrs. Issac's BP is elevated, she does not have a history of hypertension, which would be unusual for a pheochromocytoma advanced enough to produce her current symptoms. Furthermore, despite her total free catecholamines being elevated, her metanephrine level, the catecholamine most commonly elevated in pheochromocytoma, is not. Thus, pheochromocytoma is not her most likely diagnosis.

B. Acute inferior myocardial infarction (AIMI)   INCORRECT

An AIMI would not be an unlikely diagnosis for Mrs. Issac because of her symptoms, slightly elevated cardiac troponin levels, ECG findings, and echocardiography results. However, if she were having an MI, based on the location of the ST-segment elevations, it would most likely be in the anterior portion of her heart because that is the area of the heart reflected in precordial leads V_1 through V_5. An AIMI would be expected to show the ST changes in leads II, III, and aVF. Hence, this is not her most likely diagnosis.

C. Heart failure   INCORRECT

Even though she has dyspnea associated with cardiomegaly, heart failure is not her most likely diagnosis because she does not have an elevated BNP or other signs on her physical examination or CXR to support this diagnosis.

D. Takotsubo cardiomyopathy   CORRECT

Takotsubo cardiomyopathy, or apical ballooning syndrome, is a rare form of dilated cardiomyopathy that begins with an abrupt onset of severe chest pain. It generally presents with ECG changes that are consistent with an acute anterior MI; however, the coronary vessels are angiographically normal and the left ventricle exhibits the typical "octopus (or Takotsubo) pot" ballooning. It almost always follows a major release of catecholamines caused by severe physical or emotional stress, surgery, alcohol withdrawal, and certain medical conditions (e.g., hypoglycemia and hyperthyroidism). Thus, this is Mrs. Issac's most likely diagnosis from the list provided.

E. Chest pain secondary to stress reaction   INCORRECT

Chest pain secondary to stress reaction implies that no actual physical damage and/or objective findings are present to account for the pain. Therefore, in view of her physical examination and diagnostic studies, this cannot be her most likely diagnosis.

5. Treatment Plan

A. Hospitalize with telemetry and close monitoring of vital signs   CORRECT

With Mrs. Issac's degree of cardiomegaly and ventricular abnormality as well as slightly elevated troponin level, hospitalization is definitely indicated for close monitoring, further diagnostic evaluation, and treatment.

B. Repeat cTn-I and cTn-T in 4 and 8 hours   CORRECT

Repeating her cardiac troponins in 4 and 8 hours is going to permit an indirect assessment of the oxygenation status of her myocardium. A decreasing, plateauing, or insignificantly elevating level is more likely caused by ischemia secondary to the catecholamine storm effect on the epicardial vessels and/or coronary microcirculation or from skeletal muscle trauma. A significant elevation is more suggestive of an acute myocardial infarction.

C. Cardiac catheterization   CORRECT

Although Takotsubo cardiomyopathy is not associated with an obstruction of the epicardial arteries, her symptoms mandate that her coronary vasculature be evaluated to ensure that she does not have significant atherosclerosis, obstruction, or emboli. If a significant abnormality is present, then early treatment can also be instituted for that problem.

D. Meperidine 50 mg IM every 3 to 4 hours as needed   INCORRECT

Mrs. Issac should not receive meperidine for her pain because she has a history of an allergic reaction to it in the form of urticaria.

E. Nebivolol 10 mg orally once a day   INCORRECT

Beta-blockers reduce the symptoms in approximately one-third to one-half of patients with Takotsubo cardiomyopathy; however, there are no evidence-based studies or firm clinical information confirming this. Furthermore, they do not appear to be protective against sudden cardiac death. Nevertheless, because there are essentially no other treatment options available, one could be tried if her intraventricular pressure gradient is relatively normal. However, it should not be nebivolol. Nebivolol, as well as fluoxetine, is metabolized by the P-450 CYP2D6 pathway; hence, a serious adverse interaction could occur. In fact, the FDA issued a letter of warning to the manufacturers of nebivolol in November 2008 because it felt an ad in a professional journal omitted and minimized this risk. A recent study was conducted on healthy patients who had been taking fluoxetine 20 mg once a day took a single dose of nebivolol 10 mg. The combination led to an area-under-curve (AUC) increase of eightfold and a maximum concentration (C_{max}) of threefold for d-nebivolol. Hence, hypotension and syncope could occur and produce very serious, and potentially fatal, consequences because of this interaction. This is an excellent example of the importance of obtaining FULL prescribing information and weigh the potential benefits of treatment against the potential adverse effects before initiating any drug therapy.

Epidemiologic and Other Data

Takotsubo cardiomyopathy is also known as Tako-Tsubo cardiomyopathy, stress cardiomyopathy, and apical ballooning syndrome. It occurs predominately in women over the age of 50 years. It is thought to be caused by an adrenergic surge resulting from severe physical and/or emotional stress that causes the release of catecholamines. The catecholamines then attack the epicardial vessels and/or coronary microcirculation. In the majority of cases, all the symptoms are resolved in 3 to 7 days without any residual effects.

CASE 1-9
Ira Jackson
1. History

A. Were there any changes in his medical condition, medication list (including medications used on an as-needed basis), or life when he began reexperiencing palpitations and having fluctuations of his INR?   ESSENTIAL

Mr. Jackson actually has two potentially unrelated complaints—a fluctuating INR and cardiac palpitations—plus he has confusion regarding the purpose of his medications. Although he takes the warfarin for his atrial fibrillation (AF), it is to prevent him from having a CVA caused by an embolus that formed in his poorly contracting and emptying atrium. His warfarin does nothing to control his ventricular response. However, it is possible that the propranolol he takes for his hypertension suppresses his ventricular rate and enables him to remain relatively asymptomatic and hemodynamically stable.

The INR is a standardized reporting mechanism to ensure better correlation and quality between prothrombin time (PT) levels, especially when the specimens are tested at different facilities. The INR is essentially the patient's measured PT divided by the mean normal PT. In Mr. Jackson's case, it is being utilized to monitor the anticoagulant effect of his warfarin.

Warfarin produces its anticoagulant effect by interfering with the body's vitamin K (which is required for the carboxylation of glutamine) conversion cycle, which in turn causes the liver to produce partially decarboxylated proteins that have decreased anticoagulant abilities.

Hence, any medication that can prevent or reduce the production of, increase the excretion of, or prevent the absorption of vitamin K can interfere with warfarin's anticoagulant properties. Such medications include second-generation cephalosporins, third-generation cephalosporins, erythromycin, penicillin, metronidazole, moxalactam, trimethoprim-sulfamethoxazole, rifampicin, sulfonamides, thyroxine, clofibrate, cholestyramine, phenylbutazone, salicylates, nonsteroidal anti-inflammatory drugs, acetaminophen, cimetidine, omeprazole, barbiturates, carbamazepine, and alcohol. Mutations/alterations in or medications metabolized by either the P-450 hepatic CYP2C9 or the VKORC1 enzyme pathways in the liver can also alter the warfarin level upward or downward. For these reasons, it is important to inquire about new medical conditions and new medications, with an emphasis on those bought without a prescription (including vitamins, supplements, and herbal preparations), which might be taken on an as-needed basis (e.g., cimetidine, acetaminophen, or ibuprofen) or taken for short periods of time (e.g., antibiotics, antifungals, and analgesics), because the effect of the combination of the medications could either elevate or decrease his warfarin level.

Even though there are significantly fewer medications that can potentially adversely affect his propranolol level, it is still important to consider this as a possible cause of his palpitations. For example, propranolol can be potentiated by medications that contain alcohol, other antihypertensives, cimetidine, chlorpromazine, central nervous system (CNS) depressants, and thyroid hormone replacement therapy. It can also be antagonized by medications such as barbiturates, NSAIDs, phenytoin, and rifampin.

Furthermore, warfarin and propranolol can adversely affect the levels of other drugs (e.g., antiarrhythmics, anticonvulsants, calcium channel blockers, digitalis, diuretics, hypoglycemics, lidocaine, and theophylline), providing them the opportunity to produce palpitations.

Other adverse influences on the regularity of the ventricle response and hence the ability to produce palpitations in some patients include, but are not limited to, individual metabolic factors, genetic factors, neurologic (especially vagal nerve) factors, NYHA functional status classification, presence of heart failure, and length of time the arrhythmia has persisted.

B. Do his medications look different since he started experiencing problems?   ESSENTIAL

The FDA permits generic drugs to be classified as "equivalent" if the amount of active ingredient is within 25% of the brand-name product. Therefore, if he was on a generic formulation that had 25% more of the active ingredients than the brand and was changed to a different company's generic that contained 25% less of the active ingredients, then, at least theoretically, it is possible that his medication dosage was cut in half. This could account for a change in his symptom control and result in a lower INR. Conversely, going in the opposite direction could potentially result in an elevated INR. Additionally, if he was being provided a different company's generic every time he had his prescription refilled, this could also produce intermittent INR fluctuations and palpitations.

Furthermore, there is always the concern regarding human error (that the wrong medication was dispensed) when the appearance of the medication suddenly changes. Hence, it is essential to know if there was any change, and if so, to discuss it with his pharmacist to determine if he is getting the right medications in the proper dosages. Even in cases where brand-name medications cannot be justified (or afforded by the patient), requesting that the pharmacist refill the patient's medication with a generic from the same company is helpful in eliminating the problem of dosage fluctuations that could potentially occur when changed from company to company.

C. Does he consume caffeine?   ESSENTIAL

In caffeine-sensitive individuals, consuming a single serving of a caffeinated beverage is enough to incite an episode of paroxysmal AF with a variable ventricle response and palpitations like Mr. Jackson is experiencing. Excessive caffeine, even in patients who are not caffeine sensitive, can cause palpitations. Therefore, it is important to inquire regarding his caffeine intake and its relationship to his symptoms.

D. Does he alter the amounts of "greens" that he consumes daily?   ESSENTIAL

Because warfarin itself is essentially a vitamin K analog, fluctuating levels of vitamin K intake can cause fluctuating levels of the INR. Additionally, it appears that the individuals who have the most difficulty with this problem are the patients who have been on warfarin for extended periods of time. The greatest food source of vitamin K is greens (e.g., spinach, lettuce, and kale). It is theorized that this occurs because essentially all vitamin K is derived from phylloquinone. Phylloquinone is then metabolized to vitamin KH_2, which prohibits the anticoagulant effect of the warfarin, hence altering the patient's INR, especially if the daily amount consumed is altered significantly.

Furthermore, if the patient was taking vitamins, supplements, or herbal preparations with large amounts of vitamin K, or only taking them "sometimes," the same problem could occur. This underscores the importance of a drug history that specifically inquires about over-the-counter medications, supplements, and herbal preparations because many patients frequently do not consider these to be medications and will not list to taking them unless specifically asked.

E. Does he alter the amount of orange juice that he drinks daily?   NONESSENTIAL

Orange juice has not been implicated as a substance that can interfere with the vitamin K synthesis pathway or the liver metabolism associated with the use of warfarin or propranolol.

2. Physical Examination

A. Nasal and pharyngeal examination   NONESSENTIAL

B. Heart examination   ESSENTIAL

Because Mr. Jackson has a history of AF and palpitations and the majority of AF is associated with underlying cardiac disease, it is very important to perform a careful heart examination as outlined in Case 1-2 not only to evaluate the AF but also to search for associated cardiac conditions that could be responsible for his intermittent palpitations.

C. Lung auscultation   ESSENTIAL

A careful lung examination as outlined in Case 1-5 is also essential to identify any pulmonary changes caused by the AF or another underlying cardiac problem (e.g., rales from heart failure) or an associated pulmonary condition that could be causing hypoxia and precipitate the AF (e.g., wheezing secondary to asthma).

D. Evaluation of JVP   ESSENTIAL

As previously stated, the height of the JVP provides a rough estimate of central venous pressure and evaluates for the presence of right atrium involvement (i.e., enlargement) which is important with his current symptoms.

E. Check for pedal edema   ESSENTIAL

Mr. Jackson should also have his feet, ankles, and lower legs examined for pedal edema. It can result from cardiac, hepatic, or renal failure as well as some cancers. However, in Mr. Jackson's case, the greatest concern would be heart failure from a poorly controlled ventricular rate caused by the AF or from an underlying cardiac disease (e.g., myocardial ischemia, acute or old silent myocardial infarction, other arrhythmia, cardiomyopathies, or valvular heart disease).

3. Diagnostic Studies

A. International normalized ratio (INR)   ESSENTIAL

Because one of Mr. Jackson's main complaints is the inability to stabilize and maintain his INR at its goal, it is important to know what his current INR and INR goal are. Essentially, unless he has a prosthetic heart valve, his INR range would be somewhere between 2 and 3, with a goal of 2.5. With a mechanical heart valve, the patient's goal would be at least 2.5.

However, as medical treatments continue to evolve and a greater emphasis is placed on evidence-based medicine, equally (if not more) important is to determine whether Mr. Jackson is still an appropriate candidate for warfarin therapy. Numerous studies have been conducted with a multitude of stroke risk assessment tools to assist in determining which AF patients are most likely to have a CVA.

The American College of Cardiology (ACC), the AHA Task Force on Practice Guidelines, and the European Society of Cardiology (ESC) Committee for Practice Guidelines all agree that based on the currently available evidence, all patients with AF require some type of anticoagulation therapy; however, it might not be warfarin.

These organizations recommend utilizing a risk stratification system in which the patient's demographics and comorbidities are placed into one of three risk categories (invalidated/very weak, moderate, and high) to determine the likelihood of an embolic phenomenon occurring from their AF and resulting in a CVA. In other words, are the benefits relative to the prevention of an ischemic stroke with warfarin going to outweigh the risks of a potential hemorrhagic stroke, intracranial bleed or other serious bleed from the medication?

The invalidated or very weak-risk factors include being female, being between the ages of 65 and 75 years, having coronary artery disease, and having thyroid disease. Moderate-risk factors are considered being age 75 years or older, being diabetic (type 1 or type 2), having hypertension, having heart failure, and having a left ventricle ejection of 35 or less. High-risk factors are a history of a previous CVA, TIA, or embolism; the presence of mitral stenosis; and the presence of a mechanical heart valve.

Obviously, many patients are going to have characteristics that fall into more than one of these three categories. When that occurs, the higher-level risk is considered to be the category in which the patient is placed. For example, if a patient had all four invalid/very weak-risk factors, then he or she would be placed into the no-risk category; however, if another patient had only one of those same invalid/very weak-risk factors but also had one high-risk factor, then that patient would be categorized as high risk despite possessing a total of only two risk factors.

Regarding treatment, if the patient is in the no-risk (very low) group, the most appropriate anticoagulant is aspirin 81 to 325 mg once a day. However, if the patient has one moderate-risk factor and falls into the moderate-risk category, then the patient and the HCP together would make the determination as to which was better for that individual patient—one aspirin 81 to 325 mg once a day or warfarin with an INR target as defined previously. However, if the patient has one or more high-risk factors (categorized as high risk) OR two or more moderate-risk factors (still categorized as moderate risk), the treatment choice would be warfarin.

The consensus group also supported utilizing a risk-only–based approach, which is also supported by current studies. This evidence-based approach is considered to be a class 1 (highest rating) recommendation. If the patient has any of the following comorbidities, regardless of age (except where noted), he or she is considered at high risk for a CVA and should be placed on warfarin with an INR goal of between 2 and 3: presence of a mechanical heart valve; prior thromboembolic event; mitral stenosis from rheumatic heart disease; heart failure and a minimum age of 65 years; and the triad of a left ventricular ejection fraction of less than 35%, fractional shortening of less than 25%, and hypertension.

After these AF patients are eliminated, then, age plays a significant role in this model. If the patient is younger than the age of 60 years and does not have any of the aforementioned conditions, regardless of whether or not any other cardiac conditions or risks exist, antithrombotic therapy is recommended with aspirin 81 to 325 mg once a day. If the patient is between the ages of 60 and 75 years and has no other risk factors, then aspirin is also the recommended therapy. However, if a patient in this age group has either diabetes or CAD, it is recommended that he or she begin warfarin. If the patient is female and older than the age of 75 years regardless of other risk factors OR is male with any other risk factors, then warfarin is again recommended. If the patient is older than the age of 75 years, is male, and has no other risk factors, then both warfarin and aspirin are considered to be appropriate treatment options.

Another risk assessment tool to determine whether the patient with AF requires warfarin therapy is a lot easier to remember because it provides a mnemonic, CHADS$_2$ (**c**ardiac failure, **h**ypertension, **a**ge older than 75 years, **d**iabetes, and previous **s**troke). For each characteristic the patient is assigned 1 point (except for stroke, which is given 2 points), for a maximum total of 6 points. A score of 0 to 2 is considered low risk and the patient should be anticoagulated with aspirin alone. A score of 3 or 4 is considered to be moderate risk and the patient and the HCP need to discuss the risks vs benefits and together determine whether aspirin or warfarin anticoagulation is more appropriate for that individual patient. A score of 5 or 6 is considered to be high risk and the patient should be instituted on warfarin therapy unless there is a contraindication.

There is a direct correlation between the numerical score and the risk of stroke with this simple system; however, the ACC, AHA, and ESC do not support it at this time because they believe it provides warfarin at too low of a risk of stroke and results in too many unnecessary adverse events, including hemorrhagic strokes.

In general, patients who have a stroke risk of less than 2% per year tend to have more adverse effects than benefits from warfarin therapy. Hence, it is not recommended for these individuals to take it. Individuals with an annual stroke risk of greater than 6% definitely benefit from warfarin therapy. It is most difficult to determine the risk vs benefit ratio for moderate-risk individuals; that is what all of these studies and guidelines are trying to accomplish. However, it is important to remember that these are not absolutes but guidelines, and need to be treated as such. Sound clinical judgment must go into the decision-making process to treat or not to treat with warfarin on an individualized basis, including the patient preference as part of that decision.

According to the initial risk assessment supported by the ACC, AHA, and ESC, Mr. Jackson would be considered moderate risk because he has two moderate-risk factors, an age older than 75 years and hypertension; therefore, he should continue his warfarin.

B. Hematocrit (HCT) and hemoglobin (Hgb), or H&H ESSENTIAL

The H&H provides confirmation of the history and physical findings that Mr. Jackson is not experiencing any bleeding.

C. Electrocardiogram (ECG) and echocardiogram, preferably transesophageal (TEE)   ESSENTIAL

The ECG is essential because it permits evaluation of not only the ventricular response rate but also the atrial rate. Although no standards have been set regarding the goals of heart rate therapy, the accepted criteria are a ventricular rate between 60 and 80 BPM at rest and 90 and 115 BPM with moderately intense exercise. Additionally, the ECG is important for Mr. Jackson as it assists in searching for other causes of his palpitations in addition to his AF.

A TEE not only provides a clear picture of all the structural and functional details of the heart as outlined in Case 1-5, but also permits an evaluation for underlying cardiac abnormalities that are associated with AF. Furthermore, if using the aforementioned risk assessment stratification system as approved by the ACC, AHA, and ECS, a accurate measurement of the left ventricular ejection fraction is necessary.

D. Thyroid panel, hepatic function, and renal function ESSENTIAL

These tests are also recommended by the ACC, AHA, and EUS as essential in evaluating AF. They are beneficial in ruling in or ruling out some of the correctable causes of AF (e.g., hyperthyroidism or hepatic damage/cirrhosis caused by excessive alcohol intake) as well as in ensuring adequate hepatic and renal functioning before instituting any medications.

E. Holter monitor (outpatient telemetry)   ESSENTIAL

According to the ACC/AHA/ECS, a Holter monitor is not indicated as part of the initial evaluation of AF. However, the ACC/AHA/ECS guidelines would support utilizing this diagnostic test for Mr. Jackson because their main recommendations in confirming AF include determining whether the ventricular response rates (at rest and with exercise) are within the recommended ranges, evaluating further the patient who fails to respond to appropriate antiarrhythmic therapy, and/or evaluating for a second arrhythmia.

4. Diagnosis

A. Recurrent paroxysmal atrial fibrillation with fluctuations in INR as a result of inconsistent dietary vitamin K intake CORRECT

AF is relatively easy to diagnose if the patient is experiencing the abnormal rhythm during evaluation. Its diagnostic criteria consist of a suspicious history, an irregularly irregular pulse on physical examination, and the identification of the abnormality on ECG.

However, because he has good rate control at rest with the propranolol and appears hemodynamically stable, but is still complaining of palpitations, an additional cause should be sought. His Holter monitoring reveals that his AF only occurs in bursts, or spasms; hence, the diagnosis of recurrent paroxysmal atrial fibrillation can be confirmed by this diagnostic test.

Regarding his INR control, the pharmacodynamics of warfarin vary significantly from one individual to another; however, usually by frequent dosage adjusting and laboratory monitoring, one can generally achieve the desired INR goal in almost all individuals. If not, attention needs to be directed towards not only other medications that utilize the P-450 hepatic CYP2C9 or the VKORC1 enzyme pathways but also of medications and foods that can have an effect on metabolism of vitamin K (which can lower the INR level, as warfarin is a vitamin K analog). In Mr. Jackson's case, the problem appears to be a significant variation in the amount of "greens" he consumes from one day to the next. Thus, this is Mr. Jackson's most likely diagnosis.

B. Atrial fibrillation with poor medical compliance INCORRECT

In general, patients who are noncompliant with their medication regimen tend to miss doses of their medication and/or take it irregularly, which would result in Mr. Jackson's INR fluctuating from low (when noncompliant) to normal (when compliant) However, there are a few patients who take more medication than prescribed, either trying to "catch up" on doses before they are due to have their INR checked, thinking it will normalize it, or when they remember they missed several doses. Additionally, some patients hold the belief that "if one is good, two is better"; therefore, they will take extra medication if they "feel like" they need it. This latter practice could result in an INR that is high, low, or normal. Regardless, this is not Mr. Jackson's most likely diagnosis because a potential food–drug interaction was identified and he denies poor compliance with his medications.

Consultation with the patient's pharmacist to see if refills are obtained on schedule can sometimes add support to the suspicion of medication noncompliance. For example, if the patient is "late" in refilling his or her medication, he or she could be taking less than prescribed. Conversely, if the patient is consistently requiring his or her medication before the refill is technically available, he or she may be taking more than prescribed. However, it is important to remember that even though the patient might obtain the prescribed medication, he or she is not necessarily taking it as directed.

C. Familial atrial fibrillation with fluctuations in INR as a result of inadequate vitamin C in diet   INCORRECT

Mr. Jackson's AF is probably a familial form because of his strong family history of AF and his lack of any other apparent cardiac abnormalities or associated conditions. Because vitamin C is not known to have a significant effect on warfarin metabolism and his daily intake of vitamin C is consistent, this is not his most likely diagnosis.

D. Atrial fibrillation with normal INR   INCORRECT

Although Mr. Jackson has AF, he does not have a normal INR (patient, 1.6; treatment goal, 2.5 [or range between 2 and 3]). Thus, this is not his most likely diagnosis.

E. Atrial flutter with excessive propranolol dosage responsible for palpitations and INR fluctuations   INCORRECT

Atrial fibrillation, not atrial flutter, was identified on Mr. Jackson's ECG. Atrial fibrillation tends to be the faster of the two arrhythmias and is characterized by the inability to visualize the P wave and an irregularly irregular rate. Atrial flutter is characterized as an atrial rate between 250 and 350 BPM and exhibits the pathognomonic flutter (or "sawtooth") appearance.

Propranolol is metabolized through one of the same pathways as warfarin. Therefore, it is possible for them to alter one another's dosage either positively or negatively depending on whichever medication binds to the most receptor sites. However, if he is on the same dose of propranolol daily and does not miss any of the doses, another factor should account for the fluctuating INR and his warfarin dosage should be able to be regulated accordingly. Thus, this is not his most likely diagnosis.

5. Treatment Plan

A. Add digoxin 0.125 mg once a day   CORRECT

When treating a patient with AF, there are three primary treatment goals: (1) rate control, (2) rhythm control, and (3) prevention of thromboembolism. Initial management of a patient who is hemodynamically stable and not in the acute phase of the onset of the illness can be either a rate-control or a rhythm-control strategy. The goal of rate control is to manage the ventricular response without any concern regarding the underlying rhythm disturbance. Rhythm control not only attempts to restore the patient to normal sinus rhythm but also assists in controlling the rate.

According the ACC/AHA/ECS guidelines, rate control is generally accomplished with a beta-blocker or a nondihydropyridine CCB. In the past, when patients failed to respond to the medication, the dosage was increased until the desired results were achieved or the patient quit taking it because of adverse events. This practice is no longer recommended.

Because Mr. Jackson does not appear to be having any difficulty with his current dosage of propranolol, it would be logical to add a medication that worked via another pathway to complement his propranolol instead of pushing the medication to the point where he discontinues it because of adverse effects. This is currently the accepted recommendation. Therefore, he should be tried on a medication for rate control. The drug of choice for this is digoxin. The combination of digoxin and either a beta-blocker (or a CCB) should control the rate during both exercise and at rest. Caution must be taken to keep from causing a bradycardia with this combination. Additionally, digoxin should not be utilized as monotherapy to achieve rate control in paroxysmal AF.

B. Schedule for nodal ablation   INCORRECT

Nodal ablation is only indicated in chronic, stable patients when they do not respond to or are intolerant of pharmacologic therapy with a combination of digoxin and a beta-blocker or a CCB. It can be done either by medication or laser ablation. The agent of choice for this procedure is IV amiodarone. Other acceptable agents include IV procainamide, disopyramide, and ibutilide. An alternative to pharmacologic ablation in a hemodynamically stable patient would be to add oral amiodarone to his current regimen.

If medications fail to control the ventricular rate or the sustained tachyarrhythmia caused a cardiomyopathy, a catheter-directed ablation is indicated. Radiofrequency ablation is the first-line choice for AV nodal ablation in very young and/or very symptomatic patients.

C. Schedule for pacemaker implantation   INCORRECT

As long as the patient with AF remains hemodynamically stable, a pacemaker is not indicated until an adequate trial of an antiarrhythmic and/or a negative chronotropic agent has been unsuccessfully tried. The patient population that appears to benefit most from the combination of AV nodal ablation and permanent pacemaker insertion is again those who have developed a cardiomyopathy from the sustained tachyarrhythmia. The combination of a permanent pacemaker following AV nodal ablation is a very effective technique to improve symptomatic tachycardia in some patients.

D. Schedule for cardioversion   INCORRECT

Cardioversion would only be recommended for Mr. Jackson if all available pharmacologic regimens and other techniques have failed to improve his ventricular rate. The main reason to avoid it with Mr. Jackson, if at all possible, is because it significantly increases the risk of thrombolic events despite pretreatment with an anticoagulant when AF has been present for more than 48 hours.

However, there are instances when a patient will require that his or her rhythm be restored to normal sinus rhythm immediately. This is most frequently done to prevent worsening of ischemia and/or angina, when hypotension and/or syncope are present, and/or for acute-onset heart failure.

Anticoagulants should always be administered preprocedurally if at all possible.

Chemical cardioversion can generally be accomplished utilizing one of the following agents IV: flecainide, dofetilide, propafenone, or ibutilide. Amiodarone is a reasonable second-line option. Electrical cardioversion is usually the preferred method when the situation is acute. Interestingly, therapy with a statin, via an unknown mechanism, has significantly worked in maintaining the patient in normal sinus rhythm once conversion has been successful.

E. Advise patient to consume the same amount of "greens" daily and adjust warfarin dose accordingly   CORRECT

If the fluctuations of Mr. Jackson's INR are caused by the significant variability of the quantity of "greens" he consumes on a daily basis, eliminating this irregularity should permit dosage adjustments that will successfully maintain his INR within the correct range of 2 to 3.

Epidemiologic and Other Data

Atrial fibrillation is considered to be the most common sustained cardiac arrhythmia. It is estimated that it will affect approximately 25% of the U.S. population older than the age of 40 years, with the vast majority (over 19%) of these patients being older than the age of 65 years. It occurs much more often in males than in females. This gender difference increases with advancing age and is approximately doubled after the age of 75 years. It generally occurs in patients with underlying cardiac disease.

It is estimated that the initial presentation of AF will be an atrial thrombus in approximately 15% of the cases. The annual CVA rate is 45% for uncoagulated patients and 14% for coagulated patients. According to the Framingham data, the risk of CVA also increases with advancing age.

There are six types of AF recognized by the American Heart Association: (1) AF without associated heart disease, (2) AF with associated heart disease, (3) familial (genetic) AF, (4) AF associated with other medical conditions, (5) AF associated with autonomic influences, and (6) reversible AF. It is important for the patient to be knowledgeable of his or her type because in some instances, medical treatments commonly used in AF are contraindicated.

AF without associated heart disease, also known as "lone AF," is most generally found in younger patients. It is estimated that 30 to 45% of paroxysmal AF and 20 to 25% of persistent AF in younger patients are idiopathic. However, as time passes, an underlying cause may identify itself in many of these cases. This is much rarer to see in the elderly because of the normal effects of aging on the heart.

AF with heart disease is the most common type. It has definitely been linked with certain cardiac conditions including mitral stenosis and/or regurgitation, heart failure, coronary artery disease, and hypertensive heart disease with left ventricular hypertrophy. It has been strongly associated with many other primary cardiac diseases such as congenital defects, hypertrophic cardiomyopathies, and dilated cardiomyopathies. Other potential comorbid diseases include pure cardiac conditions (e.g., restrictive cardiomyopathies, constrictive pericarditis, mitral valve prolapse with regurgitation, mitral valve prolapse without regurgitation, calcification of the mitral annulus, right atrial dilation, and cardiac tumors). Cardiopulmonary conditions associated with AF include cor pulmonale, right ventricular dilation, and arrhythmias produced by hypoxia.

Familial, or genetic, AF is a "lone AF" that tends to be found in family clusters. The exact cause is unknown, but patients with idiopathic AF tend to have a first-degree family member with AF. Additionally, just as a family history of AF increases the incidence of AF, so too does a family history of hypertension, diabetes mellitus, and heart failure. Work is currently under way to identify this genetic malfunction.

The next group consists of those individuals who have AF associated with other medical conditions. This group could probably be included in the reversible causes of AF because the primary one is obesity. Long-term obesity is related to left atrial dilation. Weight reduction has recently been shown to decrease the size of the left atrium; hence, it is possible that this could reduce or eliminate this form of AF and its subsequent risk of CVA.

AF associated with autonomic influences is another classification. The autonomic nervous system appears to have a significant role in the development of AF. It appears that either vagal or sympathetic predominance must exist before AF can occur. Vagal-mediated AF appears to be much more common and occurs after activities such as eating a large meal or during sleep. Adrenergically induced AF typically happens in the daytime and is often seen in patients who have organic cardiac disease. One of the primary differences between a vagally mediated AF and a nonvagally induced AF is the fact that normal medications used in AF (e.g., adrenergic blocking agents and digitalis) can worsen the symptoms; however, anticholinergic drugs (e.g., disopyramide) are often helpful to reduce the frequency or completely eliminate the AF. Beta-blockers are considered to be the treatment of choice in these neurologic-mediated cases of AF.

The final category is reversible AF. Examples include hyperthyroidism, excessive alcohol intake during a "binge," sleep apnea, myocardial infarctions, pericarditis, myocarditis, pulmonary embolism, surgery (especially pulmonary or cardiac), and electrocution.

REFERENCES/ADDITIONAL READING

The Agency for Health Care Policy and Research. Smoking cessation clinical practice guidelines. *JAMA.* 1996;275(16): 1270–1280.

Aghababian RV, ed. *Essentials of Emergency Medicine.* Sudbury, MA: Jones & Bartlett Publishers; 2006.

Aghababian RV Diop D. Acute Coronary Syndrome (ACS). 97–116.

Anderson III HL. Chest Injuries. 920–929.

Gough J. Rodriguez L. Endocarditis and Myocarditis. 127–128.

Gough JE, Allison EJ, Jr. Dysrhythmias. 134–147

Gough JE, Rodriguez LE. Cardiomyopathies. 129–130.

Lai MW. Methemoglobinemia. 870–872.

Setnik G. Khan A. Hypertension. 148–155.

American Heart Association. Correction. (Additions to AHA guidelines for prevention of infective endocarditis *Circulation.* 2007;116:1736–1754.) *Circulation.* 2007;116:e376–e377.

Antman EM, Anbe DT, Armstrong PW. et al. (writing on behalf of the American Heart Association 1999 Guidelines for the Management of Patients with Acute Myocardial Infarction Committee). ACC/AHA Guidelines for the Management of Patients with ST-segment Elevation Myocardial Infarction: a report of the American College of Cardiology/American Heart Association Task Force on Practice Guidelines Committee to revise the 1999 guidelines for the management of patients with acute myocardial infarction. *J Am Coll Cardiol.* 2004;44(3):e1–e211.

Bonow RO, Carabello BA, Chatterjee K, et al. ACC/AHA 2006 Guidelines for the Management of Patients with Valvular Heart Disease: a report of the American College of Cardiology/American Heart Association Task Force on Practice Guidelines (Writing Committee to Revise the 1998 Guidelines for the Management of Patients with Valvular Heart Disease): developed in collaboration with the Society of Cardiovascular Anesthesiologists: endorsed by the Society for Cardiovascular Angiography and Interventions and the Society of Thoracic Surgeons. *Circulation.* 2006;114:e84–e231.

Chobanian AV, Bakris GL, Black HR, et al. The Seventh Report of the Joint National Committee on the Prevention, Detection, Evaluation, and Treatment of High Blood Pressure: the JNC 7 report. *JAMA.* 2003;289(19):2560–2572.

Duke Jr JR, Good Jr JT, Hudson LD, et al. Hemoptysis. In: Duke JR Jr, Good JT Jr, Hudson LD, et al. *Frontline Assessment of Common Pulmonary Presentations.* Denver, CO: Snowdrift Pulmonary Foundation, Inc; 2000. http://www.nlhep.org/books/pul_Pre/hemoptysis.htlm. Accessed September 6, 2008.

Easton JD, Saver JL, Albers GW, et al. Definition and evaluation of transient ischemic attack: a scientific statement for healthcare professionals from the American Heart Association/American Stroke Association Stroke Council; Council on Cardiovascular Surgery and Anesthesia; Council on Cardiovascular Radiology and Intervention; Council on Cardiovascular Nursing; and the Interdisciplinary Council on Peripheral Vascular Disease. *Stroke* 2009;40; 2276–2293.

Fauci AS, Kasper DL, Longo DL , et al., eds. *Harrison's Principles of Internal Medicine.* 17th ed. New York: McGraw-Hill Medical; 2008.

  Antman EM, Braunwald E. ST-segment elevation myocardial infarction. 1532–1544.

  Antman EM, Selwyn AP, Braunwald E, Loscalzo J. Ischemic heart disease. 1514–1527.

  Braunwald E. Hypoxia and cyanosis. 229–231.

  Braunwald E. Pericardial disease. 1488–1495.

  Darwin JP, Czany-Ratajcak. Heritable disorders of connective tissue disease. 2461–2469.

  Karchmer AW. Infective endocarditis. 789–798.

  Kotchen TA. Hypertensive vascular disease. 1549–1562.

  Low PA, Engstrom. Disorders of the autonomic nervous system. 2576–2582.

  Mann D. Heart failure and cor pulmonale. 1443–1455.

  Marchlinski F. The tachyarrhythmias. 1425–1442.

  O'Gara P, Braunwald E. Valvular heart disease. 1465–1480.

  O'Rourke RA, Braunwald E. Physical examination of the cardiovascular system. 1382–1388.

  Prockop DJ, Czarny-Ratajczak M. Heritable disorders of connective tissue. 2461–2469.

  Rader DJ, Hobbs HH. Disorders of lipoprotein metabolism. 2416–2429.

  Wynne J, Brauwald E. Cardiomyopathy and myocarditis. 1481–1488.

Forest Laboratories, Inc. *Important correction of drug information about Bystolic (nebivolol) tablets.* Publication #44-1014486. St. Louis: Forest Laboratories; 2008.

Fraker TD Jr, Fihn SD (writing on behalf of the American Heart Association 2002 Chronic Stable Angina Writing Committee). 2007 Chronic angina focused update of the ACC/AHA 2002 guidelines for the management of patients with chronic stable angina: a report of the American College of Cardiology/American Heart Association Task Force on Writing Group to Develop the Focused Update of the 2002 Guidelines for the Management of Patients with Chronic Stable Angina. *Circulation.* 2007; 116:2762–2772.

Fuster V, Rydén LE, Cannom DS, et al. ACC/AHA/ESC 2006 Guidelines for the Management of Patients with Atrial Fibrillation: a report of the American College of Cardiology/American Heart Association Task Force on Practice Guidelines and the European Society of Cardiology Committee for Practice Guidelines (Writing Committee to Revise the 2001 Guidelines for the Management of Patients with Atrial Fibrillation): developed in collaboration with the European Heart Rhythm Association and the Heart Rhythm Society. *Circulation.* 2006;114:e257–e354.

Gonzales R, Kutner J. *Current Practice Guidelines in Primary Care 2009.* New York: McGraw-Hill Medical; 2009.

Gonzales R, Kutner J. Disease management: Cholesterol and lipid management in children. 135.

Gonzales R, Kutner J. Disease management: Hypertension. 148–151.

Gonzales R, Kutner J. Disease screening: cholesterol and lipid disorders. 40–41.

Gonzales R, Kutner J. Disease screening: diabetes mellitus, type 2. 49–51.

Gonzales R, Kutner J. Disease screening: hypertension, children and adolescents. 65.

Gonzales R, Kutner J. Disease screening: obesity. 72–75.

Gonzales R, Kutner J. Appendix IV: 95th percentile of blood pressure for boys and girls. 198.

Gonzales R, Kutner J. Appendix VII: Estimate of 10-year stroke risk for men. 203–204.

Grundy SM, Cleeman JI, Bairey Merz CN, et al., for the Coordinating Committee of the NCEP. Implications of recent clinical trials for the National Cholesterol Education Program Adult Treatment Panel III guidelines. *Circulation.* 2004;110(2):227–239.

Hirsh H, Fuster V, Ansell J, Halperin JL. American Heart Association/American College of Cardiology foundation guide to warfarin therapy. *Circulation.* 2003;107:1692–1711.

Johnson JL. Manifestations of hemoptysis. *Postgrad Med.* 2002;112(4):101–113.

Judge DP, Dietz HC. Marfan's syndrome. *Lancet.* 2005;366 (9501):1965–1976.

Kavey RE, Daniels SR, Lauer RL, Atkins DL, Hayman LL, Taubert K; American Heart Association. American Heart Association guidelines for primary prevention of atherosclerotic cardiovascular disease beginning in childhood. *Circulation*. 2003;107:1562–1566.

Maron BJ. Recommendations and considerations related to preparticipation screening for cardiovascular abnormalities in competitive athletes: 2007 update: a scientific statement from the American Heart Association Council on Nutrition, Physical Activity, and Metabolism. *Circulation*. 2007;115:1643–1655.

McCrindle BM, Urbina EM, Dennison BA, et al. Drug therapy of high-risk lipid abnormalities in children and adolescents: a scientific statement from the American Heart Association Atherosclerosis, Hypertension, and Obesity in Youth Committee, Council of Cardiovascular Disease in the Young, with the Council on Cardiovascular Nursing. *Circulation*. 2007;115:1948–1967.

National Cholesterol Education Program. Executive summary of the third report of the National Cholesterol Education Program (NCEP) Expert Panel on Detection, Evaluation, and Treatment of High Blood Cholesterol in Adults (Adult Treatment Panel III). *JAMA*. 2001;285:2486–2502.

Onion DK, series ed. *The Little Black Book of Primary Care*. 5th ed. Sudbury, MA: Jones & Bartlett Publishers; 2006.

Onion DK. Cardiology. 2.1 Medications. 49–68.

Onion DK. Cardiology. 2.2 ASHD. 68–93.

Onion DK. Cardiology. 2.3 Arrhythmias. 93–109.

Onion DK. Cardiology. 2.5 Endo/Peri/Myocarditis. 119–128.

Onion DK. Cardiology. 2.9 Miscellaneous. 15.

Onion DK. Endocrine/Metabolism. 5.4 Hyperlipidemias. 1104–1117.

Onion DK. Prevention and health maintenance. 14.4 Preventive maneuvers for children. 929–936.

Onion DK. Rheumatology/Orthopedics. 18.7 Inherited and Other Rheumatologic Diseases. 1104–1117.

Pagana KD, Pagana TJ. *Mosby's Diagnostic and Laboratory Test Reference*. 8th ed. St. Louis: Mosby Elsevier; 2007 (multiple pages utilized to provide normal reference values for laboratory tests).

Poston WC II, Stevens J, Hong Y, Fortmann SP, Franklin BA, et al. (American Heart Association Council on Epidemiology and Prevention, Interdisciplinary Committee for Prevention). Population-based prevention of obesity: the need for comprehensive promotion of healthful eating, physical activity, and energy balance: a scientific statement from American Heart Association Council on Epidemiology and Prevention, Interdisciplinary Committee for Prevention (formerly the Expert Panel on Population and Prevention Science). *Circulation*. 2008;118:428–464.

Sutherland JA [Onion DK, series ed. *The Little Black Book of Cardiology*. 2nd ed. Sudbury, MA: Jones & Bartlett Publishers; 2007]

Sutherland JA. Arrhythmias. 139–164.

Sutherland JA. Atherosclerotic coronary artery disease. 83–138.

Sutherland JA. Cardiomyopathies. 189–201.

Sutherland JA. Hypertension. 217–242.

Sutherland JA. Myocarditis, pericardial disease, and cardiac tumors. 203–215.

Sutherland JA. The EKG. 33–43.

Sutherland JA. Valvular heart disease. 165–188.

U.S. Department of Health and Human Services, Public Health Service, National Institutes of Health, National Heart, Lung, and Blood Institutes. *Estimation of 10-Year Cardiac Risk for Men Based on the Framingham Study*. NIH Publication #01-3305. Washington, DC: U.S. Department of Health and Human Services, Public Health Service, National Institutes of Health, National Heart, Lung, and Blood Institutes; 2001.

Wilson W, Taubert K, Gewitz M, et al. Prevention of Infective Endocarditis: Guidelines from the American Heart Association Rheumatic Fever, Endocarditis, and Kawasaki Disease Committee, Council Cardiovascular Disease in the Young, and the Council on Clinical Cardiology, Council on Cardiovascular Surgery and Anesthesia, and the Quality Care and Outcomes Research Interdisciplinary Working Group. *Circulation*. 2007;116:1736–1754.

Zipes DP, Camm AJ, Borggrefe M, et al. ACC/AHA/ESC 2006 Guidelines for Management of Patients with Ventricular Arrhythmias and the Prevention of Sudden Cardiac Death: a report of the American College of Cardiology/American Heart Association Task Force and the European Society of Cardiology Committee for Practice Guidelines (Writing Committee to Develop Guidelines for Management of Patients with Ventricular Arrhythmias and the Prevention of Sudden Cardiac Death): developed in collaboration with the European Heart Rhythm Association and the Heart Rhythm Society. *Circulation*. 2006;114:e385–e484.

CASES IN PULMONARY MEDICINE*

CASE 2-1

Jessica Keaton

Mrs. Keaton is a 66-year-old white female who presents with the chief complaint of a productive cough. It is associated with purulent, yellowish sputum; shortness of breath on exertion; fever up to 101.2°F orally; fatigue; chills; and generalized malaise for 3 to 4 days. She has some mild orthopnea and has been sleeping on two pillows for the past two nights. Normally, she only requires one. Her symptoms are worsening. She is unaware of any aggravating or alleviating factors to any of her symptoms.

She denies chest pain/pressure, shoulder or arm pain, hemoptysis, myalgias, arthralgias, nausea, vomiting, bowel changes, or abdominal pain.

She has never had any medical problems, surgeries, or hospitalizations. She's not taking any prescription or over-the-counter medications, vitamins, supplements, or herbal preparations. She is not allergic to any medications. She has never smoked or drank alcohol.

1. Based on this information, which of the following questions are essential to ask Mrs. Keaton and why?

   A. Has she experienced any pain and/or swelling in her lower extremities?
   B. Has she recently had an upper respiratory tract infection (URI)?
   C. Has she taken antibiotics recently? If yes, what and when?
   D. Has she traveled recently? If yes, where and when?
   E. Has she had the influenza and/or pneumococcal vaccine? If yes, when?

Patient Responses

Mrs. Keaton has not experienced any recent pain and/or swelling in her legs or ankles. She has not recently had a URI. The last time she took an antibiotic was more than 1 year ago. She has not done any recent traveling. She has never received the pneumonia or the influenza vaccine.

2. Based on this information, which of the following components of a physical examination are essential to perform on Mrs. Keaton and why?

   A. Nose and throat examination
   B. Heart auscultation
   C. Auscultation of the lungs
   D. Abdominal examination
   E. Evaluation for pedal edema

Physical Examination Findings

Mrs. Keaton is 5'3" tall and weighs 122 lb (body mass index [BMI] = 21.6). Other vital signs are blood pressure (BP), 116/76 mm Hg; pulse, 88 beats per minute (BPM) and regular; respirations, 24 and regular; and oral temperature, 99.8°F.

Her nasal mucosa is nonerythematous, nonedematous, and without lesions or discharge. Her pharynx is slightly injected but without postnasal discharge or erythema. There is no tonsillar enlargement or exudates.

Her heart is regular in rate and rhythm, without murmur, gallop, or rub. Her apical impulse is nondisplaced and without a thrill. She has rales in her left lower lung field that are unaffected by cough or respiration; otherwise, her lungs are clear.

Her abdominal examination is unremarkable.

She does not have any lower extremity edema.

---

*Remember, for each question, none to all of the answers could be correct/essential or incorrect/nonessential. See page 57 for Chapter 2 answers.

3. Based on this information, which of the following diagnostic studies are essential to conduct on Mrs. Keaton and why?

  A. Pulse oximetry (O_2 sat)
  B. Arterial blood gas (ABG)
  C. Chest x-ray (CXR)
  D. White blood cell count with differential (WBC w/diff)
  E. Blood and sputum cultures and sensitivities (C&S)

Diagnostic Results

Mrs. Keaton's SaO_2 was 98% (normal: ≥ 95). Her ABGs revealed a pH of 7.41 (normal: 7.35–7.45), Po_2 of 92 mm Hg (normal: 80–100), Pco_2 of 39 mm Hg (normal: 35–45), and HCO_3 of 25 mEq/L (normal: 21–28).

Her CXR revealed an infiltrate in her left lower lobe; otherwise, there are no abnormalities.

Her WBC was 5500/mm³ (normal adult: 5000–10,000) with 80% neutrophils (normal: 55–70), 12% lymphocytes (normal: 20–40), 3% monocytes (normal: 2–8), 4% eosinophils (normal: 1–4), and 1% basophils (normal: 0.5–1). Her blood and sputum cultures, as well as her Gram stains, are pending.

4. Based on this information, which one of the following is Mrs. Keaton's most likely diagnosis and why?

  A. Bronchitis
  B. Community-acquired pneumonia (CAP)
  C. Heart failure (HF)
  D. Pleural effusion
  E. Pneumothorax

5. Based on this diagnosis, which of the following are appropriate components of a treatment plan for Mrs. Keaton and why?

  A. Hospitalization
  B. Clarithromycin extended release 250 mg bid × 7 days
  C. Ciprofloxacin 750 mg bid × 14 days
  D. Pneumococcal vaccine when well and influenza vaccine at customary time
  E. Oxygen at 2 L/min per nasal canula

CASE 2-2

Kelly Lincoln

Kelly is a 9-month-old Hispanic female who presents with acute respiratory distress that started ~1 hour ago. It appeared to get somewhat better when her parents took her outdoors into the cooler air to bring her in for treatment. However, since they have gotten back indoors, her symptoms appear to be worsening. Her mother is unaware of any other aggravating or alleviating factors. According to her mother, the shortness of breath begins "all the sudden" and is occasionally associated with a high-pitched "wheezy-like" sound that is worse on expiration when her dyspnea is most severe. She has never had symptoms like this before. Prior to the onset of the dyspnea, she had a low-grade fever (99.8°F), a decreased appetite, clear rhinorrhea, and a nonproductive cough that just started this morning. She has not had any cyanosis, apnea, nausea, vomiting, diarrhea, constipation, pulling up of her legs, or tugging/rubbing of her ears.

She is the product of a full-term vaginal delivery without any difficulties with the pregnancy, delivery, or antenatal period. She has no known medical problems and has never been hospitalized or had any surgery. She is normally seen at a pediatric group practice for her regular check-ups. According to her mother, there have been no problems with her growth and/or development to date. She is up to date on all her immunizations. Her family history is unremarkable except for a cousin with atopy.

1. Based on this information, which of the following questions are essential to ask Kelly's mother and why?

  A. Do her symptoms worsen when she runs?
  B. Has she been unusually irritable or lethargic?
  C. What has her feeding history been up to date?
  D. Does she attend day care or have older siblings in day care or school?
  E. Has she experienced grunting, nasal flaring, and/or intercostal retraction or bulging?

Patient Responses

Her mother states that Kelly has not taken an unsupported step, let alone run. She has alternated between being nearly inconsolable and lethargic, with the former predominating. She has had some grunting but no nasal flaring or intracostal retractions.

Kelly is currently and has always been bottle-fed. She was switched from formula to 2% milk in her bottle when her mother started introducing "baby foods" at the age of 4 months. Now, her diet consists predominately of table foods. She is an only child but does attend a large day care 5 days per week while her mother works.

2. Based on this information, which of the following components of a physical examination are essential to perform on Kelly and why?

  A. General appearance
  B. Ear, nose, and throat examination
  C. Heart examination
  D. Lung examination
  E. Examination for pedal edema

Physical Examination Findings

Kelly is 28" long and weighs 22 lb. Her head circumference is 17.5". Other vital signs are pulse, 120 BPM and regular; respirations, 48/min and regular; and rectal temperature, 101.6°F. She appears to be in moderate respiratory distress (but is not currently exhibiting any nasal flaring, intracostal retractions, or use of other accessory muscles of breathing) and somewhat lethargic (but not toxic) appearing. She is not cyanotic nor does she show any evidence of pallor. Her cough comes in spasms with the dyspnea in between them. The audible "wheezy" sound her mother described is not heard.

Kelly and her mother appear to be interacting appropriately. Her mother is attempting very hard to comfort and console Kelly, does not appear overly stressed, and has an appropriate level of concern for her daughter's condition.

Kelly's ear canals are nonerythematous, nonedematous, and without lesions or abnormal discharge, bilaterally.

Her tympanic membranes are slightly injected but not erythematous and appear freely mobile, bilaterally. Her nasal mucosa is slightly erythematous and slightly edematous with a clear, watery discharge, bilaterally. Her pharynx is slightly injected, but not erythematous. She does not have any tonsillar enlargement or exudates. Her oral mucosa is normal color, without lesions, and moist.

Her heart is regular in rate and rhythm for age without any murmurs, gallops, or rubs. Her point of maximum intensity is not displaced. She does not have any thrills.

Her lungs reveal low-pitched, rhonchi with expiration through all lung fields. There is no wheezing. She has no intracostal, suprasternal, or supraclavicular retractions, as well as other signs of accessory respiratory muscle use or fatigue. Her chest wall moves completely and symmetrically. Percussion is normal and equal bilaterally. Tactile fremitus is also normal. She has no pedal edema.

3. Based on this information, which of the following diagnostic studies are essential to conduct on Kelly and why?

   A. Pulse oximetry (O_2 sat)
   B. Chest x-ray (CXR)
   C. Complete blood count with differential (CBC w/diff)
   D. Blood urea nitrogen (BUN)
   E. Sputum culture and sensitivity (C&S)

Diagnostic Results

Kelly's pulse oximetry was 88% (normal: $\geq$ 95%). Her CXR revealed generalized consolidation. Her CBC w/diff was normal except for a mild leukopenia with a predominance of lymphocytes. Her BUN was normal. Her sputum C&S is pending.

4. Based on this information, which one of the following is Kelly's most likely diagnosis and why?

   A. Right lower lobe pneumonia
   B. Bronchiolitis
   C. Foreign body airway obstruction
   D. Gastroesophageal reflux disease (GERD)
   E. Asthma

5. Based on this diagnosis, which of the following are appropriate components of a treatment plan for Kelly and why?

   A. Oxygen therapy via blow-by mechanism
   B. Bronchodilator via nebulizer
   C. Dexamethasone via nebulizer
   D. Amoxicillin/clavulanic acid 400 mg/kg (based on the amoxicillin component) twice a day for 10 days
   E. Immediate hospitalization

CASE 2-3
Lionel Matthews

Lionel is an 8-year-old African American male who presents with his mother for evaluation of a productive cough, shortness of breath, chest tightness, and wheezing. All of the symptoms have occurred intermittently for the past 3 to 4 months and have not changed since their onset. They only limit him when he is experiencing them causing him to stop

to "catch my breath"; otherwise, he is not bothered by the symptoms.

His symptoms appear to be worse when he visits his grandparents, both of whom are smokers, and after exercise. They seem to improve somewhat with "rest." Neither Lionel nor his mother is aware of any additional aggravating or alleviating factors. He occasionally has nocturnal symptoms. He is currently experiencing symptoms because he and his mother ran most of the way to his appointment because they were afraid they would be late.

He denies palpations, lightheadedness, vertigo, presyncope, syncope, nausea, vomiting, diarrhea, constipation, any other bowel change, abdominal pain, anorexia, malaise, fatigue, or unusual daytime sleepiness.

His only known medical problem was atopic dermatitis as an infant, which has not produced any symptoms since he was ~2 years old. He has never been hospitalized nor had surgery. He is not taking any prescription or over-the-counter medications, vitamins, supplements, or herbal preparations. His family history is positive for asthma (father). He has annual well-child check-ups and his immunizations are up to date.

1. Based on this information, which of the following questions are essential to ask Lionel and his mother and why?

   A. Does he have a fever with the episodes?
   B. How frequently is he symptomatic during the day and at night?
   C. What color is his sputum?
   D. Does he have a rash?
   E. Has he experienced any sneezing; rhinorrhea; nasal congestion; postnasal discharge; sore throat; and/or itchy, watery eyes?

Patient Responses

He has been afebrile with each episode. Daytime episodes occur 3 to 4 days per week. Nocturnal episodes occur every week to every other week. His sputum is clear to yellowish in color. He does have some intermittent, generalized itching of his skin but never develops a rash. His mother attributes this to "dry skin." He has experienced intermittent clear rhinorrhea; nasal congestion; sneezing; itchy, watery eyes; and postnasal drip. These latter symptoms can occur with or without the presence of his chief complaint symptoms. He has not had a sore throat.

2. Based on this information, which of the following components of a physical examination are essential to perform on Lionel and why?

   A. Ears, nose, and throat (ENT) examination
   B. Heart examination
   C. Lung examination
   D. Abdominal examination
   E. Skin examination

Physical Examination Findings

Lionel is 4'5" tall and weighs 74 lb. Other vital signs are pulse, 108 BPM (normal for age: 70–110) and regular; respirations,

26/min (top normal for age: 16) and regular; BP, 88/62 mm Hg (minimum systolic for age: 86); and oral temperature, 98.4°F.

His tympanic membranes are nonretracted, nonerythematous, and fully mobile. His external auditory canals are normal in color and without edema, discharge, or lesions.

His nasal mucosa is pale and boggy with a small amount of clear discharge but no lesions. There is no evidence of nasal flaring.

His oral mucosa is within normal limits. Pharynx reveals normal-sized tonsils without exudates or lesions. He has slight pharyngeal injection and a small amount of clear postnasal discharge. No "cobble-stoning" is present.

His heart is regular in rate and rhythm for age with no murmurs, gallops, or rubs. His apical impulse is nondisplaced and without a thrill.

His lungs reveal inspiratory and expiratory wheezing and rhonchi throughout all lung fields with his expiratory phase appearing slightly prolonged. His chest expansion is slightly decreased but symmetric. He does not have any intracostal, supraclavicular, or suprasternal retractions or accessory muscle usage. Percussion is hyperresonant.

His abdominal examination is unremarkable; and he does not have any visible skin lesions.

3. Based on this information, which of the following diagnostic tests are essential to conduct on Lionel and why?

  A. Chest x-ray (CXR)
  B. Oxygen saturation (O_2 sat) via pulse oximetry
  C. Arterial blood gases (ABGs)
  D. Pulmonary function test (PFT), before and after inhaled bronchodilator administration
  E. White blood count with differential (WBC w/diff)

Diagnostic Results

His CXR revealed mild generalized hyperinflation, but no other abnormalities. His oxygen saturation was 97% on room air (normal: $\geq$ 95%). His ABGs revealed a pH of 7.40 (normal: 7.35–7.45), Po_2 of 96 mm Hg (normal: 80–100), Pco_2 of 40 mm Hg (normal: 35–45), and HCO_3 of 26 mEq/L (normal: 21–28).

His spirometry revealed a forced expiratory volume in 1 second (FEV_1) of 60% of predicted (normal: > 80%), a forced vital capacity (FVC) of 76% of predicted (normal: > 80%), and an FEV_1/FEC ratio of 79% of predicted (normal: > 80%) before the administration of a bronchodilator. After bronchodilator administration, his FEV_1 was 85% of predicted, his FVC was 95% of predicted, and his FEV_1/FVC ratio was 89% of predicted. All his symptoms were resolved after the inhaled bronchodilator therapy.

His WBC w/diff was normal except for a mild eosinophilia of 7% (normal: 1–4%). His total leukocyte count was normal, as were his other differential cell counts.

4. Based on this information, which one of the following is Lionel's most likely diagnosis and why?

  A. Mild intermittent asthma
  B. Mild persistent asthma
  C. Moderate persistent asthma
  D. Severe persistent asthma
  E. Cystic fibrosis

5. Based on this diagnosis, which of the following are appropriate components of a treatment plan for Lionel and why?

  A. Patient education, symptom and peak-flow diary, written exacerbation plan based on symptoms and peak flow, and environmental controls
  B. Referral to an allergist for skin testing
  C. Short-acting β-agonist metered-dose inhaler (MDI) with spacer for as-needed usage
  D. Long-acting β-agonist MDI with spacer for regular daily usage
  E. Regular daily usage of low-dose inhaled corticosteroids with spacer

CASE 2-4
Mary Nelson

Mrs. Nelson is a 52-year-old Asian female who immigrated to the United States when she was 12 years old. She presents with a cough associated with blood-streaked, clear sputum of 1.5 months' duration. It is associated with bilateral generalized, aching-type chest pain when she coughs; fever averaging 100°F during the day and increasing to 101°F at night; and occasional chills. She is unaware of any aggravating or alleviating factors.

She has not been experiencing any headaches, ear pain, sore throat, rhinorrhea, nasal congestion, itchy/watery eyes, arthralgias, myalgias, bowel changes, or malaise.

She works as a female correctional officer. The prison's physician assistant encouraged her to get tested for tuberculosis (TB) because they have had a couple of inmates with active TB. However, Mrs. Nelson feels that she cannot acquire TB because she had several doses of the bacillus Calmette-Guerin (BCG) vaccine as a child in her native country.

She has no known medical problems. She has never been hospitalized except for the birth of her three daughters. Her only surgery was a bilateral tubal ligation (BTL) 15 years ago. She is not taking any over-the-counter or prescription medications, vitamins, supplements, or herbal preparations. She has never smoked nor drank alcohol. Her last menstrual period was 2 years ago; she has not had any bleeding or spotting since. Her family history is noncontributory.

1. Based on this information, which of the following questions are essential to ask Mrs. Nelson and why?

  A. When was her last TB test performed, what was its technique, and what was its result?
  B. Has she been having night sweats, fatigue, weight loss, or anorexia?
  C. Has she had chest pressure, pain in her arms or shoulders, diaphoresis, nausea, vomiting, or heartburn?
  D. Has she had any dyspnea or orthopnea?
  E. Has she been feeling depressed, feeling hopeless, or experiencing anhedonia lately?

Patient Responses

Mrs. Nelson states that she had a Mantoux tuberculin skin test (TST), also known as the purified protein derivative (PPD) test, when she started working at the prison 2 years ago; it has been repeated every 6 months since per worksite protocol. The last one was 4 months ago. All of her tests have been "positive" but, she is uncertain how large the reactions were. However, on each occasion, the prison physician advised her "not to worry about it" because it was a false-positive caused by the BCG vaccinations she received as a child.

She admits to having night sweats just about every night, daytime fatigue that she attributed to not sleeping well because of the night sweats, mild to moderate anorexia, and a 10-lb weight loss over the past month.

She denies chest pressure/tightness, pain in her arms or shoulders, nausea, vomiting, heartburn, dyspnea, orthopnea, anhedonia, or feeling depressed or hopeless.

2. Based on this information, which of the following components of a physical examination are essential to perform on Mrs. Nelson and why?

A. Heart examination
B. Lung examination
C. Pelvic examination to evaluate for endometrial carcinoma
D. Fibromyalgia tender-point examination
E. Brief screening test for depression

Physical Examination Findings

Her heart is regular in rate and rhythm with no murmurs, gallops, or rubs. Her lungs are clear to auscultation. Her pelvic examination is normal. She has two positive fibromyalgia tender points (bilateral shoulders) and a negative screening test for depression.

3. Based on this information, which of the following diagnostic studies are essential to conduct on Mrs. Nelson and why?

A. Tine test
B. Mantoux tuberculin skin test (TST)
C. QuantiFERON-TB Gold Test (QFT-G)
D. Chest x-ray (CXR)
E. Sputum smear and culture for acid-fast-bacilli (with susceptibility testing if the culture is positive)

Diagnostic Results

Her tine test was negative. Her TST revealed a 13-mm in duration at 48 hours (normal: depends on size per patient characteristics; please see Responses and Discussion section for more information). Her QFT-G was positive (normal: negative). Her CXR revealed multiple 2- to 20-mm round densities with mild cavitations in both her upper lobes and hilar lymphadenopathy. Her sputum smear was positive for the presence of acid-fast-bacilli (AFB). Her sputum culture and sensitivity are pending.

4. Based on this information, which one of the following is Mrs. Nelson's most likely diagnosis and why?

A. Depression
B. Previous TB infection
C. Community-acquired pneumonia (CAP)
D. Probable latent tuberculosis infection
E. Probable active tuberculosis infection

5. Based on this diagnosis, which of the following are appropriate components of a treatment plan for Mrs. Nelson and why?

A. Trial selective serotonin reuptake inhibitor (SSRI)
B. Azithromycin 250 mg two tablets initially, then one tablet daily for 4 days
C. Combination of isoniazid (INH) and rifampin (RIF) daily
D. Combination of isoniazid (INH), rifampin (RIF), ethambutol (EMB), and pyrazinamide (PZA) daily
E. Nothing until all test results are back

CASE 2-5
Norman Obermiller

Mr. Obermiller is a 45-year-old white male who presents with progressively worsening dyspnea of approximately 5 to 6 years duration. He feels it has become much worse in the past month. He notices that it has caused him to have to stop and rest after walking shorter distances, walk slower up inclines, and not be able to carry as much in terms of weight. He is unaware of any other aggravating or alleviating factors.

He has an occasional nonproductive cough. He denies wheezing, other abnormal sounds with breathing, chest pain or pressure, palpations, pedal edema, localized or generalized weakness, fatigue, tremor, fever, chills, rhinorrhea, sneezing, sore throat, postnasal discharge, sinus/nasal congestion, heartburn, easily satiety, or gastroesophageal reflux.

He has no known medical problems. He has never had any surgery or been hospitalized. He does not take any prescription or over-the-counter medications, vitamins, supplements, or herbal preparations. He has never smoked or drank alcohol. His family history is negative, including for pulmonary conditions.

1. Based on this information, which of the following questions are essential to ask Mr. Obermiller and why?

A. Has he been exposed to a significant amount of passive smoke?
B. What are his occupation and hobby histories?
C. Does he experience leg pain while walking?
D. How frequently does he experience the cough?
E. Has he been losing weight or experiencing night sweats?

Patient Responses

He denies excessive passive smoke exposure. He currently works as a glass etcher in a glass factory and has done so for the past 5 years. Prior to that, he worked highway construction. His primary job was cutting away the rock formations to build roads. He did this for approximately 20 years until he discovered he could turn his skills and fondness of etching glass into a living. He etched glass as a hobby for approximately 10 years before starting work at the glass factory; however, since he started working at the glass factory, he no longer does this for recreation. His current hobbies include watching NASCAR, hunting, and fishing.

He does not experience leg pain while walking. His cough occurs a maximum of "a dozen times a day." He has lost 5 lb in the past 2 months; however, he has been trying to lose weight in hopes it would improve his dyspnea. He does not have night sweats.

2. Based on this information, which of the following components of a physical examination are essential to perform on Mr. Obermiller and why?

    A. Heart examination
    B. Lung examination
    C. Abdominal examination
    D. Evaluation for pedal edema
    E. Evaluation of all deep tendon reflexes (DTRs)

Physical Examination Findings

Mr. Obermiller is 6'0" tall and weighs 178 lb (BMI = 24.1). Other vital signs are BP, 120/76 mm Hg; pulse, 86 BPM and regular; respirations, 24/min and regular; and oral temperature, 97.9°F.

His heart is regular in rate and rhythm without any gallops, murmurs, or rubs. His apical impulse is nondisplaced and without a thrill. His lungs are clear to auscultation; however, his breath sounds are diminished throughout. There is no evidence of intracostal, supraclavicular, or suprasternal retractions. Tactile fremitus is slightly decreased and percussion is slightly dull.

His abdomen reveals normoactive bowel sounds in all four quadrants. There are no masses, organomegaly, or tenderness.

He does not have pedal edema. All of his deep tendon reflexes are normal.

3. Based on this information, which of the following diagnostic studies are essential to conduct on Mr. Obermiller and why?

    A. Oxygen saturation (O_2 sat) via pulse oximetry
    B. Arterial blood gases (ABGs)
    C. Chest x-ray (CXR)
    D. Pulmonary function test (PFT), before and after bronchodilator administration
    E. Electrocardiogram (ECG)

Diagnostic Results

His oxygen saturation was 95% (normal: ≥ 95% on room air).

His ABGs revealed a pH of 7.36 (normal: 7.35–7.45), Po_2 of 72 mm Hg (normal: 80–100), Pco_2 of 45 mm Hg (normal: 35–45), and HCO_3 of 25 mEq/L (normal: 21–28).

His initial spirometry revealed an FEV_1 of 60% of predicted (normal: ≥ 80% predicted), an FEV_6 of 90% of predicted (normal: ≥ 80% predicted), an FVC of 90% of predicted (normal: ≥ 80% predicted), and an FEV_1/FVC ratio of 66% of predicted (normal: ≥ 80% predicted).

After bronchodilator administration, his FEV_1 was 65% of predicted, his FEV_6 was 90% of predicted, his FVC was 95% of predicted, and his FEV_1/FEC ratio was 70% of predicted.

His CXR revealed numerous small, round opacities (largest 1 cm) throughout all lung fields with the preponderance and minimal coalescing in the upper lung fields. Also, he had calcification of the periphery of some of his hilar lymph nodes.

His ECG was normal.

4. Based on this information, which one of the following is Mr. Obermiller's most likely diagnosis and why?

    A. Asthma
    B. Chronic bronchitis
    C. Complicated silicosis
    D. Lung cancer
    E. Asbestosis

5. Based on this diagnosis, which of the following are appropriate components of a treatment plan for Mr. Obermiller and why?

    A. Home oxygen therapy
    B. Inhaled short-acting β-agonist therapy on an as-needed basis
    C. Inhaled corticosteroid therapy
    D. Mantoux tuberculin skin test (TST)
    E. CT scan of chest

CASE 2-6
Olivia Peebles

Mrs. Peebles is a 36-year-old white female who presents complaining of "shortness of breath." Her symptoms began approximately 1 week ago and are progressively worsening. The dyspnea is associated with an occasional nonproductive cough, right lateral chest pain, and a fullness-like sensation in that area. Her shortness of breath occurs at both rest and activity; however, it is much worse with exertion. She coughs frequently throughout the day and it tends to increase her dyspnea. Her chest pain is mostly a dull, full-like sensation that increases in severity when she coughs or inspires deeply; however, it is unaffected by expiration. She rates her chest pain as a 2 out of a 10 on the pain scale until she coughs or breathes deeply; then, she states it increases to about a 6 out of 10. She is unaware of any other aggravating or alleviating factors.

She has been experiencing some worsening fatigue, described as tired but not sleepy, and weakness, defined as not being physically capable of doing as much as she previously could without experiencing dyspnea.

She has not experienced any fever, chills, rigors, myalgias, wheezing, other abnormal breath sounds, rhinorrhea, nasal congestion, postnasal discharge, ear or throat pain, headache, hemoptysis, nausea, vomiting, changes in her bowel movements, abdominal pain, dizziness, vertigo, presyncope, syncope, palpations, or pain in her shoulders/arms/neck.

Her medical history is positive for rheumatoid arthritis (RA). However, her arthritis symptoms have not changed and she feels they are "in good control." She has never been hospitalized nor had any surgery. Her medications consist of methotrexate, naproxen, and lansoprazole. She is not on any other prescription or over-the-counter medications, vitamins, supplements, or herbal preparations. She has never smoked nor drank alcohol.

She was an elementary school teacher for approximately 10 years; then, she was forced to quit because of the fatigue and joint pain secondary to her RA approximately 5 years ago.

She is currently on disability. She has been married for 12 years and does not have any children. Her husband is her only sexual partner. Their method of contraception is his vasectomy. Her last menstrual period was 3 weeks ago. Her family history is negative.

1. Based on this information, which of the following questions are essential to ask Mrs. Peebles and why?

    A. Has she recently been around anyone with berylliosis?
    B. Has she noticed any pedal edema?
    C. Has she noticed any icterus of her sclera or jaundice of her skin?
    D. Has she experienced any recent trauma?
    E. Has she experienced a recent weight change?

Patient Responses

She does not know anyone with berylliosis. She has not experienced any pedal edema, noticed any jaundice or icterus, suffered any recent trauma, or had a recent weight change.

2. Based on this information, which of the following components of a physical examination are essential to perform on Mrs. Peebles and why?

    A. Heart examination
    B. Lung examination
    C. Abdominal examination
    D. Pelvic examination
    E. Evaluation for pedal edema

Physical Examination Findings

Mrs. Peebles is 5'5" tall and weighs 147 lb (BMI = 24.5). Other vital signs are BP, 130/76 mm Hg; pulse, 112/min and regular; respirations, 32/min and regular; and oral temperature, 97.9°F. Her oxygen saturation via pulse oximetry is 86%.

Her heart is tachycardic but regular in rhythm and has no murmurs, gallops, or rubs. Her apical impulse is nondisplaced and without a thrill. Her lungs are clear to auscultation except for the lower half of her right lung, where her breath sounds are virtually absent. She has a mild to moderate friction rub with respirations in her right lower lung lobe. The area is also dull to percussion and associated with both vocal and tactile fremitus. She has no pedal edema.

Her abdomen has normal, active bowel sounds in all four quadrants. It is nontender to palpation. No masses, organomegaly, or ascites is present. Her pelvic examination is normal.

3. Based on this information, which of the following diagnostic studies are essential to conduct on Mrs. Peebles and why?

    A. Total serum protein, albumin, globulins, amylase, lactate dehydrogenase (LDH), aspartate aminotransferase (AST), and alanine aminotransferase (ALT) levels
    B. CXR with additional view in right lateral decubitus position
    C. Electrocardiogram (ECG)
    D. Beryllium lymphocyte proliferation test
    E. Arterial blood gases (ABGs)

Diagnostic Results

Her blood tests revealed a total serum protein of 7.5 g/dl (normal adult: 6.4–8.3), an albumin of 3.1 g/dl (normal adult: 3.5–5), a total globulin of 4.0 (normal adult: 2.3–3.4), an α_1-globulin of 1.1 g/dl (normal adult: 0.1–0.3), an α_2-globulin of 1.9 g/dl (normal adult: 0.6–1), a β-globulin of 1.0 (normal adult: 0.7–1.1), an amylase of 100 units/L (normal 30–220), an LDH of 145 units/L (normal adult: 100–190), an AST of 22 units/L (normal adult: 0–35), and an ALT of 20 units/L (normal adult/child: 4–36). Her beryllium lymphocyte proliferation test was negative (normal: negative).

Her CXR revealed a large pleural effusion in her right lower lung field associated with adjacent atelectasis, and a left shift of her mediastinum. The radiologist estimated the fluid amount to be approximately 2000 ml. Her heart shadow was normal and there is no evidence of any other abnormalities.

Her ECG was within normal limits. Her ABGs revealed a pH of 7.32 (normal: 7.35–7.45), a Po_2 of 52 mm Hg, a Pco_2 of 48 mm Hg (normal: 34–45), and a HCO_3 was 24 mEq/L (normal: 22–26).

4. Based on this information, which one of the following is Mrs. Peebles' most likely diagnosis and why?

    A. Pulmonary embolism with pneumothorax
    B. Lung cancer
    C. Heart failure (HF)
    D. Pneumonia with pleural effusion
    E. Autoimmune disease–associated pleural effusion

5. Based on this diagnosis, which of the following are appropriate components of a treatment plan for Mrs. Peebles and why?

    A. Thoracentesis of up to 1000 ml of fluid with approximately 100 ml to be sent for pleural fluid analysis (gross appearance, protein, LDH, glucose, amylase, pH, specific gravity, cytology, WBC w/diff, Gram stain, acid-fast bacteria [AFB] smear, and cultures with sensitivities), and a serum protein and LDH
    B. Thoracentesis of all fluid collectable with approximately 100 ml for pleural fluid analysis as described in choice A
    C. Mantoux tuberculin skin test (TST)
    D. Tube thoracostomy
    E. Combination of isoniazid (INH), rifampin (RIF), ethambutol (EMB), and pyrazinamide (PZA) daily

CASE 2-7
Patricia Queen

Mrs. Queen is a 36-year-old African American female who presents to the emergency department via ambulance in severe respiratory distress. Her dyspnea began suddenly while she was sitting and watching television approximately 1 hour ago. There was no precipitating event, including coughing, sneezing, or trauma. She feels that her breathing continues to worsen and has done so since its inception. She is also complaining of severe (10 out of a 10 on the pain scale), sharp, right-sided chest pain that started at approximately the same time as the dyspnea. She is not aware of any aggravating or alleviating factors.

She admits feeling anxious "like something really, really bad is going to happen" since the onset of her symptoms. She rarely (defined as once or twice a year) has such feelings. She confesses that she keeps a "little smoker's cough." It is nonproductive, occurs several times per day, and has been present for a minimum of 5 years without any change. She denies wheezing, other abnormal breath sounds, hemoptysis, fever, chills, rigors, malaise, fatigue, weight loss, rhinorrhea, postnasal discharge, sinus pressure/fullness, headache, nasal congestion, sore throat, ear ache, nausea, vomiting, changes in her bowel movements, chest pressure, pain in her arm/shoulder/hand, lightheadedness, vertigo, presyncope, or syncope.

Her only known medical problem is endometriosis, discovered during her bilateral tubal ligation (BTL) 4 years ago. Despite the gynecologist telling her it was "extensive," she has never experienced any symptoms (including pain and/or abnormal bleeding). She denies ever being diagnosed with any pulmonary condition. Her only hospitalizations were for childbirth on three occasions (all normal vaginal deliveries without complications). Her only surgery was a BTL. She is currently experiencing normal menses. She is not taking any prescription or over-the-counter medications, vitamins, supplements, or herbal preparations, including a metered-dose inhaler or nebulizer. She does not drink alcohol or use illicit substances. Her family history is negative.

1. Based on this information, which of the following questions are essential to ask Mrs. Queen and why?

A. What is her smoking history?
B. When was her previous menstrual period and was it normal?
C. Has she had any leg or foot edema, erythema, or pain?
D. Does she use hormonal contraceptives?
E. Has she recently taken a long trip via air?

Patient Responses

For the past 20 years, Mrs. Queen has smoked approximately one pack of cigarettes per week (approximately 3 pack-years). Her previous menses was ~1 month ago and normal. She does take any hormonal medications.

She denies foot or leg edema or erythema. However, she does have some pain in her right calf from where she "pulled a muscle" bicycling 2 days ago. Mrs. Queen did travel from the United States to China by air approximately 10 days ago and returned 2 days ago. She admits to sleeping in the same position for most of the flight both directions.

2. Based on this information, which of the following components of a physical examination are essential to perform on Mrs. Queen and why?

A. Evaluation for nasal septal deviation
B. Evaluation for tracheal deviation
C. Heart examination
D. Lung examination
E. Ankle and leg examination

Physical Examination Findings

Mrs. Queen is 5'2" tall and weighs 113 lb (BMI = 20.7) Other vital signs are BP, 90/62 mm Hg; pulse, 120 BPM and regular;

respiratory rate, 48/min and irregular; and tympanic temperature, 97.5°F. Her oxygen saturation is 82%. She appears to be in significant respiratory distress. She is sitting upright, bending forward at the waist, and resting her forearms on her thighs. She does not have any cyanosis, erythema, or pallor.

She does not have any nasal deviation; however, she has some mild tracheal deviation to the left.

Her heart is tachycardic and regular in rhythm and without murmurs, rubs, or gallops. Her apical impulse is nondisplaced and without a thrill. Her lungs are clear to auscultation (CTA); however, her breath sounds are significantly diminished (and in some cases absent) in the lower half of her right lung fields. Tactile fremitus is significantly decreased and percussion is hyperresonant in this area. Her chest expansion is asymmetric (decreased on the right side).

She does not have any foot/ankle/leg edema or erythema, bilaterally. Her right calf is slightly tender to palpation. The left one is nontender. The BP cuff can be inflated to 150 mm Hg on the right and 160 mm Hg on the left before equal pain is felt. Her Homan sign is negative.

3. Based on this information, which of the following diagnostic studies are essential to conduct on Mrs. Queen and why?

A. Well's criteria for pulmonary embolism (PE) risk and D-dimer
B. Sputum for Gram stain, culture, and sensitivity
C. Arterial blood gases (ABGs)
D. Chest x-ray (CXR)
E. Electrocardiogram (ECG)

Diagnostic Results

Her Well's PE risk score was 1.5 (low risk PE: ≤ 4) and her D-dimer was 370 ng/ml (normal: < 250–600).

Her sputum Gram stain was not an adequate specimen. Her C&S is pending but likely to only grow normal oral flora.

Her ABGs revealed a pH of 7.48 (normal: 7.35–7.45), PO_2 of 62 mm Hg (normal: 80–100), PCO_2 of 31 mm Hg (normal: 35–45), and HCO_3 of 25 mEq/L (normal: 21–28).

Her CXR revealed a mild to moderate tracheal and mediastinal deviation to the left. It also revealed a visceral pleural line between the middle and lower lobes of her right lungs and a large air-filled space in the lower right lung field, estimated size 35%. Her ECG revealed a sinus tachycardia.

4. Based on this information, which one of the following is Mrs. Queen's most likely diagnosis and why?

A. Pulmonary embolism
B. Pleural effusion secondary to pneumonia
C. Pneumothorax secondary to pneumonia
D. Catamenial pneumothorax
E. Iatrogenic pneumothorax

5. Based on this diagnosis, which of the following are appropriate components of a treatment plan for Mrs. Queen and why?

A. Oxygen therapy
B. Tube thoracostomy
C. Hospitalization
D. Smoking cessation
E. IV gentamicin

CASE 2-8
Quincy Rodgers

Mr. Rodgers is a 28-year-old African American male who is in for the results of his repeat CXR performed earlier today. He was initially seen approximately 4 weeks ago by your supervising physician after being ill for approximately 2 weeks with "a cold." At that time, he was diagnosed with left upper lobe (LUL) pneumonia and was started on a 5-day course of azithromycin.

He was seen again 2 weeks ago by your supervising physician. At the second visit, his upper respiratory tract infection symptoms (rhinorrhea, nasal congestion, postnasal drainage, and sneezing) were resolved. However, he was still experiencing a nonproductive cough, fever, and chills but was not bothered with wheezing, other abnormal breath sounds, dyspnea, or myalgias. His CXR revealed a partial resolution of the LUL infiltrate and he began 10 days of ofloxacin.

He is still experiencing a nonproductive cough that might be "a little" better, severe fatigue (defined as "complete exhaustion"), fever, and chills. He denies dyspnea, hemoptysis, chest pain or pressure, rigors, anorexia, nausea, vomiting, heartburn, abdominal pain, bowel changes, weight loss, neck pain or stiffness, headache, rhinorrhea, nasal/sinus congestion, postnasal discharge, sore throat, ear pain, rash, depression, change in mood, or anhedonia. His current CXR reveals no consolidation; however, it revealed a 1.5-cm, smooth, round, well-circumscribed, dense, noncalcified solitary pulmonary nodule (SPN) in his LUL.

He has no known medical problems. He has never had any surgery nor been hospitalized. His is currently on no prescription or over-the-counter medications, vitamins, supplements, or herbal preparations. He completed the entire course of both antibiotics without any difficulties. He has resided in south-central Arizona all his life, where he has worked construction for the past 10 years. He does not smoke (and never has). He drinks "a couple" of beers (defined as two or three) on most Saturday nights with his coworkers. He denies exposure to anyone with TB.

1. Based on this information, which of the following questions are essential to ask Mr. Rodgers and why?

    A. Has he ever had a CXR prior to 1 month ago?
    B. Has he had any arthralgias, bone pain, or subcutaneous knots or nodules?
    C. Has he been experiencing any night sweats?
    D. Do his symptoms increase when he drinks alcohol?
    E. What was his maximum temperature and what time of the day did it occur? Did he experience fluctuations in his temperature not associated with antipyretic therapy?

Patient Responses

He had a CXR approximately 5 years ago as part of a preemployment physical at his local hospital. As near as he knows, it was normal.

He had some generalized arthralgias, but no actual bone pain, when he first became ill; however, they resolved after a few days. He has never experienced subcutaneous nodules.

He started having night sweats a couple of days after his initial visit and continues to have them. His highest temperature was 100.6°F at 9:00 p.m. approximately 2 weeks ago. He did not tried antipyretics for his fever.

His symptoms were unaffected by alcohol intake.

2. Based on this information, which of the following components of a physical examination are essential to perform on Mr. Rodgers and why?

    A. Heart examination
    B. Lung examination
    C. Neurologic examination
    D. Skin examination
    E. Supraclavicular, infraclavicular, and axillary lymph node examination

Physical Examination Findings

Mr. Rodgers is 5'11" tall and weighs 225 lb (BMI = 31.4). Other vital signs are BP, 136/78 mm Hg; pulse, 82 BPM and regular; respirations, 10/min and regular; and oral temperature, 98.6°F.

His heart is regular in rate and rhythm and without murmurs, gallops, or rubs. His apical impulse is nondisplaced. His lungs are clear to auscultation and reveal normal and equal air flow. Tactile fremitus and percussion are normal throughout. There are no intracostal retractions, use of accessory muscles, or asymmetry of chest wall expansion.

His neurologic examination is normal. His skin examination is unremarkable. He does not have any palpable supraclavicular, infraclavicular, or axillary lymph nodes.

3. Based on this information, which of the following diagnostic studies are essential to conduct on Mr. Rodgers and why?

    A. Whole body ^{18}F-fluro-deoyx-D-glucose positron emission tomography scan (FDG-PET)
    B. Repeat CXR again in 2 weeks
    C. CT scan of chest with and without contrast
    D. Traditional tube (TP) and complement fixation (CF) assays for coccidioidomycosis
    E. Mantoux tuberculin skin test (TST)

Diagnostic Results

Mr. Rodgers CT scan revealed a 2-cm round, smooth nodule in his left upper lung field with distinct borders and no calcifications. It was not enhanced with the administration of IV contrast media. There was not any hilar, supraclavicular, or infraclavicular lymphadenopathy. His FDG-PET scan results are and his CXR is scheduled for 2 weeks.

His TP assay was positive at 1:32 (normal: negative) and his CF was positive at 1:64 (normal: negative). His TST revealed an indurated area of 7.5 cm (normal: variable; for more information, please see Case 2-4).

4. Based on this information, in addition to his obesity, which one of the following is Mr. Rodgers' most likely diagnosis and why?

    A. TB of the lungs
    B. Lung cancer

   C. Unresolved pneumonia
   D. Coccidioidomycosis
   E. Lung abscess

5. Based on this diagnosis, which of the following are appropriate components of a treatment plan for Mr. Rodgers and why?

   A. Combination therapy with isoniazid (INH), rifampin (RIF), ethambutol (EMB), and pyrazinamide (PZA) daily
   B. Referral to oncologist
   C. Hospitalization for IV gentamicin
   D. Repeat CXR (and possibly CT scan) in 3 months and repeat coccidioidomycosis CF levels in 2 weeks
   E. Initiation of triazole therapy

CASE 2-9
Rhonda Smith

Mrs. Smith is 58-year-old Asian American female who presents with the chief complaint of increasing hoarseness. It began approximately 2 months ago as an intermittent problem; however, it has gradually progressed to being constant for the past 2 to 3 weeks. There is no fluctuation or variation in the degree of hoarseness or voice quality noticed by the patient. She is unaware of any aggravating or alleviating factors. She has not experienced any trauma.

She is also complaining of being "tired all the time" and having to alter her activities secondary to this fatigue. She denies fever, chills, sore throat, postnasal drainage, rhinorrhea, sneezing, cough, itchy/watery eyes, anorexia, nausea, vomiting, heartburn, partial regurgitation, abdominal pain, neck pain, neck swelling, chest pain, cough, hemoptysis, or wheezing.

Mrs. Smith denies any medical problems, surgeries, or hospitalizations. She does not take any prescription or over-the-counter medications, vitamins, supplements, or herbal preparations. She is not allergic to any medications. She has smoked 1.5 packs of cigarettes a day for 20 years (30 pack-year history). She does not drink alcohol. Her family history is negative.

1. Based on this information, which of the following questions are essential to ask Mrs. Smith and why?

   A. What does she mean by "tired all the time" and does she experience insomnia?
   B. Has she experienced an unintentional change in her weight?
   C. Does she have a decreased mood, increased stress, anhedonia, and/or anxiety?
   D. Is she experiencing dysphagia?
   E. Does she have any warts on her hands or feet?

Patient Responses

Mrs. Smith defines her fatigue as "totally exhausted" and "tiring much easier than she used to." She denies any excessive daytime sleepiness or any type of insomnia. She has experienced an unplanned weight loss of approximately 10 lb in the past month. She denies depression, decreased mood, increased stress, anhedonia, anxiety, dysphagia, or the presence of any warts.

2. Based on this information, which of the following components of a physical examination are essential to perform on Mrs. Smith and why?

   A. Observation of hoarseness/voice
   B. Oral mucosa/pharyngeal examination, including indirect laryngoscope
   C. Heart examination
   D. Lung examination
   E. Evaluation of cervical, supraclavicular, infraclavicular, and axillary lymph nodes

Physical Examination Findings

Mrs. Smith is 5'0" tall and weighs 105 lb (BMI = 20.5). Other vital signs are BP, 102/64 mm Hg; pulse, 76 BPM and regular; respirations, 10/min and regular; and oral temperature, 98.2°F.

Her voice is very hoarse with a "breathy" quality. Her pharynx is nonerythematous and without lesions, tonsillar enlargement, exudates, postnasal discharge, and "cobblestoning." Her oral mucosa and tongue are unremarkable. Her indirect laryngoscopy reveals a moderate lack of movement of her vocal cords on the right side only. There is no erythema, edema, or lesions.

Her heart is regular in rate and rhythm without murmurs, gallops, or rubs. Her apical impulse is nondisplaced and without a thrill. Her lungs are clear to auscultation. However, she has a slightly diminished quality to her breath sounds in her right upper lobe above her clavicle. There are no changes with percussion or tactile fremitus. Vocal fremitus is difficult to assess secondary to her hoarseness; however, it appears to be normal. She does not have any accessory muscle usage, intracostal retractions, or asymmetry of chest expansion.

Her axillary, cervical, infraclavicular, and supraclavicular lymph nodes are not palpable, even with a Valsalva maneuver. Additionally, no tenderness or fullness is noted in these areas.

3. Based on this information, which of the following diagnostic studies are essential to conduct on Mrs. Smith and why?

   A. CT scan of chest, with and without contrast
   B. Chest x-ray (CXR)
   C. 24-hour pH monitoring of lower esophagus
   D. Bacterial throat culture and sensitivity
   E. Rapid strep screen

Diagnostic Tests Findings

Her CXR revealed a spiculated, irregularly shaped mass approximately 2.5 cm in size in her right apex. She also had some mild atelectasis and mediastinal widening. Her chest CT scan is pending, as is her bacterial throat culture and sensitivity. Her strep screen was negative.

Twenty-four-hour pH monitoring of her lower esophagus was normal.

4. Based on this information, which one of the following is Mrs. Smith's most likely diagnosis and why?

    A. Asthma
    B. Lung cancer
    C. Acute laryngitis
    D. Supraglottitis
    E. Laryngopharyngeal reflux

5. Based on this diagnosis, which of the following are appropriate components of a treatment plan for Mrs. Smith and why?

    A. Omeprazole 40 mg once a day for a minimum of 3 months
    B. Referral to pulmonary surgeon for tissue specimen for histologic evaluation of lung mass via fiberoptic bronchoscopy, open thoracotomy, or other method as determined appropriate by the specialist
    C. Amoxicillin 775 mg twice a day for 10 days
    D. Otolaryngologist consultation for direct laryngoscope to confirm indirect findings
    E. Repeat CXR in 3 months to determine if change has occurred in lung lesion

CASES IN PULMONARY MEDICINE

RESPONSES AND DISCUSSION

CASE 2-1
Jessica Keaton
1. History

A. Has she experienced any pain and/or swelling in her lower extremities? ESSENTIAL

In a patient with orthopnea, dyspnea, and cough, the primary diagnoses addressed by this question are either a pulmonary embolism (PE) or heart failure (HF). Although both of these conditions can be associated with a productive cough, neither tends to produce yellowish sputum. In the case of a PE, the expectorant is generally clear and associated with varying degrees of hemoptysis. With HF, it tends to be pink and frothy as a result of alveolar edema.

Fever is rarely seen with either condition unless caused by an underlying infectious process (e.g., generalized sepsis, acute bacterial endocarditis, or a septic embolism).

B. Has she recently had an upper respiratory tract infection (URI)?   ESSENTIAL

Cough with purulent sputum production and fever is most often caused by either a lower or an upper respiratory tract infection with postnasal drainage being swallowed and then "coughed" up, in the case of the latter. Additionally, it is not uncommon for a lower respiratory tract infection to be preceded by an upper respiratory tract infection.

C. Has she taken antibiotics recently? If yes, what and when? ESSENTIAL

Mrs. Keaton's symptoms are suspicious for an infectious process. If a bacterial process is suspected, antibiotic therapy is going to be initiated. The antibiotic selection is determined empirically based on the most likely organism and its resistance potential. If the patient had recently taken (or is currently taking) an antibiotic, the initial choice is virtually always different.

D. Has she traveled recently? If yes, where and when? ESSENTIAL

Inquiring about a patient's recent travel history is important not only because of the potential of acquiring an infection caused by an atypical pathogen endemic to certain localities but also because of the varied pattern of antibiotic resistance seen in different locations.

E. Has she had the influenza and/or pneumococcal vaccine? If yes, when?   ESSENTIAL

Because the symptoms that Mrs. Keaton is describing could be caused by pneumonia or influenza, it is important to know her immunization status for these two conditions.

The seasonal influenza vaccine must be updated annually. If Mrs. Keaton did not receive one the previous fall, then she is at a much greater risk of acquiring influenza, which unfortunately is associated with a significantly greater rate of hospitalization and death in individuals over the age of 65 years. The effectiveness rates of the vaccine depend on predicting the correct strains for the upcoming season; in recent years, it has ranged from a low as 36% to a high of 90%.

Because sepsis caused by pneumococcal disease can occur in as many as 25 to 30% of all individuals with pneumonia caused by this organism, knowing if Mrs. Keaton has been immunized (and when) is essential. All adults older than the age of 65 years and all adults younger than the age of 65 years if they are immunocompromised; smokers; suffering from a chronic pulmonary (except asthma), cardiac, hepatic, or renal condition; or suffering from other conditions that would place them at greater risk if they acquired pneumonia should be immunized with the pneumococcal polysaccharide vaccine (PPSV; previously known as the PPSV23). Adults older than the age of 65 years should be revaccinated in 5 years if they have never received the PPSV or if it was given more than 5 years ago. The routine immunization of infants should begin at the age of 2 months utilizing the pneumococcal conjugate vaccine ([PCV], previously known as the PCV7).

It is the pneumococcal immunization of choice for children up to 60 months of age. At five years of age, children who have been incompletely, or never, immunized can safely be vaccinated with the PPSV.

In contradiction to popular myth, the pneumonia vaccine does not offer 100% protection against pneumonia, or even pneumonia caused by a pneumococcal organism. It offers adults 60 to 70% protection from 23 of the 80+ common pneumococcal bacterial strains contained in the vaccine.

2. Physical Examination

A. Nose and throat examination   ESSENTIAL

Although Mrs. Keaton is not complaining of any upper respiratory symptoms, it is still possible that the source of her cough is postnasal discharge.

B. Heart auscultation   ESSENTIAL

Cough and shortness of breath are generally considered to be pulmonary symptoms; however, they can also be symptoms of some cardiac conditions (e.g., heart failure, arrhythmias, and valvular diseases). Therefore, a careful heart examination as outlined in Case 1-2 is essential.

C. Auscultation of the lungs   ESSENTIAL

Because Mrs. Keaton is experiencing pulmonary symptoms, careful auscultation of the lungs (as outlined in Case 1-5) is essential.

D. Abdominal examination   NONESSENTIAL

E. Evaluation for pedal edema   ESSENTIAL

This is important to evaluate for because the possibility of heart failure, pulmonary embolism, or other cardiovascular or cardiopulmonary conditions associated with pedal edema.

3. Diagnostic Studies

A. Pulse oximetry (O_2 sat)   ESSENTIAL

An O_2 sat is a quick and noninvasive technique to determine the patient's arterial blood oxygen saturation. Unless there are underlying circumstances, it generally correlates well with the patient's Po_2 and oxygen saturation level as determined by arterial blood gas testing.

Conditions that could interfere with accurate O_2 sat readings are outlined in Case 1-7.

B. Arterial blood gas (ABG)   NONESSENTIAL

Because the patient's pulse oximetry is normal and there is no reason to suspect that this is not accurate, an ABG is not indicated. However, if Mrs. Keaton's oxygen saturation were decreased, ABGs would assist in establishing the presence of true hypoxia, as well as, determining the type of acid-base disturbance that was present. That imbalance would narrow the possible causes for her hypoxemia.

The pH establishes whether the main imbalance is an acidosis or an alkalosis. In an acidosis, the pH would be decreased, whereas in an alkalosis, the pH would be elevated. Determining whether the acidosis or alkalosis is metabolic or respiratory in nature is based on the Pco_2 and the HCO_3 levels. Generally, if dealing with a respiratory cause, the HCO_3 is normal. With respiratory acidosis, the Pco_2 is generally elevated, whereas with respiratory alkalosis, it is generally

decreased. Metabolic causes generally have normal Pco_2 levels; however, the HCO_3 is elevated in metabolic alkalosis and decreased in metabolic acidosis. However, it is not uncommon to have mixed results, especially if the hypoxemia has been present for a while.

C. Chest x-ray (CXR)   ESSENTIAL

A CXR is important to perform to assist in making Mrs. Keaton's diagnosis. It can reveal numerous findings suggestive of various pulmonary and/or cardiac conditions. Localized pulmonary infiltrates that respect anatomic borders (also known as lobar infiltrates or segmental infiltrates) are often seen in bacterial pneumonia; however, these infiltrates can also be caused by a pulmonary infarction, hypersensitivity pneumonitis (HP), bronchiolitis obliterans with organizing pneumonia (BOOP), and cryptogenic organizing pneumonia (COP). Diffuse infiltrates represent diffuse parenchymal lung disease, and their potential diagnoses can include acute respiratory distress syndrome (ARDS), BOOP, COP, HP, inflammatory autoimmune diseases, viral pneumonia, atypical pneumonia, and, in rare cases, bacterial pneumonia. Cavitations suggest a destruction of the lung tissue from a noninfectious source (e.g., carcinoma or pulmonary infarction) or an unusual infectious process (e.g., tuberculosis, funguses, or bacterial lung abscess). Absence of lung markings generally indicates a pneumothorax. Effusions can be secondary to empyema or associated with a severe pneumonia. Nodules can be caused by previous infections, calcified lymph nodes, cancer, or occupational lung diseases; whether they are singular or multiple assists in determining their possible cause.

Some of the findings of cardiac disease that are evident on CXR can consist of a pleural effusion and/or enlarged cardiac shadow suggestive of HF, enlargement of the atrial appendage indicative of atrial enlargement, and generalized enlargement of the cardiac shadow suggestive of not only HF but also cardiomyopathies.

The presence of a normal CXR in the presence of symptoms can even provide useful information. For example, the signs and symptoms of pneumonia with a normal CXR could represent bronchitis, asthma, pulmonary embolism, very early pneumonia, a nonpulmonary condition, or a cardiac condition that is not evident on CXR.

D. White blood count with differential (WBC w/diff) ESSENTIAL

The WBC (or leukocyte) count w/diff is important because it can provide valuable information regarding the severity of an infection, if present, as well as clues as to whether the lung process is viral, bacterial, parasitic, or allergic in etiology predominately via the total leukocyte count and differential. For a more indepth discussion on the role of WBCs in the evaluation of an infectious process, please see Case 1-4.

E. Blood and sputum cultures and sensitivities (C&S) NONESSENTIAL

Blood and sputum cultures are not indicated for Mrs. Keaton at this time because of the mild nature of her disease. Appropriately chosen empiric antimicrobial therapy in all likelihood will have her disease improving (generally occurs in 24 to 48 hours) before the results of the cultures and sensitivities are available (generally requires 48 to 72 hours). Furthermore, it is estimated that approximately one-half of all sputum specimens are actually inadequate for culturing (generally because they are contaminated with saliva); thus, this significantly limits the information obtained from them, even if the patient does not improve with empiric therapy. The American Academy of Family Physicians (AAFP), in developing their treatment guidelines for community-acquired pneumonia, found that *Streptococcus pneumoniae* yielded positive culture isolates in only 40 to 50% of all the cases caused by this organism.

Because Mrs. Keaton does not appear to be septic, it is highly unlikely that blood cultures would be positive. The AAFP in their guidelines for the diagnosis and treatment of community-acquired pneumonia found the rate of positive blood cultures to be from slightly greater than 5% to no more than 10.5%. Additionally, they determined that there was poor correlation between the presence of positive blood cultures, illness severity, and outcome of the disease.

Nevertheless, if Mrs. Keaton's symptoms were severe enough to warrant hospitalization, blood and sputum cultures would be recommended as part of her evaluation by the American Thoracic Society's (ATS's) guidelines. Sputum cultures are also recommended by the Infectious Diseases Society of America (IDSA) if a lower respiratory tract infection is suspected, especially if the patient has a comorbid condition that could add to the severity of the disease such as an underlying structural lung disease; chronic obstructive pulmonary disease (COPD); cavitations, infiltrates, or pleural effusions present on CXR; or alcoholism. Additionally, they recommend blood cultures in cases of comorbid conditions making sepsis more likely such as immunosuppression, leukopenia, severe chronic liver disease, or asplenia.

4. Diagnosis

A. Bronchitis   INCORRECT

Based on her history and physical examination, it appears that a respiratory tract infection (RTI) is more than likely responsible for Mrs. Keaton's illness. Although bronchitis is an RTI, it is not her most likely diagnosis because technically bronchitis is an upper respiratory tract infection, and the basilar infiltrate on her CXR would indicate a lower respiratory tract problem.

B. Community-acquired pneumonia (CAP)   CORRECT

As previously stated, Mrs. Keaton's history and physical examination are consistent with an RTI. The basilar infiltrate, in conjunction with her acquiring this infection independent of a health care facility, makes CAP her most likely diagnosis.

Current terminology divides pneumonia into two primary categories: CAP and health care–associated pneumonia (HCAP). HCAP is further divided into hospital-acquired pneumonia (HAP) and ventilator-assisted pneumonia (VAP). This new classification system makes it easier to determine the most likely pathogens for the pneumonias, the likelihood of resistance organisms, and the best first-line empiric antibiotic.

C. Heart failure (HF)   INCORRECT

HF that is severe enough to produce Mrs. Keaton's symptoms should be associated with pedal edema, a displaced apical impulse, and bilateral (not unilateral) basilar dullness and rales on physical examination. Additionally, her CXR rules

out HF as her most likely diagnosis because in HF, the more consistent findings are enlarged cardiac shadow and bilateral basal effusions.

D. Pleural effusion   INCORRECT

Pleural effusions can be present with severe respiratory tract infections (e.g., empyema or pneumonia); however, the patient tends to appear very ill, or even toxic. Furthermore, the CXR will reveal the effusion. Thus, this can be eliminated as Mrs. Keaton's most likely diagnosis.

E. Pneumothorax   INCORRECT

A pneumothorax, or "collapsed lung," is characterized by dyspnea, decreased breath sounds over the affected area, evidence of "air" on the CXR, and hypoxemia. Furthermore, it is unlikely for the patient to be febrile or to have leukopenia. Thus, this is not her most likely diagnosis.

5. Treatment Plan

A. Hospitalization   INCORRECT

Because of the high mortality rate associated with severe CAP, the difficulty in correctly assessing its severity, and the increased incidence of antibiotic resistance, the ATS and the IDSA consensus guidelines for the evaluation, diagnosis, and treatment of pneumonia include recommendations for treatment setting. These guidelines advocate utilizing one of the evidence-based scoring systems to determine the severity of the patient's condition. The most common ones are the **PSI** (**P**neumonia **S**everity **I**ndex), the **PORT** (**P**atient **O**utcome **R**esearch **T**eam), and the **CURB-65**. Based on the score derived from these instruments, the determination for the necessity of hospitalization to floor, hospitalization to the intensive care unit (ICU), or outpatient treatment can be established. (The PSI and the CURB-65 can be found in their entirety in Mandell et al. [2007] and the PORT in Fine et al. [1997].)

The PSI consists of 20 variables from the patient's history (including age and comorbid conditions), physical examination findings, and diagnostic testing results. Based on the patients' scores, they are assigned to a class from 1 to 5, depending on their disease severity (with 1 being the least severe and 5 being the most severe). Class 1 and 2 patients can generally be safely treated on an outpatient basis. Class 3 patients should be admitted to an observation unit; where their improvement or deterioration determines whether they are treated as outpatients or inpatients. Class 4 and Class 5 patients require hospitalization.

The PORT risk assessment consists of 19 variables (2 demographic, 5 comorbid conditions, 5 physical examination results, and 7 diagnostic test results); the patient is assigned points ranging from a minimum of 10 points to a maximum point score equivalent to his or her age in years for each of the 19 categories. The total maximum score is the patient's age in years (minus 10 for women) plus an additional 185 points. The total sum of the patient's points then categorizes the patient into a group equivalent to the PSI class in terms of treatment setting. The one caveat is that patients younger than 55 years of age without any of the aforementioned comorbid conditions are considered to be a class 1 designation.

With the CURB-65, only five factors are evaluated: **c**onfusion, **u**remia, **r**espiratory rate, low **B**P, and age **65** or older.

Essentially, the patient is assigned 1 point for each of the following: (1) presence of mental confusion, (2) blood urea nitrogen (BUN) greater than 7 mmol/L, (3) respiratory rate of greater than or equal to 30/min, (4) systolic BP of less than or equal to 90 mm Hg and/or diastolic BP less than or equal to 60 mm Hg, and (5) being older than the age of 65 years. Patients with 0 or 1 points can generally be treated safely as outpatients. If the patient has two of the aforementioned factors, then he or she should be hospitalized. If the patient has 3, 4, or 5 points, then he or she should be hospitalized in the ICU.

Furthermore, the IDSA/ATS guidelines recommend ICU admission for any patient with septic shock severe enough to require vasopressor therapy or any patient who requires mechanical ventilation. Additionally, if the patient has three or more of the following, he or she should also be considered for ICU admission: respirations of greater than or equal to 30/min; systolic BP of less than or equal to 90 mm Hg; temperature of less than or equal to 35°C or greater than or equal to 40°C; WBC count less than or equal to 4000; platelet count less than or equal to 100,000; BUN greater than or equal to 20; PaO_2: fractionated O_2 ratio less than or equal to 250; CXR revealing multilobar infiltrates; or the presence of mental confusion.

However, it is essential to remember that regardless of the guideline followed, it is exactly what its name implies, a guideline. Guidelines are not absolutes; therefore, the application of sound clinical judgment for each patient's individual condition is essential. One must remember to always treat the patient, not the numbers.

B. Clarithromycin extended release 250 mg bid × 7 days   CORRECT

The three most likely organisms for CAP are *S. pneumoniae, Mycoplasma pneumoniae,* and *Haemophilus influenzae.* Hence, any empiric therapy utilized should provide adequate coverage for these three organisms, which clarithromycin currently does.

The IDSA/ATS guidelines also make recommendations regarding the most appropriate antibiotic for the patient depending on whether the patient is being treated in the outpatient, inpatient, or inpatient in the ICU setting; comorbidities; antibiotic usage in the past 3 months; and geographic resistance to *S. pneumoniae* by macrolides. Because Mrs. Keaton had been previously healthy and had not had antimicrobial treatment within the past 3 months, first-line treatment for her would be either a macrolide (e.g., clarithromycin) or doxycycline.

C. Ciprofloxacin 750 mg bid × 14 days   INCORRECT

The IDSA/ATS guidelines recommend a fluoroquinolone if any comorbid condition is present or the patient had been on an antibiotic in the 90 days prior to treatment. Because neither of these criteria applies to Mrs. Keaton, this choice is incorrect.

Furthermore, because of its high rates of resistance in some areas, ciprofloxacin would not be the fluoroquinolone of choice.

D. Pneumococcal vaccine when well and influenza vaccine at customary time   CORRECT

Prevention is one of the major strategies in the war on infectious diseases. Therefore, it is essential for individuals to get appropriate immunizations as indicated. The pneumococcal vaccine can be given at any time of year. The influenza vaccine is limited to the fall and winter months.

E. Oxygen at 2 L/min per nasal canula   CORRECT

As a general guideline, oxygen therapy is only required when the patient's oxygen saturation is less than or equal to 90% or Po_2 is less than or equal to 60 mm Hg. However, any patient having respiratory difficulty may benefit from oxygen therapy.

Epidemiologic and Other Data

Approximately 1% of the US population will acquire CAP annually. Individuals at the extremes of ages as well as immunocompromised people are at the greatest risk. Approximately 80% of the cases of CAP are treated on an outpatient basis.

Utilizing the PSI, the mortality rates from CAP range from 0.1% in individuals with class 1 pneumonia to 29.2% in patients with class 5 pneumonia. Regarding the PORT classification system, a class 1 patient has a 30-day mortality rate of 0.1 to 0.4%, whereas a class 5 patient's 30-day mortality rate is 27 to 31.1%. With the CURB-65 criteria, the 30-day mortality rate is 1.5% for a score of 1, 9.2% for a score of 2, and 22% for a score of 3, 4, or 5.

CASE 2-2
Kelly Lincoln
1. History

A. Do her symptoms worsen when she runs?   NONESSENTIAL

The average age for an infant to begin walking is 12 months of age. It is not impossible for Kelly to be walking at 9 months; however, it would be highly unlikely that she is capable of running, especially considering her mother reports normal development on her well-child checks.

B. Has she been unusually irritable or lethargic?   ESSENTIAL

Infants who are mild to moderately ill tend to be fussy and irritable, but still consolable. When they are moderately to severely ill, they become unusually irritable and often inconsolable despite what the mother (or other caregivers) does. Lethargy is generally seen with severe illness.

C. What has her feeding history been up to date?   ESSENTIAL

Infants who are breast-fed tend to have fewer gastrointestinal (e.g., viral and bacterial diarrhea), respiratory (e.g., otitis media, pneumonia, bronchitis, and bronchiolitis), and serious (e.g., bacteremia and meningitis) infections as well as allergies than infants who are bottle-fed. Although the greatest protection from these conditions occurs while the infant is being breast-fed, studies indicate that these benefits continue for at least one year, perhaps longer. Complete breast-feeding throughout the first 6 months confers the greatest protection.

Conversely, infants who have been completely bottle-fed have higher incidences of otitis media, meningitis, and septicemia. This pattern seems to persist for at least the first year of life. Therefore, despite Kelly being beyond the age of being fully breast-fed, it is important to know if she was and for how long.

It is theorized that colostrum in breast milk contain high concentrations of maternal immune factors including macrophages, IgA antibodies, T cells, and other immune antibodies that boost or replace the transplacental antibodies as the infant develops his or her own immune system during the first 6 months of life, probably accounting for the greatest difference between the rates of infection in these two groups.

Furthermore, there are likely some anatomic/structural factors that can contribute to this difference. For example, the more horizontal feeding position that bottle-fed infants are held in during feeding (as compared to a more vertical position for breast-fed infants) and the fact that the infant's eustachian tube lies much more horizontally than it does in older children and adults (which is angled from the ear downward) make it significantly easier for formula to enter the eustachian tube and the middle ear, causing acute otitis media in the bottle-fed infant.

D. Does she attend day care or have older siblings in day care or school? ESSENTIAL

Children in day care tend to have many more infections than those who stay at home or with a single individual. It is theorized that this is a result of the children being in close quarters, sharing of toys, infants and toddlers not being able to cover their mouths and noses when they cough or sneeze, poor hand-washing techniques in older children (and occasionally staff), infrequent hand washing, and an immature immune system.

Other factors that increase a child's risk of acquiring an infection include having an older sibling in day care or school, being exposed to passive (second-hand) cigarette smoke, being younger than the age of 2 years, possessing a history of atopy/allergies, having a chronic illness, being immunocompromised, and having ever been hospitalized.

E. Has she experienced grunting, nasal flaring, and/or intercostal retraction or bulging? ESSENTIAL

All of these are signs of respiratory distress which place the patient at risk for progression to acute respiratory failure (which in infants can happen very rapidly).

2. Physical Examination

A. General appearance ESSENTIAL

It is essential to observe the general appearance of a sick infant. Specific areas include coloring (e.g., normal pink, pale, or cyanotic); overall degree of pulmonary distress (including respiratory muscle tone, rate, and/or use of accessory muscles); overall behavior; activity level; presence of toxicity, lethargy, and/or inconsolability; the relationship between the sick child and the mother (or caregiver); and the mother's (or caregiver's) coping skills in dealing with a sick child (especially if inconsolable) and the sleep deprivation that is usually associated with a sick child. All of these factors are significant in terms of disposition and treatment of the sick infant.

B. Ear, nose, and throat examination ESSENTIAL

The ear, nose, and throat examination are essential in Kelly's evaluation because she started her illness with rhinorrhea. The presence of an upper respiratory tract infection, allergic rhinitis, and/or foreign body could be responsible for, contributing to, or coexisting with her present illness.

C. Heart examination ESSENTIAL

Because severe shortness of breath, respiratory distress, lethargy, not being easily consolable, and anorexia can be accounted for by a cardiac cause, especially an undiagnosed congenital defect, a complete heart examination is essential. (Please see Case 1-2 for details on the exam.)

Although Kelly would be considered tachycardic by adult standards, it is essential to remember when evaluating children, especially infants, that their normal vital sign values are significantly different than adults. Essentially, the younger the child is, the higher the normal values are for pulse and respirations and the lower the normal values are for BP. **Table 2-1** lists the normal range of pulse rates for children from birth to 36 months old. Between 6 and 12 months, the pulse is 80 to 140/min; therefore, Kelly's pulse of 120 beats per minute (BPM) is normal.

D. Lung examination ESSENTIAL

Obviously because Kelly's chief complaint involves dyspnea, it is essential that a careful lung examination be performed as outlined in Case 1-5.

Again, it is important to remember that normal adult respiratory rates are markedly lower than children's, especially infants. Even though 48 breaths per minute sounds extremely rapid, **Table 2-2** reveals that this is top normal for Kelly. Furthermore, the accepted "cut-off" for a "significant" respiratory distress in someone of Kelly's age is 70 breaths per minute.

E. Examination for pedal edema NONESSENTIAL

At the age of 9 months, the majority of infants do not spend a significant amount of time standing or sitting with their legs hanging over the edge of the seat; therefore, it is extremely unlikely for them to develop dependent edema in their distal lower extremities. Thus, if there was a concern that Kelly had dependent edema (although her symptoms are not very consistent with conditions that could produce this sign), evaluating her presacral area (or possibly buttocks), not her feet, ankles, and lower legs, would be much more appropriate.

3. Diagnostic Studies

A. Pulse oximetry (O_2 sat) ESSENTIAL

A pulse oximetry is indicated because it will provide a fairly accurate, noninvasive assessment of her oxygenation

Table 2-1 Normal Pulse Rates for Children from Birth to 36 Months of Age

Age	Pulse Rate in Beats per Minute
Birth to 3 months	90–180
3–6 months	80–160
6–12 months	80–140
12–36 months	75–130

Source: Komar L. Cardiac emergencies. In: Lalani A, Schneeweiss S. The Hospital for Sick Children Handbook of Pediatric Emergency Medicine. Sudbury, MA: Jones and Bartlett Publishers 2008:157.

Table 2-2 Normal Respiratory Rates for Children from Birth to 36 Months of Age

Age	Respiratory Rate in Breaths per Minute
Birth to 3 months	40–60
3–6 months	30–50
6–12 months	30–50
12–24 months	30–40
24–36 months	20–30

Source: Garrett AL. Pediatric resuscitation. In: Aghababian RV (editor-in-chief). Essentials of Emergency Medicine. Sudbury, MA: Jones and Bartlett Publishers 2006:11.

status, which is essential given her degree of respiratory difficulty. Concern of a serious respiratory illness in a patient of Kelly's age is an O₂ sat of less than 95%. However, in adults, normal O₂ sat is considered to be > 95%; and possible critical levels are defined as < 75%.

B. Chest x-ray (CXR)   NONESSENTIAL

The classic presentation and "hallmark" findings of Kelly's condition enable her diagnosis to be established on a clinical basis; therefore, a CXR is not necessary at this time.

Additionally, there are concerns that the excessive radiation exposure can lead to the development of cancer later in life and that a CXR could "confuse" the picture regarding the correct diagnosis, further strengthening the argument not to perform this procedure. Finally, this recommendation (not to perform a CXR) is supported by the guidelines set forth by the American Academy of Pediatrics (AAP) for her condition. However, if the diagnosis is unclear or the patient is not responding as expected, then a CXR might be indicated.

C. Complete blood count with differential (CBC w/diff)   NONESSENTIAL

Because Kelly's diagnosis is essentially a clinical one, a CBC w/diff is not necessary. This is supported by the AAP guidelines, which do not recommend the use of any routine laboratory studies in the diagnosis and treatment of this condition other than an O₂ sat.

D. Blood urea nitrogen (BUN)   NONESSENTIAL

Although an abnormal BUN is not diagnostic for a specific condition, it can serve as a good screening test to confirm a suspicion for certain medical problems. If abnormal, more specific tests can be justified. A BUN can be elevated in renal (e.g., renal failure, pyelonephritis, or glomerulonephritis), urologic (e.g., urethral or ureteral obstruction), gastrointestinal (e.g., bleeding or hemorrhage), cardiac (e.g., heart failure or myocardial infarction), and metabolic (e.g., dehydration, starvation, or sepsis) conditions. It can be decreased in malnutrition, malabsorption, liver failure, and nephrotic syndrome. Because none of these conditions is on the list of potential differential diagnoses for Kelly, a BUN is not necessary at this time.

It is important to remember that "normal" laboratory values represent the average level found in 95% of healthy individuals; therefore, it is possible for a patient to have a slightly abnormal laboratory value and not have a disease process. Furthermore, these reference ranges are often different for adults and children. For example, a "normal" BUN level for an adult is considered to be 10 to 20 mg/dl. In infants and children, a "normal" BUN level is 5 to 18 mg/dl. In newborns, a "normal" BUN level is 3 to 12 mg/dl.

E. Sputum culture and sensitivity (C&S)   NONESSENTIAL

In adult populations, sputum specimens for culture and sensitivity result in inadequate specimens over 50% of the time because they are frequently contaminated with saliva because it is very difficult to produce an adequate sputum specimen on demand by coughing and expelling it through one's mouth. It would be virtually impossible for Kelly to provide a sputum specimen by coughing as a result of her age. Therefore, to obtain an adequate sputum specimen, she would have to be intubated and undergo fiberoptic bronchoscope insertion or other invasive procedures. Even then, the yield of isolating a true pathogenic respiratory pathogen is far from ideal.

A sputum specimen is considered adequate for culture if it contains greater than or equal to 26 neutrophils and less than or equal to 9 squamous epithelial cells per field on Gram stain. Although not its primary purpose, the Gram stain can be used to guide initial empiric antibiotic selection.

4. Diagnosis

A. Right lower lobe pneumonia   INCORRECT

Right lower lobe pneumonia can produce a clinical picture similar to Kelly's. However, it is not generally associated with diffuse expiratory rhonchi in all lung fields. Even when associated with respiratory distress, the abnormal breath sounds should vary in the affected lobe. Furthermore, pneumonia tends to have a more gradual onset than Kelly's symptoms and is not associated with the dramatic and rapid variations in respiratory symptoms with ambient temperature and humidity changes. Therefore, this is not her most likely diagnosis.

B. Bronchiolitis   CORRECT

Bronchiolitis is an acute viral illness most frequently caused by the respiratory syncytial virus; therefore, it frequently follows what appears to be a minor viral upper respiratory tract infection. It is characterized by its very acute and rapid onset and progression of symptoms. Additionally, the physical examination's lung findings of generalized expiratory low-pitched rhonchi are the "hallmark" of this condition. Therefore, this is Kelly's most likely diagnosis.

C. Foreign body airway obstruction   INCORRECT

A foreign body lodged in the airway would certainly produce a rapid onset of respiratory distress as seen in Kelly's case. However, it can be eliminated as her most likely diagnosis because a partial obstruction generally produces true wheezing if the foreign body is lodged in the trachea and stridor on the affected side if it is partially obstructing the trachea, not generalized low-pitched rhonchi. If complete obstruction occurs, there are no breath sounds in the affected area.

D. Gastroesophageal reflux disease (GERD)   INCORRECT

GERD has been known to produce respiratory symptoms in infants; however, they are not as severe as and are much more gradual in onset than what Kelly is experiencing. Furthermore, GERD is also associated with poor weight gain and a history of regurgitation of milk. The incidence of GERD peaks at 1 to 4 months of age and is generally resolved completely by 12 months, further eliminating it Kelly's most likely diagnosis.

E. Asthma   INCORRECT

Asthma can present with an acute onset of respiratory distress and in some cases can be preceded by a mild upper respiratory tract infection. However, it tends to be a chronic disease with intermittent episodes of these symptoms, not a single, severe event. Still, every patient has to have a first episode, which this could represent. However, it can be eliminated as Kelly's most likely diagnosis because the most common lung findings on physical examination are wheezing and rales. Furthermore, unless associated with an infection, it does not produce a fever. Finally, one cannot make the diagnosis of asthma until the child reaches the age of 2 years. Before that age, the same symptoms are diagnosed as hyperreactive airway disease (HRAD).

5. Treatment Plan

A. Oxygen therapy via blow-by mechanism   CORRECT

Anytime patients without a history of chronic obstructive lung disease (COPD) present with respiratory distress and their oxygen saturation is less than 90%, they should be provided with supplemental oxygen. In patients with normal hemoglobin levels, using the oxyhemoglobin dissociation curve, an oxygen saturation of 90% is approximately equivalent to a PaO_2, of 60 mm Hg. In patients with COPD, caution must be employed when supplying supplemental oxygen because it can potentially produce respiratory arrest because their respiratory drive is dependent on carbon dioxide instead of oxygen.

To prevent upsetting the infant and causing additional crying that is going to worsen the respiratory distress, oxygen delivered by a blow-by mechanism as opposed to nasal prongs or a face mask should be used. Furthermore, it is appropriate for the mother or other caregiver to hold the infant while the oxygen is being given to provide additional comfort.

B. Bronchodilator via nebulizer   CORRECT

Studies regarding the use of bronchodilators in the treatment of bronchiolitis have yielded mixed results. Therefore, the AAP guidelines recommend a trial of one treatment. If beneficial, it can be given again at appropriate intervals as needed. However, if it does not provide significant relief, then it should not be continued.

C. Dexamethasone via nebulizer   INCORRECT

Inhaled, oral, IM, and IV corticosteroids have been utilized with mixed results in patients with bronchiolitis. Nevertheless, the AAP guidelines recommend a single-dose trial of an ORAL agent. If it produces significant relief, it should be continued at appropriate dosing intervals as needed. If the single dose is unsuccessful, it should be discontinued. However, it is important to remember that it takes approximately 3 to 4 hours before improvement is apparent from these agents. According to the AAP guidelines, there is no role for inhaled corticosteroids in the treatment of bronchiolitis.

D. Amoxicillin/clavulanic acid 400 mg/kg (based on the amoxicillin component) twice a day for 10 days   INCORRECT

Almost always, bronchiolitis is caused by the respiratory syncytial virus (RSV). Therefore, an antibiotic is not indicated unless there is a secondary bacterial infection present. Then, antibiotics should be utilized following the appropriate guidelines for that infection (as if the patient did not have bronchiolitis).

E. Immediate hospitalization   INCORRECT

Kelly may eventually need to be hospitalized; however, other therapies should be tried first. Hospitalization is indicated for those infants with very severe respiratory distress (defined as a respiratory rate > 70/min with the use of accessory muscles AND an O_2 sat that is < 95%); who are unresponsive to oxygen, inhaled bronchodilator, and oral (or injected) corticosteroid treatment; require continued oxygen therapy; are dehydrated; had an apneic episode; are younger than 2 months of age; OR who have comorbid medical conditions. Psychosocial issues must also be considered when making this decision for or against hospitalization. When treating infants with bronchiolitis, it is important to remember that the AAP guidelines on diagnosis and treatment are evidence based and require the health care provider's (HCP's) clinical input, judgment, and knowledge to apply them appropriately to each patient on an individualized basis.

Epidemiologic and Other Data

Bronchiolitis is a respiratory tract infection that is generally caused by RSV. Other less frequently involved pathogens include adenovirus, influenza, parainfluenza, and the human meta-pneumovirus. The majority of cases occur during the winter months.

It is estimated that bronchiolitis is responsible for up to 5% of all cases of children younger than the age of 2 presenting with dyspnea and wheezing. The majority of these cases are accounted for by bronchitis and pneumonia (approximately one-third to one-half) and other respiratory tract infections (approximately one-half). Rarer causes consist of cystic fibrosis, severe hypersensitivity reaction, anaphylaxis, GERD, pyloric stenosis, and aspiration of milk/food or other foreign bodies.

CASE 2-3
Lionel Matthews
1. History

A. Does he have a fever with the episodes?   ESSENTIAL

The presence of a fever could indicate an infectious cause for his symptoms. However, the degree of temperature does not indicate whether the infection is bacterial, viral, fungal, or parasitic in nature, nor is it directly correlated with the severity of the patient's illness.

B. How frequently is he symptomatic during the day and at night?   ESSENTIAL

The frequency of symptoms typically relates to the seriousness of the condition as well as the limitations it places on the patient. Furthermore, this knowledge will play a critical role in determining the most appropriate treatment of Lionel's condition.

C. What color is his sputum?   NONESSENTIAL

As previously stated, colored sputum does not necessarily mean that the patient has a bacterial infection. It can be seen in viral, fungal, and parasitic infections as well as inflammatory processes. However, pink-tinged sputum could indicate the presence of blood. Incidentally, the same is true regarding nasal secretions and postnasal discharge.

D. Does he have a rash?   ESSENTIAL

Certain rashes are characteristic of some conditions that can present with symptoms similar to Lionel's chief complaint. For example, some viruses present with typical exanthemas or more characteristic lesions, papules, vesicles, and crusting lesions (e.g., varicella); some of the serious bacterial infections present with distinctive lesions (e.g., Janeway lesions with infectious endocarditis); and asthma can present with rashes that are typically associated with allergies (e.g., atopic dermatitis, eczema, contact dermatitis, and urticaria). Thus, the presence (or absence) of these findings can assist in narrowing the list of potential differential diagnoses for Lionel.

E. Has he experienced any sneezing; rhinorrhea; nasal congestion; postnasal discharge; sore throat; and/or itchy, watery eyes?   ESSENTIAL

These are all symptoms that could be associated with an allergic or infectious process of the upper respiratory tract. Their presence and description can be helpful in narrowing Lionel's list of potential differential diagnoses. For example, a sticky eye discharge that leaves his eyelashes matted together or crusted in the morning suggests the presence of conjunctivitis, making a viral process more likely. On the other hand, a clear, thin, spontaneous epiphora with ocular pruritus but without any matting or crusting is more likely to be associated with an allergic process.

2. Physical Examination

A. Ear, nose, and throat (ENT) examination

Because Lionel is complaining of a cough, rhinorrhea, nasal congestion, postnasal discharge, and sneezing, an ENT examination is essential to evaluate for abnormalities that may be causing his present complaint, be aggravating his present condition, or be representing an unrelated disease process.

Remember that just because a patient has several complaints, it does not mean that a single diagnosis is responsible for all of them. Patients are not limited to one diagnosis per visit.

B. Heart examination   ESSENTIAL

Because chest tightness and dyspnea are present, a cardiac cause could be responsible for Lionel's symptoms. Hence, a heart examination as outlined in Case 1-2 needs to be performed.

C. Lung examination   ESSENTIAL

Because Lionel is experiencing several pulmonary symptoms, a careful lung examination as outlined in Case 1-5 is required to evaluate for potential pulmonary causes.

D. Abdominal examination   NONESSENTIAL

E. Skin examination   ESSENTIAL

A skin examination is indicated to evaluate for subtle signs of a rash that might have been overlooked by Lionel and/or his mother. Depending on the finding, it could assist in determining the cause of Lionel's chief complaint.

3. Diagnostic Studies

A. Chest x-ray (CXR)   ESSENTIAL

A CXR is indicated because of the long-standing duration of Lionel's symptoms. Furthermore, the National Heart, Lung and Blood Institute (NHLBI) of the National Institutes of Health (NIH) in their guidelines regarding the diagnosis and management of Lionel's condition recommend a CXR as part of the workup.

B. Oxygen saturation (O_2 sat) via pulse oximetry   ESSENTIAL

An O_2 sat should be performed because Lionel is experiencing respiratory difficulty. It is also recommended by NHLBI guidelines as part of the routine evaluation for his condition.

C. Arterial blood gases (ABGs)   NONESSENTIAL

An ABG measurement is not indicated for Lionel because he is not exhibiting any symptoms indicating that he is experiencing significant respiratory distress and he has a normal O_2 sat.

D. Pulmonary function test (PFT), before and after inhaled bronchodilator administration   ESSENTIAL

PFT, or spirometry, before and after a trial of inhaled bronchodilator assists in determining if an obstructive or restrictive process is present as well as whether it is reversible or not.

The primary values generally utilized in this determination are the forced vital capacity (FVC), the forced expiratory volume in 1 second (FEV_1), and the ratio of the FEV_1/FVC. Occasionally in adults the FEV_6 will be utilized instead of the FEV_1 because certain conditions are associated with a prolonged expiratory phase (e.g., asthma), causing the FEV_1 to be an inaccurate determination of actual lung volume.

In pure obstructive lung disease, the FVC, FEV_1, and FEV_1/FVC ratio are all decreased (a decreased FEV_1/FCV ratio is < 80). In a pure restrictive lung disease, the FVC is decreased, the FEV_1 is generally normal, and the FEV_1/FCV ratio is greater than 80. However, a mixed pattern can also be seen.

Regarding airway reversibility, some sources go with as low as a 10% whereas others go with as high as a 20% improvement between the prebronchodilator test results and the postbronchodilator test results. The NHLBI utilizes an improvement of 12% (or 200 ml) or more in FEV_1 15 minutes after the inhaled bronchodilator to define the presence of a reversible airway disease.

Furthermore, it is essential to remember that PFT values vary depending on age, gender, height, weight, and race;

therefore, the correct normal values must be utilized for accurate results.

E. White blood count with differential (WBC w/diff) NONESSENTIAL

A WBC w/diff is not indicated at this time because it is highly unlikely that an significant infectious process is responsible for Lionel's symptoms.

4. Diagnosis

A. Mild intermittent asthma   INCORRECT

The NHLBI's National Asthma Education and Prevention Program's Expert Panel Report 3: Guidelines for the Diagnosis and Management of Asthma provides a diagnosis classification based on three variables: (1) the frequency of daytime and nocturnal symptoms, (2) the effect on the patient's functional status, and (3) the patient's pulmonary function testing results.

PFT results being utilized to classify the patient's disease severity should be performed when the patient is asymptomatic. Although not as desirable, it is acceptable in patients with current or chronic symptoms to utilize their post–inhaled bronchodilator test if it resolves his or her symptoms.

One of the hallmarks of asthma is its reversibility. Lionel experienced a 34% improvement in his FEV_1 from his pre– to his post–inhaled bronchodilator spirometry. This is probably exaggerated because of his symptomatic state before the bronchodilator therapy. Nevertheless, it demonstrates reversibility. Thus, Lionel has asthma.

The type of asthma that a patient has depends on symptom frequency (both daytime and nocturnal), the number of occurrences of rescue inhaler usage, the effect the disease has on daily living, the FEV_1, and the FEV_1/FVC ratio. The most severe group that any of the patient's aforementioned signs and symptoms fall into is his or her category for diagnosis. For example,

if a patient's frequency of daytime and nocturnal symptoms places him into a moderate persistent category, but his functional status and PFT results place him in a mild persistent category, he is considered to have moderate persistent asthma.

Regarding the 5- to 11-year-old age group, the definitions for the various forms of asthma are outlined in **Table 2-3**.

Despite Lionel's post–inhaled bronchodilator (or assumed asymptomatic) FEV_1 being greater than or equal to 80% of predicted and his FEV_1/FVC ratio being greater than or equal to 85% of predicted, he is experiencing exacerbations three to four times per week, having nocturnal episodes two to four times per month, and having some limitations on his level of activity because of his disease. Therefore, he does not meet the diagnostic criteria for mild intermittent asthma; thus, this is not his most likely diagnosis.

B. Mild persistent asthma   CORRECT

Lionel's post–inhaled bronchodilator (or assumed asymptomatic) FEV_1 is 85% and his FEV_1/FVC ratio is 89%. He experiences exacerbations three to four times per week, has nocturnal episodes two to four times per month, and has some mild limitations on his level of activity because of his disease. Furthermore, his short-acting β-agonist (SABA) inhalation therapy is less than twice a week (primarily because he has not been prescribed one to utilize at this time). These correspond with the mild persistent asthma category (see Table 2-3); thus, this is his most likely diagnosis.

C. Moderate persistent asthma   INCORRECT

Moderate persistent asthma consists of daily symptoms, daily SABA usage, nocturnal symptoms more than once per week (but not nightly), a moderate effect on activities, an FEV_1 of 60 to 80%, and an FEV_1/FVC ratio of 75 to 80%. Because Lionel's findings do not meet any of these parameters, this is not his most likely diagnosis.

Table 2-3 Definitions for the Various Forms of Asthma

Type of Asthma	Frequency of Daytime Symptoms	Frequency of Nocturnal Symptoms	Frequency of SABA[a] Usage	Effect on Daily Activities	FEV_1[b]	FEV_1/FVC[b]
Mild intermittent	≤ 2 ×/week	≤ 2 ×/month	≤ 2 ×/week	None	≥ 80%	≥ 85%
Mild persistent	> 2 ×/week but not daily	3–4 ×/month	> 2 ×/week	Mild	≥ 80%	≥ 80%
Moderate persistent	Daily	> 1 ×/week but not daily	Daily	Moderate	60–80%	75–80%
Severe persistent	Multiple exacerbations throughout the day	Often nightly	Multiple times throughout the day	Severe	< 60%	< 75%

Source: U.S. Department of Health and Human Services National Institutes of Health's National Heart, Lung and Blood Institute's National Asthma Education and Prevent Program. *Expert Panel Report 3: Guidelines for the Diagnosis and Management of Asthma.* Washington, DC: U.S. Department of Health and Human Services; 2007:1–440.

Notes: FEV_1, forced expiratory volume in 1 second; FEV_1/FVC, ratio of forced expiratory volume in 1 second to forced vital capacity.

[a]Short-acting β-agonist delivered via metered-dose inhaler or nebulizer.

[b]Percentage of predicted normal for age, height, weight, gender, and race.

D. Severe persistent asthma   INCORRECT

Severe persistent asthma consists of multiple daily and frequent (at least once) nightly symptoms as well multiple daily SABA usage and severe limitations on activity. Additionally, the FEV_1 is less than 60% and the FEV_1/FVC ratio is less than 75%. Because Lionel's findings do not meet any of these parameters, this is not his most likely diagnosis.

E. Cystic fibrosis   INCORRECT

Cystic fibrosis is a congenital metabolic condition characterized by abnormal secretions of the exocrine glands. Its pulmonary component can be classified as an obstructive lung disease characterized by chronic persistent coughing, wheezing, and sputum production. However, it is also characterized by frequent lung infections, bronchiectasis, nonpulmonary conditions (e.g., pancreatic insufficiency, recurrent pancreatitis, intestinal obstruction, and chronic hepatic diseases), nutritional deficiencies, and a positive sweat chloride concentration. Thus, this is not Lionel's most likely diagnosis.

5. Treatment Plan

A. Patient education, symptom and peak-flow diary, written exacerbation plan based on symptoms and peak flow, and environmental controls   CORRECT

The NHLBI guideline recommends treating asthma using a step-based approach. There are some minor variations between the different age groups (0–4 years old, 5–11 years old, and ≥ 12 years old) regarding the treatment modalities. Nevertheless, there are six steps in each age group with a recommended medication and sometimes an alternative medication choice. The starting point is based on the patient's diagnostic classification (mild intermittent, mild persistent, moderate persistent, or severe persistent).

Subsequent treatment is based on how the patient is doing at follow-up, taking into account such factors as symptoms, compliance with therapy, inhaler/spacer/nebulizer technique, and environmental controls. Depending on the findings of the varibles correlated with each level, consideration can be given to "stepping up" a level if the patient is still symptomatic or "stepping down" a level if the patient has remained very stable for a minimum of 3 months.

Along with all the medications associated with each step, patient education, written exacerbation plan based on symptoms and peak flow, and environmental control are essential. Therefore, these recommendations should be presented to both Lionel and his mother.

B. Referral to an allergist for skin testing   CORRECT

The guidelines also recommend immunotherapy for patients with persistent asthma and allergic disease. Because Lionel had a history of atopy and symptoms consistent with allergic rhinitis, he should be referred to an allergist for skin testing to determine his need for immunotherapy.

Studies have shown that untreated allergic rhinitis makes the patient's asthma more difficult to control and is associated with increased exacerbations.

Other appropriate referrals include the consideration of a consult with a pulmonologist when reaching step 3 of the medication guideline. And, upon reaching step 4, a pulmonary consult should be considered mandatory, especially in the 5- to 11-year-old age group.

C. Short-acting β-agonist metered-dose inhaler (MDI) with spacer for as-needed usage   CORRECT

All patients should have a short-acting β-agonist (SABA) in an MDI with a spacer, or a nebulizer if they cannot correctly utilize (or are too young for) an MDI, to use in case of an exacerbation. A usage diary consisting of the frequency of use, the circumstances surrounding the usage, the peak flow value before and after treatment, and response to treatment should be brought to each visit as it provides valuable information regarding control, potential allergens, environmental irritants, and need for medication adjustments.

D. Long-acting β-agonist MDI with spacer for regular daily usage   INCORRECT

As previously stated, the NHLBI asthma guideline has developed a "step-based" algorithm regarding the treatment for patients with the various forms of asthma. In addition to patient education, all patients (regardless of their type of asthma) should be provided with an SABA MDI with spacer or nebulizer for exacerbations.

Long-acting β-agonists (LABAs) are not recommended for use until the patient is considered to have moderate persistent asthma. Hence, this class of medications is not indicated for Lionel at this time because his diagnosis is mild persistent asthma.

E. Regular daily usage of low-dose inhaled corticosteroids with spacer   CORRECT

Low-dose inhaled corticosteroids are indicated in Lionel's age group for mild persistent asthma because they are considered to be the next "step" in the treatment of asthma and should be provided to any patient with any type of persistent asthma. Thus, he should be prescribed one by MDI (or nebulizer) with a spacer along with instructions on usage and how to avoid fungal infections; the possibility of growth retardation and other potential adverse effects should also be explained to him and his mother. Ideally, he should be able to demonstrate correct technique before leaving the office with a prescription for an MDI.

As stated previously, patients with moderate or severe persistent asthma require not only the treatments that are indicated in the milder forms of asthma (patient education, a SABA, and an inhaled corticosteroid), but also a LABA and a higher dose of inhaled corticosteroid. The final recommended "step" is the consideration of adding an oral corticosteroid for patients who have severe persistent asthma and are not controlled by the previous treatment strategies.

It is essential to remember that these are only guidelines based on the most up-to-date medical evidence; therefore, they should guide, not dictate, patient evaluation and treatment. Clinical judgment must play an essential role in the management of each patient individually.

If these "steps" fail to control the patient's symptoms, in addition to ensuring compliance and inhaling technique (which should be done for all patients at each visit regardless of lcvel and degree of control), other options include higher-dose oral corticosteroids, leukotriene receptor blockers, cromolyn or nedocromil sodium, theophylline, and oxygen. Very unconventional (and off-label) use of other agents is sometimes effective when all of these fail to provide patients with good control of severe persistent asthma. These drugs include azathioprine, cyclosporin, methotrexate, omalizumab, and IV γ-globulins.

Alternative treatment options such as osteopathic manipulation therapy (OMT), relaxation therapy, yoga, stretching exercises, acupuncture, and speleotherapy could be considered as there are anecdotal reports that they are effective for some patients.

Epidemiologic and Other Data

Estimates place the incidence of adults with asthma in the United States at anywhere from approximately 5 to 12%. It is estimated to be higher in children, affecting approximately 15% of the entire US pediatric population. It tends to affect females at a greater rate than males. Inner-city populations, especially children, are affected at a greater rate than suburban and rural residents. Hospitalization and death rates are significantly higher for African Americans than for any other racial group.

CASE 2-4

Mary Nelson

1. History

A. When was her last TB test performed, what was its technique, and what was its result?   ESSENTIAL

Because Mrs. Nelson has symptoms that could be caused by pulmonary TB and has been exposed to active TB as a result of her employment, it is important to know when her last TB test was, what technique was utilized to perform the test, and what its results were. This information could become important if she does have TB to determine whether it is acute, old, active, or inactive. Furthermore, knowing which test was utilized provides information regarding the accuracy of the results because there are significant sensitivity and specificity among the various testing techniques.

B. Has she been having any night sweats, fatigue, weight loss, or anorexia?   ESSENTIAL

Although these symptoms are commonly seen in patients with tuberculosis, they are not specific to this disease. Other conditions that could be responsible for these symptoms range from the benign (i.e., menopause) to the potentially fatal (i.e., cancer). Nevertheless, it is important to know if the patient has been experiencing them.

C. Has she had chest pressure, pain in her arms or shoulders, diaphoresis, nausea, vomiting, or heartburn?   ESSENTIAL

Angina and myocardial infarctions can present with atypical symptoms, especially in women. Therefore, it is appropriate to inquire if Mrs. Nelson has any typical symptoms that could be suspicious for coronary artery disease (CAD).

D. Has she had any dyspnea or orthopnea?   ESSENTIAL

If present, these would indicate a more serious process regardless of whether her chief complaint is determined to be pulmonary, cardiac, neurologic, or psychiatric in origin.

E. Has she been feeling depressed, feeling hopeless, or experiencing anhedonia lately?   NONESSENTIAL

Although Mrs. Nelson has some of symptoms that are common in depression (e.g., fatigue, insomnia [possibly resulting from night sweats], anorexia, and weight loss), she also other has symptoms that are not (e.g., hemoptysis, fever, and night sweats). Because these latter symptoms could represent a serious physical condition, they must be evaluated before a psychiatric diagnosis is entertained.

2. Physical Examination

A. Heart examination   ESSENTIAL

Because Mrs. Nelson's chest pain and cough could have a cardiac cause, it is essential to perform a heart examination on her as outlined in Case 1-2.

B. Lung examination   ESSENTIAL

Equally as important because of Mrs. Nelson's chest pain, cough, hemoptysis, and fever, a complete lung examination as outlined in Case 1-5 is also indicated.

C. Pelvic examination to evaluate for endometrial carcinoma NONESSENTIAL

Because of her significant weight loss, night sweats, and hemoptysis, the possibility of a carcinoma as the cause of her chief complaint cannot be ignored. Because her symptoms are more likely to be caused by a pulmonary malignancy (cough, hemoptysis, and chest pain) than an endometrial one (most common symptom being the return of vaginal bleeding in peri- or post-menopausal women and/or irregular vaginal bleeding in premenopausal women), it is more important to explore her chest cavity than her endometrial cavity for the cause of a malignancy (if one is present) at this time.

D. Fibromyalgia tender-point examination   NONESSENTIAL

Although Mrs. Nelson is experiencing fatigue and what could be musculoskeletal chest wall pain (however it only occurs with coughing), the lack of myalgias in other areas of her body makes the diagnosis of fibromyalgia extremely unlikely.

E. Brief screening test for depression   NONESSENTIAL

As previously stated, Mrs. Nelson does have some symptoms that could be attributed to depression (e.g., fatigue, insomnia, anorexia, and weight loss). However, these symptoms could be just as easily attributed to a physical condition. Therefore, her physical symptoms must be evaluated completely before determining that she is suffering from depression or another psychological condition (e.g., somatoform illness, factitious disorder, or conversion disorder). According to the American Psychiatric Association's *Diagnostic and Statistical Manual of Mental Disorders*, 4th ed. (DSM-IV), one of the primary diagnostic criteria for virtually every mental disorder is that the symptoms cannot be otherwise accounted for by another condition/illness. Therefore, a depression screen is not necessary at this time for Mrs. Nelson.

However, if it is determined that she needed to be screened for depression, then one of the several available screening tools (e.g., Zung Self-Assessment Depression Scale or Beck Depression Inventory) could be employed. However, the U.S. Preventive Services Task Force (USPSTF) recommends asking two simple questions as a method for screening for depression in adults: (1) "Over the past 2 weeks have you felt down, depressed, or hopeless?" and (2) "Over the past 2 weeks, have you had little interest or pleasure in doing things?" In their evidence-based review of the current literature, they concluded that a positive response to either of these questions is equally as efficacious as any of the longer screening questionnaires.

It is important to remember that a positive finding on a screening tool for depression, as for any disease, does not necessarily mean that the patient has it. Essentially, it means that additional evaluation is justified to determine whether the patient has that condition.

3. Diagnostic Studies

A. Tine test   NONESSENTIAL

Some TB tests are no longer recommended because of their inability to provide accurate, reproducible results. The best known example is the multiple puncture (or tine) test. It required the tester to puncture the skin of the forearm with a disposable device that had short prongs covered with a very small amount of the *Mycobacterium tuberculosis* organism. Unfortunately, because of tester (e.g., amount of pressure and duration of time left in place) and patient (e.g., toughness of the skin or movement during the procedure) variables, the amount of *M. tuberculosis* that entered the skin cannot be accurately assessed and therefore can vary significantly from patient to patient, yielding inconsistent and sometimes inaccurate results. Therefore, this test is no longer recommended for screening in any patient.

B. Mantoux tuberculin skin test (TST)   NONESSENTIAL

The TST is an intradermal injection of purified protein derivative (PPD), which is placed on the inner aspect of the forearm. It is considered to be the "gold standard" for screening patients for infection with *M. tuberculosis*. The results are recorded as the size of the diameter of the indurated area (not surrounding erythema) across the forearm (parallel to the elbow crease) at 48 to 72 hours postinjection.

Whether or not the result is considered positive depends on both the size of the indurated area and the characteristics of the patient. A TST is considered to be positive in any patient when there is greater than or equal to 15 mm of induration.

If the patient has human immunodeficiency virus (HIV) infection or acquired immunodeficiency syndrome (AIDS), organ transplant, or other immunocompromising condition, an induration of greater than or equal to 5 mm is considered to be positive. Additionally, an induration of greater than or equal to 5 mm is considered to be positive if the patient has recently been exposed to a patient with TB (as Mrs. Nelson had) or if his or her CXR reveals fibrotic changes consistent with a prior TB infection.

An induration of greater than or equal to 10 mm is considered positive in the following high-risk groups: IV drug abusers, patients with comorbid conditions that make them more prone to develop TB (e.g., diabetes mellitus), immigrants who have been in the United States less than 5 years, mycobacterial lab personnel, employees and residents of high-risk facilities (e.g., nursing homes, hospitals, clinics, prisons,

and homeless shelters), children younger than the age of 4 years, and children and adolescents who have been exposed to high-risk adults as defined previously.

However, the TST is a screening test. Confirmatory testing will assist in determining if the positive TST represents an acute, latent, or chronic infection OR a false-positive. False-positives have been known to occur in individuals who have previously been vaccinated with bacillus Calmette-Guerin (BCG), in patients who are infected with an acid-fast bacillus (AFB) that is not *M. tuberculosis*, and in individuals to whom the test was administered and/or read incorrectly.

False-negatives can also occur. The most common cause is an incorrectly administered and/or interpreted test. Other causes include overwhelming *M. tuberculosis* infection/sepsis, being exposed to an individual's body secretions that were positive for TB within the previous 8 to 10 weeks before testing, and having TB in the past. False-negatives also occur in children younger than the age of 6 years, patients with anergy, patients currently or recently infected by some viruses (e.g., rubeola and varicella), and patients who have recently received a live-virus immunization (e.g., measles, mumps, and rubella [MMR] or smallpoxes).

As a general rule, a positive TST requires that the patient be evaluated for an active TB infection and considered for chemoprophylaxis for latent TB. Treating asymptomatic individuals with latent TB significantly reduces the likelihood that the latent TB will later develop into active TB as well as preventing the spread of the disease to others. Treating active TB prevents associated complications from TB as well as the spread to other individuals.

However, because Mrs. Nelson has had four positive TSTs in the past 2 years, assumed to be a result of prior BCG vaccination, in all likelihood a TST on her would be positive again at this time and, therefore, yield no useful information. Therefore, a TST is not indicated for Mrs. Nelson.

Furthermore, regardless of the results of a TST on Mrs. Nelson at this time, the fact that she is symptomatic requires further evaluation to determine if she has an active case of TB, a latent case of TB, a previous case of TB, or some other condition producing her symptoms.

C. QuantiFERON-TB Gold Test (QFT-G)   ESSENTIAL

The QFT-G is a blood test that was approved by the US Food and Drug Administration (FDA) in 2005. It can be used for TB screening in all individuals who are candidates for the TST if they are older than the age of 17 years, are not immunocompromised, and do not have cancer, silicosis, and/or chronic renal disease. These exclusions are made based on the lack of data in these patient populations.

It is most appropriate for screening immigrants who have previously had the BCG vaccine, health care workers, and other individuals who are undergoing frequent serial evaluation for TB. This latter group could have a false-positive test because of a "booster" effect of the multiple tests. Therefore, this would be an appropriate test for Mrs. Nelson. An additional advantage is the elimination of bias when the results are interpreted.

A positive result suggests a *M. tuberculosis* infection is likely; however, like the PPD, additional evaluation is required to confirm the result. A negative result indicates a *M. tuberculosis* infection is unlikely, but not impossible. An indeterminate result currently has no interpretation or clinical usefulness; thus, other methods are going to be required to determine the presence or absence of *M. tuberculosis* infection.

D. Chest x-ray (CXR) ESSENTIAL

Mrs. Nelson requires a CXR because she is experiencing symptoms suggestive of a potentially serious pulmonary condition, has had multiple positive TSTs in the past 2 years, and has been exposed to active *M. tuberculosis* infections.

E. Sputum smear and culture for acid-fast-bacilli (with susceptibility testing if the culture is positive) ESSENTIAL

Mrs. Nelson also requires a sputum specimen for fuchsin stain and culture for AFB because she has signs and symptoms that are consistent with TB, has a history of multiple positive TSTs, and has been exposed to active cases of TB through her employment.

Even then, a positive sputum smear for AFB is very suspicious, but not confirmatory, for the diagnosis of TB. There are other non–*M. tuberculosis* organisms that are AFB positive. Therefore, a positive culture is required to confirm the diagnosis. Positive cultures are then followed by sensitivity because of the high rate of TB resistant organisms.

From a public health standpoint, if the CXR and/or sputum smear are positive, the patient is generally treated empirically until the culture and sensitivity results are available because sputum cultures for *M. tuberculosis* can take up to 6 to 8 weeks.

Many new techniques are being developed to attempt to diagnose the presence of *M. tuberculosis* infections faster. These include new staining techniques to identify AFB utilizing N,N-dimethyl-N-(n-octadecyl)-N-(3-carboxypropyl) ammonium inner salt; different culture media including utilizing solid media and modifications of 7H9 broth; new culturing techniques including a mycobacteria metabolite that causes the release, detection, and measurement of radioactive CO_2 or the colorimetric detection of CO_2; fluorescent compound embedded in a silicone sensor that utilizes ultraviolet light to detect O_2 consumption; serologic diagnosis using immunochromatographic tests, enzyme-linked immunosorbent assays, RNA detection, and DNA detection; and interferon-γ assay tests. However, to date, none of these techniques has been proven to be any more sensitive than the currently utilized techniques; however, they are significantly more expensive. As these techniques continue to be developed, expanded, and tested, the diagnostic tests for TB could change in the near future.

4. Diagnosis

A. Depression INCORRECT

As stated previously, Mrs. Nelson's history revealed some symptoms that could be attributed to depression; however, in addition to those symptoms, she had other complaints that are not typically seen in depression (e.g. hemoptysis, cough, night sweats, and fever). Additionally, her diagnostic tests for physical disorders are positive. Therefore, depression alone is not her most likely diagnosis.

B. Previous TB infection INCORRECT

Individuals with prior TB infections may or may not have a positive QFT-G depending on how long ago their infection

occurred. Unless another condition coexists, patients with prior TB infections are asymptomatic. Furthermore, their CXR tends to reveal findings consistent with an "old" *M. tuberculosis* infection, such as fibrosis. Additionally, their sputum smear for AFB is negative. Despite Mrs. Nelson having a positive QFT-G, she is symptomatic, her CXR revealed multiple 2- to 20-mm round densities with mild cavitations in both her upper lobes and hilar lymphadenopathy, and her sputum smear is positive for AFB. Therefore, this is not her most likely diagnosis.

However, if there is no documented proof that patients with evidence of a previous TB infection received treatment for this infection, they should be treated. More than likely, they are not contagious to others, but the bacteria could still be active in their system, placing them at risk of developing an active TB infection and its complications.

C. Community-acquired pneumonia (CAP) INCORRECT

With Mrs. Nelson's fever, cough, and dyspnea, this diagnosis would be possible if she had been sick for a few days. However, she has been symptomatic for over 6 weeks. Furthermore, the physical examination on her lungs did not reveal findings consistent with an acute pulmonary infection, and her diagnostic studies revealed a positive QFT-G, multiple nodules and cavitation lesions on CXR, and an AFB-positive sputum are inconsistent with the diagnosis of community-acquired pneumonia. Therefore, CAP is unlikely to be Mrs. Nelson's most likely diagnosis.

D. Probable latent tuberculosis infection INCORRECT

This is a potential diagnosis for Mrs. Nelson because she had a positive QFT-G. However, individuals with latent TB infections tend to be asymptomatic, have a normal CXR, and have negative sputum smears and cultures. Because Mrs. Nelson does not meet those criteria (except possibly the negative culture because hers is still pending), this is unlikely to be her most likely diagnosis.

Individuals with latent TB infections cannot spread tuberculosis to other individuals; however, they still require treatment to prevent the infection from progressing into an active mycobacterium infection. Approximately 50% of those individuals who become infected with *M. tuberculosis* will eventually develop active TB. The majority do so within the first 2 years of becoming infected. Immunocompromised individuals are at the greatest risk.

E. Probable active tuberculosis infection CORRECT

Not only does she have a positive QFT-G, but she also has symptoms that are consistent with active TB, an abnormal CXR with multiple, small round densities, mild cavitations, and hilar lymphadenopathy; and a positive sputum smear for AFB. Although Mrs. Nelson cannot technically be diagnosed with active TB until she has a positive sputum culture, this is still her most likely diagnosis from the choices provided.

5. Treatment Plan

A. Trial selective serotonin reuptake inhibitor (SSRI) INCORRECT

Mrs. Nelson's working diagnosis is currently an active TB infection, not depression; hence, this is not an appropriate treatment option for her at this time.

B. Azithromycin 250 mg two tablets initially, then one tablet daily for 4 days   INCORRECT

Azithromycin is not effective against *Mycobacterium tuberculosis*; therefore, it is not indicated as part of her treatment plan.

C. Combination of isoniazid (INH) and rifampin (RIF) daily   INCORRECT

Because of the increased incidence of multidrug-resistant TB, the combination of INH and RIF alone is generally no longer effective against the *M. tuberculosis* organism.

D. Combination of isoniazid (INH), rifampin (RIF), ethambutol (EMB), and pyrazinamide (PZA) daily   CORRECT

In cases of suspected active TB, it is appropriate to begin the preferred initial phase regimen (INH, RIF, EMB, and PZA) as outlined by the ATS, the Centers for Diseases Control and Prevention (CDC), and the IDSA guidelines before the culture and sensitivity results are available.

If her culture is positive and her sensitivity reveals that her strain of *M. tuberculosis* is susceptible to traditional first-line agents, then the EMB can be discontinued.

The ATS, CDC, and IDSA have different guidelines for medication choices for patients who are coinfected with HIV, children, and individuals who are intolerant of one or more of these agents. As with any guidelines, sound clinical judgment must accompany the medication choices and selections made on an individualized basis.

If her culture is negative, then the diagnosis needs to be reevaluated. The most likely first step would be to obtain another sputum specimen for culture, because Mrs. Nelson's sputum for AFB and QFT-G was positive. It is always possible that she is infected with a non–*M. tuberculosis* organism that is AFB positive and has an old or latent TB infection. Or even less likely, she could have an additional pulmonary process occurring with these two problems.

E. Nothing until all test results are back   INCORRECT

As stated previously, it is appropriate (and recommended) to begin treatment on all suspected cases of TB. Hence, awaiting the culture results only increases the likelihood that the patient would spread the infection to others plus develop a more severe infection herself.

Epidemiologic and Other Data

Tuberculosis is caused by *M. tuberculosis*. It is classified as a pulmonary infection; however, in up to 33% of cases, other organs are involved. The CDC estimates that the current infection rate in the United States is approximately 5 individuals per 100,000 population.

The rates of TB were decreasing in the United States and other developed countries until the late 1980s, when an upward trend began. In the United States, this increase resulted primarily from two main sources. First, the emergence of HIV/AIDS produced a population of immunocompromised individuals who were susceptible to *M. tuberculosis*. Second, a large number of infected individuals immigrated to the United States from Latin American and Asia. However, in the past few years, the rate has appeared to have plateaued and perhaps even decreased slightly.

CASE 2-5
Norman Obermiller
1. History

A. Has he been exposed to a significant amount of passive smoke?   ESSENTIAL

Although Mr. Obermiller does not smoke himself, if he is exposed to a significant amount of second-hand smoke, it can have the same detrimental effects on his lungs. Pulmonary diseases associated with cigarette smoking and/or extensive exposure to passive cigarette smoke include lung cancer, acute and chronic bronchitis, emphysema, invasive pneumococcal disease, pneumonia, and asthma. Many occupational and environmental lung diseases are also worsened by cigarette smoke exposure.

B. What are his occupation and hobby histories?   ESSENTIAL

Several occupational, environmental, and recreational activities are associated with chronic pulmonary conditions (e.g., coal worker's pneumoconiosis, silicosis, asbestosis, berylliosis, byssinosis, farmer's lung, giant cell interstitial pneumonitis, and other hypersensitivity pneumonitis). Therefore, it is important to determine if he has had any exposure to potential causative agents (e.g., inorganic dust, organic dusts, chemical agents, and/or other air pollutants).

C. Does he experience leg pain while walking?   ESSENTIAL

Leg pain, especially in the calves (and occasionally the thighs), that occurs when walking and is alleviated almost immediately upon stopping is most generally claudication. It is most frequently an indication of peripheral artery disease (PAD); however, any hypoxic condition could potentially produce similar symptoms.

Noncardiovascular and pulmonary causes of ambulatory leg pain can also occur; however, they would be unlikely to be caused by his chief complaint. Examples include the following: (1) Neurogenic claudication (or "pseudoclaudication") is leg pain that occurs immediately upon standing, continues with walking, and is alleviated with sitting. It is most frequently associated with spinal stenosis. (2) Lumbar disc disease can also produce pain with walking; however, it is generally made worse by sitting. Furthermore, lumbar disc disease is almost always associated with some degree of paresthesias or dysesthesias. (3) Peripheral neuropathies (especially of the peroneal nerve) can cause pain along the lateral tibia that increases with walking and is alleviated with rest. This pain typically increases as the patient walks faster or walks up inclines.

D. How frequently does he experience the cough?   ESSENTIAL

Some respiratory conditions are known for their frequent cough (e.g., acute bronchitis, pneumonia, chronic bronchitis, cigarette smoking, other irritants, asthma, hyperreactive airway disease, and allergic rhinitis associated with frequent/chronic postnasal discharge). Nonrespiratory conditions (e.g., gastroesophageal reflux disease, Hodgkin lymphoma, and angiotensin-converting enzyme [ACE] inhibitor usage) are also associated with a chronic cough.

Other respiratory conditions can be associated with an infrequent or a frequent cough depending on the affected area and the stage of the illness. For example, lung cancer often does not produce a cough unless the tumor is compressing the bronchial tree. Many occupational lung diseases produce a minimal cough in their early stages.

E. Has he been losing weight or experiencing night sweats? ESSENTIAL

Unintentional weight loss and night sweats are very common, but not exclusive, symptoms associated with cancer. In view of his history of dyspnea, this question is important because it makes the diagnosis of lung cancer (or some other type of cancer associated with dyspnea) more likely.

2. Physical Examination

A. Heart examination ESSENTIAL

Even though Mr. Obermiller is not complaining of any other symptoms that are suspicious for a cardiac cause, dyspnea can be associated with many cardiovascular conditions (e.g., angina, arrhythmias, heart failure, and/or a cardiomyopathy). Therefore, it is important to conduct a complete heart examination as outlined in Case 1-2.

B. Lung examination ESSENTIAL

A careful lung examination, as outlined in Case 1-5, should be performed because the majority of significant pulmonary conditions are associated with dyspnea. Because of the chronicity of his symptoms, his most likely diagnosis would consist of a chronic pulmonary condition (e.g., COPD, asthma, or an occupationally or environmentally induced disease).

Other conditions that are capable of producing dyspnea including poor conditioning, neurologic/neuromuscular diseases, psychiatric illnesses, and anemia.

C. Abdominal examination NONESSENTIAL

D. Evaluation for pedal edema ESSENTIAL

Bilateral foot, ankle, or lower leg pitting pedal edema is frequently associated with HF. Unilateral edema, erythema, warmth, and tenderness can be caused by a deep vein thrombosis (DVT), which is a potential precursor of a PE. Both of these conditions can present as progressive dyspnea. However, it would be highly unlikely that either of these conditions were solely responsible for Mr. Obermiller's symptoms because of the long duration of his symptoms. Still, they (especially HF) could be responsible for his recent dyspnea increase.

E. Evaluation of all deep tendon reflexes (DTRs) NONESSENTIAL

Although there are neurologic and neuromuscular conditions that can cause dyspnea, they are highly unlikely to occur in the absence of weakness or fatigue. Furthermore, they may or may not be identifiable on the basis of DTRs. Thus, DTRs are not indicated at this time.

3. Diagnostic Studies

A. Oxygen saturation (O_2 sat) via pulse oximetry ESSENTIAL

As stated previously, an oxygen saturation is a noninvasive measurement of the patient's oxygenation status that is fairly equivalent with what is determined by arterial blood gases. It is indicated in any patient presenting with dyspnea.

B. Arterial blood gases (ABGs) NONESSENTIAL

As a general rule, ABGs are only indicated if the patient's O_2 sat is less than 90. However, if the O_2 sat does not appear to "match" the clinical appearance of the patient or other values from the ABGs are required to rule out acidosis, alkalosis, or a metabolic process, then it would be appropriate to obtain them. For more information on the O_2 sat and/or ABGs, please see Case 2-1.

C. Chest x-ray (CXR) ESSENTIAL

Because of the chronicity and progression of the patient's symptoms, it is essential to perform a CXR to look for not only the characteristics defined in Case 2-1 but also for patterns that suggest specific occupational, environmental, or hobby exposures.

D. Pulmonary function test (PFT), before and after bronchodilator administration ESSENTIAL

Ideally, a PFT should be performed when the patient is asymptomatic to establish a baseline and to provide accurate values to determine the presence of a reversible airway disease. However, in many cases, such as Mr. Obermiller's, the patient has not been asymptomatic for years; therefore, it is appropriate to perform this test when the patient is not experiencing an acute exacerbation to ascertain similar information. For information on interpreting PFTs, please see Case 2-3.

E. Electrocardiogram (ECG) NONESSENTIAL

Mr. Obermiller's history and physical examination do not support a cardiac condition being responsible for his symptoms; therefore, an ECG is not necessary at this time.

4. Diagnosis

A. Asthma INCORRECT

Characteristic features of asthma consist of a history of a disease pattern featuring of acute exacerbations, audible wheezing with dyspnea, and a reversible component. Because Mr. Obermiller's PFTs do not reveal a reversible disease process and his CXR findings are inconsistent with this diagnosis, asthma can essentially be ruled out as his most likely diagnosis.

B. Chronic bronchitis INCORRECT

Chronic bronchitis is almost always associated with a positive smoking history (including significant passive exposure). The "hallmark" symptom of this condition is a chronic cough. Because these factors are absent, it is highly unlikely that chronic bronchitis is Mr. Obermiller's most likely diagnosis.

C. Complicated silicosis CORRECT

Given his occupational history as a granite/sandstone cutter for 20 years, his hobby of glass etching for 10 years, and his current occupation as a full-time glass etcher for 5 years, Mr. Obermiller has an occupational and recreational exposure history that is consistent with silicosis. Additionally, his CXR reveals the typical findings of chronic exposure to free silica: numerous small, round opacities (largest 1 cm) throughout all lung fields with the preponderance of these lesions as well as minimal coalescing in the upper lung fields, and calcification of the periphery of some of his hilar lymph nodes ("eggshell" pattern). Because he does have some minor coalescing of the lesions, this is consistent with complicated silicosis. With advanced, complicated silicosis, these lesions continue to coalesce, forming larger and larger lesions, termed progressive massive fibrosis (PMF; also known as "bat winging" because of its configuration). Thus, from the choices provided, complicated silicosis is Mr. Obermiller's most likely diagnosis.

There are no specific blood tests, imaging studies, or sputum findings on which to establish the diagnosis of silicosis. The diagnosis is based primarily on the exposure (generally occupational) history, presence of pulmonary symptoms, and typical CXR findings. If the CXR findings are present in the absence of an occupational, recreational, or environmental exposure, the most likely diagnosis is sarcoidosis. However, in rare cases autoimmune diseases can present with similar findings. Regardless, if the CXR reveals cavitations, TB must be ruled out.

Other occupations associated with a risk of acquiring silicosis involve those in which the worker is exposed to small particles (dust) of crystalline quartz. These jobs include mining, quarrying, and cutting of stone; sandblasting; cutting of cement (especially in highway construction); manufacturing of glass, clay, stoneware, and cement; and packing silica flour.

D. Lung cancer   INCORRECT

Although the most typical radiographic finding observed with lung cancer is a solitary pulmonary nodule, it must be considered as a possible diagnosis because of his coalescing nodules and hilar lymphadenopathy on CXR. However, his lack of systemic symptoms typically associated with a carcinoma can essentially rule it out as his most likely diagnosis because they would in evidentially be present with a cancer extensive enough to produce his CXR abnormalities.

E. Asbestosis   INCORRECT

Asbestosis is a chronic pulmonary disease characterized by lung damage secondary to significant, chronic exposure to asbestos. Asbestos can be found in older facilities, including homes, schools, churches, factories, roads, playgrounds, and landfills. Additionally, there were many occupations that once played a significant role in the development of asbestosis; however, because asbestos is no longer utilized in the manufacturing of these products or the equipment utilized by these workers, the risk, theoretically, no longer exists. Nevertheless, it is possible to have older patients retired from these professions with asbestosis. These occupations consisted of manufacturers of break linings, insulation, electrical insulation, fire-extinguishing blankets, and floor tiles; ship builders; welders; pipefitters; and boilermakers. The primary occupational risk today is in asbestos abatement workers who fail to use proper protective equipment.

Even though Mr. Obermiller is probably too young to have had a significant occupational exposure to asbestos (in approximately 1975 essentially all asbestos-containing products were changed to synthetic mineral fibers or other materials), he still is at risk for an environmental exposure from the aforementioned facilities. However, his CXR findings are not typical of this disease. The initial CXR findings in asbestosis generally consist of "streaks" in the lower lung fields. This is followed by nodules of various sizes and shapes that coalesce into a "honeycomb"-looking pattern. Therefore, asbestosis is not his most likely diagnosis.

5. Treatment Plan

A. Home oxygen therapy   INCORRECT

In patients with severe pulmonary conditions, home oxygen therapy is often required to prevent them from becoming hypoxic. The need for home oxygen is generally based on the patient's PaO_2 level as determined by ABGs. Continuous home oxygen therapy is generally not indicated until the PaO_2 is less than or equal to 55% on room air while the patient is at rest. Nocturnal oxygen therapy is indicated if the PaO_2 is less than or equal to 55% on room air while the patient is asleep. Exceptions include a PaO_2 less than or equal to 60% on room air in a patient who also has concurrent polycythemia and/or heart failure. However, because Mr. Obermiller's oxygen saturation is still well above 90%, he would not be considered a candidate for home oxygen therapy.

B. Inhaled short-acting β-agonist therapy on an as-needed basis   CORRECT

A trial of an inhaled SABA delivered via an MDI, preferably with a spacer (or a nebulizer) is appropriate to see if it alleviates the patient's dyspnea despite the lack of evidence of reversibility on his spirometry testing. Clinical trials have yielded mixed results on the benefit of SABAs in patients with silicosis.

C. Inhaled corticosteroid therapy   INCORRECT

Inhaled corticosteroids should be avoided in patients with silicosis because there is no clinical evidence revealing them to be efficacious. This is important because, even inhaled corticosteroids can be associated with systemic adverse effects, especially at higher doses (e.g., osteoporosis, adrenal gland suppression, and immunosuppression).

D. Mantoux tuberculin skin test (TST)   CORRECT

Because of silica's ability to damage alveolar macrophages, patients with silicosis are at increased risk for most pulmonary infections, including those caused by *M. tuberculosis*. Therefore, Mr. Obermiller should be screened for the disease currently, and then annually if negative, with a TST. Any positive result requires additional evaluation as outlined in Case 5-4.

E. CT scan of chest   CORRECT

Because of the extensive nodular changes on Mr. Obermiller's CXR, a CT scan of the chest should be performed to rule out the possibility of a hidden lung carcinoma (despite his lack of symptoms) because of the link between silicosis and cancer. In fact, the International Agency for Research on Cancer includes silica, or crystalline quartz, as probable for being carcinogenic to the lungs.

Epidemiologic and Other Data

Silicosis is primarily considered to be an occupational lung disease that is caused by considerable exposure to free silica (SiO_2), or crystalline quartz. However, some individuals acquire the disease via hobbies or environmental exposure. Silicosis, like all organic and inorganic dust diseases, occurs at a much greater incidence in individuals who smoke cigarettes.

The exact incidence of patients with silicosis is unknown. However, as a result of the use of appropriate protective respiratory equipment in developed countries such as the United States, the incidence appears to be decreasing. Unfortunately, in developing counties, where this equipment is not available, many individuals are still acquiring this disease.

In addition to lung infections and cancer, another complication from silicosis is autoimmune diseases (e.g., scleroderma, rheumatoid arthritis, and systemic lupus erythematous).

CASE 2-6
Olivia Peebles
1. History

A. Has she recently been around anyone with berylliosis? NONESSENTIAL

Berylliosis is a pulmonary condition resulting from exposure to beryllium via inhalation. It is classified as an occupational lung disease and is not contagious. Therefore, Mrs. Peebles being exposed to someone with the disease will not impact her symptoms.

B. Has she noticed any pedal edema? ESSENTIAL

With Mrs. Peebles' complaint of dyspnea and right lateral chest pain, it is important to know if she has been experiencing any pedal edema. If present, it could represent a serious cardiovascular, renal, hepatic, or pancreatic condition with radiation of the pain into the right lateral chest.

C. Has she noticed any icterus of her sclera or jaundice of her skin? ESSENTIAL

One of the main concerns regarding patients with RA taking disease-modifying antirheumatoid drugs (DMARDs) is that of hepatotoxicity. Given the location and description of her pain, hepatotoxicity or another hepatic condition could be responsible for her symptoms despite a lack of gastrointestinal (GI) symptoms. Therefore, inquiring about icterus and jaundice is appropriate.

D. Has she experienced any recent trauma? ESSENTIAL

Blunt trauma to her chest wall can result in several conditions that could be responsible for her current symptoms including rib fractures, hemothorax, severe contusion, pneumothorax, pleural effusion, chylothorax (caused by thoracic duct rupture), and hepatic injury. Trauma to her lower leg could result in a DVT that has progressed to her lungs, causing a PE.

Because patients are occasionally reluctant to admit to any type of trauma (especially if it results from intimate partner violence substance intoxication, or "stupidity"), it is essential that this line of questioning be approached with seriousness, concern, and empathy. The patient may need to be encouraged to provide accurate information so the correct diagnosis and treatment plan can be established.

If there is a strong suspicion that the patient's symptoms are related to abuse, direct questioning should be undertaken regarding the possibility of intimate partner violence and other forms of abuse. Open-ended, nonjudgmental, empathetic statements should be used to ask about prevalence; explain that the victim's not to blame and that the victim should not be ashamed or embarrassed; and advise what services are available in the area, including where to obtain help and the location of the nearest shelter. Additionally, the HCP must be cognizant of the laws regarding domestic violence reporting in the state in which he or she is practicing. Most states do not require mandatory reporting by HCPs unless the patient is a minor, a senior citizen, or mentally incompetent.

Another concern that causes patients to be reluctant to admit to a history of trauma especially if sustained while under the influence of alcohol or other drugs or while committing a crime because of concerns of legal repercussions.

E. Has she experienced a recent weight change? ESSENTIAL

Because Mrs. Peebles is experiencing some constitutional symptoms along with her dyspnea, it is essential to determine whether she has any others, such unintentional weight loss. An unintentional weight loss is considered to be significant if the patient has lost more than 5% of his or her previous body weight in 1 month's time. Given Mrs. Peebles' other symptoms, this weight loss, if present, could represent a carcinoma, most likely of the lung, liver, or pancreas.

Hepatic and pancreatic diseases are frequently associated with a weight loss. However, heart and liver failure can cause weight increase because of fluid accumulation.

2. Physical Examination

A. Heart examination ESSENTIAL

A careful heart examination as outlined in Case 1-2 is essential for Mrs. Peebles because she is experiencing chest pain, dyspnea, and cough, which could be caused by a cardiac condition.

B. Lung examination ESSENTIAL

A careful lung examination as outlined in Case 1-5 is also indicated because her dyspnea, cough, and chest pain, suggest the presence of a possible pulmonary problem.

C. Abdominal examination ESSENTIAL

Mrs. Peebles requires a careful abdominal examination with specific focus on attempting to identify the presence of ascites and organ abnormalities (e.g., organomegaly, irregular shape, abnormal texture, and/or tenderness). If ascites is present and Mrs. Peebles' dyspnea and chest pain are caused by a pleural effusion, an even more meticulous abdominal examination is required because this combination can result from several serious intra-abdominal abnormalities including liver cancer, cirrhosis, pancreatic cancer, pancreatitis, peritoneal abscess, ovarian cancer, or Meigs syndrome.

In the absence of a pleural effusion and/or ascites, she still requires a careful abdominal examination to identify any signs of a hepatic, gallbladder, and/or pancreatic abnormality because liver, gallbladder, and pancreatic disorders can also present with these symptoms.

D. Pelvic examination NONESSENTIAL

Even though ovarian cancer and Meigs syndrome are associated with pleural effusions, it is currently unknown if Mrs. Peebles has a pleural effusion. Furthermore, if present, the associated ascites will more than likely prevent an adequate examination of the patient's ovaries by pelvic exam.

E. Evaluation for pedal edema ESSENTIAL

As stated previously, the combination of dyspnea and right lateral chest pain can represent several cardiovascular, pulmonary, renal, or gastrointestinal conditions. The presence of pedal edema can assist in narrowing her list of potential differential diagnoses.

3. Diagnostic Studies

A. Total serum protein, albumin, globulins, amylase, lactate dehydrogenase (LDH), aspartate aminotransferase (AST), and alanine aminotransferase (ALT) levels   NONESSENTIAL

Although several of these tests can provide supportive evidence for various conditions that could cause her symptoms, none are specific to a particular illness. In fact, some can be abnormal in multiple conditions that could be causing her symptoms (e.g., an elevated amylase can be seen in acute pancreatitis, chronic pancreatitis, cholestasis, and pulmonary infarction; an elevated ALT can be seen in acute or chronic pancreatitis, liver diseases [e.g., hepatitis, cirrhosis, and drug toxicity], cholestasis, severe skeletal muscle trauma, and a myocardial infarction; and γ-globulins can be elevated in cancer, infections, and inflammation).

Additionally, many of these tests can be affected by inflammation (e.g., γ-, α_1-, and α_2-globulins and albumin), which Mrs. Peebles more than likely has secondary to her RA. Furthermore, the majority of these tests are useful in diagnosing liver, gallbladder, and pancreatic problems, which fall low on Mrs. Peebles' list of potential differential diagnoses because she lacks gastrointestinal symptoms and has a normal abdominal examination and an abnormal lung examination.

Therefore, this group of tests is extremely unlikely to provide any useful information on which to formulate Mrs. Peebles' most likely diagnosis. Thus, this "shotgun" approach to diagnostic tests needs to be avoided. Diagnostic tests should serve as confirmation of the diagnosis or monitor chronic conditions. They should NOT be selected at random in hopes of identifying the patient's correct diagnosis.

B. CXR with additional view in right lateral decubitus position   ESSENTIAL

Given her chief complaints and her physical findings on her lung examination, a CXR is definitely indicated. The addition of a lateral decubitus view permits the determination of the presence of a significant pleural effusion by the "shifting" of the fluid to the dependant portion of the x-ray view, whereas a solid mass will remain essentially unchanged in this position.

C. Electrocardiogram (ECG)   ESSENTIAL

Because Mrs. Peebles is complaining of chest pain and shortness of breath, an ECG is indicated to evaluate for atypical ischemia/infarction and/or cardiac arrhythmias.

D. Beryllium lymphocyte proliferation test   NONESSENTIAL

The beryllium lymphocyte proliferation test is a blood test that is utilized in the diagnosis and surveillance of individuals exposed to inhaled beryllium (to evaluate for the presence of berylliosis). Because Mrs. Peebles does not have a history of occupational exposure, it is not necessary.

E. Arterial blood gases (ABGs)   ESSENTIAL

Because Mrs. Peebles' pulse oximetry revealed an oxygen saturation below 90% (86%), ABGs are indicated to

further evaluate her hypoxemia. For information on the interpretation of ABGs, please see Case 2-1.

4. Diagnosis

A. Pulmonary embolism with pneumothorax   INCORRECT

Mrs. Peebles' CXR reveals a pleural effusion. However, a pleural effusion is not generally considered to be a diagnosis but a complication from another disease process. These can include pulmonary (e.g., bacterial, viral, fungal, parasitic, rickettsial, and mycobacterium infections; lung cancer; asbestosis; chronic atelectasis; and pulmonary infarction), cardiovascular (e.g., post–myocardial infarction syndrome, heart failure, constrictive pericarditis, superior vena cava syndrome, and pulmonary embolism), gastrointestinal (e.g., perforated esophagus, cirrhosis, and pancreatic disorders), renal (e.g., nephrotic syndrome, uremia, and undergoing peritoneal dialysis), and miscellaneous (e.g., sarcoidosis, autoimmune diseases, myxedema, Meigs syndrome, and adverse medication reactions) disorders.

Even though a PE can cause a pleural effusion, this is not Mrs. Peebles' most likely diagnosis because she lacks the history and/or physical signs of conditions that are known to cause the precipitating emboli (e.g., venous thromboembolic event caused by a deep vein thrombosis [most common], fat from long bone fractures, amniotic fluid from a recent delivery, air from recent neurosurgery, foreign bodies from IV drug abuse, or septic event from infective endocarditis).

Additionally, there is no evidence of free air (gas) on her chest radiograph nor did she have any signs consistent with a pneumothorax on her lung examination except for the decreased breath sounds. Furthermore, a pneumothorax should be hyperresonant to percussion.

B. Lung cancer   INCORRECT

Although lung cancer can cause a pleural effusion, a primary malignant lesion is generally evident on CXR. Because Mrs. Peebles did not have such a lesion on CXR or symptoms typically seen with lung cancer (e.g., weight loss and hemoptysis), this is not her most likely diagnosis. The cytologic analysis of the pleural effusion, if done, should confirm this.

C. Heart failure (HF)   INCORRECT

Even though heart failure is the most common cause of a pleural effusion, it can essentially be eliminated as Mrs. Peebles' most likely diagnosis because of the lack of cardiomegaly on the physical examination, ECG, and CXR, as well as the absence of pedal edema.

D. Pneumonia with pleural effusion   INCORRECT

Pneumonia, from multiple types of pathogens, can cause pleural effusions. However, this can essentially be eliminated as Mrs. Peebles' most likely diagnosis because of her lack of fever, other infectious symptoms (with the exception of a cough, which was nonproductive), and other physical and/or CXR findings consistent with pneumonia. Analysis of the pleural effusion, if done, would provide additional information to support this not being her most likely diagnosis.

E. Autoimmune disease–associated pleural effusion   CORRECT

Given Mrs. Peebles' history of RA; her lack of finding to support an infectious process, a malignancy, a DVT, or HF;

and her respiratory acidosis on ABGs, from the diagnosis list provided, this is Mrs. Peebles' most likely diagnosis. This can be confirmed by the presence of multinucleated, comet-shaped cells (or "tadpoles") on pleural fluid analysis.

5. Treatment Plan

A. Thoracentesis of up to 1000 ml of fluid with approximately 100 ml to be sent for pleural fluid analysis (gross appearance, protein, LDH, glucose, amylase, pH, specific gravity, cytology, WBC w/diff, Gram stain, acid-fast bacteria [AFB] smear, and cultures with sensitivities), and a serum protein and LDH CORRECT

A therapeutic thoracentesis is indicated when there is a significant amount of fluid, significant shortness of breath, hypoxemia, effusions that are increasing in size, or effusions that are unresponsive to conservative therapy. A diagnostic thoracentesis (a thoracentesis to obtain pleural fluid for analysis) is always performed on the fluid obtained during the therapeutic thoracentesis. A diagnostic thoracentesis is also indicated if the patient has a significant unilateral effusion, an asymmetric bilateral pleural effusion, fever, or pleuritic chest pain.

The first step in the evaluation of the pleural effusion is the gross visualization of the fluid for color, thickness, turbidity, and presence of blood. Exudative pleural effusions are generally thicker, discolored, and more turbid than are transudative effusions. However, because this determination is very significant in the evaluation and treatment of the pleural effusion, Light's criteria are applied to make this determination. Essentially, an effusion can be considered exudative if the pleural fluid protein/serum protein ratio is greater than 0.5 OR the pleural fluid LDH/serum LDH ratio is greater than 0.6 OR the pleural fluid protein is greater than 3 g/dl OR the plural fluid LDH is greater than 0.66 of the upper limit of the normal serum LDH. Additional confirmation of an exudative pleural effusion is a pleural fluid specific gravity greater than 1.018.

The knowledge of the nature of the effusion assists in determining the diagnostic evaluation, most likely diagnosis, and appropriate treatment for the effusion. For example, transudative pleural effusions are almost always caused by heart failure. Other possible causes include cirrhosis, nephrotic syndrome, pulmonary embolism, and myxedema. Hence, the primary evaluation of a transudative pleural effusion are those studies necessary to establish the diagnosis of HF. If HF is not found, then the diagnostic testing would be geared toward the aforementioned alternative diagnoses. Treatment is directed toward the underlying condition.

If the pleural effusion is exudative, experts advocate performing the remaining components of the pleural fluid analysis (as outlined previously) to assist in determining the cause. This additional analysis includes a cytologic evaluation for cells that are suspicious for cancer, infection, or an autoimmune disease (e.g., multinucleated, comet-shaped cells ["tadpoles"] as seen with RA); a WBC w/diff to determine the presence (and possibly type) of infection; a Gram stain to determine the quality of the specimen and to provide clues to the potential pathogens based on staining color and organism shape and grouping (which will enable a more informed determination regarding the presumptive etiologic pathogen and a better initial empiric antibiotic selection [if a bacterial infection appears to be the cause]); a smear for AFB as a screen for tuberculosis; and other appropriate bacterial, viral, fungal, and *Mycobacterium* cultures and sensitivities based on these findings.

However, because the majority of these results are not going to be available immediately, it is recommended to base the next diagnostic testing decisions on the pleural fluid's amylase and glucose levels. If the amylase is elevated, the patient requires evaluation for lung cancer and for nonpulmonary causes such as nonlung cancer, esophageal rupture, and pancreatic diseases. If the glucose is low (defined as < 60 mg/dl), the most likely diagnoses include a malignancy, bacterial infection, or rheumatoid pleuritis. If neither of these test results is met, most experts recommend a more in-depth evaluation for a pulmonary embolism because it can be either an exudative or a transudative process. Furthermore, a PE is extremely difficult to accurately diagnose in the presence of a pleural effusion. If a PE is not the cause of the pleural effusion at this point, then the next most likely diagnosis is tuberculosis.

If all the aforementioned diagnostic studies are negative and/or the patient is not improving, then a thoracoscopy or an open biopsy should be considered to establish the diagnosis. Other less likely causes of an exudative pleural effusion include diaphragmatic hernia, sarcoidosis, asbestosis, uremia, pericardial disease, adverse medication effects, complications of radiation therapy, or status-post abdominal, coronary artery bypass, or liver transplant surgery.

B. Thoracentesis of all fluid collectable with approximately 100 ml for pleural fluid analysis as described in choice A INCORRECT

Mrs. Peebles does require a thoracentesis and subsequent pleural fluid analysis per the criteria outlined previously. However, thoracentesis of all fluid collectable is not a good treatment option for Mrs. Peebles because the radiologist estimates the amount of pleural fluid to be approximately 2000 ml, and the removal of more than 1000 ml of fluid in a given session can lead to serious complications (e.g., pneumothorax and pulmonary edema) regardless of the total size of the effusion.

C. Mantoux tuberculin skin test (TST)   CORRECT

Because of the high incidence of TB with a pleural effusion and the public health concerns regarding spread of the disease, any patient with a pleural effusion should receive a TST.

D. Tube thoracostomy   INCORRECT

A tubal thoracostomy is not recommended for Mrs. Peebles at this time. If all the fluid is not removed with the first thoracentesis or if the fluid reaccumulates, then a repeat therapeutic thoracentesis is indicated. However, if the second procedure is ineffective, the next step would be to insert a chest tube and instill one of the fibrinolytic agents (e.g., streptokinase).

An alternative to the insertion of a chest tube would be to perform a thoracoscopy for the purpose of destroying any adhesions that are present. Decortication is another possibility if none of the aforementioned treatments is effective.

E. Combination of isoniazid (INH), rifampin (RIF), ethambutol (EMB), and pyrazinamide (PZA) daily   INCORRECT

Even though it is appropriate to treat suspected cases of TB before all the diagnostic studies are completed, the TST or the AFB of the sputum should be reported as positive before treatment is initiated. This will assist in preventing the development of additional treatment-resistant strains and/or the occurrence of adverse drug effects in the patient.

Epidemiologic and Other Data

Pleural effusions are commonly seen; however, the exact incidence is unknown. It is important to remember that a pleural effusion is not a diagnosis in and of itself but a sign of another process. In order to treat the pleural effusion, the underlying cause must be established.

CASE 2-7
Patricia Queen
1. History

A. What is her smoking history?   ESSENTIAL

All patients should be asked their smoking history; however, it becomes even more critical when dealing with patients who are experiencing acute respiratory distress, dyspnea, other pulmonary symptoms, and/or chest pain.

If the patient is a nonsmoker, then he or she should be questioned regarding never smoking vs quitting smoking. If the patient is a previous smoker, then it is important to know how long ago the patient quit, how much he or she smoked, and for how long. It takes several years from ceasing smoking until the risks of CAD, cerebral vascular accident (CVA), lung cancer, and other cancers return to baseline (if they ever do). Pulmonary function tends to improve; however, if the patient had severe disease before he or she stopped smoking, it likely will never return to normal. Furthermore, risks from smoking tend to be dose dependent (i.e., the more cigarettes smoked per day and the longer the duration of smoking, the more severe the pulmonary disease and the greater the risks of complications). This total amount is described in terms of pack-years. For example, if a patient has smoked one pack of cigarettes per day for the last 5 years, that patient would have a smoking history of 5 pack-years. Since it is already known that Mrs. Queen is a smoker, the primary purpose for this question would be to calculate her pack-year history.

B. When was her previous menstrual period and was it normal?   NONESSENTIAL

When treating any woman of childbearing age, it is important to know when her last menstrual period (LMP) occurred, whether it was normal (because some women do have light periods for the first few months of pregnancy), what method of contraception she employs, and how reliably she uses it. All of this information assists in determining if there is a possibility of pregnancy.

The primary reason for acquiring this data is that there is very little information on the effects of a medication on a fetus aside from anecdotal information and animal studies. Because the first trimester of pregnancy is when the majority of medications can do the most harm to the developing fetus and is

when the mother might not be aware of her pregnancy, raising the potential is crucial. If there is a strong suspicion of a potential pregnancy and she is nearly due for her next menstrual period, then a pregnancy test can be performed with a high degree of accuracy. However, a negative test does not necessarily rule out a possible pregnancy. In such cases, medication choices need to be made on a risk vs benefit basis, trying to avoid the ones known to cause fetal harm in cases of early pregnancy.

The FDA ranks drugs by category depending on the currently known risks. Category A drugs consist of medications for which there are adequate studies to indicate that they are probably safe to take in the first trimester (or later on) in pregnancy. Category B medications include those medications for which there are no adequate human studies but animal studies have not revealed any harm to the developing fetus OR animal studies revealed adverse fetal effects but human studies have failed to reveal the problem during the first or subsequent trimesters. Category C is composed of drugs for which no adequate human studies exist OR no adequate human studies exist but animal studies revealed harm to the developing fetus. For this category, the decision to prescribe depends on the benefit vs risk ratio for each individual patient. Category D drugs have been shown to cause adverse effects to the developing fetus; however, depending on the mother's condition, its severity, and the availability of alternative treatment choices, the benefits may still outweigh the risks. Obviously the decision of whether to use these drugs must be made on a case-by-case basis. Category X medications are those for which animal and/or human studies have shown marked fetal abnormalities and/or toxicities and the risks definitely outweigh the benefits.

However, because Mrs. Queen had a BTL (which is a very effective contraceptive method) and is currently menstruating normally, additional information regarding her menstruation history is not necessary because it would not provide any useful clinical information that would affect the decision-making process. Therefore, this question does not need to be asked.

C. Has she had any leg or foot edema, erythema, or pain? ESSENTIAL

Because of her acute onset of severe dyspnea, chest pain, tachycardia, tachypnea, smoking history, and recent air travel, a PE must be included in her differential diagnoses. Because a DVT is the primary cause of a PE, it is important to determine if the patient has or had any symptoms suspicious for such.

D. Does she use hormonal contraceptives?   ESSENTIAL

Many women when questioned regarding their medications do not include birth control pills (BCPs) or other hormonal contraceptive devices (e.g., intrauterine device [IUD], vaginal ring, or patch). Therefore, women of childbearing age, especially if their chief complaint could be caused by or their treatment could be adversely affected by concurrent hormonal contraceptive usage, should be specifically asked about hormonal contraceptive usage as a routine component of the medication history. Although Mrs. Queen had a BTL, she still should be asked specifically about hormonal contraceptive usage because she might be on some formulation for her endometriosis. The primary concern for Mrs. Queen, especially considering her smoking history, would be a PE.

E. Has she recently taken a long trip via air?   ESSENTIAL

Recent studies indicate an association between long trips made by airplane, especially without getting up and moving about the cabin or at least frequent movement of the lower extremities while seated, and the risk of a DVT (which is a significant risk factor for a PE).

2. Physical Examination

A. Evaluation for nasal septal deviation   NONESSENTIAL

B. Evaluation for tracheal deviation   ESSENTIAL

Because of the sudden onset and severity of her respiratory distress, conditions such as pneumothorax, hemothorax, and rapidly developing pleural effusions must be considered in her potential differential diagnoses. These can cause tracheal deviation.

C. Heart examination   ESSENTIAL

Because of the sudden onset of her symptoms and her complaints of dyspnea and chest pain, a complete heart examination as outlined in Case 1-2 is essential.

D. Lung examination   ESSENTIAL

Because of the acute onset of her symptoms and presence of respiratory distress, a thorough lung examination as outlined in Case 1-5 is also indicated.

E. Ankle and leg examination   ESSENTIAL

Because of the sudden onset and nature of her shortness of breath, a PE must be considered among her differential diagnoses. Because the main source of a PE is a DVT, it is imperative that her lower extremities be evaluated for edema, erythema, and tenderness. Some experts feel that this evaluation should not include a Homan sign because the rapid flexion of the ankle could cause the DVT to dislodge and progress to form a PE. However, because Mrs. Queen already has symptoms consistent with a PE, this is irrelevant.

An alternative to performing a traditional Homan sign, recommended by some providers, is to place a sphygmometer cuff around the patient's calf and pump its bladder until the patient begins experiencing pain (not just compression). Then repeat the procedure on the contralateral leg. If there is a significant difference between the two measurements, a possibility of a DVT in the leg with the lower reading exists.

3. Diagnostic Studies

A. Well's criteria for pulmonary embolism (PE) risk and D-dimer ESSENTIAL

Because there are no symptoms, signs, or constellations that are specific for a PE, the Well's criteria can be utilized to estimate the likelihood of a patient's symptoms being caused by a PE. It utilizes a combination of history, physical examination, and clinical suspicion to make the determination. Points are assigned to each item and then totaled. If the score is a 4 or lower, the probability of a PE is low; if the score is higher than a 4, then a PE is likely.

Three points are assigned if the patient has signs and symptoms consistent with a PE (which is defined as a minimum

of pedal edema with tenderness to deep vein palpation). An additional 3 points are added if a PE is at the top of the patient's differential diagnosis list. One and one-half points are given if the patient is tachycardic (pulse > 100 BPM), and an additional 1.5 points are assigned if the patient has been immobile for longer than 3 days or has had any type of surgery within the past 4 weeks. One point is given if the patient has a history of a previous DVT or PE. An additional 1 point is given if the patient has hemoptysis. A final 1 point is added if the patient has an active malignancy, regardless of site (for a maximum total of 12 points).

Regarding Mrs. Queen's case, she has a few symptoms that could be associated with a PE; however, she does not have any leg/ankle edema and her right calf tenderness is not significantly different from her left calf when measured objectively by sphygmomanometer. Therefore, she does not technically meet the minimally established criteria for this item. Because other conditions are higher on her list of differential diagnoses than a PE, she does not get any points for this item either. She is tachycardic, earning her 1.5 points. The remaining items are all negative per her history; hence, they do not yield her any additional points. Thus, her final score is 1.5 points, meaning she has a low probability of a PE being the cause of her symptoms.

If the patient's Well's probability score is a 4 or lower, then a D-dimer is recommended. If the D-dimer is within normal range, a PE can essentially be ruled out as the patient's diagnosis. However, if the Well's probability score is higher than a 4, then the patient should have a spiral chest CT to evaluate for the presence of a PE. Inconclusive CT results are associated with an improbable likelihood of the patient having a PE that is clinically significant; however, observation, reevaluation, and alternative testing (e.g., lung scan) are essential.

B. Sputum for Gram stain, culture, and sensitivity NONESSENTIAL

The lack of wheezing, rales, fever, prodromal symptoms, or a productive cough in conjunction with the rapid onset of her symptoms make the likelihood of a pulmonary infection causing her symptoms extremely low.

C. Arterial blood gases (ABGs)   ESSENTIAL

ABGs are indicated because Mrs. Queen is hypoxemic, evident by an O_2 sat of less than 90%.

D. Chest x-ray (CXR)   ESSENTIAL

A CXR is definitely indicated because of the severity of her pulmonary symptoms (e.g., tachypnea and hypoxia), and the presence of tracheal deviation.

E. Electrocardiogram (ECG)   ESSENTIAL

An ECG is indicated to determine whether her tachycardia is sinus in origin or from another arrhythmia that could potentially be the cause of her current symptoms. Additionally, an ECG will be useful to determine if any cardiovascular processes are responsible for, or contributing to, her dyspnea (e.g., heart failure (HF) or an acute myocardial infarction [AMI]).

4. Diagnosis

A. Pulmonary embolism   INCORRECT

Because of Mrs. Queen's low Well's PE probability rating score, her normal D-dimer test, and lack of signs and/or symptoms suggesting a recent or current DVT, a PE is not her most likely diagnosis.

B. Pleural effusion secondary to pneumonia   INCORRECT

Although pneumonia can cause a pleural effusion, there should be evidence of both on CXR—the presence of a consolidation/infiltrate and fluid (which tends to be more opaque than air/gas), respectively. Furthermore, pneumonia is associated with symptoms of an acute infection (e.g., fever, chills, and fatigue). Thus, this is not her most likely diagnosis.

C. Pneumothorax secondary to pneumonia   INCORRECT

Even though Mrs. Queen's symptoms, physical examination findings, and CXR results are consistent with a pneumothorax, they are not consistent with the diagnosis of pneumonia, as discussed previously. Therefore, this is not her most likely diagnosis.

D. Catamenial pneumothorax   CORRECT

Mrs. Queen has a pneumothorax; therefore, the major diagnostic question is its cause. Because Mrs. Queen has a history of endometriosis and is currently menstruating, catamenial pneumothorax is her most likely diagnosis from the choices provided.

E. Iatrogenic pneumothorax   INCORRECT

An iatrogenic pneumothorax occurs as a result of a diagnostic procedure, such as subclavian line placement, thoracentesis, or pleural biopsy; because Mrs. Queen has not undergone any causative procedure, iatrogenic pneumothorax can be eliminated as her most likely diagnosis.

5. Treatment Plan

A. Oxygen therapy   CORRECT

Because of her severe dyspnea and hypoxemia, oxygen therapy is indicated.

B. Tube thoracostomy   CORRECT

Because of the marked degree of Mrs. Queen's respiratory distress and the significant size of her pneumothorax (> 15% is the current indication for this procedure), the placement of a chest tube is indicated. Nevertheless, it is essential to remember that the "15% rule" is a guideline, not an absolute. Sound clinical judgment is required to determine if and when a tube thoracostomy is required. Depending on the severity of the patient's symptoms, the HCP's level of expertise, the availability of a pulmonary surgeon, and the physical location of the patient, other alternatives could be utilized including performing a thoracentesis with a catheter-over-needle tap, performing an open thoracostomy, transporting the patient, or observing the patient.

A catheter-over-needle tap may be justified when a tension pneumothorax is present, the patient is critically ill, and the diagnosis is relatively certain, even without the availability of a confirmatory CXR.

C. Hospitalization   CORRECT

The severity of her symptoms and the need for a tube thoracostomy, oxygen therapy, frequent vital sign assessment, close observation, telemetry, and frequent CXRs make hospitalization essential.

D. Smoking cessation   CORRECT

At all visits, smoking status should be assessed. If the patient is a smoker, he or she should be advised to quit. According to a recent study, being advised by a "doctor" to quit smoking was the number one motivator for patients to stop smoking.

A good approach to smoking cessation involves utilizing the 5 A's as developed by the Agency for Health Care Policy and Research: **A**sk, **A**dvise, **A**ttempt, **A**ssist, and **A**rrange.

E. IV gentamicin   INCORRECT

Mrs. Queen does not have any signs or symptoms indicating an infection is present; therefore, she does not require an antibiotic at this time.

Epidemiologic and Other Data

A pneumothorax is air that has been trapped between the parietal pleura and the visceral pleura. In general, pneumothoraxes are caused by the rupturing of diseased lung tissue (the most common being COPD-related bullae) or penetrating trauma, including those associated with medical procedures.

In contrast to popular misperception, spontaneous pneumothoraxes are rare. A true spontaneous pneumothorax (rupture of a normal alveolus), is most generally the result of trauma, most commonly associated with rib fractures and diving accidents. They can also occur without any cause in tall, thin individuals, with the majority of these cases occurring during adolescence.

The exact incidence of pneumothoraxes is unknown. However, approximately 50% of patients who experience a pneumothorax that is related to an underlying lung abnormality will experience a second one.

CASE 2-8
Quincy Rodgers
1. History

A. Has he ever had a CXR prior to 1 month ago?   ESSENTIAL

Mr. Rodgers' current CXR exhibits a solitary pulmonary nodule (SPN). It is unknown if it was present and obscured by his pneumonia, if it was caused by his pneumonia, or even if he had pneumonia (based on the symptom history he provided—emphasizing the importance of treating the patient, not the diagnostic test). Because approximately 40% of all SPNs are malignant in nature, it cannot be assumed that it was caused by the pneumonia or some other benign process. Hence, an evaluation to rule out a malignancy is essential.

Because of the known "doubling time" of the various forms of lung cancer, it can be assumed that an SPN is non-malignant if it has remained stable in size for at least 2 years. However, on the other hand, if it has increased in size, it is almost always cancerous. A rare exception is inflammatory nodules, which can double in size in less than 20 days.

Thus, knowing if he had a previous CXR as well as when and where it was taken can be useful. If a prior CXR exists, the film could be located; and, if a SPN was present, its size could be compared with its current size to provide an indication of its potential for malignancy.

B. Has he had any arthralgias, bone pain, or subcutaneous knots or nodules?   ESSENTIAL

The majority (~60%) of SPNs are due to a benign process. Therefore, it is imperative to question the patient regarding symptoms that are associated with nonmalignant causes. The most are a prior granulomatous infection, a fungal infection, or a mycobacterium infection. Some extrapulmonary manifestations that are commonly seen in granulomatous and fungal infections include meningitis, arthralgias, frank arthritis, bone pain, erythema nodosum, erythema multiforme, toxic erythema, and other rashes. However, bone pain can also represent bony metastases.

C. Has he been experiencing any night sweats?   ESSENTIAL

Night sweats are often associated with malignant processes. However, they can also occur in nonmalignant infections such as tuberculosis, coccidioidomycosis, histoplasmosis, or babesiosis. Incidentally, night sweats that persist for more than 3 weeks are one of the criteria that suggest that antifungal therapy should be considered in patients with coccidioidomycosis.

D. Do his symptoms increase when he drinks alcohol?   NONESSENTIAL

None of the conditions on Mr. Rodgers' differential diagnosis list is worsened by alcohol intake.

E. What was his maximum temperature and what time of day did it occur? Did he experience fluctuations in his temperature not associated with antipyretic therapy?   ESSENTIAL

The "normal" oral temperature of 98.6°F was derived by measuring the oral temperatures in a large population of healthy individuals between the ages of 18 and 40 years. The range of "normal" oral temperatures from this evaluation was 98.2° ± 0.7°F. Hence, the range of "normal" oral temperatures is from 97.5° to 98.9°F. Rectal temperatures average approximately 0.5°F higher than oral temperatures and axillary temperatures average approximately 0.5°F lower.

Furthermore, the body's normal temperature has a diurnal variation, with the lowest temperature occurring at approximately 6:00 a.m. and the highest temperature occurring at 6:00 p.m. An individual's temperature can vary as much as 1.8°F throughout the day and still be considered "normal." Maximum normal body temperatures have been defined for these times of day. For 6:00 a.m., it is 98.9°F, and for 6:00 p.m., it is 99.9°F. Anything above these values is considered to be febrile in 99% of the population. Therefore, if a patient had an oral temperature of 99.6°F, he or she would be considered febrile if the temperature was taken at 6:00 a.m.; however, if it was taken at 6:00 p.m., he or she would not be considered to have a fever. Therefore, the actual temperature, time of day taken, usage of antipyretics, and method taken (not to mention consumption of hot or cold beverages or food before oral temperature is taken) can have a significant impact on the definition and degree of febrility of the patient.

2. Physical Examination

A. Heart examination   ESSENTIAL

Because of his persistent cough and fatigue, a complete heart examination (as outlined in Case 1-2) is indicated to rule out other conditions that could be coexisting with or related to his SPN (e.g., valvular heart disease, subacute bacterial endocarditis, pericarditis, or myocarditis).

B. Lung examination   ESSENTIAL

Because Mr. Rodgers is here for a follow-up of a presumed bacterial pneumonia and still has an abnormal CXR, a complete lung examination as outlined in Case 1-5 is essential.

C. Neurologic examination   NONESSENTIAL

Even though benign and malignant SPNs can be associated with brain complications (e.g., meningitis, stroke, metastatic disease, and brain abscess), Mr. Rodgers does not have any symptoms suggesting a neurologic abnormality. Thus, a neurologic exam is not necessary at this time.

D. Skin examination   NONESSENTIAL

Mr. Rodgers denies a rash and/or subcutaneous lesions; therefore, a skin examination is not currently indicated.

E. Supraclavicular, infraclavicular, and axillary lymph node examination   ESSENTIAL

The primary lymphatic channels that are associated with the chest wall, lungs, and other intrathoracic structures drain into the hilar, supraclavicular, infraclavicular, and axillary lymph nodes. Therefore, with the possibility of a malignant, infectious, or inflammatory process being responsible for his SPN, a thorough examination of these nodal areas is essential. Although the hilar lymph nodes cannot be palpated, they can be evaluated by CXR, by CT, or by cytology.

3. Diagnostic Studies

A. Whole body ^{18}F-fluro-deoyx-D-glucose positron emission tomography scan (FDG-PET)   NONESSENTIAL

The primary purpose of performing an FDG-PET is to further evaluate the mediastinum in patients with mediastinal masses or hilar lymphadenopathy before performing surgery. Because Mr. Rodgers' CXR did not reveal an abnormal mediastinum, he does not have any evidence of lymphadenopathy, and no surgery is currently being planned for him, this test is unnecessary.

B. Repeat CXR again in 2 weeks   NONESSENTIAL

His only remaining CXR abnormality is the SPN; however, a repeat CXR in 2 weeks is too soon to yield any useful clinical information regarding a change. All it would do is expose him to unnecessary radiation; therefore, a repeat CXR in 2 weeks is not indicated for Mr. Rodgers.

C. CT scan of chest with and without contrast   ESSENTIAL

A CT scan with and without contrast would provide a baseline and predictive, but not diagnostic, information. The most specific and sensitive method of determining the presence of a malignancy is via histologic examination. Unfortunately, because of the poor yield from fiberoptic bronchoscopy (~40%) and CT-guided fine needle biopsy (~50%), a major procedure such as a thoracotomy or a thoracoscopic resection is required to obtain an adequate sample for evaluation.

Hence, other methods (e.g., serial CXRs and CT scans) are often employed if the suspicion of malignancy is low (e.g., the patient is younger than 30 years old; does not have any underlying pulmonary disease; has never smoked; and has not had significant exposure to second-hand smoke, asbestos, or other known carcinogens; and the lesion has clearly defined, smooth margins, intralesional calcifications, lacks uptake of IV radiographic contrast media, and, is stable over time) to ensure that the lesion remains unchanged. However, if growth is detected or other abnormalities develop (e.g., hilar lymphadenopathy), further investigation is required.

D. Traditional tube (TP) and complement fixation (CF) assays for coccidioidomycosis ESSENTIAL

Because coccidioidomycosis can cause the symptoms and CXR findings that Mr. Rodgers is experiencing and he lives in an area where this fungus is endemic, both TP and CF antibody assays for coccidioidomycosis are indicated. The TP antibody is measurable in the serum very quickly after infection occurs and persists for weeks. The CF antibody does not begin to elevate until later on in the infection; however, it persists longer in the serum. Increasing CF antibody titers indicate clinical progression of the disease.

The TP and CF antibodies can also be identified via immunodiffusion testing known as IDTP and IDCF, respectively. The results of the TP and IDTP appear to be fairly equivalent, as do the CF and IDCF values.

Enzyme immunoassays (EIAs) for IgM and IgG of coccidioidomycosis are also commercially available. The IgM elevates in the acute phase of the infection and the IgG elevates later on. Because of the high incidence of false-positive results associated with the IgM EIA, it is not recommended as a screening test for coccidioidomycosis. However, the IgG EIA appears to be fairly equivalent to the CF assay in determining the chronicity of the disease.

E. Mantoux tuberculin skin test (TST) ESSENTIAL

Both typical and atypical *Mycobacterium* infections can produce an SPN and the symptoms Mr. Rodgers has been experiencing. Thus, a Mantoux TST is indicated.

4. Diagnosis

A. TB of the lungs INCORRECT

TB of the lungs can essentially be eliminated as Mr. Rodgers' most likely diagnosis because his TST area of induration was less than 15 cm (negative because he does not fall into any of the high-risk groups for which a lower cut-off point exists) and he has not recently been in close contact with an individual infected with TB.

B. Lung cancer INCORRECT

Lung cancer is not Mr. Rodgers' most likely diagnosis at this time because he has positive TP and CF assays and a benign appearance of the SPN on both CXR and CT. Additionally, he doesn't have any of the aforementioned risk factors for the condition.

SPNs in patients who are younger than 35 years old have a malignancy rate of less than 1%; however, for patients older than the age of 50 years, this rate increases to 60%. Still, he will require his choice of close follow-up or a histologic examination until stability or resolution is certain.

C. Unresolved pneumonia INCORRECT

Mr. Rodgers' current symptoms consist of an essentially unchanged (but definitely not worse) nonproductive cough,

night sweats, questionable fever, chills, and fatigue. Furthermore, he never experienced any characteristic signs and symptoms of pneumonia (e.g., appearing moderately to severely ill, wheezing, rales, dyspnea, tachypnea, confirmed fever, and/or chest pain), making the initial, let alone current, diagnosis suspect. Additionally, the fact that the infiltrate is resolved and an SPN persists on CXR also points to the low likelihood of this being his most likely diagnosis.

D. Coccidioidomycosis CORRECT

Coccidioidomycosis is a respiratory infection caused by inhalation of the spores of *Coccidioides immitis* or *Coccidioides posadasii* fungus. This is Mr. Rodgers' most likely diagnosis because his history, physical findings, and diagnostic studies are consistent with this illness. Furthermore, he lives in an area (southwestern United States) that is endemic to this fungal infection.

E. Lung abscess INCORRECT

Lung abscesses are associated with much more toxic-appearing patients and different qualities to the SPN on CXR and CT scanning. For example, the walls of a lung abscess tend to be distinct but thickened in appearance and surrounded by consolidation. Furthermore, an air-fluid level is usually evident within the SPN. Hence, this is not Mr. Rodgers' most likely diagnosis.

5. Treatment Plan

A. Combination therapy with isoniazid (INH), rifampin (RIF), ethambutol (EMB), and pyrazinamide (PZA) daily INCORRECT

Even though Mr. Rodgers had an indurated area from his TST, it was not considered positive in consideration of his risk factors. Therefore, initiating combination therapy with INH, RIF, EMB, and PZA daily would not be indicated.

B. Referral to oncologist INCORRECT

Referral to an oncologist would be an inappropriate choice at this time because there is no evidence that Mr. Rodgers' SPN represents a lung carcinoma.

If Mr. Rodgers is extremely concerned regarding the possibility of having lung cancer, then a referral to a thoracic surgeon would be an appropriate option. However, as discussed previously, it is highly probable that he would require a major procedure such as a thoracotomy or a thoracoscopic resection to obtain a sample that could be histologically evaluated with enough sensitivity and specificity to provide him with any degree of reassurance. Still, this is not going to be 100% conclusive.

C. Hospitalization for IV gentamicin INCORRECT

Hospitalization for IV antibiotics is an inappropriate option because there is no evidence to support the presence of a bacterial infection, lung or otherwise. Therefore, all this option would do is potentially contribute to the problem of antibiotic resistance and place Mr. Rodgers at risk for adverse effects from this somewhat toxic medication.

D. Repeat CXR (and possibly CT scan) in 3 months and repeat coccidioidomycosis CF levels in 2 weeks CORRECT

A repeat CXR and possibly CT scan in 3 months are indicated to follow the progression of the lesion, especially its size and border smoothness. If histologic examination is not performed, radiological follow-up should be undertaken every 3 months for 2 years. If the lesion regresses or remains stable at the end of 2 years, it can essentially be ruled as benign.

Even if a histologic examination is performed and is negative, some type of radiographic follow-up is still going to be required because of the aforementioned limited specificity of the various biopsying techniques for providing adequate tissue samples for histological evaluation.

Repeating the coccidioidomycosis CF assay in 2 weeks is important because an increasing level would confirm a diagnosis of coccidioidomycosis for Mr. Rodgers; unfortunately, it could also indicate a progression of the disease. A stable or decreasing titer would indicate stability of the disease, or perhaps even improvement of Mr. Rodgers' condition. Regardless of the findings, he will still need the aforementioned diagnostic studies to ensure the stability of his SPN because it is not impossible for him to have both coccidioidomycosis and lung cancer.

E. Initiation of triazole therapy   CORRECT

The majority of individuals with a localized pulmonary infection caused by *C. immitis* or *C. posadasii* do not require antifungal treatment. However, it is recommended for patients who are immunocompromised, are symptomatic for at least 2 months, have been experiencing night sweats for more than 3 weeks, have a significant weight loss (defined as > 10% of their preillness body weight), have a positive CF assay at greater than 1:16, have extensive pulmonary involvement on CXR, or are experiencing disseminated disease. Because Mr. Rodgers has been having night sweats for approximately 4 weeks now and has a CF titer of 1:64, he should be treated with antifungal therapy. The preferred antifungal for coccidioidomycosis is a triazole, such as posaconazole.

Epidemiologic and Other Data

Coccidioidomycosis, or "valley fever," is a fungal infection caused by *C. immitis* or *C. posadaiii*. Regardless of which species is involved in the patient's infection, the clinical picture, course, and outcome are identical.

Coccidioidomycosis is found in the soil in endemic areas. Those areas are typically found between 40° North and 40° South latitudes in the Western hemisphere. In the United States, the highest concentrations are found in south-central Arizona, the south San Joaquin Valley, and the southwest Rio Grande Valley. Other US regions where coccidioidomycosis is endemic are California's southern coastal areas, Nevada's southern portions, and Utah's southwestern areas.

The overall infectious rate of residents of these areas is approximately 3% per year. Approximately 60% of all infected individuals are asymptomatic, approximately 40% develop localized primary pneumonia, and less than 1% develop a diffuse pneumonia. Pulmonary sequelae (e.g., SPN, cavitation, and chronic pneumonia) occur in approximately 5% of infected individuals. Disseminated disease, with skin, soft tissue, bony, or brain (primarily meningitis) involvement, occurs in approximately 1% or fewer of all infected individuals.

Disseminated coccidioidomycosis is more common in immunocompromised patients, elderly individuals, pregnant women, and non-Hispanic whites (Filipino Americans and African Americans have the greatest rates of infection).

CASE 2-9
Rhonda Smith
1. History

A. What does she mean by "tired all the time" and does she experience insomnia?   ESSENTIAL

Due to the vast array of symptoms patient report as fatigue, it is essential to determine exactly what symptoms he or she is experiencing. Still, the complaint of fatigue can generally be categorized into one of three groups: total exhaustion due to a lack of motivation or desire (most often due to a major mood disorder); tiring much quicker or easier than usual (most often due to medical conditions); or sleepiness (seen with psychological problems, medical conditions, or inadequate sleep).

Another distinction between physical and emotional fatigue is its pattern. In general, patients who have psychological fatigue wake up in the mornings virtually as tired as they were before they retired the previous night; however, as the day progresses, the fatigue often improves. Conversely, patients with physical causes for their fatigue tend to wake up feeling at least somewhat (if not fully) refreshed and get tired as the day progresses or with exertion.

Insomnia associated with daytime sleepiness can be caused by lack of adequate sleep, sleep apnea, or some other dyssomnia. Additionally, sleep apnea could potentially cause chronic hoarseness. Any form of insomnia (but especially early morning awakening) with her complaint of fatigue could indicate the presence of depression, which could alter the quality of voice, causing it to be flatter and quieter (which some could describe as hoarseness). Insomnia in the form of difficulty getting to sleep is most often associated with anxiety. Fragmented sleep can be the result of a major mood disorder (e.g., depression and/or anxiety) or a physical illness (e.g., pain disorders, asthma, sleep apnea, other respiratory conditions, or thyroid disease).

B. Has she experienced an unintentional change in her weight?   ESSENTIAL

Unintentional weight loss can be associated with depression but is more commonly seen with physical conditions (e.g., severe chronic respiratory diseases, malabsorption syndromes, diabetes mellitus, hyperthyroidism, pituitary adenomas, and most cancers). Unintentional weight gain is the more typical pattern for depression but it is also seen in medical conditions such as hypothyroidism, HF, and azotemia.

Mrs. Smith's decrease from 115 lb to 105 lb in the past month is considered a significant weight loss because it is greater than 5% of her body weight in a 1-month period.

C. Does she have a decreased mood, increased stress, anhedonia, and/or anxiety?   ESSENTIAL

As stated previously, depression can cause "pseudohoarseness." Other psychological illnesses seen with "pseudohoarseness" include somatization disorder, conversion disorder, or factitious disorder.

On the other hand, many chronic medical conditions can also be associated with depression. This appears to be especially true of neurologic (e.g., brain tumors, benign brain lesions, multiple sclerosis, or myasthenia gravis) and cardiovascular (e.g., ischemic or hemorrhagic cerebral vascular accidents) conditions, which could be the cause of Mrs. Smith's hoarseness.

D. Is she experiencing dysphagia?   ESSENTIAL

The presence of dysphagia in conjunction with hoarseness almost always represents a neuromuscular disorder. If the hoarseness began before the dysphagia, then the neuromuscular abnormality is most likely to be one that affects the larynx. However, if the dysphagia is present before the hoarseness, then the most likely cause involves the recurrent laryngeal nerve.

E. Does she have any warts on her hands or feet?   NON-ESSENTIAL

Recurrent respiratory papillomatosis can cause chronic hoarseness. The lesions are caused by the human papillomavirus (HPV); however, respiratory papillomatosis is caused by a different strain of HPV than the one that causes verruca vulgaris, verruca plana, filiform warts, and plantar warts. Of the 100+ strains of HPV, virtually all the cases of respiratory papillomatosis are associated with HPV 6 or HPV 11 (incidentally, the same ones that cause genital warts). Dermatologic verrucae are generally caused by HPV 1. Thus, having dermatologic verrucae does not increase the patient's risk of having respiratory papillomatosis.

2. Physical Examination

A. Observation of hoarseness/voice   ESSENTIAL

An abnormal vibration of the vocal cords is generally the cause of hoarseness. If the vocal cords do not completely come together, then too much air passes between the unopposed vocal cords' larger opening, and the result is a "breathy" quality to the voice. This generally occurs with a unilateral paralysis of the vocal cords. If the vocal cords do not vibrate regularly and are stiff, then the voice has a harsh-sounding quality. This is often seen in laryngitis and laryngeal cancer.

B. Oral mucosa/pharyngeal examination, including indirect laryngoscope   ESSENTIAL

Many localized conditions can be responsible for persistent hoarseness (e.g., chronic laryngitis [most common pathogens are *M. tuberculosis, Histoplasma, Blastomyces*, and *Candida*]; laryngeal tumors, polyps, cysts, and papillomatosis; traumatic lesions affecting the vocal folds; chronic postnasal discharge; laryngopharyngeal reflux; and vocal cord paralysis).

Regardless of the cause, it is recommended by the American Academy of Otolaryngologists Head and Neck Surgery (AAO-HNS) Neurolaryngology Committee to perform an indirect laryngoscopy in addition to a complete oral and pharyngeal examination on any patient who has hoarseness that persists longer than 2 weeks. This evidence-based recommendation is to derived from the fact that all cases of acute laryngitis should be completely resolved within 2 weeks of the resolution of any other precipitating upper respiratory infection–like symptoms.

C. Heart examination   ESSENTIAL

A heart examination is indicated to assess for signs of valvular abnormalities that could place the patient at risk for developing emboli (either dependently or independently of a

cardiac arrhythmia) and reevaluate the regularity of the patient's heart rate as a possible cause of a thromboembolic phenomenon (i.e., small stroke affecting the blood supply to the recurrent laryngeal nerve). If any abnormalities are discovered, then an echocardiogram and possibly magnetic resonance imaging (MRI), magnetic resonance angiography (MRA), or ultrasound of the cranial blood vessels are indicated.

D. Lung examination   ESSENTIAL

A lung examination is indicated because pulmonary conditions such as carcinomas, tumors, and asthma can produce hoarseness, most often by compressing the recurrent laryngeal nerve.

E. Evaluation of cervical, supraclavicular, infraclavicular, and axillary lymph nodes   ESSENTIAL

These are the primary lymph nodes involved in the drainage of the neck, larynx, chest wall, lungs, and intrathoracic structures (in addition to the hilar lymph nodes [which are obviously not palpable on physical examination]); thus, it is essential to evaluate these nodes for evidence of a lymphadenopathy that can be seen with carcinomas, infections, and inflammatory conditions.

3. Diagnostic Studies

A. CT scan of chest, with and without contrast   NONESSENTIAL

A CT scan is not indicated as a first-line diagnostic procedure for hoarseness because of the amount of radiation associated with the procedure coupled with the risk of an adverse event from the contrast media. Therefore, a plain film chest radiograph is always indicated first.

If an abnormality is found on CXR, then it is appropriate to proceed with the CT scan. This technique also permits the radiologist to focus the CT examination on the area associated with the abnormality; however, it is essential to still conduct a complete examination.

B. Chest x-ray (CXR)   ESSENTIAL

A chest x-ray is indicated as a first-line diagnostic study in a patient with chronic hoarseness to rule out benign or malignant tumors compressing adjacent nerves and producing the symptoms.

C. 24-hour pH monitoring of lower esophagus   NONESSENTIAL

Despite the fact that laryngopharyngeal reflux can produce chronic hoarseness, fewer than half of the individuals with this condition are symptomatic for even lower esophageal symptoms of GERD. Furthermore, the majority of these patients fail to meet the diagnostic criteria for GERD with conventional pH monitoring of the lower esophagus.

Therefore, if there is a strong suspicion that laryngopharyngeal reflux is responsible for the patient's hoarseness (and the direct laryngoscopy and CXR do not reveal any pathology), the most appropriate test to order is dual-probe (distal and proximal) pH monitoring with manometry. However, this combination is still associated with a significantly high rate of false-negatives. Thus, the pH of the larynx might need to be directly tested.

Because of these diagnostic challenges, the AAO-HNS Committee on Speech, Voice and Swallowing Disorders' position statement on laryngopharyngeal reflux recommends treatment with a proton pump inhibitor (PPI) at full strength twice a day for a minimum of 3 to 6 months before considering any gastrointestinal testing for this condition. Additionally, they recommend careful initial and reevaluation examinations (including the use of indirect laryngoscopy) at 3 months if improvement is not seen. Often, it can take 6 months of PPI therapy before relief is appreciable.

D. Bacterial throat culture and sensitivity   NONESSENTIAL

There are no known bacterial organisms that can cause chronic laryngitis. Therefore, a plain bacterial culture with sensitivity is not going to provide any useful information, and might even confuse the "picture" if normal oral flora are grown.

However, fungal scrapings, fungal cultures with sensitivities, AFB staining, and TB cultures with sensitivities are indicated if an infectious process is suspected as the cause because these represent the primary pathogens found in chronic laryngitis as discussed previously.

E. Rapid strep screen   NONESSENTIAL

Group A β-hemolytic streptococci is not a pathogen in chronic laryngitis.

4. Diagnosis

A. Asthma   INCORRECT

Although asthma can cause chronic hoarseness, it can essentially be eliminated as Mrs. Smith's most likely diagnosis because she does not have any "typical" asthma signs and symptoms (e.g., dyspnea, cough, wheezing, rales, and fluctuations/exacerbations of her symptoms).

B. Lung cancer   CORRECT

Lung cancer is Mrs. Smith's most likely diagnosis for her chronic hoarseness because of the suspicious-appearing mass on her CXR combined with her vocal cord palsy on indirect laryngoscopy. The hoarseness is generally caused by regional expansion of the tumor mass compressing the recurrent laryngeal nerve, resulting in paralysis of the vocal cords.

C. Acute laryngitis   INCORRECT

Acute laryngitis is the most common cause for hoarseness. However, the patient should have a history of a URI preceding the onset of the hoarseness. Furthermore, the hoarseness should not persist beyond 2 weeks after the resolution of the URI. Therefore, acute laryngitis is not Mrs. Smith's most likely diagnosis.

D. Supraglottitis   INCORRECT

Supraglottitis is the more accurate term for epiglottis in adults because the epiglottis itself generally does not become edematous and lead to airway obstruction, as it can in children. Nevertheless, it can be eliminated as Mrs. Smith's most likely diagnosis because the main symptoms of supraglottitis are rapidly developing sore throat and odynophagia (not hoarseness), and the physical examination reveals pharyngeal and supraglottal erythema and edema. Furthermore, it resolves within a few days of treatment with corticosteroids and antibiotics.

E. Laryngopharyngeal reflux   INCORRECT

Laryngopharyngeal reflux can produce chronic hoarseness by the local effect of the chronic gastric acid exposure on the larynx. Only half of the patients have symptoms consistent with reflux and partial regurgitation; therefore, the lack of these symptoms does not necessarily rule this out as a potential diagnosis. However, the suspicious-appearing tumor on her CXR along with the vocal cord paralysis is not consistent with this diagnosis. Therefore, laryngopharyngeal reflux is not Mrs. Smith's most likely diagnosis.

5. Treatment Plan

A. Omeprazole 40 mg once a day for a minimum of 3 months   INCORRECT

This treatment is not indicated for Mrs. Smith because her hoarseness appears to be secondary to lung cancer, not laryngopharyngeal reflux. Even if her diagnosis is laryngopharyngeal reflux, this would still be an incorrect choice because the dose of omeprazole is inadequate. The correct dose is full-strength PPI therapy twice, not once, a day.

B. Referral to pulmonary surgeon for tissue specimen for histologic evaluation of lung mass via fiberoptic bronchoscopy, open thoracotomy, or other method as determined appropriate by the specialist   CORRECT

Because the patient has chronic hoarseness (which is probably secondary to the lung mass compressing her recurrent laryngeal nerve) of 2 months' duration, a 30 pack-year history of cigarette smoking, and a suspicious lesion on CXR, a referral to a pulmonary surgeon to obtain a tissue specimen for histologic evaluation is essential to obtain the correct diagnosis.

C. Amoxicillin 775 mg twice a day for 10 days   INCORRECT

An antibiotic is not indicated because a bacteriologic cause is highly improbable.

D. Otolaryngologist consultation for direct laryngoscope to confirm indirect findings   INCORRECT

The indirect laryngoscope findings do not need to be confirmed because the pulmonary mass is the assumed cause of the vocal cord paralysis, not a local laryngeal condition.

E. Repeat CXR in 3 months to determine if change has occurred in lung lesion   INCORRECT

This approach is not appropriate for Mrs. Smith because of her age, her smoking history, and the suspicious appearance of the lesion on her CXR. She requires prompt evaluation because of the high likelihood of her mass representing a carcinoma. For more information regarding the carcinogenic potential of lung masses, please see Case 2-8.

Epidemiologic and Other Data

Lung cancer is the second most frequently encountered cancer in both men and women in the United States. However, it is the number one cause of cancer deaths in both genders and is responsible for 29% of all cancer deaths. The overall 5-year survival rate is approximately 14%. In 2007, there were over 200,000 new cases of lung cancer diagnosed in the United States, with slightly over half of them being in males.

Technically, lung cancer is defined as tumors that arise from the epithelium of the lungs. These structures include the bronchus, bronchioles, and alveoli. For this reason, some experts recommend the term "bronchogenic carcinoma" instead of "lung cancer" to clarify that this technically does not include sarcomas, lymphomas, or mesotheliomas.

The most common types of bronchogenic cancer are adenocarcinomas (~32%), squamous cell carcinoma (~29%), small cell (oat cell) carcinoma (~18%), and large cell carcinoma (~9%).

The greatest risk factor for lung cancer is cigarette smoking, and it is dose dependent. Cigarette smoking is estimated to increase a person's likelihood of developing bronchogenic cancer by 13-fold. The risk appears to be 150% greater in women than in men. Smoking cessation decreases the risk of developing lung cancer; however, it never returns the risk to that of a nonsmoker. Still, approximately 15% of all bronchogenic carcinomas occur in nonsmokers and are presumably the result of exposure to passive smoke or other environmental carcinogens.

REFERENCES/ADDITIONAL READING

The Agency for Health Care Policy and Research. Smoking cessation clinical practice guidelines. *JAMA*. 1996;275(16): 1270–1280.

Aghababian RV, ed. *Essentials of Emergency Medicine*. Sudbury, MA: Jones & Bartlett Publishers; 2006.

  Anderson III L. Chest injuries. 920–929.

  Garrett AL. Pediatric resuscitation. 9–13.

  Manfredi R. Asthma. 679–684.

  Torrey S, Manno M. Respiratory disorders. 496–506.

  Volturo G, DeBellis RJ. Pneumonia. 691–696.

American Academy of Otolaryngologists-Head and Neck Surgery (AAO-HNS) Neurolaryngology Committee. Common movement disorders affecting the larynx: a report from the Neurolaryngology Committee of the AAO-HNS. *Otolaryngol Head Neck Surg*. 2005;133(5):654–655.

American Academy of Otolaryngologists-Head and Neck Surgery (AAO-HNS) Committee on Speech, Voice and Swallowing Disorders. Laryngopharyngeal reflux: position statement of the Committee on Speech, Voice, and Swallowing Disorders. *Otolaryngol Head Neck Surg*. 2002; 127(1):32–35.

American Academy of Pediatrics' Subcommittee on Diagnosis and Management of Bronchiolitis. Clinical practice guideline: diagnosis and management of bronchiolitis. *Pediatrics*. 2006;118(4):1774–1793.

American Cancer Society. *Cancer Facts & Figures 2008*. Atlanta, GA: American Cancer Society; 2008.

American Thoracic Society (ATS), the Centers for Disease Control and Prevention (CDC), and the Infectious Diseases Society of America (IDSA). Treatment of tuberculosis. *Am J Respir Crit Care Med*. 2003;167:603–662.

Avnon LS, Abu-Shkra M, Flusser D, et al. Pleural effusions associated with rheumatoid arthritis: what cells predominance to anticipate. *Rheumatol Int*. 2007;27(10):919–925.

Balbir-Gurman A, Yigla M, Nahir AM, et al. Rheumatoid pleural effusion. *Semin Arthritis Rheum*. 2006;35(6):368–378.

Centers for Disease Control and Prevention. Ask the experts: pneumococcal polysaccharide vaccine (PPSV). Updated October 2009. http://www.immunize.org/askexperts/experts_ppv.asp. Accessed November 24, 2009.

Centers for Disease Control and Prevention. BGC vaccine. *TB Elimination* 2006; April.

Centers for Disease Control and Prevention. QuantiFERON-TB gold test. *TB Elimination* 2007; October.

Centers for Disease Control and Prevention. Treatment of TB: American Thoracic Society, CDC, and Infectious Diseases Society of America. Errata. *MMWR* Recomm Rep. 2005;53:1203.

Centers for Disease Control and Prevention. Tuberculosis (TB) self-study modules on tuberculosis, number 3. Reviewed June 2009. http://www.cdc.gov/tb/education/ssmodules/module3/ss3infection.htm. Accessed November 28, 2009.

Centers for Disease Control and Prevention Advisory Committee on Immunization Practices. Recommendations of the Advisory Committee on Immunization Practices (ACIP), 2009 (full report). http://www.cdc.gov/vaccines/pubs/acip-list.htm. Accessed November 24, 2009.

Centers for Disease Control and Prevention Advisory Committee on Immunization Practices. Prevention and control of seasonal influenza with vaccines: recommendations of the Advisory Committee on Immunization Practices (ACIP), 2009. *MMRW*. 2009;58(RR08):1–52.

Centers for Disease Control and Prevention Advisory Committee on Immunization Practices. Recommended adult immunization schedule–United States, 2009. *MMWR*. 2009; 57(53).

Department of Health and Human Services, Centers for Disease Control and Prevention, National Institute for Occupational Safety and Health. *NIOSH Hazard Review: Health Effects of Occupational Exposure to Respirable Crystalline Silica*. 2002;April:i-147.

Duke JR Jr, Good JT Jr, Hudson LD, et al. *Frontline Assessment of Common Pulmonary Presentations*. Denver, CO: Snowdrift Pulmonary Foundation, Inc; 2000. http://www.nlhep.org/books/pul_Pre/intro-plpr.html

  Duke Jr JR, Good Jr JT, Hudson LD, et al. Pleural effusion. http://www.nlhep.org/books/pul_Pre/pleural-effusions. htlm. Accessed September 6, 2008.

  Duke Jr JR, Good Jr JT, Hudson LD, et al. Solitary pulmonary nodule http://www.nlhep.org/books/pul_Pre/pleural-nodule.html.

Fatima N. Newer diagnostic techniques for tuberculosis. *Respir Med*. 2009;CME 2:151–154.

Fauci AS, Kasper DL, Longo DL , et al., eds. *Harrison's Principles of Internal Medicine*. 17th ed. New York: McGraw-Hill Medical; 2008.

  Ampel NM. Coccidioidomycosis. 1247–1249.

  Barnes P. Asthma.1596–1607.

  Dinarello CA, Porat R. Fever and Hyperthermia. 117–121.

  Light RW. Disorders of the pleura and mediastinum. 658–1661.

  Mandell L, Wunderink R. Pneumonia. 619–1628.

  Minna JD Schiller JH. Neoplasms of the lung. 551–562.

  Raviglione MC, O'Brien. Tuberculosis. 1006–1020.

  Rubin M, Gonzales R, Sande M. Pharyngitis, sinusitis, otitis, and other upper respiratory tract infections. Neoplasms of the lung. 205–214.

  Speizer FE, Balmes JR. Environmental lung disease. 1611–1619.

Fine MJ, Auble TE, Yealy DM, et al. A prediction rule to identify low-risk patients with community-acquired pneumonia. *N Engl J Med*. 1997;336:243.

Frazier JK. Wheezing. In: Mengel MB, Schwiebert LP, eds. *Family Medicine: Ambulatory Care and Prevention.* 5th ed. New York: McGraw-Hill Medical; 2009: 435–438.

Lalani A, Schneeweiss S. *The Hospital for Sick Children Handbook of Pediatric Emergency Medicine.* Sudbury, MA: Jones & Bartlett Publishers; 2008.

    Komar L. Cardiac emergencies. 155–172.

    Schuh S. Asthma. 142–147.

    Schuh S. Bronchiolitis. 133–138.

Lutfiyya MN, Henley E, Chang LF, Reyburn SW. Diagnosis and treatment of community-acquired pneumonia. *Am Fam Phys.* 2006;73(3):442–450.

Mandell LA, Wunderink RG, Anzueto A, et al. Infectious Diseases Society of America/American Thoracic Society consensus guidelines on the management of community-acquired pneumonia in adults. *Clin Infect Dis.* 2007;44 (Suppl 2):S27–S72.

Mazurek GH, Jereb J, LoBue P, et al. Guidelines for using the QuantiFERON®-TB gold test for detecting *Mycobacterium tuberculosis* infection, United States. *MMRW.* 2005; 54(RR-15):49–55.

Onion DK, series ed. *The Little Black Book of Primary Care.* 5th ed. Sudbury, MA: Jones & Bartlett Publishers; 2006.

    Onion DK. Emergencies. 1.2 Emergency protocols. 2–25.

    Onion DK. Pulmonary Diseases. 16.1 Infections. 965–967.

    Onion DK. Pulmonary Diseases. 16.2 Asthma and interstitial lung disease. 967–988.

    Onion DK. Pulmonary Diseases. 16.4 Pulmonary tumors. 997–1001.

    Onion DK. Pulmonary diseases. 16.5 Miscellaneous. 1001–1008.

    Onion DK, Sears S. Infectious disease. 9.5 Acid-fast organisms. 579–586.

    Onion DK, Sears S. Infectious disease. 9.11 Systemic infections. 615–626.

Pagana KD, Pagana TJ. *Mosby's Diagnostic and Laboratory Test Reference.* 8th ed. St. Louis: Mosby Elsevier; 2007 (multiple pages utilized to provide normal reference values for laboratory tests).

Porcel JM, Light RW. Diagnostic approach to pleural effusions in adults. *Am Fam Physician.* 2006;73(7):1211–1220.

Ringel E . In: Onion DK, series ed. *The Little Black Book of Pulmonary Medicine.* Sudbury, MA: Jones & Bartlett Publishers; 2009.

    Ringel E. Airway diseases. 4.1 Asthma. 167–190.

    Ringel E. Pulmonary infectious disease. 213–299.

    Ringel E. Pulmonary infectious disease. 5.9 Tuberculosis (TB). 251–264.

    Ringel E. Pulmonary infectious disease. 5.14 Fungal infections. 280–292.

    Ringel E. Pulmonary malignancy. 6.1 Bronchogenic carcinoma. 301–320.

    Ringel E. Diffuse parenchymal lung disease. 7.1 Inorganic dust pneumonitis. 325–336.

    Ringel E. Pleural disease. 413–419.

Stephan MR, Chestnutt JC, Fields SA, Toffler WL. Dyspnea. In: Bengel MB, Schwiebert LP, eds. *Family Medicine: Ambulatory Care and Prevention.* 5th ed. New York: McGraw-Hill Medical; 2009:135–140.

U.S. Department of Health and Human Services National Institutes of Health's National Heart Lung and Blood Institute's National Asthma Education and Prevent Program. *Expert Panel Report 3: Guidelines for the Diagnosis and Management of Asthma, Full Report 2007.* Washington, DC: U.S. Department of Health and Human Services; 2007:1–440.

U.S. Preventive Services Task Force. U.S. Preventive Services Task Force recommendations for screening for depression in adults. http://www.ahrq.govclinic/uspstflix.htm#Recommendation. Accessed November 24, 2009.

Wells PS, Anderson DR, Rodger M, et al. Derivation of a simple clinical model to categorize patients probability of pulmonary embolism increasing the models utility with the SimpliRED D-dimer. *Thromb Haemost.* 2000;83(3):416–420.

Yataco JC, Dweik RA. Pleural effusions: evaluation and management. *Cleve Clin J Med.* 2005;72(10):854–856.

CASES IN ENDOCRINE ABNORMALITIES*

CASE 3-1

Sally Thompson

Mrs. Thompson is a 62-year-old Native American female who presents for follow-up on her type 2 diabetes mellitus. Over the past few months, her polydipsia, polyuria, and fatigue have gotten much worse. Otherwise, she states that she is doing well with her diabetes despite not following her diet or taking her medicine. She does not exercise regularly but feels that she gets adequate exercise through her routine daily activities.

Her polyuria has progressed to the point that she has nocturia one or two times every night. Then, after voiding, she experiences terrible difficulty in getting back to sleep (can take as long as 2 hours). This has caused daytime fatigue defined as being "tired all the time" and having difficulties in getting motivated and starting projects/activities. Her polydipsia is also getting worse. Despite that, she has attempted to avoid drinking any beverages after dinner to prevent the nocturia; unfortunately, this strategy is not effective.

She denies visual problems; foot lesions; pain, numbness, or swelling, especially in the lower extremities; chest pain, pressure, or discomfort; palpations; lightheadedness or vertigo; presyncope or syncope; dyspnea; nausea; vomiting; heartburn; gastroparesis; weight change; dysuria; urinary incontinence; tremors; weakness; diaphoresis; or rashes.

She was diagnosed with DM approximately 8 years ago and it is her only known medical problem. She has never been hospitalized nor had any surgery. She is not taking any prescription medications, although she is supposed to be on metformin, rosiglitazone, miglitol, and sitagliptin. She does not take any over-the-counter medications, vitamins, supplements, or herbal preparations. She is not allergic to any medications. She has never smoked or drank alcohol. Her family history is positive for type 2 diabetes mellitus (mother and older sister); premature myocardial infarction (MI; father—fatal at 48 years of age), and hypertension (mother, father, and younger brother).

Her lab results from last revealed a fasting plasma glucose (FPG) of 280 mg/dl (normal: 70-110) and a glycated hemoglobin A1 (Hgb A1C) of 10% (normal: 3.9 to 5.2).

1. Based on this information, which of the following questions are essential to ask Mrs. Thompson and why?

   A. What types of problems did she have with her medications that caused her to discontinue them, and when did she stop them?

   B. What types of difficulties has she been experiencing that caused her to be noncompliant with her diet?

   C. Has she been experiencing any problems with vulvovaginal itching or vaginal discharge?

   D. Why doesn't she see the local "medicine man" instead of coming to the clinic if she is not going to follow the healthcare provider's (HCP's) advice?

   E. Is she experiencing any depression, mood changes, changes in appetite, poor concentration, difficulty in making decisions, poor self-esteem, feelings of hopelessness, anhedonia, or thoughts of death or suicide?

Patient Responses

Mrs. Thompson states that she has not taken any of the prescribed medications because she feels they "won't do any good." For approximately the first 5 years of having diabetes, she was able to control it by avoiding sweets. But then, she started experiencing increased polydipsia, polyuria, and fatigue and was started on metformin. She took the metformin

---

*Remember, for each question, none to all of the answers could be correct/essential or incorrect/nonessential. See page 99 for Chapter 3 answers.

regularly; however, despite regular office visits and increases in her dose of metformin, her symptoms were not any better after 1 year of therapy. At that time her FPG and Hgb A1C were also poorly controlled; thus, a second medication was added (name unknown). She took both of the medications regularly for approximately 6 months. However, at that time she was still not feeling any better, so she quit taking them. Since then, her HCP has continued "checking my blood," adding medications, and recommending dosage increases, which she never adhered to because she felt "they were not going to help either." She did not tell her HCP that she was not taking her medications and her HCP never asked.

According to her, all that happened during her previous office visits was her "blood was taken," and the HCP would tell her "it was bad" and recommend either increasing the dosage of a pill or starting a new one. She claims that she did not understand what her HCP meant by her "blood being bad."

She states that she is not following the diet recommended by her last HCP because she does not like nor is used to eating the majority of the foods "on the list."

She is not having any problems with vulvovaginal itching or vaginal discharge.

She has not seen a "medicine man" because she is uncertain where to find one. Furthermore, she doesn't think that he could help her either. However, she does not blame herself, feel guilty, or think she is being punished for having diabetes (which is a prevalent belief in some Native American cultures). She denies depression, but sometimes feels "down or blue." Upon further questioning, this has been present on most days for the past 2 to 3 years. She feels hopeless in regards to controlling her diabetes because "it's too hard." She doesn't seem to enjoy the things that used to bring her pleasure, doesn't have interest in doing them, and prefers to stay at home alone instead of being with others. However, when she does agree to "do something with her friends," she moderately enjoys herself. She denies changes in her appetite. She occasionally will have problems with poor concentration and puts off making important decisions. She denies poor self-esteem and thoughts of death or suicide. She admits her mood symptoms have been present almost every day for the past several years.

2. Based on this information, which of the following components of a physical examination are essential to perform on Mrs. Thompson and why?

  A. Funduscopic examination
  B. Thyroid examination
  C. Heart examination
  D. Pelvic examination
  E. Examination for bilateral pedal edema

Physical Examination Results

Mrs. Thompson weighs 210 lb and is 5'5" tall (body mass index [BMI] = 44.9). Her other vital signs are blood pressure (BP), 136/84 mm Hg; pulse, 80 beats per minute (BPM) and regular; respirations, 14/min and regular; and oral temperature, 98.5°F. BP repeated at the end of the visit was 134/82 mm Hg. (BP at her previous visit was 138/86 mm Hg.)

Her ophthalmologic examination revealed a normal cup:disc ratio; however, her retinas were difficult to visualize but appeared to be normal.

Her thyroid is normal size and without masses or tenderness, bilaterally.

Her heart is regular in rate and rhythm and without murmurs, gallops, or rubs. Her apical impulse is located in her fifth intercostal space and approximately 8 cm from her midsternal line. There is no thrill. She does not have any pedal edema.

Her dorsalis pedis and posterior tibial pulses are normal bilaterally. Her capillary refill is less than 2 seconds and her feet are warm to touch. She appears to have normal and equal sensation on the anterior, posterior, medial, and lateral aspects of her feet via a monofilament examination.

3. Based on this information, which of the following diagnostic studies are essential to conduct on Mrs. Thompson and why?

  A. Lipid profile, serum blood urea nitrogen (BUN) and creatinine, alanine aminotransferase (ALT), fasting plasma glucose (FPG), thyroid panel, and complete blood count with differential (CBC w/diff)
  B. Electrocardiogram (ECG)
  C. Urinalysis and serial spot for microalbuminuria if protein is negative
  D. Hamilton Depression Rating Scale
  E. Glycated hemoglobin A_1 (Hgb A1C)

Diagnostic Testing Results

Mrs. Thompson's total cholesterol was 260 mg/dl (normal adult: < 200), her low-density lipoprotein cholesterol (LDL-C) was 210 mg/dl (goal for diabetic patient per American Diabetes Association [ADA] guidelines: < 100), her high-density lipoprotein cholesterol (HDL-C) was 35 mg/dl (goal for diabetic female per ADA guidelines: > 50), her very low-density lipoprotein cholesterol (VLDL-C) was 15 mg/dl (no goal established by ADA), and her triglycerides were 220 mg/dl (goal for diabetic patient: < 150).

Her BUN was 18 mg/dl (normal nonelderly adult: 10–20), serum creatinine was 0.8 mg/dl (normal for women: 0.8–1.1), and ALT was 28 units/L (normal nonelderly adult: 4–36). FPG was 280 mg/dl (normal nonelderly adult: 70–110), and Hgb A1C was 10% (normal: < 7).

Her thyroid profile consisted of a thyroid-stimulating hormone of 8.5 µU/ml (normal adult: 2–10), a free thyroxine (FT_4) of 1.8 ng/dl (normal adult: 0.8–2.8), and a triiodothyronine radioimmunoassay (T_3 by RIA) of 150 ng/dl (normal adults > 50 years old: 40–180).

Her ECG revealed a normal sinus rhythm and no abnormalities.

Her urinalysis consisted of clear, medium-yellow-colored, normal-smelling urine. Its pH was 4.5 (normal: 4.6–8) and its specific gravity was 1.035 (normal nonelderly adult: 1.005–1.030). Her dipstick was negative for protein, ketones, leukocyte esterase, and nitrites. It was positive for 2^+ glucose. The microscopic examination was within normal limits. Her spot urinalysis for microalbuminuria (MA) was 2.5 µg/mg (normal: 0.2–1.9).

Her Hamilton Depression Rating Scale score was 9 (cut-off for depression: 10 or 11 out of a possible 52 utilizing the 17-item screen).

4. Based on this information, which one of the following is Mrs. Thompson's most likely diagnosis and why?

   A. Type 2 diabetes mellitus, with prehypertension, hyperlipidemia, class I obesity, possibly mild diabetic nephropathy, and major depressive disorder
   B. Type 2 diabetes mellitus, with hypertension (stage 1), hyperlipidemia, class II obesity, possibly mild diabetic nephropathy, and major depressive disorder
   C. Diabetes mellitus with obesity, borderline BP, and hyperlipidemia lipids
   D. Type 2 diabetes mellitus, with prehypertension, hyperlipidemia, class III (extreme) obesity, possibly mild diabetic nephropathy, and dysthymia
   E. Type 2 diabetes mellitus, stage 1 hypertension, hyperlipidemia, class I obesity, possibly mild diabetic nephropathy, and dysthymia

5. Based on this diagnosis, which of the following are appropriate components of a treatment plan for Mrs. Thompson and why?

   A. Patient education and lifestyle modifications
   B. Start ramipril 2.5 mg daily
   C. Refer to ophthalmologist for complete eye evaluation stressing the importance of the visit
   D. Restart all four diabetic medications; advise of mechanisms of action, possible adverse effects, and to call office immediately if they occur
   E. Schedule for a complete examination
   F. Start selegiline transdermal patches

CASE 3-2

Theresa Umberto

Mrs. Umberto is a 36-year-old Hispanic female who presents with the chief complaint of "I think I am going through menopause." For the past 3 to 4 months, her menstrual cycles have been irregular, varying from 21 to 61 days between menses. However, her menstrual periods are normal in amount and duration when they do occur. Her last menstrual period (LMP) was 5 weeks ago. She is sexually active and uses a diaphragm with foam consistently for contraception.

Her menstrual irregularities are associated with "hot flashes," which she describes as profuse perspiring, heat intolerance, a "shaky feeling inside," restlessness, irritability, palpations, and fatigue. The fatigue is a generalized weakness, not a tiredness, sleepiness, or lack of energy/desire.

She is also bothered by insomnia that she attributes to "night sweats." She is awakened from sleep by a sensation of heat to find that her nightgown is soaked in perspiration. She'll get up, change her nightgown, and go back to bed. She is asleep again within 5 to 10 minutes (which is the typical length of time it takes her to fall asleep when first going to bed for the night). These episodes occur anywhere from one to three times per night and have also been present for the

past 3 to 4 months. She does not appear to have abnormal leg movements or other difficulties while sleeping.

Additionally, she has experienced an unintentional weight loss of 10 lb over the past 2 months, despite an increased appetite. She denies any increased stress, major life changes, crying episodes, anxiety, moodiness, fever, light-headedness, vertigo, presyncope, syncope, dysphagia, nausea, vomiting, bowel changes, abdominal pain, breast tenderness, change in breast size, or nipple discharge.

She has no known medical problems. She was hospitalized for childbirth (the last one 4 years ago). She has never had any surgery. She takes no prescription or over-the-counter medications, vitamins, minerals, or herbal preparations. She is not allergic to any medications.

She drinks two 12-oz. caffeinated beverages per day, which is not a change from her usual. She has never smoked cigarettes. She does not drink alcohol or energy drinks. Her family history is negative. Her mother went through menopause at 52 years of age.

1. Based on this information, which of the following questions are essential to ask Mrs. Umberto and why?

   A. Has she been experiencing depression, hopelessness, or anhedonia?
   B. Has she noticed any swelling in her neck or lower legs?
   C. Has she experienced any muscle cramps, muscle weakness, or tremors?
   D. Are her "hot flashes" associated with neck and/or facial erythema?
   E. Has she noticed any changes of her hair, skin, or nails?

Patient Responses

Mrs. Umberto denies depression, hopelessness, anhedonia, actual muscle weakness, tremors, or facial/neck flushing even with "hot flashes." She has noticed a mass in the center of her anterior neck and some swelling of her lower legs over her tibias. She has occasional muscle cramps without a known precipitating event. She has noticed that her skin appears warm and moist, her hair thinner, and her nails appear to be "loose" at the distal lateral edges (onycholysis).

2. Based on this information, which of the following components of a physical examination are essential to perform on Mrs. Umberto and why?

   A. Eye examination
   B. Neck examination
   C. Heart examination
   D. Abdominal examination
   E. Distal lower extremity and skin examination

Physical Examination Results

Mrs. Umberto is 5'4" tall and weighs 110 lb (BMI = 18.8). Other vital signs are BP, 128/82 mm Hg; pulse, 112 BPM and regular; respiratory rate, 12/min and regular; and oral temperature, 99.2°F.

Her eyes reveal a minimal amount of periorbital edema and proptosis. Her upper and lower eyelids just barely meet when she closes her eyes. She has a moderate degree of upper lid retraction (positive Dalrymple sign), a slight lid lag when looking down (positive von Graefe sign), and a slight delay of the globe compared to the upper eyelid when looking upward (positive Kocher sign). Otherwise, her extraocular muscle movements appear to be normal.

Her visual fields are grossly intact. Her pupils are equal in size and shape, are round, and respond to light and accommodation (PERRLA). Her funduscopic examination is normal. Her sclerae are normal in color and noninjected. Her near vision is 20/20 bilaterally and her distant vision is 20/20 in her right eye and 20/25 in her left. Her color vision is normal.

Her neck reveals a diffusely enlarged, smooth, slightly tender thyroid gland that is approximately 250% larger than normal size. No masses or nodules are present. There is a bilateral bruit to the mass. The carotid pulses are normal and without a bruit. There is no tracheal deviation or cervical or supraclavicular lymphadenopathy present.

Her heart is tachycardic but regular in rhythm. However, her heart sounds appear "louder" than normal. She does not have a murmur, gallops, or rubs. Her apical impulse is nondisplaced and she does not have a thrill.

Her abdominal examination reveals normoactive and equal bowel sounds in all four quadrants. She has no masses, organomegaly, bruit, or tenderness.

Her distal lower extremities reveal pitting edema of her ankles and anterolateral lower legs. She has a pinkish-purple, indurated, peau d'orange–appearing plaque approximately 2 cm in size over her midtibia. Her popiteal, dorsalis pedis, and posterior tibial pulses are normal bilaterally. Her feet are warm to the touch and her capillary refill is normal.

3. Based on this information, which of the following diagnostic studies are essential to conduct on Mrs. Umberto and why?

   A. Electrocardiogram (ECG)
   B. Thyroid stimulating hormone (TSH), free thyroxine (FT_4), and triiodothyronine by radioimmunoassay (T_3 by RIA)
   C. Complete blood count with differential (CBC w/diff)
   D. Quantitative serum human chorionic gonadotropin
   E. Thyroglobulin (Tg)

Diagnostic Results

Mrs. Umberto's ECG revealed a sinus tachycardia but no other abnormalities. Her CBC w/diff was normal. Her quantitative serum HCG was 0 mIU/ml (normal nonpregnant females: < 5).

Her TSH was 0.5 µU/ml (normal: 2–10). Her FT_4 was 4.2 µg/dl (normal adult: 0.8–2.8) and her T_3 by RIA was 250 mg/dl (normal adult female 20–50 years old: 70–205). Her Tg was 6.0 ng/ml (normal females over the age of 12 years: 0.5–43.0).

Reflex confirmatory testing was provided by the lab and consisted of antithyroid antibody testing with an antithyroid peroxidase antibody (TPO-Ab) titer of 1:256 (normal: < 1:100), thyroid-binding inhibitory immunoglobulin (TBII) of 40% (normal < 10%), and thyroid-stimulating immunoglobulins (TSIs) of 185% of basal activity (normal < 130%).

4. Based on this information, which one of the following is Mrs. Umberto's most likely diagnosis and why?

   A. Graves thyrotoxicosis
   B. Multinodular goiter (MNG)
   C. Jodbasedow disease
   D. De Quervain disease
   E. Depression

5. Based on this diagnosis, which of the following are appropriate components of a treatment plan for Mrs. Umberto and why?

   A. Referral to an ophthalmologist
   B. Methimazole 30 mg orally once a day; then adjust dosage based on FT_4 levels
   C. Radioactive iodine (^{131}I) treatment instead of methimazole
   D. Immediate surgical consult for thyroidectomy
   E. Duloxetine 20 mg daily

CASE 3-3

Ulysses Valez

Mr. Valez is a 28-year-old Hispanic American male who presents with the chief complaint of being "tired and weak." His symptoms began approximately 3 to 4 months ago and have progressively gotten worse. He feels best, but not well, on awakening in the morning. Then, his symptoms worsen as the day progresses. He defines "tired" as "totally exhausted," but not as a lack of motivation/desire or sleepiness. "Weakness" is explained as "tiring easier" and "being unable to do as much as I used to be able to do," but not a true loss of muscle strength. He knows of no other aggravating or alleviating factors.

He was not ill before the onset of his symptoms. However, he has lost approximately 4 to 5 lb since becoming ill because "I am just too tired to eat sometimes." He does not have any arthralgias, myalgias, paresthesias, chest pain, pressure, palpations, dyspnea, lightheadedness, vertigo, presyncope, syncope, abdominal pain, ascites, nausea, vomiting, bowel changes, polyuria, polydipsia, fever, or chills. He also denies insomnia, depression, anxiety, mood changes, feeling hopeless, anhedonia, crying episodes, irritability, increased stress, or memory problems. He has noticed that he has been having some difficulty concentrating but attributes it to "just being tired."

He has no known medical problems. He has never had surgery nor been hospitalized. He takes a multivitamin with minerals daily, which he started approximately 2 months ago at his girlfriend's insistence; however, it did not alleviate his symptoms in any manner. He does not take any other over-the-counter or prescription medications, vitamins, supplements, or herbal preparations. He quit smoking about 3 years ago; until then he smoked a half pack per day for approximately 8 years. He does not do illicit drugs. His family history is negative. He is sexually active with women only and has been with his current girlfriend in (what he believes to be) a mutually monogamous relationship for 2 years. They use condoms regularly.

1. Based on this information, which of the following questions are essential to ask Mr. Valez and why?

   A. Has he experienced any visual changes or headaches?
   B. Does he have any urethral discharge?
   C. Has he been experiencing any cold intolerance?
   D. Has he noticed any changes of his skin, hair, or nails?
   E. Did/does he have a sore throat or enlarged lymph nodes?

Patient Responses

His only visual abnormality is a nonfluctuating decrease in his peripheral vision of "several months'" duration without change. He has also been experiencing three or four headaches per week. They are generalized in location and tend to occur in the late afternoon. They have been present for "a couple" of years and have not changed. He attributes them to "looking at the computer screen too much." He describes them as a dull ache that is nonpulsating. He rates the pain as 3 out of 10 on the pain scale and generally does not take any medicine for them. They last from one-half to 4 hours. They are not accompanied by aura, photophobia, phonophobia, nausea, or vomiting.

He also states that his girlfriend tells him that he is "paler" and his hair is "thinner" than it used to be; however, he has not noticed these changes. He has experienced intermittent cold intolerance since his fatigue began. His fingernails are slightly more brittle. He has not had a sore throat or any lymphadenopathy before or since the onset of his symptoms.

2. Based on this information, which of the following components of a physical examination are essential to perform on Mr. Valez and why?

    A. Eye examination
    B. Thyroid examination
    C. Heart examination
    D. Tender points for fibromyalgia
    E. Deep tendon reflexes

Physical Examination Findings

Mr. Valez is 5'10" tall and weighs 175 lb (BMI = 24.4). Other vital signs are BP, 116/76 mm Hg; pulse, 68 BPM and regular; respirations, 10/min and regular; and oral temperature, 97.8°F.

His eye examination reveals conjunctivae and sclera that are normal color and without injection. His pupils are equal in size, are round in shape, and react to light and accommodation. His fundi show a cup:disc ratio that is top normal to enlarged in size with the edges not markedly distinct but not truly blurry/fuzzy. He appears to have bitemporal visual field defects.

His thyroid is unremarkable.

Mr. Valez's heart is regular in rate and rhythm without any murmurs, gallops, or rubs. His apical impulse is nondisplaced and without thrills.

He has 6/18 painful tender points on fibromyalgia testing. All his deep tendon reflexes (DTRs) are somewhat decreased but equal bilaterally.

3. Based on this information, which of the following diagnostic studies are essential to conduct on Mr. Valez and why?

    A. Complete blood count with differential (CBC w/diff)
    B. Thyroid panel (TSH, FT_4, and T_3 by RIA)
    C. Slit-lamp examination
    D. Mononucleosis spot test (mono spot)
    E. Electrocardiogram (ECG)

Diagnostic Results

His CBC with differential was normal. His TSH was 0.01 µU/ml (normal adult: 2–10). His free T_4 was 0.5 ng/dl (normal adult: 0.8–2.8) and his T_3 by RIA was 35 mg/dl (normal 20- to 50-year-old: 70–205). His mono spot was negative. His ECG revealed normal sinus rhythm (NSR) without any other abnormalities. His slit-lamp evaluation is pending.

4. Based on this information, which one of the following is Mr. Valez's most likely diagnosis and why?

    A. Primary hypothyroidism
    B. Secondary hypothyroidism
    C. Atypical depression
    D. Fibromyalgia
    E. Chronic fatigue syndrome

5. Based on this diagnosis, which of the following are appropriate components of a treatment plan for Mr. Valez and why?

    A. Begin levothyroxine 25 µg/day orally and recheck TSH after 1 month of therapy to see if euthyroid; if not, adjust dosage accordingly
    B. Order thyroid-releasing hormone (TRH)
    C. Order magnetic resonance image (MRI) of pituitary
    D. Start escitalopram 10 mg/day orally and titrate to 20 mg in 1 week if necessary
    E. Start amitriptyline 25 mg one at night

CASE 3-4

Vincent Wilson

Mr. Wilson is a 45-year-old African American who recently had a metabolic screening panel done through his church for its uninsured members. His results were normal except for a serum calcium of 14.5 mg/dl (normal adult: 9–10.5) and a serum phosphorous of 2.5 mg/dl (normal adult: 3–4.5). The nurse who reviewed his test results recommended he see his HCP.

He states that he feels fine and the only reason he kept his appointment for follow-up on these abnormal results is because he promised the nurse, who is also the minister's wife, that he would do so. He also states that he is not looking forward to additional blood work being done because the nurse advised him he was a "really difficult stick."

He denies any medical problems, surgeries, or hospitalizations. He is not on any prescription or over-the-counter medications, vitamins, supplements, or herbal preparations. He has never smoked, drank alcohol, or used illicit substances. He is adopted and unaware of his family history.

1. Based on this information, which of the following questions are essential to ask Mr. Wilson and why?

    A. Does he suffer from any type of bone pain or has he ever had a fracture?
    B. Has he experienced any unexplained weight loss; night sweats; fever; unusual fatigue; muscle weakness; cough; hemoptysis; abdominal pain/fullness; epistaxis; gingival bleeding with teeth brushing; bleeding with minimal trauma; easily bruising; gynecomastia (especially unilaterally); or masses in his inguinal, axillary, infraclavicular, supraclavicular, or neck areas?
    C. Has he had kidney stones or any kidney problems?
    D. Has he ever experienced any polydipsia, polyuria, anorexia, nausea, vomiting, bowel changes, abdominal

pain, ascites, hypertension, paresthesias, depression, anxiety, hypersomnia, delusions, hallucinations, dysarthria, seizures, palpations, diaphoresis, heat intolerance, muscle cramps, tetany, paresthesias, fatiguing easier than usual, or subcutaneous masses?

E. Has he ever had a sexually transmitted infection (STI)?

Patient Responses

He denies unexplained bone pain, history of a fracture, unexplained weight loss, night sweats, fever, any type of fatigue, muscle weakness, cough, hemoptysis, abdominal pain/fullness, epistaxis, gingival bleeding with teeth brushing, bleeding with minimal trauma, easily bruising, gynecomastia, any type of masses, kidney stones, renal problems, polydipsia, polyuria, anorexia, nausea, vomiting, bowel changes, abdominal pain, ascites, hypertension, paresthesias, depression, anxiety, hypersomnia, delusions, hallucinations, palpations, diaphoresis, heat intolerance, muscle cramps, tetany, paresthesias, or STIs.

2. Based on this information, which of the following components of a physical examination are essential to perform on Mr. Wilson and why?

A. Neck examination
B. Heart examination
C. Abdominal examination
D. Genital examination
E. Muscle strength testing

Physical Examination Findings

Mr. Wilson is 5'7" tall and weighs 165 lb (BMI = 24.6). Other vital signs are BP, 128/78 mm Hg in his right arm and 128/82 mm Hg in his left arm (BP repeated at the end of the visit, 128/74 mm Hg in his right arm and 126/82 mm Hg in his left arm); pulse, 84 BPM and regular; respirations, 10/min and regular; and oral temperature 99.2°F.

His heart is regular in rate and rhythm and without murmurs, gallops, or rubs. His apical impulse is not displaced and not associated with a thrill.

He has full range of motion in his neck without pain or tenderness. His thyroid is nonenlarged and without masses, tenderness, or bruits. His parathyroid glands are not palpable. His carotids are +4/4 bilaterally without bruit. He has no cervical, supraclavicular, or infraclavicular lymphadenopathy.

His abdominal examination reveals normal and equal bowel sounds in all four quadrants without tenderness, masses, organomegaly, or bruits. His genital examination was normal.

His muscle strength is equal in both his distal upper extremities without an arm drift. His hands and wrists appear slightly weaker, but equal bilaterally. His muscle strength is also equal bilaterally in his proximal and distal lower extremities. He can perform heel, toe, and tandem walk without difficulty.

3. Based on this information, which of the following diagnostic studies are essential to conduct on Mr. Wilson and why?

A. Parathyroid hormone (PTH) level
B. Vanillylmandelic acid (VMA), catecholamine, thyroid stimulating hormone (TSH), and prolactin levels
C. Vitamin D level by 1,25(OH)$_2$D and serum chloride level

D. Dual-energy x-ray absorptiometry (DEXA) scan
E. Repeat calcium and phosphorous levels
F. 24-hour urine for calcium and creatinine with serum creatinine

Diagnostic Results

His PTH was 85 ng/L (normal: 10–65). His VMA was 5.2 mg/24 hr (normal adult: <6.8/24 hr), his free catecholamines were 86 µg/24 hr (normal: <100 µg/24 hr), his TSH was 5 µU/ml (normal adult: 2–10), and his prolactin level was 5 ng/ml (normal male: 0–20). Vitamin D level by 1,25(OH)$_2$D was 25 ng/ml (normal/goal: ≥ 30 ng/ml). His serum chloride level was 103 mEq/L (normal adult: 98–106).

His 24-hour urine calcium excretion was elevated, his 24-hour urinary creatinine was normal, and his total urine volume for the 24-hour period was within normal limits. His serum creatinine was 0.8 mg/dl (normal adult males: 0.6–1.2).

His DEXA scan was normal. His repeat serum calcium was 11.5 mg/dl (normal adult: 9–10.5) and his phosphorous was 2.6 (normal adult: 3–4.5).

4. Based on this information, which one of the following is Mr. Wilson's most likely diagnosis and why?

A. Familial benign hypocalciuric hypercalcemia
B. Secondary hyperparathyroidism
C. Multiple endocrine neoplasia (MEN) syndrome type I (MEN1)
D. Multiple endocrine neoplasia (MEN) syndrome type II (MEN2)
E. Primary hyperparathyroidism

5. Based on this diagnosis, which of the following are appropriate components of a treatment plan for Mr. Wilson and why?

A. Recheck BP in 1 month; have BP checked weekly, if possible, away from the clinic
B. Vitamin D supplementation
C. Vitamin A supplementation
D. Refer to surgeon
E. Prescribe a bisphosphonate and cinacalcet 30 mg daily orally

CASE 3-5
Wilma Xiam

Mrs. Xiam is a 56-year-old Asian American who presents for the results of her DEXA scan. It was performed approximately 1 week ago at the recommendation of her orthopedic surgeon, who did a surgical repair of her severely fractured right distal ulna and radius. According to the patient, the fracture occurred when she slipped in her driveway and caught herself on her outstretched right arm and hand.

She denies any complaints, including arm pain, vasomotor symptoms, fatigue, changes in skin, alterations in the thickness of her hair, differences in her fingernails, nausea, vomiting, bowel changes, abdominal pain, arthralgias, myalgias, weakness, paresthesias, weight changes, fever, malaise, chest pain or pressure, palpitations, vertigo, lightheadedness, presyncope, syncope, polydipsia, or polyuria. She does admit to having some difficulties doing "some things for myself" since fracturing her forearm because of the cast and her being right-handed.

Mrs. Xiam has no known medical problems. Her only surgery was an open reduction with pinning of her distal forearm approximately 2 weeks ago. Her only hospitalizations were for childbirth (three times). She does not take any prescription or over-the-counter medications (including analgesics), vitamins, supplements, or herbal preparations. She is not allergic to any medications.

Mrs. Xiam has been postmenopausal for approximately 8 years; her last menstrual period (LMP) was approximately 9 years ago. She has not experienced any bleeding or spotting since. She did have some vasomotor symptoms for approximately 1 year before until about 2 years after menopause. She smokes one pack of cigarettes per day and has done so since she was a teenager. She drinks a single alcoholic beverage on "special occasions," which amounts to two to three times per year. Her mother has osteoporosis but it was not diagnosed until she was 70 years of age. The rest of her family history is negative.

Her DEXA scan reveals a T score of –2.0 in her lumbar spine and –0.8 in her femoral neck. Her Z score is –0.6.

1. Based on this information, which of the following questions are essential to ask Mrs. Xiam and why?

    A. How tall was she when she graduated from high school?
    B. How much calcium and vitamin D does she get in her diet?
    C. Does she exercise regularly? If yes, what type and how often?
    D. What does she consider to be a serving of alcohol?
    E. After she began regular menstruation, did she ever miss any menstrual periods?

Patient Responses

She was 5'1" tall when she graduated from high school. She has been lactose intolerant all her life; therefore, she avoids dairy products and does not take calcium supplements, and more likely than not, her intake of calcium is inadequate. She regularly uses sunscreen when out of doors and does not take vitamin D; therefore, her intake of vitamin D is probably also insufficient. She does aerobic exercise for 30 minutes 5 days per week. She generally drinks vodka, has no more than one drink per setting, and considers 1.5 ounces a serving. After she began menstruation she had regular menstrual cycles except for when she was pregnant and the subsequent 5 or 6 months afterward during lactation.

2. Based on this information, which of the following components of a physical examination are essential to perform on Mrs. Xiam and why?

    A. Carotid auscultation
    B. Thyroid palpation
    C. Rectal examination
    D. Evaluation of joints of the hands
    E. Spine examination

Physical Examination Findings

Mrs. Xiam is 5'0" tall and weighs 105 lb (BMI = 20.5). Other vital signs are BP, 102/60 mm Hg; pulse, 72 BPM and regular; respirations, 10/min and regular; and oral temperature, 97.9°F.

Her carotid pulses are equal bilaterally and without bruit. Her thyroid is normal sized and without masses, tenderness, or bruits.

Her rectal examination reveals good tone, no masses, no fissures, no lesions, and soft brown stool.

She has what appears to be full range of motion of all the joints of her upper digits, although it was somewhat difficult to fully assess her right hand secondary to her cast. Her joints are not enlarged and are nontender. Her sensation is intact, color normal, and temperature warm in the tips of all her fingers and thumbs. Her spine reveals full range of motion without pain or evidence of kyphosis, lordosis, or scoliosis.

3. Based on this information, which of the following diagnostic studies are essential to conduct on Mrs. Xiam and why?

    A. Thoracic spine radiographs
    B. Serum cross-linked N-telopeptide
    C. Serum vitamin D level by $1,25(OH)_2D$
    D. Serum follicular-stimulating hormone (FSH)
    E. Complete blood count with differential (CBC w/diff), serum calcium, serum bone-specific alkaline phosphatase (B-ALP), serum creatinine, and 24-hour urinary calcium

Diagnostic Results

Her thoracic spine radiographs were normal, including no evidence of kyphosis. Her serum cross-linked N-telopeptide was 19 nm bone collagen equivalents (BCE; normal female: 6.2–19.0). Her FSH was 55 IU/L (normal postmenopausal female: 19.3–100.6). Her vitamin D level [$1,25(OH)_2D$] was 20 ng/ml (normal/goal: ≥30 ng/ml). Her CBC w/diff, serum calcium, creatinine, and 24-hour urinary calcium were all within normal range. Her B-ALP was elevated to 75 units/L (normal female: 14.2–42.7).

4. Based on this information, which one of the following is Mrs. Xiam's most likely diagnosis and why?

    A. Primary osteoporosis
    B. Secondary osteoporosis
    C. Osteopenia
    D. Normal bone mineral density (BMD)
    E. Osteoarthritis

5. Based on this diagnosis, which of the following are appropriate components of a treatment plan for Mrs. Xiam and why?

    A. Smoking cessation
    B. Calcium 500 mg two to three times per day depending on dietary allowances from her nondairy sources
    C. Vitamin D 400 to 500 IU once a day
    D. Explain treatment options available and assist in selecting an appropriate one
    E. Repeat DEXA scan in 1 year

CASE 3-6
Xandria Yoakum

Ms. Yoakum is a 26-year-old Hispanic American female who presents with the chief complaint of "my skin is tanning itself." Her skin started darkening approximately 3 to 4 months ago and has gradually been progressing. Now, it is evident to her family and friends. The skin changes are present in both sun-exposed and non–sun-exposed areas. She states it is greatest over her knuckles, elbows, knees, back of her neck, creases in her hands, nipples, and areolas. She states it is also more visible on her shoulders under her bra straps, around her chest under her bra band, around her hips below her underwear's elastic top, in diagonal lines across her buttocks and abdomen beneath the elastic sides of her underpants, and in her appendectomy scar.

She is also "getting freckles" in both sun-exposed and non–sun-exposed areas. She denies spending prolonged time outdoors, utilizing indoor tanning facilities, utilizing "self-tanning" lotions, eating increased amounts or large quantities of foods with carotene, or using a different soap or lotion. She denies taking any iron pills, other supplements, vitamins, herbal preparations, or any medications, including tetracycline or doxycycline for acne. She has never experienced anything like this in the past nor does she have any blood relatives who have.

She has no other skin lesions or changes except for perhaps bruising slightly easier. Her menstrual periods occur at 28-day intervals and have not changed in duration or amount since menarche at the age of 12 years old. She has not experienced any epistaxis, hemoptysis, hematuria, or taking longer to stop bleeding following an accidental laceration or abrasion.

She admits to feeling "tired and weak" but not unusually drowsy or sleepy nor having lack of motivation or desire to do things. However, there are some days when she is "just too tired to get up." She does not have insomnia, hypersomnia, or hyposomnia. She denies increased stress or major life change except starting night classes in addition to keeping her full-time day job. She admits to occasionally feeling anxious or irritable; however, she cannot attribute this to anything specific. As near as she can tell, it is not related to her stress level or menstrual cycle. She denies feeling depressed, down, hopeless, or suicidal. She is not experiencing anhedonia and is very excited about her future.

She has lost 10 lb in the past 6 months without trying. She attributes this to her anorexia and nausea. Initially, when these symptoms first began approximately 6 months ago, they occurred intermittently and very infrequently (not even once a day); currently, they are almost constant. She is unaware of any aggravating or alleviating factors. Despite the almost continuous anorexia and nausea, she feels she is still eating the same types and quantity of food.

Occasionally she will experience vomiting (less than once a week) and will have intermittent diarrhea (also less than once per week) defined as one very soft bowel movement without abnormal color, odor, greasiness, or blood. The vomiting and the diarrhea are unrelated and she cannot identify any aggravating (including certain foods) or alleviating

factors for them either. She denies any other changes in her bowel movements, abdominal pain, or fever.

She also experiences some intermittent generalized myalgias and arthralgias, which she attributes to "overdoing it." However, after mentioning it, she thinks they are occurring with greater frequency. She denies fever, chills, night sweats, malaise, cough, wheezing, chest pain/pressure, palpitations, headaches, difficulties with memory/concentration, or insomnia.

Her only known medical problem is depression. This is her initial episode and it began approximately 9 months ago. After two failed antidepressant trials (fluoxetine and paroxetine), she responded to duloxetine. This is her only medication and she takes 60 mg twice per day. She has been on it at that dosage for approximately 4 months and claims all her depression symptoms are resolved. She takes no other prescription medication, no over-the-counter drugs, no vitamins, no supplements, and no herbal preparations. Her only surgery was an appendectomy at age 18 years. That was her only hospitalization. She has never smoked cigarettes or drank alcohol. Her last menstrual period was 2 weeks ago and normal. She has regular menstrual cycles. She has not been sexually active in over 6 months and she always uses a condom when she is. Her family history is negative.

1. Based on this information, which of the following questions are essential to ask Ms. Yoakum and why?

  A. Has she noticed any lesions or dryness of her mucous membranes?
  B. Has she noticed any changes in hearing, tasting, and/or smelling?
  C. Has she had any episodes of shakiness, sweatiness, lightheadedness, dizziness, presyncope, syncope, or orthostatic symptoms?
  D. Has she noticed any axillary or pubic hair changes?
  E. Is she experiencing any color changes of her urine?

Patient Responses

Ms. Yoakum denies any pigment changes or dryness of her mucous membranes. She has been playing the television, radio, etc., less or at a significantly lower volume for the past several months because the "noise bothers me." She is hyperacutely aware of odors, both pleasant and unpleasant. She has not noticed any change in taste. Occasionally, she will feel "lightheaded" and her vision "gets dim" when she first stands up; however, she has not experienced any true syncope or vertigo. She hasn't noticed any changes in her axillary hair; however, her public hair is definitely thinner and straighter. She has not noticed any color changes in her urine.

2. Based on this information, which of the following components of a physical examination are essential to perform on Ms. Yoakum and why?

  A. Sclera and oral mucosa examination
  B. Skin examination
  C. Examination of wrists for evidence of scarring
  D. Heart examination
  E. Abdominal examination

Physical Examination Findings

Ms. Yoakum is 5'5" tall and weighs 115 lb (BMI = 19.1). Her supine BP is 110/66 mm Hg and drops to 80/54 mm Hg on standing, which reproduced her lightheadedness. Her pulse is 76 BPM and regular while supine and increases to 108 BPM and regular on standing. Her respirations are 12/min and regular and her oral temperature is 99.1°F.

Her sclerae are white and her conjunctivae are normal pink in color. Her oral mucosa does not have any abnormalities of color or lesions.

Her skin appears uniformly "tanned" with darker brown, "dirty-looking" areas over the backs of her knuckles, knees, elbows, neck, and palmar creases. Where the elastic of her bra and underpants places pressure on her skin, it is an even darker brown, almost black, color. Her nipples and areolas are very dark brown in color. She has multiple darker brown maculae 0.5 to 2 mm in size on her trunk, extremities, neck, and face. Her wrists are without scars.

Her heart is regular in rate and rhythm and without murmurs, gallops, or rubs. Her apical impulse is nondisplaced and without thrills.

Her abdominal examination reveals normoactive and equal bowel sounds in all four quadrants. It is soft and nontender and reveals no masses or organomegaly. She does have an approximately 6-cm-long, narrow, angulated, well-healed, hyperpigmented scar in her right lower quadrant consistent with an appendectomy.

3. Based on this information, which of the following diagnostic studies are essential to conduct on Ms. Yoakum and why?

   A. Thyroid panel (TSH, FT_4, and T_3 by RIA)
   B. Complete blood count with differential (CBC w/diff) with total iron-binding capacity (TIBC), iron, transferrin, transferrin saturation, and ferritin levels
   C. Serum dehydroepiandrosterone (DHEA) level
   D. Serum electrolytes, calcium, liver transaminases, bilirubin, and glucose
   E. Plasma level of cortisol and adrenocorticotropic hormone (ACTH) at 8:00 a.m.

Diagnostic Results

Ms. Yoakum's TSH was 5.5 µU/ml (normal adult: 2–10), her free FT_4 was 1.8 ng/dl (normal adult: 0.8–2.8), and her T_3 by RIA was 150 mg/dl (normal 20- to 50-year-old: 70–205).

Her CBC with differential revealed a red blood cell (RBC) count of 4.3 × 10^6/µl (normal female: 4.2–5.4) with a mean corpuscular volume (MCV) of 81.4 µm^3 (normal adult: 80–95), a mean corpuscular hemoglobin (MCH) of 27.4 pg (normal adult: 27–31), a mean corpuscular hemoglobin concentration (MCHC) of 33.7 g/dl (normal adult: 32–36), and a red blood cell distribution width (RDW) of 12.5% (normal adult: 11–14.5). Her white blood cell (WBC) count was 12,500/mm^3 (normal adult: 5000–10,000) with 34% neutrophils (normal: 55–70), 48% lymphocytes (normal: 20–40), 2% monocytes (normal: 2–8), 15% eosinophils (normal: 1–4), and 1% basophils (normal: 0.5–1). Her hemoglobin (Hgb) was 11.8 g/dl (normal female: 12–16) and her hematocrit (HCT) was 35% (normal female: 37–47). Her platelet (thrombocyte) count was 250,000/mm^3 (normal adult: 150,000–400,000) and her

mean platelet volume (MPV) was 7.9 fl (normal: 7.4–10.4). Her smear was consistent with the aforementioned and revealed no cellular abnormalities. Her serum iron level was 70 µg/dl (normal adult female: 60–160), her TIBC was 335 µg/dl (normal: 250–460), her transferrin was 300 mg/dl (normal adult female: 250–380), her transferrin saturation was 40% (normal female: 15–50), and her ferritin level was 75 ng/ml (normal female: 10–150).

Her electrolytes revealed a carbon dioxide (CO_2) of 21 mEq (normal: 23–30), a chloride (Cl^-) of 98.6 mEq/L (normal: 98–106), a potassium (K^+) of 6.0 mEq/L (normal adult: 3.5–5.0), and a sodium (Na^+) of 125 mEq/L (normal adult: 136–145). Her serum calcium was 9.5 mg/dl (normal adult: 9–10.5). Her fasting blood sugar was 66 mg/dl (normal: 70–110).

Her ALT was 30 units/L (normal 4–36), her aspartate aminotransferase (AST) was 11 units/L (normal adult: 1–35 [however, it is not unusual for women's AST level to run slightly lower than men's]), and her γ-glutamyl transferase (GGT) was 15 units (normal: adult females under the age of 45 years: 5–27). Her total bilirubin was 0.6 mg/dl (normal 0.3–1.0) with her direct being 0.2 mg/dl (normal: 0.1–0.3) and her indirect being 0.4 mg/dl (normal 0.2–0.8).

Her DHEA was 0.9 ng/ml (normal female: 0.5–2.7). Her 8:00 a.m. cortisol level was 2.5 µg/dl (normal: 5–23) and her ACTH was 250 pg/ml (normal < 80).

4. Based on this information, which one of the following is Ms. Yoakum's most likely diagnosis and why?

   A. Primary adrenal insufficiency
   B. Autoimmune polyendocrinopathy-candidiasis-ectodermal dystrophy (APCED)
   C. Hepatotoxicity caused by duloxetine
   D. Hemochromatosis
   E. Photosensitivity reaction and other adverse effects to duloxetine

5. Based on this diagnosis, which of the following are appropriate components of a treatment plan for Ms. Yoakum and why?

   A. Antiadrenal antibodies
   B. Stop duloxetine
   C. Hydrocortisone 15 mg every morning and 7.5 mg late each afternoon
   D. Fludrocortisone acetate 0.05 mg daily
   E. DHEA 25 mg every morning

CASE 3-7
Yolinda Zimmerman

Mrs. Zimmerman is a 56-year-old white female of Mediterranean descent who presents for follow-up on her diagnostic test ordered at a visit 1 week ago. At that visit, she had multiple complaints: generalized weakness, fatigue, upper back pain, headaches, face appearing rounder and fuller, violaceous discoloration of her striae cutis distensae, and mood changes. Her BP was 138/84 mm Hg. All her symptoms began approximately 3 to 4 months ago and are worsening in both duration and severity. Her symptoms are essentially unchanged since that initial visit.

She defined her generalized weakness as "not being as strong as I used to be." Examples include not being able to lift and/or carry objects weighing as much and having to stop and rest while cleaning her home or doing the grocery shopping (which has never occurred previously).

She was also complaining of increasing fatigue described as "having to push herself" to accomplish anything. It isn't a lack of motivation, desire, or interest. She just lacks sufficient strength/energy to complete the task. She denies daytime sleepiness, requiring a nap, or insomnia. However, she is experiencing hypersomnia and is currently sleeping 10 to 12 hours per night (an increase of 3 to 4 hours for her). She awakens feeling "somewhat" rested and definitely better than before going to sleep; still, she is not her "usual self."

Her back pain is intermittent, thoracic in location, and dull in nature. She rates the pain as a 4 out of a 10 on the pain scale. It increases with movement (especially flexion), decreases with rest, and is unchanged with ibuprofen. Otherwise, she is unaware of any aggravating or alleviating factors. She denies any trauma.

Her headaches are generalized in location and feel "like a tight band around my head." She rates them as a 6 out of a 10 on the pain scale. They occur three to four times per month and she attributes them to "stress"; however, she denies any increase in current life stressors. She is unaware of any precipitating events. They are not "the worst headache of her life," pulsatile in nature, unilateral in location, or associated with photophobia, phonophobia, or any neurologic deficits.

She denies feeling depressed or sad; however, she finds herself crying without cause two or three times per week. She refutes being anxious. However, she has been somewhat more irritable with her spouse without provocation. She claims not to be experiencing anhedonia and she still enjoys previously pleasurable activities. Nevertheless, with physical activities (e.g., dancing), she has to quit after a short period of time to rest because of the fatigue. She denies feelings of hopelessness, suicidal thoughts, and/or suicidal ideations.

She has gained 20 lb in the past 3 months without a change in appetite. She is also experiencing polyuria, polydipsia, delayed healing, and bruising more easily of approximately the same duration. She has had hirsutism since her early 20s; however, it appears to be worsening. She denies any pain elsewhere (including chest, neck, arm, or shoulder), dyspnea, wheezing, cough, pedal edema, palpitations, lightheadedness, vertigo, presyncope, syncope, nausea, vomiting, abdominal pain, heartburn, bowel changes, fever, chills, night sweats, lymphadenopathy, visual problems, or changes in sensations of smell.

Her only known medical problems include hypertension and glaucoma of "several years'" duration. She has never had any problems with depression or any other psychiatric condition. She has never had surgery nor been hospitalized. Her medications are hydrochlorothiazide 25 mg one pill every morning, enalapril 10 mg one pill every morning, and betaxolol ophthalmic solution one drop in each eye twice a day. She does not take any other prescription medications, any over-the-counter medications, vitamins, supplements, or herbal preparations. She is not allergic to any medications. She experienced menopause at the age of 51 years and had

significant vasomotor symptoms for approximately 4 years; however, they have completely resolved. She has never smoked nor drank alcohol. Her family history is positive for coronary artery disease (mother—fatal MI at age 62), hypertension (mother, two older sisters), hypothyroidism (one older sister), and osteoporosis (mother). It is negative for depression or any other mental illness.

Her diagnostic test results from her last visit 1 week ago included a CBC w/diff revealing an RBC count of $5.0 \times 10^6/\mu l$ (normal female: 4.2–5.4) with an MCV of 90 μm^3 (normal adult: 80–95), an MCH of 31 pg (normal adult: 27–31), an MCHC of 34.4 g/dl (normal adult: 32–36), and an RDW of 13.5% (normal adult: 11–14.5). Her WBC count was 9500/mm^3 (normal adult: 5000–10,000) with 66% neutrophils (normal: 55–70), 22% lymphocytes (normal: 20–40), 8% monocytes (normal: 2–8), 3% eosinophils (normal: 1–4), and 1% basophils (normal: 0.5–1). Her Hgb was 15.5 g/dl (normal female: 12–16) and her HCT was 45% (normal female: 37–47). Her platelet (thrombocyte) count was 175,000/mm^3 (normal adult: 150,000–400,000) and her MPV was 8.9 fl (normal: 7.4–10.4). Her smear was consistent with the aforementioned and revealed no cellular abnormalities.

Her FPG was 120 mg/dl (normal: 70–110). Her TSH was 7.5 μU/ml (normal adult: 2–10). Her 8 a.m. cortisol level was 25 μg/dl (adult normal: 5–23). Her dexamethasone suppression test revealed an 8 a.m. cortisol level of 7.2 μg/dl (normal: < 5).

1. Based on this information, which of the following questions are essential to ask Mrs. Zimmerman and why?

    A. Has she ever had a DEXA scan?

    B. Does she own a cat?

    C. Has she experienced any salt cravings?

    D. Did her headaches begin before the onset of her other current symptoms?

    E. Has she ever been on hormone replacement therapy (HRT)?

Patient Responses

Mrs. Zimmerman has never had a DEXA scan. She does not have a cat nor is she exposed to one elsewhere. She has not been craving salt nor has she ever been on HRT. Her headaches have been present "all my life" and have not changed in any manner.

2. Based on this information, which of the following components of a physical examination are essential to perform on Mrs. Zimmerman and why?

    A. General appearance for weight distribution

    B. Thyroid examination

    C. Skin examination

    D. Back examination

    E. Neurologic examination

Physical Examination Findings

Mrs. Zimmerman is 5'1" tall and weighs of 254 lb (BMI = 48). Other vital signs are BP, 136/84 mm Hg; pulse, 92 BPM and regular; respirations, 12/min and regular; and oral temperature, 98.4°F.

Her face is slightly large and very round appearing with a mild acnelike rash in her T-zone and marked hirsutism (in both mustache and sideburns distributions). Her skin appears to be on the slightly thin side with light purplish striae on her abdomen, thighs, and breasts. She has generalized obesity with perhaps a propensity toward a centripetal distribution. Her waist measures 54" and her hips are 50". Her arms and legs also exhibit significant adiposity.

Her thyroid is not palpable, nontender, and without masses. She has small, nontender, bilateral, and equal supraclavicular fat pads; no palpable lymph nodes are noted in these areas.

She has decreased range of motion in her cervical, thoracic, and lumbar spine without the complaint of pain, probably secondary to her obesity. Her spine is nontender to palpate, as are her pressure points for fibromyalgia (for information on the location of the fibromyalgia tender points, please see Case 3-3). She has a moderate-sized, nontender, nonerythematous fat pad of normal skin temperature located over the top one third of her thoracic spine.

Her cranial nerves are grossly intact. Her gait is normal. She can heel and toe walk without difficulty. Her arm and leg muscles reveal normal strength that is equal bilaterally. Her deep tendon reflexes are normal and equal bilaterally.

3. Based on this information, which of the following diagnostic studies are essential to conduct on Mrs. Zimmerman and why?

    A. 8:00 a.m. and 4:00 p.m. cortisol levels and an 8:00 a.m. adrenocorticotropic hormone (ACTH) level

    B. 24-hour urine for free cortisol and creatinine

    C. Glucose tolerance test or equivalent assessment

    D. Dual-energy x-ray absorptiometry (DEXA) scan

    E. Magnetic resonance image (MRI) of the adrenal glands

Diagnostic Results

Mrs. Zimmerman's 8:00 a.m. cortisol level was 24 µg/dl (normal adult: 5–23) and her 4:00 p.m. cortisol was 16 µg/dl (normal adult: 4–14), making her 4:00 p.m. value approximately 66% that of her 8:00 a.m. value. Her 8:00 a.m. ACTH level was 78 pg/ml (normal: < 80). Her 24-hour urinary cortisol measurement was 90 µg/24 hr (normal adult: < 100).

Her DEXA scan revealed a T score of –1.5 and a Z score of –0.8.

Her FPG was 116 mg/dl (normal: 70–110) and her 2-hour postglucose load was 168 (normal 50- to 60-year-old adult: < 150).

Her MRI of her adrenal glands was normal.

4. Based on this information, which one of the following is Mrs. Zimmerman's most likely diagnosis and why?

    A. Extreme obesity (obesity type III), hypertension (stage 1), type 2 diabetes mellitus, and Cushing syndrome

    B. Cushing syndrome caused by a pituitary abnormality

    C. Extreme obesity (obesity type III), prehypertension, abnormal glucose tolerance, osteopenia, and pseudo-Cushing syndrome

    D. Type 2 diabetes mellitus, obesity type I, hypertension stage 1, osteoporosis, and pseudo-Cushing syndrome

    E. Abnormal glucose tolerance, obesity type II, prehypertension, and Cushing syndrome

5. Based on this diagnosis, which of the following are appropriate components of a treatment plan for Mrs. Zimmerman and why?

    A. Low-fat, low-salt, low-calorie heart-healthy diet

    B. Glycosylated hemoglobin

    C. Schedule for an age-appropriate preventive examination

    D. Refer to surgeon for bariatric surgery

    E. Refer to endocrinologist for treatment of Cushing syndrome

CASE 3-8
Zoey Armstrong

Ms. Armstrong is a 36-year-old white female with the chief complaint of amenorrhea of 4 months' duration. She began menses at age 13 years and had regular menses at 28- to 30-day intervals until approximately 2 years ago. At that time, she began "skipping" one menstrual period every 3 to 4 months; still, she never went longer than 2 months without menstruation until now.

She is not experiencing nausea, vomiting, fatigue, breast enlargement or tenderness, abdominal pain, any type of vaginal discharge (including spotting), or increased stress.

She has no known medical problems, has never had surgery, and has never been hospitalized. She is not taking any prescription or over-the-counter medications, vitamins, supplements, or herbal preparations, including hormonal contraceptives. She denies being sexually active in over 1 year. She has never been pregnant. She has never smoked, drank alcohol, or tried/used illicit substances. Her family history is unremarkable. Her mother was menopausal at age 55 years.

1. Based on this information, which of the following questions are essential to ask Ms. Armstrong and why?

    A. Does she have any nipple discharge?

    B. Has she been experiencing any problems with headaches, visual disturbances, or abnormalities of smell?

    C. Is she an athlete, dieting, or exercising excessively?

    D. Is she experiencing vaginal dryness, hot flashes, or night sweats?

    E. Does she have problems with acne, hirsutism, or deepening of her voice?

Patient Responses

Ms. Armstrong denies any nipple discharge, headaches, visual disturbances, abnormalities of smell, vaginal dryness, hot flashes, night sweats, acne, hirsutism, or deepening of her voice. She is not an athlete and is employed as a vice president of a local bank. She is not on any special type of diet or trying to lose weight. Her only exercise is a 1-hour yoga class three nights per week.

2. Based on this information, which of the following components of a physical examination are essential to conduct on Ms. Armstrong and why?

    A. Eye and nose examination

    B. Cranial nerve evaluation

C. Breast examination

D. Pelvic examination

E. Skin examination

Physical Examination Findings

Ms. Armstrong is 5'9" tall and weighs 125 lb (BMI = 18.5). Other vital signs are BP, 106/54 mm Hg; pulse, 68 BPM and regular; respiratory rate, 10/min and regular; and oral temperature, 98.4°F.

Her eyes reveal clear conjunctivae and no discharge. Her pupils are normal, round, and equal in size bilaterally; they react to light and accommodation. Her extraocular muscles and visual fields are normal. Her funduscopic examination is unremarkable. Her nasal mucosa is nonerythematous, nonedematous, and without abnormal lesions or discharge. Her sense of smell is normal. Her other cranial nerves are also intact.

Her breasts are without visible lesions, retraction, or other abnormalities in all three positions. They are normal in consistency and without masses. There is no nipple discharge. Axillary, infraclavicular, and supraclavicular lymph nodes are nonpalpable.

Her abdomen reveals normoactive and equal bowel sounds in all four quadrants. It is soft, nontender, and without masses or organomegaly.

Her external genital examination is without any discoloration, edema, lesions, excoriation, or other abnormalities. Her vaginal mucosa is normal in color, nonedematous, and without lesions or abnormal discharge. Her cervix is normal in appearance and without edema, erythema, lesions, friability, or discharge. Her uterus is normal size and shape without any tenderness. Her ovaries are normal size, smooth, without masses, and nontender, bilaterally.

She does not have acne, hirsutism, or any other skin abnormalities.

3. Based on this information, which of the following diagnostic studies are essential to perform on Ms. Armstrong and why?

    A. Urinary human chorionic gonadotropin (HCG) test

    B. Wet-mount microscopy of vaginal secretions or vaginal pH, "whiff" test for amine odor, and point-of-care testing for vaginal pathogens via DNA

    C. Pelvic ultrasound

    D. Serum prolactin level

    E. Serum follicular-stimulating hormone (FSH)

Diagnostic Test Results

Ms. Armstrong's urinary HCG was negative. Testing of her vaginal secretions was negative for an infectious process. Her pelvic ultrasound was normal. Her serum prolactin level was 18 ng/ml (normal adult female: 0–25). Her FSH was 7 IU/L (normal female [depends on timing of menstrual cycle]: follicular [1.37–9.9], ovulatory peak [6.17–17.2], luteal phase [1.09–9.2], and postmenopausal [19.3–100.6]).

4. Based on this information, which one of the following is Ms. Armstrong's most likely diagnosis and why?

    A. Polycystic ovarian syndrome (PCOS)

    B. Hypogonadotropic secondary amenorrhea

    C. Premature ovarian failure (POF)

    D. Primary amenorrhea

    E. Pituitary adenoma causing secondary amenorrhea

5. Based on this diagnosis, which of the following are appropriate components of a treatment plan for Ms. Armstrong and why?

    A. Progesterone challenge test with 10 mg of medroxyprogesterone acetate (MPA) once a day for 10 days

    B. Luteinizing hormone (LH)

    C. Thyroid stimulating hormone (TSH)

    D. Re-evaluate diet, exercise, and stress

    E. Magnetic resonance image (MRI) of her pituitary

CASE 3-9
Anne Brown

Mrs. Brown is a 24-year-old African American female who presents to the emergency department (ED) with the chief complaint, "I am afraid that I am becoming dehydrated from my morning sickness again." Her current gestational age is 12 weeks. She has been having severe nausea and vomiting since before missing a menstrual period. She states, "I can hardly keep anything down, even water." She has been hospitalized four times during this pregnancy for IV fluids for this same problem. Her last admission was 1 week ago. At her posthospitalization visit with her obstetrician 4 days ago, she weighed 130 lb. Her pre-pregnancy weight was 128 lb. Other than the hyperemesis gravidarum, her pregnancy has been unremarkable except for fatigue so severe it required her to quit her job.

She currently sleeps approximately 10 hours per night and takes two to three naps during the day of 1 to 1.5 hours each. She and her husband are happy and excited about the pregnancy, which was planned. She denies insomnia, depression, crying episodes, feelings of hopelessness, and anhedonia. She does not have diarrhea, constipation, other bowel changes, fever, abdominal/pelvic pain or cramping, back pain, edema, chest pain or pressure, or dyspnea.

She has no known medical problems. She has never had any surgeries. Her only hospitalization was for the birth of her son 2 years ago. Her only medication is prenatal vitamins. She does not take any other prescription or over-the-counter medications, vitamins, supplements, or herbal preparations. She is gravid 2, parous 1, and abortions 0. Her first pregnancy was full-term, with a normal vaginal delivery without problems, and no postnatal or neonatal problems.

She does not smoke, do drugs, or drink alcohol or caffeine. Her family history is negative.

1. Based on this information, which of the following questions are essential to ask Mrs. Brown and why?

    A. Did she experience hyperemesis gravidarum with her first pregnancy?

    B. Has she been experiencing any cardiac palpitations or tachycardia?

    C. Has she had any vaginal spotting or bleeding?

    D. Is her nausea and vomiting worse in the mornings or the evenings?

    E. Is she planning on breast- or bottle-feeding?

Patient Responses

She had minimal "morning sickness" with her first pregnancy. She has rare palpitations and tachycardia with exertion. Her nausea and vomiting persist throughout the day; however, it is not worse at any given time. She does not have vaginal bleeding/spotting. She plans to breast-feed.

2. Based on this information, which of the following components of a physical examination are essential to perform on Mrs. Brown and why?

    A. Palpation of thyroid

    B. Heart examination

    C. Abdominal examination, including uterine fundus palpation and height, and Doppler evaluation of fetal heartbeat

    D. Rectal examination

    E. Evaluation of lower extremities for pedal edema and the skin over the sternum and/or forehead for "tenting"

Physical Examination Findings

Mrs. Brown is 5'3" tall and weighs 130 lb (BMI = 23). Other vital signs are BP, 120/70 mm Hg; pulse, 98 BPM and regular; respirations, 12/min and regular; and oral temperature, 98.5°F.

Her thyroid is slightly enlarged, nontender, and without masses.

Her heart is regular in rate and rhythm without murmurs, gallops, or rubs. Her apical impulse is nondisplaced and without thrills.

Her abdominal examination reveals normoactive and equal bowel sounds in all four quadrants. She has no hepatosplenomegaly. Kidneys are nonpalpable. Her uterine fundus is palpated at the top of her pubic symphysis. There is no tenderness or tetany. Fetal cardiac rate is 150 BPM and regular per Doppler. Her rectal examination is normal.

She does not have any pedal edema. She does not have any "tenting" of the skin over her forehead or sternum.

3. Based on this information, which of the following diagnostic studies are essential to conduct on Mrs. Brown and why?

    A. Blood urea nitrogen (BUN) and electrolytes

    B. Urinalysis

    C. Quantitative serum human chorionic gonadotropin (HCG)

    D. Obstetric ultrasound

    E. Thyroid panel (TSH, FT_4, and T_3 by RIA)

Diagnostic Results

Mrs. Brown's BUN was 20 mg/dl (normal adult: 10–20). Her electrolytes revealed a CO_2 of 27 mEq (normal: 23–30), a chloride (Cl^-) of 102 mEq/L (normal: 98–106), a potassium (K^+) of 3.6 mEq/L (normal adult: 3.5–5.0), and a sodium (Na^{2+}) of 141 mEq/L (normal adult: 136–145).

Her obstetric ultrasound did not reveal any abnormalities or multiple gestations.

Her quantitative serum HCG was 200,000 mIU/ml (normal for 12 weeks' gestation: 15,000–220,000). Her urinalysis was normal.

Her TSH was 10.5 µU/ml (normal adult: 2–10). Her FT_4 was 0.6 ng/dl (normal adult: 0.8–2.8) and her T_3 by RIA was 60 mg/dl (normal 20- to 50-year-old: 70–205).

4. Based on this information, which one of the following is Mrs. Brown's most likely diagnosis and why?

    A. Normal pregnancy with false-positive thyroid function testing as a result of pregnancy

    B. Preeclampsia

    C. Hydatidiform mole

    D. Mild hypothyroidism in pregnancy

    E. Hyperemesis gravidarum with dehydration

5. Based on this diagnosis, which of the following are appropriate components of a treatment plan for Mrs. Brown and why?

    A. Hospitalize for IV fluids

    B. Observation and repeat thyroid studies in 1 month

    C. Advise that hyperemesis gravidarum is complicated by hypothyroidism and the timing of her pregnancy (at the end of the first semester) plus treating her hypothyroidism should alleviate her symptoms in the near future

    D. Small frequent meals (at least six per day) with dry foods (e.g., crackers, toast) followed 1 hour later by clear liquids (e.g., juice, broth)

    E. Start propylthiouracil or methimazole

CASES IN ENDOCRINE ABNORMALITIES

RESPONSES AND DISCUSSION

CASE 3-1
Sally Thompson
1. History

A. What types of problems did she have with her medications that caused her to discontinue them, and when did she stop them?   ESSENTIAL

Diabetes mellitus is a chronic disease that can have many significant adverse effects including microvascular (e.g., diabetic retinopathy, macular edema, and diabetic nephropathy, which can lead to end-stage renal disease [ESRD]), macrovascular (coronary artery disease [CAD], cerebrovascular accidents [CVAs], transient ischemic attacks [TIAs], and peripheral vascular disease), and neurologic (e.g., autonomic dysfunction, peripheral neuropathy, and other sensory and/or motor mono- and/or polyneuropathy) complications. The cornerstone to treating this condition and preventing these complications is good glycemic control. This cannot be achieved without adherence to medications (when required) and lifestyle modifications.

Therefore, it is essential when a patient is not taking his or her medicine to determine in a nonjudgmental, nonconfrontational, nonaccusatory nature as to the reason. It can stem from a multitude of factors that are often coexisting. They can include asymptomatic illness, limited knowledge of the disease and the importance of treatment (despite being relatively asymptomatic) to prevent complications, unawareness of potential complications of untreated disease, no explanation of mechanism of action and need for medication, no discussion of potential adverse effects from the medications and what to do if one occurs, unaddressed fear(s) of possible side effects, cost of medication, inability to afford medication, coexisting mood disorder, cognitive decline, vascular brain diseases, and literacy problems. Therefore, it is important to question patients at each visit regarding his or her medication list, compliance with medications, and the reason(s) for noncompliance (if present).

B. What types of difficulties has she been experiencing that caused her to be noncompliant with her diet?   ESSENTIAL

Because lifestyle modifications, including diet, are just as essential as medication therapy in the management of diabetes mellitus, it is again important to ascertain in a nonjudgmental, nonconfrontational, nonaccusatory manner the reason the patient is not following his or her dietary recommendations. These reasons can include not understanding the dietary recommendations and/or their importance, food preferences not taken into account with recommendations, lack of health literacy, lack of ability to prepare meals (or availability of assistance with food preparation), difficulty with shopping including the inability to afford fresh vegetables/fruits and other "healthy" foods, and comorbid conditions making the patient disinterested in caring for him- or herself (e.g., depression, vascular brain diseases, or Alzheimer disease).

Additionally, this also enables the healthcare provider (HCP) to made recommendations, modifications, and dietitian referrals when necessary to achieve good compliance with dietary recommendations.

C. Has she been experiencing any problems with vulvovaginal itching or vaginal discharge?   NONESSENTIAL

Despite the fact that women with diabetes have a greater incidence of vulvovaginal candidiasis, it is generally not necessary to ask if they are experiencing these symptoms. The majority of women with vulvovaginal candidiasis either self-medicate with over-the-counter products or schedule appointments for the problem due to the discomfort of the condition.

It is important to remember that patients who are immunocompromised for any reason are prone to recurrent vulvovaginitis due to candidiasis; therefore, it is not specific to this condition. However, in women with recurrent candidal vulvovaginitis it is appropriate to perform a plasma glucose to determine whether diabetes mellitus is the cause for the recurrences.

D. Why doesn't she see the local "medicine man" instead of coming to the clinic if she is not going to follow the healthcare provider's (HCP's) advice?   NONESSENTIAL

This question is inappropriate and should not be asked for several reasons. First, it is culturally insensitive. Second, it implies that it is the patient's fault alone that she is noncompliant. Studies have shown that noncompliance is generally the result of several factors that involve not only the patient, but also the healthcare provider and the healthcare system. Third, it suggests that alternative medicine might be better than traditional medicine. Because there is very little scientific information and virtually no evidence-based data on alternative therapies for the treatment of diabetes mellitus, this would be considered extremely inappropriate advice.

E. Is she experiencing any depression, mood changes, changes in appetite, poor concentration, difficulty in making decisions, poor self-esteem, feelings of hopelessness, anhedonia, or thoughts of death or suicide?   ESSENTIAL

Because Mrs. Thompson is complaining of fatigue (defined as "tired all the time" and having difficulties in getting motivated and starting projects/activities), there exists a concern that she could have a coexisting mood disorder because, as discussed previously, this type of fatigue is most commonly seen with psychological problems. This is especially important given Mrs. Thompson's history because depression (and other mood disorders) can frequently be a component of medical noncompliance in patients. As previously stated, medical noncompliance is often multifactorial in nature. For example, if patients feel hopeless regarding the future, they do not see a "need" to take care of medical problem(s), especially chronic one(s); if patients lack interest in anything, it frequently includes themselves (and by extension their health), so they "don't care" about the problem(s); and if patients' fatigue can make anything a major effort, including taking medications, following a diet (and other lifestyle modifications), monitoring blood glucose levels, and performing other areas of self-care. Therefore, it is important to evaluate all noncompliant patients as well as those exhibiting minimal symptoms of a mood disorder for the presence of such, especially considering that studies are revealing that diagnosing and treating depression early result in better outcomes and resolution rates.

2. Physical Examination

A. Funduscopic examination   NONESSENTIAL

Even though all patients with diabetes mellitus should have a complete eye exam (including the usage of a slit lamp) annually, the reason for her visit today is polyuria, polydipsia, and fatigue. Because she is not complaining of any visual abnormalities, it is appropriate to defer her funduscopic examination until she can be scheduled for a complete history and physical examination for her diabetes. Further disease and lifestyle modifications as well as age-appropriate health maintenance (including appropriate immunizations) should also be conducted at that visit (if Mrs. Thompson desires preventive services).

Additionally, all patients with diabetes mellitus should see an ophthalmologist annually to have an extensive complete ocular examination to screen for signs of diabetic retinopathy. If found early, these problems can generally successfully be treated and blindness (once frequently associated with diabetes) can be prevented. The American Diabetes Association's (ADA's) guidelines recommend this exam occur

within 5 years of the diagnosis of type 1 diabetes mellitus (DM) and shortly after the diagnosis of type 2 DM is established.

B. Thyroid examination   ESSENTIAL

Although Mrs. Thompson's fatigue could be due to her diabetes, it is also seen with a multitude of other conditions (e.g., hyperthyroidism and hypothyroidism). Therefore, her thyroid gland needs to be palpated for evidence of enlargement, tenderness, masses, nodules, or other abnormalities.

C. Heart examination   ESSENTIAL

Multiple cardiac conditions (e.g., heart failure, arrhythmias, valvular abnormalities, and infectious endocarditis) can cause fatigue. Therefore, it is important to perform a heart examination as outlined in Case 1-2.

D. Pelvic examination   NONESSENTIAL

E. Examination for bilateral pedal edema   ESSENTIAL

Several conditions associated with fatigue and depression-like symptoms can cause pedal edema (e.g., heart failure, nephrotic syndrome, cirrhosis, hepatitis, and myxedema).

3. Diagnostic Studies

A. Lipid profile, serum blood urea nitrogen (BUN) and creatinine, alanine aminotransferase (ALT), fasting plasma glucose (FPG), thyroid panel, and complete blood count with differential (CBC w/diff)   ESSENTIAL

The importance of the lipid profile is to reduce the risks associated with the vascular complications of DM because hyperlipidemia is also associated with the development of these complications. In fact, the ADA guidelines recommend lower goal levels for lipids as if the patient already had CAD. They recommend the low-density lipoprotein cholesterol (LDL-C) be less than 100 mg/dl, high-density lipoprotein cholesterol (HDL-C) be greater than 40 mg/dl in men and greater than 50 mg/dl in women, and triglycerides be less than 150 mg/dl. If this goal cannot be achieved via diet and exercise, then the ADA recommends that a statin be the first-line drug of choice.

The National Cholesterol Education Project's Adult Treatment Panel III (NCEP-ATP III) automatically includes individuals with DM as coronary heart disease (CHD) risk equivalent, meaning that their likelihood of having a coronary event within the next 10 years is considered to be greater than 20%. The NCEP-ATP III set the minimal goals for this group of patients to be an LDL of less than 100 mg/dl with an optimal goal of less than 70 mg/dl. Furthermore, they make the recommendation to also treat hypertriglyceridemia and low HDL levels, which has unfortunately yet to become standard of care.

Her lipid panel could have been deferred until her follow-up appointment because it is not going to directly impact on establishing her diagnosis and treatment for her chief complaint. However, by doing it today, it prevents her from having to undergo another venipuncture to obtain the specimen, plus the results will be available for review at her follow-up visit for further discussion and treatment.

The BUN and creatinine levels are indicators of renal and hepatic function; however, their primary indication is to determine whether Mrs. Thompson's diabetes has adversely affected her kidney function. An elevation of either of these tests would be suspicious for a renal problem (e.g., nephrotic syndrome or asymptomatic pyelonephritis), which could also potentially be responsible for her fatigue. This test is also important because renally excreted medications are going to require dosage adjustments if her renal function is abnormal. Abnormalities most be confirmed by additional testing.

In some cases, fatty liver disease can occur in diabetics and produce abnormal liver function test results; the ALT, which is the most sensitive of all the liver function tests, can serve as a screening tool for this condition as well as Mrs. Thompson's overall hepatic function. Essentially, if the ALT is normal, there is no reason to be concerned regarding liver damage. However, if the ALT is elevated, additional testing is necessary to determine if a hepatic etiology is responsible for Mrs. Thompson's fatigue (e.g., cirrhosis or hepatitis). Plus he patically metabolized medications may require dosage adjustments to prevent excessive drug accumulation in the body, and some medications should probably be avoided if they are known to cause hepatotoxicity (as they can further worsen the liver's functioning). Additional testing is necessary to determine the exact nature of the abnormal ALT.

A thyroid panel is indicated to ensure that the patient does not have primary or secondary hypo- or hyperthyroidism as the cause of her fatigue. Furthermore, it is included in the ADA guidelines to perform on all newly diagnosed patients with type 1 diabetes mellitus and symptomatic patients with type 2 diabetes mellitus.

The CBC w/diff is also going to rule out potential causes of fatigue such as anemia, infection, inflammation, and certain carcinomas.

This information in conjunction with the FPG is going to provide a decent "picture" of where Mrs. Thompson's glucose control is currently, whether there are any complications from her diabetes or any factors that could be adversely affecting her blood glucose level or any proposed treatments.

B. Electrocardiogram (ECG)   ESSENTIAL

The ECG can be helpful in evaluating for potential causes of her fatigue such as an arrhythmia (either a bradycardia or a tachycardia), silent ischemia (which is more common in diabetics), ventricular enlargement (which is seen in heart failure [HF]), or an electrolyte disturbance (e.g., hypokalemia). Furthermore, it will serve as a baseline study for any future comparative tests.

C. Urinalysis and serial spot for microalbuminuria if protein is negative   ESSENTIAL

Although it is most likely that Mrs. Thompson's urinary frequency is the result of her poorly controlled diabetes, it is also possible that it is the result of an asymptomatic upper or lower urinary tract infection. Therefore, a complete urinalysis should be done instead of just screening for protein, glucose, and ketones, which is all that is normally indicated for diabetic patients.

It is not uncommon for a patient with diabetes with poor glycemic control to have some minor abnormalities on his or her urinalysis. These findings can consist of a slightly acidic urine (probably due to a mild metabolic acidosis), a slightly elevated pH if glucosuria is present, and positive glucose on dipstick analysis. Ketosis might also be present even in the absence of the ketoacidosis (which is rare in type 2 diabetes) because the glucose (although elevated in the serum) cannot

be utilized for energy due to the insufficiency of insulin; thus, a fatty acid catabolism occurs instead, producing the ketones. Urinary ketosis can also occur in starvation, high-protein diets, and acute febrile illness in children. Hence, the use of screening for ketones in the urine of an essentially asymptomatic diabetic (which the ADA recommends be done on an annual basis) is another indication of the type of control that is being achieved of the diabetes.

Serial spot urine testing for microalbuminuria (MA) is much more accurate in detecting diabetic nephropathy (especially in its early stages) than the serum creatinine, a positive urine protein, or an abnormal urine sediment. However, before it can be considered positive, the patient has to have two out of three positive results performed at 3- to 6-month intervals. It is estimated that an elevated MA level can be present for a minimum of 5 years before any protein is revealed in the urine on dipstick analysis.

Furthermore, it is theorized that MA might be the earliest determinant of impending cardiovascular disease (CVD) and hypertension (HTN). An elevated MA is considered to be associated with a 5 to 10 times risk of CVD mortality, end-stage renal disease, and retinopathy in patients with diabetes.

Persistently positive serial spot urinalysis evaluation for microalbuminuria (without proteinuria or abnormal urine sediment) plus a normal serum creatinine is indicative of a very early nephropathy. Studies are currently conflicting on whether improving glycemic and hypertensive control may or may not reverse the elevated MA level.

D. Hamilton Depression Rating Scale   ESSENTIAL

Because Mrs. Thompson is having several symptoms, besides her fatigue, that could indicate the presence of a major mood disorder, further evaluation for depression is indicated. A depression rating scale (not a screening tool because the aforementioned questions have already screened her as positive for a possible depression) should be conducted on her. Because the Hamilton Depression Rating Scale is considered by many to be the "gold standard" in rating depression, it is an appropriate test to utilize. The 17-item variety consists of nine symptoms that are rated from 0 to 4 (with 0 being absent and 4 being severe) and an additional eight items rated from 0 (absent) to 2 (clearly present) by the patient with the assistance of a trained individual as a partially structured interview. If the patient has a total score of 10 to 11 out of a possible total of 52, the diagnosis of depression can be made with a high degree of probability.

E. Glycated hemoglobin A$_1$ (Hgb A1C)   NONESSENTIAL

The Hgb A1C provides a measurement of the patient's glycemic control over the 100 to 120 days before test, which incidentally correlates with the lifespan of red blood cells (RBCs). Therefore, it is technically the amount of glucose available over the lifetime of an RBC. Because this number is not expected to change significantly during the life of the RBC, it is recommended that this test be performed no more often than 3-month intervals.

4. Diagnosis

A. Type 2 diabetes mellitus, with prehypertension, hyperlipidemia, class I obesity, possibly mild diabetic nephropathy, and major depressive disorder   INCORRECT

Mrs. Thompson does have type 2 diabetes, confirmed by her history and FPG (diagnosis of diabetes is two levels above 126 mg/dl OR one level above 200 mg/dl in a symptomatic patient).

The Seventh Report of the Joint National Committee on the Prevention, Detection, Evaluation, and Treatment of High Blood Pressure (JNC-7) Report definitions of hypertension require two different BP readings to make a diagnosis. Mrs. Thompson's BP today of 136/84 mm Hg and the one from her last visit of 138/86 mm Hg classify her as having prehypertension (systolic BP of 120 to 139 mm Hg OR diastolic BP of 89 to 90 mm Hg). Please see Case 1-1 for all BP classifications.

CAD is a common macrovascular complication of DM, and of all the additional risk factors known for CAD, uncontrolled HTN appears to be the most significant. Plus, HTN also plays a role in the development of other complications from DM, including macrovascular (e.g., CVAs and TIAs) and microvascular complications (e.g., diabetic retinopathies and nephropathies). The ADA and JNC-7 guidelines for BP control have been reduced from the normal recommendation of less than 140/90 mm Hg to the same range as a patient who has chronic kidney disease, less than 130/80 mm Hg. Therefore, Mrs. Thompson's prehypertension will need to be treated to achieve her treatment goal of less than 130/80 mm Hg.

There are some experts who advocate for an even lower BP goal and have advocated for a systolic BP of less than 120 mm Hg. However, the preliminary results of the ACCORD Trial released in 2010 revealed that intensive BP control to a systolic BP of less than 120 offered no benefit to patients with type 2 diabetes mellitus that controlling systolic BP to less than in terms of cardiovascular morbidity (MI and CVA) and mortality. Nevertheless, the lower BP goal may still provide some protection against microvascular complications such as nephropathy and retinopathy.

As stated previously, the NCEP-ATP III automatically includes individuals with DM as CHD risk equivalent, meaning that their likelihood of having a coronary event within the next 10 years is considered to be greater than 20%. Therefore, the NCEP-ATP III set the minimal LDL goal for this group of patients at less than 100 mg/dl, with an optimal goal of less than 70 mg/dl. Furthermore, they make the recommendation to also treat hypertriglyceridemia and low HDL levels. Hence, her lipid levels qualify her to be diagnosed as having hyperlipidemia.

A mild diabetic nephropathy is possible as discussed further under choice D. However, the remaining diagnoses for this choice are incorrect. Her BMI of 44.9 would be categorized as class III, not class I, obesity. (Please see Case 1-1 for the class definitions.) And depression can be eliminated based on her responses provided upon further questioning and via her Hamilton Depression Rating Scale.

B. Type 2 diabetes mellitus, with hypertension (stage 1), hyperlipidemia, class II obesity, possibly mild diabetic nephropathy, and major depressive disorder   INCORRECT

For the reasons stated in response A, Mrs. Thompson can be diagnosed as having type 2 diabetes mellitus and hyperlipidemia. However, this is not her most likely diagnosis because she has prehypertension not stage 1 and her obesity is not class II obesity.

C. Diabetes mellitus with obesity, borderline BP, and hyperlipidemia lipids   INCORRECT

Technically Mrs. Thompson has all of these conditions. However, because this diagnosis fails to describe the classification/type of these conditions and another diagnosis does so correctly, this would not be considered her MOST likely diagnosis.

D. Type 2 diabetes mellitus, with prehypertension, hyperlipidemia, class III (extreme) obesity, possibly mild diabetic nephropathy, and dysthymia   CORRECT

From the discussion in response A, it is clear that Mrs. Thompson has type 2 diabetes mellitus, prehypertension, and hyperlipidemia. Class III (extreme obesity) is also correct because it is defined as a BMI of greater than 40. Hers is 44.9.

It is also apparent that she possibly has mild diabetic nephropathy. This assumption is based on the fact that she had microalbumin on a single spot test along with a normal serum creatinine, no protein on her urinalysis dipstick, and no suspicious urine sediment. However, serial spot urine testing for microalbuminuria (MA) is much more accurate in detecting diabetic nephropathy (especially in its early stages) than either a serum creatinine or proteinuria. Nevertheless, before this diagnosis can be confirmed with certainty, she must have one more additional positive test out of her next two, which should be completed in the next 3 to 6 months.

Finally, because her Hamilton depression screen is negative but she has chronic low-grade symptoms that could be consistent with depression, her most likely diagnosis is dysthymic disorder. As with any condition described in the *Diagnostic and Statistical Manual of Mental Disorders,* fourth edition, text revision (DSM-IV—TR), there is the caveat that the condition cannot be better accounted for by another mental, physical, or substance abuse disorder, and that it is causing significant distress or impairment of important areas of functioning.

The actual diagnostic criteria include the symptoms being present on most days for a minimum of 2 years (without going for a maximum of 2 months without them) in adults (1 year in children or teens) and the absence of a major depressive episode either during or shortly before the onset of the symptoms. While experiencing these mild depressive symptoms, the patient also has to exhibit two or more of the following symptoms: insomnia, decreased energy or fatigue, feelings of hopelessness, poor concentration or difficulty in making difficult decisions, increased or decreased appetite, or low self-esteem. Therefore, this choice is Mrs. Thompson's most likely diagnosis.

E. Type 2 diabetes mellitus, stage 1 hypertension, hyperlipidemia, class I obesity, possibly mild diabetic nephropathy, and dysthymia   INCORRECT

The findings that prevent this choice from being Mrs. Thompson's most likely diagnosis is the misdiagnosis of her hypertension as stage 1 and her obesity as class I. Again, to review the stages of obesity based on BMI and the definitions of type of hypertension, please see Case 1-1.

5. Treatment Plan

A. Patient education and lifestyle modifications   CORRECT

This should include extensive patient education on the disease; current lab results, lab goals, and the importance of achieving these goals; discussions of her comorbid conditions, including their significance and impact on both her other conditions and overall health as well as developing a treatment plan for each of them; the significance of the presence of microalbuminuria and need for repeat testing; all the potential complications of diabetes; the importance of following a treatment plan including lifestyle changes and medications; assisting her in making appropriate adjustments in the dietary guidelines to include foods she likes to eat (taking into account her ethnic and cultural preferences) but still including a Dietary Approaches to Stop Hypertension (DASH)-type diet with low salt, fats, and sweets; physiology of dysthymia and importance of treating it; importance of follow-up as recommended; and referral to diabetic educator and dietitian, if available.

All of this information (both verbal and written) has to be available at an educational level the patient can comprehend and follow. Furthermore, it is going to take more than one time to review all of this with her in order for her to comprehend it. If she appears to have concerns regarding the volume of information or to not fully understand the instructions, she should be encouraged to bring her spouse, child, friend, or significant other with her to assist with these details. Additionally, if a quality diabetic support group is available in the area, she should consider joining it for further support in all the details of controlling her disease. Finally, any changes that she makes, no matter how small, must be praised. Additionally, she will need to be provided with significant amounts of encouragement to make and continue all the change necessary to properly treat her host of medical conditions.

B. Start ramipril 2.5 mg daily   CORRECT

The use of an angiotensin-converting enzyme (ACE) inhibitor or an angiotensin receptor blocker (ARB) is recommended by the ADA guidelines for diabetic patients with hypertension and/or MA to prevent further renal complications.

The use of these agents is also theorized to prevent, or at least reduce, cardiovascular complications in high-risk patients; however, this has not been confirmed in clinical trials. Ramipril, which is an ACE inhibitor, has a US Food and Drug Administration (FDA) indication for this usage.

For diabetic patients who are unable to meet their BP goal with diet, exercise, smoking cessation, and alcohol reduction/cessation, the ADA guidelines recommend the addition of an ACE inhibitor if patients are type 1 and either an ACE inhibitor or an ARB if patients are type 2. Other ADA recommendations regarding treatment include an ACE inhibitor if the patient is 50 years of age or older and has at least one cardiovascular risk factor, defined as being a man age 45 years or older, a woman age 55 years or older (or postmenopausal), a BP greater than or equal to 140/90 mm Hg, currently taking an antihypertensive agent, an HDL less than 40 mg/dl, cigarette smoking, and a positive family history or a first-degree relative with premature CAD (defined as before the age of 55 in men and 66 in women).

Unless contraindicated, the ADA guidelines also recommend aspirin therapy of 75 to 262 mg/day of an enteric-coated or buffered formulation if the patient is 40 years of age or older and has at least one of the aforementioned CAD risk factors.

Furthermore, the ADA guidelines recommend the goal of diabetes treatment to be an FPG between 70 and 130 mg/dl, a peak postprandial glucose (at 1 or 2 hours) of less than 180 mg/dl,

and an A1C of less than 7.0%. There has been some discussion of recommending even lower levels for even tighter control to prevent the complications from DM; however, this can be associated with more episodes of hypoglycemia and the associated complications. The American Association of Clinical Endocrinologists has already instituted recommendations for stricter control. They recommend an FPG of less than 110 mg/dl, a peak postprandial glucose at 2 hours of less than 110 mg/dl, and an A1C of less than or equal to 6.5%.

C. Refer to ophthalmologist for complete eye evaluation, stressing the importance of the visit   CORRECT

All type 2 diabetic patients need an ophthalmologist-performed eye exam as soon as possible after diagnosis. The importance and purpose of the visit need to be explained to the patient.

D. Restart all four diabetic medications; advise of mechanisms of action, possible adverse effects, and to call office immediately if they occur   INCORRECT

Because of Mrs. Thompson's FPG and Hgb A1C levels, she is probably going to require medication in addition to lifestyle measures to control her diabetes; however, at this time, it would be appropriate to have her start just the metformin along with lifestyle modifications.

This is especially important because she has never taken the last two medications prescribed for her diabetes and only took the second one to partial dosage; thus, starting all four of the medications at once could result in a significant hypoglycemia or other adverse events. Furthermore, if all four medications were started simultaneously and Mrs. Thompson experienced an adverse or unwanted side effect, it would be extremely difficult to determine the culprit. Additionally, she would likely be more reluctant to take any medications in the future.

With any medication that is prescribed, the patient should be informed of its purpose, its mechanism of action, potential medication (including over-the-counter, vitamins, supplements, and herbal preparations) and/or food (e.g., grapefruit juice, bran, calcium rich, or iron rich) interactions, and possible common adverse effects and what to do if they occur; not to discontinue the medications if the patient has problems and/or concerns but to call; and how to contact the office/provider during and after hours if any concerns and/or problems arise.

E. Schedule for a complete examination   CORRECT

Because of the strong propensity for serious complications related to the chronic medical conditions Mrs. Thompson has, she is going to require a visit focusing on the history, physical examination, and testing that is essential for each of her medical conditions to look for signs of these related conditions and devise treatment plans to prevent them. The examination must include complete historical data, pertinent physical examination areas, and appropriate diagnostic studies. Additionally, she should be encouraged to obtain age-appropriate preventive health services at this time (e.g., mammogram, dual-energy x-ray absorptiometry [DEXA] scan, and immunizations).

F. Start selegiline transdermal patches   INCORRECT

Selegiline transdermal patches are a monoamine oxidase inhibitor (MAOI) antidepressant and are generally not an appropriate first-line treatment for major depressive episode, let alone dysthymia. If treating dysthymia medically, a selective serotonin reuptake inhibitor (SSRI) is probably the most appropriate first-line choice. Serotonin norepinephrine reuptake inhibitors (SNRIs) are an acceptable alternative. Neither are FDA-approved for this use. Psychotherapy is also beneficial.

Epidemiologic and Other Data

The term diabetes mellitus generally refers to either type 1 diabetes mellitus (DM-1) or type 2 diabetes mellitus (DM-2). DM-1 is either an immune-mediated or idiopathic condition of hyperglycemia that is caused by a near-complete or a complete loss of insulin production by the pancreas. It does not have a genetic predisposition. In the past, it was known as insulin-dependent diabetes mellitus (IDDM) because virtually all the patients with the condition require insulin therapy for treatment.

DM-2 was previously known as non–insulin-dependent diabetes mellitus (NIDDM) because the majority of patients did not require insulin therapy. It is a condition associated with hyperglycemia, abnormal insulin secretion, and insulin resistance. The term NIDDM was changed because to achieve optimal control, insulin therapy is eventually required in the majority of patients with DM-2. It tends to have a genetic and metabolic etiology. In the past, it was rare for a patient with DM-2 to be under the age of 30 years; however, because of the obesity epidemic in this country, more and more individuals, including adolescents, have DM-2.

There are additional types of diabetes mellitus that are secondary to other conditions. The most common is gestational diabetes, associated with pregnancy. Others include genetic mutations that render the pancreatic β-cell incapable of producing insulin (e.g., insulin promoter factor-1 and proinsulin conversion), genetic abnormalities in the action of insulin (e.g., lipodystrophy syndromes and leprechaunism), pancreatic diseases that affect insulin production (e.g., pancreatitis, cystic fibrosis, and hemochromatosis), other endocrine conditions (e.g., Cushing syndrome and hyperthyroidism), medications (nicotinic acid, thyroid hormones, and thiazide diuretics), infections (congenital rubella and cytomegalovirus), rare immune defects (e.g., "stiff-person" syndrome), and genetically induced conditions that occasionally can be linked with DM (e.g., Prader-Willi syndrome, Friedreich ataxia, and Huntington chorea).

It is estimated that in the United States approximately 7% of the population, or 20.8 million individuals, is diabetic. Approximately 1.5 million adults are diagnosed with the condition annually in the United States. The incidence of DM increases with age. It is seen with a slightly greater rate in men than in women. According to race in the United States, the most frequently affected population is Native Americans (especially the Pima Indians). This is followed by African Americans, Latino Americans, Asian Americans, Pacific Islanders, and non-Hispanic whites.

CASE 3-2

Theresa Umberto

1. History

A. Has she been experiencing depression, hopelessness, or anhedonia?   NONESSENTIAL

Although Mrs. Umberto has some symptoms that can be seen in depression (e.g., insomnia, weight loss, increased appetite and fatigue), their pattern is not consistent with this diagnosis. For example, insomnia associated with depression is most commonly terminal insomnia, meaning that the patient awakens early and cannot get back to sleep. Mid-night awakenings can be seen with depression but generally have no stimulus (e.g., vasomotor symptoms). Her fatigue is a weakness, not a total exhaustion with lack of desire and/or motivation. And her weight loss is not secondary to anorexia, nor is her increased eating associated with a weight gain as would generally be found in depression.

B. Has she noticed any swelling in her neck or lower legs? ESSENTIAL

Her complaints could result from a multitude of problems including endocrine abnormalities (e.g., premature ovarian failure, pituitary adenoma or carcinoma, or thyrotoxicosis), cardiac conditions (e.g., infective endocarditis with heart failure, arrhythmias, or atypical ischemia), or pulmonary problems (e.g., tuberculosis infection or lung cancer) to name a few.

Therefore, it is important to know if she has noticed any midline neck swelling that could indicate a thyroid goiter/tumor/mass or supraclavicular swelling that could be caused by a lymphadenopathy. However, it is not uncommon for thyroid dysfunction to occur in conjunction with a normal appearing thyroid gland on physical examination. Additionally, it is essential to know if she has any pedal edema of her ankles that could represent heart failure or pretibial swelling that could be caused by myxedema.

C. Has she experienced any muscle cramps, muscle weakness, or tremors?   ESSENTIAL

Muscle cramps and tremors are commonly seen with many forms of thyrotoxicosis; however, they are also seen with electrolyte abnormalities that could be inducing a cardiac arrhythmia. Furthermore, neurologic conditions, such as dysautonomias, can cause symptoms similar to what Mrs. Umberto is experiencing and can be associated with muscle weakness and occasionally loss of muscle tone.

D. Are her "hot flashes" associated with neck and/or facial erythema?   ESSENTIAL

The average age for menopause in the United States is 51 years old, with a range from 45 to 55 years. Nevertheless, it is not impossible for Mrs. Umberto to be perimenopausal; however, it would be a premature form of menopause (e.g., premature ovarian failure). Although many of her symptoms are consistent with premature menopause (e.g., night sweats, irregular menses, and irritability), her other symptoms are generally not (e.g., palpations, unintentional weight loss, warm/moist skin, and onycholysis). However, it is important to remember that she could have two (or more) conditions occurring simultaneously, further complicating her clinical picture.

Furthermore, her description of her "hot flashes" is not typical for those associated with perimenopause and menopause. The vasomotor "hot flashes" associated with menopause generally do not include a heat intolerance but a hot or warm sensation starting across the chest and progressing proximally to the top of the head; furthermore, they are generally associated with flushing. However, the warm sensations/feelings associated with dysautonomias and cardiac arrhythmias are less transitory (but start at the top of the head and move distally). Furthermore, the latter are generally associated with facial pallor.

E. Has she noticed any changes of her hair, skin, or nails? ESSENTIAL

Metabolic abnormalities, endocrine problems, anemias, and dermatologic conditions can affect a patient's hair, skin, and nails. For example, cold, dry skin is frequently associated with hypothyroidism, whereas warm, moist skin is more commonly seen with hyperthyroidism. Dry brittle nails are seen in hypothyroidism and iron deficiency anemia. Chronic thyrotoxicosis may be associated with clubbing of the nails and/or onycholysis. Hypothyroidism and hyperthyroidism can be associated with thinning of the hair.

2. Physical Examination

A. Eye examination   ESSENTIAL

Certain types of thyrotoxicosis are associated with characteristic ocular findings. The mnemonic "NO SPECS" is sometimes utilized to ensure no potential problem is overlooked and to attempt to quantify the severity of the eye changes. Although the quantification scale ranges from a score of 0 for the "N" (**N**ormal) of "**NO SPECS**" to 6 for the last "S" (**S**ight loss), it is not a completely accurate scoring system because the patient does not necessarily follow the progression of ophthalmic abnormalities in sequential numerical order.

The remainder of the mnemonic and score is 1 for "O" (**O**nly sign is a lid lag or retraction); 2 for "S" (**S**oft tissue affected causing periorbital edema); 3 for "P" (**P**roptosis, which must be more than 22 mm); 4 for "E" (**E**xtraocular muscles affected as in diplopia or nystagmus); and 5 for "C" (**C**ornea affected, e.g., dryness and/or damage, secondary to chronic sclera exposure because of eyelids not being able to fully close, abrasions, and irritations).

B. Neck examination   ESSENTIAL

Because one of the several types of thyrotoxicosis could explain all of Mrs. Umberto's symptoms, it is essential to evaluate her neck for thyroid abnormalities (e.g., goiter, nodules, masses, bruit, and/or tenderness). Additionally, the size, shape, and consistency need to be examined because if a thyrotoxicosis is responsible for her symptoms, these characteristics can provide clues to the type.

Her cervical and supraclavicular lymph nodes need to be examined for lymphadenopathy because it could indicate that an infectious, inflammatory, or malignant process is present.

C. Heart examination   ESSENTIAL

Because Mrs. Umberto is experiencing palpations, tachycardia, and leg edema, it is essential to perform a complete heart examination as outlined in Case 1-2.

D. Abdominal examination   NONESSENTIAL

E. Distal lower extremity and skin examination   ESSENTIAL

Because Mrs. Umberto is complaining of skin changes and ankle/leg edema, it is essential to evaluate her skin and lower legs for abnormalities.

3. Diagnostic Studies

A. Electrocardiogram (ECG)   ESSENTIAL

An ECG is indicated because Mrs. Umberto is complaining of palpations and is experiencing tachycardia. It can distinguish whether her current rhythm is a sinus tachycardia or some other tachyarrhythmia. The ECG can also evaluate for possible cardiomegaly, indicating heart failure could be present.

However, it is important to remember that an ECG just provides a "snapshot" of a very short interval of time (generally a few seconds) of cardiac activity. Therefore, paroxysmal or intermittent arrhythmias could easily be missed if the HCP just relied on a single ECG for identification.

Therefore, if there is concern about an unstable arrhythmia, the patient should be hospitalized on telemetry for observation. Long-term outpatient telemetry (Holter monitoring) is an acceptable alternative if a more stable arrhythmia exists.

B. Thyroid stimulating hormone (TSH), free thyroxine (FT_4), and triiodothyronine by radioimmunoassay (T_3 by RIA)   ESSENTIAL

Thyroid function studies are indicated because Mrs. Umberto's symptoms could be caused by a thyroid condition.

C. Complete blood count with differential (CBC w/diff) ESSENTIAL

A CBC w/diff is indicated because it can provide support for or against a diagnosis of an atypical infectious, inflammatory, or hematologic cause of Mrs. Umberto's symptoms.

D. Quantitative serum human chorionic gonadotropin NONESSENTIAL

Although Mrs. Umberto is utilizing her contraceptive method regularly, the diaphragm (even in conjunction with contraceptive foam) has a typical user effectiveness rating of approximately 82%. Additionally, because she is sexually active and her last menstrual period was about 5 weeks ago, there is a possibility that she could be pregnant.

However, because she is not experiencing any abdominal pain, vaginal bleeding, or spotting, a quantitative serum human chorionic gonadotropin (HCG) is not indicated because a urinary pregnancy test will provide equally as accurate results as to whether she is currently pregnant.

Pregnancy and/or its complications could account for some, if not all, of Mrs. Umberto's symptoms. Likewise, a pregnancy would cause more caution in selecting medications because of their potential risks/harm to the fetus. For more information on the US Food and Drug Administration's (FDA) classification system regarding fetotoxic risk potential from medications, please see Case 2-7.

E. Thyroglobulin (Tg)   NONESSENTIAL

Tg is primarily utilized as a tumor marker to follow patients after they have had surgery for thyroid cancer. Thus, this test is not necessary at this time.

4. Diagnosis

A. Graves thyrotoxicosis   CORRECT

Elevated thyroid hormones, FT_4, and T_3 by RIA, in the presence of a low TSH indicate a thyrotoxicosis from a primary hyperthyroidism. The majority of the time, it is secondary to Graves (or Basedow) disease. This autoimmune disease can be distinguished clinically from other causes of thyrotoxicosis because of its characteristic physical examination findings: thyroid-associated (or Graves) ophthalmopathy, thyroid dermopathy (pretibial myxedema), and a diffusely enlarged (often two to three times normal size) but smooth thyroid. This diagnosis can be confirmed serologically by the presence of elevated levels of antithyroid antibodies (thyroid peroxidase antibody [TPO-Ab], thyroid-binding inhibitory immunoglobulin [TBII], and thyroid-stimulating immunoglobulin [TSI]). Hence, this is Mrs. Umberto's most likely diagnosis.

B. Multinodular goiter (MNG)   INCORRECT

Even though MNG, or Plummer disease, is a thyrotoxicosis caused by a primary hyperthyroidism, it can be eliminated as Mrs. Umberto's most likely diagnosis because of the lack of multiple nodules on her thyroid and the marked degree of thyromegaly present on her physical examination. Additionally, it is generally not associated with any ophthalmologic symptoms.

C. Jodbasedow disease   INCORRECT

Jodbasedow disease is an iodine-induced hyperthyroidism associated with the presence of multinodular goiter. It is most frequently caused by radiographic examinations requiring iodine contrast media or exposure to iodine-based medication, most notably amiodarone. Because of her lack of a history of exposure to either of these as well as no evidence of a multinodular goiter on physical examination, Jodbasedow disease is not Mrs. Umberto's most likely diagnosis.

D. De Quervain disease   INCORRECT

De Quervain' disease, or subacute thyroiditis, is considered to be a thyrotoxicosis without hyperthyroidism (low TSH and a normal FT_4 and T_3 by RIA). It is theorized to be viral in nature. It can be eliminated as Mrs. Umberto's most likely diagnosis because of her thyroid studies.

E. Depression   INCORRECT

Depression can be ruled out based on the lack of appropriate signs and symptoms of the disease and the results of the thyroid testing. However, if some of the symptoms that could be related to mood do not resolve once Mrs. Umberto is euthyroid, then additional evaluation should be undertaken to explore for the possible presence of a coexisting mood disorder, including depression, bipolar illness, anxiety, and panic attacks.

5. Treatment Plan

A. Referral to an ophthalmologist   CORRECT

An ophthalmologist referral is indicated when the ocular condition from Graves disease is significant and/or active. The ophthalmologist should evaluate all of the following for abnormalities and to provide a baseline study: visual acuity, color vision, function of the extraocular muscles, visual fields, intraocular pressure, the optic nerve (for signs of compression or papilledema) via dilated slit-lamp examination, the cornea with fluorescein stain under ultraviolent light (for abrasions/irritations secondary to failure of the eye[s] to completely close), and the degree of proptosis (measured via an exophthalmometer).

B. Methimazole 30 mg orally once a day; then adjust dosage based on FT_4 levels   INCORRECT

Thiourea medications, such as methimazole or propylthiouracil, are effective treatments for younger patients whose hyperthyroid symptoms are mild and goiter is small. However, because of the size of Mrs. Umberto's thyroid, her extensive symptoms, and the significant elevation of her antithyroid antibodies, it is unlikely that these medications are going to be effective in treating her condition. Furthermore, they are associated with some serious adverse effects including agranulocytosis, hepatic necrosis, cholestatic jaundice, nephritic syndrome, and serum sickness, especially in higher doses as Mrs. Umberto would more than likely require.

C. Radioactive iodine (^{131}I) treatment instead of methimazole   CORRECT

Thyroid ablation with radioactive iodine is the treatment of choice for Mrs. Umberto. The majority of the patients can start it immediately, and take it along with the propranolol for symptomatic relief from autonomic complaints, without any difficulty. However, those with severe disease, those with coronary artery disease, or the elderly may require pretreatment with a thiourea to establish a euthyroid state before undergoing radioactive iodine therapy.

D. Immediate surgical consult for thyroidectomy   INCORRECT

Thyroid surgery is indicated as a first-line therapy if thyroid cancer is suspected and/or atypical or cancerous cells are discovered on the cytologic results of a needle biopsy of a thyroid nodule. Therefore, it is not an appropriate treatment option for Mrs. Umberto at this time. However, it would be an acceptable option for her if she failed or was intolerant of the aforementioned treatments or if her goiter enlarged and became an obstructive or cosmetic problem for her.

E. Duloxetine 20 mg daily

The SNRI duloxetine is not an appropriate treatment option for Mrs. Umberto at this time because she does not appear to have depression.

Epidemiologic and Other Data

Hyperthyroidism is the presence of excessive thyroid hormone. It should not be confused with thyrotoxicosis, which is the condition that occurs as a result of that excessive thyroid hormone. Thyrotoxicosis can either be primary (e.g., Graves disease, MNG, toxic adenoma, thyroid cancer, or iodine excess), secondary (e.g., TSH-producing pituitary adenoma, chorionic gonadotropin-secreting tumors, and gestational thyrotoxicosis), or without hyperthyroidism (e.g., subacute thyroiditis, ingestion of excessive thyroid hormone, or thyroid destruction secondary to radiation).

It is estimated that Graves disease is responsible for 60% to 80% of all cases of thyrotoxicosis. It is much more frequent in females than in males. The most typical age of onset is in the third to sixth decades of life.

CASE 3-3
Ulysses Valez
1. History

A. Has he experienced any visual changes or headaches? ESSENTIAL

The chief complaint of "tired and weak" can result from literally hundreds of physical and mental conditions in virtually every body system. The importance of a comprehensive history cannot be emphasized enough when dealing with nonspecific complaints such as these.

Regarding visual changes, an unambiguous description of the abnormality (e.g., decreased near, far, central, or peripheral vision; diminished, blurred, cloudy, double, or hazy vision; diplopia that is horizontal, vertical, or diagonal; unilateral or bilateral; complete or partial; constant or intermittent; sudden or gradual; and aggravating or alleviating factors) is essential to assist in narrowing the list of potential diagnoses.

Although there are very few visual changes that are pathognomonic for a particular disease, there are those that tend to be associated with certain conditions at a greater frequency. Examples include optic neuritis with multiple sclerosis, diplopia with myasthenia gravis, focal neurologic defect with migraine headaches, complete loss of sight with a brain tumor compression on the optic chiasm or nerve, and visual field loss with a pituitary adenoma/tumor.

If a headache is present, details regarding it are also necessary. This should include location, type of pain, intensity of pain, associated symptoms (e.g., focal neurologic defects, photophobia, nausea, vomiting, fever, and upper respiratory tract infection symptoms), aggravating and alleviating factors, whether it is acute or chronic, sudden or progressive onset, pattern, and duration. Headaches in association with fatigue and weakness are even less specific for identifying a certain condition; they could represent anxiety, depression, chronic viral infections, meningitis, migraines, brain tumors, hypertension, and brain aneurysms.

B. Does he have any urethral discharge?   NONESSENTIAL

Urethral discharge is generally associated with urethritis and/or prostatitis in men of Mr. Valez's age. With the exception of chronic prostatitis (which is generally present in older men), this symptom is not very often associated with fatigue and weakness, especially of 3 to 4 months' duration. Chronic prostatitis generally is associated with irritative voiding symptoms, low back pain, and perineal pain, none of which Mr. Valez has, making this a highly unlikely diagnosis. Additionally, the causative agents in men of Mr. Valez's age are almost always sexually transmitted infection, which is unlikely because his history places him in a low-risk group for acquisition.

C. Has he been experiencing any cold intolerance?   ESSENTIAL

Cold intolerance is experienced in fewer conditions, but still is nothing that would lead to a specific diagnosis. In association with fatigue and weakness, the most likely causes include hypothyroidism, anemia, vascular diseases, and psychiatric conditions.

D. Has he noticed any changes of his skin, hair, or nails? ESSENTIAL

With the exception of dermatologic conditions, there are very few conditions that have characteristic skin, hair, and/or nail changes that cannot be found in another disorder. However, the combination of this information with the other history obtained thus far can assist in narrowing the long list of potential differential diagnoses. A few examples of diseases associated with specific skin, hair, or nail changes along with

chronic fatigue and weakness include jaundice with hepatitis B, hepatitis C, or cirrhosis; brownish discoloration of the skin secondary to melanin deposition with Addison disease and pituitary tumors; grayish-bronze skin with hemochromatosis; reddish-blue skin discoloration with polycythemia; cyanosis of the skin and clubbing of the nails with chronic obstructive pulmonary disorder (COPD); cyanosis of the skin secondary to amiodarone for severe cardiac arrhythmias; purpuric lesions (petechiae and ecchymosis) with bleeding diathesis; thinning of the hair and nails with thyroid conditions and anemia; silvery-colored skin plaques and nail pitting with psoriatic arthritis; and subungual splinter hemorrhages with subacute bacterial endocarditis.

Facial skin abnormalities include a pale, edematous face with varying degrees of eyeswelling with nephrotic syndrome; dull-appearing, puffy face and periorbital edema with myxedema with hypothyroidism; enlargement of the soft tissues of the lips, ears, and nose with a general coarseness with acromegaly; "moon facies" with erythema to the cheeks and excessive hair growth in women (e.g., mustache and sideburns) with Cushing syndrome; and "masklike" stare and decreased mobility of the nasolabial folds with Parkinson disease.

E. Did/does he have a sore throat or enlarged lymph nodes? ESSENTIAL

The presence of enlarged lymph nodes and/or a sore throat also limit the potential differential diagnosis, but they do not establish the actual diagnosis. For example, they could represent a chronic viral infection (e.g., mononucleosis), a chronic bacterial infection (e.g., subacute bacterial endocarditis), a carcinoma, or a unique condition (e.g., chronic fatigue syndrome).

2. Physical Examination

A. Eye examination   ESSENTIAL

Because Mr. Valez is complaining of visual abnormalities, an eye examination is indicated.

B. Thyroid examination   ESSENTIAL

Because tiredness and weakness can both be associated with thyroid disease, it is important to carefully evaluate the patient's thyroid gland for abnormalities in size, texture, consistency, tenderness, mobility, and/or bruits. However, it is important to remember that a significant thyroid dysfunction can occur with a normal examination.

C. Heart examination   ESSENTIAL

A heart examination as outlined in Case 1-2 is important to perform on Mr. Valez because many conditions involving chronic fatigue and weakness result from a cardiac abnormality (e.g., subacute bacterial endocarditis, a valvular condition, or heart failure).

D. Tender points for fibromyalgia   NONESSENTIAL

Fibromyalgia is associated with fatigue and weakness. Because there are no diagnostic tests to confirm the diagnosis, the American College of Rheumatology (ACR) has created guidelines utilizing clinical criteria, including these 18 (9 pairs) tender points to establish the diagnosis. They are located over the suboccipital muscle insertions in the occiput, over the sternocleidomastoid muscles in the anterolateral neck at approximately the level of C-6, over the upper trapezius muscles approximately where the neck and shoulder meet, just medial to the medial border of scapulae above the scapular spine, slightly lateral to the second costochondral junctions, over the lateral epicondyles of the elbows, slightly lateral to the midscapular line over the iliac crests, slightly posterior to the greater trochanters of hips, and at the fat pads over the medial knees. If 11 of these 18 points are tender to palpation with ~8 lb of pressure, this particular criterion is met.

E. Deep tendon reflexes   ESSENTIAL

Deep tendon reflexes (DTRs) can also be affected by multiple medical conditions, some of which present as fatigue and weakness. For example, DTRs can be decreased in endocrine problems such as hypothyroidism and neurologic conditions that affect the lower motor neurons. They can be increased in hyperthyroidism and upper motor neuron diseases.

3. Diagnostic Studies

A. Complete blood count with differential (CBC w/diff) ESSENTIAL

Although it cannot definitively establish the diagnosis, a CBC w/diff is important because it can confirm the suspicion of anemia, chronic infection, or leukemia, all of which can be associated with fatigue and weakness. For more information on the CBC w/diff, please see Case 1-4.

B. Thyroid panel (TSH, FT_4, and T_3 by RIA)   ESSENTIAL

A thyroid panel should be performed because it not only provides useful information regarding the functioning of the thyroid itself, but also ensures that the hypothalamic-pituitary-thyroid pathway is intact. A problem in any of these three glands could cause Mr. Valez's symptoms.

C. Slit-lamp examination   ESSENTIAL

This test is essential for Mr. Valez because of his history of headaches and visual field defects in conjunction with the possibility of a slightly increased cup:disc ratio with mild blurring of margins on physical examination. All of these could be caused by a benign or malignant brain tumor or pituitary enlargement. Depending on the results, an ophthalmology consult may be indicated.

D. Mononucleosis spot test (mono spot)   NONESSENTIAL

Mr. Valez did not have a fever, sore throat, or cervical lymphadenopathy at any time during his illness; therefore, the diagnosis of mononucleosis is extremely unlikely.

E. Electrocardiogram (ECG)   NONESSENTIAL

Mr. Valez's history does not suggest evidence of cardiac ischemia, a cardiac arrhythmia, or a cardiomyopathy; furthermore, his physical examination does not reveal any findings suspicious for a valvular problem, cardiomegaly, or heart failure. Thus, an ECG is unnecessary.

4. Diagnosis

A. Primary hypothyroidism   INCORRECT

On laboratory analysis, primary hypothyroidism is characterized by a low FT_4 and T_3 by RIA in conjunction with an elevated TSH. Because Mr. Valez's TSH is low, primary hypothyroidism can be essentially eliminated as his most likely diagnosis.

B. Secondary hypothyroidism   CORRECT

Both primary and secondary hypothyroidisms are characterized by a low FT_4 and T_3 by RIA. Secondary hypothyroidism is distinguished from primary hypothyroidism by a suppressed TSH. Therefore, this is Mr. Valez's most likely diagnosis. However, he will require additional testing to determine whether this abnormality is pituitary or hypothalamic in origin.

C. Atypical depression   INCORRECT

Atypical depression can also present as fatigue and weakness; however, alone it cannot account for Mr. Valez's thyroid abnormalities. Thus, based on the information thus far obtained, this is not his most likely diagnosis. However, if his symptoms persist after the cause of his secondary hypothyroidism has been discovered and treated, this is a diagnosis that should be explored.

D. Fibromyalgia   INCORRECT

Fibromyalgia is a condition of unknown etiology that is characterized by chronic diffuse muscle and soft tissue aches and pains. According to the ACR established diagnostic criteria for fibromyalgia, the patient must have widespread muscle pain (in upper body, lower body, right side of body, left side of body, and spine) as well as pain (not tenderness or pressure) in 11 of the 18 established fibromyalgia tender points. Because Mr. Valez is not complaining of diffuse pain and only had 6 out of 18 positive tender points, this is not his most likely diagnosis.

E. Chronic fatigue syndrome   INCORRECT

Chronic fatigue syndrome is a disease of unknown etiology characterized by debilitating fatigue that is unresponsive to rest. The Centers for Disease Control and Prevention (CDC) has developed criteria to establish this diagnosis because there are no confirmatory tests for the condition and it is essentially a diagnosis of exclusion. The criteria fall into two main categories. First, the illness cannot be caused by another condition, caused by chronic exertion, or alleviated with rest. Furthermore, it has to be of new onset and associated with a significant decrease in functioning. Second, the patient must have a minimum of four of the following eight symptoms for a minimum of 6 months: (1) myalgias, (2) arthralgias without erythema or edema, (3) sore throat, (4) tender axillary and/or cervical lymph nodes, (5) fever, (6) headache of new quality/onset/severity, (7) fatigue that is not alleviated with sleep OR fatigue following exertion that lasts for more than 24 hours, and (8) problems with short-term memory and/or concentration.

Because an alternative diagnosis was made for Mr. Valez's condition via laboratory studies, he has not been ill for 6 months, and he only had one of the eight symptoms, chronic fatigue syndrome can be eliminated as his most likely diagnosis.

5. Treatment Plan

A. Begin levothyroxine 25 µg/day orally and recheck TSH after 1 month of therapy to see if euthyroid; if not, adjust dosage accordingly   INCORRECT

Although it is likely that Mr. Valez is going to end up on chronic daily thyroid hormone replacement, it should not be initiated until the cause of the secondary hypothyroidism has been established. There have been reported cases of deaths in the literature from this practice.

Furthermore, the initial adult dose of levothyroxine in patients with residual thyroid function and no evidence of cardiac disease is 50 to 100 µg/day. Repeat thyroid testing should not be conducted until approximately 8 weeks after the initiation of therapy (or a change in dosage) because it tends to take a minimum of 6 to 8 weeks before the diagnostic studies are normalized on the new dosage. Symptoms can take as long as 3 to 6 months to resolve.

B. Order thyroid-releasing hormone (TRH)   CORRECT

TRH assists in determining whether the secondary hypothyroidism is pituitary or hypothalamic in nature. If the TRH is elevated, the culprit is most likely the pituitary gland. If it is suppressed, then the cause is generally hypothalamic, which is extremely rare.

C. Order magnetic resonance image (MRI) of pituitary   CORRECT

Because the pituitary is the most likely source for Mr. Valez's secondary hypothyroidism, an MRI of the pituitary is indicated to evaluate his pituitary gland for adenomas, carcinomas, necrosis, ischemia, and/or other abnormalities.

D. Start escitalopram 10 mg/day orally and titrate to 20 mg daily in 1 week if necessary   INCORRECT

If Mr. Valez's most likely diagnosis was depression, fibromyalgia, or chronic fatigue syndrome, the SSRI escitalopram would be an appropriate treatment option (however, it would be considered to be "off-label" in the case of the latter two conditions). Because this is not the case, this treatment is not indicated at this time.

E. Start amitriptyline 25 mg one at night   INCORRECT

If Mr. Valez's most likely diagnosis was fibromyalgia (or even chronic fatigue syndrome or depression), the tricyclic antidepressant (TCA) amitriptyline might be an appropriate treatment option; however, this is not the case and the medication should not be prescribed. Except for depression, these are "off-label" uses of this medication.

Epidemiologic and Other Data

Hypothyroidism is the lack of adequate thyroid hormones in the serum as a result of inadequate thyroid output. It can result from primary, secondary, or temporary causes. Primary hypothyroidism consists of conditions that affect the thyroid gland itself. They include inadequate iodine in the diet; congenital (e.g., absent thyroid and dyshormonogenesis), autoimmune (e.g., Hashimoto thyroiditis and atrophic thyroiditis), iatrogenic (e.g., prior radiation therapy for hyperthyroidism or cancer and complete or total thyroidectomy), and infiltrative (e.g., amyloidosis, sarcoidosis, and scleroderma) conditions; and medications (e.g., amiodarone, lithium, and α-interferon).

Secondary causes are extrathyroid conditions that prevent adequate functioning of the thyroid. They include inactive TSH, pituitary abnormalities (e.g., adenomas, carcinomas, and Sheehan syndrome), and hypothalamic disorders (e.g., tumors, trauma, and infiltrative disease).

Temporary causes can include status post iodine treatment for Graves disease, subacute thyroiditis, silent thyroiditis, and discontinuation of thyroxine therapy for hypothyroidism.

The most common cause worldwide is inadequate dietary iodine. In the United States, the most common cause of primary hypothyroidism is Hashimoto thyroiditis, and the most common secondary cause is an adverse effect from the treatment of hyperthyroidism.

Hypothyroidism symptoms alone from an anterior pituitary problem are rare. Generally, symptoms are present representing the results from a deficiency of all the hormones produced by the anterior pituitary gland. Hence, not only is a low TSH level seen but also low prolactin, growth hormone, luteinizing hormone, follicle-stimulating hormone, gonadotropin-releasing hormone, and adrenocorticotropic hormone levels.

CASE 3-4
Vincent Wilson
1. History

A. Does he suffer from any type of bone pain or has he ever had a fracture?   ESSENTIAL

Hypercalcemia and hypocalcemia are both associated with increased risk of bone fractures. This is not surprising because the body's internal homeostasis system tends to have the electrolytes "paired"; hence, as one increases another decreases (e.g., sodium and potassium). Hypercalcemia is associated with pathologic fractures. In contrast, in osteoporosis (which is generally not a true hypocalcemia but a result of inadequate calcium intake and/or absorption) the primary abnormality is a physiologic fracture, caused by a decreased density primarily in the trabecular bone with minimal changes in the cortical bone. The fractures from hypercalcemia are caused by weakness of the cortical bone, and an actual thickness of the trabecular bone is present.

Hypercalcemia can be associated with a generalized nonarticular pain or bone pain caused by bony cysts. However, more often than not, these latter two abnormalities are asymptomatic. Therefore, it is important to know if he has been having any bone pain or a history of fractures.

B. Has he experienced any unexplained weight loss; night sweats; fever; unusual fatigue; muscle weakness; cough; hemoptysis; abdominal pain/fullness; epistaxis; gingival bleeding with teeth brushing; bleeding with minimal trauma; easily bruising; gynecomastia (especially unilaterally); or masses in his inguinal, axillary, infraclavicular, supraclavicular, or neck areas?   ESSENTIAL

Hypercalcemia can be associated with several malignancies. The most common cancers that are known to produce hypercalcemia include carcinoma of the breast, lung, bone, thyroid, and kidney; lymphoma; and leukemia. Aside from the constitutional symptoms (e.g., weight loss, night sweats, fatigue, and frequently fever) that can be seen with any of these malignancies, some of these symptoms are specific to certain types of cancer (e.g., cough and hemoptysis with lung cancer; abdominal fullness with Burkitt lymphoma; splenomegaly with leukemia; lymphadenopathy in the area affected by a lymphoma; acute bleeding with leukemia; and unilateral gynecomastia with breast cancer). Obviously any positive responses are going to require further questioning and evaluation.

C. Has he had kidney stones or any kidney problems? ESSENTIAL

One of the most common symptoms of hypercalcemia (regardless of whether it is caused by excess production or decreased elimination) is nephrolithiasis. Complications from nephrolithiasis include nephrocalcinosis, azotemia, and frank renal failure.

Furthermore, hypophosphatemia can result from renal causes such as renal tubular defects, diabetes mellitus, and hypokalemic nephropathy.

D. Has he ever experienced any polydipsia, polyuria, anorexia, nausea, vomiting, bowel changes, abdominal pain, ascites, hypertension, paresthesias, depression, anxiety, hypersomnia, delusions, hallucinations, dysarthria, seizures, palpations, diaphoresis, heat intolerance, muscle cramps, tetany, paresthesias, fatiguing easier than usual, or subcutaneous masses?   ESSENTIAL

Other nonmalignant conditions can cause hypercalcemia (e.g., hyperthyroidism, sarcoidosis, or diabetes insipidus) and hypophosphatemia (e.g., adverse effects of medications, chronic obstructive respiratory disease, asthma, hyperthyroidism, and diabetes mellitus). These symptoms are some of the more common ones associated with these conditions or the electrolyte abnormality itself.

For example, polydipsia and tiring more easily than usual can be associated with both diabetes mellitus (hypophosphatemia) and mild hypercalcemia. Both hypophosphatemia and hypercalcemia can be caused by hyperthyroidism, and symptoms can include palpations, weight loss, and fatigue. Anorexia, nausea, vomiting, bowel changes, and abdominal pain can be seen with pancreatitis, which is sometimes associated with mild hypercalcemia; however, these same symptoms can be seen with adverse medication effects from hypophosphatemia. Visual disturbances can be seen in hypophosphatemia from diabetes mellitus or band keratopathy caused by calcium deposits from hypercalcemia.

Furthermore, moderate to severe hypercalcemia can be associated with neuromuscular diseases, pruritus, calciphylaxis, and psychiatric symptoms (depression, hypersomnia, delusions, hallucinations, and the inability to "think as clearly"). If severe, it can result in coma.

E. Has he ever had a sexually transmitted infection (STI)? NONESSENTIAL

There are no known STIs that are associated with hypercalcemia or hypophosphatemia.

2. Physical Examination

A. Neck examination   ESSENTIAL

A neck examination should be performed to palpate the thyroid for enlargement, masses, tenderness, and asymmetry and to listen for bruit(s), which could suggest either hyperthyroidism or thyroid carcinoma. Cervical and supraclavicular lymph nodes need to be assessed carefully for enlargement and/or tenderness, which could indicate a malignancy. Even though hypercalcemia and hypophosphatemia are seen in

hyperparathyroid disease, it is extremely unlikely that the enlarged parathyroid glands will be palpable because of their deeper location and small size.

B. Heart examination   ESSENTIAL

A heart examination as outlined in Case 1-2 should be performed to evaluate for arrhythmias, heart failure, or other cardiac abnormalities associated with these electrolyte disturbances.

Furthermore, hypophosphatemia is associated with metabolic syndrome, which significantly increases the patient's risk of developing CAD.

C. Abdominal examination   ESSENTIAL

An abdominal examination is indicated to look for ascites, organomegaly, masses, or tenderness, which could be associated with peptic ulcer diseases, renal carcinoma, pheochromocytoma, pancreatic adenomas, pancreatitis, and other intra-abdominal causes of hypercalcemia.

Additionally, the aorta and renal arteries should be examined for bruits, which could suggest the presence of atherosclerosis, which is possible with hypophosphatemia.

D. Genital examination   NONESSENTIAL

E. Muscle strength testing   ESSENTIAL

Muscle strength testing is important to perform because true hypercalcemia is associated with a proximal muscle weakness. If it is of gradual onset, the patient may not be aware of its existence. Hence, it assists in distinguishing between asymptomatic and symptomatic hypercalcemia (as well as to provide some clue as to whether this is an acute or chronic process).

3. Diagnostic Studies

A. Parathyroid hormone (PTH) level   ESSENTIAL

Hyperparathyroidism is the most common cause for an elevated calcium and low phosphorous level; therefore, it is essential to check the PTH level. If the PTH is elevated, then the laboratory abnormalities are most likely a result of hyperparathyroidism; however, they could also be a result of one of the extremely rare multiple endocrine neoplasia (MEN) syndromes.

If the PTH is low, then the most likely diagnosis depends on the duration of the symptoms. For example, if the hypercalcemia is chronic, then vitamin D intoxication, vitamin A intoxication, granulomatous diseases, congenital defects, hyperthyroidism, or adrenal insufficiency is the more likely cause. However, if it is acute or unknown in duration, a carcinoma must be ruled out as the primary diagnosis.

B. Vanillylmandelic acid (VMA), catecholamine, thyroid stimulating hormone (TSH), and prolactin levels   NONESSENTIAL

VMA and catecholamine levels do not need to be performed at this time because Mr. Wilson's BP is essentially normal, whereas in pheochromocytoma, it would be markedly elevated. Additionally, pheochromocytoma is an extremely rare cause for hypertension. It is generally not even considered as part of the differential diagnosis unless there are significant signs and symptoms suggesting the condition or the patient's BP is not controlled despite the combination of at least three antihypertensive medications from different classes.

Likewise, TSH and prolactin levels are not necessary at this time because he does not have any symptoms suggesting that a thyroid and/or pituitary problem are responsible for his findings.

C. Vitamin D level by 1,25(OH)$_2$D and serum chloride level ESSENTIAL

The two most common causes of hypercalcemia are hyperparathyroidism and carcinoma. Hypercalcemia related to nonsyndrome carcinomas is generally also associated with a decreased 1,25(OH)$_2$D level. Plus, vitamin D intoxication can be responsible for elevated calcium levels.

A serum chloride level is an inexpensive technique for HCPs to utilize to help ensure they are not missing a significant malignancy being responsible for the patient's hypercalcemia, even in an asymptomatic patient. As a general rule, if the serum chloride–to–serum phosphorous ratio is greater than 33.1, the abnormality is caused by hyperparathyroidism, not cancer.

D. Dual-energy x-ray absorptiometry (DEXA) scan NONESSENTIAL

A DEXA scan is the "gold standard" diagnostic test for the evaluation of a patient's bone mineral density to determine if osteoporosis or osteopenia is present. However, these conditions are generally going to be associated with hypocalcemia if any electrolyte abnormality is identified. However, the majority of the time, it is just associated with an inadequate calcium intake and/or absorption.

Although individuals with hypercalcemia do have problems with frequent pathologic fractures and occasionally bone cysts, a DEXA scan is not the diagnostic test of choice to evaluate for the presence of these problems.

In osteopenia and osteoporosis, primary metabolic abnormality is a loss of trabecular bone structure; however, the cortical bone loss is minimal. Conversely, with hypercalcemia, the primary abnormality that leads to the skeletal abnormalities consists of a cortical bone loss and a trabecular bone increase. Hence, a DEXA scan would show bone that appears to be much denser than expected for age, height, gender, and race, despite its significant risk of fracture. Therefore, one is not necessary at this time.

E. Repeat calcium and phosphorous levels   ESSENTIAL

When encountering a patient with an elevated calcium level, most experts recommend repeating the level to ensure that it is an accurate finding. Causes of false hypercalcemia can include laboratory error, prolonged tourniquet time, hemoconcentration during collection, excessive intake of calcium before venipuncture, the time of day the specimen was collected (calcium has a diurnal variation, with the highest level occurring at approximately 9:00 p.m.), decreased serum pH, and elevated serum protein.

F. 24-hour urine for calcium and creatinine with serum creatinine   ESSENTIAL

Finally, any patient with probable hypercalcemia in association with hypophosphatemia requires a 24-hour urine for calcium and creatinine (along with a serum creatinine level) to evaluate for familial benign hypocalciuric hypercalcemia (FHH), or familial benign hypercalcemia. Furthermore, the creatinine clearance will provide an estimation of the glomerular filtration rate (GFR), which is a determination of renal function (because renal failure is another cause of hypercalcemia).

Creatinine clearance (CC) is normally calculated by the laboratory automatically for the HCP. However, if it is not, then it can easily be calculated with the following formula:

$$\frac{\text{24 - hr urinary creatinine excreted in mg / dl} \times \text{amount of urine collected in 24 hours in ml / min}}{\text{Serum creatinine in mg / dl}}$$

The CC also can be utilized to determine whether a complete 24 hours of urine was collected provided the patient has a normal serum creatinine level. The CC can also be estimated from the serum creatinine by utilizing the Cockcroft-Gault formula. With it, the CC is provided in terms of ml/min and is calculated as follows:

$$\frac{\text{(140 - patient's age in years)} \times \text{lean body weight in kg}}{\text{Serum creatinine in mg / dl} \times 72}$$

(Adjust for women to account for their lower muscle mass by multiplying the result by 0.85.)

4. Diagnosis

A. Familial benign hypocalciuric hypercalcemia   INCORRECT

Familial benign hypocalciuric hypercalcemia is an autosomal dominant condition involving a mutation of the gene that encodes the calcium-stimulating receptors (CaSRs), causing them not to function properly. The CaSRs on the surface of the parathyroid glands permit an erratica release of PTH, causing the kidneys to produce excessive calcium as a result of this failed feedback mechanism. Likewise, the CaSRs in the renal tubules are also malfunctioning, causing hypocalciuria. This can be ruled out as Mr. Wilson's most likely diagnosis because both his PTH and urinary calcium were elevated. In familial benign hypocalciuric hypercalcemia, the urinary calcium is decreased.

Other potential causes of hypocalciuria include thiazide diuretic usage and milk-alkali (or Burnett) syndrome. Milk-alkali syndrome is a progressive renal disease (that is reversible if discovered in the early stages, but can cause renal failure if not identified until the later stages) caused by the consumption of large amounts of milk and alkali (previously used for the treatment of peptic ulcer disease).

B. Secondary hyperparathyroidism   INCORRECT

Secondary hyperparathyroidism is associated with failure of calcium regulation and/or production to respond appropriately to PTH. Even though his PTH level is elevated, this condition is associated with hypocalcemia, not hypercalcemia. Thus, secondary hyperparathyroidism is not Mr. Wilson's most likely diagnosis.

C. Multiple endocrine neoplasia (MEN) syndrome type I (MEN1)   INCORRECT

Multiple endocrine neoplasia (MEN) syndrome type I is a rare syndrome associated with hyperparathyroidism, a pituitary adenoma, and a pancreatic adenoma. This can essentially be ruled out as Mr. Wilson's most likely diagnosis because he does not have any symptoms that are suggestive of either a pituitary adenoma or a pancreatic adenoma. Furthermore, hypercalcemia related to MEN syndrome carcinomas is generally associated with suppressed or normal PTH levels.

D. Multiple endocrine neoplasia (MEN) syndrome type II (MEN2)   INCORRECT

Multiple endocrine neoplasia (MEN2) syndrome type II is another rare syndrome that consists of hyperparathyroidism, pheochromocytomas, and thyroid cancer. It too can be ruled out as Mr. Wilson's most likely diagnosis based on his lack of symptoms for thyroid cancer and pheochromocytoma, including a near-normal BP level as well as his elevated PTH level.

E. Primary hyperparathyroidism   CORRECT

Hyperparathyroidism can present with a multitude of symptoms or, more often, it essentially is asymptomatic. It is a commonly held opinion that by excluding the symptoms of depression and fatigue, over 90% of patients with hyperparathyroidism are asymptomatic.

Regardless, the cornerstone of diagnosis includes an elevated serum calcium, a low serum phosphorous, and a high PTH level. Additional support includes an elevated urinary calcium level. Finally, his serum chloride:phosphorous ratio is 39.6 (a ratio of > 33.1 is almost always a result of primary hyperparathyroidism). Therefore, this is Mr. Wilson's most likely diagnosis.

5. Treatment Plan

A. Recheck BP in 1 month; have BP checked weekly, if possible, away from the clinic   CORRECT

According to the accepted guidelines, Mr. Wilson's BP levels would place him in the prehypertensive category. However, to truly diagnose him as prehypertensive, he needs to have two separate readings elevated. Therefore, it is imperative that his BP be checked again soon. For more information on blood pressure level classification, please see Case 1-1.

The other consideration is that Mr. Wilson suffers from "white coat syndrome," especially because he has had limited experience with the healthcare system. "White coat syndrome" causes the patient's BP to be slightly elevated in the clinical setting but normal away from the facility. Therefore, having it checked away from the clinic is helpful.

B. Vitamin D supplementation   CORRECT

Mr. Wilson will need to increase his exposure to the sun, take a vitamin D supplement, or increase the amount of vitamin D in his diet because his vitamin D level is low. In individuals without hyperparathyroidism, vitamin D supplementation is important because vitamin D is essential in the metabolism of calcium (and hence the prevention of osteoporosis/osteopenia). However, in Mr. Wilson's case, this is important because there is some evidence to suggest that vitamin D supplementation can help to prevent calcium nephrolithiasis in patients with hyperparathyroidism.

C. Vitamin A supplementation   INCORRECT

Vitamin A supplementation is contraindicated in patients with hyperparathyroidism. It has been shown to increase osteoclastic bone destruction, especially when it is a consequence of parathyroid hormone activity.

D. Refer to surgeon   CORRECT

A surgical consult is indicated for Mr. Wilson because he is under the age of 50 years. The other currently accepted criteria for a parathyroidectomy include being symptomatic, having

a serum calcium level of greater than 12 mg/dl (although his initial level was 15 mg/dl, this was more than likely caused by excessive tourniquet time or a traumatic stick per Mr. Wilson's history), having a urinary calcium of greater than 400 mg/day, having coexisting osteoporosis, having a history of nephrolithiasis, and/or being pregnant (which obviously would not apply to Mr. Wilson). If the surgeon elects to perform a parathyroidectomy, it will permit direct examination of the thyroid gland for associated nodules and/or cancer.

However, with Mr. Wilson's only surgical indication being his age, it is possible that the surgeon will just recommend monitoring his serum calcium level and symptoms every 6 months. As long as his calcium level is not increasing and/or he is not developing symptoms, continuing surveillance is an appropriate treatment option.

E. Prescribe a bisphosphonate and cinacalcet 30 mg daily orally   INCORRECT

Although not necessary as part of the diagnostic evaluation of Mr. Wilson's condition, before prescribing a bisphosphonate, a DEXA scan should be performed. As stated previously, it is highly probable that his DEXA scan would reveal good bone density because it primarily measures trabecular bone, which is generally elevated in hypercalcemia caused by hyperparathyroidism. The fracture risk Mr. Wilson needs to be concerned with is from weakened cortical bone, for which bisphosphonates have not been proven to have any effect. Thus, a biophosphonate is not indicated at this time.

Regarding the cinacalcet, even though it is indicated for the treatment of hyperparathyroidism to reduce PTH levels, it is only indicated for secondary hyperparathyroidism, not primary, as Mr. Wilson has been diagnosed.

Epidemiologic and Other Data

PTH, produced in the parathyroid glands, is the main controller of calcium functioning in the body. The primary function of PTH is to ensure that the serum calcium level remains within its normal range. As with most endocrine systems, the release of PTH from the parathyroid glands is under the control of a negative feedback loop. If the serum calcium begins to decline, then the parathyroid glands produce more PTH. Likewise, if the serum calcium increases, then the parathyroid glands produce less PTH to maintain homeostasis.

Hyperparathyroidism can be either primary (e.g., adenomas [single gland approximately 80% of the cases], multiple glands [approximately 20%], or carcinomas [< 1%]) or secondary (e.g., inappropriate PTH secretion, lithium therapy, MEN1, or MEN2). Its symptoms can be remembered by the mnemonic "**B**ones, **S**tones, abdominal **G**roans, psychic **M**oans, and fatigue **O**vertones."

CASE 3-5
Wilma Xiam
1. History

A. How tall was she when she graduated from high school? ESSENTIAL

The majority of women have achieved their maximum height by the time they graduate from high school.

This milestone serves as a good reference point for the patient to utilize in remembering that height. A patient's maximum height is important because there is a "normal" loss of height that is associated with age; however, it should be no greater than 1 to 1.5 inches.

Any greater height loss should be considered abnormal and a cause needs to be established. Without significant trauma or having a medical condition that prevents her from standing and walking, the most likely cause for this excessive reduction in height is kyphosis from vertebral fractures secondary to osteoporosis or osteopenia.

B. How much calcium and vitamin D does she get in her diet? ESSENTIAL

Inadequate dietary intake, lack of supplementation, and malabsorption of calcium and vitamin D are associated with an increased risk of osteoporosis and osteopenia. It is essential that the patient gets adequate dosages of both because the utilization of calcium by the body is dependent on vitamin D. The longer deficiency is present, the greater the risk a patient has of acquiring osteoporosis or osteopenia. Adequate intake of calcium and vitamin D should be a routine health maintenance recommendation for everyone starting in early childhood.

The number of individuals with inadequate vitamin D levels is increasing in the United States. It is theorized that despite more foods being fortified with vitamin D, this deficiency is linked to sun avoidance and/or the increased use of sunscreen for the prevention of malignant melanoma because sunlight is the best source of vitamin D.

C. Does she exercise regularly? If yes, what type and how often? ESSENTIAL

Regular weight-bearing, aerobic, and strength training exercise for a minimum of 30 minutes on most days of the week is the best exercise to prevent the development of osteoporosis. However, women who are unwilling or unable to comply with an exercise regimen should attempt to get at least 30 minutes (does not have to be continuous) of weight-bearing (i.e., walking) exercise on most days of the week. Studies have proven that a sedentary lifestyle increases one's risk of osteoporosis.

D. What does she consider to be a serving of alcohol? NONESSENTIAL

The exact amount of alcohol intake to adversely affect bone mineral density is unknown; however, it is generally termed as "excessive." Some experts have attempted to quantify "excessive" as either two or three drinks per day every day.

Normally, it makes a difference as to whether the patient drinks beer, wine, or liquor and what she considers to be a serving because the amount of alcohol consumed can vary significantly depending on these factors (as well as number of drinks). Essentially there is an equivalent amount of alcohol in 12 ounces of beer, 5 ounces of wine, and 1.5 ounces of liquor.

However, because of Mrs. Xiam's very infrequent alcohol intake of one drink, her alcohol consumption is not going to place her at a significant risk for acquiring osteoporosis.

E. After she began regular menstruation, did she ever miss any menstrual periods? ESSENTIAL

Conditions that produce prolonged amenorrhea (generally defined as longer than 1 year); such as, anorexia nervosa, sports training, and possibly some hormonal contraceptives, can adversely affect a woman's bone mineral density and future risk of acquiring osteoporosis or osteopenia.

2. Physical Examination

A. Carotid auscultation ESSENTIAL

Although Mrs. Xiam is asymptomatic regarding the possibility of a CVA or TIA, she should still have her carotid pulses palpated and auscultated for bruits because one of the groups of medications that could be considered for her condition would be estrogen and progesterone replacement therapy, which has been known to be associated with an increased risk of CVA.

B. Thyroid palpation ESSENTIAL

Hyperthyroidism is one of the more common causes of secondary osteoporosis. Therefore, patients being evaluated for possible osteoporosis should have their thyroid palpated remembering that dysfunction can occur in the presence of a normal feeling gland.

C. Rectal examination NONESSENTIAL

The majority of gastrointestinal disorders that are associated with osteoporosis are generally disorders that affect the malabsorption of calcium, vitamin D, vitamin A, and vitamin K. Because these disorders are generally limited to the small intestines, the rectum is highly unlikely to be involved and does not need to be examined.

D. Evaluation of joints of the hands NONESSENTIAL

Mrs. Xiam is not complaining of arthralgias or other chronic hand problems; therefore, it is not necessary to evaluate the joints of her hands. However, it would probably be worthwhile, although unrelated to her chief complaint, to check the temperature and sensation of the digits of her casted arm to ensure there are no signs of a compartmental syndrome developing.

E. Spine examination ESSENTIAL

Irregardless of Mrs. Xiam's DEXA scan results, since she has loss of 1 inch of height since graduating from high school, there is a concern that she has vertebral fractures and, as a consequence, kyphosis.

3. Diagnostic Studies

A. Thoracic spine radiographs NONESSENTIAL

Although she is at risk for kyphosis, Mrs. Xiam is not complaining of any upper back pain and had a normal thoracic spine examination. Thus, she does not require thoracic spine radiographs.

Furthermore, plain film radiographs are poor substitutes for screening for osteoporosis and/or osteopenia (especially because Mrs. Xiam already had a DEXA scan, which is considered the "gold standard"). It is estimated that 20% to 25% of a patient's bone mass must be lost before osteoporosis is identifiable on a plain film radiograph. Additionally, overpenetrated x-ray films cause the bones to appear thinner than they actually are; conversely, underpenetration results in films with bones that appear to be denser than they are.

A DEXA scan is based on "normals" for age, gender, height, weight, and race. It generally provides a measurement of the bone density at the hip and lumbar spine. The T score compares the patient's bone mineral density (BMD) with that of young health controls. It is the value utilized to make the actual diagnosis of normal, osteopenia, or osteoporosis. The Z score is a comparison of the density of bone in individuals of the same gender, age, race, and size.

B. Serum cross-linked N-telopeptide   NONESSENTIAL

Serum cross-linked N-telopeptide is a measurement of bone resorption. There are some studies that suggest that it can be utilized as an adjunct test in elderly women (65 years of age or older) who have essentially normal DEXA scans despite multiple risk factors. If it is elevated, it is considered to be a significant risk factor for a future fracture and treatment should be adjusted accordingly.

Currently, its primary role is to determine the patient's response to antiresorptive agents. After therapy is instituted for osteoporosis treatment or prevention, the effect on bone as measured with a DEXA scan is not accurate until approximately 2 years later. Hence, it takes 2 years before any information is available on the effects of treatment. By performing a serum (or urinary) cross-linked N-telopeptide test before initiating treatment and again in 4 to 6 months after beginning the treatment, an indication of the patient's response to the agent can be identified much earlier and appropriate treatment adjustments can be initiated, if indicated. Basically, a decrease in the serum (or urinary) cross-linked N-telopeptide on the second test indicates that the patient is likely to have a positive result from the agent, and the follow-up DEXA scan will reveal either the same or an increased, but not a decreased, BMD.

However, inaccurate results are highly likely to be seen at this time for Mrs. Xiam because of her recent ulna and radius fractures.

C. Serum vitamin D level by 1,25(OH)$_2$D   ESSENTIAL

As stated previously, vitamin D deficiency has become a significant problem in the development of either osteoporosis or osteopenia because it prevents the calcium from being utilized correctly.

Therefore, the 2008 guidelines for the prevention and treatment of osteoporosis established by the National Osteoporosis Foundation (NOF) recently added the recommendation to routinely test for serum vitamin D level [1,25(OH)$_2$D] in patients who are *at risk* of a vitamin D deficiency. Mrs. Xiam would fall into this category because of her extremely low dairy intake and lack of sun exposure.

Other patients to consider for testing would include those with chronic renal insufficiency; individuals at potential risk for poor absorption of vitamin D; individuals with any chronic medical conditions, especially if they are housebound and have limited access to sunlight; or anyone who does not get adequate sunlight exposure.

Furthermore, some experts are now advocating performing testing on every patient being evaluated for osteoporosis and/or osteopenia to obtain a baseline for each patient. The American Association of Clinical Endocrinologists (AACE) is advocating this approach.

D. Serum follicular-stimulating hormone (FSH) NONESSENTIAL

Some feel that an elevated FSH level is useful in making the diagnosis of menopause. However, caution must be employed if attempting to utilize a single reading for such because of the wide range of normal for postmenopausal females and its lower end overlapping with values consistent with ovulatory peak levels in premenopausal women. Therefore, the best method to diagnose menopause is still clinically by utilizing the standard definition—lack of menses for a minimum of 12 consecutive months in a woman over the age of 45 years. Regardless, it can reliably be assumed without any type of a diagnostic test that Mrs. Xiam is postmenopausal because she is 56 years old and her last menstrual period was approximately 9 years ago.

E. Complete blood count with differential (CBC w/diff), serum calcium, serum bone-specific alkaline phosphatase (B-ALP), serum creatinine, and 24-hour urinary calcium   ESSENTIAL

Because of the high incidence of secondary osteoporosis (20%) in postmenopausal women, the AACE Osteoporosis Task Force recommends performing these basic tests as well as a serum vitamin D level by 1,25(OH)$_2$D before instituting any treatment beyond lifestyle modifications, regardless of whether or not the patient is symptomatic. This approach can identify these secondary causes and institute appropriate treatments. Otherwise, recommended therapies are unlikely to be effective.

For example, the CBC w/diff could reveal an anemia suggesting the possibility of hyperthyroidism, cirrhosis, bone marrow failure, multiple myeloma, or a nutritional deficiency. An abnormal serum calcium level and/or 24-hour urine for calcium could represent hyperthyroidism, hyperparathyroidism, hypoparathyroidism, a primary or secondary skeletal carcinoma, a malabsorption syndrome, or a severe calcium deficiency. The serum creatinine could suggest the presence of chronic renal abnormalities, especially of the distal tubules, affecting the elimination of calcium or the presence of decreased muscle mass affecting exercise capacity and strength training. The serum B-ALP is a measurement of bone formation, and elevations indicate the presence of an underlying skeletal condition (e.g., Paget disease or multiple myeloma).

However, care must be utilized in interpreting these nonspecific test results to ensure that the findings correlate with the patient's signs and symptoms. For example, Mrs. Xiam's serum B-ALP is likely to be elevated because of her healing fracture, not an underlying bone condition. As with any diagnostic study, it is essential to remember to treat the patient, not the test result.

The AACE also recommends disease-specific testing for symptomatic and "high-risk" patients with the following tests to rule out associated conditions: thyroid hormone levels (TSH, FT$_4$, and T$_3$ by RIA) for hyperthyroidism, parathyroid hormone for hyperparathyroidism, serum protein electrophoresis for multiple myeloma, antitissue transglutaminase antibodies for celiac sprue, and any other test as indicated by history, physical examination, and/or previous diagnostic test results that could suggest a secondary osteoporosis.

At this time, no other medical groups currently make these recommendations. The majority only evaluate patients for secondary causes if the patient is symptomatic for an underlying disease process, has an abnormal Z score (results are greater than one standard deviation from the mean, or > −1.0), or fails to respond to treatment.

4. Diagnosis

A. Primary osteoporosis   INCORRECT

The World Health Organization (WHO) developed diagnostic standards for the interpretation of DEXA scans utilizing the patient's T score. A DEXA scan is considered to be normal when the T score is within one standard deviation of the expected peak bone mass (< −1.0). Osteopenia is defined as a T score between −1.0 and −2.5 standard deviation(s) from the expected peak bone mass, or within 1 to 2.5 standard deviations. Osteoporosis is defined as a peak bone mass that falls greater than 2.5 standard deviations from the expected peak bone mass, or greater than −2.5. Because Mrs. Xiam's DEXA scan reveals her T score to be −2.0, primary osteoporosis is not her most likely diagnosis.

B. Secondary osteoporosis   INCORRECT

Secondary osteoporosis can be eliminated as Mrs. Xiam's most likely diagnosis because her T score on her DEXA test is less than −2.5, therefore failing to meet the diagnostic criteria of osteoporosis, regardless of whether it is primary or secondary. Furthermore, to have secondary osteoporosis, her Z score must be greater than one standard deviation (> −1.0). Therefore, based on her initial DEXA scan results, secondary osteoporosis can be eliminated as her most common diagnosis.

Obviously, the diagnostic studies recommended by the AACE can also provide some support for this diagnosis. Secondary osteoporosis and osteopenia are also related to other medical conditions such as premature menopause; early menopause; conditions that produce amenorrhea for longer than 1 year in a premenopausal woman; alcoholism; conditions associated with frequent falls; poor eyesight; overall poor health; and a wide array of endocrine, metabolic, hematologic, nutritional, gastrointestinal, and hereditary disorders. In the majority of the cases, there exists at least a subtle symptom that one of these conditions is occurring.

C. Osteopenia   CORRECT

Based on Mrs. Xiam's DEXA results and the WHO criteria, she has low bone mass, or osteopenia (a T score < −1.0 but > −2.5). Even though her T score for her femoral neck measurement is consistent with low-normal results (> −1.0), her lumbar spine measurement falls in the low bone mass range (> −1.0 to < −2.5). Because the final diagnosis is considered to be the level that corresponds to the lowest bone mineral density, osteopenia is her most likely diagnosis.

D. Normal bone mineral density (BMD)   INCORRECT

Because of the same guidelines in response C of determining which one is the patient's actual diagnosis when the two measurements do not correspond, the more severe (or lower bone mineral density) is the patient's diagnosis. Hence, her DEXA scan is not considered to be normal. For more information on DEXA scanning and BMD, please see Case 3-4.

E. Osteoarthritis   INCORRECT

Osteoarthritis is a degenerative disease of the joints of the body often related to articular disease. It is generally diagnosed by the presence of bone space narrowing, increased density of subchondral bone, bony cysts, and osteophytes on plain film radiographs. DEXA scans do not play a role in the diagnosis of this condition; therefore, this is not Mrs. Xiam's most likely diagnosis either.

5. Treatment Plan

A. Smoking cessation   CORRECT

Smoking cessation is a sound recommendation for anyone who smokes because there is a significant link between smoking and the development of several significant health problems, including coronary artery disease, CVAs, chronic bronchitis, osteoporosis, and a multitude of carcinomas. Smoking cessation is especially important for Mrs. Xiam if she wants to prevent her osteopenia from developing into osteoporosis because smoking is a risk factor for the development of osteoporosis.

B. Calcium 500 mg two to three times per day depending on dietary allowances from her nondairy sources   CORRECT

The National Academy of Sciences (NAS) recommendation for a female over the age of 50 years is between 1200 and 1500 mg of elemental calcium daily. Because Mrs. Xiam gets very little from her diet, she is probably going to need to take 500 mg of elemental calcium two to three times per day.

The dosage has to be in divided doses because taking more than 500 mg at a time does not result in better bioavailability or enhanced benefit. Essentially, larger doses just result in greater renal excretion of the unusable calcium and can increase the patient's risk for nephrolithiasis. Of concern is a recent meta-analysis connecting the use of calcium supplements with an increased risk (approximately 50%) of myocardial infarctions. Because this finding did not appear to occur if the calcium was also supplemented with vitamin D, additional supplementation with vitamin D is even more crucial. Additionally, until it can be determined if this is a causal relationship, calcium from dietary sources should be recommended before supplements are added.

C. Vitamin D 400 to 500 IU once a day   INCORRECT

The NAS recommendation for vitamin D intake in women over the age of 50 years is a minimum of 800 to 1000 IU daily and to maintain a serum vitamin D level [1,25(OH)$_2$D] of at least 20 to 30 ng/ml (however, most experts are currently recommending a goal of ≥ 30 ng/ml). Therefore, if her diet is inadequate for this amount, supplements and/or sun exposure should be considered. If it continues to remain below 30 ng/ml, she should be encouraged to get more exposure to the sun (the best source of vitamin D), increase her supplement, or increase foods that are high in vitamin D (with the exception of dairy products because of her lactose intolerance).

Foods rich in vitamin D besides dairy products include some fortified cereals, egg yolks, liver, and some saltwater fish; therefore, depending on her intake of these foods and her cholesterol levels, she could either increase the intake of these foods or increase her supplements to meet her goal.

Although vitamin D is a fat-soluble vitamin, research from the NAS indicates that up to 2000 IU/day is not harmful.

Data from the AACE claim that doses up to 10,000 IU do not produce any adverse effect and may be required by some patients to adequately absorb their calcium.

Recent information from the NAS states that higher doses are probably safe and in some cases needed in the elderly to maintain their vitamin D levels above the recommended 30 ng/ml. The NAS also recommends that if the level is low (e.g., below 20 ng/ml), the patient is considered to be severely deficient and at significant risk for a hip fracture. The HCP might even want to perform additional testing to attempt to determine whether there is some other condition besides poor sunshine exposure, inadequate dietary vitamin D intake, and suboptimal vitamin D supplementation contributing to this low level.

D. Explain treatment options available and assist in selecting an appropriate one   CORRECT

Which patients with osteopenia to treat is a difficult and individualized decision that should be based on risk of fracture versus adverse effects of medicine. Generally, women who have one or more risk factors for osteoporosis, in addition to being postmenopausal, should be treated. However, which risk factors to be utilized in this decision-making process was always an issue. The main factors generally considered significant were non-Hispanic white race, weight less than 127 lb, cigarette smoking, premature menopause, early menopause, amenorrhea for more than 1 year while premenopausal, positive family history of osteoporosis, history of adult fractures with minimal or no trauma, or condition/medication that could cause osteoporosis.

However, recently the World Health Organization has developed the Fracture Risk Algorithm (FRAX) model to estimate a woman's 10-year fracture risk. It is based on age, gender, height, weight, adult fracture history, parental hip fracture history, alcohol intake, tobacco use, use of corticosteroids, history of rheumatoid arthritis, and history of illness associated with osteoporosis. The model recommends treatment for all women who have a 3% or greater risk of a hip fracture or 20% or greater risk of any type of fracture within the next 10 years. (This tool can be found at http://www.NOF.org or http://www.shef.ac.uk/FRAX.) Despite these better recommendations, it is essential to remember that they are only recommendations; sound clinical judgment still must be applied on an individualized basis for each patient.

Because of her risk factors, Mrs. Xiam should be placed on medication to prevent her osteopenia from becoming osteoporosis and to reduce her fracture risk because there are actually more fractures occurring in postmenopausal women with osteopenia than with frank osteoporosis, probably because of the much larger number of women with the former. Of all the medications approved for osteoporosis, only estrogen and some of the bisphosphonates are FDA approved and recommended for prevention. In view of the negative information obtained from the Women's Health Study on hormone replacement therapy, Mrs. Xiam now being postmenopausal for 8 years, and the greatest benefit from estrogen to the bones occurring immediately following menopause, the best medication for her would probably be a bisphosphonate.

However, to have the greatest chance of continued compliance with the medication, Mrs. Xiam needs to participate in the decision-making process and make an informed decision.

Therefore, she should be advised of the importance of her beginning treatment and given information on the various bisphosphonates, including mechanism of action, possible adverse events, dosage frequency, and dosage route. Following this discussion, she should be given the option of whether she wishes to take the medication and which formulation/frequency she desires or whether she would like to hear about other off-label options (e.g., calcitonin, estrogen replacement therapy, selective estrogen modular receptors [SERMs], or teriparatide). The provider's role is to recommend treatment and to assist in selecting an appropriate option with which the patient will likely comply.

E. Repeat DEXA scan in 1 year   INCORRECT

As stated previously, when utilizing a DEXA scan for monitoring the treatment response, the correct interval following the institution of medication is 2 years. If a DEXA scan is performed earlier, there exists the possibility of false-negative results. In fact, it is not uncommon for a DEXA scan performed at 1 year after therapy initiation to show a worsening BMD as a result of the medication's activity, not treatment failure.

Epidemiologic and Other Data

It is estimated that 10 million individuals in the United States have osteoporosis, with 8 million being females. Furthermore, it is estimated that 18 million individuals in the United States have osteopenia. Osteoporosis occurs more frequently in women up until the age of approximately 70 years; then, the male:female ratio is essentially equal. The group affected most frequently is women during the first 5 years following menopause. Non-Hispanic whites have the highest incidence.

Fracture rates are inversely proportional to bone mineral density. It is estimated that osteoporosis accounts for approximately 300,000 hip fractures, 700,000 vertebral crush fractures, 250,000 wrist fractures, and 300,000 other fractures annually in the United States.

Many organizations have established guidelines regarding the use of DEXA scans for the screening of osteoporosis in asymptomatic women. The majority agree that for average-risk women, screening should begin at the age of 65 years. Those organizations include the US Preventive Services Task Force (USPSTF), the NOF, the American Academy of Family Physicians (AAFP), the AACE, and the Canadian Task Force on Preventive Health Care (CTF).

The AAFP, AACE, and USPSTF recommend routine screening of high-risk women beginning at the age of 60 years. However, the NOF recommends routine screening of high-risk women beginning at menopause.

The NOF also recommends screening all men at the age of 70 years and high-risk males starting at the age of 50 years with a DEXA scan. The only other organization that has any recommendations regarding men is the American College of Physicians (ACP), which recommends considering performing a DEXA on high-risk, older males who are suitable candidates for medical treatment.

Some organizations, such as the AACE, are now making recommendations to screen for the more common causes of secondary osteoporosis before initiating any treatment beyond lifestyle modifications.

CASE 3-6

Xandria Yoakum

1. History

A. Has she noticed any lesions or dryness of her mucous membranes? ESSENTIAL

Weakness and fatigue can occur in a multitude of conditions; however, the intermittent gastrointestinal symptoms, weight loss, and discoloration of skin significantly limit the list of differential diagnoses.

There are very few conditions outside of long-term exposure to natural or synthetic ultraviolet light capable of producing generalized hyperpigmentation. Several of these can be ruled out on the basis of Ms. Yoakum's history (e.g., hypercarotenemia, chemotherapy reaction, dialysis side effect, chronic venous insufficiency, and a postinflammatory reaction). Other causes can include hepatic diseases (e.g., hepatitis and cirrhosis), adrenal disorders (e.g., Addison disease), anorexia nervosa, polyglandular autoimmune (PGA) syndrome, adrenoleukodystrophy, hemochromatosis, alkaptonuria, pseudoporphyria, porphyria cutanea tarda, and visceral leishmaniasis.

In some of these conditions, the changes are not as generalized as Ms. Yoakum's nor are they strictly a bronze, or tanned, discoloration. However, in individuals of color, the potential list of differential diagnoses for abnormal discolorations of the skin must be more inclusive than it is for whites because their underlying skin tone can affect the shade or tone of discoloration produced. Therefore, relying strictly on the color of the skin can lead to misdiagnosis and treatment.

Regardless, it is important to inquire about oral mucosal lesions or dryness because some of the conditions that can produce hyperpigmentation are associated with specific changes of the mucous membranes. For example, Sjögren syndrome which is characterized by very dry mucous membranes and occasionally purpuric lesions on the face can be associated with adult-onset type 1 PGA, and adrenal insufficiency with bluish-black pigmented changes on the oral mucosa.

B. Has she noticed any changes in hearing, tasting, and/or smelling? ESSENTIAL

Hyperacute hearing, smelling, and tasting can occur with both primary and secondary adrenal insufficiency, which are potential causes of her symptoms.

C. Has she had any episodes of shakiness, sweatiness, lightheadedness, dizziness, presyncope, syncope, or orthostatic symptoms? ESSENTIAL

Several of the aforementioned conditions can be associated with anemia, which could produce many of these symptoms from a low blood volume. Additionally, some of these conditions can be linked with electrolyte abnormalities, diabetes mellitus, hypovolemia, and hypotension, especially of the orthostatic variety, which could account for the presence of these symptoms.

D. Has she noticed any axillary or pubic hair changes? ESSENTIAL

Endocrine disorders can be either the primary or secondary cause of (or just associated with) many of the aforementioned conditions that are not endocrine in nature. Hypothyroidism, adrenal insufficiency, hypogonadism, and primary or secondary amenorrhea can be associated with a thinning of the patient's pubic and/or axillary hair.

E. Is she experiencing any color changes of her urine? ESSENTIAL

Very pale or very dark urine can be seen in conditions that are associated with defects in the kidneys' ability to adequately concentrate the urine. Dark yellow urine could also represent an excess of bilirubin and/or urobilinogen indicating a hepatic abnormality. Gross hematuria can be seen not only in infections and carcinomas of the urinary tract itself, but also with bleeding disorders. Diet can also affect urine color (e.g. excessive carotene can produce an orange, beets a red, and rhubarb a brownish discoloration to the urine). And urine that contains homogentisic acid instantaneously turns black when exposed to air.

2. Physical Examination

A. Sclera and oral mucosa examination ESSENTIAL

An examination of her sclerae can assist in determining whether her skin color change represents jaundice. Jaundice can cause the color of the skin to appear more bronze colored than yellow in persons of color; however, their sclerae will reveal the typical yellow color if a significant liver, gallbladder, biliary duct obstruction, or other jaundice-producing condition is present.

The oral mucosa should be examined for the presence of bluish-black hyperpigmented areas, petechiae, leukoplakia, or other abnormalities that the patient might not have noticed on her own, particularly if they are located under the tongue.

B. Skin examination ESSENTIAL

A dermatologic examination is essential because her chief complaint is a skin color change. In addition to alterations to color, it should be evaluated for uniformity of color, changes to scars and striae, and other lesions that could be beneficial in formulating her list of differential diagnoses.

C. Examination of wrists for evidence of scarring NONESSENTIAL

Evidence of wrist scarring is highly unlikely to provide any additional useful information in helping to determine her correct diagnosis even if it is hyperpigmented like her appendectomy scar.

Despite the fact that previous suicide attempts are a significant risk factor for a future suicide attempt (and success), the presence of wrist scarring alone is not going to provide much information, because unintentional trauma can produce the same result. Even if a history of intentional wrist cutting is given, the presence of scars provides very little information beyond the history regarding the risk of a future successful suicide attempt, with the exception of distinguishing between a serious suicidal attempt and a suicidal gesture if there is evidence of a surgical repair for long vertical incision(s). Regardless, Ms. Yoakum's depression (and hence her risk for suicide) is controlled currently with medication and is very unlikely to be related to her chief complaint.

D. Heart examination   ESSENTIAL

A heart examination is indicated because she is experiencing lightheadedness, fatigue, and weakness, as these could represent an underlying cardiac condition (e.g., valvular abnormality, arrhythmia, cardiomyopathy, or heart failure). Furthermore, the palpation of her apical impulse could indicate either a small heart, as is sometimes seen with adrenal insufficiency, or a cardiomegaly, which is sometimes associated with hepatic diseases or heart failure.

E. Abdominal examination   ESSENTIAL

An abdominal examination is indicated based on her anorexia, nausea, weight loss, occasional vomiting, and intermittent diarrhea in addition to the concern that an intra-abdominal process could be responsible for her symptoms.

3. Diagnostic Studies

A. Thyroid panel (TSH, FT_4, and T_3 by RIA)   ESSENTIAL

A thyroid panel is indicated to determine whether primary or secondary hypothyroidism or hyperthyroidism or a hereditary condition as discussed previously could account for her symptoms.

B. Complete blood count with differential (CBC w/diff) with total iron-binding capacity (TIBC), iron, transferrin, transferrin saturation, and ferritin levels   ESSENTIAL

The CBC w/diff is important to perform because many of the conditions on Ms. Yoakum's list of differential diagnoses are associated with a leukocytic abnormality or anemia. Furthermore, it will provide some confirmation that an infectious etiology is not responsible for her symptoms.

The TIBC, iron, transferrin, transferrin saturation, and ferritin levels will be useful in determining whether hemochromatosis, cirrhosis, pernicious anemia, iron deficiency anemia, or other iron formation, absorption, conversion, or utilization problem are present either as the cause of her symptoms, associated with her symptoms, or related to her symptoms.

Remember, not all of the patient's complaints must be attributable to a single diagnosis. Patients can, and do, frequently have more than one diagnosis. This can be especially true when a significant number of nonspecific symptoms are present.

C. Serum   dehydroepiandrosterone   (DHEA)   level   NONESSENTIAL

Despite a DHEA level being low in adrenal insufficiency, which is one of the conditions on Ms. Yoakum's list of differential diagnoses, this test is not useful in making the diagnosis because it is low in approximately 15% to 20% of the general population.

D. Serum electrolytes, calcium, liver transaminases, bilirubin, and glucose   ESSENTIAL

Electrolytes are indicated because of Ms. Yoakum's chronic fatigue and long-standing history of intermittent vomiting and diarrhea. Furthermore, several of the conditions on her differential diagnosis list could be associated with electrolyte abnormalities that, if severe enough, will need to be treated along with her primary disease.

A serum calcium is also indicated as a gross screen for a parathyroid problem. A primary or secondary parathyroid disease as well as an endocrine syndrome involving either

hyperparathyroidism or hypoparathyroidism is possible. Many of her symptoms would certainly be considered consistent with the hyperparathyroidism mnemonic of "**B**ones, **S**tones, abdominal **G**roans, psychic **M**oans, and fatigue **O**vertones."

As stated previously, with Ms. Yoakum's constitutional and gastrointestinal symptoms, a chronic liver disease such as hepatitis, cirrhosis, or medication hepatoxicity as well as gallbladder problems (e.g., cholecystitis, cholelithiasis, or obstructed common bowel duct) could account for many of her complaints; therefore, liver function studies are indicated.

Finally, a fasting glucose is indicated because her constitutional symptoms, weight loss, chronic nausea, shakiness, lightheadedness, and irritability, as well as some of her other symptoms, could certainly be secondary to diabetes mellitus. Therefore, it is important to remember that diabetes mellitus could be responsible for some, if not all (unlikely), of her symptoms, either as a separate condition or as part of an endocrinopathy.

E. Plasma level of cortisol and adrenocorticotropic hormone (ACTH) at 8:00 a.m.   ESSENTIAL

These tests are considered appropriate screening tests for adrenal insufficiency in symptomatic patients. Therefore, because the vast majority, if not all, of Ms. Yoakum's symptoms could be accounted for by this problem, these are appropriate tests.

However, because the early morning (8:00 a.m.) cortisol and ACTH may not be good predictors of all types of adrenal disease, many experts advocate screening for all adrenal diseases by performing a rapid ACTH stimulation test. The most commonly performed ACTH stimulation test involves obtaining a baseline cortisol level, then injecting the patient with 250 μg cosyntropin either by the IV or IM route. Then, repeat cortisol levels are obtained 30 minutes and 60 minutes postinjection.

4. Diagnosis

A. Primary adrenal insufficiency   CORRECT

Primary adrenal insufficiency is a chronic adrenal insufficiency caused by gradual adrenal destruction, usually by an autoimmune process. The most common condition is Addison disease. In a symptomatic patient, an 8:00 a.m. plasma cortisol level of less than 3 μg/dL is virtually pathognomonic for adrenal insufficiency; this correlation is even more significant if the patient has a coexisting ACTH level of greater than 200 pg/ml. However, this fails to distinguish between primary and secondary adrenal insufficiency. This is best done on the basis of the patient's symptoms, physical examination findings, and other diagnostic test results.

Ms. Yoakum's adrenal insufficiency can be confirmed as primary because the characteristic pattern of her skin hyperpigmentation is not seen in secondary adrenal insufficiency. Primary adrenal insufficiency can be further confirmed by related laboratory findings that are consistent with the diagnosis (e.g., the presence of a mild normocytic, normochromic anemia; relative lymphocytosis; and a moderate eosinophilia on her CBC w/diff). The elevated potassium and decreased sodium, bicarbonate, and chloride levels on her electrolyte panel are consistent with a more advanced form of the disease. Hence, primary adrenal insufficiency is her most likely diagnosis.

B. Autoimmune polyendocrinopathy-candidiasis-ectodermal dystrophy (APCED)   INCORRECT

APCED is one of the endocrine syndromes, also known as type 1 (or primary) polyglandular autoimmune syndrome (PGA), and is generally diagnosed in early childhood. The most common presenting symptom is recurrent oral and perineal candidal infections. This is followed by hypoparathyroidism, abnormal dentition, and dystrophia unguium. The patient almost always acquires adrenal insufficiency by mid-adolescence. It is an autosomal recessive trait.

An adult form is not unusual. However, it is generally not associated with adrenal insufficiency, but with hypothyroidism, hypogonadism, hepatitis, malabsorption, alopecia, vitiligo, and Sjögren syndrome. Ms. Yoakum's history, physical examination, and diagnostic tests virtually rule out all of these conditions except for the possibility of malabsorption. Therefore, this is not her most likely diagnosis.

C. Hepatotoxicity caused by duloxetine   INCORRECT

Duloxetine is an SNRI antidepressant. It has been associated with chronic hepatic insufficiency and/or other chronic liver disease, especially in individuals who abuse alcohol. This is a potential diagnosis in a patient of color because what appears to be a bronze hyperpigmentation could actually be jaundice. Additionally, she is taking twice the FDA-approved dosage of duloxetine; however, there is some empirical data that the hepatotoxicity may not be dosage related. Regardless, it can be eliminated as Ms. Yoakum's most likely diagnosis because she has true hyperpigmentation and normal liver function tests.

D. Hemochromatosis   INCORRECT

Hemochromatosis is an inherited disorder (autosomal recessive) of iron metabolism that involves excessive iron ingestion and/or absorption, abnormalities of transferrin (iron-binding proteins), and excessive deposition of iron in the tissue stores of the body, most frequently the liver. It also has a great affinity to accumulate in the pancreas, skin, heart, and brain, leading to constitutional symptoms and diseases of any or all of these organs (e.g., cirrhosis, diabetes, bronze discoloration to skin, heart failure, and memory/concentration difficulties).

Although hemochromatosis can produce many of Ms. Yoakum's symptoms, it can be eliminated as her most likely diagnosis because of her normal HCT, Hgb, TIBC, ferritin, transferrin, and transferrin saturation levels. In hemochromatosis, the serum iron, ferritin, transferrin, and transferrin saturation are elevated. Additionally, there is usually mild liver enzyme elevation.

E. Photosensitivity reaction and other adverse effects to duloxetine   INCORRECT

Duloxetine, like any other medication, has the potential for various adverse effects. The effects reported in clinical trials that occurred at a greater incidence than placebo are similar to the ones experienced by Ms. Yoakum (e.g., fatigue, orthostatic hypotension, weight changes, gastrointestinal disturbances, and hyponatremia). Still, Ms. Yoakum had many symptoms that were not reported as possible adverse effects. However, this could be because of her ultra-high dosage or the short time frame utilized in the trials preventing them from being identified or reported. Nevertheless, it seems like an excessive number of complaints for an adverse drug reaction to be her only diagnosis.

A photosensitivity reaction to a medication generally produces a "sunburn"-type rash, not a "tanned" appearance. Furthermore, it tends to be limited to the areas of skin exposed to the sun, not generalized as in Ms. Yoakum's case. Additionally, even if she had the classic presentation, duloxetine is not a medication that is normally associated with a photosensitivity reaction.

There are several medications that can induce a secondary adrenal insufficiency; however, duloxetine is not one of them. The most common medication is the group of corticosteroids. Other potential medications include the opiates, anticoagulants, phenytoin, ketoconazole, rifampin, and megestrol. Hence, this is not Ms. Yoakum's most likely diagnosis.

5. Treatment Plan

A. Antiadrenal antibodies   CORRECT

The antiadrenal antibodies will provide further information regarding the cause of the primary adrenal insufficiency. If they are elevated, the adrenal insufficiency would be autoimmune in nature and most consistent with Addison disease being the final diagnosis.

B. Stop duloxetine   INCORRECT

For the reasons stated previously, this is not going to have any effect on her chief complaint of hyperpigmentation of her skin. However, if her depression was not responding adequately to the duloxetine or if she was having intolerable adverse effects (which it does not appear that she is), this would be a good choice. However, it is important to remember that patients must be tapered off antidepressant medications, especially when on ultra-high doses.

C. Hydrocortisone 15 mg every morning and 7.5 mg late each afternoon   CORRECT

The treatment of adrenal insufficiency includes replacing the corticosteroids that the adrenal gland is not producing. This is best accomplished with hydrocortisone. The daily dosage is usually divided into two doses, with the morning dose being two thirds of the total dose and the late-afternoon dose being the remaining one third. This dosing regimen more closely mimics the natural diurnal rhythm of cortisol and appears to provide the patient with more symptomatic relief.

Adjustments may be made subjectively on the basis of symptoms or objectively on the normalization of the white blood cell (WBC) differential. However, the most accepted method currently being utilized is a total of 20 to 30 mg/day based on the patient's weight alone. Studies now indicate that utilizing serum and/or urinary cortisol or serum ACTH for dosage adjustment is ineffective.

However, some patients do not respond well to or are intolerant of hydrocortisone; in that case, prednisone would be the drug of choice. Patients with very mild disease can often be maintained on corticosteroids alone.

D. Fludrocortisone acetate 0.05 mg daily   CORRECT

However, because the majority of patients with Addison disease do not achieve sufficient salt retaining effects from the corticosteroids, mineralocorticoids are also necessary. Fludrocortisone is the mineralocorticoid of choice. It is generally adjusted based on subjective symptoms as well as alleviation of the orthostatic hypotension, hyperkalemia, and hyponatremia.

If the patient is still symptomatic despite the correction of these three variables, then a plasma renin level should be performed. If it is elevated, then the dosage of fludrocortisones needs to be gradually increased until the plasma renin level normalizes.

E. DHEA 25 mg every morning   CORRECT

Experts now recommend that most women with Addison disease also be treated with prescription-grade DHEA 25 to 50 mg daily. This medication at this dosage appears to improve bone mineral density, mood, and libido in the majority of the cases.

Epidemiologic and Other Data

Adrenal insufficiency is classified as primary (the adrenal glands cannot produce adequate amounts of adrenal steroids—glucocorticoids, mineralocorticoids, and adrenal androgens) or secondary (ACTH production and/or release is inadequate).

Causes of primary adrenal insufficiency consist of conditions that produce acute or chronic destruction of the adrenal glands (e.g., congenital abnormalities, autoimmune processes, infection, bleeding, carcinoma, and surgical removal), failure in the production of the adrenal hormones (e.g., congenital abnormalities, inhibitors of necessary enzymes, and exposure to cytotoxic agents), antibodies that block ACTH, genetic mutations, and other congenital defects.

Causes of secondary adrenal insufficiency can be divided into anterior pituitary failure to release ACTH as a result of a pituitary or hypothalamic problem and hypothalamic-pituitary axis failure (or suppression) as a result of endogenous production of the steroids from a malignancy or exogenous sources (e.g., corticosteroid and other medications).

Primary adrenal insufficiency is much rarer than secondary adrenal insufficiency because of the large number of individuals taking corticosteroid medications in this country. Primary adrenal insufficiency does not have any proclivity regarding age or gender. If primary adrenal insufficiency is secondary to destruction of the adrenal gland, then a minimum of 90% of the gland must be lost before the patient becomes symptomatic.

CASE 3-7

Yolinda Zimmerman

1. History

A. Has she ever had a DEXA scan?   ESSENTIAL

Hypercortisolism is associated with osteoporosis. Therefore, it is important to know whether her BMD has ever been checked, when, and the results. If she has not had it evaluated within the past 1 to 2 years, then she should have a DEXA scan. If she has had a DEXA scan in this time frame and it revealed a low BMD, treatment and follow-up as outlined in Case 3-5 should be undertaken to prevent and/or treat osteoporosis. If it was normal, it should be repeated in 2 years from the date of the scan.

Incidentally, a DEXA scan would be indicated for Mrs. Zimmerman as part of her age-appropriate health maintenance because she is postmenopausal and has a positive family history of osteoporosis.

B. Does she own a cat?   NONESSENTIAL

The two main conditions associated with cat ownership are toxoplasmosis from handling the feces of an infected cat and cat-scratch disease. Toxoplasmosis is an infection caused by the parasite *Toxoplasma gondii*. The majority of immunocompetent patients are asymptomatic. In patients who do develop symptoms, the main one is cervical lymphadenopathy. Additional symptoms may include lymphadenopathy at other sites, headache, fever, malaise, sore throat, myalgias, and maculopapular rash. Rarely, toxoplasmosis can produce more serious infections such as pneumonia, encephalitis, pericarditis, and myocarditis in immunocompetent patients.

In immunocompromised patients and neonates who acquire it congenitally, the disease is much more severe and can result in multisystem failure and death. The central nervous system (CNS) appears to be the site affected most frequently. The most common congenital conditions include microcephaly, hydrocephalus, chorioretinitis, seizures, and mental retardation. In older patients, CNS conditions such as encephalitis, brain abscesses, cerebral dysfunction, seizure disorders, altered mental status, focal neurologic defects, cranial nerve palsies, vasculitis, intracranial hemorrhage, and hydrocephalus predominate.

Cat-scratch disease is caused by the gram-negative bacteria *Bartonella henselae*. Its initial symptom is a lesion (can be a papule, nodule, or vesicle) at the site of inoculation that persists for approximately 1 to 3 weeks. This is followed by localized, but usually significant, lymphadenopathy that occurs approximately 2 to 3 weeks after the initial insult and can last as long as 3 months. It is occasionally associated with fever, anorexia, myalgias, headache, and/or abdominal pain. Therefore, cat ownership is highly unlikely to play a role in her current illness.

C. Has she experienced any salt cravings?   NONESSENTIAL

Salt cravings are a symptom of adrenal insufficiency, not adrenal excess.

D. Did her headaches begin before the onset of her other current symptoms?   ESSENTIAL

Headaches can be a separate diagnosis or a component of another disease process. Therefore, it is important to obtain additional information regarding them to ensure that a serious intracranial pathology is not overlooked as part of her primary disease process. Thus, if she has a different headache pattern, a progression of previous headaches, or a new-onset headache, she will require additional investigation and some type of imaging study because she is over 55 years of age.

Furthermore, if her headache is associated with one of the "red flags" (e.g., "worst" headache of life; an abnormal neurologic examination; first "severe" headache; mental status changes; fever and/or other signs and symptoms suggestive of an intracranial infection [e.g., meningitis, encephalitis, or brain abscess]; pain that is increased by coughing, straining, lifting, or bending; pain that awakens the patient from sleep or is present immediately upon waking up; vomiting occurring before the onset of the headache; slowly but progressively worsening pain over a period of days; or in the presence of a known chronic illness), additional evaluation is essential.

E. Has she ever been on hormone replacement therapy (HRT)? ESSENTIAL

Even though she is not currently on HRT, recent usage could account for many of her symptoms.

2. Physical Examination

A. General appearance for weight distribution ESSENTIAL

Many different body habitus exist that can fall in the range of normal. For example, individuals with primary obesity tend to have a generalized fat pattern distribution, whereas those with metabolic syndrome tend to have central adiposity. However, patients with hypercortisolism tend to have marked central obesity that is frequently protuberant and thin limbs that appear to be out of proportion. Their faces appear larger and rounder ("moon facies") than expected, even given the significant central adiposity. Additionally, they can have "fat pads" in unique locations (e.g., supraclavicular areas and over the upper thoracic spine ["buffalo hump"]).

B. Thyroid examination NONESSENTIAL

With Mrs. Zimmerman's TSH being normal, it is highly unlikely that she would have a thyroid abnormality significant enough to account for her symptoms and be palpable on examination.

C. Skin examination ESSENTIAL

The skin examination should evaluate for thickness, friability, pigment changes, rashes, lesions, contusions, ecchymosis, and SQ nodules. The type, size, and distribution of these abnormalities, if present, should be noted.

D. Back examination ESSENTIAL

A back examination is necessary because Mrs. Zimmerman is complaining of thoracic spine pain. At a minimum, it should include visualization of the spine, palpation, and range of motion.

E. Neurologic examination ESSENTIAL

A neurologic examination is indicated because Mrs. Zimmerman is experiencing headaches and weakness.

3. Diagnostic Studies

A. 8:00 a.m. and 4:00 p.m. cortisol levels and an 8:00 a.m. adrenocorticotropic hormone (ACTH) level ESSENTIAL

Because her dexamethasone suppression test was positive, additional studies are going to need to be performed to determine whether Mrs. Zimmerman's hypercortisolism is caused by Cushing syndrome or a pseudo-Cushing syndrome. Plasma cortisol levels are considered to be the "gold standard" by which to measure adrenal function.

The body's cortisol levels are greatest between 6:00 a.m. and 8:00 a.m. and gradually fall throughout the day until they reach their lowest level at approximately midnight. Because most clinics and outpatient laboratories are not open at midnight, the acceptable protocol is to perform a cortisol level at 8:00 a.m. and 4:00 p.m. If the diurnal variation is normal, the 4:00 p.m. value should be approximately one-third to two-thirds the 8:00 a.m. value. If this variation is absent or blunted, then adrenal hyperfunction is the most likely diagnosis of the hypercortisolism.

The ACTH level also assists in determining the cause of the hypercortisolism. In general, if the ACTH level is low or even undetectable, the problem is a primary adrenal abnormality, most often an adenoma or carcinoma. If the ACTH is elevated, the cause is most likely pituitary (or hypothalamic) in nature; however, if it is markedly elevated (i.e., > 200 pmol/L), then an ectopic ACTH-producing tumor is generally the cause. These tumors can be located in the pancreas, lung, thymus, or ovary. Pseudo-Cushing syndromes are generally associated with an ACTH level ranging from the upper limits of normal to slightly elevated. ACTH also has a diurnal variation. It tends to be highest in the morning (4 a.m. to 8 a.m.) and lowest in the evening (8 p.m. to 10 p.m.) If the evening sample is compared to the morning sample, it should be one-third to one-half the morning value.

B. 24-hour urine for free cortisol and creatinine ESSENTIAL

Several factors can interfere with the accuracy of the results from a dexamethasone suppression test (e.g., medications [corticosteroids, estrogen, rifampin, phenytoin, phenobarbital, carbamazepine, and fenofibrate], pregnancy, and excessive fluid intake). Therefore, if a positive result is obtained, it is essential to confirm that the result is accurate. This is generally accomplished by obtaining a 24-hour urine for free cortisol and creatinine, which provides a quantitative measurement to determine the actual cortisol production (because unconjugated [or free] cortisol is renally excreted) and the renal function.

If the urinary free cortisol level is significantly elevated OR the urinary free cortisol:creatinine ratio is greater than 95, true hypercortisolism is present.

C. Glucose tolerance test or equivalent assessment ESSENTIAL

This test is indicated because Mrs. Zimmerman's original fasting plasma glucose (FPG) of 120 mg/dl fell between the normal value of 70 to 110 mg/dl and the diagnostic value for diabetes mellitus (DM) of greater than or equal to 126 mg/dl. Therefore, it is important to distinguish whether Mrs. Zimmerman is a diabetic or has abnormal glucose tolerance.

The simplest form of this test involves obtaining an FPG for Mrs. Zimmerman followed by having her consume a 75-g glucose and then performing a random plasma glucose (RPG) at 2 hours. An acceptable alternative is to obtain an FPG and then have her eat breakfast and have a random plasma glucose drawn 2 hours later.

D. Dual-energy x-ray absorptiometry (DEXA) scan ESSENTIAL

Because Mrs. Zimmerman has never had a DEXA scan, she needs one because hypercortisolism is associated with osteoporosis, she is postmenopausal, and she has a family history of osteoporosis.

E. Magnetic resonance image (MRI) of the adrenal glands NONESSENTIAL

Although an elevated cortisol level combined with a normal ACTH level indicates autonomous endogenous excessive secretion of cortisol by the adrenal glands, the imaging study of choice to evaluate the adrenal glands for masses/tumors is a computed tomography (CT) scan, not an MRI scan.

4. Diagnosis

A. Extreme obesity (obesity type III), hypertension (stage 1), type 2 diabetes mellitus, and Cushing syndrome   INCORRECT

Extreme obesity is defined as a BMI greater than or equal to 40. (For more information on BMI calculation and classification, please see Case 1-1.) Because Mrs. Zimmerman's BMI is 48, this component is correct.

Stage 1 hypertension is defined as either a systolic blood pressure (SBP) of 149 to 159 mm Hg OR a diastolic blood pressure (DBP) of 90 to 99 mm Hg. (For more information on the classification of BP, please see Case 1-1.) Because Mrs. Zimmerman's BP is 136/84 mm Hg at this visit and was 136/84 mm Hg at her previous visit, this choice can be eliminated as her most likely diagnosis.

B. Cushing syndrome caused by a pituitary abnormality INCORRECT

Cushing syndrome is a disease of hypercortisolism; and, approximately 70% of all endogenous causes of Cushing syndrome are due to pituitary adenomas. Although Mrs. Zimmerman does have mild hypercortisolism, her cortisol diurnal fluctuation is still preserved and her 24-hour urinary cortisol level is normal. In addition, her ACTH is still in the high-normal range. Therefore, she does not have true Cushing's syndrome but an iatrogenic hypercortisolism which is actually the most common cause of hypercortisolism. Thus, this can be eliminated as her most likely diagnosis.

C. Extreme obesity (obesity type III), prehypertension, abnormal glucose tolerance, osteopenia, and pseudo-Cushing syndrome   CORRECT

As stated previously, Mrs. Zimmerman's BMI meets the World Health Organization's definition of extreme obesity and her BP levels place her in the JNC-7 prehypertension range (systolic BP of 120 to 139 mm Hg OR a diastolic BP of 89 to 90 mm Hg) making the first two components of this diagnostic cluster correct.

The American Diabetes Association's definitions for diabetes mellitus include an FPG of 126 mg/dl on two separate occasions OR an RPG (or 2 hours after a 75-g glucose load or a meal) of greater than or equal to 200 mg/dl in a symptomatic patient. Although Mrs. Zimmerman's FPG and RPG were both elevated, she does not meet these established cut-offs. Thus, she has abnormal glucose tolerance. Therefore, Mrs. Zimmerman also meets the third component of this diagnosis.

Osteopenia, or low bone mass, is diagnosed by a DEXA scan T score between –1.0 and –2.5. Because Mrs. Zimmerman's T score was –1.5 (and her Z score of –0.8 was normal for her age), she can be diagnosed with the fourth component of this diagnosis, osteopenia (for more information on interpretation of the DEXA scan, please see Case 3-5).

Finally, Mrs. Zimmerman also has what is called pseudo-Cushing syndrome. The mainstay of diagnosing this condition is the presence of a positive dexamethasone suppression test but only a mild elevation of cortisol levels. Furthermore, she has a mildly elevated 8:00 a.m. cortisol level, a normal 24-hour urine cortisol measurement, and no loss of the normal diurnal variation of the cortisol level. Additionally, it is extremely rare to find a "true" Cushing syndrome in a markedly obese individual (type II or III).

Thus, this option is Mrs. Zimmerman's most likely diagnosis because it fits with her symptoms, physical examination findings, and diagnostic study results as described.

D. Type 2 diabetes mellitus, obesity type I, hypertension stage 1, osteoporosis, and pseudo-Cushing syndrome   INCORRECT

Although Mrs. Zimmerman does meet the diagnostic criteria for pseudo-Cushing syndrome, she fails to meet the aforementioned criteria for type 2 diabetes mellitus, obesity type I, hypertension stage 1, and osteoporosis. Thus, this option cannot be her most likely diagnosis.

E. Abnormal glucose tolerance, obesity type II, prehypertension, and Cushing syndrome   INCORRECT

As previously stated, Mrs. Zimmerman meets the diagnostic criteria as established by the ADA for having abnormal glucose tolerance and the JNC-7 criteria for prehypertension. However, her obesity is type III, not type II, and she has pseudo-Cushing syndrome, not true Cushing syndrome. Thus, this is not her most likely diagnosis.

5. Treatment Plan

A. Low-fat, low-salt, low-calorie heart-healthy diet   CORRECT

This diet will hopefully be beneficial in treating not only her obesity but also her hypertension and abnormal glucose intolerance. Furthermore, controlling these factors will hopefully prevent more serious complications caused by these conditions and resolve her pseudo-Cushing syndrome.

B. Glycosylated hemoglobin   INCORRECT

Currently, glycosylated hemoglobins are only utilized to follow up on the control of diabetes and are not indicated in the evaluation and treatment of abnormal glucose tolerance.

C. Schedule for an age-appropriate preventive examination CORRECT

Each and every patient seen should be encouraged to have regular age-appropriate preventive examinations with diagnostic testing, immunizations, and patient education regardless of their chief complaint because it is sound medical practice.

D. Refer to surgeon for bariatric surgery   INCORRECT

Mrs. Zimmerman meets the accepted weight criteria for bariatric surgery: a BMI greater than 40 OR a BMI greater than 35 plus at least two cardiovascular risk factors. However, she does not meet the criterion of failed other attempts. Furthermore, she has not been counseled regarding this option, her readiness to consider it, or even her desire to lose weight. Therefore, this is not an appropriate treatment option at this time.

E. Refer to endocrinologist for treatment of Cushing syndrome   INCORRECT

Because Mrs. Zimmerman has pseudo-Cushing syndrome as a result of her obesity, not "true" Cushing syndrome, this referral is not necessary at this time. Other causes of pseudo-Cushing syndrome include depression, anorexia nervosa, alcoholism, and familial cortisol resistance.

Epidemiologic and Other Data

Obesity has reached epidemic proportions in the United States. It is estimated that 66% of all adults in the United States meet the BMI criteria to be considered overweight or obese. It is estimated that in the very near future, the number of deaths from the complications of obesity are going to surpass the number of deaths from cigarette smoking in this country. The groups that are affected the most by overweight and obesity are non-Hispanic blacks, African Americans, individuals between the ages of 40 and 60 years, people with sedentary lifestyles, families with low incomes, individuals with lower educational levels, and married (or cohabiting) couples.

A weight loss (and maintenance) of 10% of body weight will result in a significant reduction of patients' health risks caused by obesity.

CASE 3-8
Zoey Armstrong
1. History

A. Does she have any nipple discharge? ESSENTIAL

Hyperprolactinemia, a cause of both primary amenorrhea (never menstruated) and secondary amenorrhea (post-menarchal patient who has not menstruated for a minimum of 3 months if she had regular menstrual cycles OR for a minimum of 6 months if her menses was irregular), can result from multiple causes including pregnancy, acromegaly, autoimmune diseases, cirrhosis, excessive exercise, hypothalamic disease, hypothyroidism, multiple sclerosis, pituitary stalk abnormalities, spinal cord lesions, medications, or any tumor that secretes prolactin. Regardless of the cause or type, a characteristic symptom of hyperprolactinemia is galactorrhea.

B. Has she been experiencing any problems with headaches, visual disturbances, or abnormalities of smell? ESSENTIAL

Both primary and secondary amenorrhea can result from failure of the hypothalamic-pituitary-ovarian axis. Abnormalities in any one of these areas as well as the uterus and outflow tract can produce amenorrhea. Headaches in amenorrhea can be caused by a pituitary lesion, most commonly a pituitary adenoma. Because the pituitary is confined to the sella turcica, extremely small changes in the size of the gland (even before extrasellar extension occurs) can result in a headache caused by stretching of the dural plate. As the lesion enlarges, headaches tend to become more frequent and severe; however, the size of the gland and/or the amount of extrasellar extension does not correlate well with the severity of headache.

Visual disturbances and abnormalities of smell are also symptoms generally associated with a pituitary abnormality. They are caused by suprasellar (the most common direction because the dorsal sellar diaphragm is the area of least resistance) extension of the enlarging pituitary (as a result of the associated enlargement of the mass lesion) compressing surrounding structures (e.g., optic chiasm, cerebrospinal fluid flow, or arteries).

C. Is she an athlete, dieting, or exercising excessively? ESSENTIAL

Athletes (especially those involved in gymnastics, figure skating, ballet, and similar aesthetic endeavors) are at an increased risk of developing the female athlete triad. It consists of amenorrhea (either primary or secondary), an eating disorder (most commonly anorexia nervosa), and osteoporosis.

In fact, it is estimated that nearly two thirds of all female athletes experience an eating disorder and amenorrhea.

Hypocaloric diets in and of themselves can result in amenorrhea. They can also occur as a sign of depression, resulting from loss of appetite, or anorexia nervosa, resulting from a distorted body image. Strenuous and vigorous exercise can result in amenorrhea either as an entity of its own or as part of anorexia nervosa, bulimia nervosa, or hyperprolactinemia. These problems can be seen in both primary and secondary amenorrhea. Given Ms. Armstrong's very low-normal BMI, these possibilities need to be explored.

D. Is she experiencing vaginal dryness, hot flashes, or night sweats? ESSENTIAL

Although Ms. Armstrong is not near the age of average menopause (51 years in the United States) or even the lower end of the range (41–59 years), a premature menopause could be causing her symptoms. Thus, it is worthwhile to question her regarding the presence of symptoms associated with the menopause transition.

E. Does she have problems with acne, hirsutism, or deepening of her voice? ESSENTIAL

Hyperandrogenism (suspected by the appearance of these symptoms) results in primary or secondary amenorrhea caused by an excess of testosterone; conditions include adrenal hyperplasia, adrenal tumors, ovarian tumors, or polycystic ovary syndrome (Stein-Leventhal syndrome).

2. Physical Examination

A. Eye and nose examination NONESSENTIAL

The primary purpose of an eye and nose examination in the evaluation of amenorrhea would be to test for visual field defects and/or abnormalities of smell. If present without a known cause (e.g., optic neuritis, allergic rhinitis, or upper respiratory tract infection), extrasellar expansion of a pituitary abnormality should be suspected as the cause of the patient's amenorrhea. However, because Ms. Armstrong is otherwise asymptomatic in regards to symptoms related to such, the exam is unnecessary.

B. Cranial nerve evaluation NONESSENTIAL

The most common abnormalities discovered on cranial nerve testing in a patient complaining of amenorrhea are a visual field defect and an abnormal sense of smell as a result of suprasellar compression on surrounding structures from an enlarging pituitary lesion. If the extrasellar expansion occurs in a lateral direction (much rarer), it can compress the neural structures found in the cavernous sinus. This could result in diplopia, ptosis, ophthalmoplegia, and decreased facial sensation caused by compression of cranial nerves (and/or their branches) III to VI. Nevertheless, because Ms. Armstrong does not have symptoms to suggest a pituitary lesion, this evaluation is not necessary.

C. Breast examination NONESSENTIAL

Because Ms. Armstrong does not have any breast complaints, a breast examination is not essential. However, a breast examination is important to determine not only if the breasts are present but also the appropriate Tanner stage when evaluating a patient with primary amenorrhea.

However, her age does place her in an age group where a clinical breast examination (CBE) should be recommended, or at least discussed, as part of her routine health maintenance as screening for breast cancer. The American Cancer Society (ACS) recommends a CBE every 2 to 3 years for asymptomatic women between the ages of 20 and 39 years. Other organizations feel the CBE should not begin until the age of 40 years and/or only if the woman decides to have one conducted after a discussion of the risks and benefits of such because of the lack of sound clinical evidence proving its effectiveness in reducing mortality due to breast cancer.

D. Pelvic examination   ESSENTIAL

The primary purpose of a pelvic examination in a patient with secondary amenorrhea is to evaluate for any evidence of a structural abnormality or pregnancy that could account for the patient's symptoms. For example, an enlarged uterus, Hegar sign (softening of the cervical isthmus), and Chadwick sign (a bluish discoloration of the cervix and less commonly the vaginal walls) are frequently seen with pregnancy; vaginal dryness, atrophy, and thinning of the pubic hair can suggest premature ovarian failure or other hypoestrogenic states; and an adnexal mass is possible in polycystic ovarian syndrome or ovarian cancer.

However, in the evaluation of primary amenorrhea, the primary purpose of the pelvic examination is to assess the patient's hair distribution for an appropriate Tanner stage; the external genitalia for normal female development, lack of clitoromegaly, and status of the hymen (i.e., perforated); the pelvic organs for presence and normality; and evidence of pregnancy. If a highly sensitive pregnancy test has been performed and is negative, the exam should also include attempting to pass a uterine sound through the endocervical canal to ensure patency.

E. Skin examination   ESSENTIAL

The skin should be evaluated for signs of hyperandrogenism (e.g., acne, excessive oiliness, and/or hirsutism). Other abnormalities that could suggest the cause of both primary and secondary amenorrhea include purple striae associated with Cushing syndrome, excessively dry skin associated with hypothyroidism, jaundice associated with cirrhosis and other severe liver diseases, and chloasma sometimes associated with pregnancy.

Note: The patient's vital signs can provide clues suggesting certain conditions that can be responsible for either primary or secondary amenorrhea. For example, a low BMI can be seen with anorexia nervosa, excessive strenuous and/or vigorous exercise, and/or a hypercaloric diet. Short stature can be seen with growth hormone deficiency, thyroid hormone deficiency, adrenal hormone excess, or Turner syndrome, and a tall stature could indicate gigantism or eunuchoidism as the cause of primary amenorrhea. Obesity can be related to excess androgen production as seen in polycystic ovarian syndrome (PCOS) or excessive adrenal hormone as seen in Cushing syndrome. Hypertension can be associated with hyperandrogenism states.

3. Diagnostic Studies

A. Urinary human chorionic gonadotropin (HCG) test ESSENTIAL

A pregnancy test is indicated in all women presenting with amenorrhea regardless of their stated sexual activity/

contraceptive history. Pregnancy is the most common cause of secondary amenorrhea and can be responsible for primary amenorrhea.

B. Wet-mount microscopy of vaginal secretions or vaginal pH, "whiff" test for amine odor, and point-of-care testing for vaginal pathogens via DNA   NONESSENTIAL

The primary purpose of these tests is to distinguish between the most common causes of vulvovaginitis/vaginitis. Because vulvovaginitis/vaginitis does not produce amenorrhea and Ms. Armstrong lacks signs and symptoms consistent with this diagnosis, these tests do not need to be performed.

C. Pelvic ultrasound   NONESSENTIAL

A pelvic ultrasound is not currently indicated because Ms. Armstrong's pelvic organs appeared normal on physical examination. However, if other diagnostic studies suggest a possible ovarian cause for her amenorrhea (or identify another abnormality), it might be indicated at that time.

D. Serum prolactin level   ESSENTIAL

A serum prolactin level is frequently considered to be one of the first-line diagnostic tools in evaluating a female patient who has an intact uterus, normal breast development, and a negative pregnancy test but is experiencing either primary or secondary amenorrhea.

E. Serum follicular-stimulating hormone (FSH)   ESSENTIAL

An FSH is also considered to be a first-line test in the evaluation of primary and/or secondary amenorrhea in women with an intact uterus, normal breast development, and a negative pregnancy test. In fact, some experts recommend ordering the FSH (without a prolactin level) first, and then ordering the prolactin test only if this level is decreased or normal.

4. Diagnosis

A. Polycystic ovarian syndrome (PCOS)   INCORRECT

PCOS is consistent with her findings of a normal prolactin and FSH level because it is considered to be a normogonadotropic amenorrhea, and it frequently occurs with a normal adnexal examination. However, signs of androgen excess (e.g., acne, hirsutism, and deepened voice) are almost always present. Thus, PCOS is not Ms. Armstrong's most likely diagnosis.

B. Hypogonadotropic secondary amenorrhea   CORRECT

Hypogonadotropic amenorrhea is also known as hypothalamic amenorrhea and is generally caused by an exogenous stress causing gonadotropin-releasing hormone (GnRH) suppression. Therefore, it is associated with a normal or low FSH and normal prolactin level. Because Ms. Armstrong had these diagnostic test results, an essentially normal physical examination, and secondary amenorrhea (as described previously), this is her most likely diagnosis at this time.

C. Premature ovarian failure (POF)   INCORRECT

Premature ovarian failure is menopause that occurs before the age of 40 years. (If it occurs between the ages of 40 and 50 years, it is termed premature menopause.) It is characterized by an elevated FSH level of greater than 40 IU/L. Because of the wide fluctuations associated with the FSH level during normal menstrual cycles, many experts advocate repeating this test to confirm the results before making the diagnosis. Still, because of her normal FSH level and lack of menopausal symptoms, POF can essentially be eliminated as Ms. Armstrong's most likely diagnosis.

D. Primary amenorrhea   INCORRECT

As stated previously, primary amenorrhea can only be diagnosed in women who have failed to achieve menarche; therefore, this is not Ms. Armstrong's most likely diagnosis.

E. Pituitary adenoma causing secondary amenorrhea INCORRECT

A pituitary adenoma is almost always associated with hyperprolactinemia and abnormalities of vision and/or smell. Although the FSH tends to be normal, this is still not Ms. Armstrong's most likely diagnosis because she lacked the former findings.

5. Treatment Plan

A. Progesterone challenge test with 10 mg of medroxyprogesterone acetate (MPA) once a day for 10 days   INCORRECT

A progesterone challenge test consists of providing the patient with 5 to 10 mg of MPA once a day for 10 days. If positive (some type of bleeding or even spotting occurs within 10 to 14 days of completion of the MPA), it generally indicates that the patient's uterine endometrium is functioning normally and her endocervical canal and os are patent (which should have been confirmed by uterine sound in primary amenorrhea).

Previously, it was considered to be a first-line diagnostic tool (following a negative pregnancy test) in the evaluation of primary and secondary amenorrhea. However, because of its nonspecific nature and the delay in diagnosis and treatment, it is no longer frequently employed.

B. Luteinizing hormone (LH)   INCORRECT

The LH is generally not considered to be a necessary component in the evaluation of amenorrhea because it provides very little, if any, information that cannot be obtained by the FSH. However, it is sometimes ordered in patients when PCOS is suspected because an LH:FSH ratio of greater than 2 is generally considered diagnostic for the condition.

C. Thyroid stimulating hormone (TSH)   CORRECT

A TSH is indicated for Ms. Armstrong because hypothyroidism can cause hypothalamic amenorrhea.

D. Re-evaluate diet, exercise, and stress   CORRECT

A hypocaloric diet, strenuous vigorous exercise, and excessive stress are potential causes of hypothalamic amenorrhea. Thus, these areas require further evaluation because proper treatment is going to be dependent on the elimination of the cause of GnRH suppression.

E. Magnetic resonance image (MRI) of her pituitary INCORRECT

An MRI of her pituitary is unlikely to reveal any significant abnormality based on her normal FSH and prolactin levels because both are produced by the anterior pituitary gland. However, if her symptoms persist after correcting the potential cause(s) of her condition and menstruation does not return, then an MRI should be considered to evaluate her pituitary and hypothalamus for a structural abnormality that might be producing her amenorrhea.

Epidemiologic and Other Data

It is estimated that in the United States, primary amenorrhea affects less than 1% of all females, whereas secondary amenorrhea is estimated to affect 3% to 5% of all females. A single missed period occurs at least once during a woman's lifetime in the majority of all women of childbearing age. This most commonly occurs immediately after menarche and/or before menopause.

In primary amenorrhea, it is estimated that a hypothalamic problem is responsible for approximately 27% of all cases; a pituitary abnormality, polycystic ovarian syndrome (PCOS), other ovarian abnormalities, and uterine/outflow problems are responsible for approximately 2%, 7%, 43%, and 19%, respectively (due to rounding, total does not equal 100%). In contrast, in secondary amenorrhea, hypothalamic conditions, pituitary abnormalities, PCOS, other ovarian abnormalities, and uterine/outflow problems are responsible for approximately 36%, 15%, 30%, 12%, and 7%, respectively.

CASE 3-9
Anne Brown
1. History

A. Did she experience hyperemesis gravidarum with her first pregnancy?   NONESSENTIAL

Each pregnancy is distinct. Certain complications like hyperemesis gravidarum can be present in one pregnancy and totally lacking in previous or subsequent pregnancies. Thus, the presence or absence of this condition in a previous pregnancy is irrelevant. However, recent evidence reveals an associated increased risk if the patient's mother experienced hyperemesis gravidarum with her pregnancy. The association was not found with mothers-in-law.

B. Has she been experiencing any cardiac palpitations or tachycardia?   ESSENTIAL

Nausea and vomiting is associated with the vast majority of pregnancies. It can commence as early as the first missed period but tends to resolve by the end of the first trimester. However, it is not abnormal for it to persist throughout the fifth month of gestation. In fact, a few women will experience minor, nonpathologic nausea and vomiting throughout the entire pregnancy.

However, if it is severe and persistent (called hyperemesis gravidarum), the patient needs to be evaluated for secondary causes as a result of the pregnancy (e.g., gestational trophoblastic disease or multiple gestations) or coexisting conditions that may or may not be related to the pregnancy (e.g., hypothyroidism, hyperthyroidism, renal failure, adrenal insufficiency, and parathyroid disease). Because cardiac palpitations and tachycardia can be associated with some of these conditions, it is important to ask if she is experiencing them.

Furthermore, despite fatigue being a very common symptom of pregnancy, it can be a symptom in the majority of the aforementioned conditions. However, her fatigue could also be caused by other pregnancy-related complications (e.g., anemia and/or dehydration) that generally do not cause nausea and vomiting but can cause tachycardia and palpitations.

C. Has she had any vaginal spotting or bleeding?   ESSENTIAL

One of the aforementioned pregnancy complications responsible for hyperemesis gravidarum is gestational trophoblastic disease, which can range from a hydatidiform mole (or molar pregnancy) to a choriocarcinoma. Frequently, uterine bleeding is also a complication of this abnormality and can begin as early as 6 to 8 weeks' gestation. Therefore, it is important to inquire as to whether she is experiencing any vaginal bleeding or spotting not just as an indicator of a normal viable pregnancy but also as a concern for this condition.

D. Is her nausea and vomiting worse in the mornings or the evenings?   NONESSENTIAL

Even though the nausea and vomiting of pregnancy is frequently called "morning sickness," the symptoms tend to persist throughout the day with peaks in the mornings and the evenings.

E. Is she planning on breast- or bottle-feeding? NONESSENTIAL

This is a very important decision for a pregnant woman. However, this is not the optimal time for the topic to be addressed because Mrs. Brown is not feeling well; this is a problem-focused visit, not a routine prenatal visit; and she still has several months during which to make the final decision.

2. Physical Examination

A. Palpation of thyroid   ESSENTIAL

Despite the fact that the thyroid gland normally enlarges in size during pregnancy, Mrs. Brown's thyroid should still be palpated because of her hyperemesis gravidarum to determine if she has any signs of extreme enlargement (especially asymmetric), masses, nodules, or tenderness that could indicate a secondary thyroid abnormality. However, it is important to remember that many thyroid conditions are not associated with any palpable abnormality of the gland.

B. Heart examination   ESSENTIAL

A heart examination should be performed because Mrs. Brown is complaining of intermittent exertional palpations and tachycardia. Although they could be caused by the pregnancy, they could also be caused by one of the aforementioned conditions. Additionally, Mrs. Brown could have a preexisting, undiagnosed heart condition that has been exacerbated as a result of the blood volume expansion associated with pregnancy, or she could have developed a new cardiac condition.

C. Abdominal examination, including uterine fundus palpation and height, and Doppler evaluation of fetal heartbeat ESSENTIAL

An abdominal examination can assist in ruling out other causes of her nausea and vomiting in addition to hyperemesis gravidarum. These conditions include gallbladder diseases, pancreatic problems, appendicitis, hepatic disorders, or an adrenal mass.

Additionally, abdominal examination permits palpation of the uterus for contour, tenderness, and tetany and helps ensure that its size is consistent with Mrs. Brown's gestational age. The Doppler examination of the fetus' heartbeat primarily determines the fetus' heart rate. However, it occasionally can detect abnormal cardiac sounds that require immediate evaluation or the presence of more than one heart sound, indicating a multiple gestation.

The normal fetal heart rate range is 120 to 160 beats per minute. A tachycardic or bradycardic rate can be associated with potentially serious adverse consequences and even death of the fetus. Doppler examination of the fetus' heartbeat can occasionally not detect any heart sounds (even if the fetus' heart is beating). This could be a result of equipment failure, excessive ambient noise, fetal distress, position of the baby, size of the uterine cavity, or incorrect gestational age. In general, with a Doppler, fetal heart sounds should be identifiable by 9 to 12 weeks' gestation.

D. Rectal examination   NONESSENTIAL

E. Evaluation of lower extremities for pedal edema and the skin over the sternum and/or forehead for "tenting" ESSENTIAL

Ankle edema should be checked for on every pregnant woman at each of her visits. The presence of edema in conjunction with proteinuria, an elevated BP, and a significant weight gain are all signs of preeclampsia/eclampsia. However, it is rare to see preeclampsia until at least 20 weeks' gestation (unless gestational trophoblastic disease is present).

"Tenting" is the lack of normal elastic recoil causing the skin to stay "tented," or "puckered," for a few seconds after being gently pinched, before slowly returning to its original position; it is frequently associated with dehydration. The most accurate areas to evaluate for this sign are over the sternum and over the forehead.

3. Diagnostic Studies

A. Blood urea nitrogen (BUN) and electrolytes   ESSENTIAL

If Mrs. Brown had significant dehydration or malnutrition, her BUN would be elevated. Electrolytes are helpful in the evaluation of prolonged vomiting as an indication of the severity of the condition. Plus, if an abnormality exists, it can be addressed and corrected earlier.

B. Urinalysis   ESSENTIAL

An abbreviated urinalysis should be performed on all pregnant patients at every visit utilizing a dipstick to screen for the presence of protein, glucose, and leukocyte esterase. However, because this is not a routine visit but one to evaluate hyperemesis gravidarum, Mrs. Brown needs a complete urinalysis. The specific gravity, pH, and ketones are important in evaluating for dehydration. The urinalysis is also helpful in ruling in or ruling out renal disease.

C. Quantitative serum human chorionic gonadotropin (HCG) NONESSENTIAL

HCG is produced by the placental trophoblasts once the ovum is fertilized. It is generally evident in both the blood and serum 10 days later. A quantitative test provides the actual serum HCG level. This number should correspond with "normal" values provided for each week of gestation. These numbers tend to be accurate up to approximately 12 weeks' gestation.

Early in the course of the pregnancy, HCG tests can be performed approximately every 48 hours. If a doubling of the second value (compared to the first) occurs, a spontaneous abortion or ectopic pregnancy is highly unlikely to exist.

They can also be used later in pregnancy by comparing the values to estimate for fetal loss and other complications. This test is also valuable in the evaluation of possible gestational trophic disease early in the pregnancy.

Even though this is one of Mrs. Brown's possible differential diagnoses, there is no need to perform the test for this purpose because of her gestational age. The accepted level considered to be suspicious for a possible molar pregnancy is greater than 40,000 mIU/ml. At this stage of Mrs. Brown's pregnancy, her HCG could be as high as 220,000 in a normal singleton pregnancy. At her gestational age, ultrasounds essentially replace a quantitative HCG as the diagnostic study of choice for determination of the presence or absence of a molar pregnancy as well as correct gestational age and multiple gestations.

D. Obstetric ultrasound   ESSENTIAL

As stated previously, this test essentially replaces the quantitative serum HCG as the test of choice to determine the presence of hydatiform moles, multiple-gestation pregnancy, ectopic pregnancy, and fetal demise at approximately 12 weeks' gestational age.

E. Thyroid panel (TSH, FT_4, and T_3 by RIA)   ESSENTIAL

Thyroid function studies are important because hypothyroidism and hyperthyroidism are among the potential differential diagnoses for Mrs. Brown.

4. Diagnosis

A. Normal pregnancy with false-positive thyroid function testing as a result of pregnancy   INCORRECT

The increase of estrogen associated with pregnancy produces an elevation of the thyroid-binding globulin (TBG). In turn, the TBG causes an increase in the levels of total triiodothyronine (T_3) and total thyroxine (T_4) and, in many cases, thyroid enlargement. However, free triiodothyronine (FT_3), FT_4, and TSH remain normal in pregnancy. Thus, based on her diagnostic studies, this is not Mrs. Brown's most likely diagnosis.

B. Preeclampsia   INCORRECT

Preeclampsia is a precursor to eclampsia of pregnancy characterized by hypertension, edema, significant weight gain, and proteinuria. Because Mrs. Brown lacks these characteristic findings, preeclampsia is not her most likely diagnosis. Furthermore, it rarely, if ever, occurs in women at less than 20 weeks' gestational age unless gestational trophoblastic disease is present.

C. Hydatidiform mole   INCORRECT

A hydatidiform mole, or a molar pregnancy, is the most benign form of gestational trophic disease. It is characterized clinically by large-for-gestational-age uterine size, lack of fetal heartbeat by appropriate age, marked elevation of the serum HCG as discussed previously, and evidence of the abnormality on ultrasound (can either visualize "grapelike" clusters or a "snowstorm" image). Common symptoms include first (usually) trimester bleeding, passage of the "grapelike" cluster as a mass, and severe hyperemesis gravidarum. Thus, based on Mrs. Brown's clinical findings and ultrasound results, a hydatidiform mole can be eliminated as her most likely diagnosis.

D. Mild hypothyroidism in pregnancy   CORRECT

The patient's symptoms and thyroid function studies of a slightly low FT_4 and slightly elevated TSH indicate the presence of a "true" hypothyroidism. The T_3 by RIA confirms this finding. Therefore, mild hypothyroidism in pregnancy is Mrs. Brown's most likely diagnosis.

E. Hyperemesis gravidarum with dehydration   INCORRECT

Although Mrs. Brown does have hyperemesis gravidarum, this is not her most likely diagnosis because her normal BUN, electrolytes, and urinalysis are inconsistent with dehydration.

5. Treatment Plan

A. Hospitalize for IV fluids   INCORRECT

Hospitalizing Mrs. Brown for IV fluids for dehydration is not necessary at this time because she is not currently dehydrated and can take some food and liquids by mouth at this time.

B. Observation and repeat thyroid studies in 1 month INCORRECT

In hypothyroidism in pregnancy, the TSH should be normalized as soon as possible because of the risk of adverse neuropsychological development of the unborn fetus. Repeating her level in 1 month might be appropriate to adjust her levothyroxine dosage (if necessary) to ensure she is euthyroid as soon as possible.

C. Advise that hyperemesis gravidarum is complicated by hypothyroidism and the timing of her pregnancy (at the end of the first semester) plus treating her hypothyroidism should alleviate her symptoms in the near future   CORRECT

Adequate patient education regarding her illness, its significance, why it is much more severe with this pregnancy, and the hope of its resolution in the near future frequently provides relief to the patient; knowing that the condition will be alleviated soon and that the fetus should not develop any adverse harm from her illness will provide tremendous psychological relief and have an impact on the eventual resolution of the symptoms.

D. Small frequent meals (at least six per day) with dry foods (e.g., crackers, toast) followed 1 hour later by clear liquids (e.g., juice, broth)   CORRECT

This is the treatment of choice for any nausea and vomiting of pregnancy of any severity. As symptoms improve, Mrs. Brown can advance her diet as tolerated.

E. Start propylthiouracil or methimazole   INCORRECT

Starting propylthiouracil or methimazole would be inappropriate because they are treatments for hyperthyroidism, not hypothyroidism as Mrs. Brown has. Utilizing either of these agents is likely to exacerbate her symptoms and the potential adverse effects to the fetus' nervous system.

Epidemiologic and Other Data

The incidence of maternal hypothyroidism in the United States is rare. However, it is frequently associated with adverse neurogenic problems in the unborn fetus. Therefore, it must be treated as soon as it is discovered to attempt to prevent these adverse fetal complications.

REFERENCES/ADDITIONAL READING

AACE Diabetes Mellitus Clinical Practice Guidelines Task Force. American Association of Clinical Endocrinologists medical guidelines for clinical practice for the management of diabetes mellitus. *Endocr Pract.* 2007;13(suppl 1):1–68.

The ACCORD Study Group. Effects of intensive blood-pressure control in type 2 diabetes mellitus. *N Engl J Med.* 2010; 362:1575–1585.

Agency for Healthcare Research and Quality. Quality of healthcare. In: Agency for Healthcare Research and Quality. AHRQ Publication No. 08-0041. Rockville, MD: US Department of Health and Human Services; 2007:31–96.

Aghababian RV (editor-in-chief). *Essentials of Emergency Medicine.* Sudbury, MA: Jones and Bartlett Publishers; 2006.

  Braen GR. Adrenal disease. 187–188.

  Edwards RJ. Nutritional disorders. 206–207.

  Johnson G. Thyroid disease. 215–216.

American Diabetes Association. Position statement: standards of medical care in diabetes. *Diabetes Care.* 2010;33(suppl 1): S11–S61.

American Diabetes Association. Position statement: standards of medical care in diabetes. *Diabetes Care.* 2005;28(suppl 1): S4–S36.

American Diabetes Association. Standards of medical care in diabetes. *Diabetes Care.* 2008;31(suppl 1):S12–S54.

Bolland MJ, Avenell A, Baron JA, Grey A, MacLennan GS, Gamble GD, Reid IR. Effect of calcium supplementation on risk of myocardial infarction and cardiovascular events: meta-analysis. *BMJ* 2010;341:c3691.

Burns A, Lawlor B, Craig S. Depression. In: Burns A, Lawlor B, Craig S. eds. *Assessment Scales in Old Age Psychiatry.* London: Martin Dunitz; 1999:1–16.

Chobanian AV, Bakris GL, Black HR, et al. The Seventh Report of the Joint National Committee on the Prevention, Detection, Evaluation, and Treatment of High Blood Pressure: the JNC 7 Report. *JAMA* 2003;289(19):2560–2572.

Eli Lilly and Company. *Cymbalta package insert.* Indianapolis, IN: Eli Lilly and Company; 2009. (Literature revised November 19): PV 6863.

Fauci AS, Kasper DL, Longo DL, Braunwald D, Hauser SL, Jameson JL, Loscalzo J (Eds). *Harrison's Principles of Internal Medicine,* 17th ed. New York: McGraw-Hill Medical; 2008.

  Barbieri RL, Reple JT. Medical disorders during pregnancy. 44–49.

  Hall JE. Menstrual disorders and pelvic pain. 304–307.

  Hall JE. The female reproductive system: infertility and contraception. 2324–2334.

  Jameson, JL, Weetman AP. Disorders of the thyroid gland. 2224–2247.

  Kushner RF. Evaluation and management of obesity. 468–473.

  Lindsay R, Cosman F. Osteoporosis. 2397–2408.

  Melmed S, Jameson JL. Disorders of the anterior pituitary and hypothalamus. 2195–2216.

  Potts Jr JT. Diseases of the parathyroid gland and other hyper- and hypocalcemic disorders. 2377–2396.

  Powers A. Diabetes mellitus. 2275–2304.

  Williams GH, Dluhy RG. Disorders of the adrenal cortex. 2247–2369.

Findling JW, Raff H. Cushing's syndrome: important issues in diagnosis and management. *J Clin Endocrinol Metab.* 2006;91(10):3746–3753.

Frances A (Chairperson) Task Force on DSM-IV. *Diagnostic and Statistical Manual of Mental Disorders. 4th ed. Text revision.* (DSM-IV-TR). Washington, DC: American Psychological Association; 2000.

  Frances A (Chairperson) Task Force on DSM-IV. Major depressive episode. 349–356.

  Frances A (Chairperson) Task Force on DSM-IV. Dysthymic disorder. 376–381.

Gersham K. Orthopedics/Rheumatology. 10.1 Osteoporosis. In: Gersham K (Onion DK, series ed.) *The Little Black Book of Geriatrics.* 3rd ed. Sudbury, MA: Jones & Bartlett Publishers; 2006:357–361.

Gonzales R, Kutner J. *Current Practice Guidelines in Primary Care.* New York: McGraw-Hill Medical; 2009.

  Gonzales R, Kutner J. Disease management: cholesterol and lipid management in adults. 133–134.

  Gonzales R, Kutner J. Disease management: diabetes mellitus. 142–146.

  Gonzales R, Kutner J. Disease management: obesity in adults. 153.

  Gonzales R, Kutner J. Disease management: osteoporosis. 156–157.

  Gonzales R, Kutner J. Disease screening: cancer, breast. 9–13.

  Gonzales R, Kutner J. Disease screening: diabetes mellitus, type 2. 51.

  Gonzales R, Kutner J. Disease screening: obesity. 72–75.

  Gonzales R, Kutner J. Disease screening: osteoporosis. 76–80.

Hariharan RR, Reed BC, Edmonson SR. Obesity. In: Mengel MB, Schwiebert LP, eds. *Family Medicine: Ambulatory Care and Prevention.* 5th ed. New York: McGraw-Hill Medical; 2009:565–575.

Nelson AL. Menstrual problems and common gynecologic concerns. In: Hatcher RA, Trussell J, Stewart F, et al. *Contraceptive Technology.* 17th ed. New York: Ardent Media; 1998:95–140.

Hodgson SF, Watts NB, Bilezikiam JP, et al.; AACE Osteoporosis Task Force. American Association of Clinical Endocrinologists medical guidelines for the clinical practice for the prevention and treatment of postmenopausal osteoporosis: 2001 ed with selected updates for 2003. *Endocr Pract.* 2003;9(6):544–654.

Jackson RD, LaCroix AZ, Gass M, et al. Women's Health Initiative Investigators. Calcium plus vitamin D supplementation and the risk of fractures. *N Engl J Med.* 2006; 354(7):669–683.

Kaufman A. Amenorrhea. In: Mengel MB, Schwiebert LP. *Family Medicine: Ambulatory Care and Prevention,* 5th ed. New York: McGraw Hill Medical; 2009:12–18.

Libè R, Barbetta L, Dall'Asta C, et al. Effects of dehydroepiandrosterone (DHEA) supplementation on hormonal, metabolic, and behavioral status in patients with hypoadrenalism. *J Endocrinol Invest.* 2004;27(8):736–741.

National Endocrine and Metabolic Diseases Information Service. *Hyperthyroidism*. NIH Publication No. 08-5414. Washington, DC: National Institutes of Health; 2008.

National Endocrine and Metabolic Diseases Information Service. *Hypothyroidism*. NIH Publication No. 08-6180. Washington, DC: National Institutes of Health; 2008.

National Endocrine and Metabolic Diseases Information Service. *Pregnancy and Thyroid Disease*. NIH Publication No. 08-6234. Washington, DC: National Institutes of Health; 2008.

National Osteoporosis Foundation. *Clinician's Guide to Prevention and Treatment of Osteoporosis*. Washington DC: National Osteoporosis Foundation; 2008.

Onion DK, series ed. *The Little Black Book of Primary Care*, 5th ed. Sudbury, MA: Jones and Bartlett; 2006.

    Onion DK. Endocrine/metabolism. 5.1 Adrenal disorders. 247–254.

    Onion DK. Endocrine/Metabolism. 5.5 Parathyroid/calcium/magnesium disorders. 286–293.

    Onion DK. Endocrine/Metabolism. 5.7 Thyroid disease. 302–314.

    Onion DK, Gershman K. Geriatrics. 7.1 Osteoporosis. 411–415.

    Onion DK, DeJong R. Obstetrics/Gynecology. 11.4 Pregnancy-related conditions. 810–815.

    Onion DK, DeJong R. Obstetrics/Gynecology. 11.5 Miscellaneous. 831–849.

    Onion DK. Psychiatry. 15.2 Psychiatric diseases. 949–964.

Pagana KD, Pagana TJ. *Mosby's Diagnostic and Laboratory Test Reference*. 8th ed. St. Louis: Mosby Elsevier; 2007 (multiple pages utilized to provide normal reference values for laboratory tests).

The RECORD Trial Group. Oral vitamin D_3 and calcium for secondary prevention of low-trauma fractures in elderly people (Randomized Evaluation of Calcium OR vitamin D, RECORD): a randomized placebo-controlled trial. *Lancet*. 2005;365(9471):1621–1628.

U.S. Department of Health and Human Services. Agency for Healthcare Research and Quality. Quality of health care. In: Agency for Healthcare Research and Quality. National Healthcare Disparities Report 2007 (AHRQ Publication No. 08-0041). Rockville, MD: U.S. Department of Health and Human Services. Agency for Healthcare Research and Quality 2007:31–96.

Vikanes Å, Skjærven R, Grjibovski AM, Gunnes N, Vangen S, Magnus P. Recurrence of hyperemesis gravidarum across generations: population-based cohort study. *BMJ*. 2010; 340:c2050 (DOI: 10.1136/bmj.c2050).

CHAPTER 4

CASES IN EYE, EAR, NOSE, AND THROAT DISORDERS*

CASE 4-1

Brittney Crookshanks

Brittney is a 4-year-old white female who is brought in by her mother with the chief complaint of a "left earache and fever." Her symptoms began when she awoke yesterday morning. Her mother used an over-the-counter (OTC) topical ear pain solution (the name of which she doesn't remember) without much relief. The pain has increased tremendously since its onset, especially if her mother lays her down. It appears to be alleviated significantly when her mother holds Brittney upright with her left ear pressed against her mother's chest. Her mother has been up all night holding her in this position. Brittney also has a mild clear to yellowish rhinorrhea.

Her only medication is the aforementioned OTC topical ear pain solution. She is not taking any other OTC or prescription medications, vitamins, supplements, or herbal preparations. She is not allergic to any medications.

She has no known medical problems except frequent episodes of otitis media starting at the age of 6 months. Her mother cannot accurately estimate the total number of lifetime episodes. Her last episode was 3 to 4 months ago. She has never been hospitalized nor had any surgery. She has regular well-child check-ups and her immunizations are up to date. Her family's medical history is noncontributory. Her father smokes in the house, including the same room as Brittney, but always opens the window to "let the smoke out." She attends day care.

1. Based on this information, which of the following questions are essential to ask Brittney's mother and why?

   A. How high has her fever been and how was it checked?
   B. Is she eating or drinking anything?
   C. How long has she had the rhinorrhea?

   D. Does she have any eye discharge, sore throat, nasal congestion, cough, wheezing, headache, stiff/sore neck, nausea, vomiting, diarrhea, constipation, other bowel changes, abdominal pain, decreased urination, or decreased tearing?
   E. Was Brittney breast- or bottle-fed?

Patient Responses

Her highest temperature was 102.6°F with an ear thermometer in her right ear (contralateral to her symptomatic ear) at about 6:00 a.m. this morning. Her mother has been able to get Brittney to eat a few bites of ice pops and drink a little apple juice; otherwise, she has not consumed anything since becoming ill.

Her rhinorrhea started yesterday at about the same time as her otalgia. According to her mother, Brittney has not experienced any eye discharge, sore throat, nasal congestion, cough, wheezing, headache, stiff/sore neck, nausea, vomiting, diarrhea, constipation, other bowel changes, abdominal pain, decreased urination, or decreased tearing.

She was breast-fed for the first 6 months of her life.

2. Based on this information, which of the following components of a physical examination are essential to conduct on Brittney and why?

   A. Eye examination
   B. Ear examination
   C. Nose, oral mucosa, and throat examination
   D. Neck examination
   E. Lung auscultation

Physical Examination Findings

Brittney is 36" tall and weighs 32 lb. Other vital signs are blood pressure (BP), 88/54 mm Hg; pulse, 110 beats per

---

*Remember, for each question, none to all of the answers could be correct/essential or incorrect/nonessential. See page 141 for Chapter 4 answers.

minute (BPM) and regular; respiratory rate, 24/min and regular; and rectal temperature, 103.8°F.

Her ear canals are nonedematous, normal in color, without abnormal debris, and nontender to manipulation. Her left tympanic membrane (TM) is erythematous, is bulging, and appears to have fluid behind it. Her right TM is slightly injected, with normal landmarks and no evidence of effusion.

Brittney's nasal mucosa is slightly erythematous and edematous with clear discharge, bilaterally. Her pharynx is slightly injected; tonsils are slightly enlarged, but no exudates are present. Her oral mucosa is moist and normal in color. There are no petechiae on her palate.

Her neck is supple with full range of motion and without pain. Her anterior and posterior cervical lymph nodes are moderately enlarged and slightly tender, bilaterally. Her preauricular lymph nodes are slightly enlarged and tender on the left. They are unaffected on the right.

Her lungs are clear to auscultation.

3. Based on this information, which of the following diagnostic studies are essential to perform on Brittney and why?

    A. Blood urea nitrogen (BUN)
    B. Electrolytes
    C. Complete blood count with differential (CBC w/diff)
    D. Pneumatic otoscopy
    E. Audiogram

Diagnostic Results

Brittney's BUN was 8 mg/dl (normal child: 5–18), her electrolytes were normal, and her CBC was normal except for a mild lymphocytosis with a mild leukocytosis with a rare band.

Her pneumatic otoscopy was normal on the right but revealed no mobility on the left. Her audiogram revealed a mild to moderate conductive hearing loss on the left.

4. Based on this information, which one of the following is Brittney's most likely diagnosis and why?

    A. Left serous otitis media (SOM, left)
    B. Acute left otitis media (AOM, left)
    C. Chronic left otitis media (COM, left)
    D. Viral upper respiratory tract infection (URI)
    E. Fever of unknown origin (FUO)

5. Based on this diagnosis, which of the following are appropriate components of a treatment plan for Brittney and why?

    A. Acetaminophen or ibuprofen for fever and pain
    B. Observation for 48 to 72 hours before instituting antibiotics
    C. Amoxicillin 40 to 45 mg/kg twice a day for 5 days
    D. Refer for tympanostomy tubes
    E. Amoxicillin/clavulanate 40 to 45 mg/kg twice a day for 10 days
    F. Encourage her father to quit smoking (if unable or unwilling, he needs to go outside to smoke) and explain the adverse effects of passive smoke exposure, including an increased incidence of acute otitis media for Brittney

CASE 4-2
Charlene Dawson

Ms. Dawson is a 27-year-old African American female who presents with the chief complaint of "My ear infection is messing up my face." Her illness began approximately 1 month ago with a sensation of fullness in her right ear accompanied by a malodorous yellowish discharge. She was diagnosed with otitis externa and started on colistin, neomycin, hydrocortisone, and thonzonium otic suspension. Her symptoms decreased slightly during the first few days of therapy but then worsened. At that time, she was changed to ciprofloxacin and hydrocortisone otic suspension. Again, her symptoms appeared to improve slightly during the first couple of days of therapy but then worsened. Because of her failure to respond to two different topical antibiotics, she was started on oral fluconazole for a probable fungal otitis externa. Again, upon starting the medication, her symptoms appeared to be decreasing, but they increased again a few days later. At that time, her fluconazole was increased to twice a day.

At her visit today, Ms. Dawson is complaining that her right ear pain is "worse than it has ever been" (rating of 8 out of 10 on the pain scale) and describes it as a very deep, throbbing ache. Furthermore, her ear discharge is getting more malodorous and copious. She began experiencing dizziness and a fever (maximum 101.2°F, orally) with chills 2 days ago. On awakening this morning, she stated that it felt "like my face is being pulled to my ear" and "isn't working right." She has not experienced any nasal congestion, rhinorrhea, postnasal discharge, sore throat, sneezing, cough, oral lesions, facial lesions, or left ear symptoms. She denies trauma of any type.

Her only known medical problem is type 1 diabetes mellitus of 15 years' duration. She has not had any surgeries nor been hospitalized. Her medications include NPH insulin 25 units in the morning and 10 units at dinner and fluconazole 150 mg twice a day. She is not on any other prescription or over-the-counter medications, vitamins, supplements, or herbal preparations. She does not drink alcohol, use illicit substances, or smoke. Her last menstrual period was 2 weeks ago and normal. She is not sexually active. Her family history is noncontributory.

1. Based on this information, which of the following are essential to ask Ms. Dawson and why?

    A. How does she describe her "dizziness"?
    B. Does she have a dry mouth, decreased salivation, or decreased tearing?
    C. Is she experiencing decreased moods, crying episodes, or anhedonia?
    D. What does she mean by the statement her face "isn't working right"?
    E. Has she experienced headaches, visual changes, photophobia, phonophobia, abnormalities of taste, dysphagia, weakness or problems using her extremities, or other neurologic deficits?

Patient Responses

Ms. Dawson has been having brief (< 1 minute) episodes of subjective vertigo, three to four times per day, for 2 to 3 days. They are associated with moving her head quickly; however, they are not associated with any new or changed auditory symptoms.

She has not noticed any decrease in salivation and/or tearing; however, her right eye feels a little itchy and "dryer" than usual. She does not have any ocular discharge.

She describes "isn't working right" as not being able to "move the lower right part of my face and mouth like I should." She has not attempted to eat since its onset and is uncertain if she can chew properly. She denies any numbness, dysesthesias, or paresthesias. She has not had headaches, visual changes, photophobia, phonophobia, abnormalities of taste, dysphagia, problems using her extremities, weakness of her extremities, other neurologic deficits, decreased moods, crying episodes, or anhedonia.

2. Based on this information, which of the following components of a physical examination are essential to conduct on Ms. Dawson and why?

    A. Ear examination
    B. Mastoid and temporomandibular joint (TMJ) examination
    C. Skin examination
    D. Cranial nerve examination
    E. Carotid pulse

Physical Examination Findings

Ms. Dawson is 5"6" tall and weighs 135 lb (body mass index [BMI] = 21.8). Other vital signs are BP, 120/76 mm Hg; pulse, 92 BPM and regular; respirations, 12/min and regular; and temperature, 102.4°F.

Her left ear examination is completely normal. However, her right ear examination reveals an auricle that is mildly to moderately erythematous, mildly edematous, slightly warm to touch, and mildly to moderately tender to palpate. Pressing on the tragus and pulling the pinna produces excruciating pain. The auditory canal is markedly edematous, erythematous, and tender with a question of early granulation tissue in the base. It is occluded with a very malodorous, purulent, yellowish discharge.

She has moderately enlarged and tender preauricular lymph nodes on the right. Her anterior and posterior cervical lymph nodes are moderately enlarged and tender to palpate on the right side of her neck. Her contralateral nodes are normal.

Her TMJ is slightly tender to palpate on the right side only, but revealed full range of motion without any abnormal sounds or crepitus. The associated skin is not swollen, edematous, warm to the touch, or with lesions. Her right mastoid bone is mildly tender to palpate. The skin over it appears to be slightly erythematous, slightly edematous, and warm to the touch. It does not reveal any lesions, scaling, plaquing, scarring, excoriations, or other abnormalities.

Her cranial nerves are intact including the ability to wrinkle her forehead and raise her eyebrows. The only abnormalities noted are a slight weakness when trying to hold her right eye closed, the inability to "puff out" and hold her right cheek, decreased frowning on the right, mouth pulled to the left with smiling, and a slightly flat nasolabial fold on the right.

Her carotid pulse is 90 BPM and regular.

3. Based on this information, which of the following diagnostic studies are essential to perform on Ms. Dawson and why?

    A. Remove debris from canal with small catheter and suction; then, obtain small biopsy of granulated inferior canal for culture and sensitivity
    B. Remove debris from canal with warm water irrigation and send sample for culture and sensitivity
    C. Random plasma glucose (RPG)
    D. Complete blood count with differential (CBC w/diff)
    E. Computed tomography (CT) or magnetic resonance imaging (MRI) of her right mastoid/ear area

Diagnostic Results

After removing a significant amount of debris from the canal, the tympanic membrane could be visualized and verified as intact, normal in color, and nonbulging. Her inferior canal revealed some granulation of the skin. Other than erythema and edema of the ear canal, no other skin lesions/abnormalities were noted. A biopsy was performed and sent for culture and sensitivity. It is pending.

Her imaging study revealed osteomyelitis of the floor of the right middle ear canal, the right middle fossa, and the right temporal bone, including the right mastoid bone.

Her CBC w/diff revealed a red blood cell (RBC) count of $5.1 \times 10^6/\mu l$ (normal female: 4.2–5.4) with a mean corpuscular volume (MCV) of 83 μm^3 (normal adult: 80–95), a mean corpuscular hemoglobin (MCH) of 30 pg (normal adult: 27–31), a mean corpuscular hemoglobin concentration (MCHC) of 33 g/dl (normal adult: 32–36), and a red blood cell distribution width (RDW) of 12% (normal adult: 11–14.5). Her white blood cell (WBC) count was 25,750/mm³ (normal adult: 5000–10,000) with 80% neutrophils (normal: 55–70), 10% lymphocytes (normal: 20–40), 6% monocytes (normal: 2–8), 3% eosinophils (normal: 1–4), and 1% basophils (normal: 0.5–1). Her hemoglobin (Hgb) was 12.5 g/dl (normal female: 12–16) and her hematocrit (HCT) was 39% (normal female: 37–47). Her platelet (thrombocyte) count was 220,000/mm³ (normal adult: 150,000–400,000) and her mean platelet volume (MPV) was 7.6 fl (normal: 7.4–10.4). Her smear was consistent with this and revealed no cellular abnormalities except for a few bands. Her RPG was 397 mg/dl (normal: < 200).

4. Based on this information, which one of the following is Ms. Dawson's most likely diagnosis and why?

    A. Acute otitis externa (AOE), right
    B. Chronic otitis externa (COE), right
    C. Malignant (or necrotizing) otitis externa, right
    D. Mastoiditis, right
    E. Bell palsy, right

5. Based on this information, which of the following are appropriate components of Ms. Dawson's treatment plan and why?

    A. Hospitalization
    B. Intravenous piperacillin and gentamicin
    C. Topical antipseudomonal antibiotics
    D. Otolaryngologist referral
    E. Outpatient treatment with oral ofloxacin

CASE 4-3

David Estevez

Mr. Estevez is a 26-year-old Hispanic American male who presents with the chief complaint of rhinorrhea. It is clear in color and "watery" in consistency. It has been present for several years; however, it is very intermittent in nature. He can be asymptomatic for several days and then experience single or multiple distinct episodes of rhinorrhea over the course of a day to several days. Over the years, he has tried multiple OTC sprays, pills, and capsules, including diphenhydramine and loratadine, without any significant symptom relief. He presents today to get something "stronger" because his symptoms appear to be occurring more frequently.

His rhinorrhea is occasionally associated with sneezing, nasal pruritus, and itchy, watery eyes. It is intermittently followed by nasal congestion. He does not have fever, purulent eye discharge, eye edema, cough, wheezing, chest tightness, dyspnea, eczema, atopic skin changes, hives, generalized pruritus, edema, nausea, vomiting, pyrosis, or bowel changes.

He has no known medical problems, has never had surgery, and has never been hospitalized. Currently he is not taking any prescription medications, OTC medications, vitamins, supplements, or herbal preparations. He is not allergic to any medications. He has never smoked. His family history is negative, including atopic/allergic disease(s) and asthma.

1. Based on this information, which of the following questions are essential to ask Mr. Estevez and why?

    A. Do his symptoms occur seasonally or year round?
    B. Are there any aggravating factors?
    C. Is he experiencing fatigue, weight gain, or changes in his skin, hair, or nails?
    D. Does he have any tattoos?
    E. Does he drink alcohol or use any drugs/substance of abuse?

Patient Responses

Mr. Estevez's symptoms occur year round. He notices that they are more prevalent when he is eating something very spicy. They also tend to occur if he is around any "strong smells" (e.g., cigar smoke or certain perfumes) or where the ambient temperature is "really cold."

He is not experiencing fatigue, weight gain, or changes in his skin, hair, or nails. He denies having a tattoo, drinking alcohol, or using/abusing illicit substances/drugs.

2. Based on this information, which of the following components of a physical examination are essential to conduct on Mr. Estevez and why?

    A. Eye examination
    B. Ear, mouth, and pharyngeal examination
    C. Nasal examination
    D. Abdominal examination
    E. Skin examination

Physical Examination Findings

Mr. Estevez is 5'7" tall and weighs 156 lb (BMI = 24.4). Other vital signs are BP, 120/76 mm Hg; pulse, 88 BPM and regular; respiratory rate, 12/min and regular; and oral temperature, 98.5°F.

His conjunctivae and sclerae are normal in color, noninjected, and without sicca or discharge. His nasolacrimal ducts are nontender, nonerythematous, nonedematous, and without discharge. His pupils are equal (and normal) in size, are round, and react to light and accommodation.

His auditory canals are normal color and without edema, abnormal debris, or lesions. His tympanic membranes are normal in color/thickness, nonretracted, fully mobile, and without lesions/perforations. His pharynx is normal color, is slightly injected, and reveals no postnasal discharge. His oral mucosa, palate, gums, tongue, and lips are normal color and without lesions.

His nasal mucosa is moderately pale and slightly boggy but without any discharge, lesions, or septal perforation. There is no evidence of a nasopharyngeal structural abnormality. The visible portions of his turbinates are also pale and boggy and without discharge or lesions.

His abdominal examination is unremarkable. He has no skin lesions, color changes, temperature changes, or other dermal abnormalities.

3. Based on this information, which of the following diagnostic studies are essential to perform on Mr. Estevez and why?

    A. Skin testing for allergens
    B. Serum immunoglobulin E (IgE) level
    C. Complete blood count with differential (CBC w/diff)
    D. Urine drug screen
    E. Erythrocyte sedimentation rate (ESR)

Diagnostic Results

His skin testing revealed a mild reaction to grasses and trees. His IgE level was minimal (normal: minimal). His CBC w/diff was within normal limits. His urine drug screen was negative. His ESR was 2 mm/hr (normal male: < 10).

4. Based on this information, which one of the following is Mr. Estevez's most likely diagnosis and why?

    A. Seasonal allergic rhinitis
    B. Perennial allergic rhinitis
    C. Vasomotor rhinitis
    D. Food allergy
    E. Rhinitis medicamentosa

5. Based on this diagnosis, which of the following are appropriate components of a treatment plan for Mr. Estevez and why?

    A. Avoid environmental triggers as much as possible
    B. Intranasal corticosteroid
    C. Immunotherapy for trees and grasses
    D. Additional testing for specific food allergies and start immunotherapy if identified
    E. Montelukast

CASE 4-4

Ethan Frazer

Ethan is a 4-year-old white male who presents with his mother for the chief complaint of a "nasty cold" of approximately

2 weeks' duration. It began as a clear, intermittent rhinorrhea from his right nostril only. Since then, the discharge has become more malodorous, purulent, yellowish in color, and occasionally streaked with blood. His left nostril was asymptomatic until a few days ago when he began experiencing an unchanged, intermittent clear discharge from it.

His mother tried diphenhydramine at the onset of his symptoms. However, after 3 days of regular use, his symptoms were unchanged, so she discontinued it. Other than running a cool mist humidifier, which normally provides him significant relief when he is experiencing a viral upper respiratory tract infection, she has not tried any other treatments. The humidifier is not helping. She is unaware of any aggravating or alleviating factors or a history of trauma.

He has not experienced a fever, nasal congestion, sore throat, earache, coughing, wheezing, sneezing, facial edema, facial erythema, rash, nausea, vomiting, bowel changes, abdominal pain, pruritic eyes, or ocular discharge.

He has no known medical problems. He has never had surgery nor been hospitalized. Currently, he is not taking any prescription or over-the-counter medications, vitamins, supplements, or herbal preparations. He is not allergic to any medications. He is up to date on his age appropriate health check-ups (which are reported as normal by his mother) and his immunizations. His family history is negative, including for allergic/atopic conditions.

1. Based on this information, which of the following questions are essential to ask Ethan and his mother and why?

    A. Has he complained of (or appeared to have) nasal pain or a frontal headache?
    B. Does he get frequent upper respiratory tract infections or have any structural abnormality of his upper respiratory tract?
    C. Does he "pick" his nose?
    D. Has he placed a foreign body in his nose?
    E. Does he attend day care?

Patient Responses

Ethan has not complained of (nor does his mother suspect) that he has nasal pain, facial pain, or a headache. He does get frequent "colds" but has only had one episode of otitis media. As near as his mother knows, Ethan does not have any structural abnormality of his upper respiratory tract.

Ethan and his mother deny that he digitally manipulates his nose. Ethan denies placing any object in his nose. His mother is unaware of him doing such. He attends day care 2 days a week.

2. Based on this information, which of the following components of a physical examination are essential to conduct on Ethan and why?

    A. Ear examination
    B. Nasal examination
    C. Pharyngeal and oral mucosa examination
    D. Abdominal examination
    E. Hand and foot examination

Physical Examination Findings

Ethan is 38" tall and weighs 38 lb. Other vital signs are BP, 90/54 mm Hg; pulse, 112 BPM and regular; respiratory rate, 22/min and regular; and tympanic temperature, 98.6°F.

His ear canals and tympanic membranes are normal. His left nasal mucosa is normal in color, nonedematous, and without discharge. His right nasal mucosa is erythematous, edematous, and with copious amounts of malodorous, yellowish discharge. Additionally, toward the proximal end of the nasal cavity, he has an irregularly shaped bluish object. His pharynx and oral mucosa are normal in color and without lesions.

His abdominal examination is unremarkable, as is his hand and foot examination.

3. Based on this information, which of the following diagnostic studies are essential to perform on Ethan and why?

    A. Plain film radiographs of nasal area
    B. Magnetic resonance imaging (MRI) of nasal/sinus area
    C. Diagnostic nasal endoscopy
    D. Complete blood count with differential (CBC w/diff)
    E. Prothrombin time (PT) and partial thromboplastin time (PTT)

Diagnostic Findings

Plain film radiographs were negative. MRI and nasal endoscopy couldn't be performed because of Ethan's inability to remain still. They have been rescheduled with preprocedural sedation.

CBC w/diff was within normal limits. His PT was 11.5 seconds (normal: 11–12.5) and his PTT was 62 seconds (normal: 60–70).

4. Based on this information, which one of the following is Ethan's most likely diagnosis and why?

    A. Rhinosinusitis
    B. Nasal polyp, right nostril
    C. Foreign body, right nostril
    D. Anterior epistaxis, right side
    E. Allergic rhinitis

5. Based on this diagnosis, which of the following are appropriate components of a treatment plan for Ethan and why?

    A. Have his mother hold his left nostril closed and have Ethan forcefully blow his nose
    B. Diphenhydramine as needed
    C. Right nasal irrigation
    D. Provide procedural sedation (or, if not available, restrain Ethan and insert topical anesthetic and vasoconstrictor) and remove the foreign body with nasal snares or forceps
    E. Refer to otorhinolaryngologist

CASE 4-5

Fred Goodwin

Mr. Goodwin is a 75-year-old white male who presents with the chief complaint of "pus coming out of my eye." According to Mr. Goodwin, he felt fine until approximately 3 days ago when he awoke with the medial corner of his left eye being slightly erythematous, edematous, and tender to touch. It was accompanied by epiphora. He assumed it was a sty and attempted to treat it with a warm, moist tea bag with minimal relief.

When he awoke this morning, the area was more erythematous, edematous, and tender (even without touch). This was accompanied not only by the increased tearing but also a yellowish-green purulent discharge and conjunctival injection. He has never experienced similar symptoms.

He does not have rhinorrhea, nasal congestion, sinus pressure/fullness, headache, otalgia, sore throat, postnasal drainage, cough, wheezing, dyspnea, lightheadedness, vertigo, presyncope, syncope, nausea, vomiting, bowel changes, abdominal pain, chills, or malaise.

His only medical problem is presbyopia, which is corrected with reading glasses. He has never had any surgery nor been hospitalized. His only medication is a multivitamin with minerals for men over the age of 65 years. He takes no other prescription or OTC medications, vitamins or minerals, supplements, or herbal preparations. He is not allergic to any medications. He does not drink and has never smoked. He has regular age-appropriate examinations and his immunizations are up to date. His family history is noncontributory.

1. Based on this information, which of the following questions are essential to ask of Mr. Goodwin and why?

    A. Was there a history of eye trauma before the onset of symptoms?
    B. Has he had any dysuria, urinary frequency, penile discharge, arthralgias, or mucocutaneous lesions?
    C. Does he have any abnormalities of vision?
    D. Does he have a fever?
    E. Does he wear contact lenses? If yes, what type?

Patient Responses

Mr. Goodwin denies eye and facial trauma, fever, dysuria, urinary frequency, penile discharge, arthralgias, mucocutaneous lesions, or visual abnormalities. He does not wear contact lenses.

2. Based on this information, which of the following components of a physical examination are essential to conduct on Mr. Goodwin and why?

    A. Bilateral visual acuity
    B. Bilateral eye examination
    C. Nasal examination
    D. Carotid examination for bruit
    E. Heart auscultation

Physical Examination Findings

Mr. Goodwin is 5'11" tall and weighs 170 lb (BMI = 24.4). Other vital signs are BP, 132/76 mm Hg; pulse, 82 BPM and regular; respiratory rate, 12/min and regular; and oral temperature, 98.4°F.

His far vision is 20/20, bilaterally. His near vision is 20/20 in his left eye and 20/25 in his right eye with his corrective lenses. His external ocular examination reveals a normal right eye. His left eye reveals a mildly to moderately erythematous,

edematous, tender medial canthus with a thick, yellowish-greenish discharge being expelled from his lacrimal gland upon palpation. The remainder of his upper and lower eyelids is normal. He has marked epiphora from the left eye and rarely from the right. His right eye reveals a normal-colored, noninjected conjunctivae and sclera. His left eye appears the same except for some extremely mild conjunctival injection in the medial aspect. Visual fields are grossly normal and equal bilaterally. Extraocular muscles are intact (EOMI) bilaterally. Pupils are equal, are round, and react to light and accommodation without pain. Except for some mild cataract formation, his funduscopic examination is normal bilaterally.

His nasal mucosa is normal in color, nonedematous, and without lesions, bilaterally.

His carotid arteries are normal and equal bilaterally without bruits. His heart is regular in rate and rhythm and does not reveal any murmurs, gallops, or rubs. His apical impulse is normal.

3. Based on this information, which of the following diagnostic studies are essential to perform on Mr. Goodwin and why?

    A. Left orbit radiographs
    B. Culture and sensitivity of purulent lacrimal duct discharge
    C. White blood cell count with differential (WBC w/diff)
    D. Magnetic resonance imaging (MRI) of left orbit
    E. Potassium hydroxide (KOH) preparation of discharge

Diagnostic Findings

His left orbit radiographs, MRI of the left orbit, and WBC w/diff were normal. His Gram stain revealed gram-positive cocci that divide in greater than one plane forming irregular clusters. His KOH prep was negative. His culture and sensitivity are pending.

4. Based on this information, which one of the following is Mr. Goodwin's most likely diagnosis and why?

    A. Conjunctivitis, left eye
    B. Hordeolum, left eye
    C. Acute dacryoadenitis, left eye
    D. Acute dacryocystitis, left eye
    E. Anterior blepharitis, left eye

5. Based on this diagnosis, which of the following are appropriate components of a treatment plan for Mr. Goodwin and why?

    A. Doxycycline 100 mg twice a day
    B. Amoxicillin 500 mg three times a day
    C. Hospitalization for vancomycin 1 g IV every 12 hours
    D. Warm water compresses for 20 minutes four times a day
    E. Referral to ophthalmologist for possible dacryocystorhinostomy or balloon dilation of nasolacrimal system

CASE 4-6
Gloria Harris

Ms. Harris is an 18-year-old African American female who presents with the chief complaint of "an allergy to my antibiotic." She began ampicillin after visiting the emergency department

(ED) 3 days ago for a sore throat and fever, which was diagnosed clinically as "strep throat." Her "allergy" consists of a rash that was present when she awoke this morning. Initially, it was only on her chest and back; however, it has rapidly spread to involve her entire body (expect for her genitalia). It was light pink in color initially; however, as the day progressed it became "brighter." She now describes it as a "flat, pinkish-red rash." It is not pruritic.

She continues with the low-grade fever (highest 99.2°F) and sore throat. Her throat is much more painful than it was at the ED and is now associated with dysphagia. She denies rhinorrhea; nasal congestion; sneezing; itchy, watery eyes; headache; earache; cough; wheezing; dyspnea; chest pain or discomfort; nausea; vomiting; bowel changes; abdominal pain; or chills.

Ms. Harris has no known medical problems. She has never had any surgery nor been hospitalized. Her current medication consists of ampicillin 500 mg four times per day. She is not taking any other prescription or over-the-counter medications, vitamins, supplements, or herbal preparations. She has no known drug allergies, except for possibly amoxicillin. She does not drink alcohol or use drugs. She has never smoked. Her last menstrual period began 2 weeks ago and was normal. She has never been sexually active. Her family history is negative.

She is also requesting a medical release to resume playing soccer on her college's women's team. Apparently, when her coach discovered Ms. Harris had streptococcal pharyngitis, she "benched" her until she obtains medical clearance from an HCP.

1. Based on this information, which of the following questions are essential to ask Ms. Harris and why?

   A. Is she experiencing any malaise, fatigue, anorexia, myalgias, or arthralgias?
   B. Is she aware of anyone else with similar symptoms? If yes, who?
   C. Has she noticed any icterus or jaundice?
   D. What is her contraceptive method?
   E. Are her immunizations up to date?

Patient Responses

Ms. Harris has been experiencing extreme fatigue, an increased need for sleep, and slight anorexia since her sore throat began. She denies true malaise, myalgias, arthralgias, icterus, or jaundice.

Two of her friends on the soccer team began experiencing sore throat, low-grade fever, and severe fatigue yesterday. Her immunizations are up to date.

She does not require contraception because she is not sexually active.

2. Based on this information, which of the following components of a physical examination are essential to conduct on Ms. Harris and why?

   A. Ears, nose, oral mucosa, and throat examination
   B. Neck examination
   C. Heart and lung examination
   D. Abdominal examination
   E. Skin examination

Physical Examination Findings

Ms. Harris is 5'5" tall and weighs 120 lb (BMI = 20.0). Other vital signs are BP, 104/62 mm Hg; pulse, 72 BPM and regular; respirations, 12/min and regular; and oral temperature, 98.9°F.

Her auditory canals are normal in color, nonedematous, and without lesions or abnormal discharge, bilaterally. Her tympanic membranes are intact, nonerythematous, slightly injected, freely mobile, and without any evidence of a middle ear effusion or mass, bilaterally. Her nasal mucosa is normal color and without edema, lesions, or discharge, bilaterally.

Her pharynx is erythematous with marked tonsillar enlargement that is equal bilaterally and coated with whitish exudates. No masses are evident. The uvula is midline. She has petechiae on her soft palate. No other abnormalities are present.

She has full range of motion of her neck without pain. Her anterior and posterior cervical lymph nodes are markedly enlarged and tender, but equal bilaterally. Her thyroid is not enlarged, nontender, and without masses.

Ms. Harris's heart is regular in rate and rhythm and without murmurs, gallops, or rubs. Her apical impulse is nondisplaced and without a thrill. Her lungs are clear to auscultation.

Her abdomen reveals normoactive, equal bowel sounds in all four quadrants and no tenderness. She does not have any evidence of hepatomegaly; however, her spleen is enlarged and palpable approximately 3 cm below her costal margin, but it is nontender to palpation. There is dullness to percussion over the 11th intercostal space in the anterior axillary line; it remained with deep inspiration. Her uterus and kidneys are not palpable. Her aorta is nondisplaced and normal in caliber. She does not have aortic or renal bruits.

Her skin reveals a generalized, fine (1- to 2-mm), maculopapular, medium to dark pink rash that even involves the palms of her hands and soles of her feet. The only part of her body spared is her genitalia. The lesions do not blanch with diascopy. There is no temperature change, edema, underlying erythema, jaundice, or other significant abnormalities.

3. Based on this information, which of the following diagnostic studies are essential to perform on Ms. Harris and why?

   A. Rapid plasma reagin test (RPR)
   B. Ebstein Barr virus (EBV) antibody titer
   C. Complete blood count with differential (CBC w/diff)
   D. Rapid immunologic test for group A *Streptococcus* (strep screen)
   E. Ultrasound of abdomen with emphasis on spleen

Diagnostic Test Results

Ms. Harris's RPR was 1:64 (normal: < 1:4). Her monospot was 1:256 (normal: < 1:28). Her strep screen was negative.

Ms. Harris's CBC with differential revealed an RBC count of 5.0 × 10⁶/µl (normal female: 4.2–5.4) with an MCV of 88 µm³ (normal adult: 80–95), an MCH of 29 pg (normal adult: 27–31), an MCHC of 35 g/dl (normal adult: 32–36), and an RDW of 11% (normal adult: 11–14.5). Her WBC count was 4500/mm³ (normal adult: 5000–10,000) with 20% neutrophils (normal: 55–70), 70% lymphocytes (normal: 20–40), 3% monocytes (normal: 2–8), 1% eosinophils (normal: 1–4), and 1% basophils (normal: 0.5–1). Her Hgb was 14.5 g/dl (normal female: 12–16) and her HCT was 42% (normal female: 37–47). Her platelet (thrombocyte) count was 200,000/mm³ (normal adult: 150,000–400,000) and her MPV was 7.6 fl (normal: 7.4–10.4). Her smear was consistent with this and revealed approximately 10% atypical lymphocytes (larger, darker, and with vacuolated nuclei).

Her abdominal ultrasound revealed splenomegaly with the cephalocaudal diameter of the spleen measured at 16 cm (normal maximum: 13 cm). No other abnormalities were present.

4. Based on this information, which one of the following is Ms. Harris's most likely diagnosis and why?

    A. Syphilis
    B. Infectious mononucleosis (IM)
    C. Group A β-hemolytic streptococcal (strep) pharyngitis
    D. Allergic drug reaction to ampicillin
    E. Acute lymphocytic leukemia (ALL)

5. Based on this diagnosis, which of the following are appropriate components of a treatment plan for Ms. Harris and why?

    A. Fluorescent treponemal antibody test (FTA-ABS)
    B. Erythromycin 250 mg every 6 hours × 10 days
    C. Cefprozil 500 mg once daily × 10 days
    D. Rest, fluids, and acetaminophen
    E. Sign release for soccer

CASE 4-7

Hannah Issenburg

Hannah is a 14-month-old white female who is brought to the ED by her mother and father with the chief complaint of "a high fever." According to her mother, Hannah's fever has been as high as 102.8°F (by tympanic thermometer) and present for 3 days. She is also experiencing sore throat, nasal congestion, and mild rhinorrhea of 3 days' duration. Her mother's main concern is that Hannah awoke this morning "acting like she has a stiff neck and headache." A little later in the day, Hannah also started with anorexia and intermittent drooling, which her mother attributed to dysphagia from her sore throat. The only thing she has consumed today was "a little" apple juice.

Since becoming ill, she has been "fussy," more "needy," and not sleeping as well; still, her mother is able to comfort and console her. According to her mother, Hannah has not had chills, seizures, vomiting, diarrhea, constipation, other stool change, abdominal pain, cough, wheezing, stridor, or dyspnea. She is the product of a full term, uncomplicated pregnancy with a normal vaginal delivery and postpartum period. She has no known medical problems, never been hospitalized, nor had surgery. Her only medication is acetaminophen every 4 to 6 hours, which has been effective in reducing her temperature, and a daily multivitamin. She is on no other over-the-counter or prescription medications, vitamins, supplements, or herbal preparations. She has regular well-child

check-ups that have thus far been normal. Her immunizations are up to date. Her family history is noncontributory. She does not attend day care.

1. Based on this information, which of the following questions are essential to ask Hannah's parents and why?

    A. Is she urinating normally and crying tears?
    B. Does her voice sound "muffled" or abnormal to either of her parents?
    C. How much iron is in her multivitamin?
    D. Has she had head or neck trauma, including sleeping in an awkward position?
    E. Does she appear to have any photophobia; difficulty with her vision, coordination, gait, or extremity usage; or abnormalities of her regular speech?

Patient Responses

According to her mother, Hannah is urinating normally and crying tears when "fussy" or uncomfortable. Neither of her parents has noticed any change in her voice/speech, photophobia, difficulty with vision, coordination problems, changes in gait, or problems with use of an extremity. Her mother does not know how much iron is in her multivitamins. There is no history of trauma.

2. Based on this information, which of the following components of a physical examination are essential to conduct on Hannah and why?

    A. Ear, nose, throat, and oral mucosa examination
    B. Neck evaluation, including meningeal signs
    C. Lung auscultation
    D. Abdominal aorta palpation
    E. Neurologic evaluation

Physical Examination Findings

Hannah is 30" tall and weighs 22 lb. Other vital signs are rectal temperature, 102.6°F; pulse, 140 BPM and regular; and respirations, 36/min and regular (for normal infant/toddler vital signs, please see Case 2-2). She is too young to obtain an accurate blood pressure even utilizing a pediatric cuff. She is toxic appearing.

Her auditory canals are normal color and without edema or abnormal discharge. Her tympanic membranes are slightly injected but freely mobile, and reveal no evidence of middle ear effusion or masses. Her nasal mucosa is slightly erythematous, is slightly edematous, and has a small amount of clear discharge, bilaterally. Her pharynx is erythematous with marked tonsillar enlargement with whitish exudates. Her oral mucosa is slightly more pink than expected but does not have any petechiae, exudates, or other lesions.

Hannah refuses to move her neck and keeps it flexed slightly forward and to the right. It is tender to palpate in the posterior muscles and under the left sternocleidomastoid (SCM) muscle. Other than palpable anterior cervical lymph nodes, no masses are noted; however, there does appear to be some mild edema on the left. Furthermore, the lymph nodes appear to be larger and tenderer on the right compared to the contralateral side of her neck. Meningeal signs can't be performed secondary to the patient's reluctance to lay flat and/or have her neck moved.

Her lungs are clear to auscultation bilaterally and her abdominal aorta is normal in size, without masses, and without bruit.

Her conjunctivae are slightly injected with tearing when she cries. Her pupils are equal in size, are round, and react to light and accommodation. She does not appear to have photophobia. Her funduscopic examination and EOMs appear to be normal; however, the exams were suboptimal due to Hannah's inability to cooperate. The remainder of her cranial nerves appear grossly intact. She uses all four extremities equally and appears to have equal strength bilaterally. Her deep tendon reflexes are normal and equal bilaterally. She refuses to walk.

3. Based on this information, which of the following diagnostic studies are essential to perform on Hannah and why?

    A. Oxygen saturation (O_2 sat)
    B. White blood cell count with differential (WBC w/diff)
    C. Lumbar puncture
    D. Lateral neck radiographs
    E. Noncontrast CT of neck

Diagnostic Results

Hannah's O_2 sat was 95% on room air (normal: > 95%). Her leukocyte count was 35,000/mm^3 (normal for child 2 years of age and younger: 6200–17,000) with a neutrophilia and lymphocytopenia. Her lumbar puncture, including Gram stain, was normal; however, the culture results are pending.

Hannah's lateral neck films revealed a normal C-spine except for a slight loss of normal lordosis, an enlargement of the soft tissue in the prevertebral space with a questionable density in front of C-3 to C-6, and blunting of the laryngeal "step-off" separating the posterior pharyngeal wall from the posterior tracheal wall. Her noncontrast CT also revealed a questionable density in the area but did not further clarify it.

4. Based on this information, which one of the following is Hannah's most likely diagnosis and why?

    A. Epiglottitis
    B. Peritonsillar abscess
    C. Retropharyngeal infection with probable abscess
    D. Meningitis
    E. Lemierre disease

5. Based on this diagnosis, which of the following are appropriate components of a treatment plan for Hannah and why?

    A. Hospitalize and obtain CT of neck with and without contrast
    B. Outpatient treatment with amoxicillin and close follow-up
    C. Immediately start IV clindamycin and metronidazole
    D. Close observation of airway and intubation if significant deterioration occurs
    E. Immediate consultation with an otorhinolaryngologist

CASE 4-8

Ian Jackson

Mr. Jackson is a 62-year-old Asian American male who presents with the chief complaint of "dizziness." Further questioning reveals it is an intermittent, subjective vertigo of approximately 1 year's duration. Initially, he experienced an episode every 2 to 3 months; however, it has gradually increased to his current level of one to two episodes per month. The episodes have also gradually increased in intensity since their onset. The vertigo is so severe that when it occurs, Mr. Jackson "has to stop whatever I'm doing and go to bed"; however, lying down does not alleviate his symptoms. The episodes last approximately 1 to 2 hours; then, he is asymptomatic except for feeling slightly fatigued and having a sensation of aural fullness in his left ear.

The vertigo is associated with a low-pitch tinnitus, which he describes as a "blowinglike" sound, in his left ear only. It is not pulsatile nor does it ever occur when he is not experiencing vertigo. The tinnitus begins with the onset of the vertigo and resolves before the vertigo does. He also experiences nausea and frequently vomiting and diarrhea with these episodes. In between episodes he is asymptomatic, including any gastrointestinal complaints. The last episode was approximately 1.5 weeks ago. The only potentially aggravating factor that he is aware of is with the last couple of episodes have occurred almost immediately after he had eaten shellfish. He cannot remember a recent occasion of eating shellfish when he did not experience the vertigo. He is unaware of any other aggravating or alleviating factors.

He has no known medical conditions. He has never had surgery nor been hospitalized. He takes no prescription or over-the-counter medications (including aspirin), vitamins, supplements, or herbal preparations. He does not have a history of occupational or recreational exposure to loud noise. He has been married for 27 years and has two grown children and two grandchildren. He has never smoked. He does not drink alcohol. His family history is noncontributory.

1. Based on this information, which of the following questions are essential to ask Mr. Jackson and why?

    A. Does he have any concerns regarding his hearing or experience decreased hearing with the vertigo?
    B. Does he notice a nystagmus with the vertigo?
    C. Is the vertigo associated with a headache?
    D. What is his relationship like with his wife?
    E. Has he been experiencing any problems with weakness or difficulties using his extremities, problems with coordination, speech abnormalities, dysphagia, heart palpitations, chest pain/pressure/discomfort, dyspnea, wheezing, visual abnormalities, other ocular complaints, arthralgias, myalgias, or rashes either during or between the vertiginous episodes?

Patient Responses

Mr. Jackson has noticed some hearing loss that appears to be worse in his left ear; however, he attributed it to his age. It does seem to worsen when he experiences the vertigo. He is uncertain whether he experiences nystagmus with the episodes. He denies having a headache before, during, after, or between episodes of vertigo. He and his wife have a good relationship. He has noticed a few "hives" on his face with the last three or four episodes only. He does not experience them between episodes. He denies any problems with weakness or difficulties using his extremities, problems with coordination, speech abnormalities, dysphagia, heart palpitations, chest pain/pressure/discomfort, dyspnea, wheezing, visual abnormalities, other ocular complaints, arthralgias, myalgias, or rashes either during or between the vertiginous episodes.

2. Based on this information, which of the following components of a physical examination are essential to conduct on Mr. Jackson and why?

    A. Ear, nose, and throat (ENT) examination
    B. Rinne and Weber tests
    C. Evaluation for carotid bruits
    D. Neurologic examination
    E. Skin examination

Physical Examination Results

Mr. Jackson weighs 175 lb and is 6'2" tall (BMI = 22.5). Other vital signs are BP in his right arm, 126/76 mm Hg; BP in his left arm, 128/78 mm Hg; pulse, 76 BPM and regular; respirations, 12/min and regular; and temperature, 98.5°F.

His auditory canals are normal in color, nonedematous, nontender, and clear of debris and lesions. His tympanic membranes are opaque, noninjected, fully mobile, without perforations, and without any evidence of either a middle ear effusion or mass. His Weber test lateralizes to his right ear but his Rinne test reveals equal air and bone conduction.

Mr. Jackson's nasal mucosa is normal color, nonedematous, and without discharge or lesions. His oral mucosa and pharynx are normal color and without lesions. He has no tonsillar enlargements, exudates, or asymmetry. Uvula is midline and remains there upon saying "ah."

Mr. Jackson's carotid arteries are normal bilaterally and do not reveal any bruits, murmurs, or other abnormal sounds.

His cranial nerves are grossly intact except he can hear a watch tick at a maximum of 12 inches from his right ear but only 6 inches from his left ear. He has normal and equal muscle strength in his extremities. There are no abnormalities of gait or balance identified. His deep tendon reflexes are present, normal, and equal bilaterally. The Epley (canalith repositioning) and Dix-Hallpike maneuvers do not induce vertigo.

His skin is normal in color and without any abnormal lesions.

3. Based on this information, which of the following diagnostic studies are essential to perform on Mr. Jackson and why?

    A. Audiogram
    B. Caloric stimulation testing
    C. Serum IgE antibody test for shellfish
    D. Erythrocyte sedimentation rate (ESR)
    E. Computed tomography (CT) of brain, with and without contrast

Diagnostic Test Results

His audiogram revealed a low-frequency hearing loss in his left ear but normal hearing in his right. Caloric testing was normal on the right side; however, he had a diminished nystagmus response on the left. His serum IgE antibody test for shellfish antibodies was markedly elevated. His ESR was 10 mm/hr (normal males: < 15). The CT scan of his brain was normal.

4. Based on this information, which one of the following is Mr. Jackson's most likely diagnosis and why?

    A. Benign paroxysmal positioning vertigo (BPPV)
    B. Ménière disease
    C. Labyrinthitis
    D. Vestibular neuronitis
    E. Ménière syndrome

5. Based on this diagnosis, which of the following are appropriate components of a treatment plan for Mr. Jackson and why?

    A. Meclizine 25 mg orally at onset of vertigo
    B. Prochlorperazine 5 mg orally at onset of symptoms
    C. Avoid eating shellfish
    D. Refer to otorhinolaryngologist with experience in allergic diseases for confirmation of diagnosis and further treatment
    E. Refer to physical therapy for exercises to prevent/treat vertiginous episodes

CASE 4-9
James Kirkland

Mr. Kirkland is a 24-year-old Native American who presents with the chief complaint of severe left oculodynia. It has been present approximately 4 to 5 days. He describes it initially as "feeling like I had something in my eye"; this sensation persisted for approximately 2 days, and then it became "more of a pain." Since then, the painful sensation has gradually progressed; currently he rates it as a 6 out of a 10 on the pain scale. It is sharp in nature, appears moderately deep, and is generalized in location. It is not worsened by ocular movements. It is associated with a marked epiphora (but no discolored or purulent discharge) and significant injection; both have progressively worsened since the onset of his symptoms. He is unaware of any aggravating or alleviating factors.

His right eye is totally asymptomatic. He denies being ill before or since the onset of his ocular symptoms. He denies rhinorrhea, nasal congestion, postnasal discharge, ear pain, fever, chills, malaise, nausea, vomiting, or vertigo.

His medical history is negative, including never having any surgeries or hospitalizations. He does not take any prescription or OTC medications, vitamins, supplements, or herbal preparations. He has never smoked. He does not drink alcohol or do illicit substances. His family history is noncontributory.

1. Based on this information, which of the following questions are essential to ask Mr. Kirkland and why?

    A. Was there any trauma involved?
    B. Does he feel hopeful about the future?
    C. Is he sexually active? If yes, has he had new partner(s) in the previous 3 months and does he use condoms regularly?
    D. Is he experiencing any abnormality of vision?
    E. Has he tried any topical treatments or remedies?

Patient Responses

Mr. Kirkland denies any history of trauma to his eye. He feels hopeful about the future. He is sexually active and has had three new partners in the past 3 months. He uses condoms occasionally.

He is experiencing intermittent, left unilateral blurring of vision that is alleviated if he "rubs my eyes." He cannot identify a trigger for it. It is occurring more frequently, but has not increased in severity, since his symptoms began. He has not placed anything into his eye.

2. Based on this information, which of the following components of a physical examination are essential to conduct on Mr. Kirkland and why?

- **A.** Visual acuity
- **B.** External eye examination
- **C.** Funduscopic (and, if possible, slit-lamp) examination
- **D.** Ear, nose, and throat (ENT) examination
- **E.** Heart and lung auscultation

Physical Examination Findings

Mr. Kirkland is 5'8" tall and weighs 167 lb (BMI = 25.4). Other vital signs are BP, 130/74 mm Hg; pulse, 82 BPM and regular; respirations, 14/min and regular; and oral temperature, 98.4°F.

His near and distance vision are both 20/20, bilaterally (without corrective lenses). His right sclera, palpebral conjunctivae, and cornea appear normal, and there is no discharge noted. His left sclera is normal in color but reveals diffuse conjunctival injection; however, it appears to be most prominent and deepest around, but not involving, his iris. His left lower palpebral conjunctiva is erythematous and has three distinct vesicles of approximately 2 to 3 mm in size; a lid flip revealed his left upper palpebral conjunctiva to also be erythematous and contain five similar-appearing lesions. He has a moderate amount of clear discharge from his left eye.

His lacrimal ducts appear patent, nontender, and without erythema or edema. His extraocular muscles are intact with normal movements in all directions, bilaterally. His visuals fields are normal and equal bilaterally. His pupils are round, are equal in size, and respond appropriately to light and accommodation. However, he does complain of a slight photophobia in his left eye. His funduscopic/slit-lamp examination reveals normal red reflex, clear lenses, normal cup:disc ratio, normal retina, and normal fundi, bilaterally; no abnormal lesions were present in either eye.

His auditory canals are normal color and without edema or abnormal discharge/debris. His nasal mucosa and oral mucosa are normal in color and without edema, erythema, or discharge. His pharynx is normal in color with no tonsillar enlargement, lesions, or exudates.

His heart is regular in rate and rhythm and without murmurs. His lungs are clear to auscultation.

3. Based on this information, which of the following diagnostic studies are essential to perform on Mr. Kirkland and why?

- **A.** Tonometry (or equivalent) of eyes
- **B.** Color-vision testing
- **C.** Fluorescein examination of the eyes
- **D.** Serum (× 1 only) for herpes simplex virus (HSV) antibodies, types 1 and 2
- **E.** Gram stain, Tzanck smear, bacterial culture and sensitivity, and viral culture of left eye discharge

Diagnostic Result Findings

Mr. Kirkland's tonometry of his eyes revealed normal intraocular pressure bilaterally. His color vision was normal bilaterally. The fluorescein staining of his right eye was normal; however, his left eye revealed a dendritic pattern throughout his conjunctivae. His HSV-1 antibody titer was 1:16 (normal: negative) and his HSV-2 antibody titer was 1:32 (normal: negative). His Gram stain of his left eye discharge revealed numerous white blood cells but no significant quantities of other lesions. A Tzanck smear of his left eye discharge revealed numerous multinucleated giant cells. His cultures are pending.

4. Based on this information, which one of the following is Mr. Kirkland's most likely diagnosis and why?

- **A.** Acute conjunctivitis
- **B.** Acute uveitis
- **C.** Acute iritis
- **D.** Acute glaucoma
- **E.** Acute herpetic keratoconjunctivitis

5. Based on this diagnosis, which of the following are appropriate components of a treatment plan for Mr. Kirkland and why?

- **A.** Ciprofloxacin ophthalmologic drops
- **B.** Trifluridine ophthalmic solution
- **C.** Oral acyclovir
- **D.** Topical glucocorticoids
- **E.** Topical miotics and/or beta-blockers

CASES IN EYE, EAR, NOSE, AND THROAT DISORDERS

CHAPTER 4

RESPONSES AND DISCUSSION

CASE 4-1

Brittney Crookshanks

1. History

A. How high has her fever been and how was it checked? ESSENTIAL

The exact degree of a patient's temperature and the method utilized to obtain it is important in assessing the severity of the patient's infection, especially in young children. A warm or hot forehead (or other anatomic part) is not an accurate assessment of the presence of fever. In fact, when the temperature becomes excessively elevated, the patient's skin will often feel normal or cool as a result of the body's natural mechanisms to normalize the body's core temperature. Therefore, all parents should be taught how to obtain an accurate temperature measurement on their child utilizing an instrument that they are comfortable with because utilizing the thermometer incorrectly can alter the temperature reading. However, it is important to remember that an individual with an overwhelming sepsis can have a normal or subnormal temperature and an individual with a minor infection can have a markedly elevated temperature.

Body temperature has a normal diurnal fluctuation, with it being lowest early in the morning (at approximately 6:00 a.m.) and highest in the early evening (at approximately 4:00 to 6:00 p.m.). It is not unusual for an individual's body temperature to fluctuate as much as 0.5° to 1°C (or 0.9° to 1.8°F) throughout the day. A fever is technically defined as a rectal temperature of greater than 38°C (or 100.4°F). It is important to remember that an oral temperature is approximately 0.7°F lower and a tympanic temperature approximately 1.6°F lower than a rectal temperature. Some experts feel that acute inflammation involving the middle ear and the tympanic membrane associated with acute otitis media can falsely elevate a tympanic temperature if taken in the affected ear.

Temperature is sometimes important in determining a treatment plan. For example, a temperature greater than or equal to 39°C, or 102.2°F, is one of the criteria that the American Academy of Pediatrics (AAP) utilizes to define a severe (vs mild to moderate) infection in their otitis media guidelines.

Other conditions besides infection can also cause a fever. These include young children who have had an excessively "busy" day, anxiety, shivering, inflammation, central nervous system trauma, central nervous system hemorrhage, liver disease, carcinoma, and some medications. Obviously not related to Brittney's case, women of reproductive age experience a natural fluctuation of body temperature associated with the phases of their menstrual cycle.

B. Is she eating or drinking anything? ESSENTIAL

Whether the patient is eating or drinking anything provides additional information regarding the severity of the patient's present illness and provides clues to the patient's hydration status.

C. How long has she had the rhinorrhea? ESSENTIAL

One of the distinguishing characteristics of acute otitis media (AOM) compared with otitis media with effusion (OME) is the timing of the onset of the upper respiratory symptoms in relationship to the onset of the otalgia. In AOM, the symptoms begin almost simultaneously; in OME, the upper respiratory tract infection (URI) symptoms occur for several days before the onset of the otalgia. However, the presence of rhinorrhea does not mean that the patient is experiencing AOM or OME. Other potential diagnoses could include allergic rhinitis, sinusitis, or a skull fracture.

D. Does she have any eye discharge, sore throat, nasal congestion, cough, wheezing, headache, stiff/sore neck, nausea, vomiting, diarrhea, constipation, other bowel changes, abdominal pain, decreased urination, or decreased tearing? ESSENTIAL

Otalgia can indicate a problem confined to the ear (with or without complications), another medical condition with pain that radiates to the ear, or both. The presence, and in some cases the absence, of these symptoms can assist in narrowing the list of potential diagnoses to determine the most likely diagnosis. For example, a sore throat could indicate the presence of pharyngitis alone or in addition to an ear problem; a headache or stiff neck could indicate encephalitis or meningitis with pain radiating to the ear or started by a case of otitis media; and decreased urination and/or tearing could indicate the presence of dehydration in conjunction with the current diagnosis.

E. Was Brittney breast- or bottle-fed?   NONESSENTIAL

By the age of 4 years, any immunity conferred via exposure to maternal breast milk is essentially inconsequential. Furthermore, because she should no longer be using a bottle (if she was bottle-fed), the connection between the feeding position associated with its usage and otitis media (via reflux of milk though the eustachian tubes into the middle ear) is also irrelevant.

2. Physical Examination

A. Eye examination   NONESSENTIAL

B. Ear examination   ESSENTIAL

An ear examination is indicated because Brittney's chief complaint is ear pain. These findings will assist in determining if the ear is the actual source of the problem. If so, it will also assist in distinguishing an internal versus external source for the otalgia as well as an infectious versus noninfectious process. Remember, the presence of a middle ear effusion, regardless of the cause, cannot be correctly identified without the tympanic membrane immobility via pneumatoscopy.

C. Nose, oral mucosa, and throat examination   ESSENTIAL

Nose, oral mucosa, and throat examination is important in evaluating a patient with otalgia because they provide information not only regarding symptoms associated with the chief complaint but also potential conditions that could be contributing to or coexisting with it.

For example, an erythematous pharynx, with tonsillar enlargement with exudates and petechiae on the soft palate, is suspicious for streptococcal pharyngitis with pain and/or infection radiating to the middle ear cavity. Likewise, a pale, boggy nasal mucosa could indicate the presence of an underlying allergic rhinitis, which could be responsible for, or at least contributing to, Brittney's frequent episodes of AOM. However, the paleness is generally replaced by erythema when an acute infection is present.

D. Neck examination   ESSENTIAL

A neck examination evaluates for the presence of enlarged and/or tender cervical lymph nodes as would be expected with any type of an upper respiratory tract infection in a patient in this age group. Additionally, it can provide information regarding tenderness, decreased range of motion, or meningeal signs that could indicate conditions such as a muscle strain, torticollis, meningitis, or encephalitis with pain radiating to the ear or in conjunction with (or caused by) an ear problem.

E. Lung auscultation   ESSENTIAL

In small children, it is often difficult to distinguish an upper respiratory tract from a lower respiratory tract process based on history alone. Therefore, it is essential that Brittney's lungs are auscultated for signs indicating the presence of a lower respiratory tract process, which the majority of the time is a more serious condition that generally requires a different treatment.

3. Diagnostic Studies

A. Blood urea nitrogen (BUN)   NONESSENTIAL

In a child complaining of upper respiratory symptoms and a decreased appetite, BUN would be indicated to provide an objective determination of the patient's hydration status. Although Brittney has anorexia and a decreased fluid intake, she still is urinating regularly, is crying tears, and having a moist oral mucosa, indicating she is currently adequately hydrated.

B. Electrolytes   NONESSENTIAL

Electrolytes would also be indicated in a patient with Brittney's symptoms if there was significant concern regarding the potential of an electrolyte disturbance or dehydration, or if she was experiencing significant vomiting and diarrhea.

C. Complete blood count with differential (CBC w/diff)   NONESSENTIAL

A CBC w/diff is also not going to alter Brittney's treatment plan; therefore, it is not indicated. However, it would be indicated if she failed to respond to appropriate therapy or had persisting lymphadenopathy (especially unilateral), making a lymphoma, leukemia, other hematologic condition, or an immunologic problem suspect. Because of these types of potential problems, sound medical practice dictates that a patient's complaint must be followed to resolution or referral.

D. Pneumatic otoscopy   ESSENTIAL

A pneumatic otoscopy is indicated because it provides objective confirmation of a middle ear effusion (MEE). Otitis media cannot be diagnosed without the presence of an MEE.

E. Audiogram   NONESSENTIAL

An audiogram at this time would be abnormal because of Brittney's otologic findings. If she continues with frequent episodes of AOM, appears to have hearing loss, or exhibits difficulty with proper pronunciation, an audiogram should be performed. Ideally, it should be done when she does not have evidence of an MEE or alteration of her tympanic membrane mobility.

4. Diagnosis

A. Left serous otitis media (SOM, left)   INCORRECT

In SOM, the patient exhibits an effusion of the middle ear which is essentially asymptomatic, except for a possible hearing loss, feeling of fullness, or associated symptoms of allergic rhinitis. It is not associated with fever, anorexia, marked otalgia, tympanic membrane erythema, and/or cervical lymphadenopathy. Therefore, even though Brittney's condition involves a middle ear effusion (MEE), this is not her most likely diagnosis because the effusion represents a sign of her present illness, not the condition itself.

B. Acute left otitis media (AOM, left)   CORRECT

According to the AAP guidelines, a diagnosis of AOM can be made if (1) the symptoms are acute in nature (Brittney's started yesterday), (2) an MEE is present (Brittney's was visualized with the otoscope and confirmed with pneumatic otoscopy), and (3) middle ear inflammation is present (Brittney had a bulging, erythematous tympanic membrane) PLUS otalgia occurs of a sufficient nature to interfere with normal activities (Brittney's affected her ability to sleep supine and her appetite). Thus, AOM, left, is her most likely/correct diagnosis from the list provided.

An MEE caused by AOM generally resolves in 2 to 4 weeks after the infection's resolution.

C. Chronic left otitis media (COM, left)   INCORRECT

Chronic otitis media has to persist for more than 2 to 3 weeks despite appropriate therapy. Because Brittney's symptoms started yesterday, this is not her most likely diagnosis.

D. Viral upper respiratory tract infection (URI)   INCORRECT

Technically, Brittney has what could be considered a viral upper respiratory tract infection (because the majority of the cases of AOM are viral in nature); however, this is not her most likely diagnosis because AOM is a more specific and accurate description of her illness.

It is virtually impossible to determine if AOM is viral or bacterial in origin without doing a tympanocentesis to obtain MEE for culture with sensitivities. Even then, the question is often unanswered because of the low yield from a single culture. Additionally, current clinical guidelines incorporate antibiotic usage depending on the symptomatology; therefore, performing the tympanocentesis to obtain the MEE for culture and sensitivity is not going to alter the course of treatment. Hence, it is an unpleasant and unnecessary procedure to routinely utilize.

E. Fever of unknown origin (FUO)   INCORRECT

Fever of unknown origin is defined as a temperature of greater than 101.0°F on multiple occasions over a minimum of a 3-week period without a diagnosis being established despite a 1-week hospitalization. Currently, it is subdivided into classic, nosocomial, neutropenic, and human immunodeficiency virus (HIV) related. This is not Brittney's most likely diagnosis because her fever appears to have a cause and has not been present for a minimum of 3 weeks.

5. Treatment Plan

A. Acetaminophen or ibuprofen for fever and pain   CORRECT

Analgesics are an essential component of the treatment of AOM. Therefore, medications such as acetaminophen and/or ibuprofen are good first-line choices to meet this goal.

Furthermore, they provide fever reduction, which often makes the patient more comfortable. In routine viral and bacterial infections, there is no evidence to suggest that treating a fever delays healing or not treating a fever enhances healing.

Nevertheless, some experts advocate withholding antipyretics when the diagnosis is uncertain as the fever pattern (with or without the pulse pattern) can assist in making the diagnosis in unusual infectious (e.g., typhoid fever, brucellosis, tuberculosis, and malaria) and noninfectious (e.g., Still disease, Blau syndrome, hyper–immunoglobulin D [IgD] syndrome, and other autoimmune/autoinflammatory illnesses) diseases. Others recommend against routine use to prevent obscuring inadequate or partial treatment of infections, especially until culture results are available and/or other clinical signs of improvement

occur. Some infectious disease experts also recommend against routine regular use of antipyretics in patients at the extremes of age, immunocompromised patients, or those with renal failure because in these patient populations hypothermia can actually be an indication of a worsening of the infection.

B. Observation for 48 to 72 hours before instituting antibiotics   INCORRECT

Observation for 48 to 72 hours is an appropriate treatment for AOM if the healthcare provider (HCP) is uncertain of the patient's diagnosis and the patient is older than 6 months of age OR the patient is older than 2 years of age with mild symptoms. However, close follow-up, compliant parents, and the ability to initiate antibiotic therapy if symptoms worsen or persist are essential for this option. Because the AAP utilizes the definition of a temperature of greater than or equal to 39°C (or 102.2°F) and moderate to severe otalgia to indicate a severe infection, observation is not an appropriate option for Brittney.

C. Amoxicillin 40 to 45 mg/kg twice a day for 5 days   INCORRECT

Although high-dose amoxicillin is considered a first-line agent in the treatment of AOM, the AAP guidelines only recommend it if the symptoms are mild to moderate. Because Brittney's symptoms classify her infection in the severe category, this option is not appropriate for her.

D. Refer for tympanostomy tubes   INCORRECT

Currently, the use of tympanostomy tubes is an area of tremendous controversy. However, the AAP guidelines recommend a referral if the patient experiences frequent infections (defined as more than three in a 6-month period or more than four in a 12-month period) OR if the effusion has been present continuously for longer than 3 to 6 months and associated with decreased hearing.

Because the number and frequency of episodes of AOM experienced by Brittney are unknown and her current effusion has probably not been present for 3 to 6 months, a referral for tympanostomy tubes is not indicated at this time.

E. Amoxicillin/clavulanate 40 to 45 mg/kg twice a day for 10 days   CORRECT

According to the AAP guidelines, amoxicillin/clavulanate 40 to 45 mg/kg twice a day for 10 days would be considered appropriate first-line therapy for Brittney. The AAP guidelines recommend treating the infection for 10 days in children who are younger than 2 years of age or have severe disease. They recommend 5 days for healthy older children with mild to moderate disease. However, there is considerable controversy in the ENT community regarding the appropriate duration of therapy. Experts are recommending anywhere from 3 to 14 days of medication.

F. Encourage her father to quit smoking (if unable or unwilling, he needs to go outside to smoke) and explain the adverse effects of passive smoke exposure, including an increased incidence of acute otitis media for Brittney   CORRECT

It has been proven that passive smoke exposure increases the incidence of AOM in children. Therefore, Brittney's father should be encouraged to quit smoking (for his health) or at least smoke outdoors and away from Brittney (for her health and that of other family members).

Additionally, Brittney's parents must understand that opening the window in the room and blowing the cigarette smoke out the window is not adequate to prevent the sequelae associated with secondary smoke inhalation, including frequent recurrent episodes of AOM, frequent upper respiratory tract infections, exacerbations of asthma, coronary artery disease, lung cancer, and chronic bronchitis. Patient education regarding the recommendation is essential for success.

Epidemiologic and Other Data

The majority of cases of acute otitis media are viral in origin. The major pathogens include the respiratory syncytial viruses (RSVs), the influenza viruses, the rhinoviruses, and the enteroviruses. When bacteria are responsible, the main organism is *Streptococcus pneumoniae*. Other common bacterial pathogens include *Haemophilus influenzae* and *Moraxella catarrhalis*.

Risk factors for AOM include being young in age, being bottle-fed (especially in a horizontal position), attending day care, being exposed to passive smoke, having a history of allergic rhinitis, and having a coexisting immunocompromised condition.

CASE 4-2

Charlene Dawson

1. History

A. How does she describe her "dizziness"?   ESSENTIAL

Although patients often use the term "dizziness" to describe both dizziness and vertigo, they are not the same medically. Dizziness is a vague sense of lightheadedness, unsteadiness, or faintness. Vertigo is an actual sensation of rotary movement. If the patient feels like he or she is moving and the surroundings are stable, it is termed subjective vertigo. However, if the opposite is true (the patient's surroundings appear to be rotating around the patient), it is called objective vertigo. Vertigo can be seen in numerous otologic (e.g., inner ear conditions, labyrinth disorders, canalithiasis, cupulolithiasis, and cerumen compressing the tympanic membrane), cardiovascular (e.g., cerebral vascular accidents [CVAs], arteriovenous [AV] malformations, and brain stem ischemia), neurologic (e.g., brain stem lesions, cerebellar abnormalities, and multiple sclerosis), and psychogenic (e.g., somatization disorders and anxiety) conditions.

In evaluating a patient with vertigo, peripheral causes can generally (but not always) be differentiated from central causes by their distinct features. Peripheral vertigo tends to be very sudden in onset and frequently associated with decreased hearing and/or tinnitus. On the other hand, central causes are much more gradual in onset and lack hearing changes and/or tinnitus.

Further clues to assist in determining the most likely diagnosis include the presence (or absence) of hearing loss and/or tinnitus and the duration of the vertiginous episode. For example, labyrinthitis is accompanied by auditory symptoms and can last for days, whereas vestibular neuronitis also lasts for days but does not have any associated hearing loss

and/or tinnitus. Perilymphatic fistula- and cupulolithiasis-produced vertiginous episodes tend to last for only a few seconds; the former is associated with auditory complaints, whereas the latter is not.

B. Does she have a dry mouth, decreased salivation, or decreased tearing?   ESSENTIAL

Because some of Ms. Dawson's symptoms suggest a possible cranial nerve palsy (especially of the facial nerve), it is important to determine whether she is experiencing other symptoms consistent with this diagnosis. For example, if the eyelids and lips do not close fully, the patient can experience dryness in the eyes and mouth, respectively. However, the latter needs to be distinguished from a dry mouth secondary to decreased saliva production. Autonomic dysfunction, dehydration, substance abuse, and certain medications can also produce oral and ocular mucosal dryness.

C. Is she experiencing decreased moods, crying episodes, or anhedonia?   NONESSENTIAL

Although psychiatric problems can present as pain, dizziness, and neurologic symptoms, they rarely cause objective fever and otic discharge. Therefore, before a psychological cause is explored, a physical one must be eliminated.

D. What does she mean by the statement her face "isn't working right"?   ESSENTIAL

When patients supply vague descriptions of their symptoms, it is essential to obtain further clarification to ensure there is a clear description of their complaint. Neglecting to obtain or misinterpreting Ms. Dawson's actual symptoms could result in a missed or delayed diagnosis, which could have serious adverse outcomes (e.g., CVA or increased intracranial pressure, abscess, or mass compressing her cranial nerves).

E. Has she experienced headaches, visual changes, photophobia, phonophobia, abnormalities of taste, dysphagia, weakness or problems using her extremities, or other neurologic deficits?   ESSENTIAL

Because Ms. Dawson is experiencing some symptoms that could suggest a cranial nerve palsy, it is essential to determine whether she is experiencing any other symptoms that would indicate a more generalized neurologic condition (e.g., CVA, multiple sclerosis [MS], Guillain-Barré syndrome, Bannwarth syndrome, Lou Gehrig disease, or Schilder disease) is present.

2. Physical Examination

A. Ear examination   ESSENTIAL

An ear examination is essential because Ms. Dawson's chief complaint is worsening otalgia. It can assist in distinguishing a primary otologic condition (e.g., acute otitis media or acute otitis externa) from a disease that presents with radiation to the ear (e.g., temporomandibular joint syndrome, trigeminal neuralgia, or dental abscess).

B. Mastoid and temporomandibular joint (TMJ) examination   ESSENTIAL

Because Ms. Dawson is complaining of significant ear pain, fever, and neurologic symptoms, it is essential to evaluate the bony structures surrounding the ear, including her mastoid process and TMJ, to determine whether there is an otologic problem extending into a communicating bone (i.e., mastoiditis), a primary bony disease producing the symptoms (i.e., osteomyelitis), or a combination (i.e., osteomyelitis caused by direct dissemination of infectious otologic process) present.

C. Skin examination   ESSENTIAL

A skin examination is important to determine whether inflammation (rubor, calor, dolor, or tumor), lesions, discolorations, or other skin changes are present that would provide useful information as to the cause (and/or any contributing factors) of the current problem (e.g., cellulitis, eczema, psoriasis, seborrheic dermatitis, folliculitis, or herpes zoster oticus).

D. Cranial nerve examination   ESSENTIAL

A cranial nerve examination is important because Ms. Dawson's history suggests a potential neurologic abnormality involving her cranial nerves. Furthermore, some serious ear conditions can cause inflammation (e.g., invasive otitis externa) and compress the cranial nerves or extend into the cranial nerves (e.g., acoustic neuroma).

E. Carotid pulse   NONESSENTIAL

Evaluating her carotid artery for evidence of atherosclerotic or other occlusive processes might provide some useful information; however, checking her pulse in the carotid area is unlikely to provide any clinically beneficial information regarding her chief complaint.

3. Diagnostic Studies

A. Remove debris from canal with small catheter and suction; then, obtain small biopsy of granulated inferior canal for culture and sensitivity   ESSENTIAL

When confronted with an auditory canal full of purulent material, it is imperative to determine whether the debris is coming from the auditory canal; the tympanic membrane (TM), as seen with bullous myringitis; or an inner ear process via a perforated TM (e.g., acute otitis media, serous otitis media, or middle ear abscess). Because the TM cannot be visualized, a perforation cannot be ruled out. Therefore, the material should be removed by either a small catheter with suction or an ear curette instead of irrigation. Because of the significant amount of canal inflammation, the catheter with suction is probably going to be a much less painful procedure.

Once the debris is removed, a biopsy of the granulated tissue (inferior ear canal) needs to be sent for culture and sensitivity to identify the actual etiologic organism because the canal discharge is likely to be contaminated and contain nonpathogenic flora.

B. Remove debris from canal with warm water irrigation and send sample for culture and sensitivity   NONESSENTIAL

Because an intact TM cannot be visualized, manual warm water irrigation should not be used to remove the canal debris. Instilling water directly into the middle ear can cause pain and mild to moderate vertigo in the majority of patients (and a few will experience significant vertigo).

C. Random plasma glucose (RPG)   ESSENTIAL

Because Ms. Dawson appears to have a significant infection based on her history and physical examination findings and is a known diabetic, she needs to have a random plasma

glucose performed to determine the effect the infection has on her diabetes control.

D. Complete blood count with differential (CBC w/diff)   ESSENTIAL

A CBC w/diff is essential in Ms. Dawson's case because it will provide additional information regarding the nature and severity of her infection. This information, in conjunction with her RPG, imaging results, and physical examination findings, will assist in determining whether she can safely be managed as an outpatient or if she should be hospitalized.

E. Computed tomography (CT) or magnetic resonance imaging (MRI) of her right mastoid/ear area   ESSENTIAL

Because Ms. Dawson has evidence of inflammation over her mastoid bone and granulation tissue in her auditory canal, it is essential to obtain an imaging study, either CT or MRI, to determine whether the underlying bone is involved.

4. Diagnosis

A. Acute otitis externa (AOE), right   INCORRECT

In acute otitis externa, or swimmer's ear, the patient generally lacks significant fever, granulation tissue in the auditory canal, and underlying bony abnormalities. Furthermore, the pain tends not to be as severe as Ms. Dawson's. Therefore, this is not her most likely diagnosis.

B. Chronic otitis externa (COE), right   INCORRECT

Chronic otitis externa is an otitis externa that has been present for a while and may or may not have been treated. Ms. Dawson has had symptoms for approximately 1 month now; therefore, her condition could be described as chronic. However, chronic otitis externa is not associated with high fever, granulation tissue of the auditory canal, and associated skin and bone structural abnormalities as seen in Ms. Dawson's case. Therefore, this is not her most likely diagnosis. Additionally, COE is generally secondary to another condition (e.g., psoriasis, seborrheic dermatitis, eczema, or irritation by a chronic middle effusion via a perforated TM).

C. Malignant (or necrotizing) otitis externa, right   CORRECT

Malignant, or necrotizing (also known as invasive), otitis externa is a complication of an unresolved case of otitis externa that occurs almost exclusively in diabetics and other immunocompromised patients. It is associated with severe "deep" otalgia, fever, inflammatory changes of the affected skin, granulation tissue of the auditory canal, and abnormalities of the underlying bony structures. Additionally, it is not uncommon for it to cause compression of ipsilateral cranial nerve(s) as a result of the marked inflammation. The seventh (or facial) nerve is the most frequently involved. Thus, malignant otitis externa is Ms. Dawson's most likely diagnosis.

D. Mastoiditis, right   INCORRECT

Mastoiditis is generally a complication of acute otitis media that involves the direct extension of the infection into the mastoid process, causing erosion of the mastoid air cells and creating cavities filled with infectious debris. It is typically not associated with seventh cranial nerve palsy, osteomyelitis of additional bones, and granulation of the auditory canal. Thus, mastoiditis is not Ms. Dawson's most likely diagnosis.

E. Bell palsy, right   INCORRECT

Bell palsy is a possibility based on some of the neurologic findings described in Ms. Dawson's history and confirmed on her physical examination. However, it is lower motor neuron facial weakness. Hence, even though it is associated with the inability to hold the eye tightly closed, a flattened nasolabial fold, and a weakness of the lower face as found on Ms. Dawson's physical examination, it is also associated with difficulty performing fine facial movements, difficulty chewing, not being able to wrinkle the forehead, and inability to raise the eyebrow, which Ms. Dawson did not have. Her symptoms are more consistent with an upper motor neuron lesion.

Additionally, although it is often associated with otalgia, the ear pain begins at the same time as the neurologic symptoms or a couple days before. Furthermore, it is not associated with high fever, auditory canal abnormalities (unless caused by herpes zoster oticus), or osteomyelitis of the underlying bone. Thus, Bell palsy is not Ms. Dawson's most likely diagnosis.

5. Treatment Plan

A. Hospitalization   CORRECT

Because of the severity of Ms. Dawson's condition and the fact that she is immunocompromised as a result of her diabetes, she should initially be managed as an inpatient.

B. Intravenous piperacillin and gentamicin   CORRECT

Virtually all cases of malignant otitis externa are caused by a *Pseudomonas* species; thus, an antipseudomonal antibiotic (e.g., piperacillin or ceftazidime) is indicated. Because of the severity of Ms. Dawson's infection and her being immunocompromised, initially it should be given intravenously.

Frequently, the antipseudomonal antibiotic is initially combined with an aminoglycoside or a fluoroquinolone for maximum coverage of all possible pathogens until the culture and sensitivity results are available. Other possible pathogens include *Actinomyces, Aspergillus, Staphylococcus aureus, Staphylococcus epidermitis*, and other gram-negative organisms.

C. Topical antipseudomonal antibiotics   CORRECT

Because of the significant amount of auditory canal edema and skin changes coupled with the difficulty of obtaining desirable antibiotic concentration steady states in the ear canal, topical antibiotics should also be used in conjunction with the IV ones.

D. Otolaryngologist referral   CORRECT

In all probability because of the vast amount of bony involvement, Ms. Dawson is very likely to require surgery for débridement of the infected bone. Even if that were not the case, because of the severity of her disease, a consult with an otolaryngologist is appropriate.

E. Outpatient treatment with oral ofloxacin   INCORRECT

Because of the aforementioned reasons and the fact that necrotizing otitis externa is a rapidly progressing and potentially fatal disease, Ms. Dawson cannot be managed as an outpatient with oral antibiotics at this time.

Epidemiologic and Other Data

Necrotizing (or malignant) otitis externa is also known as invasive otitis externa because of its extremely aggressive nature and high potential for death. *Pseudomonas aeruginosa* is responsible for more than 90% of all cases of necrotizing (or malignant) otitis externa. Organisms implicated in the other 10% include *S. aureus, S. epidermidis, Aspergillus* species, and *Actinomyces* species.

CASE 4-3
David Estevez
1. History

A. Do his symptoms occur seasonally or year round?   ESSENTIAL

The majority of cases of chronic rhinitis are allergic in nature. Knowing whether the symptoms occur seasonally or perennially is important in determining potential allergens (e.g., pollens and grasses tend to be seasonal, whereas animal dander and dust mites tend to be continuous).

Additionally, comparing any serum or skin allergy test positives (if performed) with the seasonal nature of the symptoms (as well as the prevalence of the plants, grass types, and foliage in the geographic area) assists in determining the potential effectiveness of immunotherapy.

B. Are there any aggravating factors?   ESSENTIAL

When dealing with any complaint, knowledge of aggravating factors is important. For example, rhinitis caused by allergy (e.g., to pollen, molds, dust mites, or animal dander) tends to be most symptomatic in the locations where the allergens are the most concentrated and least symptomatic in locations where they are not as prevalent. Rhinorrhea caused by an irritant (e.g., cigarette smoke or perfumes) generally only produces symptoms when the patient is exposed to it. Gustatory rhinorrhea typically only occurs when the patient is eating. Vasomotor rhinitis results from exposures to specific stimuli (e.g., exercise and cold ambient temperatures).

C. Is he experiencing fatigue, weight gain, or changes in his skin, hair, or nails?   ESSENTIAL

Several systemic conditions can also have rhinorrhea as the prominent complaint; one of the more common diseases is hypothyroidism. Therefore, it is important to inquire about symptoms of this disease.

Other systemic disorders associated with rhinitis include asthma, cystic fibrosis, pregnancy (which obviously is not Mr. Estevez's diagnosis), nasal polyposis, gastroesophageal reflux disease (GERD), Wegener granulomatosis, and Churg-Strauss syndrome.

Medications can also induce rhinitis, including hormonal contraceptives, estrogen replacement therapy, progesterone, phosphodiesterase-5 inhibitors, beta-blockers, angiotensin-converting enzyme (ACE) inhibitors, aspirin, and nonsteroidal anti-inflammatory drugs.

D. Does he have any tattoos?   NONESSENTIAL

Allergic reactions do occur to the dye and metals contained in the pigments of tattooing ink. However, these are generally localized reactions and do not produce nasal symptoms.

E. Does he drink alcohol or use any drugs/substance of abuse?   ESSENTIAL

Some individuals have a rhinorrhea that is associated with alcohol intake. If he does drink alcohol, he might want to observe whether there is a connection between the two.

Some drugs of abuse can also cause rhinorrhea, either directly (e.g., cocaine) or as a systemic component (e.g., amphetamines).

2. Physical Examination

A. Eye examination   ESSENTIAL

An eye examination is important because Mr. Estevez is intermittently experiencing itchy, watery eyes in association with his rhinorrhea. The primary areas of focus include evaluating the sclera and conjunctivae for signs (and degree if present) of inflammation and/or injection, which can provide clues to potential differential diagnoses (e.g., allergic rhinitis, partial nasolacrimal duct obstruction, conjunctivitis, and substance abuse). The conjunctivae also need to be evaluated for the presence of keratoconjunctivitis sicca, which often causes pruritus secondary to the dryness and secondary tearing in response to manipulation of the eyes to alleviate the itching.

The eye examination also permits an objective comparison of any eye discharge with the description provided by the patient. Additionally, pupils need to be evaluated for marked dilation and/or constriction, which could indicate substance abuse. Mydriasis tends to be seen with usage of amphetamines and cocaine, whereas myosis is associated with the use of opioids.

B. Ear, mouth, and pharyngeal examination   ESSENTIAL

When a nasal complaint is present, it is imperative to evaluate the rest of the upper respiratory system to determine whether there are any associated abnormalities that could be useful in developing the patient's differential diagnoses. Attention also needs to be directed to the nasopharyngeal structure for abnormalities because they are potential sources for rhinorrhea.

C. Nasal examination   ESSENTIAL

Because Mr. Estevez's chief complaint is rhinitis, a nasal examination is indicated. The color, degree of inflammation, and presence of edema of the nasal mucosa as well as the amount and location of any discharge provide essential clues in determining the patient's most likely diagnosis. The nasal septum needs to be carefully evaluated for signs of inhalant and inhaled drug abuse (e.g., marked irritation, ulcerations, and perforations) and structural abnormalities (i.e., deviated septum) because these can be responsible for Mr. Estevez's chief complaint.

D. Abdominal examination   NONESSENTIAL

An abdominal examination is not indicated in the evaluation of rhinorrhea unless the patient's history is suspicious that GERD is responsible for this symptom. Nevertheless, the majority of cases of GERD are associated with a normal abdominal examination.

E. Skin examination   ESSENTIAL

A skin examination permits the identification of dermatologic manifestations of conditions that can cause rhinorrhea to assist in determining the patient's most likely diagnosis (e.g., atopy [allergic rhinitis], myxedema [hypothyroidism], and excoriations [allergic rhinitis, psychogenic rhinitis, or rhinorrhea

caused by substance abuse–induced pruritus and/or hallucinations]).

3. Diagnostic Studies

A. Skin testing for allergens   NONESSENTIAL

Skin testing for allergens is only indicated if the patient is being considering for immunotherapy. In the majority of the cases of allergic rhinitis, this occurs only after the patient fails avoidance and pharmacologic interventions.

B. Serum immunoglobulin E (IgE) level   NONESSENTIAL

A serum IgE level is elevated in any nonspecific allergic process. Thus, it lacks the required degree of sensitivity and specificity to be useful in establishing Mr. Estevez's diagnosis. A good history and physical examination are going to be much more useful.

If a serum test is going to be utilized in an attempt to confirm the presence of an allergic cause for Mr. Estevez's rhinorrhea, antibodies for IgE to suspected allergens is a superior option. This is essentially the basis of radioallergosorbent (RAST) testing. However, to be effective, there must be a very high index of suspicion that the selected substances are indeed the ones producing the patient's symptoms. Furthermore, considerable controversy exists regarding its sensitivity and specificity, especially when compared to skin testing, to accurately determine the presence or absence of an allergen.

C. Complete blood count with differential (CBC w/diff)   NONESSENTIAL

A CBC w/diff is not indicated because Mr. Estevez's list of potential differential diagnoses does not include a significant infection, anemia, leukemia, or other blood dyscrasias.

Essentially, the only abnormality that might be revealed that would offer some support to a diagnosis of allergic rhinitis is the presence of a mild eosinophilia. However, this is not considered to be diagnostic, nor does the absence of a mild eosinophilia rule out the condition. Eosinophilia can also be present in parasitic infections, leukemias, and autoimmune diseases (although the eosinophil count is generally higher than those seen in allergic processes).

D. Urine drug screen   NONESSENTIAL

A urine drug screen is not indicated because Mr. Estevez denies usage and there are no signs on his physical examination to indicate otherwise.

E. Erythrocyte sedimentation rate (ESR)   NONESSENTIAL

An ESR is a nonspecific measurement of inflammation. It could be elevated in several conditions capable of causing rhinorrhea (e.g., allergic rhinitis, asthma, cystic fibrosis, nasal polyposis, Wegener granulomatosis, and Churg-Strauss syndrome). Because of its nonspecific nature, a good history and physical examination would be much more likely to determine whether any of these conditions is responsible for his symptoms.

4. Diagnosis

A. Seasonal allergic rhinitis   INCORRECT

Seasonal allergic rhinitis can be eliminated as Mr. Estevez's most likely diagnosis because there is no seasonal variability to his symptoms. Furthermore, he lacks many of the associated symptoms of the condition.

B. Perennial allergic rhinitis   INCORRECT

Even though his symptoms occur year round, perennial allergic rhinitis can be ruled out as Mr. Estevez's most likely diagnosis because of his lack of significant allergic symptoms, the intermittent nature of his symptoms, the distinct episodes associated with certain "triggers," and a negative family history of atopic/allergic diseases.

C. Vasomotor rhinitis   CORRECT

Vasomotor rhinitis presents with symptoms that are suspicious for perennial allergic rhinitis but lack the eosinophilia and allergic phase reactant. Therefore, these patients typically do not have associated atopic diseases or chronicity of symptoms because their upper respiratory tract hyperresponsiveness is caused by dilation and/or vasoconstriction of the blood vessels to the nasal mucosa, resulting from "triggers" instead of an underlying allergic process. Additionally, unlike perennial allergic rhinitis, patients with vasomotor rhinitis generally lack a family history of atopic illnesses. Because Mr. Estevez's rhinorrhea is associated with "triggers" (e.g., eating spicy foods, strong scents, and cold environments), vasomotor rhinitis is his most likely diagnosis.

D. Food allergy   INCORRECT

Symptoms associated with a food allergy can occur immediately upon ingesting the causative agent or can present with a significant delay between eating and symptom onset (making the diagnosis more difficult). In general, the more rapid the onset of the symptoms following the ingestion of the offending agent, the more severe the allergy.

Food allergy typically presents with less rhinitis and more dermatologic manifestations than most other allergic conditions. Immediate symptoms of a food allergy can include generalized urticaria, severe dyspnea, wheezing, and even anaphylaxis. Delayed food allergies often present as gastrointestinal symptoms, especially diarrhea and cramping. Furthermore, a food allergy tends to get worse with each exposure to the offending substance. Therefore, based on his history and physical examination, this is not Mr. Estevez's most likely diagnosis.

E. Rhinitis medicamentosa   INCORRECT

Rhinitis medicamentosa is characterized by two primary features: (1) nasal congestion that is out of proportion to the degree of rhinorrhea present and (2) the long-term (> 1 week) usage of topical decongestants. Unlike with allergic rhinitis and vasomotor rhinitis, the physical examination of the nasal mucosa is frequently hyperemic and edematous, not pale and boggy. Because Mr. Estevez's primary symptom is rhinorrhea with rare postsymptom nasal congestion, he is not currently taking any medications for his condition, and his nasal mucosa is moderately pale and slightly boggy, rhinitis medicamentosa is not his most likely diagnosis.

5. Treatment Plan

A. Avoid environmental triggers as much as possible   CORRECT

Avoidance is Mr. Estevez's most cost-effective treatment. However, he obviously cannot avoid all exposure to his known "triggers" because some are beyond his control. Additionally, other helpful advice would include the recommendation for using a scarf over his nose and mouth when outdoors

in the cold to help warm the air before it is inhaled, because this will often reduce, if not eliminate, his rhinorrhea associated with outdoor cold air exposure.

B. Intranasal corticosteroid   CORRECT

Because complete avoidance is impossible and reducing stimuli as much as possible is unlikely to eliminate Mr. Estevez's symptoms to a satisfactory level, he will also require a medication. The best first-line agent for vasomotor rhinitis is regular use of an inhaled intranasal corticosteroid.

C. Immunotherapy for trees and grasses   INCORRECT

Because Mr. Estevez's symptoms are perennial, it is highly unlikely that they are caused by a specific tree or grass because of their life cycle. Even if he had a combination of seasonal allergic rhinitis (to trees and grasses) and vasomotor rhinitis, a fluctuating peak in his symptoms that correlated with the height of tree and grass season (i.e., spring through early to midautumn) should be evident.

Wanting to treat Mr. Estevez with immunotherapy for trees and grasses is an excellent example of failing to follow two of the basic principles for the practice of medicine. First, diagnostic studies should never be utilized unless they are going to provide useful clinical information (i.e., to confirm a diagnosis or follow up on a chronic medical condition). Skin testing is indicated for patients being considered for immunotherapy; because Mr. Estevez's clinical picture indicates that he has vasomotor rhinitis, not an allergic rhinitis, this test should never have been performed.

Even if there was an indication to perform skin testing on Mr. Estevez and it did yield the aforementioned results, it still does not mean that trees and grass are responsible for his symptomatology. It is not uncommon for the majority of individuals to have a mild reaction on a skin test to some common substances. Therefore, these results must be interpreted in the context of Mr. Estevez's symptoms—which addresses the second principle: treat the patient, not the diagnostic test.

Finally, there is much controversy regarding the actual benefit of immunotherapy even in pure allergic rhinitis. Most would consider it beneficial to patients who have moderate to severe allergic symptoms to dust mites, pollens, and molds; however, the data are not as strong when looking at specific non–pollen-producing plants such as grass and trees. There is no evidence that indicates that it is effective in vasomotor rhinitis.

D. Additional testing for specific food allergies and start immunotherapy if identified   INCORRECT

This choice is not indicated because Mr. Estevez does not appear to have a food allergy. Even if he had a mild food allergy, just to control his rhinitis, avoidance of the offending agent, not immunotherapy, would be the appropriate evidence-based decision.

E. Montelukast   INCORRECT

Montelukast is not indicated for the treatment of vasomotor rhinitis and has not been shown in any studies to be beneficial in this condition. However, there are some studies that suggest that in resistant cases of allergic rhinitis, especially if associated with asthma, the leukotriene receptor antagonists are an effective treatment. Montelukast is indicated for seasonal allergic rhinitis in patients who are 24 months of age or older, perennial allergic rhinitis in patients who are 6 months of age or older, chronic asthma in individuals who are 12 months of age or older, and the prevention of exercise-induced asthma in patients who are 15 years of age or older.

Epidemiologic and Other Data

The incidence of vasomotor rhinitis is unknown. However, seasonal and/or perennial allergic rhinitis affects approximately 7% of the entire US population. Children and adolescents are affected the most, with the incidence reaching 20% in this age group.

In individuals with seasonal allergic rhinitis, their symptoms appear to be directly correlated with the time of year associated with the pollination of their particular allergens. In the continental United States, pollination of trees generally occurs in the spring, grasses in the summer, and ragweed in the autumn.

Individuals with perennial allergic rhinitis are allergic to environmental allergens that are present year round (e.g., dust mites, animal dander, mold spores, and cockroach feces). However, in approximately 50% of these patients, a specific allergen is never identified.

There is a direct relationship between allergic rhinitis and asthma. Approximately 40% of all individuals with allergic rhinitis have some symptoms of asthma. Conversely, approximately 70% of all individuals with asthma have some symptoms of allergic rhinitis.

CASE 4-4

Ethan Frazer

1. History

A. Has he complained of (or appeared to have) nasal pain or a frontal headache? ESSENTIAL

With essentially a unilateral problem, pain confined to the nose could indicate a localized nasal process. The range of possibilities runs from a mucosal abnormality to a nasal abscess.

The presence of a headache is also important information to ascertain. Although there is controversy regarding whether fluid and/or pus-filled sinuses are capable of producing pain, many adults with sinusitis frequently complain of pain located over the affected sinuses, especially the frontal, maxillary, and sphenoid sinuses. Even though Ethan is too young to have fully developed sinuses, this is still a possibility. The bigger concern with a headache associated with his symptoms is a contingency spread of an infectious process into the surrounding bone (causing osteomyelitis) or into the brain (producing meningitis or an intracranial abscess).

B. Does he get frequent upper respiratory tract infections or have any structural abnormality of his upper respiratory tract? ESSENTIAL

The average child gets between three and eight viral URIs per year. Structural abnormalities of the nose, turbinates, sinuses, pharynx, and palate can significantly increase this incidence. Furthermore, these structural abnormalities can cause atypical URI symptoms without the presence of either an infection or an allergy.

C. Does he "pick" his nose? ESSENTIAL

Any type of nasal mucosal manipulation either by a fingernail or other instrument has the potential to disrupt the mucosa and produce a nasal discharge, especially one that is blood streaked, or even frank epistaxis (in fact, digital manipulation is the number one cause of epistaxis). Once the mucosa is disrupted, it is more susceptible to the acquisition of an infectious process, which could account for the change in Ethan's nasal discharge.

D. Has he placed a foreign body in his nose? ESSENTIAL

Foreign bodies are a common cause of unilateral nasal discharge. The thickness and odor of the discharge are directly proportional to the length of time the object has been present. However, caution must be employed regarding the provided response because the patient is often reluctant to reveal (or has forgotten) the event and the parent may truly be unaware of the incident.

E. Does he attend day care? ESSENTIAL

Day care attendance increases the likelihood of acquiring an upper respiratory tract infection and provides opportunity for insertion of objects into the nose without parental knowledge.

2. Physical Examination

A. Ear examination   ESSENTIAL

Because of the communication between the areas of the upper respiratory system, any patient presenting with rhinorrhea should have an ear examination.

B. Nasal examination   ESSENTIAL

Because the patient has a nasal complaint, a carefully conducted nasal examination is indicated.

C. Pharyngeal and oral mucosa examination   ESSENTIAL

Because of the communication and the close proximity of the pharynx to the nasal passageways, it is essential to evaluate the pharynx and oral mucosa in patients with rhinorrhea.

D. Abdominal examination   NONESSENTIAL

E. Hand and foot examination   NONESSENTIAL

3. Diagnostic Studies

A. Plain film radiographs of nasal area   NONESSENTIAL

Ethan's diagnosis has been established clinically based on the findings of his history and physical examination. Thus, diagnostic studies are not indicated.

If a high nasal foreign body is suspected, a plain film radiograph is generally not useful because the majority of foreign bodies are radiolucent. The exception is if there is a suspected metallic object; then, plain film radiographs are a very beneficial and cost-effective imaging technique.

B. Magnetic resonance imaging (MRI) of nasal/sinus area NONESSENTIAL

Ethan's diagnosis was established clinically; therefore, an MRI is not necessary. Considerations for an MRI in his case would include suspicion of a nasal or intracranial abscess; a breach in the bony structure involving the nasal cavity as a result of prolonged exposure to a nonmetallic, rough-edged foreign body; or an insect/larvae infestation. An imaging study would also be indicated for the insertion of a button battery that is not visible clinically; however, because it is a metallic object, a plain film radiograph or a CT is preferable to MRI.

C. Diagnostic nasal endoscopy   NONESSENTIAL

A nasal endoscopy is not indicated because the diagnosis has already been confirmed clinically.

D. Complete blood count with differential (CBC w/diff)   NONESSENTIAL

Because Ethan's diagnosis has been made clinically and a significant infection is not a concern, a CBC w/diff is not indicated.

E. Prothrombin time (PT) and partial thromboplastin time (PTT)   NONESSENTIAL

Although Ethan had blood-streaked nasal discharge, it was neither spontaneous nor significant. Therefore, there is not a concern regarding a bleeding disorder or a need for these tests.

4. Diagnosis

A. Rhinosinusitis   INCORRECT

Rhinosinusitis can produce a copious, purulent nasal discharge; however, it is almost always bilateral and associated with other upper respiratory tract symptoms and fever. It can further be eliminated as Ethan's most likely diagnosis by the foreign body being present in his nostril.

B. Nasal polyp, right nostril   INCORRECT

Nasal polyps can present as bluish-appearing masses protruding into the nostril or located in the turbinates. However, they are generally smooth in shape and tend to be a more purplish-blue than distinct blue in color. Nasal polyps are generally asymptomatic until they become of sufficient size to produce obstructive symptoms. They tend to be associated with allergic disease and a family history of such. Therefore, a nasal polyp is not Ethan's most likely diagnosis.

C. Foreign body, right nostril   CORRECT

Unless they present as an acute problem, nasal foreign bodies are typically associated with a unilateral, purulent, malodorous nasal discharge but minimal other symptoms coupled with visualization of the object on examination. Despite Ethan's denial of inserting a foreign body in his nostril, this is his most likely diagnosis because a foreign body is evident in his right nostril.

D. Anterior epistaxis, right side   INCORRECT

Although Ethan did experience some intermittent blood streaking of his nasal discharge, he did not experience true epistaxis; therefore, anterior epistaxis is not his most likely diagnosis.

E. Allergic rhinitis   INCORRECT

Allergic rhinitis can be ruled out as Ethan's most likely diagnosis because he did not have any symptoms (or a positive family history) that would indicate an allergy process was responsible for his chief complaint, except for some intermittent mild nasal congestion. Furthermore, the description of his discharge was very atypical for allergic disease.

5. Treatment Plan

A. Have his mother hold his left nostril closed and have Ethan forcefully blow his nose   INCORRECT

Although this is an effective technique to remove a foreign body in an older child, Ethan is probably too young to clearly understand the instructions for this procedure to work effectively. Therefore, attempting this procedure could result in his inhaling (instead of expelling) the foreign body, causing the foreign body to move to a higher location (e.g., the turbinates) or even aspiration of the foreign body. Aspiration could lead to respiratory obstruction, respiratory distress, suffocation, hypoxic brain damage, and a more complicated procedure for the removal of the foreign body.

B. Diphenhydramine as needed   INCORRECT

Diphenhydramine is an antihistamine used in allergic diseases. It is unlikely to have an effect on Ethan's symptoms, as his mother proved when she tried it. However, it could lead to dryness of the nasal mucosa, making extraction of the foreign body more difficult and traumatic.

C. Right nasal irrigation   INCORRECT

Right nasal irrigation is an inappropriate treatment for Ethan, or any patient with a nasal foreign body, because it can actually force the object farther into the nasal cavity, resulting in greater difficulty in removal or even aspiration of the foreign body.

D. Provide procedural sedation (or, if not available, restrain Ethan and insert topical anesthetic and vasoconstrictor) and remove the foreign body with nasal snares or forceps   CORRECT

Because his foreign body is clearly visible and irregular in shape, it is likely to be able to be effectively removed utilizing this technique. However, care must be employed to prevent damage to the nasal mucosa by the instruments and/or forcing the object farther into the nasal cavity. Therefore, it should only be done by someone who is trained and has experience in this procedure. It is poor medical practice for any HCP to perform a procedure on a patient if it is not within his or her comfort level or scope of practice.

E. Refer to otorhinolaryngologist   CORRECT

A referral to an otorhinolaryngologist could not be considered an incorrect treatment option, especially if the staff and equipment necessary to perform the aforementioned procedure were unavailable. Furthermore, one could easily argue that the inability to provide procedural sedation would necessitate otorhinolaryngologist referral because removal utilizing restraints and topical agents is going to be traumatic for Ethan. And, if the initial extraction is unsuccessful, endoscopy in the skilled hands of an otorhinolaryngologist may be necessary to facilitate the removal anyway.

Epidemiologic and Other Data

Although the exact incidence of nasal foreign bodies is unknown, it is considered to be a common problem especially in young children and individuals with limited mental capacity.

The most common location for a nasal foreign body is below the inferior turbinate and anterior to the middle turbinate on the floor of the nasal cavity.

Most nasal foreign bodies are relatively benign unless they are aspirated (and cause respiratory obstruction and respiratory distress), remain in place for an extended period of time and lead to an infection (especially if perforation of the thin nasal cavity or the nasal septum occurs), involve button batteries (because they produce immediate, marked localized tissue inflammation and necrosis that rapidly leads to septal perforation, localized stenosis, and/or adhesions), or consist of insects and/or larvae (which in rare cases can lead to nasal bone and/or cartilage destruction).

CASE 4-5
Fred Goodwin
1. History

A. Was there a history of eye trauma before the onset of symptoms?   ESSENTIAL

Any time a patient is seen with a localized area of inflammation, especially if tenderness and edema are significant symptoms, it is important to inquire regarding a history of trauma because some patients will be reluctant to self-report this information, especially if abuse was involved. In Mr. Goodwin's case it is imperative to keep elder abuse in mind as a possible coexisting problem, especially if there is a discrepancy between his history and physical findings/diagnosis.

B. Has he had any dysuria, urinary frequency, penile discharge, arthralgias, or mucocutaneous lesions?   NONESSENTIAL

The triad of urethritis, arthralgias, and conjunctivitis (or iritis or uveitis) is known as Reiter syndrome (or reactive arthritis). Mucocutaneous lesions are also often present. However, Mr. Goodwin is experiencing a medial canthus discharge, not a red eye, so this diagnosis is unlikely.

C. Does he have any abnormalities of vision?   ESSENTIAL

Any time a patient presents with an ocular complaint, it is ideal to not only question the patient regarding his or her vision but also test visual acuity before manipulating the eye if possible. In addition to an overall decrease in vision or complete blindness, this question also includes partial vision loss (e.g., central, peripheral, or other visual field defects). Changes in clarity of colors, abnormalities of light versus dark, diplopia, blurring of vision, dimness/haziness of vision, and the appearance of wavy lines, black dots, spots, "flashes" or "floaters" can represent a significant ocular, vascular, or neurologic abnormality. If any problems are identified, a distinction needs to be made between bilateral versus unilateral (and if so, is it the ipsilateral or contralateral eye from the one with the symptoms?), continuous versus intermittent (and if so, are there any known aggravating or alleviating factors?), and sudden versus gradual onset.

D. Does he have a fever?   NONESSENTIAL

The lack of systemic symptoms, as well as those of a significant infectious process, makes the presence of a fever very unlikely. Thus, this question is unimportant in determining his correct diagnosis and treatment.

E. Does he wear contact lenses? If yes, what type?   ESSENTIAL

Symptoms such as those Mr. Goodwin is experiencing can often be the result of a severe acute bacterial conjunctivitis; a subacute bacterial, viral, or fungal ocular infection; or acute exacerbations of chronic dacryocystitis. Contact lens use, especially extended-wear soft lenses, is a significant risk factor for bacterial, viral, fungal, and amebic corneal infections.

Hard contact and nondisposable soft lenses can also cause ocular infections if proper sterilization, removal, and/or insertion procedures are lax or not performed under optimal hygienic conditions. Furthermore, the reuse of disposable contact lenses is another potential cause for corneal abrasions and infections as well as conjunctivitis. Therefore, because he has corrective lenses in the form of glasses, it is essential to inquire about the usage of contact lenses as well.

2. Physical Examination

A. Bilateral visual acuity   ESSENTIAL

The evaluation of any eye complaint should begin with testing of bilateral far and near visual acuity, unless contraindicated (i.e., caustic or similar materials in eye demanding immediate irrigation to prevent further ocular damage). This should be done before any examination, manipulation, and especially instillation of drops for anesthesia, pupillary dilation, and/or staining to obtain accurate results. If the affected eye has worse vision than the unaffected eye, a reason for that discrepancy must be identified. However, it is important to remember that vision is often not equal in both eyes, and this difference could represent a preexisting refraction error.

B. Bilateral eye examination   ESSENTIAL

Any eye complaint, regardless if unilateral or bilateral, requires a complete examination of both eyes including the external appearance, the visual fields, extraocular muscles (EOMs), pupillary responses, and funduscopic evaluation to discern both gross and subtle abnormalities.

C. Nasal examination   ESSENTIAL

If a discharge is a component of the eye complaint, a nasal examination is important to perform to look for evidence of an obstruction of the nasolacrimal duct or a coexisting upper respiratory problem that could be responsible for the symptoms.

D. Carotid examination for bruit   NONESSENTIAL

Although a carotid examination for bruit would be indicated in an age-appropriate preventive examination for an 85-year-old male, it is not indicated in this problem-focused encounter because Mr. Goodwin's symptoms are not consistent with a cardiovascular cause.

However, if his visual symptoms included sudden painless unilateral vision loss, the evaluation of the carotid artery for a bruit would be indicated as it could represent a central retinal artery occlusion, which can be an embolic phenomenon from carotid atherosclerosis.

E. Heart auscultation   NONESSENTIAL

Cardiac auscultation would be indicated in an age-appropriate preventive examination for an 85-year-old male. However, it is not essential in dealing with his eye problem today. Ideally, it is sound medical practice to always listen to the heart and lungs of every patient seen; however, because of the limited time and need to focus on the presenting complaint, this is often not possible.

3. Diagnostic Studies

A. Left orbit radiographs   NONESSENTIAL

A radiograph of Mr. Goodwin's orbit is not necessary because his symptoms are inconsistent with and he denied a history of trauma; therefore, a fracture is unlikely to be present.

B. Culture and sensitivity of purulent lacrimal duct discharge ESSENTIAL

A purulent discharge from the nasolacrimal duct mandates that a culture and sensitivity be obtained to hopefully identify the causative organism and assist with antibiotic selection.

C. White blood cell count with differential (WBC w/diff) NONESSENTIAL

A WBC w/diff is not indicated because he does not appear to have a significant infection.

D. Magnetic resonance imaging (MRI) of left orbit NONESSENTIAL

The primary indications for an MRI of Mr. Goodwin's left orbit would be history of severe trauma, especially penetrating; signs and symptoms of cellulitis and the possibility of an underlying periosteal infection or osteomyelitis; and/or sudden unilateral visual field loss, making a venous or arterial occlusion a possibility. Because none of these conditions are present, an MRI is unnecessary.

E. Potassium hydroxide (KOH) preparation of discharge ESSENTIAL

Viewing a sample of Mr. Goodwin's nasolacrimal duct discharge under microscopy (after mixing with KOH) for budding yeast, hyphae, or yeast spores is indicated because a fungal infection, especially *Candida albicans*, can cause his symptoms. These findings in conjunction with the Gram stain results from the bacterial culture and sensitivity are going to be very beneficial in determining his first-line empiric anti-infective therapy.

4. Diagnosis

A. Conjunctivitis, left eye   INCORRECT

Conjunctivitis is an inflammation of the conjunctiva most frequently caused by an infectious process that can be viral, bacterial, or fungal in nature. Although generally bilateral, it can be unilateral. It is frequently associated with pruritic eyes, some degree of conjunctival injection, and a discharge of varying color and consistency. Although the discharge is frequently found in the medial canthus, it does not come from the nasolacrimal duct or produce erythema, edema, or tenderness of the area. Thus, conjunctivitis is not Mr. Goodwin's most likely diagnosis.

B. Hordeolum, left eye   INCORRECT

A hordeolum, or sty, is a small, distinct-edged abscess of a hair follicle or a sweat gland that is located on either the upper or lower eyelid. The opening of the lesion is toward the outside of the lid. However, it can be ruled out as Mr. Goodwin's most likely diagnosis because it does not cause medial canthus inflammation or discharge to be expelled from the nasolacrimal duct.

C. Acute dacryoadenitis, left eye   INCORRECT

Acute dacryoadenitis is an inflammatory process of the lacrimal gland caused by an infection, or occasionally penetrating trauma. It most frequently involves the glands on the temporal aspect of the eye. The inflammation and edema can be so severe that the upper eyelid becomes deformed. In adults, if acute dacryoadenitis occurs in the absence of a penetrating trauma or bacterial conjunctivitis, it is almost exclusively caused by *Neisseria gonorrhoeae*. In children, dacryoadenitis will infrequently occur as a complication of a rubeola, mumps, or influenza infection. Nevertheless, this is not Mr. Goodwin's most likely diagnosis.

D. Acute dacryocystitis, left eye   CORRECT

Dacryocystitis is an infection of the lacrimal gland that generally results from an obstruction of the nasolacrimal duct. Acute infections are characterized by inflammation of the nasolacrimal duct, epiphora, medial lacrimal gland inflammation, and tenderness; and almost always production of a purulent discharge with palpation. Chronic dacryocystitis often presents just as tearing and purulent discharge. Therefore, acute dacryocystitis is Mr. Goodwin's most likely diagnosis.

E. Anterior blepharitis, left eye   INCORRECT

Anterior blepharitis is an infection of the distal portion of the eyelids. The associated inflammation causes the lids to appear to be lined in red and scales can frequently be seen in the lashes. It can be distinguished from dacryocystitis because it involves the lids, not just the medial canthus; is associated with generalized inflammation, not a discrete area of inflammation; does not cause lacrimal gland discharge with palpation; and instead of being tender or painful is often itchy and burning. Hence, anterior blepharitis is not Mr. Goodwin's most likely diagnosis.

5. Treatment Plan

A. Doxycycline 100 mg twice a day   CORRECT

Because of the most likely pathogens involved (please see Epidemiologic and Other Data section that follows), the first-line, empiric outpatient antibiotics are doxycycline or trimethoprim-sulfamethoxazole.

B. Amoxicillin 500 mg three times a day   INCORRECT

Amoxicillin is not considered to be a first-line, empiric outpatient antibiotic because of its poor coverage for methicillin-resistant *Staphylococcus aureus* (MRSA).

C. Hospitalization for vancomycin 1 g IV every 12 hours INCORRECT

Hospitalization and vancomycin IV would only be indicated if the patient has a severe infection, septicemia, or underlying osteomyelitis.

D. Warm water compresses for 20 minutes four times a day CORRECT

Warm compresses are indicated to help with the edema, drainage, and pain related to his illness.

E. Referral to ophthalmologist for possible dacryocystorhinostomy or balloon dilation of nasolacrimal system CORRECT

An ophthalmologist consultation for possible dacryocystorhinostomy or balloon dilation of the nasolacrimal system is indicated to correct any underlying defects in the nasolacrimal system; otherwise, Mr. Goodwin is at risk of developing chronic dacryocystitis.

Epidemiologic and Other Data

In acute cases of dacryocystitis, the most common causative organisms are *S. aureus, S. pneumoniae, Streptococcus pyogenes, Haemophilus influenza,* and *P. aeruginosa.* Rarely other bacteria, viruses, and funguses are implicated.

CASE 4-6
Gloria Harris
1. History

A. Is she experiencing any malaise, fatigue, anorexia, myalgias, or arthralgias?   ESSENTIAL

The presence of certain systemic symptoms in a patient with what appears to be an infectious process can provide useful information to assist in discerning between a bacterial and a viral cause. Although far from absolute, malaise, fatigue, anorexia, and myalgias are more common with viral infections, whereas arthralgias are generally seen in bacterial infections.

B. Is she aware of anyone else with similar symptoms? If yes, who?   ESSENTIAL

If other individuals are experiencing similar symptoms, the probability of Ms. Harris's illness being an infectious process increases tremendously.

Furthermore, who is symptomatic and the proximity of their relationship to her assist in determining the degree of infectivity of the illness. If no one else is ill and she has an infectious process, it would be minimally contagious. Moderately contagious infections require intimate contact (a minimum of touching the other person) to be transmitted. Highly contagious infectious processes only require being in general contact with the patient (e.g., in the same room or the same crowded facility [e.g., college dormitory or military housing]) to acquire it.

This information is important because it assists in excluding or including some of the potential differential diagnoses for Ms. Harris. Additionally, it is important from a public health standpoint because certain diseases that are transmitted by general contact with the patient may require isolation, vaccination, immunoglobulin, or other prophylactic measures to prevent a pandemic situation from developing (e.g., rubeola and influenza). Also, depending on the illness, if transmission of infection is via an intimate route (as defined previously), the contact(s) may require testing and/or treatment for the disease or some of the aforementioned prophylactic treatments (e.g., sexually transmitted infections or varicella). Furthermore, with many infections, these measures often can be limited to contacts that are high risk or immunocompromised.

C. Has she noticed any icterus or jaundice?   NONESSENTIAL

Because Ms. Harris was not tested for strep and a throat culture was not obtained before treatment was instituted for presumptive strep pharyngitis, her actual diagnosis is unknown. Possibilities include a streptococcal infection that is slow in responding to the antibiotic therapy, another bacterium, a viral pathogen, a fungal infection, or a noninfectious cause for her sore throat.

Icterus and/or jaundice are signs of hepatic involvement that can be seen in conjunction with a few illnesses (predominately those with a viral origin) in which a sore throat is a predominate symptom. However, before the patient develops jaundice/icterus from a hepatic process (regardless of the cause), he or she generally has some symptoms suspicious for liver involvement (e.g., nausea, vomiting, anorexia, or abdominal pain). Because Ms. Harris lacks these symptoms, it is not necessary to inquire about jaundice/icterus unless skin discoloration is noted during the visit. However, as stated previously, identifying the presence of jaundice in dark-skinned individuals is more difficult, especially when it is mild, because the skin tone changes are more subtle.

D. What is her contraceptive method?   NONESSENTIAL

When treating a female patient of reproductive age, it is important to know if there is a possibility of pregnancy, especially if medications are going to be prescribed or recommended to the patient, because many medications can be harmful to the fetus, especially during the first trimester. (For more information regarding the US Food and Drug Administration [FDA] pregnancy categories, please see Case 2-7.)

Inquiring directly about sexual activity, contraceptive choice including consistency of usage, and last menstrual period are good determinates as to the potential of an undiagnosed pregnancy. However, because Ms. Harris states that she has never been sexually active, she does not need a contraceptive method. Even if she was not being truthful in her initial response, it is highly unlikely that she would name a contraceptive method after denying sexual activity.

E. Are her immunizations up to date?   ESSENTIAL

Inquiring about her immunization status is important because it permits, with a fair degree of certainty, exclusion from Ms. Harris's differential diagnosis list of those diseases that are theoretically prevented by appropriate immunization (e.g., *Corynebacterium diphtheria* or *Haemophilus influenzae* causing her pharyngitis and rubella or rubeola producing her rash, with her sore throat as a prodromal symptom [or even a separate illness]).

2. Physical Examination

A. Ears, nose, oral mucosa, and throat examination   ESSENTIAL

Because Ms. Harris is complaining of a sore throat and fever, in addition to her pharynx, her entire upper respiratory tract should be inspected for clues to her most likely diagnosis.

B. Neck examination   ESSENTIAL

A neck examination should be performed on any patient complaining of a sore throat. It permits evaluation not only of the cervical lymph nodes but also for other abnormalities representing conditions where the pain can radiate to the throat (e.g., thyroiditis, neck abscesses [e.g., submandibular or parapharyngeal], muscle strains, and cervical palsies).

C. Heart and lung examination   ESSENTIAL

Severe fatigue in addition to fever and sore throat should compel a thorough examination of the heart and lungs so that a serious diagnosis (e.g., infectious endocarditis, pericarditis, myocarditis, pneumonia, or pleural effusion) is not overlooked.

D. Abdominal examination   ESSENTIAL

Because Ms. Harris does not have any abdominal pain or gastrointestinal symptoms, it would be very unusual for an intra-abdominal process to be responsible for her symptoms. However, there are some conditions (primarily viral illnesses) that could be causing her symptoms that can be associated with splenomegaly and hepatomegaly. Thus, an abdominal examination is indicated. The presence of this organomegaly will assist in confirming these diagnoses; however, the absence of splenomegaly and hepatomegaly do not rule these conditions out.

E. Skin examination   ESSENTIAL

It is important to perform a skin examination to thoroughly evaluate her rash, including color, lesion type, texture, distribution, variability, blanching, temperature change, and excoriations.

3. Diagnostic Studies

A. Rapid plasma reagin test (RPR)   ESSENTIAL

Although Ms. Harris denies being sexually active, it is not unusual for individuals in her age group to not be totally honest when discussing sensitive/private issues with older authority figures, including HCPs, especially on the initial visit or until a good rapport can be established.

Because so few conditions can produce a rash on the palms of the hands and the soles of the feet (e.g., Rocky Mountain spotted fever, syphilis, erythema multiforme, contact dermatitis, toxic shock syndrome, hand-foot-mouth disease, scabies, and occasionally infectious mononucleosis) and Ms. Harris's age falls within the range associated with the greatest incidence of sexually transmitted infections, an RPR should be performed so early treatment can be initiated to prevent the sequela of this disease as well as spread to others.

B. Ebstein Barr virus (EBV) antibody titer   ESSENTIAL

Infectious mononucleosis (IM) could certainly be the causative agent of Ms. Harris's condition considering her age, her symptoms (e.g., sore throat and severe fatigue), her physical findings (e.g., splenomegaly and significant cervical lymphadenopathy), and her development of a rash (possibly caused by ampicillin). Therefore, a Monospot test (also known as a mononuclear heterophil test or a heterophil antibody test) is indicated.

C. Complete blood count with differential (CBC w/diff) ESSENTIAL

A CBC w/diff is indicated to assist in determining whether her condition is caused by an infection (and if so, its severity and probable nature, i.e., bacterial or viral) and/or a myeloproliferative disorder.

D. Rapid immunologic test for group A *Streptococcus* (strep screen)   NONESSENTIAL

A rapid strep screen is not indicated at this time because Ms. Harris has been on antibiotic therapy for over 48 hours and any antibiotic usage can cause the test to produce a false-negative result. Plus, because her antibiotic was ampicillin and there have been no documented cases of penicillin resistance to group A β-hemolytic *Streptococcus*, a positive result would likely represent a false-positive or noncompliance with her antibiotic therapy and only confuse the clinical picture.

E. Ultrasound of abdomen with emphasis on spleen ESSENTIAL

An abdominal ultrasound is indicated to obtain an accurate baseline measurement of Ms. Harris's spleen. This is especially important in Ms. Harris's case because she is a competitive college soccer player. Serial ultrasounds are probably going to be necessary to ensure that her spleen is back to normal size before she is released to compete. An abdominal injury to an enlarged spleen could result in splenic rupture and its associated consequences, including death.

4. Diagnosis

A. Syphilis   INCORRECT

Even though Ms. Harris's RPR was positive, it does not mean that she has syphilis. Nontreponemal tests (like the RPR) are utilized to screen for syphilis. A positive nontreponemal test must be confirmed by a treponemal test (such as the fluorescent treponemal antibody test [FTS-ABS]) before the diagnosis of syphilis can be made. Furthermore, false-positives can occur with nontreponemal tests, including acute bacterial and viral infections (including streptococcal infections and infectious mononucleosis), malaria, autoimmune diseases, and pregnancy. Additionally, recent alcohol consumption can alter the results. Also, Ms. Harris has signs and symptoms that are not typically seen in syphilis. Thus, syphilis is not her most likely single diagnosis.

B. Infectious mononucleosis (IM)   CORRECT

Given Ms. Harris's predominate symptoms (fatigue, sore throat, and a nonallergic rash while on penicillin), her physical examination findings (tonsillar enlargement with exudates, cervical lymphadenopathy, and splenomegaly), and diagnostic test results (a positive monospot, a leukopenia with leukocytosis, and 10% atypical leukocytes), IM is her most likely diagnosis.

C. Group A β-hemolytic streptococcal (strep) pharyngitis INCORRECT

It is always possible that Ms. Harris has a coexisting group A β-hemolytic *Streptococcus* infection in addition to IM; however, that will remain unknown because a strep screen and/or throat culture were not performed prior to instituting antibiotics (see previous discussion). However, given her degree of fatigue, marked cervical lymphadenopathy, splenomegaly, and laboratory findings, this is unlikely and certainly not her most likely single diagnosis. Furthermore, strep pharyngitis is generally associated with a leukocytosis of predominately neutrophils.

D. Allergic drug reaction to ampicillin   INCORRECT

Because Ms. Harris's rash did not have a typical allergic appearance and was not associated with pruritus, an alternative diagnosis should be sought before establishing this as her diagnosis. Given that the vast majority (95 to 100%) of patients with infectious mononucleosis who are given ampicillin or amoxicillin will develop a nonallergic rash and approximately 5% of all patients with IM will develop a maculopapular rash (rubeola-like rash generally confined to the arms and/or trunk) without being on antibiotic therapy, an allergic drug reaction to ampicillin is not Ms. Harris's most likely diagnosis.

E. Acute lymphocytic leukemia (ALL)   INCORRECT

Ms. Harris's findings of fatigue, nonresolving/frequent infections, splenomegaly, lymphadenopathy, and lymphocytosis could be suggestive of ALL; however, acute lymphocytic leukemia is generally associated with a leukocytosis, band cells, anemia, and thrombocytosis (none of which Ms. Harris had on her WBC count). Therefore, ALL is not her most likely diagnosis.

5. Treatment Plan

A. Fluorescent treponemal antibody test (FTA-ABS)   CORRECT

Because Ms. Harris has a positive nontreponemal test for syphilis, she is going to need a treponemal test to confirm (or refute) this result as discussed previously.

B. Erythromycin 250 mg one pill every 6 hours × 10 days   INCORRECT

Erythromycin is considered to be an acceptable second-line antibiotic for treating pharyngitis caused by streptococcus despite some areas of the country revealing that over one third of all cases of group A β-hemolytic *Streptococcus* are resistant. However, because Ms. Harris does not have laboratory-confirmed strep pharyngitis and does have IM, this is not an appropriate alternative for her at this time.

C. Cefprozil 500 mg once daily × 10 days   INCORRECT

Cefprozil is an appropriate second-line agent for group A β-hemolytic *Streptococcus*; however, even if Ms. Harris had confirmed strep pharyngitis and an allergic reaction to ampicillin, this drug should be avoided, if at all possible, because of the potential of cross-sensitivity between cephalosporins and penicillins.

D. Rest, fluids, and acetaminophen   CORRECT

Infectious mononucleosis generally only requires supportive measures unless a significant complication occurs; thus, rest, fluids, and acetaminophen are an appropriate recommendation.

E. Sign release for soccer   INCORRECT

Ms. Harris cannot go back to playing soccer, or any contact sport, until her splenomegaly (and other symptoms) is resolved; therefore, providing her with a medical release to do so is inappropriate.

Epidemiologic and Other Data

IM is a viral infection caused by the Epstein-Barr virus (EBV), a member of the Herpesviridae family. It is estimated that over 90% of all American adults have antibodies to EBV indicating a prior infection. IM has two predominate peaks—one in early childhood and a second one in late adolescence. The majority of cases occur between the ages of 10 and 35 years. It is generally transmitted via saliva; however, it is possible for it to be acquired via blood transfusions and bone marrow transplantations.

Within 2 to 4 weeks, essentially all the symptoms are generally resolved with the exception of fatigue and concentration difficulties. Unfortunately, they can remain for several months after the other symptoms have subsided.

Serious sequelae include meningitis, encephalitis, hemiplegia, Guillain-Barré syndrome, transverse myelitis, ataxia, peripheral neuropathies, Bell palsy, other cranial nerve weaknesses, psychosis, upper respiratory tract obstruction, pneumonia, hepatitis, autoimmune hemolytic anemia, vasculitis, myocarditis, pericarditis, pneumonia, other secondary bacterial infections, and splenic rupture; however, these complications are rare.

CASE 4-7
Hannah Issenburg
1. History

A. Is she urinating normally and crying tears?   ESSENTIAL

Because Hannah has anorexia and has only been drinking minimally, it is important to determine if she is becoming dehydrated. Knowing if she is urinating normally and crying tears is a simple gross assessment. Generally, unless a child has tearless crying and/or goes for longer than 8 hours without urinating, he or she is sufficiently hydrated.

Other clinical indictors of the hydration status clinically observable include skin turgor (gently pinching the skin over her abdomen resulting in "tenting" of skin could indicate dehydration), observation of her anterior fontanelle (if is not closed) while she is sitting up and not crying (a "sunken" appearance could be associated with dehydration), and degree of moistness of the oral mucosa (decreased saliva and a "dry" appearance could indicate dehydration).

B. Does her voice sound "muffled" or abnormal to either of her parents?   ESSENTIAL

Because Hannah's sore throat is so severe that she is experiencing dysphagia and occasional drooling, conditions associated with pharyngeal masses/obstruction (e.g., epiglottitis, peritonsillar abscess, retropharyngeal abscess, parapharyngeal infection, or Ludwig angina) must be included in her differential diagnoses. A symptom common to these illnesses is a "muffled"-sounding voice.

C. How much iron is in her multivitamin?   NONESSENTIAL

The amount of iron does not vary significantly from product to product in infants' and toddlers' vitamin preparations. What is much more important is whether she is receiving the right dosage and formulation for her weight. This is equally important regarding her acetaminophen.

D. Has she had head or neck trauma, including sleeping in an awkward position?   ESSENTIAL

Any time that a patient complains of pain (or appears to be in pain), it is essential to inquire about the possibility of trauma. Because Hannah's head and neck were apparently asymptomatic before retiring last night but symptomatic upon awakening this morning, sleeping in an abnormal position could be a potential "trauma" accounting for her apparent discomfort in these areas.

In dealing with children and pain, it is imperative to always be alert to the potential of child abuse as the cause. The presence of additional symptoms (e.g., fever, sore throat, rhinorrhea) does not rule out this possibility. In fact, it could be argued that an ill infant (or young child) is at additional risk of abuse because someone (most generally a caregiver) lacking in the skills necessary to cope with the added, chronic stress of dealing with the demands of an ill child resorts to child abuse out of his or her own frustration.

Warning signs of child abuse include conflicting information regarding the cause and/or duration of the injury, the "story" changes, the injury is inconsistent with the history, frequent visits to the emergency department or multiple providers for injuries, child labeled as "accident prone," or a history of multiple fractures (especially if identified by radiography and not by history).

E. Does she appear to have any photophobia; difficulty with her vision, coordination, gait, or extremity usage; or abnormalities of her regular speech?   ESSENTIAL

Because her mother feels that Hannah is suffering from a stiff neck and headache, all potential causes must be considered including serious, life-threatening conditions. Given her age, the mostly likely cause for Hannah would be an infectious process (e.g., meningitis, encephalitis, or deep neck structure infections/abscesses).

Other potential causes would include torticollis and congenital or acquired defects (e.g., AV malformations, benign brain lesions, cranial dystonia, or a premature complete cranial suture fusion). In older children and adults, other conditions to consider would include a primary headache condition (e.g., atypical migraines or muscle contracture headaches), a brain tumor (either benign or malignant), or a brain hemorrhage (e.g., aneurysm or a subdural hematoma). Most of these would produce some type of neurologic symptoms.

2. Physical Examination

A. Ear, nose, throat, and oral mucosa examination ESSENTIAL

Because Hannah's illness began as symptoms of an upper respiratory tract infection and fever, it is essential to examine her ears, nose, throat, and oral mucosa for abnormalities that would either eliminate (or possibly add) conditions to Hannah's list of potential differential diagnoses.

B. Neck evaluation, including meningeal signs   ESSENTIAL

Because a possible headache and stiff neck are included in Hannah's symptoms, it is essential to evaluate the neck for skin color changes, asymmetry, and discrete lesions; palpate it for masses, tenderness (including over the internal jugular veins, carotid arteries, and thyroid), abnormalities of muscle tone, temperature differences, and thyroid abnormalities; and perform range-of-motion (ROM) and meningeal sign testing (including Kerning and Brudzinski signs).

C. Lung auscultation   ESSENTIAL

Because several of the conditions on Hannah's list of differential diagnoses have the potential to cause full or partial airway obstruction, respiratory suppression/depression, dyspnea, and tachypnea, it is important to evaluate her lower airways for signs of these complications.

D. Abdominal aorta palpation   NONESSENTIAL

E. Neurologic evaluation   ESSENTIAL

Because Hannah might be experiencing a stiff neck and headache, it is essential that Hannah has a neurologic evaluation to look for signs of potentially life-threatening neurologic conditions. As stated previously, the most likely one would be an infectious process.

3. Diagnostic Studies

A. Oxygen saturation (O_2 sat)   ESSENTIAL

An O_2 sat needs to be performed on Hannah to provide a noninvasive objective measurement of her oxygenation status because she currently is experiencing a mild tachypnea. Additionally, it can serve as a baseline measurement for monitoring her respiratory status.

B. White blood cell count with differential (WBC w/diff) ESSENTIAL

A WBC w/diff is necessary for Hannah because it can provide some objective data to incorporate with the subjective data acquired via the history and physical examination to assist in determining the severity of her infectious process.

C. Lumbar puncture   ESSENTIAL

If Hannah were older, she would be better able to describe her own symptoms and cooperate more fully with neurologic testing (including signs to evaluate for meningeal irritation); then, a lumbar puncture might not be considered as an essential first-line diagnostic test. However, because of these limitations, her toxic appearance, her unwillingness to move her neck, and her mother's impression that she is suffering from a headache, Hannah needs a lumbar puncture to evaluate for the possibility of a neurologic infection (despite it being an invasive procedure).

D. Lateral neck radiographs   ESSENTIAL

Lateral neck films are indicated because Hannah is experiencing drooling (although they might also provide some insight as to why she is refusing to move her neck). With drooling, it is essential to evaluate the radiographs for soft tissue structure abnormalities the neck for specific signs of conditions that could result in airway obstruction (e.g., "the thumbprint" sign seen with epiglottitis; blunting of the laryngeal "step-off" common in retropharyngeal abscesses; or a soft tissue mass or enlargement that could represent an abscess or lesion in the retropharyngeal, parapharyngeal, or submandibular spaces).

However, a positive finding is not in and of itself diagnostic for any of its associated conditions; still, it raises the index of suspicion even higher and assists in determining what the next appropriate diagnostic or therapeutic step should include. Furthermore, a negative examination does not necessarily mean the condition is not present. It is essential in cases like this one to remember to treat the patient, not the test.

E. Noncontrast CT of neck   NONESSENTIAL

A noncontrast CT of the neck is unlikely to provide any further information than a plain film radiograph; therefore, it is not indicated because of the extra radiation exposure involved and the need to sedate Hannah for the procedure.

However, with a very strong clinical suspicion and/or an abnormal neck radiograph, a contrast CT could be very useful in further identifying the cause of a mass (or other abnormalities) of the deep neck structures.

4. Diagnosis

A. Epiglottitis INCORRECT

Epiglottitis is an inflammatory process of the epiglottis most frequently caused by an infectious process. Even though epiglottitis can produce a high fever, sore throat, headache, and drooling, it can be ruled out as Hannah's most likely diagnosis because it typically is not associated with neck symptoms (e.g., pain, decreased range of motion, or torticollis). On a lateral neck radiograph, epiglottitis is characterized by thickened aryepiglottic folds, known as the "thumbprint sign."

B. Peritonsillar abscess INCORRECT

A peritonsillar abscess is an abscess formation that occurs as a result of an extension of tonsillitis beyond the tonsillar cavity (most commonly in a superior/posterior direction). It is frequently associated with many symptoms that Hannah is experiencing. However, it can be ruled out as her most likely diagnosis because of her physical examination findings. In general, only the affected tonsil is enlarged; a mass, or at least an asymmetry, can be identified between the ipsilateral superior tonsillar capsule and the ipsilateral superior constrictor muscles; and the uvula is deviated away from the affected side. Neck radiographs might reveal a mass in the involved location.

C. Retropharyngeal infection with probable abscess CORRECT

A retropharyngeal infection is a deep cellulitis-type inflammatory infection without a distinct wall separating it from the surrounding tissue, whereas a retropharyngeal abscess is a true "walled-off" mass in the retropharyngeal space. A retropharyngeal infection and/or abscess begins as an upper respiratory tract infection followed by a moderate to high fever and dysphagia, often with drooling, torticollis, and Bolte sign (limited range of motion of the neck in extension).

Hannah's presentation is fairly typical for either of these conditions. Additionally, her neck x-ray findings are consistent with either of these two conditions. Thus, from the choices provided, this is Hannah's most likely diagnosis. A contrast CT of her neck is generally able to distinguish between these two conditions.

D. Meningitis INCORRECT

Meningitis is an inflammation of the meninges covering the brain (and occasionally the spinal cord), which is generally caused by a bacterial infection. It frequently presents as a headache, neck stiffness, and a fever, and can often follow an upper respiratory tract infection. However, it can be ruled out as Hannah's most likely diagnosis based on the normal findings on the lumbar puncture. Additionally, dysphagia and drooling are generally not associated with meningitis.

E. Lemierre disease INCORRECT

Lemierre disease, also known as postanginal septicemia, can present with similar symptoms and illness course as Hannah's. However, it generally has symptoms that Hannah did not have (e.g., pulmonary infiltrates and septic arthritis). Its distinguishing characteristic is its spread into the lateral pharyngeal space where the infection and inflammation can cause a thrombophlebitis of the internal jugular vein. Therefore, based on the information thus far obtained, this is not her most likely diagnosis. It can generally be diagnosed by a contrast CT of the neck.

5. Treatment Plan

A. Hospitalize and obtain CT of neck with and without contrast CORRECT

Because of Hannah's toxic appearance, her leukocytosis, and the potential for airway obstruction and other complications from her illness, hospitalization is essential.

As stated previously, a contrast CT of the neck is essential because it can generally identify the presence of a retropharyngeal mass (abscess) and its exact location, if present, versus a retropharyngeal infection without abscess formation. Furthermore, it evaluates the lateral pharyngeal space for evidence of thrombophlebitis of the internal jugular vein suggesting Lemierre disease instead of, or in addition to, a retropharyngeal abscess and/or infection.

B. Outpatient treatment with amoxicillin and close follow-up INCORRECT

Outpatient treatment is not appropriate for Hannah because of the severity of her infection, the strong likelihood of a polymicrobial cause, the potential of airway obstruction, and the possibility of severe, life-threatening complications. Furthermore, because of the probable polymicrobial bacterial cause, amoxicillin is not an acceptable antibiotic choice.

C. Immediately start IV clindamycin and metronidazole INCORRECT

Despite the facts that the majority of cases of retropharyngeal infections and/or abscesses are caused by a polymicrobic combination consisting of both anaerobes and aerobes and IV clindamycin and metronidazole are excellent initial antibiotics of choice, this option is still incorrect at this time because empiric antibiotics should not be instituted until sampling for cultures, sensitivities, and Gram stains is completed. Because biopsy, drainage, and/or surgical excision of the area may be necessary to obtain these specimens, antibiotics should not be instituted until after the patient has been evaluated by the otorhinolaryngologist, if possible.

D. Close observation of airway and intubation if significant deterioration occurs CORRECT

Airway obstruction is a possible complication in patients with retropharyngeal infections and/or abscesses; therefore, Hannah needs to be observed closely for this potentially fatal complication. If her O_2 sat significantly decreases and/or she develops stridor and/or wheezing, then intubation must be strongly considered.

E. Immediate consultation with an otorhinolaryngologist CORRECT

Hannah should be under the care of an otorhinolaryngologist because of the potential seriousness and relative rarity of her condition. Furthermore, because biopsy, drainage, and/or surgical excision may be necessary to not only treat Hannah but also to obtain an initial sample for Gram staining, culturing, and sensitivity testing, the consult should be immediate.

Epidemiologic and Other Data

Retropharyngeal infections and/or abscesses are generally polymicrobial in nature involving both anaerobes and aerobes. The most common organisms are group A β-hemolytic *Streptococcus*, *S. aureus*, and *Eikenella corrodens*.

It generally occurs as a severe complication of pharyngitis/tonsillitis. However, it can also result from oral/dental infections, penetrating trauma to the posterior pharynx, otitis media, vertebral osteomyelitis, and Ludwig angina.

Once a deep neck infection is established, it can easily progress to an infection of the meninges, basilar skull, mediastinum, and sheath of the ipsilateral carotid artery. If one of these complications occurs, the mortality rate is estimated to be between 20 and 50%.

CASE 4-8

Ian Jackson

1. History

A. Does he have any concerns regarding his hearing or experience decreased hearing with the vertigo?   ESSENTIAL

Mr. Jackson's symptoms are suspicious for several vestibular syndromes and other medical conditions that have vertigo and tinnitus as part of their symptomatology. These range from relatively benign causes (e.g., benign paroxysmal positioning vertigo [BPPV], migraine headaches, Ménière disease, and Ménière's syndrome) to potentially life-threatening conditions (e.g., vertebrobasilar insufficiency, Cogan syndrome, or CNS lesions). (For more information regarding the classification and distinguishing characteristics of vertigo and various conditions, please see Case 4-2.) The presence or absence of an associated hearing loss can assist in limiting the differential diagnoses to fewer possibilities. However, it is important to remember that a hearing loss may be caused by presbyacusia and unrelated to the chief complaint.

Frequently elderly individuals are very sensitive regarding any suggestion that they might be suffering from any hearing loss. Many are inclined to deny its existence, even when it is obvious in attempting to obtain historical information from the patient. Therefore, it is important when questioning patients about hearing problems that it is done in a sensitive, nonthreatening manner. The wording of this question accomplishes that task.

An even less threatening approach is to inform the patient that presbyacusia is a normal aging process and the US Preventive Services Task Force (USPSTF) recommends that all older adults be questioned periodically regarding any hearing concerns, hence the reason he or she is being asked. (The recommendations go on to state that the HCP should advise the patient regarding the availability of hearing-enhancing devices and refer him or her for appropriate evaluation if there is a concern.)

B. Does he notice a nystagmus with the vertigo? NONESSENTIAL

Even though the presence of a nystagmus (and whether it is horizontal, vertical, or rotary) and the direction of its "fast phase" are essential to accurately evaluate a patient complaining of vertigo, the evaluation for this sign involves observation of the patient for abnormal eye motions in response to EOM testing and head rotation. Because there is generally a visual fixation that prevents nystagmus, it is virtually impossible to test oneself for this condition or even notice it while looking in the mirror.

Questions that could heighten the suspicion for the presence of a nystagmus include whether vertigo worsened with lateral head movements (especially if rapid), whether focus on a particular object/spot inhibited the vertigo, and whether diplopia was present. In the latter, patients with diplopia caused by weakness and/or paralysis of one or more ocular muscles will often experience vertigo when focusing in the direction where the image's disconvergence is greatest.

C. Is the vertigo associated with a headache?   ESSENTIAL

The presence of a headache is important to ask because if he is experiencing one, it increases the likelihood that a neurologic or neurovascular process is responsible for the vertigo instead of a vestibular disorder. Examples include a CNS lesion, a CNS bleed, migraine headaches, other primary headache disorders, transient ischemic attack (TIA), or vasospastic conditions.

D. What is his relationship like with his wife?   NONESSENTIAL

Questions regarding the patient's social situation are always beneficial to enhance the patient–provider relationship and provide clues to indicate whether an underlying psychological process is responsible for his symptoms. However, before suspecting that a stress conversion disorder or other somatization disorder (which may or may not be connected to his relationship with his wife) is responsible for his vertigo, one must rule out the possibility of a physical cause.

E. Has he been experiencing any problems with weakness or difficulties using his extremities, problems with coordination, speech abnormalities, dysphagia, heart palpitations, chest pain/pressure/discomfort, dyspnea, wheezing, visual abnormalities, other ocular complaints, arthralgias, myalgias, or rashes either during or between the vertiginous episodes? ESSENTIAL

The presence of any of these symptoms could indicate that Mr. Jackson's vertigo is related to a nonvestibular cause (e.g., CVA, TIA, vertebrobasilar insufficiency, intracranial masses [both benign and malignant], intracranial hemorrhage, autoimmune diseases, vasculitis, syphilis, or allergic reactions) and where to focus follow-up questions.

Obtaining a blood pressure reading in both arms is another technique to assist in distinguishing whether a potential nonvestibular condition is present (either as the problem or in addition to it). A significant difference between the two measurements would raise concern regarding a large vessel vasculitis (e.g., temporal arteritis, Behçet disease, or Takayasu arteritis).

2. Physical Examination

A. Ear, nose, and throat (ENT) examination   ESSENTIAL

Because Mr. Jackson does have some aural fullness, hearing loss, and tinnitus with his vertigo, an inner ear, or more specifically a vestibular, condition could easily be responsible for his complaints. Therefore, examination of the ears and their communicating organs is essential.

B. Rinne and Weber tests   ESSENTIAL

The Rinne and Weber tests assist in determining whether Mr. Jackson's hearing loss is the result of a conductive problem (e.g., occluded auditory canal, tympanic membrane perforation and/or scarring, or a middle ear effusion) or a sensorineural problem (e.g., acoustic neuroma, Ménière disease, or labyrinthitis). In a pure conductive hearing loss, the Weber test lateralizes to the affected ear and the Rinne test reveals bone conduction as greater than air conduction in the affected ear. In a pure sensorineural hearing loss, the Weber test will lateralize to the good ear and the Rinne test will reveal air conduction greater than bone conduction in the affected ear.

C. Evaluation for carotid bruits   ESSENTIAL

The presence of a carotid bruit, cardiac murmur with radiation to the neck, or other abnormal vascular sounds could indicate the presence of a cardiovascular cause for Mr. Jackson's vertigo (e.g., TIA, CVA, temporal arteritis, or Takayasu arteritis).

D. Neurologic examination   ESSENTIAL

A complete neurologic examination is required in any patient complaining of vertigo. The findings can provide a wealth of information to assist in ruling in or ruling out various problems.

E. Skin examination   NONESSENTIAL

Because Mr. Jackson only experiences urticaria with his vertigo (and is not currently vertiginous) and denies any other dermatologic manifestation, a skin examination is unnecessary.

3. Diagnostic Studies

A. Audiogram   ESSENTIAL

An audiogram is indicated to confirm and quantify the hearing loss in the affected ear as well as to compare it to the contralateral ear.

B. Caloric stimulation testing   ESSENTIAL

Caloric stimulation testing is simple to perform and will provide a gross evaluation of oculovestibular function. (However, it is important to ensure that both TMs are fully visualized and without perforation before performing the procedure.)

Normally, the introduction of ice water into the auditory canal will induce a few minutes of a rotary nystagmus with the slow component deviating toward the ear instilled with the ice water. The instillation of hot water into the auditory canal will produce a jerking nystagmus with the slow phase deviating toward the contralateral ear. In a vestibular, a labyrinth, or an eighth cranial nerve abnormality, this response is blunted or absent.

C. Serum IgE antibody test for shellfish   ESSENTIAL

This test is indicated because Mr. Jackson has noticed that at least some of his episodes of vertigo have occurred almost immediately after he has consumed shellfish. Combined with the nausea and vomiting (which could be caused by the vertigo itself), diarrhea and urticaria are suspicious that he is experiencing an allergic reaction to shellfish which is causing (or contributing to) his condition.

D. Erythrocyte sedimentation rate (ESR)   ESSENTIAL

Although an ESR is a nonspecific measure of inflammation caused by autoimmune diseases, vasculitis, carcinomas, infections, and tissue necrosis to name a few, it is still indicated in Mr. Jackson's case as a gross screen for the presence

of an autoimmune disease (which is unlikely to present at his age) or a vasculitis that could account for his symptomatology.

E. Computed tomography (CT) of brain, with and without contrast   NONESSENTIAL

A CT scan of the brain, with and without contrast, is not indicated at this time because there is insufficient evidence to suspect that the cause of Mr. Jackson's vertigo is an ischemic or hemorrhagic CVA, an intracranial hemorrhage from another source, or a mass lesion. Furthermore, if any of these conditions were suspect, an MRI would be a better imaging study because of the chronicity of his symptoms and the enhanced visualization of these problems via MRI.

4. Diagnosis

A. Benign paroxysmal positioning vertigo (BPPV)   INCORRECT

The typical history for a patient with BPPV (or benign positioning vertigo, BPV) is a clustering of multiple recurrences of severe vertigo, associated with head movement (generally in the lateral position), which occurs over a period of a few days. The vertigo tends to resolve within a few seconds (generally no longer than 1 minute); however, the patient tends to feel "unbalanced" for several hours following the episode of vertigo. On physical examination, the vertigo is generally reproducible with either the Epley or Dixie-Hallpike maneuvers. For these reasons, BPPV is not Mr. Jackson's most likely diagnosis.

B. Ménière disease   INCORRECT

Ménière disease (or endolymphatics hydrops) characteristically involves subjective vertigo, tinnitus, aural fullness, and a sensorineural hearing loss that follows a pattern essentially identical to Mr. Jackson's. However, it can be ruled out as his most likely diagnosis because his symptoms do not appear to be idiopathic (as is required with the definition of Ménière disease).

C. Labyrinthitis   INCORRECT

Labyrinthitis involves inflammation of the labyrinth of the inner ear. It is also typically characterized by vertigo, tinnitus, and hearing loss. However, with labyrinthitis, the acute vertigo tends to be severe and constant for the first several days to a week; then, it gradually regresses and resolves completely over a several-week period. Because Mr. Jackson's vertigo typically resolves within 1 to 2 hours of onset, labyrinthitis is not his most likely diagnosis.

D. Vestibular neuronitis   INCORRECT

Vestibular neuronitis is associated with a very acute onset of vertigo that tends to last for several days to weeks. It is not associated with hearing loss, tinnitus, or aural fullness. Furthermore, it typically affects young to middle-aged individuals, frequently following an upper respiratory tract infection. Therefore, it can be ruled out as Mr. Jackson's most likely diagnosis.

E. Ménière syndrome   CORRECT

The following criteria must be present to make the diagnosis of either Ménière syndrome or Ménière disease: episodic spontaneous attacks of subjective vertigo that last at least 20 minutes but no longer than 5 days (average range 20 minutes to a few hours), low-tone tinnitus and/or aural fullness, and a low-frequency sensorineural hearing loss (without the air–bone gap).

The primary distinction between these two entities is that Ménière disease is an idiopathic primary condition, whereas Ménière syndrome is secondary to another condition. Because Mr. Jackson's symptoms appear to follow shellfish consumption and are associated with other symptoms suspicious for an acute allergic food reaction as well as an elevated IgE antibody to shellfish, his most likely diagnosis is Ménière syndrome secondary to a shellfish allergy.

5. Treatment Plan

A. Meclizine 25 mg orally at onset of vertigo   CORRECT

Because Mr. Jackson cannot identify any nonmedical interventions that alleviate his symptoms, pharmacologic agents are indicated. Meclizine is an antihistamine that is FDA approved for vestibular origin vertigo (and the prophylaxis of motion sickness) and is generally very effective in the treatment of vertigo caused by Ménière syndrome.

As with any medication being prescribed, the patient should be advised of the name of the medication, its indications for him or her, whether it is FDA approved for that usage, the dosage and frequency, the importance of taking it as directed, its most common potential adverse effects, and what to do if an adverse event occurs. In the case of meclizine, this would include advising Mr. Jackson of the possibility of drowsiness and not to drive after taking it (which he should not be doing anyway with acute vertigo).

B. Prochlorperazine 5 mg orally at onset of symptoms CORRECT

An additional component of the pharmacologic therapy includes the use of prochlorperazine for his nausea and vomiting. Prochlorperazine is a phenothiazine that is indicated for perioperative nausea and vomiting as well as motion sickness and schizophrenia.

Again, he will need to be made aware of the aforementioned information regarding this medicine, including its potential for drowsiness, not to drive while under the influence of it (or with the vertigo), and its off-label (albeit frequently done) usage for this purpose.

C. Avoid eating shellfish   CORRECT

Because his syndrome appears to be related to the consumption of shellfish, avoidance of shellfish should be effective in reducing the frequency of, if not totally eliminating, his vertigo.

Additionally, he should eliminate shellfish because his associated allergic symptoms appear to be increasing in frequency. Further exposure is likely to result in reactions that are more severe, including anaphylaxis and death. If he feels he cannot avoid shellfish or would have a significant risk of exposure via other means, then he should consider immunotherapy.

D. Refer to otorhinolaryngologist with experience in allergic diseases for confirmation of diagnosis and further treatment CORRECT

Because Ménière syndrome can be related to a multitude of medical conditions and is capable of mimicking many medical problems, it would be sound medical practice to refer Mr. Jackson to an otorhinolaryngologist with experience in allergic diseases for confirmation of the diagnosis and further treatment if indicated (e.g., immunotherapy for shellfish, decompression of the endolymphatic sac, and/or labyrinthectomy).

E. Refer to physical therapy for exercises to prevent/treat vertiginous episodes   INCORRECT

A referral to a physical therapist for exercises to prevent/treat vertiginous episodes is not indicated because there are no adequate studies or even case reports to indicate physical therapy is effective in the treatment Ménière syndrome. Hence, it is not considered to be standard of care for Ménière syndrome. However, it does appear to be effective in the treatment of BPPV.

Epidemiologic and Other Data

The actual incidence of Ménière disease and/or Ménière syndrome is unknown. However, it is estimated that idiopathic Ménière disease (also known as endolymphatic hydrops, auditory vertigo, and labyrinthine vertigo) is more common than Ménière syndrome, which must be secondary to another cause.

The primary defect in Ménière syndrome is suspected to be a result of an endolymphatic system distortion that accompanies this condition. Although most agree that the distortion is probably secondary to an endolymphatic sac dysfunction, the exact cause of this dysfunction is speculative (e.g., infectious, inflammatory, traumatic, and/or autoimmune cause).

CASE 4-9
James Kirkland
1. History

A. Was there any trauma involved?   ESSENTIAL

Any time a patient presents with a painful red eye, it is essential to inquire as to whether there was any trauma involved. This includes major trauma (e.g., being involved in a motor vehicle accident or punched in the eye during an altercation) and minor trauma (e.g., piece of dust or insect getting into the eye, accidentally scratching the eye with a fingernail, or coughing/sneezing hard).

B. Does he feel hopeful about the future?   NONESSENTIAL

This is one of the two brief screening questions (other one is "Does he feel down or depressed more days than not?") designed to determine whether additional evaluation for depression is indicated. It would be wonderful to be able to screen all patients at all visits with both questions; however, in the time constraints associated with the practice of medicine today, that is generally not feasible.

C. Is he sexually active? If yes, has he had new partner(s) in the previous 3 months and does he use condoms regularly? ESSENTIAL

Several sexually transmitted infections (STIs, e.g., chlamydia, gonorrhea, and genital herpes) can produce ocular symptoms (most frequently via inadvertent autoinoculation with infected genital secretions), which can result in serious visual problems (e.g., corneal scarring, corneal keratopathy, corneal perforation, and blindness). Because most STIs occur in adolescents and young adults, this is a relevant question to ask Mr. Kirkland because of his age.

The 3-month period is an arbitrarily chosen time frame; however, it is pertinent because most sexually transmitted bacterial and protozoan infections reveal themselves within a few weeks from exposure. Viral infections tend to require a slightly longer time period. STIs are either symptomatic or able to be identified via screening techniques by this time.

Inquiring about condom usage is important because condoms can reduce, but not eliminate, the transmission of STIs; hence, usage makes an STI a less likely, but still possible, cause. Frequency of condom usage is indirectly proportional to risk of acquiring an STI. However, failure to wash one's hands thoroughly after removing and disposing of a condom can increase the risk of an ocular infection as a result of accidental inoculation with infected genital secretions.

D. Is he experiencing any abnormality of vision?   ESSENTIAL

Any time a patient presents with an ocular complaint, it is essential to inquire regarding any abnormality of vision. And as with any symptoms, further details are required when present. (For a list of potential problems, please see Case 4-5.) This must also include inquiring about the need for and current usage of corrective lenses and what type as well as pre-existing visual difficulties to ensure that an old refractory error is not attributing to the current complaint.

E. Has he tried any topical treatments or remedies? ESSENTIAL

It is important to know if the patient has instilled any foreign substances, including traditional medical and/or homeopathic remedies, into the eye. This could include ordinary items (e.g., contact lenses, contact saline solution, eye irrigants, OTC medications) and atypical objects (e.g., evaporated milk ["home remedy" for conjunctivitis], acids, irritants, or feces).

In addition to knowing what was placed in the eye, it is essential to know for what purpose. Other pertinent information includes amount, frequency, last instillation, and duration of use. This assists in determining whether other conditions (e.g., irritation/infection/allergic reaction from contact lenses, contact supplies, medications, home remedies, and/or other substances; Munchausen syndrome; or deliberate self-harm) are present. Furthermore, irrigation might be indicated if limited time has passed since the most recent instillation.

2. Physical Examination

A. Visual acuity   ESSENTIAL

The first step in the evaluation of patients with an eye complaint, unless they are having difficulty with their ABCs (airway, breathing, and circulation) or require immediate and continuous irrigation to prevent further ocular damage, is to objectively measure their visual acuity for both near and far vision utilizing a Snellen chart (or similar age-appropriate instrument). If this must be delayed because of the aforementioned problems, then it should be done as soon as possible. If the patient wears corrective lenses, the visual acuity should be measured with and without them, if possible. This is useful to obtain baseline vision and objective data regarding any vision loss.

B. External eye examination   ESSENTIAL

Because the patient is complaining of an ocular problem, a complete examination of the external structures, including "flipping" of the upper and lower lids to evaluate the palpebral conjunctivae, is essential.

C. Funduscopic (and, if possible, slit-lamp) examination ESSENTIAL

Ocular complaints also require that a comprehensive internal eye examination be performed. If a thorough examination is not possible utilizing a funduscope, then a slit-lamp examination is mandatory. Many experts argue that a slit-lamp exam is required for all ocular complaints.

D. Ear, nose, and throat (ENT) examination   ESSENTIAL

Because of the anatomic proximity and the communication via the nasolacrimal duct, any patient who presents with an ocular complaint associated with epiphora and/or a discharge should have an ENT examination to evaluate for possible causes and/or complications.

E. Heart and lung auscultation   NONESSENTIAL

Although it would be ideal to perform a heart and lung examination on every patient, time constraints associated with the practice of medicine today make this virtually impossible.

3. Diagnostic Studies

A. Tonometry (or equivalent) of eyes   ESSENTIAL

Several conditions can cause a painful red eye. One serious condition that needs to be diagnosed in a timely manner to prevent complications is glaucoma. In the medical office setting, tonometry is still the diagnostic method most often utilized to evaluate intraocular pressure. When performing a tonometry, it is important to check the asymptomatic eye first not only to obtain what would probably be the patient's normal intraocular pressure but also to prevent the spread of a possible infection to the unaffected eye by utilizing contaminated equipment. For this reason, it is essential that the tonometer be appropriately sterilized/cleaned between patients.

There are newer, more convenient, simpler techniques to measure intraocular pressure; however, because of the expense and limited usage of the much more expensive equipment, it is generally not readily available in the majority of medical practices.

B. Color-vision testing   NONESSENTIAL

C. Fluorescein examination of the eyes   ESSENTIAL

Fluorescein examination of the eyes is essential in the evaluation of the red eye because it assists in determining the presence of foreign bodies; corneal abrasions and/or lacerations; potential differentiation between fungal, bacterial, and viral infections; excessive ultraviolet, both natural and man-made, exposure; welding injuries; and inadequate closure of the eyes. It is essential to remember to evaluate the nonexposed areas of the conjunctivae for abnormalities as well by retracting the lower eyelid and "flipping" the upper eyelid.

D. Serum ($\times$ 1 only) for herpes simplex virus (HSV) antibodies, types 1 and 2   NONESSENTIAL

A single serum sampling for HSV-1 and HSV-2 antibodies is not going to provide much useful clinical information.

To establish the presence of a primary HSV infection, both acute and convalescent titers are required (generally 2 weeks apart), and the convalescent titer must be at least a fourfold increase over the acute specimen's level. Recurrent infections tend not to reveal such a dramatic titer increase; in fact, they may not cause any elevation.

An additional difficulty associated with a single serum antibody testing for the HSV is the large percentage of individuals who are already seropositive (an estimated 50 to 90% of adults for HSV-1 and 15 to 50% for HSV-2). Increased prevalence for HSV-2 antibodies is found in individuals who are sexually active, have a greater number of lifetime partners, participate in "high-risk" sexual behaviors, and have another (current or prior) STI.

E. Gram stain, Tzanck smear, bacterial culture and sensitivity, and viral culture of left eye discharge   ESSENTIAL

If a discharge is present in a significantly red and painful eye (greater than expected with uncomplicated acute conjunctivitis), then an evaluation for the presence of an infection is mandatory. Even if the patient only has epiphora, if there is a high index of suspicion for an infection, a minimum of a Gram stain with bacterial culture and sensitivity should be performed.

However, with Mr. Kirkland, a viral culture and Tzanck smear are also indicated because of the vesicles discovered on his palpebral conjunctivae. The dendritic pattern throughout his conjunctivae on fluorescein staining is nearly pathognomonic for an HSV infection. Given his history and physical examination findings, an HSV infection must be considered in his differential diagnoses. The viral culture is still considered the "gold standard" to diagnose HSV. However, it is associated with an extremely high sensitivity but only a moderate specificity. Therefore, if it is positive, the diagnosis can be confirmed. However, if it is negative, it does not necessarily mean the patient does not have a herpetic infection.

4. Diagnosis

A. Acute conjunctivitis   INCORRECT

Acute conjunctivitis characteristically involves only the superficial conjunctiva resulting in mild inflammation and injection of the blood vessels; therefore, the eye is more pink (hence the layman's term "pink eye") than red in color. It is most often caused by an adenovirus infection; however, with a purulent, colored discharge, a bacterial cause must also be considered.

Additionally, itching or very mild pain is associated with acute conjunctivitis, not the moderate pain like Mr. Kirkland is experiencing. Acute conjunctivitis also tends not to be associated with any visual abnormalities, unless blurring occurs from the discharge, which is alleviated by "wiping" the eye. Therefore, acute conjunctivitis is not Mr. Kirkland's most likely diagnosis.

B. Acute uveitis   INCORRECT

Acute uveitis is inflammation of the uveal tract of the eye, including the anterior portion of the eye consisting of the iris, ciliary body, and choroid. It can produce a painful, red eye. However, it tends to be moderately to severely painful and associated with a decrease in visual acuity as a result of significant

(virtually constant) blurring of the vision, circumcorneal conjunctival injection, miosis, poor pupillary response, keratic precipitates on the cornea, and the cellular precipitates (most often inflammatory in nature) drifting in the aqueous humor. Furthermore, it tends not to be associated with an ocular discharge or epiphora. Therefore, acute uveitis can be ruled out as Mr. Kirkland's most likely diagnosis.

C. Acute iritis   INCORRECT

Acute iritis can be ruled out as Mr. Kirkland's most likely diagnosis because it is essentially another term for acute uveitis; therefore, it would have the same symptoms and distinctions.

D. Acute glaucoma   INCORRECT

Acute glaucoma is characterized by an elevated (often significantly so) intraocular pressure, a steamy-looking cornea, moderately mydriatic and unresponsive pupil, severe pain, severely blurred vision, and no discharge. Thus, it can be ruled out as Mr. Kirkland's most likely diagnosis.

E. Acute herpetic keratoconjunctivitis   CORRECT

Keratoconjunctivitis is an infection that involves not only the conjunctivae but also the cornea, producing a red, painful eye. The pain is typically mild to moderate in nature and associated with intermittent blurring of vision (but no other visual abnormalities), epiphora (and occasionally a slightly discolored thin discharge), and conjunctival injection to (but not including) the iris. Hence, Mr. Kirkland's symptoms and physical exam findings are certainly consistent with this diagnosis. The vesicles on his palpebrate conjunctivae and the Tzanck stain (or smear) revealing multinucleated giant cells are almost pathognomonic for a herpes simplex infection.

5. Treatment Plan

A. Ciprofloxacin ophthalmologic drops   INCORRECT

The lack of organisms on the Gram stain makes it unlikely that Mr. Kirkland has a bacterial cause for his ocular complaints. Therefore, antimicrobial therapy, even topical, is not indicated at this time. However, if the culture reveals an organism, then the patient would require re-evaluation of signs, symptoms, and response to treatment. Consideration would need to be given to the reported organism; and a determination regarding the presence of a true bacterial infection or a contaminated specimen would need to be made.

B. Trifluridine ophthalmic solution   CORRECT

However, this same lack of organisms combined with the numerous WBCs on the Gram stain as well as the presence of numerous multinucleated giant cells on the Tzanck smear make a viral process, especially HSV, an extremely likely cause. Hopefully, the viral culture will confirm this diagnosis. Thus, trifluridine solution is an appropriate choice at this time. It is an antiviral eye drop that is indicated in the treatment of herpes simplex virus (types 1 and 2), acute keratoconjunctivitis, and recurrent epithelial keratitis.

C. Oral acyclovir   CORRECT

Again, based on the lack of organisms combined with the numerous WBCs on the Gram stain, the multinucleated giant cells on the Tzanck smear, and the vesicles on Mr. Kirkland's palpebral conjunctiva, a viral process (especially one caused by HSV) is the most likely cause at this time. Hopefully, the viral culture will confirm this diagnosis. Therefore, oral acyclovir (as well as the other oral antivirals that are effective against HSV) is an appropriate recommendation. Furthermore, the patient should be advised of the advantages versus disadvantages of continuing the acyclovir for a minimum of 1 year to prevent further damage and recurrences.

D. Topical glucocorticoids   INCORRECT

Topical glucocorticoids should never be used by an HCP unless he or she practices in ophthalmology. They can actually cause a superficial eye infection to worsen and spread to deeper structures, causing adverse complications. This is especially true in acute herpetic keratoconjunctivitis.

E. Topical miotics and/or beta-blockers   INCORRECT

Topical miotics and/or beta-blockers are not indicated for Mr. Kirkland because they are indicated in the treatment of glaucoma, which was ruled out as outlined previously.

Epidemiologic and Other Data

Acute herpetic keratoconjunctivitis is most commonly caused by HSV-1 or HSV-2. However, it can occasionally be caused by varicella zoster virus (VZV). Because HSV corneal infections are the number one cause of blindness in the United States, it is essential to diagnose this condition correctly and treat it promptly before complications occur. Because of this high rate of blindness, it is mandatory to obtain an ophthalmologic consult on every patient with an HSV-1, HSV-2, or VZV infection (despite this not being an option in the aforementioned treatment plan).

Complications can include herpetic stromal keratitis (for which it is theorized that the destruction of the deeper layers of the cornea are caused by T cells), herpes chorioretinitis (which appears to be related to the immune status of the patient as it is more commonly seen in patients who are immunocompromised), and necrotizing retinitis (which can be caused by either of the HSVs or VZV). Serious complications such as these tend to be seen in recurrent cases. However, the first few episodes of acute herpetic conjunctivitis and/or keratoconjunctivitis can be asymptomatic or only mildly symptomatic and resolve spontaneously without incident. Therefore, these severe conditions can occur with what appears to be the patient's initial episode.

REFERENCES/ADDITIONAL READING

Aghababian RV (editor-in-chief). *Essentials of Emergency Medicine.* Sudbury, MA: Jones and Bartlett Publishers; 2006.
Alexander JL, Samadi RR, Burton J. Nose/Sinus. 228–236.
DeFlitch CJ. Throat and oropharynx. 237–241.
Guerguerian R, Singh AJ, Brunell TA. Viral infections. 341–364.
Krause RS. Hypersensitivity. 301–306.
Leaming J. External Eye. 242–253.
Lee L. Disorders of the External Ear. 223–224.
Lee L. Disorders of the Internal Ear. 225–227.
American Academy of Pediatrics (AAP) and the American Academy of Family Physicians (AAFP) Subcommittee on Management of Acute Otitis Media. Clinical practice guideline: diagnosis and management of acute otitis media. *Pediatrics.* 2004;113(5):1451–1465.
Fauci AS, Braunwald E, Kasper DL, Hauser, SL, Longo DL, et al. *Harrison's Principles of Internal Medicine*, 17th ed. New York: McGraw-Hill Medical; 2008.
Austen KF. Allergies, anaphylaxis, and systemic mastocytosis. 2061–2070.
Cohen JL. Epstein–Barr virus infections, including infectious mononucleosis. 1106–1109.
Corey L. Herpes simplex viruses. 1095–1102.
Daroff RB. Dizziness and vertigo. 144–147.
Dinarello CA, Porat R. Fever and hyperthermia. 117–121.
Gelfand JA, Callahan MV. Fever of unknown origin. 130–134.
Henry PH, Longo D. Enlargement of lymph nodes and spleen. 370–375.
Horton JC. Disorders of the eye. 180–195.
Lalwani AK. Disorders of smell, taste, and hearing. 196–204.
Rubin MA, Gonzales R, Sande MA. Pharyngitis, sinusitis, otitis, and other upper respiratory tract infections. 205–214.
Gilbert ND, Moellering Jr. RC, Eliopoulos GM, and Sande MA.(eds.) The *Sanford Guide to Antimicrobial Therapy 2008*, 38th ed. Sperryville, VA: Antimicrobial Therapy, Inc. 2008.
Gilbert ND, Moellering Jr. RC, Eliopoulos GM, and Sande MA. (eds.) Clinical approach to initial choice of antimicrobial therapy. 4–58.
Gilbert ND, Moellering Jr. RC, Eliopoulos GM, and Sande MA. (eds.) Suggested management of suspected or culture-positive community-acquired phenotype of methicillin-resistant s. aureus (CA-MRSA) infections. 73.
Lalani A, Schneeweiss S. *The Hospital for Sick Children: Handbook of Pediatric Emergency Medicine.* Boston: Jones & Bartlett Publishers; 2008.
Lalani A. Foreign bodies. 463–470.
Lalani A. Otitis media. 114–118.
Pirie J. Oropharyngeal infections. 124–130.
Nelson HS. Advances in upper airway diseases and allergen immunotherapy. *J Allergy Clin Immunol.* 2006;117(5): 1047–1053.
Onion DK, series ed. *The Little Black Book of Primary Care*, 5th ed. Sudbury, MA: Jones and Bartlett; 2006.
Onion DK. Ear, Nose, and Throat. 4.1 Ear. 221–233.
Onion DK. Ear, Nose, and Throat. 4.2 Nose/Throat. 234–240.
Onion DK, Sears S. Infectious disease. 9.21 Viral infections. 666–706.
Onion DK. Ophthalmology. 12.2 Miscellaneous. 857–863.
Pagana KD, Pagana TJ. *Mosby's Diagnostic and Laboratory Test Reference.* 8th ed. St. Louis: Mosby Elsevier; 2007 (multiple pages utilized to provide normal reference values for laboratory tests).
Ridder GJ, Technau-Ihling K, Sander A, Boedek CC. Spectrum and management of deep neck space infections: an 8-year experience of 234 cases. *Otolaryngol Head Neck Surg.* 2005;133(5):709–714.

Rosenfeld RM, Brown L, Cannon CR, et al. American Academy of Otolaryngology—Head and Neck Surgery Foundation. Clinical practice guideline: acute otitis externa. *Otolaryngol Head Neck Surg*. 2006;134(suppl 4):S4–S23.

Rosenstein N, Phillips WR, Gerber MA, Marcy SM, Schwartz B, Dowell SF. The common cold: principles of judicious use of antimicrobial agents. *Pediatrics*. 1998;101(suppl): s181–s184.

US Preventive Services Task Force. Screening for hearing impairment. In: US Preventive Services Task Force. *Guide to Clinical Preventive Services: Report of the U.S. Preventive Services Task Force*. 2nd ed. Baltimore: Williams & Wilkins; 1996:393–404. (Note: This recommendation is in the process of revision.)

CHAPTER 5

CASES IN GASTROENTEROLOGY AND NUTRITION*

CASE 5-1

Kathy Lemons

Mrs. Lemons is a 44-year-old white female who presents with the chief complaint of "constipation." It started during her adolescence and has gradually worsened. Currently, she has approximately one bowel movement (BM) per week, which requires a normal saline enema to induce. She estimates that for most of her adult life, she has experienced a maximum of two spontaneous BMs per week. This gradually decreased until approximately 1 year ago, when she started experiencing only one spontaneous BM per week. Then, about 6 months ago, the interval between her bowel movement increased to every 10 to 14 days. Because of this prolonged interval, she started using an occasional normal saline enema. For the past 3 to 4 months, she has regularly utilized one enema every Saturday evening to induce a BM. She feels that if she did not use the enema, she would not have a BM.

Despite the enema, for the past 3 to 4 months, she has found it necessary to digitally evacuate her rectum of very hard 1/2"- to 1"-sized, round or oval-shaped pieces of normal-colored feces before she is able to have a BM. (This prompted her to schedule today's appointment.) She strains "a lot" during her bowel movements; however, after experiencing a BM, she feels that she has completely evacuated her bowels. Her stool is medium brown in color and extremely hard and lumpy in consistency. She has not noticed them being narrower in their caliber, flat on one side, or "oily" or "tarry" in appearance. Her BMs are not accompanied by mucus, bright red bleeding, or a variation in stool color. She has been afebrile and has not experienced any weight change. She has not had any associated nausea, vomiting, or heartburn.

She has not altered her diet or exercise program in the past 1 to 2 years. She has unsuccessfully tried increasing her

water consumption, adding dietary fiber, and trying fiber supplements, bulk laxatives, over-the-counter (OTC) stool softeners, and multiple OTC laxatives. Her only medication consists of using a normal saline enema once a week for the past 3 to 4 months. She is not taking/using any other OTC products, prescription medications, vitamins, supplements, or herbal preparations. She has never taken iron supplements. She has no known medical problems. Her only hospitalizations have been for childbirth (vaginal delivery × 2). Her only surgery has been a bilateral tubal ligation approximately 10 years ago. Her last menstrual period was 2 weeks ago and normal. Her menstrual cycles are regular. Her family history is negative, including for colon cancer and inflammatory bowel disease (IBD).

1. Based on this information, which of the following questions are essential to ask Mrs. Lemons and why?

A. Has she eaten anything that could have been under-cooked, inadequately stored, inappropriately cooled after bulk cooking, or infected with bacteria?

B. Does she experience abdominal pain, cramps, bloating, or other abdominal discomfort with the constipation? If yes, does a bowel movement (BM) alleviate the symptom(s)?

C. Has she had difficulty in the past or currently with depression, sadness, anhedonia, anxiety, and/or feelings she must be "in control"?

D. Has she been experiencing any fatigue, weakness, paresthesias, difficulty utilizing her extremities, problems with balance, abnormalities of gait, visual disturbances, heat or cold intolerance, and/or changes in the texture of her hair or skin?

E. Does she feel the urge to defecate or experience fecal incontinence?

---

*Remember, for each question, none to all of the answers could be correct/essential or incorrect/nonessential. See page 178 for Chapter 5 answers.

Patient Responses

Mrs. Lemons denies consuming any food(s) likely to produce a food-borne illness. She has not had any abdominal pain, cramps, bloating, or other abdominal discomfort associated with her constipation. She also denies depression, sadness, anhedonia, anxiety, needing to be "in control," fatigue, weakness, paresthesias, trouble using her extremities, problems with balance, difficulties with gait, visual disturbances, heat or cold intolerance, and/or changes in the texture of her hair or skin. She does not feel the urge to defecate most of the time nor does she experience fecal incontinence.

2. Based on this information, which of the following components of a physical examination are essential conduct on Mrs. Lemons and why?

- **A.** Heart and lung examination
- **B.** Abdominal examination
- **C.** Visual inspection of anorectal area, with and without straining mimicking defecation
- **D.** Digital rectal examination, including testing of muscle strength and occult testing of feces for blood
- **E.** Anocutaneous sensation and reflex

Physical Examination Findings

Mrs. Lemons is 5'6" tall and weighs 130 lb (body mass index [BMI] = 21). Other vital signs are blood pressure (BP), 128/72 mm Hg; pulse, 78 beats per minute (BPM) and regular; respirations, 14/min and regular; and oral temperature, 97.9°F.

Her heart is regular in rate and rhythm and without murmurs, gallops, or rubs. Her lungs are clear to auscultation. Her abdomen reveals normoactive and equal bowel sounds in all four quadrants. It is soft, nontender, and without masses or organomegaly. Renal and abdominal aortic bruits are absent. Her external anorectal examination does not reveal any evidence of rectal prolapse, rectocele, skin tags, hemorrhoids, masses, fissures, tears, or other lesions at rest. With straining mimicking defecation, she has a mild rectal prolapse and paradoxical contraction of the rectum; however, no other abnormalities were noted with this maneuver. Her anocutaneous sensation and reflex are normal. Her digital rectal examination reveals a slightly enlarged rectal vault with a moderate amount of hard, brown stool that tests negative for occult blood. These are no palpable masses, polyps, internal hemorrhoids, or lesions. Her rectal tone appears slightly weak on insertion of and with having her contract her rectal muscles around the examiner's finger. Digital rectal examination also revealed a mild weakness with rectal pushing and perineal descent when she was asked to expel the examiner's finger from her rectum. She has normal relaxation of her sphincter upon removal of the examiner's finger.

3. Based on this information, which of the following diagnostic studies are essential to perform on Mrs. Lemons and why?

- **A.** Colonoscopy
- **B.** Complete blood count with differential (CBC w/diff)
- **C.** Thyroid-stimulating hormone (TSH), free thyroxine (FT$_4$), and triiodothyronine by radioimmunoassay (T$_3$ by RIA)
- **D.** Serum calcium
- **E.** Serum electrolytes

Diagnostic Results

Mrs. Lemons' colonoscopy was completely normal.

Her CBC w/diff revealed a red blood cell (RBC) count of $5.1 \times 10^6/\mu l$ (normal female: 4.2–5.4) with a mean corpuscular volume (MCV) of 84 μm^3 (normal adult: 80–95), a mean corpuscular hemoglobin (MCH) of 29 pg (normal adult: 27–31), a mean corpuscular hemoglobin concentration (MCHC) of 34 g/dl (normal adult: 32–36), and a red blood cell distribution width (RDW) of 13.5% (normal adult: 11–14.5). Her white blood cell (WBC) count was 7500/mm^3 (normal adult: 5000–10,000) with 60% neutrophils (normal: 55–70), 34% lymphocytes (normal: 20–40), 2% monocytes (normal: 2–8), 3% eosinophils (normal: 1–4), and 1% basophils (normal: 0.5–1). Her hemoglobin (Hgb) was 14.5g/dl (normal female: 12–16) and her hematocrit (HCT) was 42% (normal female: 37–47). Her platelet (thrombocyte) count was 250,000/mm^3 (normal adult: 150,000–400,000) and her mean platelet volume (MPV) was 7.9 fl (normal: 7.4–10.4). Her smear was consistent with these results and revealed no cellular abnormalities.

Her TSH was 7 μU/ml (normal: 2–10). Her free T$_4$ was 10 μg/dl (normal adult female: 5–12) and her T$_3$ by RIA was 175 mg/dl (normal adult 20–50 years of age: 70–205).

Her serum calcium was 10 mg/dl (normal adult: 9.9–10.5). Her electrolytes revealed a carbon dioxide (CO_2) of 26 mEq/L (normal: 23–30), a chloride (Cl^-) of 102 mEq/L (normal: 98–106), a potassium (K^+) of 4.5 mEq/L (normal adult: 3.5–5.0), and a sodium (Na^{2+}) of 140 mEq/L (normal adult: 136–145).

4. Based on this information, which one of the following is Mrs. Lemons' most likely diagnosis and why?

- **A.** Primary constipation, probably dysergic defecation
- **B.** Primary constipation, probably normal transit
- **C.** Secondary constipation, probably caused by hypothyroidism
- **D.** Irritable bowel syndrome, constipation predominant (IBS-C)
- **E.** Normal bowel movements

5. Based on this diagnosis, which of the following are appropriate components of a treatment plan for Mrs. Lemons and why?

- **A.** Continue weekly saline enemas
- **B.** Refer to gastroenterologist for possible anorectal manometry, defecography, colon transit study with radiopaque markers, and/or other diagnostic studies deemed necessary
- **C.** Daily mineral oil, titrated to produce one bowel movement per day
- **D.** Lubiprostone 24 mg twice a day
- **E.** Tegaserod 6 mg twice a day

CASE 5-2

Larry Myers

Larry is a 5 ½-month-old white male who presents with his mother for the chief complaint of "he's just not himself." His mother explains that Larry is normally a "very good" baby; however, for the past 2 days he has been having intermittent episodes of screaming and crying inconsolably. These episodes last for approximately 10 to 30 minutes and are followed by a single incidence of vomiting; then, he is asymptomatic until the next episode occurs. They happen approximately four to five times per day and do not appear to be increasing in severity or frequency.

The emesis consists of "curded milk"; however, it is free of visible blood, a "coffee-grounds" appearance, or bile. Today, his mother noticed a small amount of blood in his morning bowel movement, which prompted her to bring Larry in for evaluation. This is the only time she has noticed the blood. His stools are a brownish yellow and unchanged in color. She has never noticed dark, "tarry"-appearing stools; pale-looking stools; or any other color changes.

He has experienced a slight decrease in appetite as well. However, he has not had constipation, diarrhea, and apparent discomfort/pain before or during his bowel movements. Additionally, he has not been febrile or experiencing rhinorrhea, nasal congestion, perceptible sore throat, noticeable ear pain, apparent headache, suggestion of a stiff neck, wheezing, stridor, or shortness of breath. He has never been ill or taken an antibiotic.

He is not on any prescription or OTC medications, vitamins, supplements, or herbal products. He has no known drug allergies or medical problems. He has never been hospitalized nor had any surgeries, including a circumcision. He is the product of a normal, full-term pregnancy without any complications during the pregnancy, delivery, or perinatal period. He is on breast milk only. No other foods have been introduced. Larry has had regular age-appropriate health examinations with no abnormalities reported. His immunizations are up to date and were administered on schedule. His family history is noncontributory.

1. Based on this information, which of the following questions are essential to ask Larry's mother and why?

A. When was his first rotavirus vaccination given?
B. Has he been flexing his knees and hips over his abdomen during these episodes?
C. Is he urinating normally and still crying tears?
D. Is there any mucus in his bowel movements or do they look like "currant jelly"?
E. Why has she not introduced "food" into Larry's diet?

Patient Responses

According to Larry's mother, his initial rotavirus vaccine was given on schedule at 2 months of age and his last was given approximately 6 weeks ago during his 4-month well-child visit.

She has noticed him flexing his legs up tightly and thinks he could be having abdominal pain. He is urinating normally and crying tears. There has been a small amount of clear mucus in his bowel movements since the onset; otherwise, except the one with a small amount of blood this morning, his stools have been normal in appearance.

Larry's mother has not supplemented his diet because his pediatrician recommended exclusive breast-feeding until the age of 6 months.

2. Based on this information, which of the following components of a physical examination are essential to conduct on Larry and why?

A. Ear, nose, and throat examination
B. Lung auscultation

C. Abdominal examination
D. Rectal examination with testing for occult blood
E. Examination of posterior fontanelle

Physical Examination Findings

Larry weighs 20 lb. A height is not obtainable because he is experiencing an episode of pain and would not permit full extension of his legs. His other vital signs are pulse, 140 BPM and regular; respiratory rate, 40/min and regular; and rectal temperature, 100.8°F.

His auditory canals are normal in color, without edema or abnormal discharge. His tympanic membranes (TMs) are normal bilaterally. His nasal mucosa is normal in color and reveals no edema, discharge, or lesions bilaterally. His oral mucosa is normal in color, moist, and without lesions. His pharynx is normal in color and without edema, tonsillar enlargement, or exudates. His uvula is midline.

His lungs are clear to auscultation.

His abdominal exam reveals hyperactive bowel sounds in the right upper quadrant and hypoactive bowel sounds in the remaining quadrants. His abdomen is somewhat firm and reveals a tender, "sausage-shaped" mass in his right upper quadrant. His right lower quadrant appears "empty" (positive Dance sign). There are no other abnormalities noted. His rectal examination is normal with soft brown stool in the rectal vault. It tests positive for occult blood.

His posterior fontanelle is closed.

3. Based on this information, which of the following diagnostic studies are essential to perform on Larry and why?

A. Complete blood count with differential (CBC w/diff)
B. Urinalysis, including microscopic examination
C. Blood urea nitrogen (BUN)
D. Electrolytes
E. Kidneys, ureters, and bladder (KUB) radiograph

Diagnostic Findings

His CBC, including his white blood count, hematocrit, and hemoglobin; BUN; and electrolytes were within normal limits for his age. His urinalysis was unremarkable.

His abdominal radiograph revealed a decreased gas pattern in the cecal area but a pocket of increased gas in the colon with a soft tissue mass projecting into it (positive crescent sign) and what appears to be a double lumen in that area (positive target or doughnut sign).

4. Based on this information, which one of the following is Larry's most likely diagnosis and why?

A. Appendicitis
B. Early urinary tract infection
C. Perforated small intestine
D. Early viral gastroenteritis
E. Intussusception

5. Based on this diagnosis, which of the following are appropriate components of a treatment plan for Larry and why?

A. Surgical consult
B. Contrast air barium enema

C. Hospitalization
D. Oral ampicillin
E. BRAT (bananas, rice, applesauce, and toast) diet

CASE 5-3
Michael Nestor

Mr. Nestor is a 37-year-old African American male who presents with the chief complaint of abdominal pain. It has been present for approximately 6 months and is described as a burning, gnawing, "hunger-like" epigastric pain. He estimates that it occurs four to five times per day. Typically the pain begins approximately 2 to 3 hours after he has eaten. It occasionally awakens him at night (approximately two to three times per month). It appears to be alleviated by eating food or taking two OTC calcium-based antacid tablets (which he averages two to three doses per day). However, for the past week, the antacid has not been providing him with the full relief that it previously afforded.

He is not experiencing any fever, chills, anorexia, nausea, vomiting, hematemesis, jaundice, icterus, diarrhea, constipation, hematochezia, melena, or other bowel changes. The pain does not radiate to his back, shoulders, or arms. He has no associated lower abdominal pain, chest pain/pressure, dyspnea, orthopnea, or pedal edema.

He has no known medical problems. He has never been hospitalized nor had surgery. His only medication is the OTC calcium-based antacids. He is not taking any other OTC or prescription medications, vitamins, supplements, or herbal therapies.

He smokes one pack of cigarettes per day and has done so for the past 20 years. He rarely drinks alcohol (defined as two to three beers per weekend). He denies the use of illicit substances. He is single and lives alone. His family history is noncontributory, including any gastrointestinal (GI) malignancies or conditions.

1. Based on this information, which of the following questions are essential to ask Mr. Nestor and why?

A. Is the pain associated with dysphagia?
B. Has he been experiencing any depression/sadness, anhedonia, changes in sleep (aside from the awakenings secondary to his epigastric pain), increased stress, or dissatisfaction with life in general?
C. Has he experienced a recent unintentional weight change?
D. Is he experiencing any pyrosis or reflux of stomach contents?
E. How often does he have a bowel movement?

Patient Responses

He denies dysphagia, pyrosis, gastric content reflux, weight change, depression/sadness, anhedonia, additional sleep changes, increased stress, or dissatisfaction with life in general. He has a bowel movement every morning after breakfast.

2. Based on this information, which of the following components of a physical examination are essential to conduct on Mr. Nestor and why?

A. Palpation of thyroid
B. Palpation of cervical lymph nodes

C. Abdominal examination
D. Rectal examination with occult blood testing of stool
E. Skin and sclera examination for discolorations

Physical Examination Findings

Mr. Nestor is 6'2" tall and weighs 225 lb (BMI = 28.9). Other vital signs are BP, 128/68 mm Hg; pulse, 84 BPM and regular; respirations, 14/min and regular; and oral temperature, 98.5°F.

His thyroid is midline and normal in size, shape, and texture. There are no palpable masses or tenderness. His cervical lymph nodes are normal in size, not enlarged, and nontender.

His abdomen reveals normoactive and equal bowel sounds in all four quadrants; slight tenderness without rebound or rigidity in his epigastric area only; and no organomegaly or masses. His rectal examination was normal except his stool tested positive for occult blood.

His skin and sclera were normal in color.

3. Based on this information, which of the following diagnostic studies are essential to perform on Mr. Nestor and why?

A. Upper GI endoscopy with biopsy for *Haemophilus pylori*
B. Barium upper GI radiographic series
C. Colonoscopy
D. Complete blood count with differential (CBC w/diff)
E. Serum *H. pylori* antibodies; amylase and gastrin levels

Diagnostic Results

Mr. Nestor's upper endoscopy was normal except for a superficial duodenal ulceration of ~0.75 cm × 0.75 cm in size with minor bleeding. His histology and rapid urea testing were both positive for *H. pylori*. Histology was negative for precancerous or cancerous changes.

His barium upper GI series was normal except for a superficial duodenal ulceration of ~0.75 cm in diameter.

His colonoscopy did not reveal any abnormalities.

His CBC was within normal limits.

His serum *H. pylori* antibodies were positive (normal: negative). His amylase and gastrin levels were normal.

4. Based on this information, which one of the following is Mr. Nestor's most likely diagnosis and why?

A. Duodenal ulcer, secondary to *H. pylori* infection
B. Gastric ulcer, secondary to *H. pylori* infection and smoking
C. Zollinger-Ellison syndrome
D. Gastroesophageal reflux disease (GERD), secondary to *H. pylori* infection
E. Gastritis, secondary to *H. pylori* infection

5. Based on this diagnosis, which of the following are appropriate components of Mr. Nestor's treatment plan and why?

A. Omeprazole 20 mg twice a day for 14 days, then decreased to once a day for 1 to 2 months
B. Clarithromycin 500 mg twice a day plus amoxicillin 1 g twice a day for 14 days
C. Metronidazole 250 mg four times a day plus tetracycline 500 mg four times a day for 14 days

D. Retest for *H. pylori* with serology 1 week after completion of the antibiotic component of the treatment
E. Retest for *H. pylori* with either stool antigen assay or urea breath test after completion of the antibiotic portion of the treatment

CASE 5-4
Norma Olsen

Mrs. Olsen is a 58-year-old African American female who presents with the chief complaint of abdominal pain. For the past 10 months, she has been experiencing intermittent, crampy, right and left lower abdominal pain with diarrhea. It comes in distinct episodes that begin as a mild lower abdominal discomfort; then, within 10 to 60 minutes, it has progressed to its maximum (6 out of 10 on the pain scale) intensity. Shortly after her pain has reached its peak, she experiences one loose, watery BM. After the BM, the pain is resolved and she is asymptomatic except for her underlying symptoms of fatigue and arthralgias, which have been present for "years" without change. She attributes these to "a little arthritis."

When her GI symptoms commenced, she experienced the abdominal pain and diarrhea approximately four or five times per day in cycles lasting from 3 to 7 days with ~1 to 1 ½ months between occurrences. They have been gradually increasing in frequency and duration, but not in intensity. She currently experiences ~5 to 10 BMs per day for 10 to 14 days; however, the interval of ~1 to 1 ½ months between episodes has remained consistent. She is not aware of any precipitating factors. She is also unaware of any aggravating factors, including specific foods (especially dairy intake), or any alleviating factors except for the BM following her abdominal pain. She has currently been experiencing her gastrointestinal symptoms continuously for 10 consecutive days.

She has never passed any bright red blood per rectum, with or without a bowel movement. Her stools are not "tarry" or "oily" appearing. She does have some clear to brownish mucoid discharge in conjunction with some, but not all, of the diarrheal episodes. She is unable to identify a precipitating factor for the occurrence of the mucus. She has not noticed her stools being paler in color. There has been no change in her stool's consistency except for when she is experiencing the diarrhea.

She does have some lower abdominal bloating and fecal urgency; however, she has never experienced fecal incontinence or abnormal flatulence. Occasionally, she feels like she is febrile on her symptomatic days; however, she has never checked her temperature with a thermometer. Her symptoms are not associated with anorexia, eating more, nausea, vomiting, or constipation. She has never experienced dysuria, urinary urgency or frequency, hematuria, or vaginal discharge. She has not been sexually active since her husband died approximately 1 year ago. She feels that she has accepted that loss.

Mrs. Olsen has no known medical problems. Her only surgeries include a total abdominal hysterectomy with bilateral ovariosalpingectomy (TAH/BSO) approximately 18 years ago for uterine fibroids and an appendectomy approximately 25 years ago for acute appendicitis. Otherwise, she has never been hospitalized. She takes no prescription or over-the-counter medications, vitamins, supplements, or herbal preparations.

She has not been on an antibiotic for a minimum of 2 years. She has never smoked or drank alcohol. She does not have regular age-appropriate preventive health examinations or diagnostic tests. Her family history is positive for both of her parents dying from ischemic cerebral vascular accidents in their late 70s. Otherwise, her family history is negative, including for colon cancer, IBD, and any other gastrointestinal disorders.

1. Based on this information, which of the following questions are essential to ask Mrs. Olsen and why?

A. Does she ever have to get up at night to have a bowel movement?
B. Has she experienced any unintentional weight change since her illness began?
C. Had she acquired a pet before the onset of her symptoms?
D. What joints tend to be involved with the "arthritis"?
E. Has she ever been diagnosed with iritis, uveitis, episcleritis, sclerosing cholangitis, pyoderma gangrenosum, thromboembolic disease, erythema nodosum, urinary calculi, urinary obstruction, osteoporosis, endocarditis, myocarditis, and/or interstitial lung disease?

Patient Responses

Occasionally, Mrs. Olsen will experience a nocturnal bowel movement. She estimates it occurs approximately once or twice per week when she is experiencing symptoms. It never occurs between the clusters of her symptoms.

She has experienced a 6-lb weight loss in the past 4 months; however, she is actively trying to lose weight by eating "smarter."

She does not have any pets nor did she have any before the onset of her symptoms.

The joints that are most affected by her "arthritis" are her knees, ankles, and proximal-interphalangeal (PIP) joints. The arthritis appears to be present and equal bilaterally.

She has never been diagnosed with iritis, uveitis, episcleritis, sclerosing cholangitis, pyoderma gangrenosum, thromboembolic disease, erythema nodosum, urinary calculi, urinary obstruction, osteoporosis, endocarditis, myocarditis, and/or interstitial lung disease.

2. Based on this information, which of the following components of a physical examination are essential to conduct on Mrs. Olsen and why?

A. Thyroid palpation
B. Abdominal examination
C. Rectal examination with fecal occult blood testing
D. Pelvic examination
E. Hand examination

Physical Examination Findings

Mrs. Olsen is 5'3" tall and weighs 176 lb (BMI = 31.2). Other vital signs are BP, 120/64 mm Hg; pulse, 78 BPM and regular; respirations, 10/min and regular; and oral temperature, 99.8°F.

Her thyroid is midline and normal in size, shape, and consistency. It has no palpable masses or tenderness.

Her abdominal examination reveals normoactive and equal bowel sounds in all four quadrants. Her abdomen is soft.

She does have some mild right and left lower quadrant tenderness, with the right being slightly greater; however, there is no rebound or rigidity. There are no masses or organomegaly noted. She has a diagonal surgical scar approximately 5 cm in length in her right lower quadrant consistent with her history of a previous appendectomy and a 14-cm horizontal suprapubic surgical scar consistent with her history of a previous TAH/BSO.

Her rectal examination reveals a small fissure at 12 o'clock but no other abnormalities. With straining mimicking defecation, her fissure is more pronounced and she experiences a clear to moderate brownish mucoid discharge. No rectal prolapse, paradoxical contraction of the rectum, or other abnormalities are noted with this maneuver. Her digital rectal examination (DRE) is normal except for being able to feel a mass just at the tip of the examining finger. Her stool tested negative for occult blood. Her rectal tone appears normal.

Her pelvic examination is unremarkable except her uterus and ovaries are not palpable.

Her hands reveal a slight amount of joint enlargement over her PIPs, with minimal edema and no increased warmth or erythema bilaterally. She has full range of motion bilaterally. Her muscle strength in her hands is normal and slightly greater on the right (she is right-handed). She does not have any discoloration of her fingers, abnormal capillary refill, or clubbing of her nails.

3. Based on this information, which of the following diagnostic studies are essential to perform on Mrs. Olsen and why?

    A. Complete blood count with differential (CBC w/diff)
    B. Thyroid-stimulating hormone (TSH), free thyroxine (FT$_4$), and triiodothyronine by radioimmunoassay (T$_3$ by RIA)
    C. Antiendomysial antibodies
    D. Colonoscopy
    E. Stool sample or rectal biopsy for immunoassays for *Clostridium difficile* toxins A and B

Diagnostic Results

Mrs. Olsen's CBC w/diff revealed an RBC count of 4.4×10^6/µl (normal female: 4.2–5.4) with an MCV of 81 µm^3 (normal adult: 80–95), an MCH of 28 pg (normal adult: 27–31), an MCHC of 33 g/dl (normal adult: 32–36), and an RDW of 11.5% (normal adult: 11–14.5). Her WBC count was 10,000/mm^3 (normal adult: 5000–10,000) with 55% neutrophils (normal: 55–70), 40% lymphocytes (normal: 20–40), 2% monocytes (normal: 2–8), 2% eosinophils (normal: 1–4), and 1% basophils (normal: 0.5–1). Her Hgb was 12.2 g/dl (normal female: 12–16) and her HCT was 38% (normal female: 37–47). Her platelet (thrombocyte) count was 200,000/mm^3 (normal adult: 150,000–400,000) and her MPV was 7.8 fl (normal: 7.4–10.4). Her smear was consistent with these results and revealed no cellular abnormalities.

Her TSH was 8 µU/ml (normal: 2–10). Her FT$_4$ was 9 µg/dl (normal adult female: 5–12) and her T$_3$ by RIA was 150 mg/dl (normal adult 20–50 years old: 70–205).

Her BUN was 20 mg/dl (normal adult: 10–20). Her electrolytes revealed a carbon dioxide of 25 mEq/L (normal: 23–30), a chloride of 99 mEq/L (normal: 98–106), a potassium of 3.6 mEq/L (normal adult: 3.5–5.0), and a sodium of 137 mEq/L (normal adult: 136–145).

Her antiendomysial antibodies were negative (normal: negative).

Her colonoscopy confirmed the presence of a small rectal fissure at 12 o'clock (as seen on her physical examination). Additionally, it revealed segmental involvement with stellate and linear ulcerations throughout the distal one half of her colon and upper one third of her rectum. She also had three large (3–4 cm in size), round, slightly irregular-surfaced, pedunculated masses in her descending colon. The most distal nearly borders on the anal verge. Repeat testing for occult blood was positive. Histology of the ulcerations revealed granulomatous, but no neoplastic, changes. The pedunculated masses were excised and their histology revealed adenomatous polyps without any precancerous or malignant changes.

4. Based on this information, which one of the following is Mrs. Olsen's most likely diagnosis and why?

    A. Irritable bowel syndrome (IBS) with polyps
    B. Crohn disease with polyps
    C. Ulcerative colitis with polyps
    D. Familial adenomatous polyposis
    E. Celiac disease

5. Based on this diagnosis, which of the following are appropriate components of a treatment plan for Mrs. Olsen and why?

    A. Colectomy
    B. Well-balanced, heart-smart diet
    C. Trial of avoidance of dairy products
    D. Cholestyramine 2 to 4 mg two to three times per day before meals
    E. Prednisone 10 mg bid

CASE 5-5

Oscar Phillips

Mr. Phillips is a 43-year-old Asian American male who presents with intermittent, right upper quadrant pain. He describes it as being "sharp but crampy" in nature and rates it as a 6 out of a 10 on the pain scale during its maximum intensity. It is associated with nausea, vomiting, malaise, fatigue, low-grade fever (maximum oral temperature, 99.2°F), generalized myalgias, enlarging abdominal girth, and slight pedal edema. He vomits "acidy-watery stuff" approximately three to four times a day; however, it is unrelated to his pain. He has not noticed any gross blood, "coffee ground"-looking materials, or fecal matter in his emesis. His symptoms are unrelated to eating or fasting. He is unaware of any aggravating or alleviating factors. His has been ill for approximately 1 month and his symptoms are worsening in frequency, duration, and severity.

His only other symptoms are halitosis (despite brushing his teeth more frequently, using breath mints, and chewing gum) and dysgeusia. He denies having flulike symptoms, a serum sickness–type illness, or any prodromal symptoms within the 3 months prior to the onset of his symptoms. He is not experiencing any reflux of his stomach contents into his esophagus and/or oropharynx, constipation, diarrhea, melena, hematochezia, other bowel changes, fever, chills, or arthralgias.

He has not noticed any color change of his bowels, urine, skin, or eyes.

His history is negative for medical problems, hospitalizations, surgeries, or blood transfusions. He is not currently taking (or was taking at the time of his illness onset) any prescription or over-the-counter medications, vitamins, supplements, or herbal preparations. He drinks two to six glasses of wine per day. He denies any substance abuse or use. He has never smoked cigarettes or done any foreign traveling. He admits to having unprotected sex with men, but never with male prostitutes. He has been in a monogamous relationship with one male partner (who is not ill) for the past 2 months. During the year before that, he "rotated" among six different men. He estimates his total number of lifetime male partners to be more than 100. None of his previous partners is ill to his knowledge. His family history is noncontributory.

1. Based on this information, which of the following questions are essential to ask Mr. Phillips and why?

   A. Has he noticed a change in his weight and/or appetite?
   B. Has he ever had a tattoo?
   C. Does he consume raw seafood?
   D. Has he noticed any mental status, cognitive, or mood changes?
   E. When was the last time he was sexually active with a woman?

Patient Responses

Mr. Phillips has gained 8 lb since the onset of his illness despite a moderate decrease in appetite. He does not eat seafood.

He and his current partner got matching tattoos approximately 2 months ago; however, they were done at a tattoo parlor that was supposedly certified by the local health department.

He hasn't noticed any mental status, cognitive, or mood changes; however, he states that his partner has been complaining that he has been more irritable and forgetful lately.

He has never been sexually active with women.

2. Based on this information, which of the following components of a physical examination are essential to conduct on Mr. Phillips and why?

   A. Oropharyngeal examination
   B. Heart and lung auscultation
   C. Abdominal and rectal examination
   D. Skin and sclera examination
   E. Gastro-omental, gastric, colic, and superior mesenteric lymph node palpation

Physical Examination Findings

Mr. Phillips is 5'8" tall and weighs 167 lb (BMI = 25.3). Other vital signs are BP, 138/78 mm Hg; pulse, 90 BPM and regular; respiratory rate, 18/min and regular; and oral temperature, 99.1°F.

His oral mucosa, tongue, gingivae, and pharynx are free from erythema, edema, and abnormal lesions. His teeth appear to be normal and in good repair. However, he does have malodorous breath consistent with the unique odor of fetor hepaticus.

His heart is regular in rate and rhythm without murmurs, rubs, or gallops. His lungs are clear to auscultation.

His abdomen reveals normoactive and equal bowel sounds in all four quadrants; however, in all areas, they display a distant resonance. His abdomen is soft and moderately distended and appears to have fluid present, which is confirmed by placing the patient in the left lateral decubitus position. He has superior right upper quadrant tenderness that is similar to, but not as intense as, the pain he has been experiencing. Hepatosplenomegaly also appears to be present; however, because of the ascites it is difficult to accurately assess the organ's size. Additionally, he has varicose veins that start at his umbilicus and extend outward (caput medusae) and multiple spider telangiectasias.

His external rectal examination is normal except for the presence of anal fissures in the 12 and 6 o'clock positions. He has small internal hemorrhoids and slight decreased muscle tone; otherwise, his rectal examination, including his stool testing, is normal. (For more information regarding false-negative results from a single stool test for occult blood, please refer to Cases 5-1 and 5-2.) His prostate is normal sized, smooth, and nontender.

His skin reveals a hint of mild jaundice, which is confirmed by a yellowish discoloration of his sclera. He has multiple spider telangiectasias all over his body; they are worse on his trunk and face. He also has palmar erythema and bilateral Dupuytren contractures, but no asterixis. He has 1+ pedal edema in his ankles and feet that is equal bilaterally. Additionally, he has mild gynecomastia. His skin is warm and moist to touch and without areas of increased or decreased temperature. His capillary refill is normal and equal bilaterally in his hands and feet. His pulses are normal and equal bilaterally.

Gastro-omental, gastric, colic, and superior mesenteric lymph nodes are not palpable.

3. Based on this information, which of the following diagnostic studies are essential to perform on Mr. Phillips and why?

   A. Alanine aminotransferase (ALT), aspartate aminotransferase (AST), and α-glutamyl transferase (GGT)
   B. Prothrombin time (PT), total protein, albumin, and bilirubin (total, direct, and indirect)
   C. Hepatitis B surface antigen (HBsAg), hepatitis B surface antibody (HBsAb), hepatitis B core antibody total (HBcAb total), hepatitis B core antibody immunoglobulin M (HBcAb IgM), hepatitis B e-antigen (HBeAg), and hepatitis B e-antibody (HBeAb)
   D. Abdominal ultrasound
   E. Serum α-fetoprotein (AFP)

Diagnostic Results

Mr. Phillips' ALT was 170 units/L (normal: 4–36), his AST was 165 units/L (normal: 0–35), and his GGT was 107 units/L (normal: 8–38). His PT was 24 seconds (normal: 11–25).

His total protein was 4 g/dl (normal adult: 6.4–8.3) and his albumin was 1.5 g/dl (normal adult: 2.3–3.4). His total bilirubin was 6 mg/dl (normal: 0.3–1.0), his direct bilirubin was 0.5 mg/dl (normal: 0.1–0.3), and his indirect bilirubin was 5.5 mg/dl (normal: 0.2–0.8).

His HBsAg was negative, HBsAb was negative, HBcAb was positive, HBcAb IgM was negative, HBeAg was positive, and HBeAb was positive.

His abdominal ultrasound confirmed the presence of moderate ascites and hepatosplenomegaly. His AFP was 45 ng/ml (normal adult male: < 40).

4. Based on this information, which one of the following is Mr. Phillips' most likely diagnosis and why?

  A. Acute hepatitis B
  B. Chronic hepatitis B, immune tolerant phase
  C. Chronic hepatitis B, immune active phase
  D. Chronic hepatitis B, inactive (or remission) phase
  E. Liver cancer

5. Based on this diagnosis, which of the following are appropriate components of a treatment plan for Mr. Phillips and why?

  A. Liver biopsy
  B. Hepatitis B virus (HBV) DNA levels
  C. Hepatitis A virus antibody (HAV-Ab) IgM and IgG
  D. Interferon alfa-2b, peginterferon alfa-2a, or lamivudine starting 6 months after his HBeAg becomes negative
  E. Hepatitis D virus antigen (HDV-Ag), hepatitis D virus antibody total (HDV-Ab total), and hepatitis D virus antibody IgM (HDV-Ab IgM)

CASE 5-6

Pricilla Queens

Ms. Queens is a 46-year-old Hispanic American female who presents for an initial visit with the chief complaint of abdominal pain. She describes it as epigastric in location, severe (10 out of 10 on the pain scale), steady, boring, and radiating into her back. The pain started immediately after she ate lunch, approximately 4 hours ago, and has continued to worsen in intensity. For lunch she had two slices of pepperoni and cheese pizza with a regular cola. Three of her co-workers shared the pizza with her and they are completely asymptomatic. She does not have any food allergies or problems with the consumption of dairy products. Her pain is alleviated slightly by sitting up and hugging her knees against her chest. It intensifies when she is supine or walking. Otherwise, she is not aware of any aggravating or alleviating factors. She denies having any symptoms before the onset of the pain or any previous episodes of similar-type pain.

Her pain is associated with anorexia, nausea, vomiting, fever (although she has not verified this with a thermometer), and diaphoresis. She has now vomited six times. Her emesis initially consisted of undigested food particles; currently it is "pure acid." There is no visible blood, "coffee grounds"-appearing material, mucus, fecal-looking substances, or other abnormalities in her emesis. She is not currently (or previously) experiencing any pain elsewhere in her abdomen, diarrhea, constipation, hematochezia, melena, pale or "clay-colored" stools, passage of mucus with or without a BM, or other bowel changes.

She denies chest pain/pressure, shortness of breath, wheezing, vertigo, lightheadedness, presyncope, syncope, headache, arthralgias, myalgias, fatigue, weakness, recent weight changes, hematuria, dysuria, urinary urgency, polydipsia, polyuria, or neuropathies.

Her only known medical problem is migraine headaches. She has never been hospitalized. Her only surgery was a bilateral tubal ligation (BTL) performed at the age of 26 years. Her medications consist of valproic acid 600 mg twice a day for prophylaxis of migraines and sumatriptan IM as needed for breakthrough headaches. She takes no other prescription or OTC medications, vitamins, supplements, or herbal preparations. She denies drinking alcohol, taking illicit drugs/substances, or smoking cigarettes. Her last menstrual period was 1 week ago and normal; she has regular menstrual cycles. She has been cohabitating with her current partner, in what she understands to be a mutually monogamous relationship, for the past 26 years. He accompanies her today and refuses to leave the examination room during any portion of the visit despite multiple staff requests. Ms. Queens provides written consent for him to remain with her during the entire visit. Her family history is noncontributory.

1. Based on this information, which of the following questions are essential to ask Ms. Queens and why?

  A. Where in her back does the pain radiate?
  B. Has she noticed any skin discolorations, rashes, and/or lesions?
  C. How old is her youngest child?
  D. How often does she have a "breakthrough" headache? When did she take her last dose of sumatriptan? Does the sumatriptan always work? If yes, how many doses are required? If not, what is effective?
  E. Has she had any recent trauma?

Patient Responses

Her pain radiates into her intrascapular area and bilateral flanks. She denies any dermatologic manifestations or recent trauma. She has approximately two to three "breakthrough" headaches per year. The last one was approximately two months ago. They are always alleviated with a single dose of sumatriptan and sleep. She does not have any children.

2. Based on this information, which of the following components of a physical examination are essential to conduct on Ms. Queens and why?

  A. Evaluation of salivary glands and ducts
  B. Eye examination
  C. Heart and lung auscultation
  D. Abdominal examination
  E. Skin examination

Physical Examination Findings

Ms. Queens is 5'5" tall and weighs 150 lb (BMI = 25.0). Other vital signs are BP, 100/56 mm Hg; pulse, 112 BPM and regular; respirations, 20/min and regular; and oral temperature, 101.2°F. She is sitting on the exam table, slightly bent forward, with her legs flexed tightly against her chest and her arms wrapped tightly around her legs, crying. She appears to be in acute distress.

Her oral mucosa is slightly dry appearing but without erythema or lesions. Her salivary glands and ducts are normal.

The conjunctivae and sclera of her eyes are normal in color and noninjected. Her pupils are normal in size and react appropriately to light and accommodation bilaterally. She does not appear to have photophobia. Her funduscopic examination is normal bilaterally.

Her heart is regular in rate and rhythm; it is without murmurs, rubs, or gallops. Her apical impulse is nondisplaced and without a thrill. Her lungs are clear to auscultation.

Her bowel sounds are slightly hypoactive and equal in all four quadrants. Her abdomen appears mildly distended but without ascites. She has marked epigastric and moderate left upper gastric tenderness with significant guarding but no rebound tenderness. She has no masses or organomegaly. Her rectal examination is unremarkable and her stool tested negative for blood.

Her skin turgor is slightly decreased. She has no evidence of jaundice, other discolorations (including contusions), rashes, lesions, nodules, or edema.

3. Based on this information, which of the following diagnostic studies are essential to perform on Ms. Queens and why?

   A. Amylase, lipase, fractionated lactate dehydrogenase (LDH), and random plasma glucose (RPG)
   B. Complete blood count with differential (CBC w/diff) and PT
   C. Computed tomography (CT) of the abdomen
   D. Liver function testing (LFT), blood urea nitrogen (BUN), and electrolytes
   E. Urinary human chorionic gonadotropin (HCG) test

Diagnostic Results

Ms. Queens' amylase was 180 Somogyi units/dl (normal: 60–120). Her lipase was 520 units/L (normal: 0–160). Her total LDH was 275 units/L (normal: 100–190). Her low-density lipoprotein-1 (LDL-1) was 17% (normal: 17–27), her LDL-2 was 27% (normal: 27–37), her LDL-3 was 18% (normal: 18–25), her LDL-4 was 31% (normal: 3–8), and her LDL-5 was 7% (normal: 0–5). Her RPG was 204 mg/dl (normal: < 140).

Her CBC w/diff revealed an RBC count of $5.4 \times 10^6/\mu l$ (normal female: 4.2–5.4) with an MCV of 91 μm^3 (normal adult: 80–95), an MCH of 29 pg (normal adult: 27–31), an MCHC of 35 g/dl (normal adult: 32–36), and an RDW of 13.5% (normal adult: 11–14.5). Her WBC count was 21,000/mm³ (normal adult: 5000–10,000) with 50% neutrophils (normal: 55–70), 46% lymphocytes (normal: 20–40), 2% monocytes (normal: 2–8), 1% eosinophils (normal: 1–4), and 1% basophils (normal: 0.5–1). Her Hgb was 16 g/dl (normal female: 12–16) and her HCT was 50% (normal female: > 37–47). Her platelet (thrombocyte) count was 120,000/mm³ (normal adult: 150,000–400,000) and her MPV was 7.2 fl (normal: 7.4–10.4). Her smear was consistent with these results and revealed no cellular abnormalities. Her PT was 24 seconds (normal: 11–25).

Liver function studies revealed an ALT of 50 units/L (normal: 4–36), an AST of 45 units/L (normal: 0–35), and a GGT of 52 units/L (normal: 8–38).

Her BUN was 23 mg/dl (normal adult: 10–20). Her electrolytes revealed a carbon dioxide (CO_2) of 23 mEq/L (normal:

23–30), a chloride (Cl^-) of 99 mEq/L (normal: 98–106), a potassium (K^+) of 3.4 mEq/L (normal adult: 3.5–5.0), and a sodium (Na^{2+}) of 137 mEq/L (normal adult: 136–145).

Her urine HCG was negative (normal: negative).

Her abdominal CT revealed a mildly enlarged pancreas, without any pseudocysts, cysts, masses, streaking, or necrosis. No other abnormalities were identified.

4. Based on this information, which one of the following is Ms. Queens' most likely diagnosis and why?

   A. Ectopic pregnancy
   B. Acute pancreatitis secondary to valproic acid with mild dehydration
   C. Perforated duodenal ulcer with mild dehydration
   D. Acute cholelithiasis
   E. Factitious abdominal pain with drug-seeking behavior

5. Based on this diagnosis, which of the following are appropriate components of a treatment plan for Ms. Queens and why?

   A. Hospitalize with IV fluids
   B. Determine presentation (initial) Ranson criteria score
   C. IV morphine as needed for pain
   D. Initiate antibiotic therapy
   E. Refer for immediate total pancreatectomy

CASE 5-7

Quillain Rogers

Mr. Rogers is a 72-year-old white male who presents with the chief complaint of abdominal pain. It is left lower quadrant in location, intermittent and achy in nature, and mild (3 out of 10 on the pain scale) in severity. It has been present for approximately 5 days without any change. It does not radiate outside his left lower quadrant. It has awakened him at night. He experienced three or four episodes of a very loose, thin stool on the first day of his illness; however, he has not had a bowel movement since. He is also experiencing some mild nausea and rare vomiting. He estimates he has vomited two to three times since the onset of his pain. The last episode occurred yesterday evening after eating dinner. The emesis consists of "stomach acid." There is no blood, "coffee grounds"-appearing materials, fecal-like substances, mucus, or other abnormalities. None of his symptoms appear to be affected by food intake or fasting. He is unaware of any aggravating or alleviating factors for any of his symptoms.

He feels that he has been running a fever; however, he has not checked his temperature with a thermometer. He had some mild hematochezia with the diarrhea; however, he has not experienced any rectal bleeding in the absence of a bowel movement. Normally, he has one BM per day with a soft, light brown stool. He is not experiencing anorexia, melena, or other stool changes. He also denies dysuria, urinary urgency or frequency, hematuria, and penile discharge.

His past medical history is negative, including no surgeries or hospitalizations. He does not take any prescription or over-the-counter medications, vitamins, supplements, or herbal preparations. He is allergic to ciprofloxacin, which caused urticaria and perioral edema, but no dyspnea or wheezing. He has never consumed alcohol nor smoked cigarettes.

He does not have regular age-appropriate preventive health examinations. His family history is noncontributory.

1. Based on this information, which of the following questions are essential to ask Mr. Rogers and why?

  A. Does he drink untreated water from a lake, stream, spring, or other natural sources?
  B. Does he have a girlfriend?
  C. Has he been on an antibiotic recently?
  D. Does he thoroughly wash all fruits and vegetables before eating? Does he completely cook all meats to recommended temperature before consuming? Does he store his food and leftovers properly?
  E. Has he traveled outside the United States recently?

Patient Responses

Mr. Rogers states that he only drinks water from his tap that is supplied by the municipal water company. There has not been any recent "bans" or "boil water" advisories issued.

He does not have a girlfriend; however, he has been married for 50 years to the same spouse in what he assumes is a mutually monogamous relationship. His wife prepares all of their meals; however, he is certain she cleans, handles, cooks, and stores their food properly.

He last took an antibiotic 4 to 5 years ago. He has never traveled outside of the United States.

2. Based on this information, which of the following components of a physical examination are essential to conduct on Mr. Rogers and why?

  A. Thyroid examination
  B. Abdominal examination
  C. Rectal examination with occult blood testing of obtained stool (if present)
  D. Skin examination for jaundice
  E. Neurologic examination

Physical Examination Findings

Mr. Rogers weighs 188 lb and is 6'1" tall (BMI = 24.8). Other vital signs are BP, 126/72 mm Hg; pulse, 86 BPM and regular; respirations, 12/min and regular; and oral temperature, 99.8°F.

His thyroid is normal in size and equal bilaterally. There are no abnormalities in consistency, masses, or tenderness.

His abdominal examination reveals slightly hypoactive bowel sounds in the left lower quadrant; however, the remainder of his abdomen revealed normoactive bowel sounds. His abdomen is soft and nondistended. He has a palpable left lower quadrant mass of approximately 3 cm by 5 cm in size over his descending colon that is slightly tender to palpation; however, there is no rebound or guarding. He does not have any other masses or organomegaly. His rectal examination is essentially normal and his stool tests negative for occult blood.

His skin does not reveal any evidence of jaundice and his neurologic examination is within normal limits (wnl).

3. Based on this information, which of the following diagnostic studies are essential to perform on Mr. Rogers and why?

  A. Complete blood count with differential (CBC w/diff)
  B. Immediate colonoscopy

  C. Stool for culture and sensitivity (C&S) and *Clostridium difficile* toxins
  D. Flat-plate radiograph of the abdomen
  E. Computed tomography (CT) of the abdomen

Diagnostic Test Results

Mr. Rogers' CBC w/diff was normal except for a mild leukocytosis and lymphopenia. His stool samples are all pending. His colonoscopy, flat-plate radiograph, and CT of the abdomen were negative for perforation, obstruction, ileus, and acute changes.

4. Based on this information, which one of the following is Mr. Rogers' most likely diagnosis and why?

  A. Acute appendicitis
  B. Diverticulosis
  C. Diverticulitis
  D. Large bowel perforation with acute peritonitis
  E. Irritable bowel syndrome (IBS)

5. Based on this diagnosis, which of the following are appropriate components of a treatment plan for Mr. Rogers and why?

  A. Levofloxacin 750 mg once a day with metronidazole 500 mg four times a day orally for 7 to 10 days
  B. Trimethoprim-sulfamethoxazole double strength (DS) twice a day plus metronidazole 500 mg four times a day orally for 7 to 10 days
  C. Hospitalization
  D. Clear liquid diet
  E. Avoidance of fruits with seeds, nuts, corn, broccoli, cauliflower and other foods that might pass as small undigested food particles that could get "stuck" in a bowel pouch

CASE 5-8
Richard Stevenson

Mr. Stevenson is a 23-year-old white male who presents with the chief complaint of "I can't get rid of these hemorrhoids." He started experiencing anal itching, which appears to be slightly worse in terms of frequency and duration (but not intensity) since its onset, 1 month ago. His symptoms are not worse at night. He is unaware of any aggravating or alleviating factors.

He has not noticed any protruding masses, anogenital lesions, and/or bright red rectal bleeding with or without a bowel movement. He is experiencing occasional tenesmus and defecatory urgency, but it rarely results in a bowel movement. However, the majority of the time, it does result in the passage of a light yellowish-colored mucoid discharge that is frequently (but not always) blood tinged. He does not have any diarrhea. In fact, he states that he has been "constipated" (further defined as approximately two slighter harder and lumpier than his normal BMs per week) since the onset of his symptoms. He denies any other changes in the number, frequency, color, or consistency of his bowel movements. Before becoming ill, he had a daily BM that was soft and medium brown in color. He is not experiencing abdominal pain, nausea, vomiting, fever, chills, anorexia, or weight loss.

He saw another healthcare provider (HCP) approximately 2 weeks ago for this problem. Based on an external examination and a cellophane tape test, it was concluded that he did not have pinworms and the itching was caused by internal hemorrhoids. It was recommended that he try an OTC hemorrhoidal suppository. When this did not provide Mr. Stevenson with any relief, he tried various OTC creams, ointments, suppositories, and pads for hemorrhoids. None of these products provide him with any symptomatic improvement.

He has no known medical problems. He has never had surgery or been hospitalized.

Other than the aforementioned hemorrhoidal preparations (consisting of the pharmacy's own brand and Mr. Stevenson being unaware of their brand equivalent and/or active ingredients), which he quit using 2 to 3 days ago, he does not take any prescription or OTC medications, vitamins, supplements, or herbal preparations. He admits to drinking alcohol occasionally (which he further defines as drinking one or two drinks an average of twice a week). He denies cigarette smoking and illicit substance use/abuse. His family history is negative.

1. Based on this information, which of the following questions are essential to ask Mr. Stevenson and why?

   A. Has he visualized any *Enterobius vermicularis*?
   B. Has he noticed any jaundice or icterus?
   C. What are his sexual history and practices?
   D. Has he noticed any genital lesions?
   E. Is he experiencing a penile discharge, dysuria, urinary urgency, and/or urinary frequency?

Patient Responses

Mr. Stevenson has not noticed any *E. vermicularis*. He also denies the presence of jaundice, icterus, penile discharge, dysuria, urinary urgency, urinary frequency, and genital lesions.

He is sexually active with both women and men and only uses condoms when his partner insists. He is frequently the receptive partner when he has intercourse with men. His sexual practices involve oral–genital/anal contact; however, neither he nor his partners have ever utilized a dental dam. He is indiscriminate with his choice of partners and has innumerable lifetime partners. He does not have a current stable partner.

2. Based on this information, which of the following components of a physical examination are essential to conduct on Mr. Stevenson and why?

   A. Oropharyngeal examination
   B. Abdominal examination
   C. Rectal examination
   D. Genital examination
   E. Skin and eye examination for jaundice and/or icterus

Physical Examination Findings

Mr. Stevenson is 6'0" tall and weighs 170 lb (BMI = 23). Other vital signs are BP, 124/74 mm Hg; pulse, 82 BPM and regular; respirations, 13/min and regular; and oral temperature, 98.8°F.

His oropharyngeal mucosa is normal in color and moistness and does not reveal any lesions, ulcerations, or exudates.

On abdominal examination, his bowel sounds are normoactive and equal in all four quadrants. There is no tenderness, rigidity, abnormal masses, or organomegaly.

His external rectal examination is normal and without any anorectal erythema, ulcerations, lesions, or discharge. His digital rectal examination reveals marked tenderness, spontaneous tightening of his rectal and anal sphincter muscles, and a blood-streaked mucoid discharge remaining on the examiner's glove (which tests positive with occult blood testing).

His genital examination reveals normal-sized, descended testicles with a normal scrotum, including no abnormal masses, tenderness, or fluid. No penile lesions, ulcerations, skin discoloration, or discharge is present. Additionally, the application of acetic acid does not produce any gross or microscopically visible lesions.

He had no evidence of jaundice and/or icterus.

3. Based on this information, which of the following diagnostic studies are essential to perform on Mr. Stevenson and why?

   A. Anoscopy
   B. Rapid plasma reagin (RPR)
   C. Dark-field microscopy of the rectal discharge
   D. Complete blood count with differential (CBC w/diff)
   E. Rectal swab for immediate microscopic examination, Gram stain, Tzanck stain, viral culture for herpes simplex virus (HSV), and cultures (and/or DNA probe testing) for *Neisseria gonorrhoeae* and *Chlamydia trachomatis*

Diagnostic Test Results

Mr. Stevenson's anoscopy revealed a slightly erythematous and friable rectal mucosa with a rare superficial ulceration of approximately 2 to 3 mm in size. These abnormalities extended distally approximately 5 cm above the dentate line.

His RPR and dark-field microscopy were negative for syphilis (normal: negative). His CBC w/diff was unremarkable.

Microscopic examination of his rectal discharge revealed too numerous to count (TNTC) WBCs (normal: < 5), 3+ bacteria (normal: ≤ 1+), and no trichomonads, hyphae, or budding yeast (normal: none). His Gram stain also revealed numerous leukocytes in addition to gram-negative intracellular diplococci. His Tzanck testing was negative for multinucleated giant cells.

His cultures are pending.

4. Based on this information, which one of the following is Mr. Stevenson's most likely diagnosis and why?

   A. Anal condylomata lata
   B. Ulcerative colitis
   C. Thrombosed hemorrhoid
   D. Genital and rectal herpes simplex
   E. Gonococcal proctitis

5. Based on this diagnosis, which of the following are appropriate components of a treatment plan for Mr. Stevenson and why?

   A. Gemifloxacin 320 mg once a day for 7 days
   B. Single dose of ceftriaxone 125 mg IM plus doxycycline 100 mg twice a day for 7 days
   C. Benzathine penicillin G 2.4 million units IM

D. Open the affected vein and remove the thrombosis

E. Rectal cryotherapy

CASE 5-9

Samantha Thompson

Ms. Thompson is an 18-year-old white female who presents with the chief complaint of lower abdominal pain. It is located in her right lower quadrant and is described as a severe (10 out of 10 on the pain scale), constant, "dull ache" that has been progressively worsening since its sudden onset approximately 4 hours ago. The pain radiates into her right flank. It increases if she coughs, sneezes, or walks. She does not know of any alleviating factors. It began while she was sitting in a classroom taking a written examination. She has never experienced any pain remotely similar to this.

It is associated with anorexia, nausea, and one episode of mild vomiting. The emesis consisted of a small amount of clear "stomach acid"; there were no undigested food particles, blood, "coffee grounds"-appearing material, fecal-looking substances, or other abnormalities noted. She has not eaten since last night. However, she had a 32-ounce diet cola for her breakfast (approximately 2 hours before the onset of her symptoms). She is not experiencing constipation, diarrhea, melena, hematochezia, rectal mucus, other bowel changes, eructation, bloating, pyrosis, fever, chills, diaphoresis, myalgias, or arthralgias.

She reached menarche at the age of 16 years. Her menstrual cycles have been irregular since their onset. Typically, she has a menstrual period every 2 to 3 months. Her last menstrual period was 6 weeks ago and it was normal. She has never been sexually active.

She has no known medical problems, hospitalizations, or surgery. She takes no over-the-counter or prescription medications, vitamins, supplements, or herbal preparations. She does not drink, smoke cigarettes, or use any illicit substances. She had a preventive health examination with immunizations (for college admission) 2 months ago. Her family history is negative.

1. Based on this information, which of the following questions are essential to ask Ms. Thompson and why?

A. Did the pain start elsewhere and migrate to the right lower quadrant?

B. Was she able to complete the test? How does she feel about her performance on it?

C. What course/class was the test in?

D. What is the relationship between the anorexia and vomiting and the pain?

E. Has she experienced urinary urgency, urinary frequency, dysuria, hematuria, vaginal discharge, or unusual vaginal bleeding/spotting?

Patient Responses

Ms. Thompson states that the pain has always been in the right lower quadrant. It began before the onset of her anorexia, nausea, and vomiting. The episode of vomiting did not appear to alter the pain in any manner. She is not experiencing urinary urgency, frequency, dysuria, hematuria, vaginal discharge, or unusual vaginal bleeding/spotting.

She was able to complete the test in her abnormal psychology course and felt she did well.

2. Based on this information, which of the following components of a physical examination are essential to conduct on Ms. Thompson and why?

A. Abdominal examination

B. Digital rectal examination

C. Pelvic examination

D. Evaluation for costovertebral angle (CVA) tenderness

E. Right hip and leg examination

Physical Examination Findings

Ms. Thompson is 5'3" tall and weighs 108 lb (BMI = 19.1). Other vital signs are BP, 134/78 mm Hg; pulse, 96 BPM and regular; respiratory rate, 16/min and regular; and oral temperature, 99.8°F.

Her bowel sounds are present in all four quadrants, but a slight decrease is noted in her right lower quadrant. She has right lower quadrant tenderness at the McBurney point, with rebound and guarding. There is a question of a right lower quadrant mass; however, it cannot be fully assessed secondary to guarding, even with the patient's knees flexed and employing distraction techniques. No other masses or organomegaly are appreciated. She has a small amount of increased pain at the McBurney point when her left lower quadrant is palpated (positive Rovsing sign). Passive flexion of her right hip while internally rotated causes her pain to increase (positive obturator sign), as does passive extension of her right hip (positive psoas sign).

Her rectal examination is normal except for a complaint of increased pain when palpating the right lateral wall. Her stool tests negative for occult blood.

Her pelvic examination reveals normal external genitalia. Her cervix is normal in color and without discharge or lesions. Movement of the cervix does not produce pain (negative chandelier sign). Her uterus appears nontender and normal size. Palpation of her right vaginal wall produces an increase in her pain. Her left adnexal area is nontender and without any masses. Her right adnexal area is painful to palpate and appears to reveal a mass; however, it is difficult to adequately assess the area secondary to Ms. Thompson's discomfort and guarding.

She does not have costovertebral angle tenderness. No abnormalities are identified on her right hip and leg examination.

3. Based on this information, which of the following diagnostic studies are essential to perform on Ms. Thompson and why?

A. Abdominal/intravaginal ultrasound

B. Complete blood count with differential (CBC w/diff)

C. Urinalysis

D. Urine culture and sensitivity (C&S)

E. Urinary human chorionic gonadotropin (HCG) test

Diagnostic Test Results

An abdominal ultrasound was attempted on Ms. Thompson; however, it had to be discontinued because she was experiencing a significant increase in her pain secondary to the procedure. Although painful, especially in examining the right intra-abdominal structures, an intravaginal ultrasound examination was able to be performed. It revealed slight enlargement and edema of her right ovary. Doppler study revealed a mild decrease in blood flow to the right ovary. Her appendix is visualized and measures 12 mm in diameter. There was some question regarding possible wall edema; however, there was no evidence of an appendicolith.

Her CBC w/diff revealed an RBC count of $5.2 \times 10^6/\mu l$ (normal female: 4.2–5.4) with an MCV of 90 μm^3 (normal adult: 80–95), an MCH of 28 pg (normal adult: 27–31), an MCHC of 33 g/dl (normal adult: 32–36), and an RDW of 12.5% (normal adult: 11–14.5). Her WBC count was 16,000/mm³ (normal adult: 5000–10,000) with 84% neutrophils (normal: 55–70), 10% lymphocytes (normal: 20–40), 3% monocytes (normal: 1.2–8), 2% eosinophils (normal: 1–4), and 1% basophils (normal: 0.5–1). Her Hgb was 13 g/dl (normal female: 12–16) and her HCT was 40% (normal: 37–47). Her platelet (thrombocyte) count was 180,000/mm³ (normal adult: 150,000–400,000) and her MPV was 8.4 fl (normal: 7.4–10.4). Her smear was consistent with these results and revealed no cellular abnormalities.

Her urinalysis was normal and her urinary HCG was negative (normal: negative). Her urinary C&S is pending.

4. Based on this information, which one of the following is Ms. Thompson's most likely diagnosis and why?

    A. Pelvic inflammatory disease (PID)
    B. Pyelonephritis
    C. Acute appendicitis
    D. Ovarian torsion and acute appendicitis
    E. Mittelschmerz

5. Based on this diagnosis, which of the following are appropriate components of a treatment plan for Ms. Thompson and why?

    A. Reassurance, ovulatory pain will resolve without intervention
    B. Naproxen as needed, return if symptoms increase or persist after 2 days
    C. Hospitalization
    D. Immediate gynecologic/surgical consult
    E. Single dose of ceftriaxone 250 mg IM plus doxycycline 100 mg twice a day and metronidazole 500 twice a day for 14 days

CASES IN GASTROENTEROLOGY AND NUTRITION

RESPONSES AND DISCUSSION

CASE 5-1

Kathy Lemons

1. History

A. Has she eaten anything that could have been under-cooked, inadequately stored, inappropriately cooled after bulk cooking, or infected with bacteria?   NONESSENTIAL

Food-borne illnesses are usually associated with diar-rhea, not constipation. Plus, the chronic nature of her symp-toms is not consistent with food-borne illnesses, which are usually acute.

B. Does she experience abdominal pain, cramps, bloating, or other abdominal discomfort with the constipation? If yes, does a bowel movement (BM) alleviate the symptom(s)?   ESSENTIAL

In addition to primary (idiopathic) and secondary (caused by another disease or condition) constipation as diseases, there are other gastrointestinal disorders that have constipation as a symptom (e.g., irritable bowel syndrome [IBS], colon can-cer, colon polyps, volvulus, and rectal prolapse). The presence of associated symptoms as well as their descriptions are help-ful in differentiating these conditions. For example, irritable bowel syndrome, constipation predominate (IBS-C) tends to be associated with abdominal pain, cramping, bloating, or some other type of abdominal discomfort; additionally, the patient gets relief of these symptoms upon having a BM.

C. Has she had difficulty in the past or currently with depres-sion, sadness, anhedonia, anxiety, stress, and/or feelings she must be "in control"?   ESSENTIAL

Psychiatric conditions (e.g., depression, "control" issues, and eating disorders) are a frequent cause of secondary consti-pation; hence, this possibility should be explored as part of her history.

Because of the stigmata society still perpetrates regarding mental illness and some healthcare providers (HCPs) quickly attributing any long-term complaint to anxiety, depression,

and/or "stress," particularly if the patient already has a history of a psychiatric illness, some patients are reluctant to disclose these symptoms (and even current antidepressant usage), es-pecially during the initial encounter with a new HCP. There-fore, to obtain accurate answers, the HCP needs to address these symptoms in a sensitive, nonjudgmental, and profes-sional manner. This is crucial because the presence of these symptoms, and especially current antidepressant medication usage (which is frequently associated with chronic constipa-tion because of their anticholinergic properties), can alter the initial diagnostic and therapeutic plan for the patient.

Regardless, open and honest dialogue is an essential component of any medical encounter to ensure that accurate information is obtained on which to base diagnostic and ther-apeutic decisions. Because the most frequent cause of sec-ondary constipation is adverse medication effects, it is essential to have an accurate medication list. In addition to antidepressants, iron, opioids, anticholinergics, and calcium channel blockers have been linked with constipation.

D. Has she been experiencing any fatigue, weakness, pares-thesias, difficulty utilizing her extremities, problems with bal-ance, abnormalities of gait, visual disturbances, heat or cold intolerance, and/or changes in the texture of her hair or skin? ESSENTIAL

There are many other potential causes of secondary con-stipation (endocrine abnormalities [e.g., hypothyroidism, dia-betes mellitus, and Addison disease], neurologic diseases [e.g., Parkinson disease, dysautonomias, and multiple sclerosis], gy-necologic conditions [e.g., pregnancy, uterine leiomyomas ex-ternally compressing the colon, and endometriosis], and systemic diseases [e.g., scleroderma and progressive systemic sclerosis]). Therefore, questions to screen for these and other potential conditions are important to determine whether the patient has an associated condition presenting as constipa-tion. These questions primarily screen for the possibility of a neuroendocrine abnormality that could be responsible for the patient's symptoms.

E. Does she feel the urge to defecate or experience fecal incontinence?   ESSENTIAL

The lack of an urge to defecate helps not only to distinguish the various causes of primary constipation but also to differentiate primary from secondary causes. The urge to defecate can be absent in slow-transit and dysergia types of primary constipation. Generally, it is present in chronic constipation secondary to other conditions. Fecal incontinence is often caused by the passage of a softer or liquid stool around a fecal impaction or a neurologic abnormality.

2. Physical Examination

A. Heart and lung examination   NONESSENTIAL

B. Abdominal examination   ESSENTIAL

An abdominal examination is essential in attempting to establish Mrs. Lemons' differential diagnoses.

A comprehensive abdominal examination includes inspection of (1) the overlying skin for scars, lesions, discolorations, and venous dilation (for evidence of prior surgeries/trauma, potential coexisting or contributing conditions and/or infections, the presence of inferior vena cava obstruction, and other dermatologic abnormalities that could indicate a systemic condition is responsible for the patient's constipation); (2) the contour of the abdomen for shape, symmetry, and masses (generalized protuberant abdomens are predominately a result of obesity and/or ascites; asymmetric areas and/or protruding masses generally represent an abnormality/enlargement of the underlying structure [e.g., uterus, bladder, or splenic flexure of the colon]); (3) visible peristalsis (can be normal in thin individuals; otherwise, it generally indicates the presence of an intestinal obstruction); and (4) pulsations (if not obscured by fat, the aortic pulsation should be visible in the epigastric area; pulsations in other areas are considered to be abnormal).

It also includes auscultating the bowel sounds in all four quadrants for symmetry and over the epigastric area (where they should be slightly louder and prolonged [borborygmi]). Increased bowel sounds are often associated with increased peristalsis or an early intestinal obstruction; later on the bowel sounds from an obstruction are more high pitched in the affected area. Decreased bowel sounds are seen in hypomotility disorders, ileus, and peritonitis.

The costal margins should be auscultated for the presence of a friction rub associated with the liver and/or spleen. If there is concern of a vascular disease, the renal arteries and abdominal aorta should be auscultated for bruits and the aorta palpated for intensity and size.

Light palpation, followed by deeper palpation, should be performed to evaluate all areas of the abdomen for possible tenderness, masses, and/or organomegaly. With a few exceptions, the location of the abnormality generally indicates the affected area (e.g., suprapubic masses are most often the result of enlargements of the bladder or uterus, right upper quadrant abnormalities are generally associated with hepatomegaly, and epigastric tenderness is more than likely the result of an abnormality of the stomach). Regardless, any abnormality should be described in detail, including comparison of tenderness to presenting discomfort, type of sensation experienced, radiation to other areas, and presence of rebound tenderness. Masses should be described in terms of location, size, shape, consistency, tenderness, pulsations, and any other noted characteristics. Organomegaly should be described in terms of degree (size) of the finding (including location of measurement provided), the presence and characteristics of any tenderness, texture of the organ, smoothness of its edges, and other related features.

Percussion should ideally be performed over all four quadrants, the epigastric area, and the suprapubic area for appropriate dullness and tympany. However, it frequently is only performed clinically to assist in evaluating the size of an organomegaly.

Special maneuvers may be required to properly assess the abdomen and any possible abnormalities. For example, distraction (having the patient interlock his or her fingers with elbows flexed and attempting to "pull them apart" while the HCP is palpating the abdomen) may be useful in patients who are extremely "ticklish" or who are displaying marked guarding of an area. Having the patient raise his or her head up to tighten the abdomen muscles may make a hernia, diastasis recti, or abdominal wall mass more prominent. Placing the patient in the left lateral decubitus position may make ascites or splenomegaly easier to detect.

C. Visual inspection of anorectal area, with and without straining mimicking defecation   ESSENTIAL

Visual inspection of the anorectal area is essential because it can assist in identifying some secondary causes of constipation (e.g., suppression of defecation urge caused by pain associated with having a bowel movement in the presence of rectal fissures, hemorrhoids, genital warts, and genital herpes lesions); structural abnormalities such as rectocele, rectal strictures, rectal prolapse, and uterine prolapse; or other gastrointestinal disorders (e.g., rectal polyps), as well as their severity.

With straining, many of these conditions are more prominent (e.g., hemorrhoids, sessile rectal polyps, rectal polyps, or other lesions located close to the anal verge; rectal prolapse; and uterine prolapse). Additionally, this maneuver can identify the presence of paradoxical contraction of the rectum, which is suggestive of dysfunction of the pelvic floor.

D. Digital rectal examination, including testing of muscle strength and occult testing of feces for blood   ESSENTIAL

The digital rectal examination (DRE) also provides information regarding the possibility of secondary causes of chronic constipation (e.g., rectal carcinoma, large rectal polyp[s], spinal cord injuries, multiple sclerosis, and other neurologic conditions) and dysergic primary constipation.

Additionally, the stool obtained as part of the DRE can be tested for the presence of occult blood. However, if there is significant concern regarding the possibility of occult blood being present (or if using a combination of DRE and highly sensitive occult blood testing for colorectal cancer screening), the patient needs to collect three separate BM specimens at home. Care must be given to ensure the patient understands the dietary and medication restrictions as well as their importance before and during the testing procedure.

The presence of occult blood is considered to be a "red flag" (or "alarm symptom") when dealing with constipation and should immediately result in the patient being scheduled for a colonoscopy. Other "red flags" for constipation include new-onset constipation in middle-aged or older adults, unintentional weight loss, anemia, or hematochezia.

E. Anocutaneous sensation and reflex   ESSENTIAL

Although Mrs. Lemons does not have significant historical findings that would be consistent with a neurologic disease, a neuromuscular condition, or a spinal cord injury, she does admit to having to digitally stimulate her rectum to have a BM. Although this can be seen in primary constipation, it can also represent a neurologic or neuromuscular problem; therefore, Mrs. Lemons should be evaluated for decreased anocutaneous sensation or an abnormal "wink" reflex.

3. Diagnostic Studies

A. Colonoscopy   NONESSENTIAL

This test is not indicated at this time because her evaluation has not identified any "red flags" (as defined above), a strong suspicion for colon cancer or inflammatory bowel disease (IBD) and she has not reached the age (50 years for average-risk individuals) of routine colon cancer screening. (Surveillance should start younger if the patient has a positive family history of premature colon cancer or adenomas in a first-degree relative; has multiple first-degree relatives with colon cancer or adenomas, IBD, or specific inherited syndromes [e.g., familial adenomatous polyposis]; and/or is of African American or Hispanic descent [because of the earlier age of disease and increased mortality in these racial groups]).

B. Complete blood count with differential (CBC w/diff)   ESSENTIAL

The American College of Gastroenterology (ACG) recommends several "routine" diagnostic tests in the evaluation of chronic constipation. The CBC w/diff is one of them. Its primary purpose is to evaluate for asymptomatic, undiagnosed anemia, which is a "red flag" requiring immediate colonoscopy to evaluate for bleeding. It can also suggest inflammation when a mild leukocytosis is present, indicating that systemic illness (especially autoimmune conditions) capable of producing chronic constipation and/or IBD needs to be considered in the differential diagnosis.

C. Thyroid-stimulating hormone (TSH), free thyroxine (FT_4), and triiodothyronine by radioimmunoassay (T_3 by RIA)   ESSENTIAL

Because asymptomatic (or mildly symptomatic) hypothyroidism can cause secondary constipation, the ACG guidelines recommend screening for this disorder.

D. Serum calcium   ESSENTIAL

A serum calcium level is also recommended on all patients with chronic constipation per the ACG guidelines. The primary purpose is to screen for the possibility of hypoparathyroidism being responsible for the problem. Additionally, hypercalcemia can be present in tumor lysis (indicating that further evaluation for colorectal [and/or other] cancer) and in some neurologic conditions that could be responsible for secondary constipation (indicating the need for additional evaluation and testing for neurologic abnormalities and associated conditions).

E. Serum electrolytes   ESSENTIAL

These are also indicated per the ACG guidelines for the evaluation of chronic constipation. Electrolyte abnormalities can indicate problems related to chronic laxative use/abuse, eating disorders, and other conditions that could be related to chronic constipation.

4. Diagnosis

A. Primary constipation, probably dysergic defecation   CORRECT

Constipation is technically defined as having less than one spontaneous bowel movement per week. However, most experts expand this definition (despite the patient having a normal number of BMs [accepted as three or more per week]) to include a decrease in the number of BMs (from patient's normal), significant straining with defecation, sensation of incomplete bowel evacuation after a bowel movement, lower abdominal fullness, and/or the presence of hard stools. Mrs. Lemons technically meets the criteria established by this definition because she is currently experiencing only one induced BM per week. Additionally, her history indicates the presence of some of the criteria identified in the expanded definition (e.g., hard stools and significant straining). Given the long history she provides for the problem, she can easily be considered to have chronic constipation.

Because Mrs. Lemons is not on any medications that can cause chronic constipation and does not have any signs or symptoms suggestive of a secondary cause, she most likely has primary constipation. Primary constipation is divided into dysergic (lack of expulsion of the stool from the proximal to distal rectum because of incoordination of the pelvic floor musculature), slow transient time (delay of stool being moved from the cecum to the rectum because of decreased or incoordinated contractions in the colonic lumen), and lifestyle induced (inadequate fiber and/or fluid consumption).

Because of the findings on Mrs. Lemons' history (rarely having an urge to defecate, marked straining with BMs, digital disimpaction necessary before having a bowel movement, enema usage required to stimulate the passage of feces, and lack of abdominal discomfort with her constipation) and physical examination (paradoxical contraction of the rectum and mild rectal prolapse with straining on anorectal visualization; weak rectal muscle tone, inadequate rectal pushing, inadequate descent, slightly enlarged vault, and stool consistency on DRE), her most likely diagnosis at this time is dysergic primary constipation.

B. Primary constipation, probably normal transit   INCORRECT

The definition of this condition can be inferred by the previous rationale. This term is sometimes utilized in patients complaining of constipation who have a misperception of their actual number of BMs. Rarely it is utilized as a diagnosis for patients who are experiencing three or more BMs per week but are experiencing significant straining with BMs, very hard or lumpy stools, a sensation that the bowels are not fully evacuated following a BM, an awareness of lower abdominal fullness, and/or painful BMs in the absence of an identifiable secondary cause for the complaint, because in the majority of these cases, an identifiable cause can be established. Examples include neurologic (e.g., spinal cord injury or multiple sclerosis), gastrointestinal (e.g., IBS, rectal obstruction caused by a mass lesion, or rectal stricture), or psychogenic (e.g., "control issues," depression, or conditioned behavioral response to avoid the urge to defecate [and prevent defecation] because of the fear of reproducing a previously experienced pain with a bowel movement) conditions. Thus, primary constipation with normal transit of stool can be eliminated as Mrs. Lemons' most likely diagnosis because it would imply that she is having a normal number of BMs (three or more per week).

C. Secondary constipation, probably caused by hypothyroidism   INCORRECT

Secondary constipation, probably caused by hypothyroidism, can be ruled out as Mrs. Lemons' most likely diagnosis because of her normal thyroid function testing.

D. Irritable bowel syndrome, constipation predominant (IBS-C)   INCORRECT

IBS-C shares many of the same characteristics as chronic constipation. However, it can be eliminated as Mrs. Lemons' most likely diagnosis because she is not experiencing abdominal pain, which is required to make the diagnosis of IBS-C.

The diagnostic criteria for IBS (called Rome II) requires that the patient must be experiencing at least two of the following three characteristic symptoms for a minimum of 6 months (with symptoms occurring on at least 3 days per week for the past 3 months): (1) presence of abdominal pain/discomfort alleviated by a BM, (2) onset of the abdominal pain associated with a change in the number of BMs (increase or decrease), and (3) onset of the abdominal pain associated with a change in stool consistency (harder, softer, liquidlike, lumpy, or a combination).

E. Normal bowel movements   INCORRECT

Normal bowel movements defined in terms of frequency means three or more BMs per week. This can be eliminated as Mrs. Lemons' most likely diagnosis because she is only experiencing one BM per week.

5. Treatment Plan

A. Continue weekly saline enemas   INCORRECT

Osmotic laxatives, like normal saline enemas, are not a good long-term treatment option because they can be associated with electrolyte disturbances.

B. Refer to gastroenterologist for possible anorectal manometry, defecography, colon transit study with radiopaque markers, and/or other diagnostic studies deemed necessary   CORRECT

According to the ACG guidelines for the management of chronic constipation, in addition to patients with "red flags," those patients suspected to have dysergia should be referred to a gastroenterologist to confirm the diagnosis. The initial treatment is generally biofeedback.

C. Daily mineral oil, titrated to produce one bowel movement per day   INCORRECT

Mineral oil is unlikely to be very effective for Mrs. Lemons because its primary mechanism of action is to coat the stool in oil, making them more slippery and hence easier to pass. Because Mrs. Lemons' problem is dysergia, its usage is unlikely to result in spontaneous BMs.

Additionally, it has been associated with leakage of liquid feces and/or the mineral oil itself around the constipated stool. Furthermore, it has been associated with the malabsorption of fat-soluble vitamins, including vitamin D, which is essential to maintain her bone health and may prevent other serious conditions (e.g., hypertension, metabolic syndrome, myocardial infarction, peripheral artery disease, diabetes mellitus, dementia, and some cancers).

D. Lubiprostone 24 mg twice a day   INCORRECT

Lubiprostone is not considered to be a first-line agent in the management of primary constipation of the dysergic type. However, if biofeedback, lifestyle changes, and stimulant laxatives are ineffective in alleviating Mrs. Lemons' constipation, then lubiprostone is considered to be the next most likely treatment option. It activates select chlorine channels in the lining of the gut to increase intraluminal fluid production, resulting in increased gastrointestinal (GI) motility and softer feces.

E. Tegaserod 6 mg twice a day   INCORRECT

Tegaserod, a partial 5-HT_4 receptor agonist, is an inappropriate choice for Mrs. Lemons because it is only approved by the US Food and Drug Administration (FDA) for very restricted use for IBS-C or chronic idiopathic constipation in women 65 years of age or younger. Furthermore, it is only currently available on an investigational basis because it was voluntarily withdrawn from the market in early 2007 after a meta-analysis suggested an increase in ischemic cardiovascular events in patients taking it.

Epidemiologic and Other Data

Population-based studies conducted in the United States estimate that the incidence of constipation is 12 to 19%. The female-to-male ratio of those affected is 2:1. Approximately 33% of those affected will seek medical attention for the condition. Constipation is much more prevalent in developed countries than undeveloped and developing areas.

CASE 5-2
Larry Myers
1. History

A. When was his first rotavirus vaccination given?   ESSENTIAL

The current rotavirus vaccine is a series of three injections given 2 months apart. The first injection should be administered between the ages of 6 and 12 weeks. Because of safety concerns based on adverse events reported with the original formulation of this product, it should not be administered outside of the recommended age window (6 to 32 weeks old), and the first dose should not be administered after the age of 12 weeks.

The primary adverse event leading to the withdrawal of the original product from the US market was intussusception associated with the initial vaccine dose. Subsequent analysis of the data revealed that the cases of intussusception reported appeared to be limited to children receiving the initial immunization dose after the age of 12 weeks.

Although Larry's mother reported that his were provided on schedule, it is still worthwhile to specifically inquire about this vaccine given Larry's symptoms to ensure his initial dose was not postponed for some reason (e.g., staff didn't want to administer too many vaccines at once, parental hesitancy about giving, or vaccine unavailability).

B. Has he been flexing his knees and hips over his abdomen during these episodes?   ESSENTIAL

Flexing of the legs at the hips (and generally at the knees as well) during an inconsolable crying episode frequently equates with an intense, cramping abdominal pain, especially in an infant.

C. Is he urinating normally and still crying tears?   ESSENTIAL

Because of his decreased appetite, vomiting, and extreme of age, the possibility of dehydration is a justifiable concern. Generally, if the patient has urinated in the previous 8 hours and produces tears when crying, he or she is not significantly dehydrated. The absence of urination for greater than 8 hours and the loss of tears when crying typically do not occur unless the patient has a greater than 5% fluid loss.

D. Is there any mucus in his bowel movements or do they look like "currant jelly"?   ESSENTIAL

Mucus in the stool generally indicates an inflammatory cause, whereas "currant jelly"-looking stools are almost pathognomonic for intussusception (however, it is generally a late sign).

E. Why has she not introduced "food" into Larry's diet? NONESSENTIAL

The American Academy of Pediatrics (AAP) guidelines regarding infant nutrition/feeding recommend exclusive breast-feeding until 6 months of age. Because Larry is only 5 ½ months old, food should not have been introduced at this age.

Furthermore, asked in this manner, this question could actually discourage exclusive breast-feeding until age 6 months. It has an accusatory tone that could be misinterpreted to imply that she is doing something "wrong" by delaying the introduction of food; therefore, it could cause her to introduce food immediately instead of waiting until the recommended age.

2. Physical Examination

A. Ear, nose, and throat examination   ESSENTIAL

Because of Larry's age, he cannot adequately verbalize or even indicate "what is bothering him" or "where it hurts." The presence of a low-grade fever, mild anorexia, inconsolable crying, and vomiting without many other symptoms can indicate an infection of the upper respiratory tract.

B. Lung auscultation   ESSENTIAL

Because Larry cannot communicate what is causing his current discomfort and/or its location, it is essential to examine his lungs because pulmonary conditions including bronchitis, pneumonia, or aspiration of milk and/or a foreign body could be responsible for his symptoms.

C. Abdominal examination   ESSENTIAL

An abdominal examination is essential to assist in narrowing the possible differential diagnoses for Larry because he is experiencing vomiting, blood-streaked feces, and probably abdominal pain. The pattern of his bowel sounds; the location, degree, and characteristics of tenderness and/or masses; and the size of his abdominal organs are all essential

information to obtain to assist in the determination of his correct diagnosis. (For more information regarding the abdominal examination, please see Case 5-1.)

D. Rectal examination with testing for occult blood ESSENTIAL

A rectal examination is important to evaluate for the presence of rectal fissures, strictures, masses, or other structural abnormalities that can be associated with a blood-streaked stool. It also permits his stool to be evaluated for color, consistency, and gross blood or mucus.

Occult blood testing of the stool, if positive, can help to narrow the potential list of differential diagnoses for Larry; on the other hand, a negative result does not provide much useful information because of the possibility of false-negative results, even with highly specific tests.

False-positives can also occur but are extremely unlikely in Larry's case because of his age and diet. In older children and adults, false-positives can occur from strenuous exercise; consumption of red meat, certain fish, turnips, and horseradish; and some medications (e.g., colchicine, iodine, and boric acid).

E. Examination of posterior fontanelle   NONESSENTIAL

The posterior fontanelle is generally closed by 2 months of age; therefore, palpation of the posterior fontanelle is unlikely to provide any useful information because Larry is 5 ½ months old.

However, the anterior fontanelle typically does not close until the infant is between the ages of 7 and 19 months (however, it can occur as early as 4 months or as late as 26 months) and might provide some useful information regarding Larry's condition. The anterior fontanelle will often bulge in cases of increased intracranial pressure, including central nervous system (CNS) infections. Other causes include tumors, other space-occupying mass lesions, and ventral circulation obstruction. The anterior fontanelle is generally depressed when the intracranial pressure is low; this finding could represent dehydration. However, when evaluating the anterior fontanelle, it is important to ensure that the child is resting comfortably because crying, coughing, sneezing, and vomiting can cause temporary bulging of the anterior fontanelle.

3. Diagnostic Studies

A. Complete blood count with differential (CBC w/diff) ESSENTIAL

A CBC w/diff provides two main pieces of information to assist in determining Larry's correct diagnosis. First, his white blood cell (WBC) count and differential provide clues regarding the presence or absence, as well as the degree, of an infectious and/or inflammatory process. Still, a normal count does not absolutely rule out the possibility of these entities because early in the course of the illness, or with a milder disease process, the WBC count and differential can be normal. Also, a marked leukocytosis can occur with perforation of the intestines or intra-abdominal organs.

The second piece of useful information that could be provided is the presence or absence of gastrointestinal hemorrhage and/or anemia. This is primarily based on his hematocrit (HCT) and hemoglobin (Hgb) levels. An anemia and/or blood loss produces a reduction of these values. However, when interpreting these values in acute hemorrhage, an important caveat to remember is that the HCT and Hgb levels can be normal or only slightly decreased early in the process because the changes in these levels lag behind the actual blood loss.

If an anemia is present, his red blood cell (RBC) indices (mean corpuscular volume [MCV], mean corpuscular hemoglobin [MCH], mean corpuscular hemoglobin concentration [MCHC], and RBC distribution width [RDW]) can provide important clues regarding the cause of anemia. For example, a normocytic (RBCs are normal in size), normochromic (RBCs are normal in color) anemia is most frequently associated with acute hemorrhage, early iron deficiency, sepsis, malignancy, aplastic anemia, and acquired hemolytic anemia. A microcytic (small-sized RBCs), hypochromic (lighter-colored RBCs) anemia is most often caused by an iron deficiency, thalassemia, or lead poisoning. A macrocytic (larger than normal RBCs), normochromic anemia is often present with a vitamin B_{12} deficiency, a folic acid deficiency, hydantoin therapy, and chemotherapy.

Hence, a chronic GI blood loss typically results in a microcytic, hypochromic anemia, whereas an acute blood loss can be associated with either no anemia or a normocytic, normochromic anemia. In both cases, the cause of the anemia is an iron deficiency.

B. Urinalysis, including microscopic examination   ESSENTIAL

A urinalysis, including microscopic examination, is indicated to evaluate Larry for objective signs of dehydration as well as the presence of an upper (e.g., pyelonephritis or glomerulonephritis) or a lower (e.g., cystitis or urethritis) urinary tract infection.

As previously stated, dehydration is a potential complication of Larry's present illness because of his extremely young age and his vomiting. Urinalysis findings associated with dehydration include a darker yellow color, a high specific gravity, and possibly ketones.

A urinary tract infection can cause symptoms similar to what Larry is experiencing (i.e., fever, abdominal pain, vomiting, and irritability). Urinalysis findings possibly associated with a urinary tract infection include gross changes such as a darker red discoloration (if gross hematuria is present) and a cloudy appearance; a foul odor; the presence of leukocyte esterase and/or nitrites on the dipstick examination; and bacteruria associated with an increased number of WBCs on the microscopic examination. Upper urinary tract infections can also produce epithelial, granular, hyaline, waxy, WBC, and/or RBC casts.

C. Blood urea nitrogen (BUN)   ESSENTIAL

A BUN is most commonly ordered to evaluate renal function. However, it is also elevated in other conditions, including dehydration and gastrointestinal bleeding/hemorrhage.

D. Electrolytes   ESSENTIAL

Electrolyte abnormalities can be seen in patients with significant dehydration and/or vomiting. Because of Larry's extreme of age, he is more susceptible to dehydration and its consequences.

E. Kidneys, ureters, and bladder (KUB) radiograph   ESSENTIAL

A KUB radiograph is another term for a plain film radiograph of the abdomen. Although Larry's symptoms could represent a number of abnormal intra-abdominal processes, his physical findings are consistent with a specific condition. By evaluating his KUB radiograph for possible abnormal air-fluid levels, unusual gas patterns, colonic dilatation caused by air and/or feces, intraluminal masses (particularly soft tissue), and the appearance of a double lumen, significant support can be provided for (if present) or against (if absent) his most likely diagnosis.

4. Diagnosis

A. Appendicitis   INCORRECT

Despite the atypical presentation of appendicitis in infants and children, it can still be ruled out as Larry's most likely diagnosis based on his abdominal examination findings and diagnostic study results. On abdominal examination the typical finding of appendicitis is a right lower quadrant (or a periumbilical) tenderness. If a mass is present, it is also generally located in the right lower quadrant. Furthermore, a positive Dance sign is generally not seen in appendicitis.

However, a number of other signs (which are much less sensitive in infants than in older children and adults) can often be identified in patients with appendicitis. These signs include psoas (extension of the right thigh when the patient is lying on his or her left side reproduces the abdominal pain), obturator (internal rotation of the flexed right hip with the patient lying supine reproduces the pain), Aaron (epigastric and/or chest pain or discomfort when pressure is continually applied to the McBurney point), Bassler (localized pain when the appendix is compressed against the iliac muscle), Blumberg (abdominal pain is reproduced by rapid removal of the examiner's hand after compression over the McBurney point for a few seconds), McBurney (pain is reproduced by applying pressure over the McBurney point), Rovsing (abdominal pain is elicited by palpation over the McBurney point), and Sumner (gentle palpation in the right or left lower quadrants results in involuntary tightening of the abdominal muscles).

Although a paucity of gas in the cecum can be visualized on plain film abdominal radiographs in appendicitis if perforation has occurred, crescent and doughnut (or target) signs are not present unless another condition coexists with the appendicitis. In general, the findings of appendicitis on abdominal plain film radiographs are subtle, if present at all. They may include a dilated cecum with an air-fluid level or a right spinal curvature. Occasionally a calcified appendicolith can be visualized on the plain film.

B. Early urinary tract infection   INCORRECT

An early urinary tract infection (UTI) can essentially be eliminated as Larry's most likely diagnosis because of the lack of findings to support the presence of a UTI on urinalysis.

C. Perforated small intestine   INCORRECT

Although a perforated small intestine can produce the radiographic findings of minimal gas in the cecum, his other radiographic findings are inconsistent with this being his most likely diagnosis. Furthermore, with a perforation, Larry should appear more acutely ill and not experience fluctuation from severe symptoms to an asymptomatic state. Also, the abdominal examination would likely yield a generalized tenderness, no mass, and the Dance sign would not be present.

D. Early viral gastroenteritis   INCORRECT

Early viral gastroenteritis, by definition, has diarrhea as a symptom. The lack of this symptom, in addition to his physical examination and abdominal x-ray findings being inconsistent with viral gastroenteritis, makes this extremely unlikely to be his most likely diagnosis.

E. Intussusception   CORRECT

In this condition, the bowel invaginates itself (generally proximally to distally). It is characterized by a triad of episodic, severe, cramping abdominal pain; vomiting without diarrhea; and a positive test for fecal occult blood. Unfortunately, this triad is estimated to be present in only 20% of the infants and toddlers with this condition.

What is considered more characteristic of intussusception is the presence of intermittent, severe, cramping abdominal pain associated with flexion of the legs; a marked reduction of symptoms (or even the absence of symptoms) between episodes; bilious vomiting; and "currant jelly"-appearing stools. These symptoms are found in over 50% of all cases. However, the appearance of "currant jelly" stools and bilious emesis are late findings of the condition. The presence of crescent and doughnut (or target) signs on the plain film abdominal radiograph and the "sausage-like" mass on physical examination are also nearly exclusive for intussusception. Therefore, intussusception is Larry's most likely diagnosis.

5. Treatment Plan

A. Surgical consult   CORRECT

A surgical consult is essential because not all infantile cases of intussusception have therapeutic resolution with the performance of a diagnostic air contrast barium enema. The resolution rate ranges from 59 to 90%. Thus, a surgical team needs to be prepared for possible intervention.

B. Contrast air barium enema   CORRECT

This is considered to be the "gold standard" diagnostic procedure for intussusceptions. Additionally, as stated previously, it is also therapeutic in many cases.

C. Hospitalization   CORRECT

Because of the potential complications (e.g., GI hemorrhage, bowel perforation, and sepsis) and Larry's young age, he should be hospitalized for further evaluation, observation, and treatment.

D. Oral ampicillin   INCORRECT

Antibiotics, such as ampicillin, are not indicated unless perforation and peritonitis occur; then, the means of administration would be IV, not PO (per os, or orally). Additionally, an antibiotic with a broader spectrum of antimicrobial coverage than ampicillin would be indicated.

E. BRAT (bananas, rice, applesauce, and toast) diet INCORRECT

A BRAT diet is used in the treatment of viral gastroenteritis and is not indicated in patients being treated for intussusception. Furthermore, it would involve the introduction of "new" foods to Larry while he is ill because he is exclusively breast-fed at this time.

In general, patients with intussusception are initially not permitted to take anything by mouth (NPO [nothing per os]).

IV fluids are provided for hydration and caloric intake. A nasogastric (NG) tube may be required for decompression.

Epidemiologic and Other Data

Primary intussusception (without a structural abnormality) occurs almost exclusively in children. It has a male-to-female ratio of 4:1. Recurrence rates are approximately 5% regardless of whether the patient was treated with a mechanical or surgical procedure.

On the other hand, secondary intussusception (caused by a structural defect) occurs primarily in adults. The most common abnormality is a carcinoma located on its leading edge. Treatment in adult cases almost always requires surgical intervention.

CASE 5-3
Michael Nestor
1. History

A. Is the pain associated with dysphagia?   ESSENTIAL

The presence or absence of other GI symptoms can assist in developing an appropriate differential diagnosis list for Mr. Nestor. This particular symptom is also significant because it represents one of the "red flag" (warning or alarm) symptoms mandating a more comprehensive evaluation to ensure that a serious medical condition is not missed (e.g., erosive esophagitis, carcinoma, perforated ulcer, hemorrhagic gastritis, and/or esophageal stricture).

The other "red flag" symptoms associated with the complaint of epigastric pain and/or dyspepsia include new-onset symptoms in patients older than the age of 55 years, weight loss, persistent vomiting, hematemesis, hematochezia, melena, occult blood in the stool, palpable abdominal mass, organomegaly, jaundice, icterus, constant and/or severe pain, coexisting anemia, and/or age older than 45 years in patients who are born in regions associated with a higher incidence of gastric cancer.

B. Has he been experiencing any depression/sadness, anhedonia, changes in sleep (aside from the awakenings secondary to his epigastric pain), increased stress, or dissatisfaction with life in general?   ESSENTIAL

Depression can present, especially in primary care settings, with physical complaints instead of mood symptoms. Some of the most common complaints are gastrointestinal in origin, with dyspepsia and epigastric pain being reported frequently. Others include headache, back pain, generalized pain, paresthesias, fatigue, and/or weakness. Furthermore, there appears to be a relationship between peptic ulcer disease, stress, and type A personality.

C. Has he experienced a recent unintentional weight change? ESSENTIAL

As stated previously, weight loss is a "red flag" symptom that requires a more extensive evaluation because it could result from significant esophageal and/or gastric conditions (including cancer) and/or pathology of other upper intra-abdominal organs (e.g., pancreatitis, pancreatic carcinoma, hepatitis, cirrhosis, hepatic carcinoma, metastatic hepatocellular disease). A weight increase could indicate that he is attempting to alleviate and/or prevent his discomfort with food (either consciously or subconsciously). Any weight change could indicate the presence of a major mood disorder.

D. Is he experiencing any pyrosis or reflux of stomach contents? ESSENTIAL

The presence of reflux of gastric contents into the esophagus and/or oropharynx is also important to inquire about because if present, esophageal conditions (e.g., gastroesophageal reflux disease [GERD], erosive esophagitis, and/or esophageal lesions [including carcinomas and strictures]) will need to be added to Mr. Nestor's list of potential differential diagnoses. However, it is important to remember that it is possible to have an esophageal condition, especially GERD, in addition to another benign or serious gastrointestinal disorder(s).

E. How often does he have a bowel movement? NONESSENTIAL

Because Mr. Nestor has already denied experiencing diarrhea, constipation, or other bowel changes and his discomfort is confined to the epigastric area, knowing the frequency of his bowel movements is not likely to provide any useful information to assist in establishing the cause of his chief complaint.

2. Physical Examination

A. Palpation of thyroid   NONESSENTIAL

B. Palpation of cervical lymph nodes   NONESSENTIAL

The term "cervical lymph nodes" denotes the preauricular, postauricular, occipital, tonsillar, submaxillary, submental, superficial cervical, poster cervical chain, and deep cervical chain lymph nodes. These structures are responsible for the lymphatic flow from the structures of the head and neck. Therefore, because Mr. Nestor does not have any symptoms associated with these areas, palpation of the cervical lymph nodes is unlikely to provide any useful information.

However, if the supraclavicular lymph nodes are also included in this definition (as a few references indicate), then palpating them in conjunction with the infraclavicular lymph nodes might be beneficial.

C. Abdominal examination   ESSENTIAL

The abdominal examination is essential because Mr. Nestor is complaining of abdominal pain/discomfort. (For more information regarding the abdominal examination, please see Case 5-1.)

D. Rectal examination with occult blood testing of stool ESSENTIAL

A rectal examination is important to perform in a patient with an abdominal complaint. It can assist in identifying rectal abnormalities, motility disorders, and obstructions. Furthermore, it can provide information regarding the color and consistency of the stool, when present. Occult blood testing can also be performed on the stool; however, it is important to remember that both false-negatives and false-positives can occur with a single test. (For more information, please see Cases 5-1 and 5-2.)

E. Skin and sclera examination for discolorations   ESSENTIAL

A skin and sclera examination is necessary to evaluate for signs of jaundice and/or icterus. Good lighting and being alert for subtle changes are necessary to properly evaluate a patient for the presence of jaundice, especially in its early stages. Additionally, the palpebral conjunctivae and skin should be carefully evaluated for evidence of pallor (which could indicate that an underlying anemia caused by upper gastrointestinal tract hemorrhage is present).

3. Diagnostic Studies

A. Upper GI endoscopy with biopsy for *Haemophilus pylori* ESSENTIAL

Mr. Nestor requires an upper endoscopy because he has a "red-flag" symptom on his physical examination (positive occult blood testing of his stool). Biopsy specimens need to be obtained of any lesion to look for precancerous or malignant cells as well as the organism *H. pylori*. Biopsies should also be collected from the antrum and greater curvature of the stomach, regardless of the presence of other lesions, to identify the presence of *H. pylori* because it has been implicated as the causative agent in 90 to 95% of all cases of peptic ulcer disease.

The "gold standard" for the identification of the presence of the bacterium *H. pylori* is via microscopic identification of the organism on a biopsy specimen. Cultures are almost as accurate and can be performed on the biopsied specimens; however, cultures take several weeks before the results are available. The most rapid result is obtained by testing a biopsy specimen for urease; if positive, the presence of an *H. pylori* infection is assumed because of the production of massive amounts of the urease enzyme by the bacterium.

In the absence of "red flag" symptoms, the current standard of care for the evaluation of patients who are not taking a nonsteroidal anti-inflammatory drug (NSAID) presenting with new-onset dyspepsia and/or epigastric pain is to perform a noninvasive test for *H. pylori* via a serum (antibody based), feces (antibody based), or breath l (urease based). The most common technique employed is serum testing for *H. pylori* antibodies because it does not require dietary and/or medication restrictions to ensure accurate results.

If that test is positive, therapy directed at *H. pylori* is employed. Four weeks after completion of therapy, a urea breath test (considered the "gold standard" for evaluating the resolution of *H. pylori*) is performed. If the patient is still symptomatic or still tests positive for *H. pylori* at that time, an upper endoscopy is indicated.

If the patient has been taking an NSAID or his or her noninvasive test for *H. pylori* was negative, an empiric trial of a histamine-2 (H₂) blocker or proton pump inhibitor (PPI) is considered to be the treatment of choice. If the patient is still symptomatic after 1 month of therapy, an upper endoscopy is indicated. Obviously, if any "red flag" symptom appears during the treatment period, an immediate upper endoscopy is indicated.

B. Barium upper GI radiographic series   NONESSENTIAL

Once the diagnostic test of choice for epigastric pain/discomfort associated with dyspepsia, this test is no longer considered to be an appropriate diagnostic tool for the evaluation of this complaint and has essentially been replaced with upper

GI endoscopy. Upper GI endoscopy has a higher sensitivity and specificity than a barium upper GI radiographic series; furthermore, it permits immediate biopsying capabilities and photographic opportunities of abnormalities identified.

C. Colonoscopy   NONESSENTIAL

A colonoscopy is not indicated at this time for Mr. Nestor as his history and physical examination did not reveal any signs of a lower GI disorder, with the possible exception of his stools testing positive for occult blood (which can occur in either an upper or lower gastrointestinal bleed).

Therefore, if his upper GI endoscopy fails to reveal a cause for the presence of the occult blood, further evaluation is going to be necessary to determine one. A colonoscopy could be part of that evaluation. Additionally, a colonoscopy could be indicated for colorectal cancer (CRC) screening if Mr. Nestor were older. (For more information, please see Case 5-1.)

D. Complete blood count with differential   (CBC w/diff) ESSENTIAL

Mr. Nestor requires a CBC w/diff to evaluate for the presence of anemia associated with a GI bleed. (For additional discussion regarding GI bleeding and anemia, please refer to Case 5-1.)

E. Serum *H. pylori* antibodies; amylase and gastrin levels NONESSENTIAL

Serum *H. pylori* antibodies are not necessary to obtain on Mr. Nestor because the biopsies obtained during the upper GI endoscopy will more effectively evaluate for the presence of the *H. pylori* organism.

Because pancreatitis is not included on Mr. Nestor's differential diagnosis list, an amylase level is not indicated at this time. However, an elevated amylase level is not specific for this condition. It can be seen with other GI disorders (e.g., penetrating peptic ulcer disease, perforated peptic ulcer, perforated upper or lower intestines, necrosis of the bowels, proximal upper intestinal obstruction, and acute cholecystitis). However, it is generally not utilized for diagnosing these other disorders because of its lack of specificity and sensitivity.

A serum gastrin level is not indicated at this time because Mr. Nestor's symptoms are mild, he has not been treated for a more common condition, and his upper GI endoscopy findings are inconsistent with conditions associated with excessive gastrin secretion (e.g., Zollinger-Ellison Syndrome [most common], other gastrinomas, pyloric obstruction, atrophic gastritis, stomach cancer, and G-cell hyperplasia). Plus, his antacid usage can result in a false-positive level.

Gastrin levels are generally not indicated as part of an initial diagnostic evaluation unless there is a significant family history of peptic ulcer disease or cancer of the pancreas, pituitary, or parathyroid; recurrence of symptoms after surgical resection for an ulcer; inexplicable diarrhea and/or steatorrhea; endoscopic findings of multiple ulcers, ulcers in atypical locations, and/or prominent folds of the mucosa; hyperchlorhydria; or hypercalcemia.

4. Diagnosis

A. Duodenal ulcer, secondary to *H. pylori* infection   CORRECT

Upper gastrointestinal (or peptic) ulcers are defined as a greater than 5-mm break in the mucosa of either the stomach or duodenum that reveals at least the submucosa. Because Mr. Nestor's upper GI endoscopy revealed such a finding in his duodenum and his biopsy tested positive for the presence of an *H. pylori* infection, this is his most likely diagnosis.

B. Gastric ulcer, secondary to *H. pylori* infection and smoking INCORRECT

Although they have essentially the same symptoms and can both be positive for an *H. pylori* infection, a gastric ulcer is located in the stomach, not the duodenum (as Mr. Nestor's was).

Smoking is a risk factor for both gastric and duodenal ulcers; therefore, regardless of the ulcer's location, Mr. Nestor must be counseled on cigarette cessation.

C. Zollinger-Ellison syndrome   INCORRECT

Zollinger-Ellison syndrome consists of peptic ulcer disease (frequently found in atypical locations and multiple in number), hypersecretion of gastric acid, and non–beta cell tumors of the pancreatic islet cells resulting in the overproduction of gastrin.

It can be ruled out as Mr. Nestor's most likely diagnosis because of his lack of significant symptoms, weight loss, diarrhea, steatorrhea, and other "atypical" symptoms. Additional support against this diagnosis includes a negative family history of GI disease and/or malignancy in addition to the presence of a single ulcer in an expected location on his upper GI endoscopy.

D. Gastroesophageal reflux disease (GERD), secondary to *H. pylori* infection   INCORRECT

GERD secondary to *H. pylori* infection can essentially be eliminated as Mr. Nestor's most likely diagnosis because *H. pylori* does not cause GERD. Furthermore, Mr. Nestor does not exhibit any symptoms suggestive of GERD nor was there evidence of reflux visualized on his upper GI endoscopy.

E. Gastritis, secondary to *H. pylori* infection   INCORRECT

Gastritis is an inflammation of the lining of the stomach that can present with dyspepsia and/or epigastric pain/discomfort. Although it is frequently associated with an *H. pylori* infection, it is not characterized by the presence of peptic ulcer disease. However, it can occur in conjunction with one. Nevertheless, it can be ruled out as Mr. Nestor's most likely diagnosis because of the lack of erythema of the gastric mucosa on his endoscopy, which is characteristic of the disease.

5. Treatment Plan

A. Omeprazole 20 mg twice a day for 14 days, then decreased to once a day for 1 to 2 months   CORRECT

A PPI is indicated twice a day for the first 7 to 14 days of treatment, then once a day for an additional 4 to 8 weeks to ensure complete healing of the ulcer. Because no single PPI has been proven superior, omeprazole is an appropriate choice.

B. Clarithromycin 500 mg twice a day plus amoxicillin 1 g twice a day for 14 days   CORRECT

Combination antibiotic therapy for 7 to 14 days is indicated to eradicate the *H. pylori* infection; this is an accepted regimen.

C. Metronidazole 250 mg four times a day plus tetracycline 500 mg four times a day for 14 days   INCORRECT

This choice is incorrect because metronidazole 250 mg four times a day plus tetracycline 500 mg four times a day for

14 days is not effective in the eradication of *H. pylori*; however, the addition of bismuth subsalicylate, 2 tabs, four times a day would make this regimen effective and an appropriate option. Other acceptable alternatives include clarithromycin plus tetracycline and clarithromycin plus metronidazole.

D. Retest for *H. pylori* with serology 1 week after completion of the antibiotic portion of the treatment   INCORRECT

Retesting for *H. pylori* to ensure the eradication of the infection should not be performed any sooner than a minimum of 1 week after the completion of the last dose of the PPI, not the antibiotic. Furthermore, testing with serology to determine whether the infection has been eradicated after completion of the antibiotic portion of the treatment is an inappropriate choice because up to 40% of all patients with an *H. pylori* infection will have a positive serology to *H. pylori* 1 year after the associated condition has been successfully treated. Therefore, testing by serology after the end of the antibiotic therapy will frequently result in a false-positive test and concerns that the infection is still present despite treatment.

E. Retest for *H. pylori* with either stool antigen assay or urea breath test after completion of the antibiotic portion of the treatment   INCORRECT

Retesting for *H. pylori* with either stool antigen assay or urea breath test after completion of the antibiotic portion of the treatment, but while the patient is still on PPI therapy, can produce false-negative results because of the PPI. This could also lead to the incorrect assumption that the infection has been eradicated. As stated previously, the ultimate time to retest for eradication is at least 1 week after the completion of the last dose of the PPI utilizing either a stool antigen assay or urea breath test (preferred method).

If it appears that the patient is going to require maintenance PPI therapy for a longer period of time, then the PPI should be stopped for 1 week, the test performed, and the medication resumed.

Epidemiologic and Other Data

Duodenal ulcers (DUs) are estimated to affect approximately 6 to 15% of adults residing in the United States. Over 95% of them occur in the most proximal segment of the duodenum, with approximately 90% being located within the first 3 cm of the duodenum. In general, they are less than or equal to 1 cm in size; however, ulcers as large as 6 cm have been reported.

The bacterium *H. pylori* has been implicated as the causative agent in the majority (90 to 95%) of cases of DUs. It is believed that the treatment for this bacterial infection has significantly reduced not only the incidence but also the morbidity (including frequent recurrences and the need for surgical interventions) and mortality related to duodenal ulcer disease. The other two most frequent causes of DUs are NSAID usage and overproduction of gastric acid, as seen in conditions such as Zollinger-Ellison syndrome.

Duodenal ulcers and gastric ulcers (GUs) collectively are termed peptic ulcer disease (PUD). The lifetime incidence of developing PUD for an individual residing in the United States is estimated to be approximately 10% for females and 12% for males. The ratio of DU to GU is considered to be approximately 5:1.

Gastric ulcers are associated with a significantly higher rate of gastrointestinal malignancy mortality when compared to DUs. Further, GUs tend to be associated with an older age at onset and a male predominance.

CASE 5-4
Norma Olsen
1. History

A. Does she ever have to get up at night to have a bowel movement?   ESSENTIAL

The presence of nocturnal bowel movement(s) is significant because individuals with functional bowel disorders rarely have nocturnal bowel movements, whereas patients with organic causes frequently experience nocturnal symptoms.

B. Has she experienced any unintentional weight change since her illness began?   ESSENTIAL

A significant (defined as > 10 lb in 1 month) weight loss in conjunction with diarrhea and lower abdominal pain can result from serious gastrointestinal conditions, including carcinomas. In fact, unintentional weight loss is considered to be one of the "red flag" (warning or alarm) symptoms (although some are signs) for patients presenting with abdominal pain and diarrhea.

The other "red flag" symptoms include elderly age, anemia, gross or occult blood in the stool, fever, severe diarrhea (especially if nocturnal), progressive worsening of symptoms, acute onset of symptoms, unremitting pain, being unresponsive to conservative treatment, and positive family history of colon cancer or IBD.

C. Had she acquired a pet before the onset of her symptoms?   NONESSENTIAL

There are so few zoonoses that cause abdominal pain with diarrhea that this is generally not a consideration. The most frequently encountered is probably the transmission of *Salmonella* from miniature turtles; however, this should be an acute, short-duration illness.

D. What joints tend to be affected with the "arthritis"?   ESSENTIAL

Because the majority of IBDs are considered to be "immune mediated," other symptoms frequently observed in "autoimmune" conditions, such as fatigue and arthralgias, need to be fully evaluated to determine whether the symptom is related to the chief complaint (making the possibility of an IBD more likely) or belongs to a coexisting condition.

Regarding arthralgias, which joints and the number affected are important distinguishing characteristics that can assist in ruling in or ruling out potential differential diagnoses. Although there is some overlap, many conditions have specific disease patterns. For example, osteoarthritis, technically classified as a monoarthritis, is most frequently a polyarthritis involving the distal interphalangeal (DIP), proximal interphalangeal (PIP), first carpometacarpal, first metatarsophalangeal, knee, hip, lumbar vertebral, and cervical vertebral joints; acute gouty arthritis is typically a monoarticular disease most frequently involving the first metatarsophalangeal, tarsal, ankle, and knee joints; and rheumatoid arthritis is a polyarthritis most commonly affecting the PIP, metacarpophalangeal, wrist, and knee joints. The joints most frequently involved in patients with IBD are the knee, ankle, and PIP.

E. Has she ever been diagnosed with iritis, uveitis, episcleritis, sclerosing cholangitis, pyoderma gangrenosum, thromboembolic disease, erythema nodosum, urinary calculi, urinary obstruction, osteoporosis, endocarditis, myocarditis, and/or interstitial lung disease?   ESSENTIAL

This is a list of other conditions that commonly occur with IBD. Their presence could add additional support toward a diagnosis of IBD being Mrs. Olsen's most likely diagnosis.

2. Physical Examination

A. Thyroid palpation   ESSENTIAL

Hyperthyroidism has been implicated as a cause of diarrheal disease. Therefore, a thyroid examination might provide clues to her diagnosis. However, it is important to remember that both hyperthyroidism and hypothyroidism can occur with a completely normal thyroid examination.

B. Abdominal examination   ESSENTIAL

An abdominal examination is essential because Mrs. Olsen is complaining of abdominal pain and diarrhea. Areas of tenderness and masses as well as organomegaly in relationship to their location are important in developing her differential diagnosis list. (For more information regarding the abdominal examination, please see Case 5-1.)

C. Rectal examination with fecal occult blood testing ESSENTIAL

A rectal examination with fecal occult blood testing is also important to perform on Mrs. Olsen because abnormalities of the external anal area can provide clues to certain conditions (e.g., hemorrhoids, fissures, and fistulas can be associated with IBD; rectal masses can be a polyp, rectal carcinoma, or other tumor; and poor sphincter tone and/or weak abdominal, pelvic, and/or rectal muscles can be seen with a variety of neurologic conditions).

The presence (or absence) of occult blood discovered in the stool must be interpreted with caution because of the significant number of false-positives and false-negatives associated with this single test. (Please see Cases 5-1 and 5-2 for additional information.)

D. Pelvic examination   NONESSENTIAL

A pelvic examination is not indicated on Mrs. Olsen at this time because she had a complete hysterectomy with bilateral ovariosalpingectomy several years ago and has not been sexually active in over 1 year. That removes the potential for the majority of gynecologic disorders that can present as abdominal pain (e.g., pelvic inflammatory disease, uterine leiomyomas, endometritis, ovarian torsion, ovarian cysts, and ectopic pregnancy).

E. Hand examination   ESSENTIAL

A hand examination is important to determine whether Mrs. Olsen's arthralgias are a "true" arthritis versus joint pain from another cause. Furthermore, it permits the examiner to evaluate for the presence of clubbing of the nails, abnormalities of the fingernails, Raynaud disease or syndrome, and

circulatory problems. Arthritic changes in the PIP and clubbing of the nails can be seen in IBD.

Although PIP arthritis and nail clubbing can be seen with IBD, their presence is only supportive, not pathognomonic, for this diagnosis. Other coexisting medical condition(s) can be responsible for these findings. The presentation or discovery of multiple signs and symptoms during a single encounter does not necessarily indicate that they are all connected to a single diagnosis. Patients can have multiple diagnoses identified during a single clinical visit.

3. Diagnostic Studies

A. Complete blood count with differential (CBC w/diff) ESSENTIAL

A CBC w/diff should be performed on Mrs. Olsen to assist in determining whether there is any evidence of an infectious, inflammatory, or anemic process associated with her condition.

B. Thyroid-stimulating hormone (TSH), free thyroxine (FT_4), and triiodothyronine by radioimmunoassay (T_3 by RIA) ESSENTIAL

Thyroid function studies should also be done because hyperthyroidism, a pituitary abnormality, or a hypothalamic condition could all present as diarrhea, fatigue, and weight loss.

C. Antiendomysial antibodies   NONESSENTIAL

Celiac disease, which can present as intermittent abdominal pain and diarrhea, is generally associated with positive antiendomysial antibodies. This is the only test recommended by the ACG for patients with frequent diarrhea who do not have "red flag" symptoms. However, Mrs. Olsen has "red flag" symptoms making this test unnecessary at this time.

D. Colonoscopy   ESSENTIAL

A colonoscopy is indicated in Mrs. Olsen's case for several reasons: (1) the presence of a rectal mass discovered during her DRE; (2) the presence of several "red flag" symptoms (fever [low grade on examination and possibly present per history], nocturnal symptoms, severe diarrhea [defined as six or more BMs per day; mild is defined as less than four and moderate as four to six] when it does occur, progressive nature to her symptoms, and their acute onset); and (3) colorectal cancer (CRC) screening because of her age and the lack of previous screening.

The latest recommendations from the American Cancer Society (ACS) state that appropriate screening techniques include colonoscopy every 10 years OR sigmoidoscopy every 5 years **with** highly sensitive fecal occult blood testing performed on three separate stool specimens, taken on 3 different days, every 3 years OR highly sensitive fecal occult blood testing of three separate stool specimens, taken on 3 different days, annually. These recommendations are for average-risk individuals between the ages of 50 and 75 years. Because of the more advanced stages of CRC at diagnosis and the earlier age of presentation, the ACS recommends screening African Americans earlier (e.g., 45 years of age if normal risk).

E. Stool sample or rectal biopsy for immunoassays for *Clostridium difficile* toxins A and B   NONESSENTIAL

C. difficile colitis is generally associated with antibiotics causing a disruption of the normal intestinal flora, permitting this organism to produce its toxins. Its onset typically occurs after the patient has received antibiotic therapy for a few days to shortly after completion of the course of antibiotics; occasionally it does not manifest until several weeks after the antibiotic therapy has been completed. The majority of cases of *C. difficile* colitis are self-limiting; however, in rare cases, it can be complicated by peritonitis, septic shock, and death.

Because Mrs. Olsen lacks a history of antibiotic usage for at least 2 years and her diarrheal illness has been present for 10 months, this diagnosis is highly unlikely. However, some experts feel that prior gastrointestinal infection(s) with *C. difficile* (and/or another organism) may be responsible for IBD. Other postulated "triggering" organisms for IBD include *Escherichia* sp., *Salmonella* sp., *Shigella* sp., *Campylobacter* sp., *Lactobacillus* sp., *Taenia suis,* and *Saccharomyces boulardii*.

4. Diagnosis

A. Irritable bowel syndrome (IBS) with polyps   INCORRECT

Even though Mrs. Olsen has colonic polyps identified on her colonoscopy and her symptoms would meet the Rome III diagnostic criteria for IBS (symptoms present for a minimum of 6 months AND within the last 3 months experiencing on a minimum of 3 days per month an intermittent abdominal pain accompanied by two of the following three conditions: pain alleviated with a BM, pain onset associated with a change in BM frequency, and/or pain onset linked to a change in stool consistency), her history (e.g., presence of nocturnal diarrhea), other findings on colonoscopy (e.g., ulcerations), and the histology of her biopsy specimens are not consistent with this diagnosis; therefore, this is not Mrs. Olsen's most likely diagnosis.

B. Crohn disease with polyps   CORRECT

Crohn disease (CD) is one of the two major forms of IBD. The other is ulcerative colitis (UC). Although some symptoms are more prevalent in one of the conditions (e.g., UC is almost always accompanied by the appearance of gross blood and mucus in the stool, whereas they rarely occur with CD; conversely, patients with CD frequently have systemic symptoms and pain, whereas patients with UC rarely have these symptoms), their initial presentation can be very similar. Often histologic examination of the intestinal mucosa (which will reveal granulomatous changes in CD) is required to differentiate the two conditions. The appearance of a distinct separation of abnormal lesions/ulcerations by normal tissue (known as "cobblestoning") is considered pathognomonic for CD, whereas UC's involvement is almost always continuous. Although CD can occur anywhere from the mouth to the perineal area, the lack of rectal involvement is also more consistent with a diagnosis of CD because the disease process in UC almost always involves the rectum. Finally, UC is only found in the large intestine.

Mrs. Olsen's symptoms, physical examination findings, and diagnostic test results are consistent with the diagnosis of Crohn disease. The identification of polyps on the colonoscopy and their confirmation by histology examination establish the remaining half of this diagnosis.

C. Ulcerative colitis with polyps   INCORRECT

As stated previously, UC is the second major type of IBD. Despite Mrs. Olsen having several signs and symptoms that are suggestive of this condition, UC can be ruled out as her most likely diagnosis because her colonoscopy findings are inconsistent with this diagnosis. The typical colonoscopy findings seen in UC include a colonic mucosa that has generalized erythema, edema, and a mild granular appearance (often referred to as "sandpaper"-like). Small localized hemorrhages can also be visible as well as ulcerations of varying sizes. As the disease progresses, the hemorrhages and ulcerations increase in size and frequently involve the entire colon (starting distally and extending proximally). Megacolon and perforations are also possible late findings.

Furthermore, Mrs. Olsen's histologic findings are also inconsistent with this diagnosis. The histology of the biopsied tissue in UC generally reveals crypt abnormalities, including a decrease in total number and cryptal separation, and cellular abnormalities, which can include inflammation as a result of the invasion of plasma cells, macrophages, lymphocytes, and neutrophils. Additionally, she lacked a bloody diarrhea, which is almost always a clinical feature of UC, and experienced abdominal pain, which is generally not seen in UC.

D. Familial adenomatous polyposis   INCORRECT

Familial adenomatous polyposis (FAP) is a hereditary syndrome caused by a chromosomal abnormality related to a germline mutation. It is characterized by numerous (frequently hundreds to thousands) adenomatous colorectal polyps, of which a few will develop atypical histologic findings and a very small percentage of these will develop into full malignancies.

It can be ruled out as Mrs. Olsen's most likely diagnosis because she lacks a family history of colorectal polyps and colorectal cancer. Additionally, she only had three large polyps on examination, not the hundreds to thousands that are typically seen in this disease.

E. Celiac disease   INCORRECT

Celiac disease (also known as celiac sprue, nontropical sprue, and gluten-sensitive enteropathy) is the most common malabsorption syndrome in Americans. It can encompass an entire spectrum of symptomatology ranging from asymptomatic (diagnosed via serologic or small bowel biopsy) to diarrhea with steatorrhea, weight loss, and severe malnutrition with resultant anemia and osteoporosis.

Despite the fact that the symptoms can be intermittent and the diagnosis can be made in adulthood, it is extremely unlikely for the initial presentation of celiac disease to be diarrhea in a 58-year-old. Furthermore, although it can present as diarrhea, abdominal pain is not a typical feature of celiac sprue. Finally, because nontropical sprue is a disorder of the small intestinal mucosa, it is not going to be associated with any large intestinal and/or rectal abnormalities as discovered on Mrs. Olsen's colonoscopy. Thus, this is not her most likely diagnosis.

5. Treatment Plan

A. Colectomy   INCORRECT

Although a colectomy is a treatment for severe Crohn disease, Mrs. Olsen's history, physical examination, and diagnostic test findings are not severe enough to justify this drastic surgical procedure as a first-line treatment component for her disease.

B. Well-balanced, heart-smart diet   CORRECT

A well-balanced, heart-smart diet is indicated for any patient. However, because of the special nutritional needs associated with CD (plus the patient's desire to lose weight), it is essential.

C. Trial of avoidance of dairy products   CORRECT

Very few limitations are placed on the diet of a patient with Crohn disease; however, because of the high incidence of associated lactose intolerance with this condition, it is worth a trial of dairy product elimination to see whether any improvement of symptoms could be achieved, despite Mrs. Olsen not being able to link the ingestion of dairy products to her symptoms.

D. Cholestyramine 2 to 4 mg two to three times per day before meals   CORRECT

Cholestyramine 2 to 4 mg two to three times per day before meals is often effective to absorb moisture out of the stool and cause it to be firmer. Because of this ability, it is considered to be a first-line treatment for mild to moderate Crohn disease, despite not having a US Food and Drug Administration (FDA)-approved indication for this condition.

E. Prednisone 10 mg bid   INCORRECT

Although prednisone is a very effective drug for the treatment of Crohn disease, this choice would be inappropriate at this time for Mrs. Olsen because it is indicated only in moderate to severe disease, or mild to moderate disease that is unresponsive to other treatment modalities.

Epidemiologic and Other Data

The incidence of individuals residing in the United States to acquire Crohn disease is estimated to range from 3.1 to 14.6 per 100,000 patient-years. It has two primary peaks of onset: the first peak occurs during the latter half of the second to the end of the third decades of life, and the second peak is during the seventh and eighth decades of life. It tends to occur more frequently in women, individuals of higher socioeconomic status, urban dwellers, and smokers.

Ethnicity and race tend to also influence the rate of CD. Individuals of Jewish descent have the highest overall incidence of CD (estimated to be two to four times greater). The lowest prevalence tends to be in Asian Americans. African Americans and Hispanic Americans have slightly lower rates than non-Hispanic, non-Jewish Caucasians.

Individuals residing in various parts of the world have significant differences in the incidence of CD. The highest incidences are seen in Europe (including the United Kingdom) and North America (including the United States).

CASE 5-5
Oscar Phillips
1. History

A. Has he noticed a change in his weight and/or appetite? ESSENTIAL

Because of his symptoms, his differential diagnosis list can be quite extensive. It can range from **a**lcohol-related conditions (e.g., gastritis, cirrhosis, hepatitis, or mood disorders) **to z**oonotic infections because of an underlying immune deficiency. A significant weight increase in conjunction with his

symptoms could result from ascites and pedal edema caused by an underlying infectious, inflammatory, or malignant process of the liver or pancreas. Likewise, these symptoms, a weight increase, and pedal edema could represent a cardiovascular or renal abnormality in conjunction with a hepatic, hepatobiliary, or pancreatic disease. Furthermore, a weight gain could represent excessive eating to ease gastritis, anxiety, or depression.

On the other hand, the aforementioned gastrointestinal conditions and mood disorders can be responsible for a significant weight loss. Other potential causes include a cachetic state from a noncancerous liver or pancreas condition, a hepatic infection, an underlying immune deficiency, a thiamine deficiency, other nutritional deficiency, chronic alcoholism, avoidance of eating because of pain (e.g., gastritis, esophagitis, or esophageal strictures), or reduced food intake secondary to dysgeusia and/or anorexia).

Likewise, dysgeusia can be caused by any of the aforementioned gastrointestinal conditions; however, it can also result from a wide array of other disease processes that may or may not be related to his present illness. These potential abnormalities including localized oropharyngeal conditions (e.g., fungal infection, viral infection, or xerostomia), upper respiratory conditions (e.g., bacterial or viral sinusitis or allergic rhinitis), other gastrointestinal conditions (e.g., gastroesophageal reflux disease or postvagectomy), neurologic disorders (e.g., heavy metal intoxication, cerebral vascular accidents, and facial nerve palsies), autoimmune conditions (e.g., Sjögren syndrome or Wegener granulomatosis), metabolic conditions (e.g., renal diseases), endocrine disturbances (e.g., hypothyroidism and diabetes mellitus), and adverse effects of medications (e.g., tetracycline, antithyroid drugs, and chemotherapy).

B. Has he ever had a tattoo?   ESSENTIAL

In addition to Mr. Phillips' previously identified risk factors for acquiring a blood-borne infection, having a tattoo is an additional risk factor that should be sought. Tattooing is not always performed under sterile conditions. Hence, there is the concern of typical and atypical (if the patient is immunocompromised) organisms causing an acute dermatologic infection that could lead to sepsis and multiorgan failure. The practice of reusing needles or an accidental needlestick to an infected artist during the procedure can also place the patient at risk for blood-borne infections that can cause malaise, fatigue, and abdominal pain. These infections include the human immunodeficiency virus (HIV), hepatitis B virus (HBV), hepatitis C virus (HCV), hepatitis D virus (HDV), and *Mycobacterium leprae*. Additionally, there is the rare possibility of lead toxicity from the colored ink that can lead to intermittent colicky abdominal pain.

C. Does he consume raw seafood?   ESSENTIAL

Consumption of undercooked or raw contaminated seafood can also lead to gastrointestinal and/or hepatic illnesses that can present with symptoms similar to Mr. Phillips'. Some of the offending organisms that might require testing to identify include HBV, *Vibrio parahaemolyticus*, *Entamoeba histolytica*, and occasionally *Plesiomonas* sp.

D. Has he noticed any mental status, cognitive, or mood changes?   ESSENTIAL

In conjunction with Mr. Phillips' previously identified symptoms, the appearance of alterations (and their severity)

in any of these areas could represent anything from a coexisting mood disorder to a metabolic encephalopathy. Encephalopathies can include a wide range of neuropsychiatric symptoms from mild memory loss, depression, and anxiety to psychosis, stupor, and coma.

Encephalopathy can be associated with several conditions. Of particular concern in Mr. Phillips' case would be HIV dementia (dementia caused by an underlying acquired immunodeficiency syndrome [AIDS]); a hepatic, or portal-systemic, encephalopathy (neuropsychiatric symptoms resulting from the reflux of nitrogenous toxins from the portal to systemic circulation caused by a hepatic disease); Wernicke syndrome (a psychosis caused by toxins produced from a thiamin deficiency usually secondary to chronic alcohol use/abuse); and Korsakoff syndrome, or alcoholic amnestic syndrome (alcohol use/abuse resulting in confusion and significant recent memory loss frequently compensated by telling of untruths).

E. When was the last time he was sexually active with a woman?   NONESSENTIAL

Questions regarding Mr. Phillips' sexual history should only serve to determine his risk status in regards to the possibility of a sexually transmitted infection being responsible for his current illness. The provided history is sufficient to determine he is at high risk.

Furthermore, questioning him about this sensitive subject in this manner can be detrimental to the patient–provider relationship and the honesty of information reported by the patient, because the "tone" of this question could be interpreted as judgmental to the patient in regards to his sexual orientation if he is not bisexual.

2. Physical Examination

A. Oropharyngeal examination   ESSENTIAL

Because Mr. Phillips is complaining of unremitting halitosis and dysgeusia, a comprehensive oropharyngeal examination needs to be performed to evaluate for lesions, discolorations, atrophy, dryness, edema, signs of infection, and other abnormalities of his oral cavity, pharynx, lips, tongue (including the dorsal surface where the majority of oral carcinomas are located), gingivae, and teeth.

In addition to the visualization of the area, his breath should be evaluated for foul and distinct odors (e.g., fruity odor [caused by the production of ketones and acetone from the destruction of stored fat cells in patients with diabetic ketoacidosis], almondlike odor [associated with cyanide poisoning], or fetor hepaticus [caused by the aromatic substances that develop in the blood and urine of patients with chronic hepatic disease]).

The tongue, floor and lateral aspects of the mouth, gingival surfaces, and lips should be palpated for masses that are not visible. The teeth should be palpated for tenderness and abnormal motion that could represent an underlying dental, gingival, or bony structural defect.

B. Heart and lung auscultation   ESSENTIAL

Auscultation of the heart is important to evaluate for distant heart sounds and/or ventricular enlargement that could suggest the presence of a cardiomyopathy and/or heart failure (HF) because Mr. Phillips is complaining of pedal edema.

Additionally, the heart valves need to be evaluated for murmurs that could suggest a structural valvular defect and/or endocarditis. Lung auscultation is necessary to evaluate for signs consistent with HF.

C. Abdominal and rectal examination   ESSENTIAL

An abdominal examination should be conducted as outlined in Case 5-1 because Mr. Phillips' chief complaint is abdominal pain.

A rectal examination is almost always indicated in a patient with severe GI symptoms in order to assist in the determination of the correct diagnosis, prevent missing a serious condition (for more information regarding the rectal examination, please see Case 5-1), and test the stool specimen for occult blood (for more information on limitations of a single stool specimen obtained during the physical examination, please see Cases 5-1 and 5-2). Furthermore, because of complications for the receptive participant of men who have sex with men, the rectal examination should evaluate for certain conditions (e.g., rectal fissures, poor sphincter tone, internal and external human papillomavirus [HPV] lesions, and minor rectal abnormalities that could suggest HPV [because of its apparent association with rectal cancer]), other signs suggestive of a sexually transmitted infection (e.g., rectal discharge and tenderness associated with gonococcal proctitis; painless, single ulcer associated with primary syphilis; and painful papules, vesicles, and/or ulcerations as can be seen with herpes simplex infections), and any other visible lesions.

D. Skin and sclera examination   ESSENTIAL

A skin and sclera examination is indicated for Mr. Phillips to evaluate for the presence of jaundice and/or icterus that could indicate that a hepatic or hepatobiliary ductal abnormality is the cause of his complaint. This is important despite his denial of skin color changes because it is not unusual for minimal changes not to be noticed by patients and/or their close contacts, especially if these findings are mild and gradual in onset and/or occur in an individual of color or with tanned skin. When evaluating for skin color changes in individuals of color or with tanned skin, jaundice (especially if mild) is frequently easier to identify on the palms of the hands because they tend to be lighter in color than the remaining skin, so changes are more apparent. Furthermore, conducting the examination in a location with a good light source is key to early identification.

Additionally, the skin examination should also evaluate for other clues to assist in confirming or refuting the most likely differential diagnoses and/or identifying coexisting or comorbid conditions. For example, some liver conditions are associated with other specific and nonspecific skin changes (e.g., palmar erythema, spider telangiectasias, contusions, caput medusae, and Dupuytren contracture).

In a correctly performed dermatologic examination, the HCP would not randomly evaluate areas of the body that are most likely to demonstrate abnormalities in overall color, segmental color variations, lesions, edema, and venous dilatation that could be associated with the patient's chief complaint but would conduct an organized, comprehensive skin evaluation to ensure that related (and unrelated) abnormalities are not missed.

The visual portion of the examination evaluates for asymmetry between right and left sides of the body as well as the presence of generalized color changes, localized color variations, lesions, and/or edema. Any abnormality should be described in terms of location, whether it is unilateral or bilateral (and if bilateral, whether it is equal or unequal), pattern of distribution, size, and type (e.g., macule, papule, wheal, vesicle, contusion, or ulcer). Special attention needs to be paid to pigmented lesions, utilizing the ABCs established to identify potential malignant melanoma (**A**symmetry, **B**order irregularity, **C**olor changes, **D**iameter of larger size, and **E**levated areas).

Further, the skin examination should include palpation of the skin for superficial texture (e.g., oiliness, moistness, dryness, and other abnormalities). If lesions are present, the HCP should use examination gloves unless he or she is absolutely certain the abnormalities are noninfectious. Lesions should be palpated for tenderness, texture, consistency, blanching, and histamine release. If suspicious for an infection (e.g., cellulitis, folliculitis, abscess, or furuncle) or malignancy, a regional lymph node examination should also be performed.

Edematous areas should be evaluated for symmetry within the area and with the contralateral aspect of the body, tenderness, temperature changes, and "pitting." Finally, the skin should be examined for temperature changes. Any abnormalities should be further evaluated by obtaining additional history, determining if a vasodilatation or vasoconstriction is present, testing capillary refill, and checking associated pulses.

E. Gastro-omental, gastric, colic, and superior mesenteric lymph node palpation   NONESSENTIAL

The enlargement of these lymph nodes could provide useful information regarding the potential location of the patient's problem as well as whether it could be an infectious or malignant process. However, because these lymph nodes are located deep in the abdominal cavity near their corresponding vein, they cannot be evaluated via palpation, even in very thin individuals.

3. Diagnostic Studies

A. Alanine aminotransferase (ALT), aspartate aminotransferase (AST), and γ-glutamyl transferase (GGT)   ESSENTIAL

Because Mr. Phillips' symptoms and findings on his physical examination are very suspicious of either an intrahepatic or hepatobiliary abnormality, liver function tests are indicated. The ALT is almost entirely specific for hepatic problems, whereas the AST can also be elevated in cardiac ischemia. Viewed together, these two tests can provide very useful information. If both are essentially equally elevated, it almost always indicates the presence of a hepatic problem. If the elevation is less than five times the upper limit of normal, conditions such as chronic viral hepatitis, medication adverse effects, autoimmune hepatitis, cirrhosis, and alcohol-related hepatic injury lead the list of possible diagnoses. If the values are more than five times the upper limit of normal, then the most common diagnoses include acute ischemic hepatitis and acute bile duct obstruction.

The ratio of these tests to each other can provide additional support regarding the presence of hepatocellular disease. The ALT/AST ratio (De Ritis ratio) is almost always less than 1.0 in patients with a hepatocellular condition, with the exception of viral hepatitis. In both acute and chronic viral hepatitis, this ratio is generally greater than 1.0.

The GGT is generally the most sensitive of these tests to indicate the presence of a biliary obstruction; however, it can also be elevated in alcohol-related conditions.

B. Prothrombin time (PT), total protein, albumin, and bilirubin (total, direct, and indirect)   ESSENTIAL

Many of the clotting factors are produced in the liver; therefore, with severe liver disease they will be produced in much lower concentrations, leading to increased bleeding times and an increased PT. However, obstructive biliary disease can also cause the PT to elevate via fat malabsorption from failure of the bile to enter the GI tract in response to eating. Other nonhepatic causes can include taking aspirin or warfarin, disseminated intravascular coagulation (DIC), intrinsic factor or vitamin K deficiency, or large blood transfusions.

Albumin is the primary protein made in the liver. Therefore, in hepatic disease the protein and albumin are often decreased.

Bilirubin is a component of the bile metabolized by the liver and stored in the gallbladder to be expelled when the patient eats. Therefore, the total bilirubin can be elevated in both hepatic and obstructive gallbladder disease. However, breaking it down into its direct (conjugated) and indirect (unconjugated) components can assist in establishing the patient's diagnosis. An increase in direct bilirubin tends to be associated with cholelithiasis, duct obstruction, or adverse medication reactions. An increase in indirect bilirubin is generally associated with a primary hepatic disease (e.g., hepatitis, cirrhosis, or hemolytic jaundice). However, other rarer conditions that can affect the liver and/or the red blood cells can account for these abnormalities as well.

C. Hepatitis B surface antigen (HBsAg), hepatitis B surface antibody (HBsAb), hepatitis B core antibody total (HBcAb total), hepatitis B core antibody immunoglobulin M (HBcAb IgM), hepatitis B e-antigen (HBeAg), and hepatitis B e-antibody (HBeAb)   ESSENTIAL

These tests are important in determining the patient's HBV status. The presence or absence of these antigens and antibodies can not only determine if a patient has a current or previous HBV infection but also, if an infection is present, whether it is acute or chronic. **Table 5-1** indicates the typical postexposure appearance, postexposure disappearance and significance of each of these tests.

D. Abdominal ultrasound   ESSENTIAL

The first-line imaging study for Mr. Phillips to determine the size, composition, regularity, and presence of tumors/masses of his liver and spleen (especially because they could not be accurately assessed via physical examination) as well as to evaluate the ascites is an abdominal ultrasound.

E. Serum α-fetoprotein (AFP)   ESSENTIAL

Serum AFP levels are most commonly used in obstetrics to screen maternal blood for possible fetal abnormalities (e.g., Down syndrome and fetal wasting are suspected by a decreased AFP level, whereas an increased level is suspicious for neural tubal defects, abdominal wall defects, congenital anomalies, threatened or incomplete abortion, fetal distress, or multiple gestation).

However, AFP is an oncofetal protein; therefore, it can also be utilized as a tumor marker and/or for screening for

Table 5-1 Typical Serological Findings in Hepatitis B

Test	Appearance	Disappearance	Significance
HBsAg	4–12 weeks	1–3 months	Acute infection, often present before prodromal symptoms occur If persists, considered to be a chronic carrier
HBsAb	3–10 months	6–10 years	Prior infection/immunity assumed
HBcAb	3–12 weeks	Never	Prior infection/convalescent stage
HBcAb IgM	2–12 weeks	3–6 months	Acute infection present
HBeAg	1–3 weeks	6–8 weeks	Early acute infection with highest possibility of transmission If persists, increased risk of chronic infection
HBeAb	4–6 weeks	4–6 years	Acute infection almost resolved or no longer present; risk of transmission now low If persists, increased risk of chronic infection

Adapted from Pagana KD, Pagana TJ. Hepatitis virus studies. Pagana KD, Pagana TJ. *Mosby's Diagnostic and Laboratory Test Reference*. 8th ed. St. Louis: Mosby Elsevier; 2007:526–530.

certain malignancies in high-risk individuals. Because AFP is produced by the fetus' liver and yolk sac, an elevated value could indicate hepatic carcinomas or tumors arising from germ cells (e.g., ovarian, testicular, renal cell, lymphoma, and Hodgkin disease). The degree of elevation appears to be proportional to the severity of the tumor burden. Additionally, it can be mildly elevated in noncancerous conditions that are associated with hepatic necrosis (e.g., hepatitis, cirrhosis, and ischemia).

4. Diagnosis

A. Acute hepatitis B   INCORRECT

Hepatitis is an inflammatory hepatic disease that is characterized by some degree of hepatic insufficiency, hepatic cell necrosis, Kupffer cell hyperplasia, and cholestasis. Because the symptoms can frequently be the same in acute (generally defined as present for < 6 months) and chronic (generally defined as present for > 6 months) hepatitis, it is frequently difficult to distinguish between the two based on the clinical picture alone. In dealing with viral causes (which almost exclusively cause acute hepatitis), this differentiation is generally made based on the results of the various serologic markers.

Regarding hepatitis caused by an HBV infection, both acute and chronic hepatitis can be associated with positive serologic markers for HBeAg and HBeAb. Nevertheless, acute HBV hepatitis can be eliminated as Mr. Phillips' most likely diagnosis because his laboratory testing does not reveal a positive HBsAg or HBcAb IgM, which are almost always present in an acute HBV infection. Furthermore, he has a positive result for the HBcAb, which generally indicates a prior or chronic HBV infection. (Please see Table 5-1.)

B. Chronic hepatitis B, immune tolerant phase   INCORRECT

Distinguishing between the types of chronic infection can also generally be done based on serologic testing. The results typically used in this determination are HBeAg, HBeAb, HBV DNA, ALT, and AST. Even though Mr. Phillips' HBeAg is positive and his levels of HBV DNA are elevated, this is not his most likely diagnosis because he also has elevated liver function tests (LFTs). In the immune tolerant phase the LFTs are generally normal.

C. Chronic hepatitis B, immune active phase   CORRECT

The hallmark of this phase includes a positive HBeAg, elevated levels of HBV DNA, and active liver disease based on LFTs. Thus, this is Mr. Phillips' most likely diagnosis.

D. Chronic hepatitis B, inactive (or remission) phase   INCORRECT

Even though the HBeAb is positive in the inactive phase of chronic HBV infection, this is not Mr. Phillips' most likely diagnosis because the inactive phase is characterized by normal liver enzymes and a low level (or even undetectable levels) of HBV DNA.

However, regardless of which phase the patient is currently diagnosed in, he or she requires frequent monitoring because it is not unusual for the patient to alternate between stages and even revert from an inactive disease to one of the more active forms of chronic hepatitis caused by HBV.

E. Liver cancer   INCORRECT

Although liver cancer can occur as a complication of both acute and chronic hepatitis caused by HBV, it can essentially be ruled out as Mr. Phillips' most likely diagnosis because there was no evidence of a mass or lesion disrupting the architecture of the liver on his abdominal ultrasound. Furthermore, his AFP level was only slightly elevated indicating hepatitis, cirrhosis, or other benign liver diseases in comparison to hepatomas, which tend to significantly elevate AFP levels.

5. Treatment Plan

A. Liver biopsy   CORRECT

Because estimates of survival in patients with chronic HBV are frequently determined by the degree of liver damage identified as necroinflammatory activity and fibrosis on the histologic examination of the hepatic tissue, a liver biopsy is essential to determine the classification/grade (degree of necroinflammatory activity) and stage (severity of fibrosis) of his disease.

There are two primary systems for determining the classification/grade of chronic hepatitis infections. They are the Histological Activity Index (HAI) score and the less extensive METAVIR scale. Regardless of which system is utilized, the patient is either classified as having no (inactive carriers), mild, moderate, or severe disease. In general, the severity of the disease is directly correlated to the elevation of the total score (i.e., lower scores are associated with mild disease, whereas the highest scores are associated with the most severe disease).

In the HAI system, the necroinflammatory activity, or grade, is given a score by assigning points based on the degree of periportal necrosis (ranging from 0 [if none] to 4 [if severe necrosis is present]), confluent intralobular necrosis (ranging from 0 [if none] to 6 [if panacinar/multiacinar cells are present]), focal intralobular necrosis (ranging from 0 [if none] to 4 [if more than 10 foci are found under a 10 × microscopic field]), and portal inflammation (ranging from 0 [if none] to 4 [if marked portal inflammation is present]).

In contrast, the METAVIR system does not consider the degree of portal inflammation in assessing the severity of the necroinflammatory activity. Further, it does not distinguish between confluent and focal intralobular necrosis when evaluating the extent of intralobular necrosis; however, when evaluating periportal necrosis, the METAVIR system separates piecemeal necrosis from bridging necrosis. It provides a score of 0 (mild) to 3 (severe) when defining the degree of piecemeal necrosis; a score of 0 (none or mild) to 2 (severe) for the degree of intralobular necrosis; and a "present" or "absent" regarding bridging necrosis.

The disease's stage is determined by the severity of the fibrosis (ranging from 0 points [none] to 6 points [cirrhosis present] in the HAI classification scheme and ranging from 0 points [none] to 4 points [cirrhosis present] in the METAVIR system) on histologic examination.

B. Hepatitis B virus (HBV) DNA levels   CORRECT

Although classification and stage are important to determine survival in patients with HBV infections, the decision to treat (or not) depends more on the level of viral replication; therefore, it is very important to obtain an HBV DNA level on Mr. Phillips.

In chronic hepatitis caused by HBV, generally the severity of the infection is directly proportional to the degree of HBV DNA elevation. Thus, the greater the viral replication (as indicated by the HBV DNA level), the more severe the disease process is going to be.

C. Hepatitis A virus antibody (HAV-Ab) IgM and IgG   CORRECT

Experts recommend immunizing all patients with hepatitis caused by HBV, especially if chronic, with the HAV vaccine if they test negative for an HAV infection. Therefore, Mr. Phillips needs to be tested for the presence of a past or current HAV infection before proceeding with the vaccination.

If both his HAV-Ab IgM and HAV-Ab IgG are negative, then Mr. Phillips is at risk for acquiring HAV and requires the immunization. If his HAV-Ab IgM is positive and his HAV-Ab IgG is negative, he is suspected of having an acute HAV infection and appropriate evaluation and possibly treatment are indicated. If his HAV-Ab IgM and HAV-Ab IgG are positive, he is considered to have an HAV infection of indeterminate age and again appropriate treatment and follow-up are indicated. Furthermore, he would be considered immune to HAV and not require HAV immunization. However, if his HAV-AB IgG is positive and his HAV-Ab IgM is negative, he would be considered to have previous HAV exposure and immunity; therefore, he would not require the immunization.

D. Interferon alfa-2b, peginterferon alfa-2a, or lamivudine starting 6 months after his HBeAg becomes negative   INCORRECT

Interferon alfa-2b, peginterferon alfa-2a, and lamivudine are all considered to be effective drugs for patients with chronic HBV infections; however, if they are indicated in the patient's treatment plan, they should be initiated immediately after his liver biopsy results are available.

Although the appearance of the HBeAg typically indicates that the acute phase of the infection is nearly or completely resolved, persistent elevations of the HBeAg are a risk factor for chronic HBV infection; furthermore, it is currently unknown if the HBeAg will ever revert to negative in these cases. Therefore, withholding treatment until his HBeAg has been negative for at least 6 months would not be a practical approach for this reason alone. Additionally, based on his history, physical examination, and diagnostic findings, Mr. Phillips already has a chronic HBV infection. This indicates that aggressive therapy needs to be considered immediately to prevent further hepatic damage and complications, not if and when his HBeAg becomes negative.

E. Hepatitis D virus antigen (HDV-Ag), hepatitis D virus antibody total (HDV-Ab total), and hepatitis D virus antibody IgM (HDV-Ab IgM)   CORRECT

Although hepatitis D virus (HDV) is an RNA virus, it appears to almost exclusively occur in the presence of the hepatitis B virus, a DNA virus. Patients simultaneously infected with both HBV and HDV do not appear to have any change in the outcome of their disease. However, if HDV is acquired in a patient with chronic HBV infection, a significantly more severe disease outcome can occur. Therefore, it is important to attempt to determine if he has a coexisting acute HDV infection, has a coexisting chronic HDV infection, or is an HDV carrier.

In general, the presence of a positive HDV-Ag, a positive or negative HDV-Ab IgM, and a negative HDV-Ab total indicates an acute infection. If all three tests are positive, it represents an HDV infection of indeterminate age; however, it is still extremely likely that the patient has an acute HDV infection (because the HDV-Ag is generally undetectable within 1 week postexposure). Likewise, if the patient's HDV-Ag is negative, HDV-Ag IgM is positive, and HDV-Ab total is negative, more than likely the patient has an acute HDV infection because the HDV-Ab IgM generally reverts to negative in 30 to 90 days after exposure to the virus; however, the HDV-Ag total is not generally identifiable in the serum until 60 to 90 days postexposure. If the patient's HDV-Ag is negative, HDV-IgM is positive, and HDV-Ag total is elevated, he either had an HDV infection in the past 14 to 15 months or he had a previous infection and is an HDV carrier. Likewise, a negative HDV-Ag in conjunction with a positive HDV-Ab IgM and HDV-Ab total most likely represents an infection in the past 60 to 90 days or a chronic carrier state for HDV.

Furthermore, most experts agree that it is prudent to evaluate any individual being considered for antiviral therapy, any patient who has a prolonged acute illness from an HBV infection, and any person who develops unexplainable jaundice for the presence of a coexisting HDV infection.

Epidemiologic and Other Data

Hepatitis is an inflammatory process that affects the liver. It is attributed to RNA viruses (hepatitis A, C, D, and E), a DNA virus (hepatitis B), bacterial sepsis, alcohol, toxins, medications, or an autoimmune process. Although hepatitis G and TT viruses exist as blood-borne pathogens, they do not appear to cause hepatic disease.

In acute hepatitis, the cause is almost exclusively a viral process as a result of one of the five hepatitis viruses: HAV, HBV, HCV, HDV, or hepatitis E virus (HEV). Furthermore, HDV is virtually never identified except in the presence of an HBV infection. Some consider the RNA virus hepatitis D to be an exclusive agent of the DNA virus hepatitis B. In chronic hepatitis, the cause is most frequently a viral process (HCV, HBV, and/or HDV).

Hepatitis caused by the hepatitis B virus (previously known as serum hepatitis) is transmitted via blood, semen, salvia, and other bodily fluids. Although it is endemic in some areas of the world (e.g., China, Southeast Asia, and Northern Africa), with over 50% of the population infected with HBV, it is relatively rare in the United States, with an estimated lifetime prevalence of approximately 5%. The estimated lifetime prevalence of chronic HBV infection is estimated to be approximately 0.35% in the United States.

However, this lower prevalence does not appear to be attributable to HBV immunization. After its introduction, the incidence of HBV infection actually increased in the United States. Experts believe this was because the vaccine was initially recommended only for "high-risk" individuals. Studies indicated that more than 90% of individuals who were considered "high risk" never received the vaccine. Furthermore, nearly one third of all the individuals with an acute HBV infections did not meet the "high-risk" criteria. Therefore, universal vaccination starting at birth was instituted.

Unprotected sexual intercourse is the primary means of transmission of HBV in the United States. Vertical transmission (from mother to infant), blood transfusions, dialysis, and nosocomial infections account for a minuscule number of cases in the United States. Known risk factors include unprotected intercourse, IV drug abuse/use (especially if needles are shared), and occupational exposure to blood and body fluids.

The estimated incubation period for HBV is approximately 5 weeks to 6 months. Prodromal symptoms and/or acute hepatitis from HBV may be so mild that they are unnoticed by the patient or are attributed to the "flu." However, infections with HBV (as well as HCV and HDV) can also be extremely severe, producing illness including fulminant cirrhosis, hepatocellular carcinoma (HCC), and even death.

CASE 5-6
Pricilla Queens
1. History

A. Where in her back does the pain radiate?   ESSENTIAL

Although far from specific, the pattern of upper abdominal pain radiation provides important clues to the possible diagnosis. Radiation into the intrascapular area is often seen in conditions that affect the liver, gallbladder, stomach, duodenum, esophagus, and pancreas. Radiation into the flanks can be seen in pancreatic diseases. Radiation to the shoulder or neck is suggestive of an intestinal, gastric, or esophageal perforation as well as a cardiac (e.g., angina, acute myocardial infarction, or pericarditis) or pulmonary (e.g., pulmonary infarction and pneumonia) condition.

However, caution must be taken not to assume that pain in another anatomic location is absolutely caused by radiation from the primary source; it could represent a coexisting condition. This is especially true when dealing with abdominal and thoracic conditions.

B. Has she noticed any skin discolorations, rashes, and/or lesions?   ESSENTIAL

Several types of acute and chronic dermatologic manifestations can be seen in patients with gastrointestinal complaints. Although they are not pathognomonic for a specific disease process, they can provide useful clues in assisting to establish the correct diagnosis.

Discolorations can be seen in a variety of conditions. Jaundice is frequently associated with hepatocellular liver diseases and obstructive biliary diseases. Although rare in pancreatic diseases, it can occur if the pancreatic head compresses the intrapancreatic segment of the common bile duct. Multiple contusions in varying stages of healing can be seen in hepatocellular liver diseases and obstructive biliary diseases that can prevent the formation of the coagulation factor and multiple traumas, including intimate partner violence. A light bluish discoloration around the umbilicus (Cullen sign) can be seen if there is blood in the peritoneal cavity. A purplish or greenish-brown discoloration over the flanks (Turner sign) is sometimes evident in abdominal conditions that are associated with the breakdown of hemoglobin.

Erythematous subcutaneous nodules secondary to fat necrosis can occasionally be seen in necrotizing pancreatitis. Yellowish-colored elongated plaques (xanthomas) can be visualized on the extensor surfaces of the knees and elbows, on the upper eyelids, and medial to the inner canthus of the eyes in conditions related to marked hypertriglyceridemia (i.e., secondary to pancreatitis) and hypercholesterolemia (i.e., as a result of cirrhosis caused by biliary obstruction [Rayer disease]). Erythematous maculae and papules, representing a viral exanthem, can be present in some viral infections that produce gastrointestinal symptoms.

C. How old is her youngest child?   NONESSENTIAL

Because a viable intrauterine pregnancy following a bilateral tubal ligation (BTL) is unlikely (especially given her history of never being hospitalized) and her BTL was performed approximately 20 years ago, it can be inferred with a high degree of accuracy that her youngest child, if she has any, is older than the age of 20 years. Regardless, it is irrelevant to her present illness and does not need to be asked.

Although it is rare to find an ethical gynecologist who would perform a BTL on a single, childless female, especially of 26 years of age, it is not impossible. Still, asking the age of a child, instead of inquiring about the existence of children, makes some assumptions regarding the role of women and could be interpreted as judgmental by the patient and adversely affect the patient–provider relationship.

D. How often does she have a "breakthrough" headache? When did she take her last dose of sumatriptan? Does the sumatriptan always work? If yes, how many doses are required? If not, what is effective?   ESSENTIAL

Normally in a problem-focused medical examination, questions regarding unrelated conditions are not indicated. However, these questions are relevant in Ms. Queens' case because sumatriptan, a 5-HT receptor agonist, can cause both cardiovascular and colonic ischemia resulting in symptoms similar to hers. Additionally, these vasoconstrictive properties potentially could be attenuated if the medication is utilized in more frequent intervals and/or quantities than prescribed. Hence, the frequency of usage and number of injections per headache are pertinent.

Knowing what medications are effective in alleviating Ms. Queens' headache in the event of sumatriptan failure is also important. Ergotamines can potentially enhance the vasoconstrictive properties of sumatriptan, increasing the possibilities of cardiovascular and/or colonic ischemia. Taking extra dosages of valproic acid to alleviate her headache can enhance potential adverse effects including nausea, vomiting, diarrhea, hepatotoxicity, pancreatitis, and thrombocytopenia. Concomitant usage of aspirin, and potentially other NSAIDs, can increase the serum level of valproic acid and its associated adverse effects. Furthermore, severe gastritis, peptic ulcer disease (especially penetrating and perforating peptic ulcers), and hepatic insufficiency/failure can occur in NSAID therapy, including aspirin.

Additionally, if narcotic analgesics are the only effective treatment for her breakthrough migraine headaches, the HCP would need to maintain some degree of suspicion that perhaps her complaint of severe abdominal pain today stems from an attempt/desire to obtain narcotics. This behavior is more frequently seen in patients who present complaining of severe pain on their initial visit. Other suspicious findings include a history of a chronic pain disorder that is unresponsive to current therapy and requires frequent supplement narcotics to achieve pain relief, multiple allergies to nonnarcotic pain medications, and requesting a specific pain medication by name. However, just because these "suggestive" findings are present, it does not absolutely mean that the patient is seeking narcotics and is not physically ill. Hence, all prejudices and initial impressions must be set aside while the patient's complaints are being adequately evaluated.

E. Has she had any recent trauma?   ESSENTIAL

Any time a patient presents with acute pain, it is essential to inquire about the possibility of trauma as a causative factor. The addition of trauma can significantly alter the potential differential diagnoses as well as the diagnostic studies employed. One of the most common reasons that adults do not report a precipitating traumatic event is if the trauma was a result of intimate partner violence. This is a concern for Ms. Queens because she has some "red flags" that could possibly indicate that she is a victim of intimate partner violence (e.g., partner refusing to leave the examination room, her not disagreeing with that decision, this being her initial visit, cohabitating for a number of years without marriage, and having multiple pain disorders [especially involving headaches, abdominal pain, and pelvic pain]).

Nevertheless, the presence of these "red flags" is not definite for intimate partner violence. The findings could be attributed to a multitude of other factors (e.g., anxiety concerning her current condition, previous negative healthcare experience, being new to the area or desiring a different HCP, prior personal [or parental and/or close acquaintance] marital/relationship difficulties, or previous interpersonal problems). Still, a high index of suspicion is mandatory.

2. Physical Examination

A. Evaluation of salivary glands and ducts   ESSENTIAL

Ms. Queens' salivary glands and ducts need to be evaluated because serum amylase and lipase levels are likely to be performed as part of the diagnostic evaluation for her acute upper abdominal pain. Salivary gland abnormalities (including parotiditis and acute bacterial sialadenitis) and salivary duct abnormalities (e.g., obstruction from a sialolithiasis or a mucous plug secondary to acute bacterial sialadenitis) can cause elevations of these enzymes. Thus, by knowing the status of her salivary gland and/or ducts, her laboratory results can be analyzed utilizing this information, thereby preventing elevated values (if present) from being misinterpreted and the patient to be misdiagnosed.

B. Eye examination   ESSENTIAL

An eye examination is essential for Ms. Queens to evaluate for the presence of icterus, which would add support to a hepatic or hepatobiliary cause for her acute abdominal pain.

Her eye examination should also include a funduscopic examination to observe for early signs of retinopathy (e.g., diabetic retinopathy [which would be unlikely to exist before the diagnosis of diabetes mellitus was established] or Purtscher retinopathy [which is also unlikely because it typically presents as a sudden, acute vision loss or even blindness]) because it could occur secondary to conditions that can produce pancreatic inflammation, infection, and/or masses.

Finally, the pupils should be evaluated for mydriasis or miosis, which could indicate the presence of substance use/abuse because drug-seeking behavior is a potential concern.

C. Heart and lung auscultation   ESSENTIAL

Because it is difficult to distinguish between thoracic and abdominal conditions in patients presenting with epigastric pain, especially when it radiates to their back, it is essential to look for any signs of a cardiac or pulmonary abnormality. The most likely abnormality that could be identified by cardiac auscultation is the presence of a friction rub, which could indicate that acute pericarditis is responsible for Ms. Queens' epigastric pain. Other findings could include a displaced apical impulse indicative of cardiomegaly and/or abnormal heart sounds/murmurs resulting from structural defects; depending on their cause, they may or may not be associated with pain that radiates to the epigastric area. Other possible cardiac causes for her symptoms include myocardial ischemia or angina, which typically are not going to be associated with any specific cardiac (or pulmonary) findings on physical examination.

Although pulmonary findings are more difficult to interpret because severe intra-abdominal conditions can be associated with pulmonary abnormalities (e.g., unilateral [most commonly left-sided] or bilateral basilar rales, atelectasis, and pleural effusions) and pulmonary conditions (e.g., pulmonary embolism, pneumonia, pleural effusions, and asthma) can result in epigastric pain, it is still essential to auscultate Ms. Queens' lungs for any abnormalities.

D. Abdominal examination   ESSENTIAL

Because Ms. Queens is complaining of epigastric pain, an abdominal and rectal examination (as outlined in Case 5-1) is indicated to evaluate for signs to narrow her current differential diagnosis list.

E. Skin examination   ESSENTIAL

A dermatologic examination (as outlined in Case 5-5) is indicated with specific emphasis looking for the abnormalities described previously. Additionally, skin turgor should be assessed as a gross determination of Ms. Queens' hydration status.

3. Diagnostic Studies

A. Amylase, lipase, fractionated lactate dehydrogenase (LDH), and random plasma glucose (RPG)   ESSENTIAL

The amylase, lipase, fractionated LDH, and RPG are important tests to perform as part of the evaluation of a patient with epigastric pain/discomfort, especially if there is radiation to his or her back. These diagnostic studies are useful in supplying supporting evidence for the presence (or absence) of pancreatic, hepatobiliary, hepatic, and cardiovascular causes for the pain.

The amylase has a high sensitivity, but a low specificity, for pancreatic disease. In addition to pancreatic abnormalities, the amylase can also be elevated in other GI conditions (e.g., perforated bowel, perforated ulcer, intestinal infarction, and intestinal obstruction) and non-GI disorders (e.g., ectopic pregnancy, parotiditis, and diabetic ketoacidosis [DKA]). However, significant elevations (more than three times the upper end of normal) reduce the list of potential diagnoses to essentially four: pancreatitis, intestinal perforation, bowel infarction, and salivary gland diseases. The degree of elevation is not proportional to the severity of the disease.

The lipase is more sensitive for pancreatic disorders than the amylase. Nevertheless, it can also be elevated in other conditions (e.g., perforated gastric ulcers, perforated intestines, obstructed bowels, parotiditis, peptic ulcer disease, gallbladder disease, and renal disease). However, it is the degree of elevation (along with history, physical examination, and other diagnostic test results) that can assist in distinguishing between these various conditions. In pancreatic disease, the lipase level is generally elevated 5 to 10 times the upper end of normal, whereas in other conditions, it frequently does not rise above three times the upper end of normal. Furthermore, the degree of elevation of the amylase and the lipase are equal in acute pancreatitis.

A fractionated LDH can provide additional confirmation of a pancreatic disease. LDH-4 is specific for pancreatic, renal, and placental tissue; therefore, a significant elevation of the amylase and lipase along with an elevated LDH with LDH-4 predominance increases the likelihood of a pancreatic condition causing the patient problem. Still, the history, physical examination, and diagnostic test results play a significant role in the diagnosis of the patient.

Because the LDH can be elevated in a variety of other conditions that can present as acute abdominal pain, a fractionation is essential to assist in making the correct diagnosis. The LDH-1 is generally elevated in cardiac conditions. The LDH-2 is predominately associated with the abnormalities of the reticuloendothelial system. The LDH-3 is most often elevated because of pulmonary diseases. The LDH-5 is generally increased with hepatic and striated muscle abnormalities.

An elevated plasma glucose is frequently seen with pancreatitis because of the beta cell dysfunction; however, it can also be seen in DKA. This emphasizes the need to keep the patient's entire clinical picture in view when assessing a medical complaint or test result.

B. Complete blood count with differential (CBC w/diff) and PT   ESSENTIAL

A CBC w/diff can provide useful clues to the presence of an infection, sepsis, inflammation, and/or hemoconcentration secondary to dehydration.

A PT is frequently elevated in hepatocellular liver disease (e.g., hepatitis, cirrhosis, and hepatomas) and obstructive hepatobiliary duct disease (e.g., cholelithiasis, intraductal tumors, intrahepatic cholestasis secondary to sepsis or drugs). Still, an elevated PT in conjunction with abdominal pain is not specific for hepatic disease. It is also elevated in hereditary bleeding disorders, disseminated intravascular coagulation, vitamin K deficiency, aspirin overdose, and excessive alcohol ingestion (without evidence of hepatic dysfunction and/or disease). Drugs can cause the PT to be elevated; however, valproic acid and sumatriptan are not among the offending agents.

C. Computed tomography (CT) of the abdomen NONESSENTIAL

Most experts agree that the initial imaging study for a patient with acute upper abdominal pain is an abdominal ultrasound. It permits visualization of the architectural structure and size of the abdominal organs and aorta, distinguishes between cystic and solid masses, evaluates for ascites, and is superior to CT in identifying gallstones. If after this examination there is still concern regarding a perforation or obstruction, a plain film radiograph is the imaging study of choice.

CT scans are indicated in patients who have a significant abnormality identified on the aforementioned imaging studies, severe disease, or a poor (or no) response to traditional therapy.

D. Liver function testing (LFT), blood urea nitrogen (BUN), and electrolytes   ESSENTIAL

Liver function testing should be performed in all patients complaining of upper abdominal pain to provide additional information to rule in or rule out the presence of a hepatic, hepatobiliary duct, and/or gallbladder abnormality. The LFT panel should include at least the measurement of ALT, AST, and GGT.

The vast majority of ALT in the human body is located in the liver; therefore, an elevation of this enzyme almost always indicates a hepatocellular problem. However, because there are minor amounts in the skeletal muscle, heart, and kidneys, it can be elevated in other conditions that can present as epigastric pain including pancreatitis, myocardial infarction, abdominal wall muscle trauma, and infectious mononucleosis. Nevertheless, the degree of elevation can assist in the differentiation of hepatic versus nonhepatic causes. In hepatic conditions, the ALT is almost always more than three times the upper end of normal.

The AST is found predominately in the heart and liver; however, it also exists in small quantities in the skeletal muscles. Therefore, when viewed independently in a patient with acute epigastric pain, an elevation would most likely represent a myocardial infarction or a hepatic abnormality. However, other conditions that could be responsible for Ms. Queens' chief complaint that could be associated with an elevated AST include pancreatitis, infectious mononucleosis, and abdominal muscle trauma. However, the degree of damage to the organ is directly proportional to the degree of elevation of the AST. Significant elevations almost always represent a cardiac or hepatic injury.

Hepatic disease can further be confirmed as the cause of the patient's problem if the AST and ALT are essentially equally elevated. Utilizing these enzymes to distinguish between hepatocellular damage and obstructive hepatocellular disease is discussed in Case 5-5.

The GGT is found in the greatest concentrations in the liver and hepatobiliary ducts; hence, it is generally the most sensitive liver enzyme to indicate the presence of a biliary obstruction. However, it is not hepatic and/or hepatobiliary specific and can be found in smaller concentrations in the heart, intestine, kidney, spleen, prostate gland, and brain. Therefore, nonhepatic and hepatobiliary conditions can present with epigastric pain and an elevated GGT (e.g., pancreatitis, pancreatic cancer, benign pancreatic lesions, myocardial infarction, infectious mononucleosis, cytomegalovirus infections, and Reye syndrome). Finally, it is estimated to be elevated in approximately 75% of all individuals who consume alcohol on a regular, long-term basis.

Medications have been associated with elevations of one, two, or all three of these liver enzymes; however, valproic acid and sumatriptan are generally not known for this alteration.

A BUN and electrolytes are also indicated for Ms. Queens because of her history of vomiting and slightly dry-appearing mucous membranes on physical examination to determine whether she is dehydrated. Dehydration would be most suspicious with a combination of an elevated BUN and a low potassium level. However, an elevated BUN can also be seen in conditions capable of producing epigastric pain (e.g., gastrointestinal bleeding and acute myocardial infarction). A decreased BUN can be seen in liver failure, among other diseases.

E. Urinary human chorionic gonadotropin (HCG) test NONESSENTIAL

Ovulation occurs 14 days before the onset of menses and HCG levels cannot be detected until at least 10 days after conception, or approximately 4 days before the onset of menses. Ms. Queens has regular menstrual cycles and her last menstrual period was 1 week ago and normal; thus, it would be virtually impossible for her to have a significantly detectable level of HCG as a result of an intrauterine pregnancy let alone an extrauterine pregnancy (which would be more likely with her history of a BTL). Thus, it would be impossible to distinguish a true-negative from a false-negative at this time without additional diagnostic studies. Because a pregnancy complication is low on her differential diagnosis list and her BTL essentially eliminates prescribing concerns with a potential pregnancy, this test is not indicated.

Additionally, even if her HCG level was sufficiently elevated to produce a positive test result, further testing would be required to determine if her finding represented a true elevation or a false-positive as a result of her valproic acid. False-positives can occur with medications from the following drug categories: anticonvulsants, hypnotics, sedatives, tranquilizers (especially the typical antipsychotic agents), and antiparkinsonian agents.

4. Diagnosis

A. Ectopic pregnancy   INCORRECT

Ectopic (or extrauterine) pregnancies are responsible for the vast majority of the few pregnancies that occur after bilateral tubal ligation. Still, an ectopic pregnancy is typically asymptomatic until approximately 6 to 8 weeks after a missed menstrual period (or 2–4 weeks after a missed or significantly lighter menstrual period). Because Ms. Queens had a normal menstrual period 1 week ago and her history is inconsistent with that of an ectopic pregnancy (i.e., right or left lower quadrant pain [depending the ectopic pregnancy's location] that is crampy in nature and associated with vaginal bleeding), an ectopic pregnancy is not her most likely diagnosis.

B. Acute pancreatitis secondary to valproic acid with mild dehydration   CORRECT

Acute pancreatitis is generally defined at the initial painful episode of pancreatic inflammation. Conversely, chronic pancreatitis is diagnosed when the patient has multiple episodes of pain (or constant pain caused by the effects the chronic inflammation has on the underlying structure of the pancreatic cells). It is not uncommon for it to also be associated with hyperlipidemia (especially hypertriglyceridemia), diabetes mellitus (as a result of beta cell destruction), malnutrition (most frequently as a result of a loss of exocrine and its resultant malabsorption), peptic ulcer disease (theorized to result from an overproduction of gastric acid because the inhibitory feedback loop is disrupted by the lack of pancreatic enzymes entering the gut), hepatobiliary cirrhosis, pancreatic cancer, gastrointestinal perforation and/or hemorrhage, and splenic vein thrombosis.

Although Ms. Queens' history and physical examination are consistent with the diagnosis of acute pancreatitis, some would incorrectly discount this diagnosis because her amylase level is only 1.5 times the upper end of normal (whereas more than three times is considered diagnostic) and her lipase level is only approximately 3.5 times the upper end of normal (not the 5 to 10 times that is considered diagnostic). However, these levels (as with the results of any diagnostic study) must be interpreted in the context of the clinical picture. Ms. Queens presented approximately 4 hours after the onset of her pain, and significant elevations of amylase do not occur until approximately 24 hours after the onset of symptoms; therefore, this level of amylase would be considered consistent with the diagnosis of acute pancreatitis. Likewise, her lipase is proportionally much more elevated than her amylase, which is not consistent with a classic presentation of acute pancreatitis. However, this finding is consistent with this diagnosis because lipase levels rise faster than amylase levels in acute pancreatitis. Elevations of the lipase usually begin within 4 hours of the onset of symptoms and tend to peak at approximately 8 hours; then, they remain relatively constant for 8 to 14 days. Therefore, acute pancreatitis is a very viable diagnosis for Ms. Queens.

Regarding the cause of her acute pancreatitis, idiopathic is the most common; however, it can only be the diagnosis when all other potential causes have been eliminated. The second most common cause is medications. Because she is on a drug (valproic acid) that has a "black box" warning for the possibility of pancreatitis, this is highly likely to be the cause. Other medications implicated include estrogens, codeine, NSAIDs, salicylates, acetaminophen, erythromycin, tetracycline, sulfonamides, nitrofurantoin, metronidazole, corticosteroids, antiretroviral drugs, furosemide, thiazides, angiotensin-converting enzyme (ACE) inhibitors, cimetidine, famotidine, and some chemotherapeutic agents.

Mild dehydration is probably the easiest portion of this diagnosis to establish. Her history of vomiting, the presence of a slightly dry oral mucosa and decreased skin turgor on her physical examination, and her diagnostic findings of a slightly elevated BUN, a slightly low potassium level, and evidence of hemoconcentration on her CBC essentially confirm this portion of the diagnosis. Thus, from the list provided, acute pancreatitis secondary to valproic acid with mild dehydration is Ms. Queens' most likely diagnosis.

C. Perforated duodenal ulcer with mild dehydration INCORRECT

Although a perforated duodenal ulcer could present with symptoms similar to Ms. Queens' and she does have documented mild dehydration (please see response B), this can still be ruled out as her most likely diagnosis primarily because she is hemodynamically stable.

Additionally, her diagnostic findings are inconsistent with this diagnosis unless she has a coexisting condition to account for them. Although it is essential to treat the patient and not the diagnostic studies, the diagnostic findings should still provide some support for the diagnosis. The most significant discrepancy is that her CBC w/diff reveals a high normal Hgb and a slightly elevated HCT. A perforated peptic ulcer should result in low (or low-normal) Hgb and HCT levels after 4 hours of acute gastrointestinal bleeding, even considering the fact that the actual amount of blood loss is not accurately represented by these values in acute bleeding.

Other discrepancies include an elevated amylase (should only occur if the peptic ulcer is penetrating into the pancreas), a lipase that is elevated more than three times its upper normal limit (peptic ulcer disease can cause an elevation of lipase; however, nonpancreatic causes rarely, if ever, result in elevations that are greater than three times), an elevated GGT (although GGT is found in intestinal tissue, it does not generally increase in response to a peptic ulcer perforation), an elevated ALT (should only occur in peptic ulcer perforation without a coexisting condition if shock is present), and a slightly elevated AST.

D. Acute cholelithiasis   INCORRECT

Despite a similar history and clinical picture, gallstones can be ruled out as Ms. Queens' most likely diagnosis because the pain from cholelithiasis tends to almost always involve the right upper quadrant (either alone or in addition to the epigastric area). Also, acute cholelithiasis is inconsistent with her diagnostic findings unless she has a coexisting condition present.

Although an elevated lipase level can be seen with acute cholelithiasis, the amylase is generally normal. The LDH could be elevated with acute cholelithiasis; however, the elevation would more than likely occur in the LDH-5, not the LDH-4, group. Also, her liver enzymes with acute cholelithiasis should be elevated to a greater degree and represent an obstructive pattern (especially if cholestasis is also present). Plus, this diagnosis ignores the signs, symptoms, and diagnostic test findings consistent with mild dehydration in conjunction with her current illness.

E. Factitious abdominal pain with drug-seeking behavior INCORRECT

Despite her having some signs and symptoms that could be consistent with drug-seeking behavior, this can be eliminated as her most likely diagnosis because her physical examination and diagnostic studies indicate actual physical pathology, not a factitious disorder.

5. Treatment Plan

A. Hospitalize with IV fluids   CORRECT

Ms. Queens needs to be hospitalized for additional evaluation, hydration, pain control, and early detection and treatment of possible complications from her pancreatitis. IV fluids are essential to treat her dehydration, maintain normal intravascular volume (which can become depleted as a result of the decreased secretion of pancreatic enzymes), and provide some nutritional support because she should also be placed on complete bowel rest. Enteral nutrition/feedings may be required, especially if she develops chronic pancreatitis.

B. Determine presentation (initial) Ranson criteria score CORRECT

The Ranson criteria scoring system was established to attempt to determine the patient's prognosis (in terms of mortality risk) due to acute pancreatitis based on established criteria identified during the patient's presentation and again at 48 hours. The initial score (completed at presentation and/or hospitalization) evaluates five risk factors associated with an unfavorable outcome and assigns 1 point for each positive risk factor that the patient has present. The risk factors are (1) age older than 55 years, (2) random plasma glucose (RPG) greater than 200 mg/dl, (3) white blood cell count greater than 16,000/mm³, (4) LDH greater than 350 IU/L, and (5) AST level greater than 250 units/L.

From these preliminary findings, patients who meet two or fewer of these criteria (Ranson score ≤ 2) are estimated to have a 1% mortality rate from the condition. Patients who meet three or four of these criteria (Ranson score of 3 or 4) have an estimated mortality rate of approximately 15%. Individuals with all five of the criteria (Ranson score of 5) have an estimated mortality rate of nearly 100%. Obviously, these classifications can also assist in determining which patients are going to require more aggressive therapy to hopefully prevent severe complications and death.

The repeat Ranson criteria incorporates six additional risk factors (also worth 1 point for each positive item) in a reevaluation that occurs 48 hours after the initial scoring. The additional second surveillance criteria are (1) serum calcium less than 8 mg/dl, (2) elevation of the BUN by greater than 5 mg/dl over baseline on presentation/admission, (3) decrease of hemoglobin by greater than 10% from presentation/admission, (4) pO_2 less than 60 mm Hg, (5) fluid sequestration greater than 6 L, and (6) base deficit greater than 4 mEq/L. Even though the second score contains six additional criteria (for a possible total score of 11), the total numerical score and its associated mortality risk remains the same (i.e., score of ≤ 2, ~1% mortality; score of 3 or 4, ~15% mortality; and score of ≥ 5, nearly 100% mortality).

Although most experts agree that the Ranson score is an accurate predictor of mortality from acute pancreatitis regardless of its cause, there are some who feel it is only applicable to patients with alcoholic pancreatitis. Therefore, two additional classification schemes have been established to estimate the patient's mortality risk. These classification systems include the Glasgow criteria (designed exclusively for patients with pancreatitis caused by cholelithiasis) and the APACHE-II scoring system. The advantage of the APACHE-II is its design to evaluate the patient's risk daily (thereby hopefully identifying deterioration and instituting appropriate treatment measures sooner); however, it is more cumbersome to administer.

C. IV morphine as needed for pain INCORRECT

Although IV morphine is clearly an effective analgesic agent, it has essentially been replaced by meperidine as the first-line treatment for pain control in individuals with pancreatitis. Unlike morphine, meperidine is not associated with the potential risk of producing a spasm of the sphincter of Oddi (which would obviously increase the patient pain and complication risk).

D. Initiate antibiotic therapy INCORRECT

The utilization of antibiotics in the treatment of acute pancreatitis has met with mixed results in the current literature. Meta-analyses reveal that prophylaxis antibiotics might offer some benefit in reducing the overall mortality and rate of sepsis in patients with necrotizing pancreatitis. However, antibiotic prophylaxis was not associated with a decreased incidence of surgical interventions, multiorgan failures, extrapancreatic infections, fungal infections, and length of hospitalization, even in these patients. In patients with early mild to moderate acute pancreatitis (where necrosis has not yet developed), antibiotic prophylaxis has failed to demonstrate a consistent benefit and should not be utilized.

E. Refer for immediate total pancreatectomy INCORRECT

If Ms. Queens' symptoms worsen, she might require a surgical procedure; however, it is more likely going to consist of the drainage of a pancreatic cyst and/or the treatment of

necrosis, not a total pancreatectomy, especially because her precipitating medication should have been discontinued.

Furthermore, surgery within the first few days of the onset of symptoms is associated with a much higher mortality rate; therefore, if surgery is required, it is best to delay it approximately 2 weeks (unless it became an emergent situation).

Epidemiologic and Other Data

It is estimated that there are approximately 200,000 new cases of acute pancreatitis diagnosed each year in the United States, making its incidence nearly 80 per 100,000 individuals.

The cause of inflammation of the pancreas is unknown. Some experts theorize that there is a triggering event that causes the proteolytic enzymes to become activated in the pancreas instead of the normal location inside the small intestine. Some of these more common theorized triggers include medications, alcohol ingestion, hypertriglyceridemia, obstruction of the pancreatic and/or biliary ducts (e.g., cholelithiasis and microlithiasis), dysfunction of the sphincter of Oddi, trauma, and complications following medical procedures (e.g., abdominal surgery or endoscopic retrograde cholangiopancreatography [ERCP]).

Other less common proposed triggers include hereditary conditions, abnormalities of the pancreas (e.g., carcinomas, multiple stones, diverticula, and pancreas divisum), hypercalcemia, renal failure, cystic fibrosis, autoimmune diseases, viral syndromes (e.g., cytomegalovirus, echovirus, coxsackievirus, and Rubulavirus), and parasitic infections.

CASE 5-7
Quillain Rogers
1. History

A. Does he drink untreated water from a lake, stream, spring, or other natural source? ESSENTIAL

Natural water sources can become contaminated with animal and/or human feces. Consumption of this water (without treatment to destroy potential pathogens) can result in a bacterial gastroenteritis with symptoms similar to Mr. Rogers'. The most commonly implicated organisms include enterotoxigenic *Escherichia coli*, *Vibrio cholerae*, *Campylobacter jejuni*, *Shigella* sp., and *Yersinia enterocolitica*.

Attempting to determine which of these organisms is the most likely cause of a patient's illness requires a detailed patient history, especially in terms of symptom severity, associated problems, and time lapse since exposure. Still, microscopic examination and cultures of the stool are often necessary to identify the causative pathogen.

B. Does he have a girlfriend? NONESSENTIAL

The primary reason to obtain a sexual history on a patient in a problem-focused visit is to establish his or her risk of acquiring a sexually transmitted infection (STI) that could be responsible for his or her presenting illness. However, left lower quadrant abdominal pain, in the absence of genitourinary symptoms and the presence of gastrointestinal symptoms, in a patient of Mr. Rogers' age is extremely unlikely to be caused by a sexually transmitted infection.

Regardless, the formatting of this question is inappropriate and could be considered insulting to some patients. A better initial screening question is to inquire about Mr. Rogers' marital status; then, appropriate follow-up questions could be crafted based on his response.

C. Has he been on an antibiotic lately?   ESSENTIAL

Antibiotics have the ability to alter the normal bacterial flora in the intestines. In some cases, these alterations can result in an "overgrowth" infection with lower abdominal pain, bloody diarrhea, and fever as a result of an overgrowth of naturally occurring intestinal organisms and their subsequent toxin formation (e.g., *Clostridium difficile* and *Escherichia coli*).

D. Does he thoroughly wash all fruits and vegetables before eating? Does he completely cook all meats to recommended temperature before consuming? Does he store his food and leftovers properly?   ESSENTIAL

Foods that have not been adequately washed, prepared, or stored can become infected with organisms (that generally produce toxins) and potentially produce symptoms similar to those described by Mr. Rogers. The most common pathogens include *Bacillus cereus, Campylobacter jejuni, Clostridium botulinum, Escherichia coli, Salmonella* sp., *Shigella* sp., *Staphylococcus* sp., *Streptococcus lactis, Vibrio cholerae, Vibrio parahaemolyticus,* and *Yersinia enterocolitica.* Hence, these questions are important to ask the patient.

The identification of the most probable organism(s) responsible for the patient's symptoms depends significantly on the patient's history in terms of severity of symptoms, associated symptoms, and time lapse since exposure. The actual causative organism may not be identifiable without stool microscopic examination and cultures on appropriate media.

E. Has he traveled outside the United States recently?   ESSENTIAL

Travel to foreign countries can expose the patient to many food-borne and oral–fecally transmitted organisms that could produce symptoms very similar to those Mr. Rogers is experiencing. Some of the more common pathologic organisms can include *Aeromonas, Campylobacter* sp., *Cryptosporidium, Cyclospora, Endamoeba histolytica, Escherichia coli, Giardia lamblia, Plesiomonas, Salmonella typhi, Salmonella* sp., *Shigella dysenteriae* type 1, other *Shigella* sp., *Vibrio cholerae,* caliciviruses (including noroviruses), and rotaviruses.

2. Physical Examination

A. Thyroid examination   NONESSENTIAL

Although hyperthyroidism has been known to produce diarrhea, it is generally a chronic problem that is not associated with (possible) fever and hematochezia followed by no bowel movements.

B. Abdominal examination   ESSENTIAL

Because Mr. Rogers' chief complaint is abdominal pain, a comprehensive abdominal examination as outlined in Case 5-1 is essential.

C. Rectal examination with occult blood testing of obtained stool (if present)   ESSENTIAL

A rectal examination is essential to perform on Mr. Rogers because he is experiencing lower abdominal pain with a bowel change as well as hematochezia. Despite the limitations of testing a single stool specimen for occult blood (as discussed in Cases 5-1 and 5-2), any stool obtained should be tested in hopes of detecting whether microscopic bleeding is also present in addition to the hematochezia that Mr. Rogers experienced on the first day of his illness. A positive test for occult blood is considered to be a "red flag" (or warning) symptom (includes signs) in lower abdominal pain indicating that further evaluation is required to ensure a serious condition (e.g., cancer or IBD) is not present. The other "red flags" are significant weight loss, elderly age, anemia, gross blood in the stool, fever, severe diarrhea (especially if nocturnal), progressive worsening of symptoms, acute onset of symptoms, unremitting pain, being unresponsive to conservative treatment, and positive family history of colon cancer or IBD.

D. Skin examination for jaundice   NONESSENTIAL

Hepatic, hepatobiliary, gallbladder, and occasionally pancreatic diseases can produce jaundice; however, these conditions are primarily associated with upper abdominal pain. Therefore, because Mr. Rogers is experiencing lower abdominal pain, does not have any risk factors for abnormalities of these organs (e.g., significant alcohol intake, medications that could be hepatotoxic or capable of producing pancreatitis, previous episodes of upper abdominal pain and/or vomiting, high risk for acquiring a blood-borne or sexually transmitted infection, or known [or a positive family history] of any hereditary conditions associated with cholestasis, hyperbilirubinemia, and/or hemolysis), and is not complaining of skin color changes, the likelihood of discovering a clinically significant jaundice is extremely small.

E. Neurologic examination   NONESSENTIAL

Although bowel changes (and abdominal pain) can be present in some neurologic conditions, Mr. Rogers' history does not provide any evidence to suggest the presence of one.

3. Diagnostic Studies

A. Complete blood count with differential (CBC w/diff)   ESSENTIAL

A CBC w/diff is indicated to provide additional information regarding the severity of his condition, especially in terms of infection, inflammation, and hemodynamic stability. (For additional information regarding the interpretation of the CBC w/diff, please see Case 1-4.)

Many experts consider the leukocyte count to be a significant factor in determining whether a patient with Mr. Rogers' condition can be safely managed as an outpatient or not.

B. Immediate colonoscopy   NONESSENTIAL

Because of the high risk of intestinal perforation associated with performing a colonoscopy in patients with Mr. Rogers' condition, a colonoscopy is not indicated at this time. However, if it was determined that he had significant rectal bleeding, anemia, and/or hemodynamic instability, the decision to proceed with the procedure would need to be made considering the potential risks versus benefits for his individual situation. Regardless, a colonoscopy is indicated approximately 6 to 8 weeks after the resolution of his inflammation not only to confirm his diagnosis but also to evaluate his hematochezia and screen him for colorectal cancer.

C. Stool for culture and sensitivity (C&S) and *Clostridium difficile* toxins   NONESSENTIAL

Although bacterial gastroenteritis and antibiotic-related (formerly pseudomembranous) colitis caused by *Clostridium difficile* can present with symptoms similar to Mr. Rogers', stool specimens for C&S and *Clostridium difficile* toxins are not indicated at this time because his history is incompatible with the acquisition of causative pathogens.

D. Flat-plate radiograph of the abdomen   ESSENTIAL

A flat-plate (plain film) radiograph of the abdomen is the most appropriate imaging study for Mr. Rogers at this time. It eliminates, with a relatively high degree of certainty, serious complications (e.g., ileus, colonic perforation, or bowel obstruction) that could be present.

E. Computed tomography (CT) of the abdomen NONESSENTIAL

A CT of the abdomen would be the best initial imaging study for Mr. Rogers if he were exhibiting severe symptoms and/or a significant leukocytosis on his CBC w/diff. Additionally, it would be the imaging study of choice if his condition worsens or is unresponsive to conservative therapy.

4. Diagnosis

A. Acute appendicitis   INCORRECT

Acute appendicitis is an inflammatory condition involving the vermiform appendix. Although acute appendicitis can initially begin as a left lower quadrant (or periumbilical) pain, it migrates to (and remains in) the right lower quadrant within a few hours of symptom onset. Any type of (or no) bowel movement changes can be seen with acute appendicitis; nevertheless, the complaint of bloody diarrhea followed by a several-day absence of bowel movements is an extremely unlikely scenario. Its hallmark feature is anorexia that does not begin until after the onset of the abdominal pain. Furthermore, by the fifth day of the illness, the leukocytosis should be much more pronounced and the patient much more ill than Mr. Rogers'. Thus, acute appendicitis can be eliminated as Mr. Rogers' most likely diagnosis.

B. Diverticulosis   INCORRECT

Diverticulosis is a large bowel disease (generally confined to the sigmoid colon) that consists of defects in the colon wall resulting in pouch-like formations. It can be divided into two main forms: true diverticulosis and pseudodiverticulosis. True diverticula disease affects all the layers of the intestine, whereas pseudodiverticula disease affects only the intestinal mucosa (and does not extend into the muscular layer). The number of diverticular pouches can vary from a couple to hundreds. In diverticulosis, these anatomic defects are asymptomatic. Therefore, this condition can be ruled out as Mr. Rogers' most likely diagnosis.

C. Diverticulitis   CORRECT

When the "outpouching" of the intestinal wall in diverticulosis becomes inflamed and/or infected, the resulting condition is known as diverticulitis. Of the conditions provided, this is Mr. Rogers' most likely diagnosis. His history (intermittent, aching left lower quadrant abdominal pain; bloody diarrhea followed by obstipation; mild nausea and vomiting; and low-grade fever), physical examination findings (a palpable left

lower quadrant mass with tenderness, and slightly hypoactive bowel sounds but without rebound or guarding), and diagnostic finding of a mild leukocytosis are characteristic for mild diverticulitis.

When an infection is present, the primary organism is almost exclusively *Enterobacteriaceae*. Rarely *Pseudomonas aeruginosa* or a *Bacteroides* sp. can be present.

D. Large bowel perforation with acute peritonitis   INCORRECT

Peritonitis is an inflammatory process involving the peritoneum. Although it can result from both infectious and noninfectious causes, virtually all cases of acute peritonitis are caused by an infectious process. When an intra-abdominal abnormality (i.e., colonic perforation) is identifiable as the source of the infection, it is designated as secondary infectious peritonitis. If an intra-abdominal source is not identifiable, it is referred to as spontaneous, primary, or iatrogenic infectious peritonitis.

If peritonitis results from a colonic perforation, it is most frequently caused by a ruptured diverticulum (as a complication of diverticulitis) or appendix (as a complication of appendicitis). Penetrating trauma affecting the colon is also a major cause. Depending on the severity and duration of the condition, the associated pain and abdominal tenderness can be either localized or generalized. Regardless, there is generally abdominal wall rigidity (with or without rebound) and absent bowel sounds on abdominal examination. Other findings can include fever, dehydration, tachycardia, and hypotension. Plain film abdominal radiographs generally reveal the presence of free air under the diaphragm but can also show large and/or small bowel dilatation with edema of the intestinal walls. Because Mr. Rogers did not reveal the characteristic findings on his physical examination and abdominal radiographs, large bowel perforation with acute peritonitis is not his most likely diagnosis.

E. Irritable bowel syndrome (IBS)   INCORRECT

Despite Mr. Rogers having the requisite two out of the three symptoms (the onset of abdominal pain associated with a change in the number of bowel movements AND linked to an alteration in the consistency of his stool) necessary to establish the diagnosis of IBS, he still fails to meet the diagnostic criteria because the duration of his symptoms has been much less than the required 6 months, plus he has not been experiencing symptoms on a minimum of 3 days per week for the past 3 months. (Please see Case 5-1 for a more in-depth discussion of the Rome II criteria for IBS diagnosis.) Furthermore, IBS is considered to be a functional bowel disease; therefore, it is extremely unusual for nocturnal symptoms to be present. Thus, IBS is not Mr. Rogers' most likely diagnosis.

5. Treatment Plan

A. Levofloxacin 750 mg once a day with metronidazole 500 mg four times a day orally for 7 to 10 days   INCORRECT

Levofloxacin 750 mg once a day with metronidazole 500 mg four times a day for 7 to 10 days orally is an appropriate first-line antibiotic regimen for a patient with diverticulitis. However, because Mr. Rogers experienced urticaria and perioral edema on another fluoroquinolone, all fluoroquinolones should be avoided, if at all possible, to prevent a similar (or worse) allergic reaction.

B. Trimethoprim-sulfamethoxazole double strength (DS) twice a day plus metronidazole 500 mg four times a day orally for 7 to 10 days   CORRECT

Trimethoprim-sulfamethoxazole DS twice a day plus metronidazole 500 mg four times a day for 7 to 10 days orally is an acceptable first-line antibiotic option for the treatment of diverticulitis. It is a better alternative for Mr. Rogers given his previous adverse reaction to a fluoroquinolone.

C. Hospitalization   INCORRECT

Hospitalization is not necessary because Mr. Rogers' symptoms are mild, his leukocytosis is minimal, and he has no signs or symptoms of dehydration and/or any other complications. Thus, outpatient treatment with proper advice and frequent follow-up is appropriate at this time.

D. Clear liquid diet   CORRECT

A clear liquid diet is indicated to allow his gut some "rest" without having to utilize IV therapy.

E. Avoidance of fruits with seeds, nuts, corn, broccoli, cauliflower, and other foods that might pass as small undigested food particles that could get "stuck" in a bowel pouch   INCORRECT

Until recently, it was theorized that the reason diverticula became inflamed and subsequently infected was because undigested food particles became lodged in one of the intestinal outpouches. As a result, the patient was placed on lifelong dietary restrictions eliminating foods with portions that might not be completely broken down during the digestive process (e.g., seeds in blackberries and strawberries, kernels from popcorn and fresh corn on the cob, and florets in cauliflower and broccoli). However, this theory has been disproven, and the only current dietary recommendations (with the exception of eliminating any food that has been known to cause an exacerbation) is to ensure that the patient is getting adequate fluids and fiber in his or her diet.

Epidemiologic and Other Data

Although diverticular disease is rare in underdeveloped countries, it has a significant incidence in developed countries. It is theorized that this significant difference is a result of the lack of adequate fiber in the diet of individuals residing in developed countries like the United States. Increasing age is a risk factor for colonic diverticular disease, with the number of individuals affected by the disease increasing proportionally with advancing age. It is estimated that in the United States, the incidence for individuals in their 40s is less than 10%; however, by the time an individual reaches his or her 60s, the incidence increases to approximately 50%. Still, symptomatic disease (diverticulitis) is limited to approximately 20% of all the patients affected with this condition.

Risk factors for bleeding, and even frank hemorrhage, caused by diverticulitis appear to be increased in patients with comorbid hypertension, those with cardiovascular disease, and those who regularly take NSAIDs.

CASE 5-8
Richard Stevenson
1. History

A. Has he visualized any *Enterobius vermicularis?*   NONESSENTIAL

An *Enterobius vermicularis* (or common "pinworm") infestation frequently presents as rectal itching. However, the itching tends to be much more intense at night. Because Mr. Stevenson lacks an increased nocturnal pruritus and recently had a negative cellulose tape mount examination for the identification of the eggs (and occasionally the nematode itself), it is highly unlikely that this helminthic infection is responsible for his symptoms.

B. Has he noticed any jaundice or icterus?   NONESSENTIAL

Rectal symptoms (even with constipation) in the absence of abdominal pain/discomfort (and other signs of a hepatic, hepatobiliary, gallbladder, and/or pancreatic disease) are highly unlikely to be associated with a condition that could produce jaundice.

C. What are his sexual history and practices?   ESSENTIAL

Sexually transmitted infections (STIs), especially those due to herpes simplex virus (HSV), *Treponema pallidum, Neisseria gonorrhoeae,* and *Chlamydia trachomatis,* can cause proctitis, proctocolitis, enterocolitis, and enteritis. Because the majority of STIs occur in individuals during mid- to late adolescence and young adulthood, Mr. Stevenson's age places him "at risk" for acquiring one. Thus, his sexual history is important to determine whether he has additional risk factors, which would increase the possibility that an STI is responsible for his symptoms.

Sexually transmitted proctitis is most frequently diagnosed in the receptive partner of men who have sex with men (MSM); however, it can result from being the receptive partner in heterosexual relationships. Sexually transmitted proctocolitis, enterocolitis, and enteritis can also result from oral–anorectal contact by either men or women.

Sexually transmitted infections that commonly present as genital lesions can also produce perianal and rectal lesions in individuals who are the receptive partner in rectal intercourse or who practice oral–genital intercourse. These conditions include genital herpes, syphilis, condyloma acuminata, lymphogranuloma venereum, and chancroid.

Organisms that are traditionally considered to be non–sexually transmitted can also be transmitted to either partner (although the receptive partner is at greater risk [especially in a heterosexual encounter]) and cause gastrointestinal (GI) tract infections. These potential organisms include *Campylobacter* sp., *Shigella* sp., *Entamoeba histolytica,* and *Giardia lamblia.*

Patients (especially MSM) who are immunocompromised, secondary to AIDS or another condition, have a greater potential for acquiring a GI infection caused by a traditional, nontraditional, or other enteric pathogen.

D. Has he noticed any genital lesions?   ESSENTIAL

Because of the aforementioned association of STIs, including those that present as genital ulcer disease and gastrointestinal infections, as well as Mr. Stevenson's "higher-risk" category, it is important to inquire whether he had any other signs of STIs. If he does, it is imperative to obtain a description of not only the appearance of the lesion but also the course of the lesion, because in many cases this information can assist in directing diagnostic studies toward the most likely pathogens.

Furthermore, it is not uncommon for an individual with one STI to have a second. Thus, the presence of a genital lesion also could represent a coinfectious STI.

E. Is he experiencing a penile discharge, dysuria, urinary urgency, and/or urinary frequency?   ESSENTIAL

Some of the aforementioned STIs capable of causing gastrointestinal infections are also significant pathogens for urethritis, most notably *Neisseria gonorrhoeae* and *Chlamydia trachomatis*. Because it is possible for an individual to be infected at more than one site by these organisms, more "typical" symptoms (e.g., those associated with urethritis) should also be sought.

Additionally, as stated previously, because it is not uncommon for a patient with one STI to have a second one at the same or an alternative site, these questions can also be utilized to identify the possibility of a coinfection.

2. Physical Examination

A. Oropharyngeal examination   ESSENTIAL

An oropharyngeal examination is unlikely to identify any signs of a gastrointestinal disorder (e.g., mucosal and dental damage secondary to chronic vomiting and/or gastric acid refluxing into the oropharynx) because Mr. Stevenson does not have any upper gastrointestinal tract symptoms and has only had symptoms for 1 month. Nevertheless, an oropharyngeal examination is necessary to look for evidence suggesting the presence of a sexually transmitted infection (e.g., pharyngitis caused by gonorrhea or the chancre of primary syphilis) because he practices both fellatio and cunnilingus.

B. Abdominal examination   ESSENTIAL

Even though Mr. Stevenson is not experiencing abdominal pain/discomfort, an abdominal examination (as outlined in Case 5-1) is essential not only because he is experiencing constipation but also to evaluate for any abnormalities that could indicate other portions of the colon besides the rectum are affected.

C. Rectal examination   ESSENTIAL

Because his chief complaint involves rectal symptoms, both external inspection and a digital rectal examination (as outlined in Case 5-1) are essential to perform on Mr. Stevenson.

D. Genital examination   ESSENTIAL

A genital examination is also indicated because of his sexual practices and preferences as well as the association between STIs and proctitis/proctocolitis as discussed previously.

E. Skin and eye examination for jaundice and/or icterus NONESSENTIAL

Even though Mr. Stevenson's chief complaint is gastrointestinal in nature, because of his lack of upper GI complaints and constitutional symptoms, it is highly unlikely that an abnormality of his liver, hepatobiliary tree, gallbladder, or pancreas is producing his symptoms.

3. Diagnostic Studies

A. Anoscopy   ESSENTIAL

Because Mr. Stevenson's symptoms could be caused by an inflammatory process of the rectum, an anoscopy is indicated to visually inspect the rectal mucosa for masses, lesions, vesicles, ulcerations, breaks in integrity, and incongruity of the mucosal pattern. Furthermore, it will ensure that the process in confined to the rectum.

B. Rapid plasma reagin (RPR)   ESSENTIAL

Although the chancre associated with primary syphilis tends to be asymptomatic, a rectal location of this lesion could produce localized discomfort, tenesmus, and defecatory urgency. Additionally, if Mr. Stevenson had another STI producing his symptoms, it would not be uncommon for syphilis to also be present.

Very early in the course of primary syphilis, it is possible for a patient to develop a chancre without having an elevation of the RPR. This is because the nontreponemal tests (RPR and venereal disease research laboratory [VDRL]) are based on antibodies to a specific response to a phospholipid (reagin) and cannot yield a positive result until a sufficient quantity is manufactured. Therefore, these tests generally do not become positive until approximately 2 weeks after the patient has been infected with syphilis; still, the chancre can appear as early as 9 days (to as long as 90 days) postinoculation. If there is a high index of suspicion that the patient's symptoms are caused by syphilis and the disease cannot be diagnosed by another method, then it is appropriate to repeat the RPR in 1 week in a compliant patient. This should not be a concern because Mr. Stevenson has been symptomatic for approximately 1 month.

Still, false-negatives can occur mandating diagnostic procedures be employed if there is a high index of suspicion that his symptoms are caused by syphilis. Additionally, because of the potential for false-positives, any positive result must be confirmed with a treponemal test such as the fluorescent treponemal antibody absorption test (FTA-ABS). These tests measure the antibody formation to the *Treponema*.

C. Dark-field microscopy of the rectal discharge   ESSENTIAL

A dark-field examination is principally utilized to evaluate painless ulcerations (both genital and nongenital) when there is a high index of suspicion that the lesion is a syphilitic chancre to identify the presence of the spirochetes in the discharge. However, rectal discharge that is caused by a *Treponema pallidum* infection can also have spirochetes identifiable on dark-field microscopy.

On rare occasions, immunofluorescence antibody staining has also been successfully employed to identify spirochetes in a sample of discharge obtained from a suspicious lesion. Silver staining of the tissue can also be employed to identify the spirochete; however, care must be instituted to ensure that the individual performing the procedure is very proficient in doing such because an extremely high number of artifacts can cause very similar changes.

D. Complete blood count with differential (CBC w/diff) NONESSENTIAL

Because Mr. Stevenson's history and physical examination findings are not consistent with a severe infection, sepsis, hemorrhage, and/or hemodynamic instability, a CBC w/diff is unnecessary.

E. Rectal swab for immediate microscopic examination, Gram stain, Tzanck stain, viral culture for herpes simplex virus (HSV), and cultures (and/or DNA probe testing) for *Neisseria gonorrhoeae* and *Chlamydia trachomatis*   ESSENTIAL

A microscopic examination provides a good indication that an infectious process is occurring by the identification of an increased leukocyte count. Furthermore, the type of infection can be determined with a high degree of certainty. A bacterial process is associated with an increased amount of bacteria, a trichomoniasis infection is characterized by mobile trichomonads, and a yeast infection is identified by the presence of hyphae and/or budding yeast cells.

The Gram stain is traditionally the initial step in a bacterial culture. As stated previously, its primary function is to evaluate the specimen to ensure it is adequate for a culture. However, it also provides additional information regarding potential bacterial pathogens by determining their shape, formation, and classification (gram negative or gram positive). However, in some cases, it is not followed by a culture. For example, in a male patient with a urethral discharge, the presence of gram-negative, intracellular diplococci on a Gram stain is considered to be pathognomonic for an infection caused by *Neisseria gonorrhoeae*. Still, a confirmatory test should be conducted. Although special media are required to culture *Neisseria gonorrhoeae* and *Chlamydia trachomatis*, it is still considered to be the "gold standard" for diagnosis. However, because of the need for specific media and care in transporting the specimen, DNA amplification testing is rapidly replacing the use of cultures for these two organisms because of its superior sensitivity, making the Gram stain obsolete or at least a separate procedure from a culture.

A Tzanck smear evaluates for the presence of multinucleated giant cells, which are frequently found in a herpes simplex virus (HSV) infection. However, viral cultures still are considered the "gold standard" for identifying a HSV infection. False-positives are very unlikely, but false-negatives occur at a significant rate.

Despite the high rates of false-negative results for many of these tests, the combination of these tests plus a dark-field microscopy will successfully lead to identification of the organism in over 90% of the cases of proctitis caused by an STI.

4. Diagnosis

A. Anal condylomata lata   INCORRECT

Condylomata lata (or "flat warts") are flat, brownish-colored plaques caused by a secondary syphilis infection. This can be ruled out as Mr. Stevenson's most likely diagnosis because he does not have any anal/perianal lesions on his physical examination and his RPR is negative.

B. Ulcerative colitis   INCORRECT

Ulcerative colitis (UC) is one of major forms of inflammatory bowel disease (for a more in-depth discussion, please see Case 5-4) that produces a noninfectious inflammation of the colonic mucosa. Although early in the illness it can present as defecatory urgency, tenesmus, and the passage of blood-tinged mucus per rectum, it can be eliminated as Mr. Stevenson's most likely diagnosis because its hallmark characteristic symptom is bloody diarrhea (which he does not have).

Furthermore, a Gram stain of the rectal discharge from a patient with UC is not going to reveal an elevated number of bacteria, especially gram-negative diplococci. Additionally, UC is virtually always associated with some degree of left lower quadrant pain/discomfort as a result of involvement of the distal colon and frequently weight loss and fever.

C. Thrombosed hemorrhoid   INCORRECT

Hemorrhoids are essentially a varicose vein of one of the internal or external rectal veins. A thrombosed hemorrhoid is one that has a thrombosis (or clot formation) located inside the affected vein. Thus, a thrombosed hemorrhoid tends to present with pain, not just anal pruritus. Because the majority of thromboses do not involve internal hemorrhoids (formed above the dentate line), it is essentially a disease of external hemorrhoid (formed below the dentate line).

The classic physical examination is the identification of smooth, roundish, bluish masses protruding from the anus. They generally are easily identifiable by visual inspection of the external anal verge, especially when the patient is asked to bear down as if simulating a bowel movement. They are visible and identifiable via anoscopy.

Because they tend to be an acute problem, a single thrombosed hemorrhoid is unlikely to persist without significant alteration in symptoms over the course of 1 month. Typically the pain resolves and the mass decreases in size over a period of a few days, with or without treatment. Therefore, because no hemorrhoids (either thrombosed or not) were discovered on Mr. Stevenson's external rectal and anoscopy examinations, a thrombosed hemorrhoid can essentially be ruled out as Mr. Stevenson's most likely diagnosis.

D. Genital and rectal herpes simplex   INCORRECT

As stated previously, some STIs are capable of producing both genital and nongenital infections, either simultaneously or individually. One of these organisms is the HSV. The typical manifestation is a dysesthesia followed by the appearance of small clusters of pinkish to erythematous papules, generally on an erythematous base, associated with mild localized edema. These initial lesions evolve into vesicles. These vesicles then rupture, creating extremely small ulcers that can coalesce to produce a larger ulcer formation. Then, it spontaneously heals and resolves most generally within 7 to 10 days from the appearance of the initial lesion. Localized lymphadenopathy can occur with both genital and anal/rectal herpes; however, it is most common with the initial episode. The initial episode, which tends to be the most severe the patient will experience, can also be associated with a "flulike" syndrome.

Because a large percentage of individuals infected with HSV will experience subclinical or very mild initial infections with even milder exacerbations, they may not realize that they are infected. Therefore, this would explain Mr. Stevenson's ability to have both a genital and anal/rectal HSV infection without his awareness (or identifiable signs on physical examination) of any genital lesions. Unfortunately, because of these subclinical and extremely mild cases, it is much easier for infected individuals to unknowingly transmit the infection to sexual partners. Thus, despite not being able to identify any of the signs and symptoms of a genital herpes infection, this could theoretically be Mr. Stevenson's diagnosis because his anoscopy results are very similar to those seen in the latter stages of herpes proctitis. However, a rectal herpes simplex infection can be eliminated as Mr. Stevenson's most likely diagnosis because examination of the associated rectal discharge revealed an increased bacteria count of gram-negative intracellular diplococci but no multinucleated giant cells on his Tzanck smear, making all three tests inconsistent with the diagnosis.

E. Gonococcal proctitis   CORRECT

Proctitis is an inflammatory condition that affects the rectal mucosa, regardless of whether the cause is infectious or noninfectious. Its characteristic symptoms consist of rectal pain, bloody rectal discharge, tenesmus, and constipation. In comparison, proctocolitis (inflammation of both the colon, or at least the distal colon, and the rectum) tends be associated with all the same symptoms, except the constipation is replaced by diarrhea (and the tenesmus is absent). In enterocolitis, the inflammation affects both the large and small bowels, and in enteritis, the inflammation is limited to the mucosa of the small bowel alone. These latter two conditions tend to present as a diarrheal illness, regardless of whether the underlying pathology is an infectious or noninfectious process.

Mr. Stevenson's sexual history and practices place him at an increased risk for an STI. With the significant number of WBCs and bacteria on his rectal discharge microscopy plus his Gram stain revealing gram-negative diplococci, Mr. Stevenson's most likely diagnosis is gonococcal proctitis.

Regarding STIs and gastrointestinal infections, in general, proctitis is from direct inoculation of the rectal mucosa with the causative organism. In proctocolitis, the STI can be a result of either direct rectal inoculation and ascension of the organism into the distal segment of the colon or ingestion of the organism through the practice of fellatio and/or cunnilingus. In enterocolitis and enteritis, the STI is virtually transmitted via oral–genital/anal intercourse.

5. Treatment Plan

A. Gemifloxacin 320 mg once a day for 7 days   INCORRECT

Quinolones are no longer indicated in the treatment of gonococcal infections because of the high rates of resistance in many areas. Furthermore, gemifloxacin is only indicated in the treatment of mild to moderate bacterial pneumonia, acute bacterial bronchitis, and acute exacerbations of chronic bronchitis when a bacterial pathogen is suspected as the causative factor.

B. Single dose of ceftriaxone 125 mg IM plus doxycycline 100 mg twice a day for 7 days   CORRECT

A single dose of ceftriaxone should be effective in eradicating Mr. Stevenson's *Neisseria gonorrhoeae* infection; however, because of the large number of individuals with gonorrhea who are coinfected with *Chlamydia trachomatis*, it is recommended by the Centers for Disease Control and Prevention (CDC) to also provide antibiotic coverage that is effective against *Chlamydia trachomatis*.

Doxycycline is currently a CDC-recommended drug for chlamydia, making this choice correct.

C. Benzathine penicillin G 2.4 million units IM   INCORRECT

The clinical use of benzathine penicillin G, especially in the outpatient setting, is predominately limited to the treatment of syphilis. Therefore, this is not indicated as part of

Mr. Stevenson's current treatment regimen because both his dark-field microscopy examination of his rectal discharge and his RPR were negative, making it unlikely that he has primary or secondary syphilis causing his symptoms (or is occurring asymptomatically in conjunction with his symptoms).

D. Open the affected vein and remove the thrombosis INCORRECT

If Mr. Stevenson had an acutely thrombosed external hemorrhoid, this would be a very appropriate treatment option, especially if done early in course of the condition.

E. Rectal cryotherapy   INCORRECT

Rectal cryosurgery has been utilized on condyloma acuminatum affecting the rectum and as an alternative treatment for hemorrhoids. However, it has no role in the treatment of gonococcal proctitis. Furthermore, rectal cryosurgery should only be performed by someone who has extensive training and experience in this technique to minimize the potential complications of perforation, strictures, loss of rectal flexibility, and damage to rectal and anal sphincter muscles.

Epidemiologic and Other Data

The incidence of proctitis in the United States is unknown. However, it does occur more commonly in males than in females. Furthermore, it appears limited primarily to adults but is seen rarely in children. Risk factors include a history of radiation therapy, an immunosuppressing condition, an autoimmune disease, high-risk sexual practices, and rectal fistulas. The most frequently encountered sexually transmitted organisms that can cause proctitis include HSV, *Neisseria gonorrhoeae*, *Chlamydia trachomatis*, and *Treponema pallidum*.

CASE 5-9
Samantha Thompson
1. History

A. Did the pain start elsewhere and move to the right lower quadrant?   ESSENTIAL

Right lower quadrant abdominal pain can result from an extensive array of gastrointestinal, gynecologic, urologic, neurologic, and psychological disorders. Additionally, there have been rarer cases of metabolic conditions producing right lower quadrant pain as well as toxins, medications, and heat-related illnesses. A comprehensive history (and physical examination) is crucial to limit the number of potential diagnoses as well as to reduce the number of potential diagnostic tests required to adequately evaluate the complaint.

Therefore, focused and specific questions related to the unique aspect of specific conditions are important to assist in differentiating the numerous potential diagnoses. For example, the pain in appendicitis frequently begins in the periumbilical, or occasionally the epigastric, area and then moves to and remains in the right lower quadrant. It is estimated that the sensitivity and specificity of this migratory pain is ~80% for acute appendicitis. However, the presence (or absence) of these distinct features does not automatically rule in (or rule out) the condition, but it does supply supporting evidence for one diagnosis over another.

B. Was she able to complete the test? How does she feel about her performance on it?   ESSENTIAL

These questions are important because they not only provide some indication of the severity of her pain early in the course of her illness but also afford important clues regarding the possibility of a somatoform disorder. In a somatoform disorder, physical symptoms can be subconsciously produced, generally as the result of overwhelming stress (e.g., early somatization disorder or conversion disorder), or consciously fabricated (e.g., early factitious illness and malingering) to get out of an unpleasant task or undesired duty.

C. What course/class was the test in?   NONESSENTIAL

This question, along with a host of other social/personal questions, is terrific for establishing rapport with the patient. However, such questions do not provide relevant information toward establishing the diagnosis and/or treatment plan for the patient. Unfortunately, with the time constraints currently associated with medical practice, attempts to establish good rapport with the patient often have to be sacrificed to obtain essential clinical information.

D. What is the relationship between the anorexia and vomiting and the pain?   ESSENTIAL

As previously alluded to, the list of potential differential diagnoses for an adolescent female who is complaining of acute-onset right lower quadrant pain is quite extensive. Questions must be focused to attempt to differentiate the various conditions. One distinction that could supply additional support in favor of a potential diagnosis involves the sequencing of symptoms. For example, in acute appendicitis, the abdominal pain virtually always precedes the onset of the anorexia and vomiting. Or, vomiting is associated with a decrease (or possibly a complete resolution) of abdominal pain that is caused by a small intestinal obstruction. Conversely, pain caused by cholecystitis and pancreatitis is unaffected by vomiting.

E. Has she experienced urinary urgency, urinary frequency, dysuria, hematuria, vaginal discharge, or unusual vaginal bleeding/spotting?   ESSENTIAL

Nongastrointestinal conditions (e.g., pelvic inflammatory disease, ovarian cysts, urinary tract infections, and ureterolithiasis) can also cause right lower quadrant pain; thus, inquiring about symptoms specific to these common disorders is paramount in attempting to establish Ms. Thompson's diagnosis.

2. Physical Examination

A. Abdominal examination   ESSENTIAL

Because Ms. Thompson is complaining of abdominal pain, a complete abdominal examination as outlined in Case 5-1 is essential.

B. Digital rectal examination   ESSENTIAL

Some experts feel that digital rectal examination (DRE) and pelvic assessment should be considered compulsory in any female patient who complains of abdominal pain. In some conditions, striking tenderness can be elicited when the affected organ is palpated through the rectal wall on DRE. In the majority of cases, this serves as additional support toward a particular differential diagnosis. Furthermore, when the affected intra-abdominal structure is more posterior in location, the abdominal examination may fail to identify any significant localized tenderness or other suspicious findings, especially in obese patients. This marked tenderness can be extremely useful in ensuring that potentially serious conditions are not overlooked. Some of the more common conditions that can present with right lower quadrant tenderness and pain upon palpation of the affected organ rectally include pelvic inflammatory disease (especially when the uterus is retroverted), ovarian cyst, ovarian torsion, ectopic pregnancy, diverticulitis, and appendicitis (especially when it extends more posteriorly off the cecum).

Furthermore, because the majority of cases of right lower quadrant pain have a gastrointestinal cause, it is prudent to examine and obtain information regarding as much of the gastrointestinal tract as possible. Therefore, a rectal examination with testing of any stool obtained for occult blood is an essential component of the physical examination. If a pelvic examination is done prior to the rectal examination (or vice versa), it is essential to use a new examination glove to prevent autoinoculation and/or containment of specimen(s) obtained.

C. Pelvic examination   ESSENTIAL

Because gynecologic conditions can also produce right lower quadrant abdominal pain, it is important to perform a pelvic examination on all postmenarche females with this complaint. A gynecologic cause is less likely in premenarchal girls; therefore, the decision to perform a pelvic examination must be decided on a case-by-case basis.

D. Evaluation for costovertebral angle (CVA) tenderness   ESSENTIAL

Because Ms. Thompson's pain radiates into her flank, it is important to evaluate for costovertebral tenderness. If present, it could suggest a renal cause for her pain (e.g., pyelonephritis and/or renal calculi).

E. Right hip and leg examination   NONESSENTIAL

Specific diagnostic maneuvers (e.g., obturator and psoas signs) are generally performed in patients with right lower quadrant abdominal tenderness that involves the passive movement of the right hip and/or leg to evaluate for possible appendicitis (please see Case 5-2). However, performing a complete musculoskeletal survey of the right hip and leg is probably not going to yield any useful clinical information.

3. Diagnostic Studies

A. Abdominal/intravaginal ultrasound   ESSENTIAL

Although an ultrasound is not as sensitive as a spiral (helical) CT scan (85 to 90% vs 96 to 98%) for confirming the diagnosis of acute appendicitis, it is more sensitive in evaluating other intra-abdominal structures for abnormalities that could be producing the pain. Because it does not require contrast media or radiation, many experts are advocating that it should be the first-line imaging technique in patients presenting with acute right lower quadrant pain.

B. Complete blood count with differential (CBC w/diff)   ESSENTIAL

Although an elevated WBC count, especially with neutrophilia, would be consistent with several potential diagnoses (e.g., acute appendicitis, pelvic inflammatory disease, ovarian torsion, psoas abscess, intestinal abscess of distal ileum, bowel obstruction, and Crohn disease), it is far from specific for any one condition. Nevertheless, it is essential to perform on Ms. Thompson to evaluate for the presence (and degree of severity, if applicable) of infection, inflammation, and/or blood loss.

C. Urinalysis   ESSENTIAL

Because urinary tract conditions (e.g., pyelonephritis and nephrolithiasis) can present as right lower quadrant abdominal pain without any evidence of irritative symptoms (i.e., dysuria, urinary frequency, and urinary urgency), a urinalysis is necessary to evaluate for the presence of these conditions. The urinalysis will also provide some basic information regarding the hydration status of the patient.

However, it is important to note that some patients with appendicitis have microscopic hematuria that is not related to a urinary tract (including renal) abnormality.

D. Urine culture and sensitivity (C&S)   NONESSENTIAL

A urine culture and sensitivity is not necessary in the evaluation of right lower quadrant pain unless the patient's signs, symptoms, and/or urinalysis are suspicious for an infection.

E. Urinary human chorionic gonadotropin (HCG) test ESSENTIAL

Most experts agree that any woman of reproductive age who presents with right lower quadrant pain (regardless of what she states about her possibility of pregnancy) should have a urinary human chorionic gonadotropin test to evaluate for a possible intra- or extra-uterine pregnancy.

4. Diagnosis

A. Pelvic inflammatory disease (PID)   INCORRRECT

PID is a general term indicating an infection anywhere in the upper female reproductive tract; therefore, it would include endometritis, salpingitis, and a tubo-ovarian abscess. The CDC minimal criteria require the presence of one or more of the following three findings on pelvic examination: cervical motion tenderness, uterine tenderness, or adnexal tenderness. Despite the fact that Ms. Thompson appeared to be experiencing adnexal tenderness, this is not her most likely diagnosis because she fails to meet the expanded CDC criteria (established to enhance the sensitivity of the diagnosis of PID): physical examination findings of a temperature greater than 101°F and the presence of a mucopurulent cervical discharge.

The other expanded criteria involve the presence of positive findings on diagnostic tests (that were not performed on Ms. Thompson). These include a significantly elevated WBC count on the microscopic examination of the vaginal and/or cervical discharge, a positive objective measurement of systemic inflammation (e.g., elevated C-reactive protein [CRP] and/or erythrocyte sedimentation rate [ESR]), and laboratory confirmation (either culture or DNA probe) of the presence of a gonorrhea or chlamydia reproductive tract infection. Furthermore, Ms. Thompson's intravaginal ultrasound and Doppler studies failed to reveal evidence of PID (e.g., free pelvic fluid, fallopian tube edema, intraluminal fallopian tube fluid, or a tubo-ovarian complex).

B. Pyelonephritis   INCORRECT

Pyelonephritis is inflammation of the proximal-most portion of the upper urinary tract located inside the kidney. It is most frequently caused by a bacterial infection. It can be ruled out as Ms. Thompson's most likely diagnosis because of her normal urinalysis and lack of CVA tenderness.

C. Acute appendicitis   INCORRECT

Acute inflammation of the appendix is a very likely diagnosis given her history, presentation, physical examination findings, and diagnostic test results of a leukocytosis with neutrophilia, a normal urinalysis, and a negative urinary HCG. Further support for this diagnosis can be obtained via her ultrasound results of a possible appendical wall edema and an enlarged appendical diameter of 12 mm. An appendix diameter of greater than 6 mm in size on ultrasonography is considered to be very suspicious for acute appendicitis.

Additionally, this diagnosis is supported by an Alvarado score of 9. The Alvarado scoring system is a tool designed to assist in determining the probability that the patient has acute appendicitis. It assigns a point value to eight clinical findings. Those obtained by history include nausea and/or vomiting (1 point), anorexia (1 point), and migratory pain (1 point). The physical examination findings consist of a temperature of greater than 99.1°F (1 point), tenderness at the McBurney point (2 points), and a positive Rovsing sign (1 point). Diagnostic test findings of a total leukocyte count greater than 10,000/mm^3 (2 points) and a neutrophil count of greater than 75% (1 point) are the last two criteria, making a total of 10 points possible. The interpretation of the total (sum of the points assigned to any positive items identified during the patient's evaluation) score is as follows: less than 4, acute appendicitis unlikely; 5 to 6, possible acute appendicitis; 7 to 8, probable acute appendicitis; and 9 to 10, very high probability of acute appendicitis.

However, this diagnosis alone does not account for the finding of a probable adnexal mass on Ms. Thompson's physical examination or her right ovarian abnormalities identified by her intravaginal ultrasound study. Thus, appendicitis alone is not her most likely diagnosis.

D. Ovarian torsion and acute appendicitis   CORRECT

Ms. Thompson's history and physical findings, as well as her diagnostic test result of a leukocytosis with neutrophilia, a normal urinalysis, and a negative urinary HCG, are consistent with both conditions. The potential that she has both conditions occurring simultaneously is significantly increased by her ultrasound findings. First, the appearance of any degree of ovarian enlargement, edema, and decreased blood flow via Doppler is consistent with the diagnosis of ovarian torsion. Likewise, her ultrasound findings of possible appendical wall edema and an enlarged appendical diameter of 12 mm are consistent with the diagnosis of acute appendicitis. Thus, from the list of potential diagnoses provided, this is Ms. Thompson's most likely diagnosis.

E. Mittelschmerz   INCORRECT

Mittelschmerz is the pain that accompanies ovulation. Because Ms. Thompson's menstrual cycles are irregular, this diagnosis cannot be eliminated based on her menstrual history. However, it can be ruled out as Ms. Thompson's most likely diagnosis because of the severity of her symptoms, abdominal and pelvic examination findings, and diagnostic test results.

5. Treatment Plan

A. Reassurance, ovulatory pain will resolve without intervention   INCORRECT

Although Mittelschmerz does generally resolve spontaneously, that is not relevant advice to provide to Ms. Thompson because this is not the cause of her symptoms.

B. Naproxen as needed, return if symptoms increase or persist after 2 days   INCORRECT

Outpatient management with an NSAID is not an appropriate treatment option for acute appendicitis or ovarian torsion.

C. Hospitalization   CORRECT

Because Ms. Thompson has two conditions that would classify her as having an acute abdomen that will likely require emergency surgery, hospitalization is definitely indicated.

D. Immediate gynecologic/surgical consult   CORRECT

Acute appendicitis is unlikely to resolve without intervention (most commonly surgical) to prevent complications (e.g., peritonitis and sepsis). Likewise, an ovarian torsion rarely results in spontaneous resolution and generally requires surgery to prevent necrosis and death of the affected ovary. Therefore, an immediate consultation with a surgeon who is skilled in the management of both conditions is necessary.

E. Single dose of ceftriaxone 250 mg IM plus doxycycline 100 mg twice a day and metronidazole 500 twice a day for 14 days   INCORRECT

Although this is acceptable outpatient treatment for a patient with mild to moderate PID, it is not an acceptable treatment option for an ovarian torsion or acute appendicitis, let alone both.

Epidemiologic and Other Data

The incidence of acute appendicitis in the United States is a little over 1 per 1000 individuals per year. The lifetime prevalence is approximately 7%. It is most likely to affect individuals who are in their late teens and 20s. It is rare in infants and toddlers as well as the extreme elderly. It tends to affect both sexes at equal rates.

Acute appendicitis is theorized to occur when appendiceal lumen obstruction leads to appendiceal wall inflammation and edema. The most common cause of this obstruction is a fecalith. Other proposed causes include viral infections, helmintic infections, alterations of normal colonic bacteria flora that results in a bacterial overgrowth that affects the wall of the appendix, and adverse effects as a result of a medical procedure (e.g., retained barium).

REFERENCES/ADDITIONAL READING

Aghababian RV, ed. *Essentials of Emergency Medicine*. Sudbury, MA: Jones & Bartlett Publishers; 2006.

Blanchard J, Rosenbaum T. Rectum and Anus. 89–94.

Brinsfield K. Female genital tract. 713–722.

DeIorio N. Large bowel. 84–88.

Dischner KR, Teferah L, Riviello RJ. Liver. 58–65.

Karasch S, Alexander J, Monyota A, Galletta G. Gastrointestinal disorders. 507–528.

Knopp R, Hokanson J. Small bowel. 75–83.

Moorhead JC, Halvorson DS. Esophagus and Stomach. 46–57.

Prince LA, Hehir DR, Peikert M. The Pancreas. 70–74.

American Association for the Study of Liver Diseases. Practice guidelines for chronic hepatitis B. *Hepatology*. 2007;45: 507–539.

American Gastroenterological Association medical position statement: evaluation of dyspepsia. *Gastroenterology*. 2005;129:1753–1755.

Brandt LJ, Prather CM, Quigley EM, et al. Systemic review on the management of chronic constipation in North America. *Am J Gastroenterol*. 2005;100(suppl 1):S5–S21.

Brandt LJ, Prather CM, Quigley EM, et al. Systemic review on the management of irritable bowel syndrome in North America. *Am J Gastroenterol*. 2002;97(suppl 11):S7–S26.

Carroll JK, Herrick B, Gipson T, Lee SP. Acute pancreatitis: diagnosis, prognosis, and treatment. *Am Fam Physician*. 2007;75:1513–1520.

Centers for Disease Control and Prevention. Sexually transmitted diseases treatment guidelines, 2006. *MMWR*. 2006;55:1–94.

Centers for Disease Control and Prevention. Update to CDC's sexually transmitted diseases treatment guidelines, 2006: fluoroquinolones no longer recommended for treatment of gonococcal infections. *MMWR*. 56;(14):332–336.

Chey W. American College of Gastroenterology guideline on the management of Helicobacter pylori infection. *Am J Gastroenterol*. 2007;102:1808–1825.

Drossman DA. The functional gastrointestinal disorders and the Rome III process. *Gastroenterology*. 2006;130:1377–1390.

Fauci AS, Kasper DL, Longo DL, et al., eds. *Harrison's Principles of Internal Medicine*. 17th ed. New York: McGraw-Hill Medical; 2008.

Camilleri M, Murray JA. Diarrhea and constipation. 245–255.

Del Valle J. Peptic ulcer disease and related disorders. 1855–1872.

Dienstag JL. Acute viral hepatitis. 1932–1949.

Dienstag JL. Chronic hepatitis. 1955–1969.

Friedman S, Blumberg RS. Inflammatory bowel disease. 1886–1899.

Gearhart SL. Diverticular disease and common anorectal disorders. 1903–1909.

Gearhart SL, Silen W. Acute appendicitis and peritonitis. 1914–1917.

Ghany M, Hoofnagle JH. Approach to the patient with liver disease. 1918–1923.

Greenberger NJ, Toskes PP. Acute and chronic pancreatitis. 2005–2017.

Hall J. Menstrual disorders and pelvic pain. 304–307.

Holmes K. Sexually transmitted infections: overview and clinical approach. 821–835.

Pratt DS, Kaplan MM. Evaluation of liver function. 1923–1926.

Ram S, Rice P. Gonococcal infections. 914–920.

Toskes PP, Greenberger. Approach to the patient with pancreatic disease. 2001–2005.

Gilbert ND, Moellering RC Jr., Eliopoulos GM, and Sande MA. (eds.) Clinical approach to initial choice of antimicrobial therapy. In: Gilbert ND, Moellering RC Jr, Eliopoulos GM, Sande MA, eds. *The Sanford Guide to Antimicrobial Therapy 2008*. 38th ed. Sperryville, VA: Antimicrobial Therapy, Inc; 2008: 4–58.

Gordon S. Blacks at greater risk of precancerous colon polyps. *US News and World Reports Health Day; 2008*. http://health.usnews.com/health-news/managing-your-healthcare/articles/2008/09/23/health-highlights-sept-23—2008.html. Accessed September 25, 2008.

Harrington L. Abdominal emergencies. In: Lalani A, Schneeweiss S, eds. *The Hospital for Sick Children: Handbook of Pediatric Emergency Medicine*. Boston: Jones & Bartlett Publishers; 2008: 196–201.

Hay EW. In: Onion DK, series ed. *The Little Black Book of Gastroenterology*. 2nd ed. Sudbury, MA: Jones & Bartlett Publishers; 2006.

Hay EW. Approaching common clinical problems (1.7 Constipation). 17–22.

Hay EW. Stomach and duodenum (3.3 Peptic ulcer disease). 114–120.

Hay EW. Inflammatory, functional, and other intestinal disorders. (4.4 Colonic diverticulosis and diverticulitis). 165–172.

Hay EW. Inflammatory, functional, and other intestinal disorders (4.6 Appendicitis). 174–177.

Hay EW. Inflammatory, functional, and other intestinal disorders (4.7 Crohn's disease). 177–190.

Hay EW. Inflammatory, functional, and other intestinal disorders. (4.8 Ulcerative colitis). 190–197.

Hay EW. Anorectal disorders (7.8 Intussusception). 300.

Hay EW. Pancreas. (9.1 Acute pancreatitis). 311–322.

Hay EW. Infections of the liver (11.2 Hepatitis B). 362–376.

Locke GR 3rd, Pemberton JH, Phillips SF. American Gastroenterological Association technical review on constipation. *Gastroenterology*. 2000;119:1766–1778.

Maconi G, Manes G, Porro GB. Role of symptoms in diagnosis and outcome of gastric cancer. *World J Gastroenterol*. 2008;14(8):1149–1155.

Mengel MP, Schwiebert LP. *Family Medicine: Ambulatory Care and Prevention*. 5th ed. New York: McGraw-Hill Medical; 2009.

Ramakrishnan K. Abdominal complaints. 1–9.

Ramakrishnan K. Perianal complaints. 352–358.

Minderhound IM, Oldenburg B, Wismeijer JA, et al. IBS-like symptoms in patients with inflammatory bowel disease in remission: relationships with quality of life and coping behavior. *Dig Dis Sci*. 2004;49:469–474.

Onion DK, series ed. *The Little Black Book of Primary Care*. 5th ed. Sudbury, MA: Jones & Bartlett Publishers; 2006.

Onion DK, Sahn E. Dermatology. 3.2 Infectious dermatitis. 191–195.

Onion DK. Gastroenterology. 6.1 Upper GI diseases. 325–338.

Onion DK. Gastroenterology. 6.2 Pancreatic diseases. 338–346.

Onion DK. Gastroenterology. 6.4 Hepatic diseases. 352–373.

Onion DK. Gastroenterology. 6.5 Small bowel diseases. 373–384.

Onion DK. Gastroenterology. 6.6 Large bowel diseases. 384–395.

Onion DK. Gastroenterology. 6.7 Miscellaneous. 395–401.

Pagana KD, Pagana TJ. *Mosby's Diagnostic and Laboratory Test Reference*. 8th ed. St. Louis: Mosby Elsevier; 2007 (multiple pages utilized to provide normal reference values for laboratory tests).

Rao SS, Ozturk L, Laine L. Clinical utility of diagnostic tests for constipation in adults: a systemic review. *Am J Gastroenterol*. 2005;100:1605–1615.

Taveras EM, Ruowei L, Gummer-Strawn L, et al. Opinions and practices of clinicians associated with continuation of exclusive breastfeeding. *Pediatrics*. 2004;11(4):e283–e290.

U.S. Preventive Services Task Force. Screening for colorectal cancer: U.S. Preventive Services Task Force recommendation statement. *Ann Intern Med*. 2008;149(9):627–637.

Weinbaum CM, Williams I, Mast EE, et al.; Centers for Disease Control and Prevention. National Center for HIV/AIDS, Viral Hepatitis, STD, and TB Prevention. Division of Viral Hepatitis. Recommendations for identification and public health management of persons with chronic hepatitis B virus infection. *MMWR*. 2008;57(RR08):1–20.

Wilson JF. In the clinic: irritable bowel syndrome. *Ann Intern Med*. 2007;147:ITC7-1-ITC7-16.

CASES IN GENITOURINARY DISEASES*

CASE 6-1

Thomas Underwood

Mr. Underwood is a 58-year-old African American male who presents with the chief complaint of "having to get up a lot at night to urinate." The nocturia began approximately 2 years ago and consisted of having to get up once at night to urinate; however, for the past month this has increased to three to four times per night. It interferes with the quality and quantity of his sleep, leaving him drowsy at work the following day. In addition, he is experiencing urinary urgency, urgency frequency, sensation of incomplete bladder emptying after voiding, difficulty starting stream, straining to continue stream, weaker force and diameter of the stream, and postvoid dribbling. He has not noticed an abnormal or unusual odor to his urine. He is not having any abdominal pain, back pain, flank pain, fever, nausea, vomiting, urinary incontinence, urethral discharge, bowel changes, leg weakness, or paresthesias affecting the trunk or lower extremities.

Mr. Underwood's only known medical problem is mild seasonal allergic rhinitis, which is currently controlled with diphenhydramine 50 mg at bedtime. He initiated this therapy approximately 1 month ago. He takes no other prescription or over-the-counter (OTC) medications, vitamins, supplements, or herbal preparations. He has never been hospitalized nor had any surgeries. He smokes one pack per day (PPD) and has done so for the past 40 years. He drinks alcohol on occasion (defined by him as two drinks every 2 to 3 months). He does not have regular age-appropriate preventive medical evaluations. His family history is unremarkable, including prostate or bladder cancer.

1. Based on this information, which of the following questions are essential to ask Mr. Underwood and why?

A. Has he recently had anorexia, weight loss, night sweats, or true fatigue?

B. Has he noticed any gross hematuria?

C. What is his bedtime routine?

D. Does he have any problems with erectile dysfunction (ED)?

E. How much caffeine does he consume in the average day?

Patient Responses

Mr. Underwood denies any recent anorexia, weight loss, night sweats, true fatigue, gross hematuria, or ED. He normally goes to bed at 10 p.m. and watches television until midnight. He does not consume any beverages during this time period. However, he does admit that in the past month he has increased his caffeinated beverage intake to 5 to 10 drinks during work hours to "stay awake and alert."

2. Based on this information, which of the following components of a physical examination are essential to conduct on Mr. Underwood and why?

A. Heart and lung examination

B. Abdominal examination

C. Rectal and prostate examination

D. Genital examination

E. Skin examination

Physical Examination Findings

Mr. Underwood weighs 175 lb and is 5'10" tall (body mass index [BMI] = 25.1). Other vital signs are blood pressure (BP), 130/72 mm Hg; pulse, 88 beats per minute (BPM) and regular; respirations, 16/min and regular; and oral temperature, 97.9°F.

---

*Remember, for each question, none to all of the answers could be correct/essential or incorrect/nonessential. See page 223 for Chapter 6 answers.

His heart is regular in rate and rhythm and without murmurs, gallops, or rubs. His apical impulse is nondisplaced and does not exhibit a thrill. His lungs are clear to auscultation.

His abdomen reveals normoactive and equal bowel sounds in all four quadrants. It is soft, nontender, and without masses or organomegaly. His rectal examination is normal except for a slightly enlarged, smooth prostate with a shallow medial furrow. It is normal in consistency and does not reveal any masses or indentations.

His genital examination shows both testicles to be descended and without masses; scrotal sacs as nontender and with abnormal masses; midline urethra; and status postcircumcision. No lesions, lymphadenopathy, or hernias are identified.

His skin is normal in color and temperature; there is no edema, masses, or lesions.

3. Based on this information, which of the following diagnostic studies are essential to perform on Mr. Underwood and why?

    A. Postvoid residual (PVR) urine measurement
    B. Prostatic ultrasound
    C. Prostate-specific antigen (PSA), if the patient desires after being advised of the pros, cons, and various organizational recommendations regarding testing as well as his personal risk factors for prostate cancer
    D. Urinalysis
    E. Serum creatinine

Diagnostic Results

Mr. Underwood's PVR was 155 mL (normal: < 100–200). His prostatic ultrasound was normal. His PSA was 4.5 ng/ml (normal: < 4). His urinalysis was unremarkable and his serum creatinine was 0.8 mg/dl (normal male: 0.6–1.2).

4. Based on this information, which one of the following is Mr. Underwood's most likely diagnosis and why?

    A. Acute prostatitis
    B. Benign prostatic hypertrophy, symptoms worsened by antihistamine usage
    C. Prostate cancer
    D. Nephrolithiasis
    E. Neurogenic bladder

5. Based on this diagnosis, which of the following are appropriate components of a treatment plan for Mr. Underwood and why?

    A. Decrease or, if possible, eliminate caffeine, and avoid fluids 4 to 6 hours before bedtime
    B. Watchful waiting and repeat American Urological Association Symptom Index (AUA SI) in 3 months to determine symptom progression
    C. Stop diphenhydramine and try topical cromolyn sodium for allergic rhinitis
    D. Tamsulosin 0.4 mg one-half hour before bed; can increase to 0.8 mg if patient tolerates and continues to be symptomatic
    E. Prostatic ultrasound

CASE 6-2
Umberto Valentino

Mr. Valentino is a 19-year-old African American male who presents with the chief complaint of dysuria. It is associated with a thin, clear to pale yellow penile discharge. The pain on urination appears to be located at his meatus. His symptoms have been present and unchanged for 2 days. He knows of no aggravating or alleviating factors. He does not have any urgency, frequency, genital pain, abdominal pain, back/flank pain, nausea, vomiting, chills, or fever.

He has no known medical problems, surgeries, or hospitalizations. He is not taking any over-the-counter or prescription medications, vitamins, supplements, or herbal products. He does not smoke, drink alcohol, or use illicit substances. His family history is noncontributory.

1. Based on this information, which of the following questions are essential to ask Mr. Valentino and why?

    A. What is his sexual history?
    B. Is he currently experiencing or has he recently experienced any skin or mucous membrane lesions?
    C. Is he currently experiencing or has he recently experienced any ocular symptoms or arthralgias?
    D. Is he currently experiencing or has he recently experienced a sore throat?
    E. Is he currently experiencing or has he recently experienced a cough?

Patient Responses

Mr. Valentino states that he is sexually active with women only. He has never had sex with men. He always has used and continues to use latex condoms regularly. He estimates that he has had over 100 lifetime sexual partners, including approximately 10 new partners in the last 30 days. The majority of these partners are women he met through his employment at the local coffee shop. He does not have a "regular" partner.

He has not experienced (nor does he currently have) a rash, other skin lesions, mucosal lesions, eye complaints, arthralgias, sore throat, or cough.

2. Based on this information, which of the following components of a physical examination are essential to conduct on Mr. Valentino and why?

    A. Oropharyngeal examination
    B. Lung auscultation
    C. Abdominal examination
    D. Digital rectal examination
    E. Genital examination

Physical Examination Findings

Mr. Valentino weighs 155 lb and is 5'8" tall (BMI = 23.6). Other vital signs are BP, 122/66 mm Hg; pulse, 88 BPM and regular; respirations, 12/min and regular; and oral temperature, 98.9°F.

His oral mucosa, pharynx, and tongue are normal in color and without lesions. He does not have tonsillar enlargement or exudates.

His lungs are clear to auscultation bilaterally.

His abdominal examination reveals normoactive and equal bowel sounds in all four quadrants. There is no tenderness, masses, or organomegaly. His perineum is without abnormal discoloration or lesions. His anus is without any lesions, fissures, or other visual abnormalities. His anal sphincter tone is normal. He has no rectal masses or palpable lesions. His prostate is normal in size, contour, and consistency; there is no tenderness or masses.

His genital examination reveals normally developed genitalia without any lesions or erythema. He has a small amount of a thin, slightly yellowish discharge from his urethra. His testicles are descended bilaterally, normal sized, and nontender to palpation. He does not have any abnormal scrotal masses, tenderness, or edema. There is no evidence of an inguinal hernia.

3. Based on this information, which of the following diagnostic studies are essential to perform on Mr. Valentino and why?

A. Sample of the urethral discharge for microscopic examination with normal saline and Gram staining
B. Penile swab for nucleic acid amplification test for *Neisseria gonorrhoeae* and *Chlamydia trachomatis*
C. Urine culture
D. Rapid plasma reagin (RPR)
E. Complete blood count with differential (CBC w/diff)

Diagnostic Test Results

Mr. Valentino's microscopic examination of his urethral discharge revealed 25 to 50 white blood cells (normal: < 5), 3+ bacteria (normal: < 1+), no mobile trichomonads (normal: none), no budding yeast or hyphae (normal: none) per high-power field, and rare mobile sperms.

His Gram stain revealed 10 to 20 polymorphonuclear neutrophils (PMNs) per oil immersion field (normal: < 5), rare bacteria (normal: < 1+), and no gram-negative diplococci (normal: none).

His RPR was positive at 1:32 (normal: nonreactive). His CBC w/diff was normal. His penile swab *N. gonorrhoeae* and *C. trachomatis* and urine culture results are pending.

4. Based on this information, which one of the following is Mr. Valentino's most likely diagnosis and why?

A. Gonococcal urethritis (GU)
B. Nongonococcal urethritis (NGU)
C. Urethritis and syphilis
D. Cystitis
E. Acute prostatitis

5. Based on this diagnosis, which of the following are appropriate components of a treatment plan for Mr. Valentino and why?

A. Single dose of ceftriaxone 125 mg IM and azithromycin 1 g orally
B. Have patient's partners evaluated and treated for current illness and encourage patient and all partners to be tested for other sexually transmitted infections (STIs)

C. Valacyclovir 1 g orally every 8 hours for 10 days
D. Fluorescent treponemal antibody absorption test (FTA-ABS)
E. Ciprofloxacin 500 mg bid for 5 days plus a single dose of azithromycin 1 g orally

CASE 6-3
Vincent White

Mr. White is a 72-year-old white male who presents with the chief complaint of "I need to get some of those blue triangle pills." Further questioning confirms that Mr. White is having difficulty with erectile dysfunction (ED). His primary problem is not being able to achieve an erection suitable for intercourse. According to him, the problem started approximately 9 months ago and has gradually worsened. At the onset, it just occurred rarely. Now, it happens almost every time he tries to have intercourse.

He isn't experiencing any problems with urination, including starting or maintaining his stream, narrowing or decreased force of his stream, dribbling after finishing urinating, incontinence, dysuria, urgency, frequency, or hematuria. He does not have fever, chills, weight loss, night sweats, nausea, vomiting, bowel changes, abdominal pain, perineal pain, flank pain, difficulty with gait, leg weakness, dysesthesias, claudication, or fecal incontinency.

His only known medical problems are angina and hypertension. He has not had a myocardial infarction, been hospitalized, or had any surgery or surgical procedures. His medications consist of transdermal nitroglycerine 0.4 mg/hr on for 12 hours, then off for 12 hours; metoprolol 50 mg twice a day; aspirin 81 mg once a day; and sublingual nitroglycerine tablets as needed (he estimates that he uses one tablet approximately every 3 to 4 months). He is not taking any other prescription or over-the-counter medications, vitamins, supplements, or herbal preparations.

He quit smoking 40 years ago after smoking one pack per week for approximately 15 years. He has not drunk any alcoholic beverages in 40 years. He denies ever using (or currently using) any illicit substances or abusing drugs. He has regular age-appropriate preventive check-ups and his last one was 6 months ago. He stated that it included a prostate examination and a prostate-specific antigen (PSA), which were reported to him as normal.

He has been married for 53 years and is in a mutually monogamous relationship. They have not recently experienced any significant life changes, increased stress, or interpersonal relationship problems. His wife is in good health and desires to be sexually intimate with him. His family history is noncontributory.

1. Based on this information, which of the following questions are essential to ask Mr. White and why?

A. Does he experience nocturnal or early morning erections?
B. When he gets an erection, is he able to sustain it, achieve an orgasm, and ejaculate?
C. Has he had individual sexual therapy?

D. Does he have problems with premature ejaculation?

E. Has he noticed any changes in his libido, sleep, appetite, activities, interests, mood, or outlook on life?

Patient Responses

Mr. White occasionally experiences nocturnal and/or early morning erections. If he does achieve an erection, it is sustained and he can complete the act, achieve an orgasm, and ejaculate without difficulty. He denies premature ejaculation, loss of libido, or changes in his sleep habits, appetite, activities, interests, mood, or positive outlook on life. He has not had any sex therapy.

2. Based on this information, which of the following components of a physical examination are essential to conduct on Mr. White and why?

A. Thyroid examination

B. Genital and prostate examination

C. Penile blood pressure

D. Examination of the aorta and lower extremities for vascular changes

E. Neurologic examination of the genitalia, perineum, and lower extremities

Physical Examination Findings

Mr. White weighs 172 lb and is 5'11" tall (BMI = 24.0). Other vital signs are BP, 128/72 mm Hg; pulse, 78 BPM and regular; respirations, 14/min and regular; and oral temperature, 98.6°F.

His thyroid is palpable, normal in size, nontender, and without masses bilaterally.

His penile systolic blood pressure is 122/68 mm Hg. His genitalia are normal in appearance without any discoloration, lesions, or other abnormalities. He is circumcised. His urethra is normal in location and without any gross abnormalities. He is able to determine temperature change and vibration in his penis. His testicles are normal in size, shape, and consistency; descended bilaterally; and without tenderness or masses. He has no abnormal scrotal masses, increased warmth, or tenderness. There is no evidence of a hernia. His perineum is without lesions and with intact sensation to sharp and dull touch that is equal bilaterally. His bulbocavernosus reflex is normal and equal bilaterally. His prostate is slightly enlarged, nontender, slightly boggy, and without masses. His rectal and anal sphincter tone are normal.

His abdominal aorta is normal in size and pulsation. He does not have an aortic, renal, or femoral bruit. His femoral, popliteal, dorsalis pedis, and posterior tibial pulses are normal and equal bilaterally. There are no skin, temperature, or hair changes of his lower extremities.

Mr. White's muscle strength is normal and equal bilaterally in his legs. His gait is normal. Sharp and dull sensation is intact and equal in both legs. Knee jerk, ankle jerk, and plantar response are normal and equal bilaterally. No pedal edema is present.

3. Based on this information, which of the following diagnostic studies are essential to perform on Mr. White and why?

A. Urinalysis

B. Fasting plasma glucose (FPG) and lipid panel

C. Serum testosterone (total), prolactin, follicle-stimulating hormone (FSH), and luteinizing hormone (LH) levels

D. Nocturnal penile tumescence and rigidity study

E. Scrotal ultrasound

Diagnostic Test Results

Mr. White's urinalysis was normal. His fasting plasma glucose was 102 mg/dl (normal: 70–126). His total cholesterol was 174 mg/dl (normal healthy adult: < 200). His high-density lipoprotein (HDL) was 64 mg/dl (normal healthy male: > 45), his low-density lipoprotein (LDL) was 85 mg/dl (normal healthy adult: 60–180), and his very low-density lipoprotein (VLDL) was 25 mg/dl (normal healthy adult: 7–32). His triglycerides were 142 mg/dl (normal healthy adult male: 40–160).

His total testosterone level was 204 ng/dl (normal adult male: 280–1080). His prolactin was 17 ng/ml (normal adult male: 0–20). His FSH was 20.2 IU/L (normal adult male: 1.42–15.4), and his LH was 10.7 IU/L (normal adult male: 1.24–7.8).

Nocturnal penile tumescence and rigidity study revealed 3 to 5 erections per episode of rapid eye movement (REM) sleep (normal: 3–5) and a total erection time of 102 minutes (normal: > 90). His scrotal ultrasound was normal.

4. Based on this information, which one of the following is Mr. White's most likely diagnosis and why?

A. Erectile dysfunction caused by primary hypogonadism

B. Erectile dysfunction caused by secondary hypogonadism

C. Erectile dysfunction caused by a psychological condition

D. Erectile dysfunction caused by a pituitary adenoma

E. Erectile dysfunction due to normal male aging

5. Based on this diagnosis, which of the following are appropriate components of a treatment plan for Mr. White and why?

A. Desvenlafaxine 50 mg once a day

B. Testosterone topical patch 2.5 mg; apply one patch once a day to dry skin (after obtaining copy of his PSA level to ensure it is normal)

C. Change metoprolol to clonidine 0.1 mg twice a day

D. Sildenafil 50 mg approximately 1 hour before planned intercourse

E. Referral to urologist for implantation of inflatable penile prosthesis

CASE 6-4

Wilson Xandiaver

Mr. Xandiaver is a 32-year-old white male who presents to the emergency department complaining of intermittent left flank pain radiating to his groin. The pain begins as a mild ache (1 out of 10 on the pain scale) and progresses over the next 45 to 60 minutes to become a severe, intolerable (10 out of 10 on the pain scale), "cramping spasmlike" pain. Then, it spontaneously resolves in 20 to 30 minutes, only to occur again in another 15 to 60 minutes. It started approximately 6 hours ago and awoke him from sleep. It does not appear to be worsening in severity or frequency. He is unaware of any aggravating or alleviating factors. He denies any trauma or back injury (both acute and chronic). He claims that he has never experienced the same or similar symptoms in the past.

When severe, the pain is associated with nausea and diaphoresis. He experienced vomiting during the pain's peak with the last episode of pain, prompting his visit. The emesis consisted of clear, thin, "bitter" fluid. It did not contain any blood, "coffee grounds"-appearing materials, or other abnormal substances, including fecal material. He denies fever, chills, malaise, abdominal pain, myalgias, arthralgias, constipation, diarrhea, other bowel changes, or flulike symptoms. He has not had a sore throat or a viral infection within the past few weeks. However, approximately 2 weeks ago he thought he was getting a cold but "fought it off."

He is not on any prescription medications. He has no known medical problems and has never had surgery nor been hospitalized. However, he admits he is severely claustrophobic. He denies drinking alcohol, using illicit substances/drugs, or smoking cigarettes. He is sexually active with his wife of 10 years. As near as he knows, they have a mutually monogamous relationship. For contraception, his wife takes birth control pills. His family history is negative.

1. Based on this information, which of the following questions are essential to ask Mr. Xandiaver and why?

A. Does he take any over-the-counter medications, vitamins, supplements, or herbal preparations?
B. Is he on any special "diet"?
C. Has he experienced any hematuria, discolored urine, dysuria, urinary urgency, urinary frequency, difficulty initiating urination, incontinence, decrease in caliber or strength of his stream, or urethral discharge?
D. Is he really monogamous?
E. Has he ever practiced or experimented with sex with men?

Patient Responses

He has been taking 2000 mg/day of vitamin C for the past 2 weeks in an effort to "fight off a cold." He is not taking any other medications, supplements, vitamins, or herbal preparations. He is not on any type of diet; however, he admits to not eating "as healthy as I should."

He noticed his urine being a "little darker" than usual for the past 1 to 1.5 weeks. Yesterday, he noticed that he was having some difficulty initiating urination and a slight reduction in the caliber and strength of his stream. He denies any hematuria, dysuria, urinary urgency, urinary frequency, incontinence, or urethral discharge.

He is adamant that he has only been sexually active with his wife since their marriage. He denies ever having sex with a man.

2. Based on this information, which of the following components of a physical examination are essential to conduct on Mr. Xandiaver and why?

A. Oral examination to evaluate dentition
B. Abdominal examination
C. Prostate examination
C. Genital examination
E. Evaluation for costovertebral angle (CVA) tenderness

Physical Examination Findings

Mr. Xandiaver weighs 198 lb and is 6'2" tall (BMI = 26.9). Other vital signs are BP, 140/82 mm Hg; pulse, 98 BPM and regular; respirations, 18/min and regular; and oral temperature, 99.0°F.

His teeth are clean and in good condition and repair.

His abdominal examination reveals normoactive and equal bowel sounds in all four quadrants. It is soft, nontender, and nondistended. No masses, organomegaly, or bruits are noted. His rectal and prostate examinations are unremarkable.

His genitalia are normal in appearance and without discoloration, rashes, lesions, or urethral discharge. His testicles are normal size without masses, descended bilaterally, and nontender. His scrotum has no abnormal masses and is nontender. There is no evidence of a hernia.

He has no CVA tenderness.

3. Based on this information, which of the following diagnostic studies are essential to perform on Mr. Xandiaver and why?

A. Urinalysis and urine culture and sensitivity (C&S)
B. Electrolytes
C. Baseline serum calcium, phosphate, uric acid, and creatinine levels
D. Plain x-ray film of the abdomen
E. Spiral computed tomography (CT) of abdomen and pelvis with contrast and sedation

Diagnostic Test Results

Mr. Xandiaver's urine was pale pink in color, clear, and with normal odor. His pH was 4.5 (normal: 4.6–8.0) and his specific gravity 1.015 (normal: 1.005–1.030). His dipstick was negative for glucose, protein, nitrites, ketones, and leukocyte esterase (normal: negative). His microscopic examination revealed 4 white blood cells (WBCs) per low-power field (normal: 0–4), no WBC casts (normal: none), 20 to 25 red blood cells (RBCs) per low-power field (normal: ≤ 2), no RBC casts (normal: none), 0 to 3 calcium oxalate crystals (normal: none), and no casts (normal: none) per low-power field. His urine C&S is pending.

His electrolytes revealed a carbon dioxide of 26 mEq/L (normal: 23–30), a chloride of 102 mEq/L (normal: 98–106), a potassium of 4.5 mEq/L (normal adult: 3.5–5.0), and a sodium of 140 mEq/L (normal adult: 136–145).

His serum calcium was 10 mg/dl (normal adult: 9.9–10.5), phosphate was 3.5 mg/dl (normal adult: 3.0–4.5), uric acid was 4.3 mg/dl (normal adult male: 4.0–8.5), and creatinine was 1.1 mg/dl (normal adult male: 0.6–1.2).

His abdominal radiograph was normal. His spiral CT revealed a 4.75-mm, slightly irregularly shaped mass in the distal portion of the proximal one third of his left ureter.

4. Based on this information, which one of the following is Mr. Xandiaver's most likely diagnosis and why?

A. Acute pyelonephritis
B. Calcium nephrolithiasis, produced by excessive vitamin C intake
C. Struvite calculi
D. Uric acid nephrolithiasis
E. Phlebolith

5. Based on this diagnosis, which of the following are appropriate components of a treatment plan for Mr. Xandiaver why?

  A. Enteric-coated naproxen 500 mg twice a day
  B. Stop vitamin C
  C. Increase water intake to a minimum of 2 liters/day
  D. Strain urine and bring in any sediment for analysis
  E. Hospitalize, initiate IV lines for hydration, and obtain a urology consultation

CASE 6-5

Xavier Yount

Mr. Yount is a 21-year-old African American male who presents with the chief complaint of "a hernia." Approximately 2 hours ago, he attempted to lift a 50-lb box from the floor to his workstation. Before getting the box 6 inches off the floor, he began experiencing a sharp pain in his left testicle. It was so severe that he dropped the box and "collapsed" to the floor. Since then, the pain has increased (currently, 10 out of 10 on the pain scale) and is radiating into his ipsilateral flank. He is also complaining of scrotal edema and discoloration. The company's onsite nurse advised him to elevate his genitalia with a towel and apply an ice pack to the area. When the pain increased despite this maneuver, she advised him to have it evaluated immediately. One of his co-workers accompanied him to the emergency department. He denies any direct trauma to his testicle.

He is nauseated and diaphoretic. He is not experiencing vomiting, abdominal pain, diarrhea, constipation, other bowel changes, penile discharge, hematuria, urinary urgency, urinary frequency, dysuria, fever, chills, sore throat, oral lesions, headache, myalgias, arthralgias, lightheadedness, or vertigo.

He has no known medical problems and has never had any surgery nor been hospitalized. He takes no prescription or over-the-counter medications, vitamins, supplements, or herbal products. He denies ever smoking cigarettes, drinking alcohol, or using illicit substances.

He is sexually active in what he assumes to be a mutually monogamous relationship with a female for the previous 9 months. Because it is an exclusive relationship and his girlfriend takes oral contraceptives, he has not used condoms for the past 6 months. They do not practice oral–genital/anal intercourse. His number of lifetime partners is three. He denies ever having sex with a male.

1. Based on this information, which of the following questions are essential to ask Mr. Yount and why?

  A. Did he have any symptoms before the pain began or has he experienced the same or similar pain in the past?
  B. What does he mean by "collapsed"?
  C. Is his other testicle symptomatic?
  D. Has he recently had parotitis?
  E. Did anyone see him lift the box?

Patient Responses

Mr. Yount states that he was totally asymptomatic before attempting to lift the box. He has never experienced any type of genital pain in the past. He defines "collapsed" as "dropping to the floor and rolling in pain." He did not lose consciousness or experience a presyncopal or syncopal episode. Several of his co-workers witnessed him attempting to lift the box.

He does not have contralateral testicular and/or scrotal pain or tenderness, and his contralateral scrotum is not enlarged or discolored. He has never experienced parotitis.

2. Based on this information, which of the following components of a physical examination are essential to conduct on Mr. Yount and why?

  A. Oropharyngeal evaluation
  B. Palpation of parotid and submandibular glands
  C. Abdominal examination
  D. Genital examination
  E. Evaluation for CVA tenderness

Physical Examination Findings

Mr. Yount weighs 150 lb and is 5'9" tall (BMI = 22.2). Other vital signs are BP, 148/88 mm Hg; pulse, 98 BPM and regular; respirations, 20/min and regular; and oral temperature, 98.9°F. He is diaphoretic and appears to be in significant pain.

His oral mucosa and pharynx are normal in color and without masses, ulcerations, exudates, or other lesions. His parotid and submandibular glands are normal size and nontender.

His abdomen reveals normoactive and equal bowel sounds in all four quadrants. There are no masses, organomegaly, tenderness, bruits, or distension. No bulges are identified with the patient supine or with the unsupported elevation of his head and shoulders at approximately 15°.

His external rectal examination reveals no lesions, fissures, or other abnormalities. He has good sphincter tone. His rectal vault is normal and has a small amount of soft, brown stool in it. His prostate is normal size, without masses, and slightly tender on the left.

His genital examination reveals a left scrotum that is moderately purplish red in color, slightly warm to touch, extremely tender to palpate, approximately twice the size of his contralateral one, and with dependent edema. Despite its size and dependent edema, his left scrotum still appears to be more proximal in location than the right one. Additionally, his left testicle appears to be elevated and his epididymis anterior in location; both are extremely tender to any touch. His pain is unchanged with his scrotum being raised above the level of his pubic symphysis (negative Prehn sign). No blue dot sign is identified (a blue dot sign is a pinpoint bluish area that can sometimes be visualized through the scrotal skin over the proximal testes and is generally associated with a torsed testicular appendage).

His right testicle is descended; normal in size, shape, and consistency; and nontender to palpation. He has no abnormal right scrotal masses, edema, tenderness, discoloration, or temperature change. He has no other genital abnormalities, masses, lesions, rashes, discolorations, or penile discharge. There is no inguinal lymphadenopathy or evidence of an inguinal hernia. His cremasteric reflex is present on the right but absent on the left.

3. Based on this information, which of the following diagnostic studies are essential to perform on Mr. Yount and why?

    A. Scrotal color Doppler ultrasound

    B. Urinalysis

    C. Penile swab for Gram stain and nucleic acid amplification test for *N. gonorrhoeae* and *C. trachomatis*

    D. Testicular scintigraphy

    E. Complete blood count with differential (CBC w/diff)

Diagnostic Test Results

Mr. Yount's color Doppler ultrasound of his left scrotum revealed a moderate-size hydrocele and a more horizontal and medial testicular rotation of approximately 180° on its spermatic cord. It appeared to be associated with a decreased blood flow of approximately 75%. No testicular appendages were identified. His left epididymis was anterior in location and appeared slightly edematous. Otherwise, the examination was normal.

His urine was clear and normal in color and odor. His pH was 6.5 (normal: 4.6–8.0) and his specific gravity was 1.015 (normal: 1.005–1.030). His dipstick was negative for nitrites, leukocyte esterase, glucose, protein, and ketones (normal: negative for all). His microscopic examination revealed 0 to 2 WBCs (normal: 0–4), no WBC casts (normal: none), 0 to 2 RBCs (normal: ≤ 2), no RBC casts (normal: none), trace bacteria (normal: none), and no crystals or casts (normal: none) per low-power field.

His Gram stain revealed 0 to 1 PMNs per oil immersion field and no gram-negative diplococci. His penile swab for *N. gonorrhoeae* and *C. trachomatis* are pending.

His CBC w/diff was normal except for a very mild leukocytosis (WBC count of 10,500/mm³ [normal adult: 5000–10,000]) with a predominance of neutrophils (75% [normal: 55–70]).

4. Based on this information, which one of the following is Mr. Yount's most likely diagnosis and why?

    A. Urinary tract infection

    B. Left gonococcal epididymitis

    C. Left testicular torsion

    D. Left traumatic hydrocele and inguinal hernia

    E. Cryptorchidism

5. Based on this diagnosis, which of the following are appropriate components of a treatment plan for Mr. Yount and why?

    A. Bed rest with scrotal elevation

    B. Naproxen 500 mg twice a day

    C. Ceftriaxone 250 mg IM × one dose plus doxycycline 100 mg orally twice a day for 10 days

    D. Immediate surgical consultation

    E. If surgeon is not immediately available, attempt manual detorsion

CASE 6-6

Yolinda ("Lindy") Zickafoose

Lindy is a 34-month-old Native American female who presents with her mother for the chief complaint of "swelling around her eyes." Her mother first noticed it when she awoke 2 days ago. She attributed it to "allergies" because they had been outdoors on a picnic the day before its onset. However, last night when she was helping Lindy with her bath, her mother noticed Lindy had some mild labial edema. On awakening this morning, Lindy's mother noticed that the edema around her eyes and her labia was even more pronounced. In addition, she had also developed bilateral ankle edema. She does not have any swelling elsewhere in her body. However, her mother did remember that Lindy's face started looking "puffy" approximately 1 week ago.

The edema does not appear to fluctuate. There are no aggravating or alleviating factors that her mother is aware of. Lindy has gained about 2 lb since the onset of her illness. She has not experienced any rhinorrhea, nasal congestion, sneezing, itchy/watery eyes, conjunctival injection, icterus of sclera, coughing, wheezing, shortness of breath, pruritus, jaundice, skin erythema, urticaria, or any other type of rash or skin lesions. She has not been ill otherwise. Her last illness was a viral upper respiratory tract infection approximately 4 months ago.

She has no known medical problems. She has never been hospitalized nor had surgery. She is on no prescription or over-the-counter medications, vitamins, supplements, or herbal preparations. Furthermore, she has not taken any in several months according to her mother. She has regular age-appropriate health maintenance physical examinations and her immunizations are up to date. Her mother denies any trauma. Lindy's father is 29 years old and was diagnosed with hyperlipidemia several years ago, and she has a paternal cousin with "some kind of kidney problem." Otherwise, her family history is negative.

1. Based on this information, which of the following questions are essential to ask Lindy's mother and why?

    A. Has her mother recently changed soaps, lotions, detergents, fabric softeners, or any other product that could come in contact with Lindy's skin?

    B. Does she attend day care?

    C. Has there been any change in her urine's appearance or urination patterns?

    D. Does her diet contain consumption of a lot of salt, unwashed fruits/vegetables, or any new or unusual foods?

    E. Was she stung by a bee within the last 3 weeks?

Patient Responses

Her mother has not changed soaps, lotions, detergents, or other products that are in contact with Lindy's body. Lindy does not attend day care. Her mother has not noticed any irritative or obstructive urinary symptoms. However, she has observed that Lindy's urine appears "foamy" and possibly slightly darker in color, and that Lindy might be urinating less often. Otherwise, Lindy's mother has not noticed any changes in Lindy's urine and/or voiding habits.

There has not been a change in Lindy's diet (including unusual or new foods), consumption of any unwashed fruits/vegetables, or utilization of excessive salt. As near as her mother knows, Lindy has never suffered a bee envenomation.

2. Based on this information, which of the following components of a physical examination are essential to conduct on Lindy and why?

    A. Eyes, ears, nose, mouth, and throat examination

    B. Heart and lung examination, including blood pressure

C. Abdominal examination

D. External genital and rectal examination

E. Evaluation of the skin for additional sites of edema plus discoloration, urticaria, rashes, and/or other lesions

Physical Examination Findings

Lindy weighs 30 lb and is 36.5" tall. Other vital signs are BP, 110/68 mm Hg in right arm and 111/69 mm Hg in left arm (for more information on normal BP for age, please see discussion in answer section); pulse, 108 BPM and regular (for more information on normal cardiac rates in children younger than the age of 3 years, please see Table 2-1); respirations, 22/min and regular (for more information on normal respiratory rates in children younger than the age of 3 years, please see Table 2-2); and oral temperature, 98.7°F.

Lindy has generalized facial edema that is worse periorbitally; however, there is no eversion of her eyelids. Her sclera and conjunctivae are normal in color, noninjected, and without discharge. There is no edema or tenderness around or over her lacrimal ducts. Her pupils are round, normal in size, and equal. They react to light and accommodation. Her funduscopic examination is normal.

Her ear canals are normal shape and size without edema, erythema, or abnormal discharge, bilaterally. Her tympanic membranes are nonerythematous and noninjected, exhibit normal movement, and do not reveal any evidence of a middle ear effusion or mass, bilaterally. She does not have any edema or eversion of her lips. Her nasal mucosa, oral mucosa, tongue, and pharynx are normal in color and without edema, lesions, ulcers, exudates, or other discharge. Her tonsils are normal bilaterally.

Her heart is regular in rate and rhythm. She does not have any murmurs, gallops, or rubs. Her apical impulse is nondisplaced and without a thrill. Her lungs are clear to auscultation.

Her abdomen reveals normoactive and equal bowel sounds in all four quadrants. It is soft, nondistended, and without masses, organomegaly, or tenderness. Her external genital examination reveals mildly edematous labia without any abnormality of color, rashes, or lesions. Her hymen is intact. Her perineal area and lower buttocks reveal mild pitting edema. There is no discoloration, rash, or lesions. Her anal sphincter is normal in appearance (no fissures, masses, or lesions) and her rectal tone is normal.

She has mild pitting edema of her feet and ankles. There does not appear to be any edema involving her legs, hands, or arms.

3. Based on this information, which of the following diagnostic studies are essential to perform on Lindy and why?

A. Urinalysis

B. Serum albumin, globulin, and total protein

C. Serum blood urea nitrogen (BUN) and creatinine

D. Strep screen

E. Lipid panel

Diagnostic Test Results

Lindy's urine was yellow in color, frothy appearing, and normal in odor. Her pH was 6.0 (normal: 4.6–8.0) and her specific gravity 1.030 (normal: 1.005–1.030). Her dipstick was positive for 4+ protein but negative for glucose, nitrites, leukocyte esterase, and ketones (normal: negative for all). Her microscopic examination revealed 2 to 4 WBCs (normal: 0–4), no WBC casts (normal: none), 0 to 2 RBCs (normal: ≤ 2), 3 to 5 RBC casts (normal: none), rare bacteria (normal: none), "grapelike" clusters of fatty casts (or oval "fat bodies"), and hyaline casts, but no crystals (normal: no crystals or casts) per low-power field.

Her serum albumin was 1.25 g/dl (normal child: 4–5.9), her globulin was 4.5 g/dl (normal: 2.3–3.4), and her total protein was 5.75 g/dl (normal child: 6.2–8). Her BUN was 2 mg/dl (normal child: 5–18), her serum creatinine was 0.4 mg/dl (normal child: 0.3–0.7), and her BUN/creatinine ratio was 5.0.

Her strep screen was negative.

Her total cholesterol was 286 mg/dl (normal child: 120–200), her LDL was 214 (normal: 60–180), her HDL was 35 mg/dl (normal female: > 45), her VLDL was 37 mg/dl (normal: 7–32), and her triglycerides were 185 (normal female child 0–5 years of age: 32–99).

4. Based on this information, which one of the following is Lindy's most likely diagnosis and why?

A. Acute glomerulonephritis

B. Acute pyelonephritis

C. Nephrotic syndrome

D. Child abuse

E. Allergic reaction to unknown agent

5. Based on this diagnosis, which of the following are appropriate components of a treatment plan for Lindy and why?

A. Hospitalization

B. Nephrology consultation for evaluation, possible renal biopsy, and treatment

C. Furosemide 0.5 g/kg IV followed by 25% salt-deficient albumin 0.5 g/kg IV

D. Prednisone 2 mg/kg/day orally

E. Complete blood count with differential (CBC w/diff)

CASE 6-7
Zelda Armstrong

Ms. Armstrong is a 22-year-old Hispanic female who presents with the chief complaint of "I think I have a urinary tract infection again." She has been experiencing one about every 2 weeks for the past 3 months. She's had dysuria with minimal urgency and frequency for the past 3 to 4 days. Her symptoms have been unchanged since their onset. She denies hematuria, urinary incontinence, nausea, vomiting, abdominal pain, back pain, flank pain, pelvic pain, constipation, diarrhea, other bowel changes, chills, or fever. She has been drinking a lot of cranberry juice without any improvement of her symptoms. She is unaware of any aggravating or alleviating factors.

She has no known medical problems. She has never been hospitalized nor had any surgeries. Her only medication is oral contraceptives. She denies taking any other prescription or over-the-counter medications, vitamins, supplements, or herbal preparations. Her last menstrual period (LMP) was 2 weeks ago and normal. She has not missed any pills. She does not drink alcohol or smoke cigarettes. Her family history is negative.

1. Based on this information, which of the following questions are essential to ask Ms. Armstrong and why?

    A. When during voiding does her dysuria begin and where is her pain located?

    B. Has she noticed any vaginal discharge or genital lesions?

    C. What is her sexual history?

    D. Has she passed any kidney stones?

    E. Has she noticed any changes in the color and/or odor of her urine?

Patient Responses

Her dysuria begins toward the end of voiding and is external in location. She does have a small amount of thin, vaginal discharge; however, she states that it is "normal" for her when she has a urinary tract infection (UTI). The vaginal discharge is yellowish in color and slightly malodorous. She has not noticed any genital lesions. She is sexually active and has been in what she assumes to be a mutually monogamous relationship with her current boyfriend for approximately 6 months. They quit using condoms about 2 months ago. She has never had sex with a female and this is only her second male partner. As near as she knows, he is asymptomatic. She has not noticed any kidney stones or stone fragments in her urine; however, she has noticed it having a slightly malodorous smell.

2. Based on this information, which of the following components of a physical examination are essential to conduct on Ms. Armstrong and why?

    A. Heart examination

    B. Lung examination

    C. Abdominal examination

    D. Pelvic examination

    E. Evaluation for CVA tenderness

Physical Examination Findings

Ms. Armstrong weighs 125 lb and is 5'5" tall (BMI = 20.8). Other vital signs are BP, 112/70 mm Hg; pulse, 78 BPM and regular; respirations, 12/min and regular; and oral temperature, 98.9°F.

Her heart is normal in rate and rhythm and without murmurs. Her lungs are clear to auscultation.

Her abdominal examination reveals normoactive bowel sounds in all four quadrants without any evidence of rigidity, distension, tenderness, organomegaly, or masses. She does not have any CVA tenderness.

Her external genitalia are normal in color, nonedematous, and without any rashes/lesions. Her vaginal mucosa is mildly erythematous and covered with a small amount of minimally frothy yellowish-white discharge. No vaginal or cervical lesions are present. Her cervix is nonerythematous and without discharge. On bimanual examination, her pelvic organs are normal in shape and size. She does not have any cervical motion tenderness.

3. Based on this information, which of the following diagnostic studies are essential to perform on Ms. Armstrong and why?

    A. Urinalysis

    B. Urine culture and sensitivity (C&S)

    C. Urinary human chorionic gonadotropin (HCG) test

    D. Wet-mount microscopy of vaginal secretions

    E. Vaginal pH, "whiff" test for amine odor, and point-of-care testing for vaginal pathogens via DNA

Diagnostic Test Results

Ms. Armstrong's urine was light yellow in color, clear, and with a slightly foul odor. Her pH was 6.0 (normal: 4.6–8.0) and her specific gravity was 1.020 (normal: 1.005–1.030). Her dipstick was positive for 2+ leukocyte esterase and 1+ nitrites; and, it was negative for glucose, protein, and ketones (normal: negative for all). Her microscopic examination revealed 5 to 10 WBCs (normal: 0–4), no WBC casts (normal: none), 0 to 1 RBCs (normal: ≤ 2), no RBC casts (normal: none), 4+ bacteria (normal: none), 4+ epithelial cells, and no casts or crystals per low-power field (normal: no crystals or casts). Her urine C&S is pending.

The wet-mount microscopy of Ms. Armstrong's vaginal secretions revealed 25 to 35 WBCs per high-power field (normal: < 5), 3+ bacteria (normal: <1+), 2+ epithelial cells that are normal in appearance (normal: no clue cells), and motile trichomonads (normal: none). Her vaginal pH was elevated to 5.5 (normal: 3.5–4.5) and her whiff amine test was slightly positive (normal: negative). Her point-of-care test results are pending.

4. Based on this information, which one of the following is Ms. Armstrong's most likely diagnosis and why?

    A. Cystitis

    B. *Trichomonas* vaginitis

    C. Candidal vulvovaginitis

    D. Vaginitis caused by bacterial vaginosis

    E. Pelvic inflammatory disease

5. Based on this diagnosis, which of the following are essential components of Ms. Armstrong's treatment plan and why?

    A. Metronidazole 2 g orally × one dose

    B. Azithromycin 500 mg, 2 pills stat, then 1 pill a day for 4 days

    C. Tinidazole 2 g once a day for 5 days

    D. Advise the patient not to take her medication after drinking alcohol or with an alcoholic beverage, and not to drink alcohol for a minimum of 72 hours after finishing the medication

    E. Provide expedited partner treatment

CASE 6-8
Alex Bing

Mr. Bing is a 31-year-old Asian American male who presents with dull, aching, generalized perineal pain. It began approximately 2 weeks ago and has been gradually getting worse. He rates it as 3 out of 10 on the pain scale at its maximum intensity; currently, it is 3 out of 10. The pain does not radiate; however, he does experience mild, intermittent right testicular aching. The pain worsens slightly if Mr. Bing sits for long periods of time; however, it quickly returns to its baseline intensity after he has been standing for a few minutes. It is alleviated temporarily by sitting in a bathtub of hot water. He knows of no other aggravating or alleviating factors. He denies a history of trauma.

He has mild dysuria, once-a-night nocturia, slight straining to urinate, minimal hesitancy upon initiating urination, and a sensation of incomplete bladder emptying following urination. He has not had hematuria, change in color of his urine, difference in odor of his urine, urinary urgency, urinary frequency, dribbling of urine after voiding, a decrease in the caliber or strength of his urine's stream, or urinary incontinency. Mr. Bing also denies flank pain, abdominal pain, nausea, vomiting, diarrhea, constipation, other bowel changes, malaise, fever, and/or chills.

He has no known medical problems, has never been hospitalized, and has never had surgery. He takes no prescription or over-the-counter medications, vitamins, supplements, or herbal preparations. He does not smoke, drink alcohol, or use illicit substances. He has been sexually active with women only. He estimates his lifetime number of partners to be 10. He has been married for the past 3 years and, to his knowledge, their relationship is mutually monogamous. He does not use condoms. For contraception, his wife takes oral contraceptives.

1. Based on this information, which of the following questions are essential to ask Mr. Bing and why?

   A. Has he noticed any lesions, swelling, itching, or other abnormalities of his genital and/or perineal areas?
   B. Does he have penile pain and/or a urethral discharge?
   C. Does he experience pain with ejaculation?
   D. Does he carry a lot of pennies or other copper items in his front pockets?
   E. Does he have a history of urinary tract infections, urethritis, or prostatitis?

Patient Responses

He has not noticed any perineal or genital lesions, swelling, itching, paresthesias, or other abnormalities. He does not have penile pain or discharge. He has a mild burning sensation with ejaculation. He does not carry excessive copper in any of his pockets. He has never been diagnosed with a UTI, urethritis, or prostatitis; however, he has experienced similar symptoms in the past, which spontaneously resolved in a few days.

2. Based on this information, which of the following components of a physical examination are essential to conduct on Mr. Bing and why?

   A. Eye examination for icterus
   B. Thyroid palpation
   C. Abdominal examination
   D. Perineal and rectal examination
   E. Genital examination

Physical Examination Findings

Mr. Bing weighs 170 lb and is 5'9" tall (BMI = 25.1). His other vital signs are BP, 120/72 mm Hg; pulse, 68 BPM and regular; respirations, 13/min and regular; and oral temperature, 98.5°F.

His eyes do not reveal any icterus.

His thyroid is normal in size, location, and consistency. There is no evidence of nodules, tenderness, or other abnormalities.

His abdomen has normoactive and equal bowel sounds in all four quadrants. It is soft to palpation and does not reveal any masses or organomegaly. His perineal area is normal in appearance and without lesions, erythema, or excoriations. His rectal tone is slightly increased. He has a normal-sized prostate gland of normal consistency without any masses; however, it is slightly tender to palpate. Palpation/massage of his prostate gland does produce a penile discharge. Otherwise, his rectal examination is normal.

His genitalia are normal in appearance. There is no evidence of erythema, lesions, or rash. He did not have any spontaneous penile discharge. His testicles are normal in size, shape, and consistency and without masses or tenderness. His scrotum reveals no abnormal masses or areas of tenderness. There is no evidence of an inguinal hernia or inguinal lymphadenopathy.

3. Based on this information, which of the following diagnostic studies are essential to perform on Mr. Bing and why?

   A. Prostate-specific antigen (PSA)
   B. Midstream pre– and post–prostate massage urinalyses
   C. Expressed prostatic secretions (EPSs) for microscopy evaluation and culture
   D. Culture and sensitivity (C&S) on both urine specimens
   E. Blood cultures

Diagnostic Test Results

Mr. Bing's PSA was 1.2 ng/ml (normal: < 4).

His pre-examination urine was light yellow in color, clear, and without an abnormal odor. His pH was 6.0 (normal: 4.6–8.0) and his specific gravity was 1.020 (normal: 1.005–1.030). His dipstick was negative for leukocyte esterase, nitrites, glucose, protein, and ketones (normal: negative for all). His microscopic examination revealed 0 to 2 WBCs (normal: 0–4), no WBC casts (normal: none), 0 to 1 RBCs (normal: ≤ 2), no RBC casts (normal: none), no bacteria (normal: none), and no casts or crystals per low-power field (normal: no crystals or casts).

His post-examination urine was light yellow in color, clear, and without an abnormal odor. His pH was 6.5 (normal: 4.6–8.0) and his specific gravity was 1.020 (normal: 1.005–1.030). His dipstick was negative for leukocyte esterase, nitrites, glucose, protein, and ketones (normal: negative for all). His microscopic examination revealed 0 to 2 WBCs (normal: 0–4), no WBC casts (normal: none), 0 to 1 RBCs (normal: ≤ 2), no RBC casts (normal: none), no bacteria (normal: none), and no casts or crystals per low-power field (normal: no crystals or casts). His cultures are pending.

4. Based on this information, which one of the following is Mr. Bing's most likely diagnosis and why?

   A. Acute bacterial prostatitis
   B. Chronic bacterial prostatitis
   C. Inflammatory chronic pelvic pain syndrome (CPPS-I)
   D. Noninflammatory chronic pelvic pain syndrome (CPPS-NI)
   E. Epididymitis

5. Based on this diagnosis, which of the following are appropriate components of a treatment plan for Mr. Bing and why?

    A. Trimethoprim-sulfamethoxazole double strength, twice a day for 1 to 3 months

    B. Diclofenac 50 mg three times a day

    C. Ceftriaxone 250 mg IM × one dose plus doxycycline 100 mg orally twice a day for 14 days

    D. Erythromycin 250 mg four times a day for a minimum of 2 (to a maximum of 6) weeks

    E. Terazosin 1 mg/day

CASE 6-9

Bsharma Caudwell

Mrs. Caudwell is an 84-year-old Pakistan native who is brought in today by her daughter because "she seems to be confused." Despite living in the United States for over 50 years, she still does not speak much English. Because of her confusion, the language barrier, and a qualified interpreter not being available, her daughter is serving as her primary history giver and interpreter.

According to her daughter, she first noticed Mrs. Caudwell's confusion when the patient awoke yesterday morning. Prior to that time, Mrs. Caudwell was asymptomatic and did not have any cognitive difficulties. Throughout the day yesterday, her daughter noticed that Mrs. Caudwell was forgetting the names of common objects, the location of rooms in her home of 50 years, the date of her son's last visit, and eating meals. Yesterday evening, Mrs. Caudwell also experienced an episode of urinary incontinence while attempting to locate the bathroom.

This morning, Mrs. Caudwell started complaining of nausea and vomited once. The emesis consisted of a small amount of undigested food from her breakfast and "normal stomach acid." There was no blood, "coffee grounds"-appearing substances, fecal-looking materials, or any other abnormalities. She appeared to be experiencing chills for approximately 1/2 hour following the episode of vomiting. Her daughter noticed that Mrs. Caudwell felt "warm" earlier today; however, she did not take her temperature. Her daughter doesn't think Mrs. Caudwell is experiencing a headache, malaise, weight loss, weight gain, edema, constipation, diarrhea, abnormal-appearing stools, rectal bleeding, abdominal pain, incontinence of bowel, or skin lesions. Furthermore, her daughter states that Mrs. Caudwell has not complained of any of these symptoms and denied their presence when directly questioned during this visit by her daughter. However, her daughter states that Mrs. Caudwell also denies feeling ill or experiencing memory difficulties.

Also according to her daughter, Mrs. Caudwell does not have any known medical problems. She has never been hospitalized except to have her five children. Her only surgery was an appendectomy approximately 25 years ago. She takes no prescription or over-the-counter medications, vitamins, supplements, or herbal preparations. Her daughter has never known her to smoke or drink alcohol. Mrs. Caudwell's husband died approximately 15 years ago; her daughter and her family moved in with Mrs. Caudwell at that time.

1. Based on this information, which of the following questions are essential to ask her daughter if she has noticed and to have her interpret for Mrs. Caudwell and why?

    A. Has she been experiencing any difficulties with speech, using facial muscles, walking, coordination, weakness in her extremities, or dysphagia?

    B. Has she had any urinary urgency, frequency, dysuria, hematuria, abdominal pain, or flank pain?

    C. Does her confusion appear to remain constant or does it fluctuate?

    D. Has she had a vaginal discharge?

    E. Has she had chest pain, cough, wheezing, dyspnea, palpations, arm pain, dyspepsia, vertigo, presyncope, syncope, or diaphoresis?

Patient Responses

According to her daughter, Mrs. Caudwell's memory appeared to be much worse last evening than it was during the day yesterday or even this morning. Her daughter has noticed Mrs. Caudwell going to the bathroom more often than usual and rubbing her right flank occasionally over the past couple of days. However, according to her daughter, Mrs. Caudwell denies these observations when questioned about them.

Her daughter has not noticed Mrs. Caudwell experiencing any problems with her speech, facial muscle usage, walking, coordination, weakness in her extremities, dysphagia, urinary urgency, dysuria, hematuria, abdominal pain, flank pain, vaginal discharge, chest pain, cough, wheezing, dyspnea, palpations, arm pain, dyspepsia, vertigo, presyncope, syncope, or diaphoresis. According to her daughter, Mrs. Caudwell denies all of these symptoms as well.

2. Based on this information, which of the following components of a physical examination are essential to conduct on Mrs. Caudwell and why?

    A. Thyroid palpation

    B. Heart and lung examination

    C. Abdominal examination

    D. Neurologic examination, including evaluation of mental status

    E. Evaluation for costovertebral angle (CVA) tenderness

Physical Examination Findings

Mrs. Caudwell weighs 205 lb and is 5'0" tall (BMI = 40). Other vital signs are BP, 126/72 mm Hg; pulse, 104 BPM and regular; respirations, 16/min and regular; and oral temperature, 101.2°F. Her oxygen saturation (O_2) is 99% on room air (RA). She is slightly ill appearing.

Her heart is slightly tachycardic but regular in rhythm. No murmurs, gallops, or rubs are noted. Her apical impulse is nondisplaced and without a thrill. Her lungs are clear to auscultation.

Her abdomen is protuberant and soft and reveals normoactive and equal bowel sounds in all four quadrants. There are no masses or organomegaly noted. She does not have any tenderness or guarding. Her aorta is normal in diameter. She does not have any aortic or renal artery bruits. Her rectal examination is normal and her stool tested negative for occult blood.

Her pelvic examination is normal except for the presence of atrophic vaginitis.

Her cranial nerves appear grossly intact. Her gait is normal. Her hand, arm, foot, and leg strength are normal and equal bilaterally. Her reflexes are also normal.

The mini-mental status examination (MMSE) and confusion assessment method (CAM) cannot adequately be administered because of the language barrier. However, according to responses provided via her daughter as interpreter during the MMSE, Mrs. Caudwell is oriented to person only, could only remember one of three objects at 5 minutes, and could not perform serial 7's. Mrs. Caudwell's language skills are intact when her daughter speaks to her and she writes in her native language.

She has marked CVA tenderness on the right; however, none is present on the left.

3. Based on this information, which of the following diagnostic studies are essential to perform on Mrs. Caudwell and why?

    A. Complete blood count with differential (CBC w/diff)
    B. Blood urea nitrogen (BUN) and creatinine
    C. Urinalysis
    D. Urine culture and sensitivity (C&S)
    E. Blood culture and sensitivity (C&S)

Diagnostic Results

Mrs. Caudwell's CBC w/diff revealed an RBC of $5.2 \times 10^6/\mu l$ (normal female: 4.2–5.4) with a mean corpuscular volume (MCV) of 89 μm^3 (normal adult: 80–95), a mean corpuscular hemoglobin (MCH) of 30 pg (normal adult: 27–31), a mean corpuscular hemoglobin concentration (MCHC) of 35 g/dl (normal adult: 32–36), and a red blood cell distribution width (RDW) of 12.5% (normal adult: 11–14.5). Her WBC count was 25,500/mm³ (normal adult: 5000–10,000) with 82% neutrophils (normal: 55–70), 9% lymphocytes (normal: 20–40), 5% monocytes (normal: 2–8), 3% eosinophils (normal: 1–4), and 1% basophils (normal: 0.5–1). Her hemoglobin (Hgb) was 12.8 g/dl (normal female: 12–16) and her hematocrit (HCT) was 42% (normal female: 37–47). Her platelet (thrombocyte)

count was 225,000/mm³ (normal adult: 150,000–400,000) and her mean platelet volume (MPV) was 7.9 fl (normal: 7.4–10.4). Her smear was consistent with these results and revealed no cellular abnormalities except for a few bands.

Her BUN was 29 mg/dl (normal adult: 10–20; elderly patients might be slightly higher) and her creatinine was 1.3 mg/dl (normal adult female: 0.5–1.1; elderly patients might be slighter lower because of decreased muscle mass).

Mrs. Caudwell's urine was dark yellow in color, clear, and with a foul odor. Her pH was 7.5 (normal: 4.6–8.0) and her specific gravity 1.025 (normal: 1.005–1.030). Her dipstick was 4+ positive for leukocyte esterase and 3+ positive for nitrites but negative for glucose, protein, and ketones (normal: negative for all). Her microscopic examination revealed too numerous to count (TNTC) WBCs (normal: 0–4), 5 to 8 WBC casts (normal: none), 1 to 4 RBCs (normal: ≤ 2), 0 to 2 RBC casts (normal: none), 4+ bacteria (normal: none), 1+ epithelial cells, and no casts or crystals (normal: no crystals or casts) per low-power field. Her urine C&S and blood C&S are pending.

4. Based on this information, in addition to class III obesity, which one of the following is Mrs. Caudwell's most likely diagnosis and why?

    A. Alzheimer disease
    B. Pneumonia
    C. Pyelonephritis
    D. Interstitial cystitis
    E. Heart failure

5. Based on this diagnosis, which of the following are appropriate components of a treatment plan for Mrs. Caudwell and why?

    A. Trial donepezil 5 mg once a day
    B. Hospitalization
    C. IV ampicillin and gentamicin until C&S results available, then continue or change based on her response and C&S findings
    D. Stat intravenous pyelogram (IVP)
    E. Promethazine suppositories 12.5 mg every 8 to 12 hours as needed for nausea

CASES IN GENITOURINARY DISEASES

RESPONSES AND DISCUSSION

CASE 6-1

Thomas Underwood

1. History

A. Has he recently had anorexia, weight loss, night sweats, or true fatigue?   ESSENTIAL

Many urologic conditions can be responsible for Mr. Underwood's symptoms, including prostate cancer. Therefore, it is essential to inquire as to whether he has been experiencing any constitutional symptoms that could indicate the presence of an associated malignancy.

B. Has he noticed any gross hematuria?   ESSENTIAL

Gross hematuria can be associated with several urologic conditions (e.g., nephrolithiasis, bladder cancer, or urinary tract infection). Regardless of other symptoms, patients who have painless hematuria in conjunction with risk factors for bladder cancer are considered to have a bladder carcinoma until proven otherwise.

Accepted risk factors for bladder cancer include male gender, Caucasian race, advancing age, cigarette smoking, aniline dye (found in fabric dye, hair coloring, and wood stains) exposure, some medications (e.g., phenacetin and chloranaphazine) usage, and previous radiation therapy (especially external beam).

C. What is his bedtime routine?   NONESSENTIAL

Mr. Underwood's bedtime routine is highly unlikely to affect his symptoms. However, inquiring about his evening activities (in particular, how much fluid he consumes after dinner until he goes to bed) might provide a clue to assist in improving his symptomatology. Excessive fluid intake during the late evening hours can exacerbate nocturia regardless of its cause.

D. Does he have any problems with erectile dysfunction (ED)?   ESSENTIAL

Because his symptoms could be caused by prostatic tissue hypertrophy and the currently accepted theory is that prostate gland enlargement, which is associated with the normal aging process, results from decreasing testosterone levels (which also occur with the normal aging process), it is important to determine whether the patient is experiencing symptoms suggestive of a decreased testosterone state. One of the primary symptoms caused by hypotestosteronism is ED.

However, ED is not specific for prostate enlargement, regardless of the cause (i.e., benign prostatic hypertrophy or prostate cancer). It can also occur with other urologic conditions (e.g., urinary tract infections and urethritis) and nonurologic conditions (including cardiovascular [e.g., atherosclerosis and hypertension], neurologic [e.g., spinal cord injury, multiple sclerosis, or peripheral neuropathies], endocrine [e.g., diabetes mellitus and hyperprolactinemia], and psychogenic [e.g., performance anxiety, victim of childhood sexual abuse, or relationship conflicts]). Medication adverse effects can also produce ED (e.g., anticholinergics, antidepressants, antihypertensives, histamine-2 [H_2] antagonists, and hormones).

E. How much caffeine does he consume in the average day?   ESSENTIAL

Caffeine is considered to be not only a bladder irritant but also a diuretic. Therefore, excessive caffeine intake can increase urinary output and frequency of voiding, including at night.

2. Physical Examination

A. Heart and lung examination   NONESSENTIAL

Ideally, a heart and lung examination should be performed on all patients regardless of the reason for the clinical encounter; however, in the "real world" time constraints associated with the practice of medicine unfortunately force the healthcare provider (HCP) to focus only on the areas that are going to provide the greatest "bang for the buck." Therefore, the only essential components of the history and physical examination are those that are going to provide useful clinical information to guide diagnostic studies and formulate the correct diagnosis and treatment plan.

B. Abdominal examination   ESSENTIAL

Despite Mr. Underwood's denial of abdominal pain, an abdominal examination is still indicated because it can identify abnormal findings (e.g., presence of a distended bladder, irregularities to the shape of the bladder, or a renal mass), which can provide useful information in formulating his list of differential diagnoses and evaluating him for complications related to these conditions.

C. Rectal and prostate examination   ESSENTIAL

The digital rectal examination (DRE) is very important because it permits abnormalities in the size, consistency, contour, and tenderness of the prostate gland to be identified. However, it is important to remember that when the prostate gland is responsible for the patient's symptoms, its overall size does not correlate well with the severity of these symptoms.

Furthermore, specific attention needs to be focused on the muscle tone of Mr. Underwood's anal sphincter. It is generally accepted that strength of the anal sphincter tone correlates with the strength of the urinary bladder sphincter tone.

D. Genital examination   ESSENTIAL

A genital examination is also indicated when men present with symptoms like Mr. Underwood's. It can identify abnormalities that lend support for or against the conditions on his list of potential diagnoses as well as provide information regarding coexisting conditions (e.g., phimosis, hypospadias, epididymitis, or urethritis) that might be contributing to his nocturia.

E. Skin examination   NONESSENTIAL

Outside of a few sexually transmitted infections, there are very few urogenital conditions that are associated with dermatologic manifestations, especially in nongenital areas.

3. Diagnostic Studies

A. Postvoid residual (PVR) urine   measurement   NONESSENTIAL

The PVR volume can be measured by ultrasound or Foley catheterization. Most experts agree that it is indicated when there is a high index of suspicion that an obstructive uropathy (most suggestive findings include continuous [but can be intermittent] suprapubic pain/discomfort with radiation into the flanks [or low back], oliguria, obstructive urinary symptoms [e.g., difficulty starting and/or maintaining urinary stream, decreased caliber of urinary stream, "dribbling" after voiding, feeling of incomplete postvoid bladder emptying, and urinating at intervals < 2 hours in length], palpable bladder distension, and an elevated serum blood urea nitrogen [BUN] and creatinine with an elevated BUN/creatinine ratio) is producing, coexisting with, and/or complicating the patient's condition.

Because marked benign prostatic hypertrophy (BPH) can cause an obstructive uropathy, some experts maintain that this test should be performed on all patients with known or suspected BPH with moderate to severe symptoms as indicated by his American Urological Association Symptom Index (AUA SI) score (see later). However, other experts maintain that if the patient's history and physical examination are consistent with the diagnosis of BPH (without evidence of an obstructive uropathy), this test is not required as part of the diagnostic workup.

Furthermore, there are varying opinions regarding what is considered normal and what is considered indicative of an obstructive uropathy. The majority of experts consider a PVR volume of less than 200 mL to be normal; however, some experts believe this volume should be less than 100 mL. Regarding the definition of urinary obstruction, expert opinions range from a PVR volume of greater than 100 to one that is greater than or equal to 350 mL as the cutoff. Regardless of the actual volume of PVR, studies have failed to reveal a correlation between PVR, symptom severity, and/or urodynamic study results.

In view of this information and the fact that the results of a PVR are not going to assist in determining Mr. Underwood's correct diagnosis or alter his treatment plan, one is not necessary at this point in his evaluation.

The AUA SI is a self-assessment questionnaire that asks the patient to assign a numerical value to the severity of seven symptoms of BPH (feeling of incomplete bladder emptying after voiding, urinating within 2 hours of last urination, difficulty maintaining urine stream, difficulty postponing urination, straining to urinate, weakening of urine stream, and experiencing nocturia) during the past month on a scale of 0 (never experiences) to 5 (almost always occurs) to obtain a quantitative measure of the patient symptom severity and their impact on the patient's quality of life. Scores ≤ 7 are considered to be mildly symptomatic, scores from 8 to 19 moderately symptomatic, and scores ≥ 19 severely symptomatic. This measurement is then utilized to assist in determining the most appropriate therapy for the individual patient as well as in serving as a tool to monitor therapeutic response to the intervention.

B. Prostatic ultrasound   NONESSENTIAL

A prostatic ultrasound is not indicated because there were no distortions of contour, overt masses, or marked hardness of consistency identified on Mr. Underwood's DRE of his prostate. As a general rule, a prostatic ultrasound is not indicated unless a prostatic biopsy for one of these abnormalities is being considered.

C. Prostate-specific antigen (PSA), if the patient desires after being advised of the pros, cons, and various organizational recommendations regarding testing as well as his personal risk factors for prostate cancer   ESSENTIAL

There is considerable controversy regarding the value of utilizing the PSA as a modality to detect early prostate cancer because of the associated psychological and physiologic consequences connected with an elevated value. Studies have documented varying levels of increased stress and anxiety in patients who have a positive screening test for cancer. This anxiety is greatest during the period following the notification of a positive result until the final (usually pathology) report is relayed to the patient. However, even in the presence of a disease-free confirmatory test result, some patients experience continued anxiety and/or other mood disorders because of concerns regarding the validity of the confirmatory results (and whether they are truly disease free).

Prostate cancer is associated with a greater potential for mood disorders because of its physiologic characteristics. Generally, prostate cancer is a very slow-growing malignancy. In some patients, a recommendation is made not to treat the patient's prostate cancer because his estimated life expectancy is shorter than the predicted time for significant problems to develop as a result of the carcinoma. Some patients have a difficult time dealing with both the knowledge of having an untreated malignancy in their bodies and their inevitable mortality.

Another physiologic characteristic of prostate cancer that has been utilized in arguments for and against the screening of asymptomatic older men with a PSA test is that occasionally the carcinoma is not slow growing but very aggressive and could progress and metastasize at a much faster rate. These concerns are further complicated by the fact that autopsy results revealed that over 90% of all men in their eighth decade of life had evidence of hyperplastic changes to their prostatic tissue; and over 70% had cancerous prostatic changes regardless of their cause of death.

Furthermore, there are problems with using the PSA as a screening tool primarily because the PSA is specific to prostate tissue but not prostate cancer. Elevations can occur as a result of normal aging (probably as a result of increased prostate size), BPH, prostatitis, recent ejaculation, and possibly vigorous DRE. This is further complicated by the occurrence of false-negative results as well as certain medications (e.g., 5α-reductase inhibitors) being able to decrease the PSA level. Additionally, there are conflicting results regarding the reduction in mortality in asymptomatic men whose cancer was diagnosed by PSA versus men whose diagnosis of cancer was delayed until they became symptomatic.

Most experts agree that if the PSA is less than 4, the likelihood of that patient having prostate cancer is very small. Likewise, if the PSA is greater than 10, the likelihood of that patient having prostate cancer is very high. However, there is no consensus regarding the most appropriate management for men with PSA levels between 4 and 10. PSA density, age-adjusted PSA values, blind prostate biopsy, percent free PSA (%FPSA), and prostatic-specific membrane antigen are all tests that are being utilized to attempt to determine if a malignancy is present when the PSA is elevated and the DRE and prostatic ultrasound are both normal.

Therefore, it is no wonder that different "expert groups" have reached different recommendations regarding testing. The AUA guidelines recommend an annual PSA in all men starting at the age of 50 years; however, if there is a positive family history or if the patient is African American, then his prostate cancer screenings should start at age 40 years. The American Cancer Society recommendations state that all men should be offered an annual PSA starting at the age of 50 years if their life expectancy is greater than 10 years. However, individuals who have a first-degree relative with prostate cancer before the age of 65 years or are African American should start their screening at age 45 years, if desired. Additionally, individuals with a strong family history (multiple first-degree relatives with prostate cancer before the age of 65 years) might want to start annual screenings as early as 40 years old. The Centers for Disease Control and Prevention's (CDC's) viewpoint is that the benefits of screening for early prostate cancer might not outweigh the harms of a false-positive test. Therefore, they recommend providing the patient with the currently available data and letting him make the decision to be tested. The US Preventive Services Task Force has a similar recommendation. They advise against screening anyone older than the age of 75 years; and for men younger than 75 years, they recommend discussing the pros and cons of screening before testing is performed and letting them make

the decision to have it done or not. Their recommendations for men younger than the age of 75 years are based on what they term "insufficient evidence" to recommend for or against.

Risk factors for prostate cancer include advancing age, positive family history, African-American heritage, cigarette smoking, consuming an unhealthy diet (e.g. containing a high fat content, large quantities of red meat [probably due to the release of polycyclic aromatic hydrocarbons with cooking], and low quantities of vegetables [especially of the cruciferous variety and those high in retinoids, like lycopene]).

D. Urinalysis   ESSENTIAL

A urinalysis is recommended to provide clues to systemic diseases that could be causing nocturia (e.g., diabetes mellitus, diabetes insipidus, or heart failure), an infectious process of the urinary tract (e.g., urethritis, cystitis, prostatitis, pyelonephritis), a renal abnormality (e.g., glomerulonephritis, carcinoma, staghorn calculus, or renal trauma), or other urogenital abnormality (e.g., bladder carcinoma, lower urinary tract trauma, or nephrolithiasis).

E. Serum creatinine   ESSENTIAL

Because the patient's serum creatinine is generally directly proportional to his or her renal function, it should be performed on all older men with urinary symptoms to ensure that their kidney function is not compromised by (or contributing to) their condition (e.g., urinary tract obstruction, pyelonephritis, diabetic nephropathy, or reduced renal blood flow).

4. Diagnosis

A. Acute prostatitis   INCORRECT

Acute prostatitis is generally the result of a bacterial infection causing the prostate gland to become inflamed. On DRE, the prostate is very tender, boggy, and enlarged. The patient is often ill appearing, febrile, and experiencing perineal and/or low back pain. Additionally, the urinalysis may show evidence of an infection, especially if performed after DRE. Because Mr. Underwood only had one of these primary findings (prostatic gland enlargement on DRE), it is unlikely that acute prostatitis is his most likely diagnosis.

B. Benign prostatic hypertrophy, symptoms worsened by antihistamine usage   CORRECT

Mr. Underwood's symptoms are classic for BPH. In view of the negative findings on his additional history questions, physical examination, and diagnostic results, this is his most likely diagnosis. Additionally, the symptoms of BPH can be worsened by the patient taking antihistamines. Because his symptom escalation occurred at approximately the same time he began the diphenhydramine, it is very suspicious that this medication was responsible. Other medications that can increase the symptoms of BPH include anticholinergics, decongestants, tranquilizers, and α-adrenergic agonists.

C. Prostate cancer   INCORRECT

Although prostate cancer can present with essentially the same symptoms that Mr. Underwood is complaining (not to mention that he does possess some risk factors for the disease [e.g., African American race, age older than 50 years, and a 40-pack-year smoker]), it can still be eliminated as his most likely diagnosis at this time because his history failed to reveal any symptoms suggestive of malignancy and his DRE did not detect any suspicious abnormalities.

In order for prostate cancer alone to be his most likely diagnosis, he would need to have a large enough malignant prostatic lesion to produce the symptoms. Therefore, it would be highly unlikely that he did not have some palpable abnormality of his prostate gland on DRE (i.e., mass, nodules, and/or indurated areas). Despite men with a PSA level in his range having an estimated incidence of prostate cancer of ~25%, it is still unlikely that he does because the degree of elevation of the PSA level directly correlates with the size and stage of the disease.

D. Nephrolithiasis   INCORRECT

Nephrolithiasis, or kidney stones, can produce some of the symptoms experienced by Mr. Underwood. However, he does not have the classic symptoms of severe, colicky abdominal and/or flank pain with hematuria. Therefore, nephrolithiasis is not his most likely diagnosis.

E. Neurogenic bladder   INCORRECT

A neurogenic bladder can present with some, but not all, of the symptoms Mr. Underwood is experiencing. However, if it is significant enough to present as an obstructive uropathy, it should be associated with some findings consistent with that condition (see earlier). Furthermore, because it involves some interference with the normal enervation of the spine, it is expected that symptoms of such (e.g., leg weakness, paresthesias, or incontinence) or a condition associated with such (e.g., diabetes mellitus, multiple sclerosis, or a spinal cord injury) would be identified through his history. Because of the lack of the findings on his history and physical examination of evidence of an obstructive uropathy, neurologic defect, or associated medical condition plus his normal serum creatinine level, a neurogenic bladder is not his most likely diagnosis.

5. Treatment Plan

A. Decrease or, if possible, eliminate caffeine, and avoid fluids 4 to 6 hours before bedtime   CORRECT

As stated previously, caffeine can increase urinary frequency because it is both a bladder irritant and a diuretic. This urinary frequency can occur both during the day and at night; hence, eliminating caffeine from his diet is likely to reduce the frequency of his nocturia. Additionally, eliminating fluids (especially those that contain caffeine and alcohol) 4 to 6 hours before bedtime will make less urine during the night and hopefully also reduce the frequency of his nocturia.

B. Watchful waiting and repeat American Urological Association Symptom Index (AUA SI) in 3 months to determine symptom progression   INCORRECT

Watchful waiting is not an appropriate option for Mr. Underwood because of the severity of his symptoms and their impact on his life. Some experts advocate that "watchful waiting" is only indicated when the patient has an AUS IS score of less than or equal to 7.

C. Stop diphenhydramine and try topical cromolyn sodium for allergic rhinitis   CORRECT

Stopping the diphenhydramine and trying topical cromolyn sodium for allergic rhinitis is an appropriate treatment

option for Mr. Underwood because antihistamines can increase the symptoms of BPH and cromolyn sodium, a topical mast cell stabilizer, is antihistamine free and not known to produce this adverse effect. Because it is not associated with some of the adverse effects seen with topical steroids (i.e., epistaxis), tolerability as well as compliance should be increased.

D. Tamsulosin 0.4 mg one-half hour before bed; can increase to 0.8 mg if patient tolerates and continues to be symptomatic   CORRECT

Tamsulosin, as well as any other alpha-blocker, is an appropriate first-line agent to treat BPH. If maximum dosage does not produce the desired results (or is not tolerated by the patient), then the addition of a 5α-reductase inhibitor, which is generally considered a second-line agent, should be considered. However, it would not be totally incorrect to begin a patient with severe symptoms on both. If this combination fails, a urology consult is indicated for additional evaluation, confirmation of diagnosis, the addition of an anticholinergic agent, and/or a surgical intervention.

E. Prostatic ultrasound   CORRECT

Mr. Underwood's PSA level is slightly elevated; however, considering his symptoms and DRE findings, it is most likely caused by his BPH. However, because this slightly elevated PSA could represent an early prostate carcinoma in addition to his BPH and Mr. Underwood does have positive risk factors for prostate cancer, a prostatic ultrasound is indicated.

Epidemiologic and Other Data

The incidence of benign prostatic hypertrophy increases with advancing age. It is rare in men younger than the age of 40 years. In the United States, it affects approximately 8% of men in their 40s, and this number dramatically increases to affect 40 to 50% of men in their 50s. The US incidence in men older than the age of 80 years is at least 80%.

CASE 6-2
Umberto Valentino
1. History

A. What is his sexual history?   ESSENTIAL

A spontaneous urethral discharge in a young man is most frequently the result of a sexually transmitted infection (STI); therefore, it is important to know about Mr. Valentino's sexual history, including his practices and preferences. First, it needs to be established whether he is currently sexually active. If he isn't, then it needs to be determined whether he has been recently or remotely sexually active. If he has not, then he requires a comprehensive evaluation of his entire genitourinary system to evaluate for potential causes of his dysuria and urethral discharge.

It should never be assumed that a patient is heterosexual; therefore, the next question in his sexual history (provided he is sexually active) is to inquire whether he is sexually active with women, men, or both. This is a nonjudgmental approach and will frequently result in an honest response. This is important because men who have sex with men (MSM) can have a urethral discharge from not only the typical pathogens but also enteric organisms.

Questioning the patient regarding his total number of current and lifetime sexual partners provides an assessment of his risk for acquiring a sexually transmitted infection, including human immunodeficiency virus (HIV). The number of new sexual partners in the previous 30 days is also significant because it is directly proportional to the probability that the patient's urethral discharge is a result of an STI (the majority of sexually transmitted pathogens responsible for a urethral discharge are generally symptomatic within 2 to 3 weeks postexposure). If the patient has a single, regular partner, it is essential to know if the relationship is mutually monogamous and for how long. This information also addresses Mr. Valentino's possibility of having an STI.

Whether his sexual practices include anal intercourse and/or oral–genital/anal intercourse is important because these practices can introduce nontraditional sexually transmitted pathogens (i.e., acquired enteric organisms). The use of condoms for vaginal and anal intercourse as well as a dental dam for oral–genital/anal practices significantly decreases the likelihood of acquiring a sexually transmitted infection; however, it does not eliminate it completely. Nevertheless, it is important to inquire not only about the utilization of these protective devices but also about the frequency of their usage (i.e., regular or sporadic).

B. Is he currently experiencing or has he recently experienced any skin or mucous membrane lesions? ESSENTIAL

Several STIs present as genital lesions and/or ulcerations (e.g., genital warts [condyloma acuminatum], genital herpes, syphilis, chancroid, granuloma inguinale, and lymphogranuloma venereum). However, in order for one of these infections to produce dysuria in men, the lesion(s) needs to be confined to the urethra and/or the urethral meatus. Typically, this limits the list to genital warts, genital herpes, and syphilis. Furthermore, in order for the lesion to also be associated with a urethral discharge, it has to be an ulcerated, draining, urethral or urethral meatus lesion. This further limits the potential conditions to essentially genital herpes (although rarely syphilis and condyloma acuminatum can). Therefore, unless the lesion extends beyond the urethral meatus, the patient is not going to be able to visualize it. Thus, asking about genital lesions/ulcerations is not so much to identify the causative organism as to identify associated STIs because it is not unusual for more than one to occur simultaneously.

Reiter syndrome (a reactive arthritis) is a constellation of symptoms including urethritis, iridocyclitis, arthritis, and mucocutaneous lesions. In a few cases diarrhea is also present. Although this condition can occur as a result of pathogens not typically considered sexually transmitted infections (e.g., *Salmonella* sp., *Shigella* sp., *Campylobacter* sp., *Mycoplasma* sp., and *Yersinia* sp.), it can also result from sexually transmitted organisms, particularly *Chlamydia trachomatis*. The rash of Reiter syndrome looks very similar to psoriasis in many cases; therefore, any patient with a psoriatic-like rash and arthritis should be evaluated for this syndrome and psoriatic arthritis.

Additionally, some STIs can produce a generalized rash; the two most common are secondary syphilis and disseminated gonococcal infection (DGI). Genital herpes can also present as a disseminated infection in immunocompromised individuals. Furthermore, the herpes simplex virus can also produce localized nongenital infections (e.g., herpes labialis, herpes gingivostomatitis, and herpes whitlows). Therefore, when considering the diagnosis of an STI, it is important not to limit the questions regarding rashes and skin lesions to just the genital area.

C. Is he currently experiencing or has he recently experienced any ocular symptoms or arthralgias? ESSENTIAL

Some STIs are associated with eye and/or joint symptoms. For example, Reiter syndrome, as previously discussed, consists of urethritis, iridocyclitis, arthritis, and mucocutaneous lesions. DGI is often associated with arthralgias and/or tenosynovitis. Septic arthritis (generally monoarticular) can result from a gonococcal infection. Syphilis can be associated with uveitis, iritis, and neuroretinitis, especially if permitted to progress to tertiary syphilis. Herpes simplex virus (HSV) can cause scarring of the conjunctivitis; however, unless there is involvement over the pupil, it rarely produces visual abnormalities, but a dry, gritty, or itchy sensation may be present.

D. Is he currently experiencing or has he recently experienced a sore throat? ESSENTIAL

A sore throat and/or an oropharyngeal irritation/pain can occur in conjunction with a number of STIs. As alluded to previously, some STIs can cause infections in nongenital locations, and the mouth is the most common. Reiter syndrome can cause mucocutaneous lesions, including in the oropharynx. Gonorrhea can produce pharyngitis. Although the chancre of primary syphilis is usually painless, an oral lesion can be noticed. Any STI that can infect mucous membranes can produce oropharyngeal lesions; the risk is increased with the practice of oral–genital intercourse.

E. Is he currently experiencing or has he recently experienced a cough? NONESSENTIAL

Cough is an extremely rare manifestation of the typical organisms responsible for dysuria and a urethral discharge. Although chlamydia is a common pathogen in pneumonia, it is caused by *Chlamydia pneumoniae*, not *Chlamydia trachomatis*, the organism responsible for the STI.

2. Physical Examination

A. Oropharyngeal examination ESSENTIAL

A pharyngeal and oral mucosal examination is essential to evaluate for abnormalities that could provide clues to the presence of (and most likely pathogen related to) an STI.

B. Lung auscultation NONESSENTIAL

C. Abdominal examination ESSENTIAL

Despite Mr. Valentino's dysuria appearing to be confined to his urethral meatus only, it is still important to ensure that he does not have a palpable bladder abnormality.

D. Digital rectal examination NONESSENTIAL

A digital rectal examination (DRE) is not indicated at this time for Mr. Valentino because of the low incidence of it yielding any useful information since he is a sexually active young male with a urethral discharge and dysuria but no gastrointestinal symptoms. However, if he were not sexually active and had the dysuria and penile discharge, he would require a DRE to assist in the evaluation for a possible prostate or bladder infection as the cause of his symptoms.

Additionally, if Mr. Valentino were middle-aged or older, he would require a prostate examination to evaluate for conditions that are more likely to produce his symptoms in these older age groups (e.g., acute prostatitis and chronic prostatitis in middle-aged men and benign prostatic hypertrophy and prostate cancer in older men).

E. Genital examination   ESSENTIAL

A genital examination is indicated not only to visualize but also to obtain appropriate diagnostic specimens of the urethral discharge. It is important to inspect the genitalia and perineal areas for signs of STIs (e.g., ulcers, vesicles, other lesions, masses, and/or lymphadenopathy). Furthermore, the genital examination evaluates for contributing and/or coexisting conditions (e.g., epididymitis, balanitis, or phimosis).

3. Diagnostic Studies

A. Sample of the urethral discharge for microscopic examination with normal saline and Gram staining   ESSENTIAL

A microscopic examination of the penile discharge is indicated to determine the number of white blood cells that are present (elevation indicates an infectious process), the amount of bacteria that is present (increased associated with a bacterial cause), and the presence of other abnormalities (e.g., motile trichomonads [diagnostic for trichomoniasis] and/or budding yeast/hyphae [suggestive of a fungal infection, especially of the *Candida* sp.]).

The Gram stain of the discharge confirms the presence of an infectious process if it reveals greater than or equal to 5 polymorphonuclear neutrophils (PMNs) per oil immersion field. Additionally, it evaluates for the presence of bacteria, including gram-negative intracellular diplococci (GNID). If GNID are present, it can be assumed with a high degree of certainty that Mr. Valentino has a *Neisseria gonorrhoeae* infection. However, in women, the presence of GNID is not conclusive for the diagnosis of gonorrhea because some of the normal vaginal flora are (or mimic) GNID.

B. Penile swab for nucleic acid amplification test for *Neisseria gonorrhoeae* and *Chlamydia trachomatis*   ESSENTIAL

A penile swab for nucleic acid amplification testing for *N. gonorrhoeae* and *C. trachomatis* (or cultures on appropriate media) is necessary because these two organisms account for the majority of the cases of urethral discharge with and without dysuria in sexually active young men. Furthermore, it is not uncommon for them to coexist.

C. Urine culture   NONESSENTIAL

A urine culture is not indicated because it should only be performed if the urinalysis results and/or the patient's signs and symptoms are suggestive for a urinary tract infection (UTI).

D. Rapid plasma reagin (RPR)   ESSENTIAL

An RPR is indicated to screen for the possibility of syphilis because of the high incidence of this disease coexisting with other STIs, the high probability that an STI is causing Mr. Valentino's symptoms, and the slight possibility that *Treponema pallidum* is the causative organism of his symptoms.

E. Complete blood count with differential (CBC w/diff) NONESSENTIAL

Although Mr. Valentino appears to have an infection, its presentation is not significant enough to warrant a CBC w/diff because he lacks signs and symptoms consistent with a severe infection/septicemia. Furthermore, there is nothing in his history or physical examination to indicate that he might be anemic, leukemic, experiencing another hematological abnormality, or affected by a condition associated with significant inflammation, because these are the other primary indications for a CBC w/diff.

4. Diagnosis

A. Gonococcal urethritis (GU)   INCORRECT

Urethritis is an inflammation of the urethra most commonly caused by an infectious process. In men, its most common presentation is a penile discharge and distal dysuria. Nevertheless, based on the currently available data, gonococcal urethritis (GU) can be eliminated as Mr. Valentino's most likely diagnosis because his microscopic examination failed to reveal any bacteria and, more specifically, his Gram stain did not reveal GNID (which is a hallmark finding for GU in men). Although the result of his DNA amplification test (or culture plated on Thayer-Martin media) is not yet available, a negative result will essentially confirm the absence of gonorrhea. A positive result will require reevaluation of the patient, a review of the causes of false-negative microscopy and Gram stains (the most obvious being human error) and false-positives for DNA amplification (or culturing) for GU, and consideration of the possibility of a coinfection.

B. Nongonococcal urethritis (NGU)   CORRECT

As stated previously, urethritis is an inflammatory condition of the urethra most commonly caused by an infection. NGU is characterized by a penile discharge, varying degrees of dysuria (especially limited to the meatus), and 5 or more PMNs per oil immersion field without any gram-negative diplococci on Gram staining. Thus, this is Mr. Valentino's most likely diagnosis.

C. Urethritis and syphilis   INCORRECT

As discussed previously, Mr. Valentino has urethritis. However, despite his positive RPR result, he may or may not have syphilis. The RPR is a fairly sensitive nontreponemal antibody test utilized to screen for syphilis. However, because it reacts positively to phospholipids that are similar to the lipids found on the *Treponema pallidum* membrane, it can also react positively to other phospholipids caused by unrelated conditions (e.g., hyperlipidemia, autoimmune diseases, malaria, and pregnancy). Therefore, a confirmatory procedure must be performed utilizing a treponemal test (e.g., fluorescent treponemal antibody absorption test [FTA-ABS]) before the diagnosis of syphilis can be made. Thus, this cannot be considered his most likely diagnosis at this time.

D. Cystitis   INCORRECT

Although Mr. Valentino is complaining of dysuria, cystitis can essentially be ruled out as his most likely diagnosis because he lacked other irritative urinary symptoms (i.e., urinary urgency and urinary frequency) that are generally found in cystitis. Furthermore, his dysuria was confined to the urethral meatus and he had a urethral discharge, which are both unusual in an uncomplicated urinary tract infection (cystitis). Additionally, the microscopy and Gram stain evaluation of his urethral discharge revealed a significant number of PMNs (which would also not be found in an uncomplicated cystitis). Finally, cystitis is extremely rare in young males.

E. Acute prostatitis   INCORRECT

Prostatitis can be eliminated as Mr. Valentino's most likely diagnosis because he lacks the characteristic symptoms (e.g., perineal/abdominal/back pain, fever, and ill appearing) and because of his age (this condition is extremely rare in men younger than the age of 30 years).

5. Treatment Plan

A. Single dose of ceftriaxone 125 mg IM and azithromycin 1 g orally   CORRECT

The majority of cases of nongonococcal urethritis (NGU), especially in sexually active young men, are caused by *Chlamydia trachomatis*. The CDC recommends a single dose of azithromycin 1 g orally as a first-line treatment to cover this infection.

However, despite not identifying any GNID on his Gram stain, the CDC STI treatment guidelines still recommend that sexually active young men with a presumed *Chlamydia trachomatis* also be treated for *Neisseriae gonorrhoeae* because of the high incidence of coinfection with these two organisms. Because *Neisseriae gonorrhoeae* is currently responsive to a single dose of ceftriaxone 125 mg IM and this combination is one of the CDC's first-line treatment choices for NGU in sexually active young men, this choice is appropriate for Mr. Valentino.

B. Have patient's partners evaluated and treated for current illness and encourage patient and all partners to be tested for other sexually transmitted infections (STIs)   CORRECT

Because of public health concerns and the potential for the patient to get reinfected, it is imperative that all the patient's partners be identified, evaluated, and treated to prevent complications from a *Chlamydia trachomatis* and/or a *Neisseriae gonorrhoeae* infection. Furthermore, because of the potential for coexisting STIs, it is important to encourage the patient and all of his contacts to be evaluated for other potential STIs and appropriately treated if any are diagnosed. Mr. Valentino should abstain from having intercourse with any previous partners until their evaluation and treatment plan have been completed.

It is important to remember that in many states, the vast majority of STIs have mandatory reporting requirements for HCPs (i.e., the HCP is required by law to report any confirmed STI to the appropriate governmental agency). Therefore, it is imperative to be knowledgeable of and follow the reporting regulations in the state of practice.

C. Valacyclovir 1 g orally every 8 hours for 10 days   INCORRECT

This treatment would only be indicated if Mr. Valentino also had an initial episode of genital herpes.

D. Fluorescent treponemal antibody absorption test (FTA-ABS)   CORRECT

Mr. Valentino needs a treponemal test, like the FTA-ABS, to either confirm or negate his positive RPR. (For additional information regarding the need for a confirmatory test, please see the additional discussion available on this subject in Cases 4-6 and 5-8.)

E. Ciprofloxacin 500 mg bid for 5 days plus a single dose of azithromycin 1 g orally   CORRECT

As stated previously, azithromycin should be adequate to treat Mr. Valentino's NGU. The purpose of the ciprofloxacin would be to "cover" the patient against the possibility of a gonorrhea co-infection. Despite this being a very slight possibility, ciprofloxacin is still not indicated as part of Mr. Valentino's treatment plan because of the high incidence of gonococcal resistance to the fluoroquinolones.

Epidemiologic and Other Data

It is estimated that there are over 4 million cases of male urethritis annually in the United States. The majority of these cases occur in men in their teens and 20s. The preponderance of these cases are sexually transmitted.

Urethritis is divided into gonococcal (caused by *Neisseria gonorrhoeae*) urethritis (GU) and nongonococcal urethritis (NGU). Slightly more than half of all cases of NGU are caused by an infection with *Chlamydia trachomatis*. The remaining cases are caused by other typical sexually transmitted organisms (predominately *Herpes simplex virus [HSV]* and *Trichomonas vaginalis*) and atypical sexually transmitted organisms (predominately *Ureaplasma urealyticum, Mycoplasma hominis, Mycoplasma genitalium,* and the adenoviruses).

Rarely does nonsexually transmitted urethritis occur. Hence, the greatest risk factors for acquiring urethritis are being sexually active, having multiple partners, being men who have sex with men, and not utilizing condoms.

CASE 6-3
Vincent White
1. History

A. Does he experience nocturnal or early morning erections? ESSENTIAL

Even though psychological causes are only responsible for a very small percentage of all the cases of ED, they still need to be separated from physiologic conditions of the genitourinary tract (e.g., benign prostatic hypertrophy, chronic prostatitis, or hypogonadism), systemic illnesses (e.g., prostate cancer, arterial insufficiency, diabetes mellitus, and hypothalamic/pituitary abnormalities), and medication adverse effects (see later) before treatment for ED is initiated for the greatest potential of successful therapy.

Although not absolute, there are characteristics of ED that suggest that a psychological cause is more likely than a physiologic abnormality. For example, deep sleep tends to suppress psychological issues that can be related to ED; therefore, the preservation of nocturnal and/or early morning erections makes a psychological cause more likely than a physiologic one. However, it is essential not to base the final diagnosis on the response to a single question. Furthermore, in any patient with long-standing ED, there is a high probability that some degree of a psychological component is going to be present because of the impact the condition has on the patient's self-esteem and stress level and the resultant performance anxiety. Still, a gradually worsening problem is more often related to a physiological cause than a psychological one.

B. When he gets an erection, is he able to sustain it, achieve an orgasm, and ejaculate?   ESSENTIAL

Because Mr. White's symptoms are intermittent, there is a concern that he could have a psychological cause or at least a psychological overlay (as previously discussed) contributing to his ED. Although not absolute, knowing which components of the male sexual response (i.e., true ED [inability to achieve and sustain adequate penile rigidity to have intercourse] vs difficulties with libido, orgasm, and/or ejaculation) are affected can also provide clues as to whether the cause is more likely to be psychological or physiologic. In general, if the patient can get an erection but cannot sustain it, then the cause is more frequently an organic problem (most commonly a vascular problem, a neurologic abnormality, or an adverse drug effect [including alcohol and recreational drugs]); however, psychological problems can occasionally present in this manner.

The inability to have an orgasm is generally related to a psychological problem. Whereas the inability to ejaculate is generally a result of retrograde ejaculation that can be caused by conditions such as diabetes mellitus, medications (see later), or prostate or other pelvic surgery.

As previously stated, any of these components of the male sexual response can be attributed to an adverse medication effect. Although not all agents in these general therapeutic groups have the potential to produce ED, it is essential when evaluating a patient with ED to determine if the patient is currently on (or has recently been taking) any medications that would fall within these most commonly implicated therapeutic classes: anticholinergics, anticonvulsants, antidepressants, antihyperlipidemics, antihypertensives, antipsychotics, anxiolytics, cytotoxic agents, H_2 blockers, hormones, narcotics, and tranquilizers. Individual drugs (e.g. digoxin, lithium, and ketoconazole) have also been implicated.

If present, a more comprehensive look at the individual drugs and their effect on the sex hormones, sexual desire, arousal, and orgasm needs to be undertaken to assess the likelihood of the medications attributing to or causing ED. Furthermore, the risks versus benefits versus acceptable alternatives of these drugs must be explored on an individualized basis before stopping or substituting these agents.

Tobacco, alcohol, and other substances of abuse ([most commonly cocaine, marijuana, 3,4-methylenedioxymethamphetamine [MDMA], amphetamines, and phencyclidine [PCP]) can cause and/or contribute to ED. If present, the offending substance should be stopped. Depending on the agent, amount, frequency, and duration of usage, inpatient management may be necessary to control withdrawal symptoms and enhance the potential of the patient remaining substance free.

C. Has he had individual sexual therapy?   NONESSENTIAL

Sex therapy is only indicated when there appears to be interpersonal relationship issues that are severe enough to be producing the ED. Therefore, it should always include both partners when the patient has a single, regular, long-term partner (as Mr. White does).

D. Does he have problems with premature ejaculation? ESSENTIAL

Premature ejaculation is an associated characteristic that must be differentiated from true ED (as defined earlier).

It also provides some support for or against a psychological (vs physiologic) cause of the patient's problem. In general, premature ejaculation is associated with a psychological problem, most commonly anxiety (including performance anxiety). However, it can be caused by substance abuse including alcohol, cocaine, and marijuana.

E. Has he noticed any change in his libido, sleep, appetite, activities, interests, mood, or outlook on life?   ESSENTIAL

Libido is another associated characteristic of ED that must be differentiated from true ED. A change in libido is usually related to an androgen deficit; however, it can also be caused by a psychological problem, most commonly depression. Therefore, it is important to determine whether there are other signs or symptoms of a major mood disorder (MMD) present that might provide additional support toward a psychological cause for Mr. White's chief complaint.

Depression, anxiety, and other mood disorders (as well as the medications used to treat them) can result in, contribute to, or result from ED or associated conditions of sexual arousal.

2. Physical Examination

A. Thyroid examination   NONESSENTIAL

A primary thyroid condition is extremely unlikely to cause ED. However, secondary hypo- or hyperthyroidism can be present if a pituitary or hypothalamic problem is responsible for the patient's ED.

B. Genital and prostate examination   ESSENTIAL

Because the majority of cases of ED are organic in origin, a careful physical examination to evaluate for abnormalities is essential. Because this is a male reproductive tract problem in an older man, a genital examination and a prostate examination are essential to identify any abnormalities that could be causing and/or contributing to the problem (e.g., penile plaques or scarring; testicular atrophy or masses; or changes in the consistency, texture, or size of the prostate gland).

C. Penile blood pressure   ESSENTIAL

The penile blood pressure (BP) is an essential component of the physical examination to determine if arterial insufficiency could be responsible, in part or totally, for the patient's ED. Normally the ratio of the penile systolic BP to the brachial systolic BP is greater than 0.75. If the ratio is less than 0.6, then significant penile arterial insufficiency exists.

The penile BP is measured by inflating a pediatric sphygmomanometer cuff around the base of the penis, then using a Doppler stethoscope over the corpora cavernosa slowly deflate the cuff to determine the systolic penile BP (i.e., the number when the first arterial beat is heard). The diastolic value is determined by the disappearance of the arterial beat; however, it has no clinical utility.

In the absence of risk factors for peripheral arterial disease (e.g., coronary artery disease, hyperlipidemia, and/or diabetes), adverse medication effects can cause an abnormal penile BP.

D. Examination of the aorta and lower extremities for vascular changes   ESSENTIAL

Because primary and secondary atherosclerotic arterial disease can cause ED as a result of arterial insufficiency, the pulses from the aorta distally need to be evaluated for decreased intensity and bruits, where appropriate. Additionally, the skin needs to be visualized and palpated for color changes, lesions, temperature changes, and edema that could be related to circulatory problems.

E. Neurologic examination of genitalia, perineum, and lower extremities   ESSENTIAL

Primary (e.g., multiple sclerosis, spinal cord injuries, and some peripheral neuropathies) and secondary (e.g., caused by diabetes mellitus, alcoholism, or previous pelvic surgery) neurologic conditions can also cause ED; therefore, it is essential to evaluate the genitalia, perineum, and legs for signs of any neurologic abnormality.

3. Diagnostic Studies

A. Urinalysis   ESSENTIAL

A urinalysis is indicated to evaluate for abnormalities (e.g., leukocyte esterase, nitrites, white blood cells, and red blood cells and casts) that could indicate that a urinary tract problem (e.g., cystitis, prostatitis, or ureteral obstruction) is causing, exacerbating, or coexisting with his ED.

B. Fasting plasma glucose (FPG) and lipid panel   ESSENTIAL

Because arterial insufficiency is responsible for a large number of the cases of ED, it is important to screen for conditions that could be causing it (e.g., diabetes mellitus, hyperlipidemia, and hypertriglyceridemia), especially considering that Mr. White already has coronary artery disease (angina) and hypertension. Additionally, diabetes mellitus can be responsible for neurogenic ED.

C. Serum testosterone (total), prolactin, follicle-stimulating hormone (FSH), and luteinizing hormone (LH) levels   ESSENTIAL

Hypogonadism is the third most common cause of ED (following vascular insufficiency and neurogenic problems). A serum testosterone level is important in the evaluation of this condition. The prolactin, FSH, and LH levels primarily serve to determine whether a primary or secondary hypogonadism is the cause if the testosterone level is decreased.

D. Nocturnal penile tumescence and rigidity study   NONESSENTIAL

The nocturnal penile tumescence and rigidity study measures the number of erections per episode of rapid eye movement (REM) sleep as well as the total erection time per night. It is no longer routinely performed in the evaluation of ED because of the effectiveness of the phosphodiesterase-5 (PDE-5) inhibitors in a wide array of ED causes. It is occasionally utilized if the preliminary evaluation fails to reveal a cause for the ED and there are still significant questions regarding whether the patient's ED has a psychological or physiologic basis.

E. Scrotal ultrasound   NONESSENTIAL

The primary indications for this test are to evaluate for undescended testicles, measure testicular size, evaluate testicular masses, provide ultrasonic guidance for needle biopsy of testicular masses, evaluate free fluid in the scrotum, evaluate scrotal masses/pain, screen for damage following significant scrotal trauma, and follow up on testicular carcinomas and/or infections.

4. Diagnosis

A. Erectile dysfunction caused by primary hypogonadism   CORRECT

Based on his history, physical examination, and diagnostic studies, Mr. White's most likely diagnosis is ED secondary to primary hypogonadism. The classic diagnostic findings include a low serum testosterone level, an elevated FSH, an elevated LH, and a normal prolactin level.

B. Erectile dysfunction caused by secondary hypogonadism   INCORRECT

Secondary hypogonadism is primarily caused by a pituitary adenoma; however, any pituitary or hypothalamic condition could cause it. This can be ruled out as Mr. White's most likely diagnosis based on his laboratory studies. In a secondary hypogonadism, the patient's serum testosterone level is low (like Mr. White's), but the serum prolactin level is also low and the FSH and LH are either low or normal (in contrast to Mr. White's elevated findings).

C. Erectile dysfunction caused by a psychological condition   INCORRECT

Because a physiologic condition was diagnosed via his laboratory findings and no signs or symptoms of an underlying psychopathology were identified, ED caused by a psychological condition can be ruled out as his most likely diagnosis at this time.

D. Erectile dysfunction caused by a pituitary adenoma   INCORRECT

ED caused by a pituitary adenoma is considered to be a secondary form of hypogonadism. Therefore, it can be eliminated as Mr. White's most likely diagnosis based on his diagnostic test results as discussed earlier.

E. Erectile dysfunction due to normal male aging   INCORRECT

Despite the incidence of ED increasing with age, it is not acceptable to attribute it to the normal aging process. Therefore, this is not Mr. White's most likely diagnosis.

5. Treatment Plan

A. Desvenlafaxine 50 mg once a day   INCORRECT

Desvenlafaxine, a serotonin-norepinephrine reuptake inhibitor (SNRI), is indicated for the treatment of depression. Because Mr. White's ED has an identifiable physiologic cause and he has no signs or symptoms suggestive of depression, this is not an appropriate choice for him.

B. Testosterone topical patch 2.5 mg; apply one patch once a day to dry skin (after obtaining copy of his PSA level to ensure it is normal)   CORRECT

Because Mr. White's ED is most likely caused by primary hypogonadism, it would be appropriate to start him on androgen therapy. However, it is imperative to have the results of his PSA to ensure that they are normal before initiating therapy and to serve as a baseline level. Androgen replacement therapy can produce elevations of the patient's PSA level presumably by increasing the prostate volume. Thus, there is a concern that testosterone can cause an undetected prostate cancer to proliferate at an enhanced rate. However, there is no current evidence available to suggest that androgen replacement therapy can actually cause prostate cancer. Nevertheless, these potential adverse effects need to be discussed thoroughly and honestly with the patient. If he chooses to go with the replacement therapy, a plan should be formulated for frequent screening for the development of prostate cancer.

Regardless, testosterone should never be used in men with a history of breast or prostate cancer. It is also contraindicated in men with an abnormal DRE or an elevated PSA level that has not been thoroughly evaluated and prostate cancer definitely eliminated. Additionally, it should not be given to men with marked benign prostatic hypertrophy (BPH), defined as an AUA BPH symptom score of greater than 19. (For more information regarding the AUA score to quantify the symptoms of BPH, please see Case 6-1.) Other contraindications include a New York Heart Association functional classification of a class III or IV [PMS2], sleep apnea, severe chronic obstructive pulmonary disease (COPD), and polycythemia

Testosterone is the treatment of choice for primary hypogonadism. It is available as a daily patch, an injection given every 3 weeks, a gel that is applied daily, and a daily pill. The oral preparation is not frequently prescribed because it can cause hepatotoxicity (especially cholestatic jaundice). Most men prefer the patch and/or gel to the injection primarily because they do not have to return to the clinic every 3 weeks for an injection. The patch is less messy and associated with less dosage fluctuation than the gel. Furthermore, the patch mimics normal testosterone physiology closer than any of the other methods; however, there are no currently available data to indicate whether this is beneficial.

Despite the fact that low-normal testosterone levels generally alleviate ED caused by primary hypogonadism, the goal of treatment is to normalize the patient's testosterone levels to the midrange of normal. This recommendation stems from the fact that replacing testosterone to only low-normal levels does not prevent/improve the low bone density and decreased muscle mass that are associated with hypogonadism. To adequately address these associated problems, levels must be restored to the midrange of normal. When correcting androgen deficiency with the testosterone patch, a repeat serum level should be obtained after 2 to 3 months of therapy and within 3 to 12 hours after putting on a new patch. If the level is not in the midrange of normal, the dosage needs to be adjusted accordingly.

C. Change metoprolol to clonidine 0.1 mg twice a day INCORRECT

Beta-blockers have been known to cause ED. This is obviously not Mr. White's entire problem (although it might be a contributing factor) because primary hypogonadism (which is unrelated to the physiologic effects of beta-blockers) was identified. Additionally, his ED onset does not correlate with the initiation of his metoprolol; thus, it makes it less suspect.

Furthermore, in many patients with cardiovascular disease, especially coronary artery disease, beta-blockers are an integral component of their treatment plan to prevent complications. The pros and cons of discontinuing this therapy would have to be carefully weighed before cessation. Thus, because a treatable cause was uncovered to account for his ED, it would be prudent to first treat that condition. If his symptoms do not resolve when his hypogonadism is corrected,

then other treatment options, such as changing his medicine, would be considered.

However, if the decision to substitute his beta-blocker was made, it would be prudent to change to an antihypertensive that was not associated with ED. Because clonidine also has this potential adverse effect, it would not be an appropriate substitution. Other antihypertensives that have been implicated either as a group or individually to cause ED include calcium channel blockers (CCBs), thiazide diuretics, spironolactone, guanethidine, methyldopa, and reserpine.

D. Sildenafil 50 mg approximately 1 hour before planned intercourse INCORRECT

Sildenafil is one of three PDE-5 inhibitors that are currently approved by the US Food and Drug Administration (FDA) for the oral treatment of ED. The other two are tadalafil and vardenafil. These agents have been shown to be effective in treating ED from a variety of causes, including vascular, neurogenic, and psychogenic. However, they have not been proven to be very effective in patients with ED caused by hypogonadism in the absence of one of these conditions.

Additionally, none of these medications should be prescribed for Mr. White because of his coronary artery disease and nitrate therapy. PDE-5 inhibitors cause peripheral vasodilatation that can accentuate this effect from the nitroglycerine and result in marked hypotension.

E. Referral to urologist for implantation of an inflatable penile prosthesis INCORRECT

Although the inflatable penile prosthesis is still a viable option for men who suffer from ED, it is now only recommended and used in refractory ED because of the availability of less invasive treatment options. Hence, it would not be considered to be an appropriate first-line therapy.

Epidemiologic and Other Data

It is estimated that sexual dysfunction affects between 10 and 25% of all middle-aged and older men and women in the United States. In order of frequency, the most common causes of ED are vascular insufficiency, neurogenic problems, and hypogonadism. Medication adverse effects are estimated to cause one quarter of all the cases. The incidence of ED increases with age and with the existence of other chronic medical conditions.

More individuals are being seen, diagnosed, and treated for sexual dysfunction than ever before. This is theorized to be related to the increased awareness of the disease, the patient's and HCP's awareness that this is not part of normal aging, more treatment options being available, and improved insurance coverage pertaining to this condition.

CASE 6-4
Wilson Xandiaver
1. History

A. Does he take any over-the-counter medications, vitamins, supplements, or herbal preparations? ESSENTIAL

When inquiring about a patient's medication history, it is important to specifically inquire about nonprescription products, including medications, vitamins, supplements, and herbal preparations, because many patients do not consider these "medications" and will not volunteer this information. Additionally, this must be approached in a routine, nonjudgmental fashion because patients tend to want to seek the approval of their HCP. If they feel admitting to the usage of these products is going to be perceived negatively by the HCP, they are reluctant to admit to using them, even when specifically asked. This is unfortunate because many of the products, including the "natural" ones, are associated with significant drug-to-drug interactions and adverse effects that could cause symptoms similar to what Mr. Xandiaver is experiencing.

B. Is he on any special "diet"?   ESSENTIAL

Flank pain with radiation into the groin can be caused by nephrolithiasis. Because diet is an important feature regarding the formation and/or risk of developing this condition, it is essential to inquire as to whether the patient is on a specific diet (and if yes, which one and for how long). Diets that are high in protein, contain significant amounts of purine, are high in sodium, are rich in dairy products, include excessive alcohol, and/or are high in caffeine have been linked to the various types of nephrolithiasis.

C. Has he experienced any hematuria, discolored urine, dysuria, urinary urgency, urinary frequency, difficulty initiating urination, incontinence, decrease in caliber or strength of his stream, or urethral discharge?   ESSENTIAL

The presence of urinary tract symptoms is important in developing Mr. Xandiaver's list of potential differential diagnoses. Hematuria, both gross and microscopic, can be caused by a wide array of activities and/or conditions (e.g., excessive exercise, intercourse, hemorrhagic cystitis, urethritis, pyelonephritis, glomerulonephritis, nephrolithiasis, bladder cancer, prostate cancer, foreign bodies in the urethra or bladder, sickle cell disease, and medications [e.g., warfarin and aspirin]).

Additionally, color changes can be the result of hematuria, a urinary tract infection, increased urinary concentration, prescription and over-the-counter medications, and diet. Odor changes can result from variations in urinary concentration, a urinary tract infection, or ketosis. Dysuria can be the result of a whole host of infectious, inflammatory, or cancerous causes.

Irritative symptoms consist of urinary urge, incontinence (generally urge), urinary frequency, and/or nocturia. They are seen in such conditions as urge incontinence, excessive fluid intake, bladder carcinoma, nephrolithiasis that is in or near the bladder, urinary tract infections, foreign bodies, urethral irritation, prostatitis, and occasionally benign prostatic hypertrophy (BPH). Polyuria can also be seen with nephrotic syndrome, diabetes mellitus, diabetes insipidus, and heart failure.

Incontinence is also considered to be an obstructive symptom, with the majority of cases resulting from overflow, not urge or muscle weakness (stress). Other obstructive symptoms include difficulty initiating urination, straining to urinate, decrease in size or strength of stream, dribbling after completing urination, and sensation of bladder not fully emptied after urinating. These symptoms can be seen in acute and chronic, infectious and noninfectious, obstructions caused by BPH, prostate cancer, nephrolithiasis, and other urinary tract masses. Urethral discharges are most commonly seen in urethritis but can also be present with acute prostatitis.

D. Is he really monogamous?   NONESSENTIAL

Reasking this question in this manner is unlikely to produce a different response and could be considered insulting to patient as well as harmful to the patient's relationship with his spouse and/or the healthcare provider.

E. Has he ever practiced or experimented with sex with men?   NONESSENTIAL

This question is not pertinent to his current complaint because Mr. Xandiaver and his wife have, to the best of his knowledge, been in a mutually monogamous relationship for the past 10 years. Thus, if he ever had sex with men, it was over 10 years ago. Because it is virtually impossible that an STI acquired more than 10 years ago could be producing his current symptoms, regardless of his sexual partner's gender, this question is irrelevant. Furthermore, with the possible exception of acquired immunodeficiency syndrome (AIDS) and hepatitis, it would be highly improbable that he would develop any symptoms as a result of an STI acquired more than 10 years ago.

2. Physical Examination

A. Oral examination to evaluate dentition   NONESSENTIAL

B. Abdominal examination   ESSENTIAL

Despite Mr. Xandiaver not complaining of abdominal pain, he does have some obstructive urinary symptoms; therefore, it is important to evaluate his abdomen for the presence of a suprapubic mass, indicating a distended bladder. An evaluation for renal bruits ensures that renal arterial insufficiency and/or thrombosis are not responsible for his back pain. And evaluation of the abdominal aorta provides some assurance that his back pain is not caused by an abdominal aortic aneurysm.

C. Prostate examination   ESSENTIAL

Several prostatic conditions can present with symptoms similar to Mr. Xandiaver's; therefore, a prostate examination is necessary to evaluate for conditions such as acute prostatitis, chronic prostatitis, BPH, prostatic masses, and prostate cancer.

D. Genital examination   ESSENTIAL

Because Mr. Xandiaver's pain is radiating from his flank to his groin, a genital examination is required to evaluate for evidence of trauma, urethral obstruction, phimosis, epididymitis, or other conditions that could account for his symptoms.

E. Evaluation for costovertebral angle (CVA) tenderness   ESSENTIAL

CVA tenderness is most commonly associated with renal and/or upper urinary tract problems (e.g., proximal ureter stricture, nephrolithiasis, and pyelonephritis), which can cause his symptoms.

3. Diagnostic Studies

A. Urinalysis and urine culture and sensitivity (C&S)   ESSENTIAL

Because Mr. Xandiaver's symptoms are consistent with a urinary tract abnormality including an obstructive uropathy or an upper urinary tract infection, a urinalysis and culture (with sensitivity) are essential to assist in better determining his correct diagnosis.

Normally, a urine culture is only performed when the leukocyte esterase and/or the nitrites are positive on the dipstick and there are a minimum of 5 white blood cells per field on microscopy; however, in the case of suspected nephrolithiasis, because of the potential coexistence of a urinary tract infection, a culture and sensitivity should always be performed.

B. Electrolytes ESSENTIAL

Electrolytes should be performed on Mr. Xandiaver to evaluate for evidence suggesting the presence of renal abnormalities, coexisting conditions, and/or complications from his chief complaint (e.g., dehydration, renal failure, diabetes insipidus, renal tubular acidosis, and medical conditions associated with electrolyte abnormalities that could result in nephrolithiasis [such as hypokalemia occurring in hypocitraturic calcium nephrolithiasis]).

C. Baseline serum calcium, phosphate, uric acid, and creatinine levels ESSENTIAL

Because Mr. Xandiaver has symptoms consistent with an obstructive uropathy, baseline serum calcium, phosphate, uric acid, and creatinine levels are required. They will determine whether his renal function is normal and whether he has any associated metabolic abnormalities that could result in elevations of his serum calcium, phosphate, and uric acid levels, which in turn could be responsible for the production of nephrolithiasis as a cause of an obstructive uropathy (e.g., hypercalcemia, gout, uric acid–producing carcinomas, hyperparathyroidism, or alterations of renal tubular absorption).

D. Plain x-ray film of the abdomen NONESSENTIAL

A plain abdominal radiograph when used to evaluate the urinary tract is often referred to as a KUB (**k**idneys, **u**reters, and **b**ladder). However, it has essentially been replaced by spiral computed tomography of the abdomen and pelvis in the evaluation of patients presenting with Mr. Xandiaver's symptoms.

The KUB's current role in urology is as an inexpensive technique for monitoring the progression of kidney stones provided they are of sufficient size to be visualized; not obscured behind pelvic bones; and composed of either calcium, cystine, or struvite because they are radiopaque (compared to uric acid stones, which are radiolucent).

E. Spiral computed tomography (CT) of abdomen and pelvis with contrast and sedation ESSENTIAL

Spiral CT of the abdomen and pelvis with contrast is the most sensitive and specific imaging technique currently available for identifying all sizes (including very small) of urinary tract masses. Because Mr. Xandiaver has obstructive symptoms in conjunction with severe flank pain, this is the best imaging study for him. However, because of his severe claustrophobia, he needs to be provided with some type of sedation not only for his comfort but also to complete the procedure and obtain quality images for the evaluation of his chief complaint.

4. Diagnosis

A. Acute pyelonephritis INCORRECT

Pyelonephritis is an inflammation of the upper urinary tract (predominately the renal pelvis, calyces, and parenchyma) most commonly caused by an infection. The diagnosis of pyelonephritis can essentially be eliminated as Mr. Xandiaver's most likely diagnosis via history and physical examination because he lacks several of the key features of this condition (i.e., fever, CVA tenderness, and possibly irritative urinary symptoms). His urinalysis also failed to reveal evidence of an infection (e.g., positive leukocyte esterase and nitrites on dipstick examination and significant pyuria and bacteria on his microscopic examination) as well as the characteristic findings of white blood cell casts on microscopic examination of the urine sediment.

B. Calcium nephrolithiasis, produced by excessive vitamin C intake CORRECT

Mr. Xandiaver's history, physical examination, and diagnostic studies are fairly classic for diagnosis of nephrolithiasis. The calcium oxalate crystals identified on the microscopic examination of his urine significantly increase the likelihood that his kidney stone is composed of calcium. Excessive vitamin C (defined as > 1 g/day) can increase the levels of oxalate in the urine, resulting in calcium nephrolithiasis. Therefore, from the choices provided, the most likely diagnosis for Mr. Xandiaver is calcium nephrolithiasis, produced by excessive vitamin C intake.

Other over-the-counter products that have been implicated in the formation of nephrolithiasis include high-protein supplements, sulfur-containing amino acid formulations, and salt tablets.

C. Struvite calculi INCORRECT

Calculi are stones that become too large to pass from the renal pelvis into the ureter. They can distend into the renal calyces and produce staghorn calculi. In many cases, the formations are asymptomatic until renal function has been significantly compromised. Because they are generally composed of magnesium, ammonium, and phosphate, they should not produce the calcium oxalate crystals that were noted in Mr. Xandiaver's urine. Also, struvite stones tend to be associated with an alkaline urinary pH, not an acidic one as seen in this case.

In addition to being rare, they are almost exclusively seen in women with a history of frequent urinary tract infections or in any patient who requires chronic catheterization of the bladder. It is theorized to be caused by bacteria that produce urease, the most common being the *Proteus* sp. Finally, they were not visualized on his spiral CT. Thus, this is not Mr. Xandiaver's most likely diagnosis.

D. Uric acid nephrolithiasis INCORRECT

As stated previously, Mr. Xandiaver's history, physical examination, and diagnostic studies are fairly classic for a diagnosis of nephrolithiasis. However, nephrolithiasis caused by uric acid is not his most likely diagnosis. This is based on his low-normal serum uric acid level and lack of urea (but the presence of calcium oxalate) crystals in his urine.

E. Phlebolith INCORRECT

A phlebolith is a small calcium deposit that can be seen in the vascular wall or in a thrombus formation on an imaging study of the abdomen. It can be ruled out as Mr. Xandiaver's most likely diagnosis because phleboliths are generally much smaller in size than his mass, not located in the ureter, and asymptomatic.

5. Treatment Plan

A. Enteric-coated naproxen 500 mg twice a day   CORRECT

A nonsteroidal anti-inflammatory drug (NSAID) is an appropriate first-line medication for the outpatient management of nephrolithiasis provided that the patient has normal renal function and no other contraindications to the medication. Some experts suggest that NSAIDs are more effective than narcotics for the treatment of pain caused by nephrolithiasis. Still, if they are not effective for the individual patient, then a narcotic analgesic is considered appropriate second-line therapy and should be prescribed.

B. Stop vitamin C   CORRECT

Because Mr. Xandiaver's excessively high doses of vitamin C likely resulted in the formation of his calcium nephrolithiasis, it is essential to discontinue it and advise him accordingly.

C. Increase water intake to a minimum of 2 liters/day   CORRECT

Increasing water consumption is an important component for the treatment of nephrolithiasis. However, it is not to "flush" the stone out of the urinary tract but to dilute the urine and prevent further stone formation.

Other fluids can probably be utilized; however, caffeine and alcohol should be avoided. Grapefruit juice has conflicting data as to whether or not it leads to the formation of stones; therefore, it should in all probability also be eliminated. It also has the potential of creating significant drug interactions. Cranberry juice has been shown to be helpful. Other beverages are most likely acceptable alternatives.

D. Strain urine and bring in any sediment for analysis   CORRECT

Straining the urine and performing analysis of the sediment is an important component of Mr. Xandiaver's treatment. Hopefully, this analysis of the stone and/or its fragments will confirm the suspicion of their composition. Based on these findings, additional testing can be directed toward determining the precise cause responsible for the nephrolithiasis formation and instituting appropriate measures with the goal of preventing recurrences.

E. Hospitalize, initiate IV lines for hydration, and obtain a urology consultation   INCORRECT

Although Mr. Xandiaver is experiencing significant (but intermittent) pain, he has no evidence of dehydration, coexisting urinary tract infection, sepsis, or other factors requiring hospitalization.

Nevertheless, he should have frequent follow-up to ensure he is improving and has passed the stone(s). There is no consensus on the exact size of a stone that will pass without difficulty; however, it is generally considered to be a maximum of ~4 to 6 mm. Regardless, most agree that if a stone is larger than 10 mm, it is likely going to require some type of intervention.

Thus, in a stone that is less than 10 mm in size, as long as there is no sign of infection, worsening of renal functioning, or increasing symptoms, most experts feel that conservative measures can be utilized for up to 6 weeks. At that time (or before if complications develop or the patient's condition deteriorates), a decision needs to be made regarding the most appropriate technique to remove the stone based on the provider's skill and expertise level, the patient's preference, and the location of the stone. Choices would include shock wave or ureteroscopic lithotripsy with or without stent placement; ureteroscopic stone retrieval with basket; and percutaneous, laparoscopic, or open surgical extraction.

Epidemiologic and Other Data

The lifetime incidence for nephrolithiasis in the United States is approximately 7% for females and 13% for males. The incidence increases with advancing age. Non-Hispanic whites have the highest incidence of nephrolithiasis.

Patients who have recurrent episodes of nephrolithiasis generally do so at a rate of one episode approximately every 2 to 3 years. The recurrence rate appears to be highest in patients with calcium-based stones; within 10 years of experiencing their first episode of nephrolithiasis, approximately one half have developed at least one additional episode of nephrolithiasis.

In the United States, stones composed of calcium oxalate and/or calcium phosphate account for the vast majority of all kidney stones (approximately 75 to 85%). Stones composed of uric acid account for an additional 5 to 10% of all kidney stones. Struvite-based stones account for another 5 to 10%. Cystine stones account for approximately 1% of all cases of nephrolithiasis. Other rare causes comprise less than 1% of all stones.

CASE 6-5

Xavier Yount

1. History

A. Did he have any symptoms before the pain began or has he experienced the same or similar pain in the past?   ESSENTIAL

The presence of prodromal symptoms in the few days preceding his presentation or a history of similar testicular pain (but generally not as severe) assists in narrowing Mr. Yount's list of potential differential diagnoses. For example, in epididymitis, the patient frequently will experience a dull ache for several days before the onset of acute pain. Orchitis, when presenting as a complication of a viral illness (e.g., mumps), is generally preceded by the symptoms of that viral process.

Likewise, a hydrocele, epididymitis, and/or orchitis can result from lymphatic filariasis. In this nematode infestation, the patient frequently experiences acute lymphangitis before experiencing inflammation, edema, or lymphatic obstruction peripherally from the affected lymph nodes. However, patients can experience a mild episode of spontaneous resolving acute lymphangitis with minimal associated peripheral symptoms. This can result in a chronic process with rare (at several-month intervals) acute exacerbations of the lymphangitis and associated symptoms or even filarial fevers (acute exacerbations of the associated symptoms [of varying severity] without lymph node involvement). Thus, with this condition, the patient can present with either an acute lymphangitis prior to the onset of the genital symptoms or intermittent mild genital symptoms with or without associated lymphangitis for a several-year period before the symptoms become sufficiently severe and/or prolonged enough for the patient to seek treatment.

A previous episode of epididymitis could suggest complications from the disease. The most common are a granulomatous disease (most frequently caused by *Mycobacterium tuberculosis*) and testicular torsion. Additionally, testicular torsion (whether related to a previous epididymitis or not) is frequently characterized by multiple episodes of similar (albeit not generally as severe) episodes of testicular pain. In fact, up to 50% of the patients who present with acute testicle torsion have had less severe episodes in the past that resulted in spontaneous correction.

B. What does he mean by "collapsed"?   ESSENTIAL

The term "collapsed" connotes a wide array of potential events including a pulseless, apneic episode; a syncopal episode with or without a loss of consciousness; a state of severe prostration; falling down (generally on knees) because of the marked intensity of the pain; or just having to sit down because of the pain's severity. Thus, it is extremely important to determine which one of these definitions, if any, Mr. Yount is utilizing when stating he "collapsed" in order to formulate an appropriate differential diagnosis list and not overlook a potential life-threatening condition. Obviously, if a true syncopal episode, acute circulatory compromise, or loss of consciousness occurred, further evaluation is required to identify the reason for that problem in addition to his chief complaint.

C. Is his other testicle symptomatic?   NONESSENTIAL

Because of the anatomy of the male pelvic area, it is extremely unlikely for an acute, extremely painful, bilateral testicular process to occur. In the rare cases where this is possible, the patient will complain of bilateral involvement (even if one side is significantly more painful). Plus, this information is easily obtainable via the physical examination of the patient's genitalia.

D. Has he recently had parotitis?   ESSENTIAL

Paramyxovirus mumps can produce orchitis (which is frequently unilateral in location and thus would result in unilateral testicular pain and swelling) in approximately 20% of the postpubertal males who acquire the condition. Because the most prominent symptom in patients with mumps is generally parotitis, it is important to ask if this condition has recently been present in patients complaining of scrotal pain in association with scrotal tenderness and edema.

E. Did anyone see him lift the box?   NONESSENTIAL

From a medical standpoint, this question is not essential because it is not going to direct diagnostic studies or assist in establishing a diagnosis or treatment plan. However, if the patient plans on filing a worker's compensation claim (or taking other legal action against his employer) because he feels his condition is the direct result of a workplace injury, this is an important component of that claim.

2. Physical Examination

A. Oropharyngeal evaluation   NONESSENTIAL

The primary purpose of an oropharyngeal examination on a patient with a genital complaint but no oropharyngeal symptoms is to evaluate for signs of an asymptomatic or mildly symptomatic coexisting site of nongenital infection. Although Mr. Yount's age falls into the range where the vast majority of STIs occur, it is highly unlikely that an STI is responsible for his symptoms primarily because he has only had one sexual partner for the past 9 months and virtually all STIs that can present as testicular pain and/or oropharyngeal lesions occur within 4 to 6 weeks postinfection. Furthermore, his STI risk is relatively lower because of his limited number of lifetime partners, and his lack of participating in oral–genital/anal intercourse further reduces the likelihood of a sexually transmitted oral lesion being present.

B. Palpation of parotid and submandibular glands NONESSENTIAL

Because Mr. Yount did not experience any prodromal symptoms or a recent episode of parotiditis, it is extremely unlikely that his current complaint is related to mumps (the most likely cause for the combination of scrotal pain with swelling and parotiditis).

C. Abdominal examination   ESSENTIAL

Although Mr. Yount is not experiencing any abdominal pain, he does have genital and flank pain. Therefore, it is important to perform an abdominal examination to evaluate for signs of a suprapubic mass (a smooth one would likely be caused by a distended bladder, whereas an irregular one could possibly represent a bladder carcinoma). Additionally, his midlateral abdomen also requires palpation for enlarged kidneys and auscultation for renal bruits (indicating a potential renal problem as the cause of or complication of his chief complaint). Because he is tachycardic and diaphoretic, his abdominal aorta should also be palpated and auscultated for signs indicating the rare possibility of an occlusion or an aneurysm producing his symptoms.

D. Genital examination   ESSENTIAL

Because this is the area involving his chief complaint, he needs a comprehensive genital examination.

E. Evaluation for CVA tenderness   ESSENTIAL

Because he is experiencing ipsilateral flank pain in addition to his genital pain, evaluating for CVA tenderness can assist in determining if his problem is limited to the scrotum/testicle or if it appears to be accompanied by an upper urinary tract abnormality as well.

3. Diagnostic Studies

A. Scrotal color Doppler ultrasound   NONESSENTIAL

The color Doppler ultrasound is considered to be the diagnostic test of choice for the evaluation of scrotal masses because it has a sensitivity and specificity of greater than or equal to 90% (when performed by an experienced operator) and the results are generally available in "real time." It is indicated when the diagnosis cannot be established with a high degree of certainty clinically OR if the patient's testicular pain has been present for 12 hours or longer. Mr. Yount meets neither of these conditions.

B. Urinalysis   ESSENTIAL

This quick test should be performed on Mr. Yount because it can provide support for or against his most likely diagnosis; plus, it can provide support for the assumption that there is no renal problem responsible for (or associated with) his flank pain. Gross or microscopic hematuria could indicate the presence of a nephrolithiasis, renal calculi pyelonephritis, or glomerulonephritis. Bacteruria or pyuria could be caused by urethritis, cystitis, pyelonephritis, prostatitis, or epididymitis.

C. Penile swab for Gram stain and nucleic acid amplification test for *N. gonorrhoeae* and *C. trachomatis*   NONESSENTIAL

Because Mr. Yount's history and physical examination are inconsistent with a sexually transmitted urethral infection and suggest a noninfectious condition with a high degree of certainty, this test is unnecessary at this time.

D. Testicular scintigraphy   NONESSENTIAL

Although this diagnostic test provides the greatest sensitivity (~90%) and specificity (100%) for evaluating the blood flow to the testicles (increased in epididymitis and testicular appendiceal torsion and decreased in testicular torsion), it is not indicated in Mr. Yount's case because of the amount of time it takes to perform the procedure and obtain the results. For example, if a testicular torsion is responsible for Mr. Yount's symptoms, this delay to surgery could have a significant impact on the salvage rate of his testicle, especially because he has already been symptomatic for 4 hours. If the time from symptom onset to surgical completion occurs within 6 hours, the salvage rate is 80% or higher. However, by 8 hours, this rate decreases to approximately 55 to 85%, and at longer than 24 hours, the salvage rate is near 0%.

E. Complete blood count with differential (CBC w/diff) ESSENTIAL

Although Mr. Yount's vital sign abnormalities and severe pain are probably related to his most likely diagnosis, a CBC w/diff should still be performed to ensure that a significant infectious, inflammatory, or hemorrhagic condition is not present.

4. Diagnosis

A. Urinary tract infection   INCORRECT

The phrase "urinary tract infection," or UTI, is most commonly utilized to indicate an infection of the bladder (cystitis). However, technically a UTI could be considered to be an infection anywhere from the urethral meatus to the kidneys. Nevertheless, a UTI generally does not present with testicular pain/edema and alone will not produce abnormal genital findings (as Mr. Yount has). Additionally, the lack of irritative voiding symptoms and a normal urinalysis are inconsistent with this diagnosis. Therefore, a UTI is not Mr. Yount's most likely diagnosis.

B. Left gonococcal epididymitis   INCORRECT

Epididymitis is an inflammation of the epididymitis most generally caused by an infectious process, in this case gonorrhea. It can present as testicular pain and scrotal swelling; however, its onset is generally more insidious. Also, it tends to be associated with a fever and moderate leukocytosis. Furthermore, unless another condition is also present, the cremasteric reflex is preserved and the patient tends to have a positive Prehn sign (the testicular pain is alleviated, or at least decreased, when the testicle is raised above the pubic symphysis). Therefore, left gonococcal epididymitis can essentially be ruled out as Mr. Yount's most likely diagnosis.

However, it is important to remember that the presence or absence of the Prehn sign is not considered sufficiently reliable enough to rule in or rule out the patient's most likely diagnosis. It is just another factor to consider as part of the accumulated data.

C. Left testicular torsion   CORRECT

Testicular torsion is the rotation of the testicle in an upward medial direction on the spermatic cord. It is generally associated with a defect in the testicle's attachment to the tunica vaginalis. This is Mr. Yount's most likely diagnosis because of the acute onset of his symptoms, the severity of his pain without direct genital trauma, his genital examination findings characteristic for the condition (i.e., testicular elevation and medial rotation, epididymis located in the anterior scrotum, hydrocele, lack of cremasteric reflex, and negative Prehn sign), and his essentially normal CBC w/diff and urinalysis results.

D. Left traumatic hydrocele and inguinal hernia   INCORRECT

A traumatic hydrocele can essentially be eliminated as Mr. Yount's mostly diagnosis because he did not experience any direct injury to his genitalia. An inguinal hernia can also be fairly accurately ruled out because no bulges were identified on his physical examination suggesting its presence. Occasionally, mild to moderate scrotal swelling can be evident if the bowel protrudes into the scrotal sac with an inguinal hernia; however, marked enlargement of the testicle as well as the presence of a significant hydrocele is extremely rare in this condition.

E. Cryptorchidism   INCORRECT

Cryptorchidism, or undescended testicles, can essentially be ruled out as Mr. Yount's most likely diagnosis because both of his testicles are palpable and descended on physical examination.

5. Treatment Plan

A. Bed rest with scrotal elevation   INCORRECT

This is an inappropriate treatment option for Mr. Yount because any delay to surgery is only going to result in a higher probability of scrotal hypoxia and subsequent decreased fertility.

B. Naproxen 500 mg twice a day   INCORRECT

This option is incorrect because it is unlikely that an NSAID, such as naproxen, is going to provide Mr. Yount with any significant pain relief. Furthermore, he should not be allowed anything by mouth because his condition calls for emergency surgery.

C. Ceftriaxone 250 mg IM × one dose plus doxycycline 100 mg orally twice a day for 10 days   INCORRECT

Antibiotics are not going to have any impact on Mr. Yount's primary diagnosis of testicular torsion. Even though he may require prophylactic and postoperative antibiotics, this decision (including drug selection, dosage, route, and duration) should be determined by the surgeon.

D. Immediate surgical consultation   CORRECT

Because the time to surgical correction is directly proportional to the ability to salvage his testicle, an immediate surgical consult for emergency surgery is indicated.

E. If surgeon is not immediately available, attempt manual detorsion   CORRECT

If the surgeon (or surgical suite) is not immediately available, attempts to manually detorse the testicle are indicated in hopes of salvaging the testicle within the critical time frame.

The detorsion procedure is sometimes referred to as "opening the book" because the majority of testicular torsions tend to be upward and medially around the spermatic cord and manual detorsion involves rotating the testicle inferiorly and outward approximately 180° (similar to the movement utilized when opening a book).

Epidemiologic and Other Data

In the United States, the incidence of testicular torsion is approximately 0.25 per 1000 cases annually. Testicular torsion has a bimodal presentation, with the majority occurring within the first 6 weeks of life and a second peak around puberty. It is rare for the condition to occur in men older than the age of 30 years. The incidence of a male having either unilateral or bilateral torsion of a testicle or a testicular appendage by the age of 25 years is slightly over 0.6%.

Risk factors include the presence of the "bell-clapper deformity" (the testicle is suspended loosely within the scrotal sac [because of its lack of adhesion with the tunica vaginalis] resembling the clapper in a bell); congenital absence of scrotal ligaments; incomplete descent of the testicles; testicles that are small in size or atrophied; testicular trauma; previous manual (or spontaneous) detorsion of testicle; attempted inguinal hernia reduction; straining with urination, defecation, exercise, or lifting; sexual activity; immersion in cold water; spasm of the cremasteric muscle; or a sudden scare.

CASE 6-6

Yolinda ("Lindy") Zickafoose

1. History

A. Has her mother recently changed soaps, lotions, detergents, fabric softeners, or any other product that could come in contact with Lindy's skin?   NONESSENTIAL

Contact allergic reactions generally present as a pruritic rash (contact dermatitis) in exposed areas. Occasionally, contact urticaria with surrounding erythema, slightly increased skin temperature, and/or nonpitting localized edema occurs. Because Lindy's only symptom is edema, it is highly unlikely that it could result from a contact allergic reaction.

Intermittent generalized edema can also be seen in rare conditions (e.g., hereditary angioedema). Unlike Lindy's presentation, the edema generally occurs suddenly in all body locations (most commonly the extremities and mucosal surfaces of the respiratory and gastrointestinal tracts), is nonpitting, and resolves within 24 hours.

B. Does she attend day care?   ESSENTIAL

Because of the confined space, close contact with other children who could be ill or harboring organisms, and potential for poor hand-washing hygiene, day care attendance increases the risk of acquiring an infection that is transmitted via respiratory droplets, the fecal–oral route, and/or skin-to-skin contact. Although the majority of these illnesses are self-limiting viral syndromes, serious viral and bacterial infections can occur.

Some of these viruses (e.g., parvovirus, hepatitis B, and hepatitis C) and bacteria (e.g., group M *Streptococcus, Streptococcus viridans, Streptococcus bovis, Staphylococcus aureus,* and *Enterococcus*) have the potential to cause either glomerulosclerosis or glomerulonephritis, which should be a concern because Lindy is essentially asymptomatic except for the edema and her cousin has "some type" of renal condition. Illnesses that are rare in the United States but can be transmitted via close contact with others can also produce glomerular disease (e.g., malaria, leprosy, and schistosomiasis). Thus, knowing whether Lindy attends day care is important because it would expand her list of potential differential diagnoses to include these infectious processes.

Unfortunately, day care attendance can also increase the patient's risk of child abuse, including psychological, physical, and sexual. Physical abuse (i.e., forcing the child to consume excessive quantities of salt) with or without sexual abuse could account for Lindy's symptoms.

C. Has there been any change in her urine's appearance or her urination patterns?   ESSENTIAL

Generalized edema (especially if it includes dependent edema [which could be labial and/or ankle in location in a patient of Lindy's age]) primarily occurs from problems in three organs: the heart, the kidneys, and the liver. Obstruction to lymphatic flow, increased capillary permeability, hypoproteinemia, hypothyroidism, hyperadrenocortism, pregnancy, some malignancies, and medication adverse effects (e.g. estrogens, NSAIDs, vasodilators, and diuretics) can also produce some form of generalized edema. Hence, it is essential to determine if her mother has noticed any change in Lindy's urinary patterns (e.g., increased or decreased frequency, increased or decreased quantity, urgency, incontinence, or increased enuresis) or urine's appearance (indicating an increase or a decrease in concentration or the presence of blood, pus, or bilirubin). This information is important in evaluating for potential renal abnormalities.

D. Does her diet contain consumption of a lot of salt, unwashed fruits/vegetables, or any new or unusual foods?   ESSENTIAL

There is the potential for a diet that contains excessive sodium to produce minor edema and weight gain. However, it would be unusual for it to be as much as Lindy's (6% of total body weight).

Foods (and their preservatives) can cause angioedema, which can present as an asymptomatic nonpitting edema. This can occur alone or in conjunction with urticaria and gastrointestinal symptoms. The most frequently implicated foods include shellfish, fish, peanuts, other nuts, chocolate, and dairy products. Angioedema can also occur from the consumption of improperly washed fruits and/or vegetables that could contain pesticides, fertilizers, preservatives, or other chemicals.

E. Was she stung by a bee within the past 3 weeks?   NONESSENTIAL

Hymenoptera envenomation can produce various symptoms, including edema, during three potential stages of the disease. The immediate reaction (initial phase reaction) occurs within a few seconds to a couple of hours post-sting.

It is typically characterized by a slightly erythematous papule or plaque at the site of the sting that is often surrounded by a hypopigmented area, varying degrees of localized edema, increased skin temperature, and pruritus. However, it can also involve an anaphylactic reaction that potentially results in edema elsewhere on the body (primarily the face and respiratory tract). The faster the onset of symptoms postenvenomation occurs, the greater the potential for a serious reaction.

In some individuals, a second stage reaction occurs approximately 4 to 6 hours post-sting and generally consists of the return of symptoms from the initial phase reaction. In an even smaller percentage of patients, a delayed hypersensitivity reaction can occur approximately 10 to 14 days after the initial sting. It can consist of minor symptoms (e.g., subcutaneous firm nodule with mild localized edema and pruritus) or a serious "serum sickness"-type reaction with constitutional symptoms and arthralgias.

Regardless, Lindy's pattern of edema (i.e., gradual onset, involving the face first, no localized lesion, no respiratory symptoms, and no pruritus) makes a bee sting extremely unlikely to be the causative agent for her symptoms even with a history of hymenoptera envenomation.

2. Physical Examination

A. Eyes, ears, nose, mouth, and throat examination ESSENTIAL

Because Lindy's symptoms technically began as mild facial edema that progressed to a periorbital involvement, an examination of her face and eyes, including an evaluation for lacrimal duct edema and tenderness, ptosis, exophthalmos, conjunctival injection, and other ocular abnormalities, is indicated. Furthermore, her ears, mouth, and throat also need to be examined for evidence of involvement from either an associated allergic or infectious process.

B. Heart and lung examination, including blood pressure ESSENTIAL

Cardiac diseases can be responsible directly (i.e., heart failure) or indirectly (i.e., glomerular involvement following subacute bacterial endocarditis) for the presence of edema. Therefore, her heart needs to be examined with attention to size, clarity of heart sounds, and murmurs.

Because heart failure frequently has coexisting pulmonary signs (e.g., bibasilar rales or pleural effusions), chronic allergic rhinitis is often associated with asthma, and acute allergic reactions are affiliated with respiratory tract inflammation, it is essential to auscultate her lungs.

Pediatric Blood Pressure

According to The Fourth Report on the Diagnosis, Evaluation, and Treatment of High Blood Pressure in Children and Adolescents, the determination of normal versus abnormal BP is based on the patient's gender, age, height, and associated percentile of blood pressure. As with adults, BP measurements must be performed on two separate occasions and the average of those two readings must be elevated to correctly establish the diagnosis of hypertension. If the patient's blood pressure falls below the 90th percentile

for both systolic blood pressure (SBP) and diastolic blood pressure (DBP), then it is considered normal. If the patient's SBP and/or DBP is the 90th percentile or above but below the 95th percentile, then he or she is considered to have prehypertension. If the patient's SBP and/or DBP is the 95th percentile or above but less than the 99th percentile + 5 mm Hg, then he or she is considered to have stage 1 hypertension. If the patient's SBP and/or DBP is the 99th percentile or above + 5 mm Hg, then he or she is considered to have stage 2 hypertension.

Because the age ranges are in years, not months, Lindy would still be considered 2 years old. With her height at approximately the 50th percentile for her age, her BP levels (in mm Hg) per percentiles are listed in **Table 6-1.**

C. Abdominal examination   ESSENTIAL

The abdominal examination is essential not only to look for signs of distention and/or ascites that could represent an additional site of edema but also to evaluate the size of the kidneys and the liver. Conditions that can result in enlargement or atrophy of the liver and/or kidneys (e.g., glomerulonephritis, chronic renal failure, cirrhosis, and hepatitis) can also produce edema.

D. External genital and rectal examination   ESSENTIAL

Despite her mother's denial of trauma and/or skin discoloration, multiple locations of swelling (especially labial) should arouse some degree of suspicion for child abuse, including sexual assault. Therefore, the genital and rectal areas must be examined closely not only to determine the degree of labial edema but also to look for any labial, vaginal, perineal, and rectal trauma or lesions that could be caused by sexual assault and/or a sexually transmitted infection.

However, it is important to remember than an intact hymen and normal rectal sphincter do not eliminate the possibility of sexual abuse because the perpetrator could only be fondling, kissing, licking, or biting the genitalia. Penetration could have occurred with a single finger and/or other small objects. Conversely, hymen tears are not proof of sexual assault.

Table 6-1 Blood Pressure (BP) Levels (in mm Hg) per Percentiles for a 2 y.o. at the 50th percentile of height

	50th	90th	95th	99th
Systolic BP	88	101	105	112
Diastolic BP	45	59	63	70

Source: National High Blood Pressure Education Program Working Group on High Blood Pressure in Children and Adolescents. Blood pressure tables. *The Fourth Report on the Diagnosis, Evaluation, and Treatment of High Blood Pressure in Children and Adolescents.* (NIH Publication No. 05-5267). Washington, DC: US Department of Health and Human Services, National Institutes of Health, National Heart, Lung, and Blood Institute; 2005:8-15. http://www.nhlbi.nih.gov/health/prof/heart/hbp/hbp_ped.pdf.

E. Evaluation of the skin for additional sites of edema plus discoloration, urticaria, rashes, and/or other lesions   ESSENTIAL

A comprehensive evaluation of her edema as well as the presence and location of mild or undetected edema elsewhere could provide clues to potential differential diagnoses. Care must be take to detect any discolorations (even subtle) that could be present; these include jaundice (indicating the potential for hepatic involvement), erythema (suggesting an inflammatory, infectious, allergic, or autoimmune process), and contusions, especially in various stages of healing and located near the swollen areas (suggesting child abuse, bleeding diathesis, and/or hepatic involvement significant enough to affect the patient's prothrombin time). The presence of rashes and other lesions, depending on their location and distribution, could indicate an allergic, infectious, or autoimmune cause for her edema.

3. Diagnostic Studies

A. Urinalysis   ESSENTIAL

Because there are several renal conditions that are associated with edema and hypertension (even though technically Lindy cannot be diagnosed with hypertension [despite an elevated BP for age at this visit] because it can only be diagnosed after the average of two readings on two separate visits falls into the age and height-determined hypertensive range), a urinalysis is essential.

B. Serum albumin, globulin, and total protein   ESSENTIAL

Total protein is essentially composed of albumin (~60%) and globulin (~40%). Because the majority of total protein consists of albumin, the terms "hyperproteinemia" and "hyperalbuminemia" are frequently used interchangeably. Likewise, hypoproteinemia and hypoalbuminemia are often considered to be the same condition. Because albumin is produced in the liver and eliminated by the kidney, the ratio of albumin to globulin and its relationship to the total protein level assists in the measurement of hepatic function and to a lesser degree renal function. The normal albumin-to-globulin ratio is greater than 1. If this ratio is decreased, it almost always indicates chronic liver failure.

Renal disease, if associated with a significant proteinuria, generally has a decreased serum albumin level, a low-normal (or slightly decreased) total protein level, and an increased serum globulin level. However, this pattern can also be seen in severe/end-stage hepatic disease as well. To determine the exact cause of this pattern, protein electrophoresis is required to differentiate the γ-globulin components.

C. Serum blood urea nitrogen (BUN) and creatinine   ESSENTIAL

Although these two tests are commonly referred to as renal function studies, this combination evaluates not only renal function but also hepatic function. Urea is produced in the liver and eliminated by the kidneys, whereas creatinine is produced in the skeletal muscles and is excreted renally. Hence, the levels of these two substances in the blood in conjunction with their ratio to each other are excellent indicators of both renal and hepatic function.

A normal BUN/creatinine ratio is considered to be 15.5, with the actual range being from 6 to 25. An elevated ratio (in conjunction with an elevation of both the BUN and creatinine) is most commonly a result of a decrease in renal function, whether it is prerenal (e.g., dehydration, gastrointestinal bleeding, hypovolemia, sepsis, shock, or starvation), renal (e.g., pyelonephritis, glomerulonephritis, or staghorn calculi), or postrenal (e.g., nephrolithiasis, ureter stricture, or urethra obstruction). Whereas a decrease in the BUN/creatinine ratio (and/or a decreased BUN with a normal serum creatinine level) is primarily a result of hepatic failure; however, these findings can also be seen with nephrotic syndrome.

D. Strep screen   NONESSENTIAL

Strep screens are rapid antigen tests to detect the presence of Group *A Streptococcus* (GAS, or *Streptococcus pyogenes*) in throat/tonsillar specimens. Although estimated to be greater than 95% specific for GAS pharyngitis, they have no role in the identification of a GAS infection at other sites. Without throat symptoms, a positive test indicates a carrier state that is not indicative as the cause of an infection elsewhere in the body.

E. Lipid panel   ESSENTIAL

Because of the feedback mechanism to preserve the serum's osmotic pressure (primarily maintained by albumin, and to a much lesser degree globulin), when significant protein losses occur, the decreasing albumin levels prompt the liver to not only produce albumin but also to manufacture all of its protein, including the lipoproteins. Therefore, a lipid profile is indicated (especially considering Lindy's family history) because renal problems, such as nephrotic syndrome, are characterized by an accompanying hyperlipidemia.

4. Diagnosis

A. Acute glomerulonephritis   INCORRECT

Acute glomerulonephritis is an acute, generally noninfectious glomerular disease that results in significant inflammation of these structures. Although it can present as edema and assumed hypertension (see earlier), it can be eliminated as Lindy's most likely diagnosis because it is not associated with the significant proteinuria and hypoalbuminemia that was discovered on Lindy's diagnostic studies. Furthermore, acute glomerulonephritis almost always presents with hematuria, renal insufficiency, and red blood cell (and possibly white blood cell) casts in a microscopic urinalysis.

B. Acute pyelonephritis   INCORRECT

Acute pyelonephritis is an inflammatory process involving the upper urinary tract (predominately the renal pelvis, calyces, and parenchyma) most commonly caused by an infection. It can be eliminated as Lindy's most likely diagnosis because it is infrequently associated with edema, presumed hypertension (see earlier), significant proteinuria, and hypoalbuminemia. However, it is frequently associated with signs of an upper urinary tract infection (e.g., fever, chills, nausea, vomiting, flank pain, abdominal pain, and/or possibly diarrhea and/or irritative urinary symptoms). Furthermore, the urinalysis in patients with an upper urinary tract infection reveals leukocyte esterase, nitrites, bacteriuria, pyuria, and white blood cell casts.

C. Nephrotic syndrome   CORRECT

Nephrotic syndrome is characterized by proteinuria (generally ≥ 3 g/day), hypoalbuminemia (defined as serum albumin level of < 3.0 g/dl), and red blood cell casts on urinalysis as well as edema and hypertension. Oliguric renal failure, hyperlipidemia, headache, flank pain, malaise, nausea, vomiting, and anorexia can also be present. The majority of cases involving children are primary nephritic syndrome; hence, only one kidney is involved.

D. Child abuse   INCORRECT

Child abuse, as a lone entity, can be eliminated as Lindy's most likely diagnosis based on the findings from her physical examination (e.g., presumed hypertension [see earlier]; pitting nature to her edema; and the lack of ecchymosis, various stages of contusion healing, abrasions, lacerations, and/or other suspect lesions) and diagnostic studies (e.g., abnormal urinalysis with proteinuria, hypoalbuminemia, and hyperlipidemia).

E. Allergic reaction to unknown topical agent   INCORRECT

A contact allergic reaction is generally associated with pruritus and/or a rash (and occasional surrounding erythema and increased skin temperature), none of which Lindy has. Furthermore, it is generally not associated with the probable hypertension, proteinuria, hypoalbuminemia, and hyperlipidemia; therefore, this is not Lindy's most likely diagnosis.

5. Treatment Plan

A. Hospitalization   CORRECT

Being that this is the initial diagnosis of nephrotic syndrome for Lindy, she should be hospitalized for additional evaluation, monitoring, and treatment.

B. Nephrology consultation for evaluation, possible renal biopsy, and treatment   CORRECT

Because of the potential seriousness of the condition and its potential complications, Lindy should be promptly evaluated by a nephrologist who will attempt to determine the type, classification, and cause of her nephrotic syndrome. This information will provide more information on which to base her individual treatment plan and prognosis.

C. Furosemide 0.5 g/kg IV followed by 25% salt-deficient albumin 0.5 g/kg IV   INCORRECT

If Lindy were adequately hydrated and had severe edema (which she does not) in combination with her current serum albumin level, she would be given albumin followed by furosemide (not furosemide followed by albumin).

D. Prednisone 2 mg/kg/day orally   INCORRECT

Although prednisone is a useful treatment for nephrotic syndrome, it should not be given until all potential sources of infection can be identified/treated or ruled out, including a test for tuberculosis.

E. Complete blood count with differential (CBC w/diff)   CORRECT

A CBC w/diff is indicated to provide additional clues to the presence of an infectious, inflammatory, or anemic process causing Lindy's nephrotic syndrome. Furthermore, it evaluates for hemoconcentrated and the presence of "S" hemoglobin on the smear as found in sickle cell disease (which is unlikely given her ethnicity).

Other indicated diagnostic tests include a 24-hour urine for protein and creatinine, liver function testing (LFT), chest x-ray (CXR), prothrombin time (PT), partial thromboplastin time (PTT), electrolytes, sickle cell trait (if indicated), and erythrocyte sedimentation rate (ESR).

Additional testing that should be considered on an individualized basis to attempt to establish the type/classification of nephrotic syndrome includes fasting plasma glucose (FPG), C-reactive protein (CRP), antinuclear antibodies (ANAs), hepatitis antibody/antigen screening, HIV testing, complement levels, serum and urinary protein electrophoresis, vitamin D levels, zinc levels, copper levels, bone marrow biopsy, colonoscopy, thyroid ultrasound, thyroid nuclear scan, intravenous pyelogram (IVP), and CT and magnetic resonance imaging (MRI) of the abdomen.

Epidemiologic and Other Data

In the United States, the annual incidence of nephrotic syndrome in children is estimated to be approximately 0.02 to 0.05 per 1000. The majority of these cases are considered to be primary (affecting only one kidney) and an estimated 70 to 90% are caused by minimal change disease (MCD). In contrast, MCD accounts for only 10 to 15% of all cases in adults.

Other causes of primary nephrotic syndrome include primary (idiopathic) focal segmental glomerulosclerosis, membranous glomerulonephritis, and membranoproliferative nephritis.

Secondary nephrotic syndrome typically involves both kidneys and is secondary to another medical condition. The majority of these cases are caused by secondary focal segmental glomerulosclerosis, which can result from medication adverse effects (e.g., NSAIDs, other analgesics, ampicillin, and immunizations), viral infections (including parvovirus, HIV, and hepatitis B), sickle cell disease, Alport syndrome, reflux nephropathy, and familial podocytopathy.

Other secondary causes include secondary membranous glomerulonephritis, most commonly caused by breast, colon, esophageal, lung, and renal cancers; infections with hepatitis B, hepatitis C, syphilis, and malaria; medications such as NSAIDs, probenecid, and older antirheumatoid arthritis agents; and autoimmune diseases. Coexisting autoimmune conditions such as Crohn disease, Fanconi syndrome, Guillain-Barré syndrome, Weber-Christian syndrome, and diabetes mellitus. Glomerular deposition diseases (including light chain deposition disease, renal amyloidosis, and fibrillary-immunotactoid glomerulopathy), anaphylactoid purpura, Fabry disease, Wilms tumor, lymphoma, obesity, metabolic syndrome, atopy, and asthma have also been implicated.

CASE 6-7
Zelda Armstrong
1. History

A. When during voiding does her dysuria begin and where is her pain located?   ESSENTIAL

Knowing when the dysuria begins and whether the patient perceives it as internal or external in location provides essential information that assists in making the distinction between urinary and genital sources. Dysuria from cystitis frequently occurs immediately upon initiation of voiding and is often described as a sharp subpubic pain. The pain associated with urethritis in women generally starts shortly after the patient begins voiding and gradually increases in intensity as she continues to urinate. It is frequently defined as "internal" but not abdominal or pelvic in location. The dysuria associated with vulvovaginitis, genital ulcer disease, or other conditions causing a disruption in the vaginal or labial mucosal surface generally occurs toward the end of voiding or shortly thereafter and is defined as being external in location. The latter is theorized to be caused by contact of the acidic urine with the inflamed mucosa.

B. Has she noticed any vaginal discharge or genital lesions? ESSENTIAL

Although dysuria is one of the defining symptoms of cystitis (along with urinary urgency and frequency), as previously stated, dysuria (and in some cases urinary urge and frequency) is also a common presenting symptom in women with conditions causing disruption of the genital mucosa (e.g., vulvovaginitis, genital ulcer disease). This latter group can have these symptoms.

Some women are uncertain as to whether their vaginal discharge (especially if minimal) is physiologic or pathologic; therefore, they are reluctant to mention it as a symptom. When directly questioned regarding the presence of a vaginal discharge, they might respond with a vague, noncommittal response; this should be interpreted as an affirmative response.

C. What is her sexual history?   ESSENTIAL

Dysuria caused by a urethritis, vulvovaginitis, or vaginitis can be the result of a sexually transmitted infection (e.g., gonorrhea, chlamydia, and trichomoniasis). Because Ms. Armstrong is in the age range where the majority of sexually transmitted infections occur, it is imperative to inquire about her sexual history. (For more information regarding the sexual history, please see Case 6-2.)

D. Has she passed any kidney stones?   NONESSENTIAL

Kidney stones large enough to be visible with the naked eye (especially without straining the urine) are going to produce more significant symptoms (e.g., hematuria, abdominal and/or flank pain, and obstructive urinary symptoms) than what Ms. Armstrong is complaining.

E. Has she noticed any changes in the color and/or odor of her urine?   ESSENTIAL

Malodorous urine can be associated with infection, enterobladder fistula, increased concentration, medications, and occasionally consumption of certain foods (e.g., garlic). Diabetic ketoacidosis is associated with "sweet"-smelling urine.

Pale-appearing urine is frequently a result of it being dilute, whereas dark urine occurs with concentration and the presence of blood, urobilinogen, or bilirubin. Other conditions, foods, medications, and infections can result in abnormal-colored urine (e.g., gross hematuria, excessive consumption of beets, or docusate calcium laxative use can result in a pink to red discoloration of the urine [depending on the quantity]; eating rhubarb or taking nitrofurantoin can result in brown-colored urine; taking multivitamins and/or vitamin B can produce a brighter yellow urine discoloration; *Pseudomonas* sp. infection occasionally produces a greenish discoloration to the urine; and the diuretic triamterene can occasionally give the urine a pale bluish hue).

2. Physical Examination

A. Heart examination   NONESSENTIAL

B. Lung examination   NONESSENTIAL

C. Abdominal examination   ESSENTIAL

An abdominal examination should be performed on all patients complaining of dysuria. The primary focus would be the suprapubic area to evaluate for bladder abnormalities (e.g., tenderness, distension, and/or irregular shape). Although unlikely to provide much information, palpation of the kidneys and evaluation for renal bruits should be done as well.

The abdominal examination could also provide clues regarding the source of vaginal discharge. If it is associated with salpingitis or a tube-ovarian abscess, it can reveal tenderness and possibly a mass in the ipsilateral lower quadrant. Endometritis tends to be associated with suprapubic tenderness. However, these conditions are generally associated with abdominal pain and the findings more pronounced and identifiable on a pelvic examination. Vulvovaginitis is generally associated with a negative abdominal examination.

D. Pelvic examination   ESSENTIAL

Because Ms. Armstrong is complaining of vaginal discharge in addition to her dysuria, a pelvic examination is indicated. The external pelvic examination permits examination of the area for signs of conditions that could produce these symptoms. For example, erythema, edema, and/or excoriations could be associated with an allergic vulvovaginitis, vulvovaginal candidiasis, trauma, Bartholin duct abscess and/or obstruction, Skene duct abscess/and or obstruction, or another infectious process. Ulcers could result from sexually transmitted infections, including syphilis or genital herpes. Excoriations and lichenification are seen with lichen sclerosis. Atrophy is seen in women with severe atrophic vulvovaginitis.

The speculum examination provides visual inspection of the walls of the vagina and the cervix. In vulvovaginitis or vaginitis, the discharge (unless disturbed from douching, tampon use, intercourse, etc.) covers the entire vaginal surface and some degree of erythema and/or edema could be present. Ulcerations, lacerations, discolorations, and other lesions could represent coinfection or trauma. Cervicitis tends to present as erythema, edema, os discharge, and increased friability of the cervix. The presence of cervical lesions/ulcerations could represent a more severe infection, a coinfection, trauma, or carcinomas. Therefore, any cervical abnormality requires follow-up to ensure resolution and/or testing for a malignancy.

The bimanual examination permits evaluation of the internal pelvic structures. It enables the size, location, consistency, and presence of tenderness or masses involving the uterus, fallopian tubes, and ovaries to be identified.

E. Evaluation for CVA tenderness   ESSENTIAL

Because Ms. Armstrong's chief complaint is a "urinary tract infection" yet she lacks significant irritative urinary symptoms, it is important to determine whether CVA tenderness is present. If present, it that could indicate involvement of the upper urinary tract. Upper urinary tract infections generally are not associated with the irritative urinary symptoms seen with lower urinary tract infections.

3. Diagnostic Studies

A. Urinalysis   ESSENTIAL

A urinalysis is indicated because Ms. Armstrong is complaining of a "urinary tract infection" and dysuria. It will assist in confirming the presence (or absence) of UTI and distinguish between upper or lower urinary tract involvement (if an infection is present).

B. Urine culture and sensitivity (C&S)   NONESSENTIAL

A urine culture is only indicated if the initial urine is suspicious for a UTI. This generally consists of a positive test for leukocyte esterase and nitrites on the dipstick, greater than 5 white blood cells (WBCs) per low-power field, and significant bacteria on microscopy. Although Ms. Armstrong's urinalysis does meet these criteria, a urine culture is not indicated based on the numerous epithelial cells that are also present, which typically indicates a genital contaminant.

Therefore, if there was a strong suspicion that her symptoms were caused by a UTI, she should be reinstructed on how to correctly obtain an uncontaminated, clean-catch midstream urine. If that specimen is also contaminated, ideally she should be catheterized to obtain a sterile specimen for examination and subsequent culture and sensitivity. In fact, some laboratories will reject urine specimens for culture if any epithelial cells are present because of the high rate of false-positives due to growth of normal vaginal or skin flora and not true urinary pathogens.

C. Urinary human chorionic gonadotropin (HCG) test   NONESSENTIAL

A urinary HCG, or pregnancy, test is not indicated for Ms. Armstrong because she regularly and reliably uses a highly effective contraceptive method and had a normal menstrual period 2 weeks ago.

D. Wet-mount microscopy of vaginal secretions   ESSENTIAL

Traditionally, the diagnosis of vulvovaginitis (or vaginitis) has been made based on the results of a normal saline wet mount of the vaginal secretions viewed under low-power microscopy. A positive test would be indicated by the presence of greater than 5 WBCs per low-power field and the identification of signs of one of the three primary causes of vulvovaginitis: bacterial vaginosis, candidiasis, and trichomoniasis. A potassium hydroxide (KOH) prep, in addition to the saline mount, is considered essential by some experts because the addition of KOH to the vaginal secretions makes the appearance of yeast and the odor of amines more prominent.

Despite the fact that the wet-mount microscopy, with or without the KOH prep, results in a lower specificity and sensitivity compared to the combination of a "whiff" test, pH testing, and point-of-care testing, it should still be performed whenever possible as confirmation of the latter findings. The "gold standard" for identifying any of the aforementioned organisms is still considered to be identification via appropriate culture (which is rarely performed in clinical practice).

E. Vaginal pH, "whiff" test for amine odor, and point-of-care testing for vaginal pathogens via DNA   ESSENTIAL

This combination of tests provides a higher sensitivity and specificity rate in determining the pathogen responsible for vulvovaginitis than wet-mount microscopy. It is especially important in facilities that do not have access to the equipment and/or an individual trained to perform immediate microscopy on vaginal secretions.

The vaginal pH is measured utilizing Nitrazine paper. The "whiff" test is to determine the presence of an amine odor to the discharge. The point-of-care testing involves polymerase chain reaction (PCR) testing for the DNA of the pathogens responsible for the three most common causes of vaginitis (bacterial vaginosis, candidiasis, and trichomoniasis).

4. Diagnosis

A. Cystitis   INCORRECT

Although Ms. Armstrong is complaining of a "urinary tract infection" and has dysuria and a urinalysis suspicious for cystitis, this is not her most likely diagnosis because she lacks the other two characteristic symptoms (urinary urgency and frequency). Furthermore, there is vaginal contamination of her urinalysis, as well as positive findings on the diagnostic test of her vaginal discharge.

Additionally, urinary tract infections, without the presence of a significant structural abnormality or immunosuppression of the patient, generally do not recur at 2-week intervals. The majority of UTIs (and their symptoms) will worsen over a 3- to 4-day time period.

B. *Trichomonas* vaginitis   CORRECT

Based on her history of a vaginal discharge and dysuria, her physical examination findings of erythema of her vaginal mucosa and discharge adherent to her vaginal walls, and her diagnostic test results of a contaminated urine but an abnormal wet-mount, pH, and "whiff" amine test, Ms. Armstrong's diagnosis is much more consistent with a vaginitis than a UTI.

The causative organism of her vaginitis should be identifiable based on the results of her wet-mount microscopy, point-of-care testing, and vaginal pH and whiff amine test **(Table 6-2)**. The presence of motile trichomonads on microscopy, an alkaline vaginal pH, and a whiff amine test being slightly positive make *Trichomonas* vaginitis her most likely diagnosis.

Petechial lesions can sometimes be visualized on the speculum examination (but most of the time require colposcopy) in patients who have trichomoniasis. If the cervix is infected, these lesions cause it to resemble a "strawberry," hence the origin of the term "strawberry cervix."

C. Candidal vulvovaginitis   INCORRECT

Candidal vulvovaginitis is a vulvovaginitis caused by one of the candidal species, with *Candida albicans* the most common. This can be ruled out as Ms. Armstrong's most likely diagnosis because of the lack of vulvar involvement and typical vaginal findings of a thick, white, "curd"-like vaginal discharge on a more erythematous mucosa. Furthermore, the lack of hyphae and/or budding yeast on her saline and KOH wet mounts, her alkaline vaginal pH, and the slightly positive "whiff" amine test are also inconsistent with this diagnosis. Finally, the presence of the protozoans on microscopy provides more evidence that this alone is not her most likely diagnosis.

D. Vaginitis caused by bacterial vaginosis   INCORRECT

It is theorized that bacterial vaginosis results from an overgrowth of the normal vaginal flora. Its characteristic findings

Table 6-2 Summary of Diagnostic Findings of Vulvovaginitis/Vaginitis

Causative agent	Common symptom(s)	Clinical appearance of discharge	Characteristic microscopic findings	"Whiff" test	pH test
Bacterial vaginosis	Odor and discharge	Very thin white, gray, or slightly yellow	"Clue" cells	Positive and "fish"-like odor	> 4.5
Candidiasis	External genitalia itching	Thick, "curd"-like, and white	Hyphae and/or budding yeast	Negative	≤ 4.5
Trichomoniasis	Relative asymptomatic to copious discharge	"Foamy" yellow to green	Motile trichomonads	Slightly positive or negative	≥ 5.0

on wet-mount microscopy are the presence of "clue cells" (WBCs that have the appearance of "black pepper" being applied to them). The associated vaginal pH is generally normal to alkaline, and the whiff amine test is positive. Despite Ms. Armstrong's history and physical examination being consistent with a vaginal infection, these characteristics eliminate vaginitis caused by bacterial vaginosis as her most likely diagnosis.

E. Pelvic inflammatory disease   INCORRECT

Pelvic inflammatory disease (PID) is an inflammatory response, most generally caused by an infectious process, of the upper female reproductive tract. It can be eliminated as Ms. Armstrong's most likely diagnosis because she lacks the characteristic physical finding of cervical motion tenderness (positive Chandelier sign). Furthermore, her physical examination does not reveal any uterine or adnexal tenderness, which is almost always present in this condition.

5. Treatment Plan

A. Metronidazole 2 g orally × one dose   CORRECT

Metronidazole, a nitroimidazole, is considered by the CDC guidelines to be one of the first-line therapies for the treatment of trichomoniasis at the dosage of a single oral dose of 2 g. The CDC guidelines also approve the use of metronidazole at 500 mg twice a day for 7 days as an alternative first-line treatment; however, this dosage is generally reserved for cases in which the single dose is ineffective or if the patient has frequent recurrences.

B. Azithromycin 500 mg, 2 pills stat, then 1 pill a day for 4 days   INCORRECT

The antibiotic azithromycin has no activity against the protozoa *Trichomonas vaginalis*.

C. Tinidazole 2 g once a day for 7 days   INCORRECT

Tinidazole, another nitroimidazole, is also CDC approved for first-line therapy for trichomoniasis. However, the correct dosage is a single oral dose of 2 g. Despite the fact that this is considered to be a first-line treatment by the CDC, most HCPs still only utilize this medication when the patient fails to respond to metronidazole. It is also indicated for the treatment of bacterial vaginosis. The dosage for bacterial vaginosis condition is 1 g daily for 5 days.

D. Advise the patient not to take her medication after drinking alcohol or with an alcoholic beverage, and not to drink alcohol for a minimum of 72 hours after finishing the medication   CORRECT

The combination of metronidazole (or tinidazole) with alcoholic beverages can result in severe nausea, vomiting, and flushing (similar to the reaction seen when alcohol is combined with the alcohol deterrent disulfiram). Furthermore, there have been rare cases of acute psychotic episodes if nitroimidazole is taken within 2 weeks of disulfiram.

E. Provide expedited partner treatment   CORRECT

Ideally, Ms. Armstrong's partner should be tested before being treated for trichomoniasis; however, because it is very difficult to get partners evaluated and treated in a timely fashion (especially if they are asymptomatic), expedited partner treatment for trichomoniasis is considered to be appropriate. Because trichomoniasis is generally not associated with other STIs and is rarely associated with any complications or serious sequelae, the primary purpose of partner treatment is to prevent reinfection of the patient.

Expedited partner treatment consists of providing the patient with the medication (and directions for use as well as patient education) for his or her partner without the partner coming in for an examination. Randomized controlled trials found the behavioral and clinical outcomes similar to those of traditional treatment regimens; however, it is imperative to be aware of state regulations regarding this option when treating other STIs, especially those that are reportable.

Epidemiologic and Other Data

In the United States, over 10,000,000 clinical visits are generated annually by women complaining of a vaginal discharge. The majority of these cases are caused by vulvovaginitis/vaginitis. Bacterial vaginosis (generally caused by one of the following organisms: *Haemophilus vaginalis*, *Gardnerella vaginalis*, *Mycoplasma hominis*, *Atopobium vaginae*, *Mobiluncus* sp., *Prevotella* sp., and anaerobes) accounts for nearly half of all of these presentations (40–50%), vulvovaginal candidiasis (most frequently caused by *Candida albicans*; significantly less frequently involved are *Candida glabrata* or *Candidal tropicalis*) is responsible for approximately one fourth (20–25%) of these visits, and *Trichomonas* vaginitis (caused by *Trichomonas vaginalis*) is responsible for an additional 15 to 20%.

Cervicitis (inflammation of the cervix most frequently caused by an infectious process) can also cause a vaginal discharge and accounts for another 20 to 25% of all visits. Most frequently, it is caused by *Trichomonas vaginalis, Neisseria gonorrhoeae, Chlamydia trachomatis,* and HSV.

The majority of noninfectious conditions causing women to present complaining of a vaginal discharge are due to either atrophic vaginitis or allergic vaginitis (most frequently caused by tampons, spermicides, latex condoms, douches, soaps, bathing products, and perfumes).

However, even after eliminating the patients with noninfectious causes for their vaginal discharge, it is argued that 10 million is an underestimation of the total number of vulvovaginitis/vaginitis cases. Possible reasons include the large number of women who present complaining of urinary tract symptoms instead of a vaginal discharge, the availability of over-the-counter products to treat vaginal infection (especially those caused by *Candida albicans*), homeopathic remedies, and the resolution of symptoms despite nontreatment.

In men, the majority of *Trichomonas vaginalis* infections are asymptomatic. However, it can cause urethritis, epididymitis, and prostatitis. In rare cases, periodontitis, gastroenteritis, colitis, proctocolitis, and proctitis can result from a *Trichomonas* infection.

CASE 6-8
Alex Bing
1. History

A. Has he noticed any lesions, swelling, itching, or other abnormalities of his genital and/or perineal areas? ESSENTIAL

Because Mr. Bing's symptoms are consistent with a urogenital problem, it is appropriate to inquire if he has noticed any abnormalities in his genital area. If so, it is equally important to obtain information regarding appearance, duration, course, location, and pain description.

Lesions anywhere on the genitalia, perineum, and/or anal area could indicate a sexually transmitted infection (e.g., genital herpes, condyloma acuminatum, or syphilis). Swelling, depending on its location and characteristics, could be an inguinal hernia, hydrocele, scrotal and/or testicular mass, or inguinal lymphadenopathy. Pruritus could represent a fungal infection, an allergic process, or a healing genital lesion. Erythematous scaly skin could be tinea cruris. Paresthesias could occur before the onset of a herpes (simplex or zoster) infection.

B. Does he have penile pain and/or a urethral discharge? ESSENTIAL

Penile pain is associated with a variety of conditions. If present, a description regarding its location, type, intensity, radiation, duration, course, and associated symptoms is essential, as it would be with any type of pain. Causes of penile pain include trauma, a sexually transmitted infection (e.g., genital herpes or chancroid), dysesthesias before the onset of a herpes infection, chronic prostatitis, chronic pelvic pain syndrome (CPPS), and a psychological condition.

If a urethral discharge is present, additional questioning should address its duration, appearance, consistency, and whether it is spontaneous. A purulent, discolored urethral discharge is most commonly associated with urethritis; however, this finding can also be present in prostatitis. The absence of urethral discharge does not eliminate these conditions. Urinary incontinence can present as a urethral discharge composed of urine; it can occur as a result of a bladder neck, urethral, or meatal obstruction or mass. An enlarged prostate is frequently associated with postvoid "dribbling" of urine. In patients without a coagulopathy, a bloody discharge (especially if it is spontaneous) almost always represents a traumatic process. However, infectious conditions that can produce ulcers in the urethra and urethral meatus can also present in this fashion; the most common is probably genital herpes.

Spontaneous urethral discharge can be seen with sexually transmitted infectious (e.g., gonorrhea, chlamydia, or trichomoniasis), nonsexually transmitted infections (a rare condition generally found almost exclusively in immunocompromised patients), or inflammatory reactions (e.g., foreign body or instrumentation). Spontaneous discharge occasionally does occur with prostatitis; however, in the majority of the cases it has to be expelled via prostatic massage.

C. Does he experience pain with ejaculation? ESSENTIAL

Pain with ejaculation can occur with a variety of conditions including chronic prostatitis, inflammatory CPPS, noninflammatory CPPS, and certain psychological conditions (e.g., history of sexual abuse, history of sexual assault, relationship difficulties, or delusions).

D. Does he carry a lot of pennies or other copper items in his front pockets? NONESSENTIAL

Copper-containing substances, large quantities of items, or significant weight from objects carried in his front pants pockets are highly unlikely to account for Mr. Bing's symptoms.

E. Does he have a history of urinary tract infections, urethritis, or prostatitis? ESSENTIAL

A history of frequent UTIs, urethritis, or prostatitis is often associated with an anatomic defect of the urinary tract (especially if it permits retrograde flow of urine), chronic prostatitis, or chronic pelvic pain syndrome (CPPS).

2. Physical Examination

A. Eye examination for icterus NONESSENTIAL

Unless Mr. Bing has a coexisting condition of his liver, hepatobiliary system, gallbladder, or pancreas (which is highly unlikely because he lacks symptoms of such), he should not have icterus.

B. Thyroid palpation NONESSENTIAL

C. Abdominal examination ESSENTIAL

An abdominal examination is important to perform on Mr. Bing to evaluate for any intra-abdominal pathology that could be responsible for or contributing to his symptoms. The most common finding would be an enlarged bladder caused by urinary obstruction.

D. Perineal and rectal examination ESSENTIAL

The perineal examination is important to evaluate for visible causes of perineal pain (e.g., genital warts, genital herpes, other lesions, and rectal fissures). The rectal examination is essential to not only evaluate for lesions, masses, and other abnormalities that could produce Mr. Bing's symptoms but also to evaluate his prostate. Additionally, gentle prostatic massage can produce expressed prostatic secretions (EPSs) for viewing microscopically, Gram staining, culturing, or other testing.

Vigorous prostatic massage is contraindicated, especially in men who appear to have acute bacterial prostatitis, because it has the potential to cause bacterial sepsis.

E. Genital examination ESSENTIAL

A genital examination is necessary to evaluate for urethral discharge, color changes of the skin, skin lesions, masses, and lymphadenopathy to assist in narrowing his differential diagnosis list.

3. Diagnostic Studies

A. Prostate-specific antigen (PSA) NONESSENTIAL

The primary purpose of the PSA test is to follow men with prostate cancer for effectiveness of treatment and signs of recurrence. With a significant amount of controversy (please see Case 6-1), it is also utilized to screen for prostate cancer. Because Mr. Bing does not have a history of prostate cancer, any symptoms suggestive of prostate cancer, an identifiable mass or hard glandular consistency on prostate examination suggesting a potential carcinoma, nor reached the age to consider asymptomatic prostate cancer screening, a PSA is not indicated. Furthermore, benign prostate conditions can cause a mild elevation of a patient's PSA. Therefore, if Mr. Bing's symptoms are caused by a prostate problem and a PSA was performed and elevated, this would be the most probable reason. Nevertheless, it likely would lead to undue anxiety and unnecessary testing in an attempt to ensure that there is no underlying malignancy present.

B. Midstream pre– and post–prostate massage urinalyses ESSENTIAL

When a man complains of urinary tract symptoms that are suggestive of prostatitis, midstream pre– and post–prostatic massage urinalyses are essential to assist in determining if the symptoms are prostatic in nature as well as infectious in origin.

C. Expressed prostatic secretions (EPSs) for microscopy evaluation and culture NONESSENTIAL

Normally, this is essential in evaluating men with urinary tract symptoms suggestive of prostatitis. However, because no EPSs were obtained on Mr. Bing's exam, it cannot be performed.

D. Culture and sensitivity (C&S) on both urine specimens ESSENTIAL

The pre- and posturine specimens should be sent for C&S testing, regardless of their results. A positive culture would assist in confirming an infectious cause. Which results are positive helps to clarify the location of the infection. Generally, if the pre–prostatic massage urine culture is positive and the post–prostatic massage urine culture is negative, then the most likely causes include cystitis, contamination of the

initial urine specimen, or nongrowth of the second culture. If the post–prostatic massage urine culture is positive and the pre–prostatic massage urine culture is negative, then the most likely causes include acute bacterial prostatitis, chronic bacterial prostatitis, contamination of the second specimen, or nongrowth of the first culture. If they are both positive, the most likely cause is acute bacterial prostatitis. However, chronic bacterial prostatitis, coexisting bacterial prostatitis with a lower urinary tract infection (e.g., cystitis or urethritis), and contamination of both specimens are rarer possibilities.

Regardless of the results, they must be correlated with the clinical picture and other test findings.

E. Blood cultures NONESSENTIAL

Blood cultures are not indicated for Mr. Bing because he is afebrile and not toxic appearing.

4. Diagnosis

A. Acute bacterial prostatitis INCORRECT

Acute bacterial prostatitis is an inflammatory condition of the prostate gland caused by an acute bacterial infection. *Escherichia coli* is the most common organism; however, other uropathogens have also been implicated. Generally the patient appears acutely ill or even toxic and has dysuria, fever, and chills, in addition to the perineal discomfort. On physical examination, the prostate gland tends to be uniformly enlarged, excruciatingly tender, and "mushy" in consistency. Furthermore, the EPSs and post–prostatic massage urine specimens yield significant pyuria and bacteria (as well as positive cultures). The pre–prostatic massage urinalysis is generally unremarkable; however, it can reveal pyuria and bacteriuria, and its culture can be positive. Therefore, acute bacterial prostatitis is not Mr. Bing's most likely diagnosis.

B. Chronic bacterial prostatitis INCORRECT

Although Mr. Bing does have both irritative and obstructive urinary symptoms, chronic bacterial prostatitis is not his most likely diagnosis. He lacks the history of frequent episodes of prostatitis (or even cystitis); a post–prostatic massage urine revealing positive findings for leukocyte esterase, nitrates, pyuria (defined as > 10 WBCs per low-power field [WBCs/LPF]), and bacteriuria; and an EPS that is positive for greater than 5 WBCs/LPF and bacteria. Additionally, the post–prostatic massage urine and EPS cultures tend to be positive for *Escherichia coli, Klebsiella* sp., *Proteus sp.*, or other uropathogens. Regardless of the total leukocyte count identified in the specimens, the amount of bacteria in the EPS and the post–prostatic massage urine should be greater than the amount of bacteria in the pre–prostatic massage urine in the case of chronic bacterial prostatitis.

C. Inflammatory chronic pelvic pain syndrome (CPPS-I) INCORRECT

Chronic pelvic pain syndrome is a newer diagnostic term for nonbacterial prostatitis. It consists of the symptoms of prostatitis; minimal physical examination findings; and negative cultures for the pre–prostatic massage urine, the post–prostatic massage urine, and the EPSs. It is further divided into inflammatory and noninflammatory. Inflammatory CPPS (CPPS-I) is characterized by the presence of pyuria in the absence of bacteriuria on the EPS and post–prostatic massage urinalysis. This is further delineated by CPPS-I being associated with a post–prostatic massage urinalysis that has at least 10-fold the number of leukocytes when compared to the initial urinalysis; and/or the EPS revealing greater than or equal to 1000 leukocytes per microliter.

Although CPPS-I was previously referred to as nonbacterial prostatitis, it is now suspected that it might have a bacterial cause. Additionally, it is suspected that this bacterial process is caused by a sexually transmitted infection because the majority of the cases occur in young, sexually active men with a history of recent nongonococcal urethritis in the absence of chlamydia or another causative organism. Still, the suspected organisms are *Chlamydia trachomatis* and *Ureaplasma urealyticum*. Although Mr. Bing meets the diagnostic criteria established for CPPD, his laboratory findings are not consistent with the criteria for CPPD-I; thus, this is not his most likely diagnosis.

D. Noninflammatory chronic pelvic pain syndrome (CPPS-NI) CORRECT

CPPS-NI is the newer term for prostatodynia. It is theorized to be the result of an inadequacy of the internal sphincter and/or the pelvic floor muscles. Its diagnostic criteria consist of no evidence of prostatic inflammation (defined as no leukocytosis on the post–prostatic massage urinalysis and the EPS) and no abnormal amounts of bacteria in the post–prostatic massage urine and the EPS. Culture of both the postprostatic massage urine and the EPS should be negative. Because Mr. Bing meets the criteria established for CPPS (as previously defined) and his laboratory studies are consistent with the noninflammatory form, CPPS-NI is his most likely diagnosis.

E. Epididymitis   INCORRECT

Epididymitis is an inflammation of the epididymitis most generally caused by an infection. It can be ruled out as Mr. Bing's most likely diagnosis because he does not have epididymal tenderness. Generally it is also associated with the presence of a fever and moderate leukocytosis. Furthermore, the prostate examination should be normal unless a prostatic condition is also present.

5. Treatment Plan

A. Trimethoprim-sulfamethoxazole double strength, twice a day for 1 to 3 months   INCORRECT

CPPS-NI does not appear to have a bacterial cause; thus, antibiotic therapy is not indicated. However, 1 to 3 months of double-strength trimethoprim-sulfamethoxazole twice a day is an appropriate treatment for chronic bacterial prostatitis. The other first-line agents for chronic bacterial prostatitis consist of the fluoroquinolones, levofloxacin or ciprofloxacin, for 4 weeks.

B. Diclofenac 50 mg three times a day   CORRECT

NSAIDs are considered to be a first line treatment option for pain management in patients with CPPS-NI. However, as with any NSAID, gastrointestinal protection with a proton pump inhibitor (PPI) should be considered if the patient is going to be on the medication long term. Furthermore, it is recommended that patients taking diclofenac have liver function studies performed within the first 4 weeks of initiating therapy and periodically thereafter. Warm sitz-baths should also be employed by the patient to assist with pain relief.

C. Ceftriaxone 250 mg IM × one dose plus doxycycline 100 mg twice a day for 14 days   INCORRECT

As stated previously, because CPPS-NI is not linked with a bacterial pathogen, antibiotic therapy is contraindicated. However, ceftriaxone 250 mg IM × one dose plus doxycycline 100 mg twice a day for 14 days is considered an appropriate first-line treatment option for the outpatient management of milder cases of acute bacterial prostatitis in men younger than the age of 35 years. In men older than the age of 35 years, the use of fluoroquinolones (e.g., levofloxacin or ciprofloxacin) for 10 to 14 days is considered to be first-line treatment. Double-strength trimethoprim-sulfamethoxazole twice a day for 10 to 14 days is also considered to be an acceptable first-line treatment for men older than the age of 35 years. However, some experts advocate an even longer treatment time. Regardless of the antibiotic selection, outpatient management of acute bacterial prostatitis must include close follow-up and only be utilized in proven compliant patients. Otherwise, hospitalization should be considered. Severe cases of acute bacterial prostatitis require hospitalization and IV antibiotics.

D. Erythromycin 250 mg four times a day for a minimum of 2 (to a maximum of 6) weeks   INCORRECT

Again, because CPPS-NI is not considered an infectious process, antibiotic therapy is not indicated. However, it is considered to be an acceptable treatment for patients with CPPS-I. If the patient is receiving some benefit from this therapy, it should be continued for 4 more weeks.

E. Terazosin 1 mg/day   INCORRECT

The alpha-blocker terazosin is indicated for the treatment of both hypertension and BPH. However, it is considered an appropriate off-label treatment option for men with CPPS-NI who have moderate to severe obstructive symptoms. The usual starting dose is 1 mg daily; then, it is titrated as tolerated until symptoms are alleviated or until a maximum of 20 mg has been reached. Because of the mildness of Mr. Bing's obstructive symptoms, it is appropriate to evaluate his response to the NSAID and warm Sitz baths before initiating this therapy. As with any medication, the risks and benefits must be carefully considered, explained to the patient (including if the indication is off-label), and individualized for that person.

Other treatments that have been utilized successfully include diazepam, biofeedback, and pelvic floor muscle transcutaneous electrical nerve stimulation. In men older than the age of 40 years with obstructive symptoms, the 5α-reductase inhibitors (e.g., finasteride and dutasteride) may also provide the patient with relief. All of these medication options are off-label uses in CPPS-NI.

Epidemiologic and Other Data

It is estimated that approximately one half of all men in the United States will experience urologic complaints consistent with some type of prostatitis. Prostatitis is now classified into five diagnostic categories based on age of presentation, symptoms, and diagnostic test findings.

The most common category is CPPS-I, formerly known as nonbacterial prostatitis; it accounts for approximately 40 to 65% of all cases. The next most common prostatitis is CPPS-NI, formerly known as prostatodynia; it accounts for approximately

20 to 40% of all cases. Chronic bacterial prostatitis (~7%), acute bacterial prostatitis (≤ 5%), and asymptomatic inflammatory prostatitis (incidence unknown) are the remaining types.

Risk factors for any type of prostatitis include previous episode(s) of prostatitis, cystitis, urethritis, or epididymitis; history of urogenital tract abnormalities; history of urinary tract surgery; reflux of urine back into the bladder or ureters; frequent or recent urinary catheterization; and anal intercourse (with men and/or women).

CASE 6-9
Bsharma Caudwell
1. History

A. Has she been experiencing any difficulties with speech, using facial muscles, walking, coordination, weakness in her extremities, or dysphagia?   ESSENTIAL

Acute confusion in the elderly can be caused by a vast array of conditions, ranging from normal cognitive decline associated with aging to a serious septicemia. Cerebrovascular accidents, encephalitis, meningitis, hydrocephalus, Parkinson disease, hepatic encephalopathy, and many other neurologic conditions can present as acute confusion. Thus, questioning about symptoms of a neurological impairment is essential in the evaluation of a patient presenting with acute confusion.

B. Has she had any urinary urgency, frequency, dysuria, hematuria, abdominal pain, or flank pain?   ESSENTIAL

Approximately one third of elderly patients with a urinary tract infection (UTI) will present with confusion; however, only ~20% of those with a UTI will present with the typical signs of urinary urgency or frequency. Furthermore, in patients with an upper urinary tract infection, these characteristic findings are typically not present. On the other hand, flank pain is generally noticed by the patient or found upon physical examination. Hematuria (both gross and microscopic) can be present in both an upper and a lower urinary tract infection. New-onset urinary incontinence is sometimes the only urinary symptom an elderly patient might have with an acute urinary tract infection.

C. Does her confusion appear to remain constant or does it fluctuate?   ESSENTIAL

In evaluating an elderly patient with confusion, it is important to determine if the process represents changes accompanying the normal aging process, dementia, or delirium. All three of these conditions can exhibit some fluctuations in the degree of impairment; however, delirium is more likely to be worsened in the evenings and at night (known as the "sunsetting" phenomenon).

Furthermore, these conditions can be further delineated by the nature of their onset. Dementia and memory loss as a result of normal aging are generally gradual in onset. Delirium tends to have a much more rapid onset.

D. Has she had a vaginal discharge?   NONESSENTIAL

Vaginal discharges are most frequently caused by an infection of the vagina and/or cervix. However, atrophic vaginitis and allergic vaginitis are also potential causes. Nevertheless,

none of these conditions should cause a change in the patient's mental status.

E. Has she had chest pain, cough, wheezing, dyspnea, palpations, arm pain, dyspepsia, vertigo, presyncope, syncope, or diaphoresis?   ESSENTIAL

Pneumonia, pulmonary embolism, pneumothorax, myocardial infarction, cardiac arrhythmia, heart failure, and cerebral ischemia caused by cardiac emboli, as well as other cardiac and pulmonary conditions, can produce acute confusional states. Thus, questioning about symptoms of such is essential in the evaluation of a patient presenting with acute confusion.

2. Physical Examination

A. Thyroid palpation   ESSENTIAL

Because hypothyroidism and hyperthyroidism can cause acute confusion and delirium, the thyroid gland should be palpated for possible enlargement, tenderness, and irregularities in contour and consistency. However, the lack of an abnormality does not exclude a thyroid condition.

B. Heart and lung examination   ESSENTIAL

Auscultation of the heart is important to determine whether valvular heart disease, cardiomegaly, or distance heart sounds are present indicating the possibility of atrial emboli formation, endocarditis, subacute endocarditis, heart failure, pericarditis, or other less common cardiac conditions that can be associated with acute confusion. The presence of arrhythmias can be discovered during cardiac auscultation as well as by evaluating the patient's pulse. Furthermore, the blood pressure will provide additional clues to potential causes of acute confusional states including dehydration, hypotension, and hypertension.

Lung auscultation is important to evaluate for rales, rhonchi, wheezing, absent breath sounds, decreased breath sounds, and other abnormalities that could be responsible for potential cardiopulmonary and pulmonary causes of acute confusion such as heart failure, pulmonary embolism, pneumonia, and pneumothorax. Respiratory rate and oxygen saturation should also be performed to evaluate for the presence of hypoxemia, hypercapnia, hypocapnia, hypopnea, and hyperpnea that could represent the existence of a respiratory, pulmonary, or metabolic abnormality.

C. Abdominal examination   ESSENTIAL

The abdominal examination is essential to evaluate for the presence of any masses, organomegaly, tenderness, or bruits that could assist in the identification of the cause of Mrs. Caudwell's mental status changes (i.e., urinary retention, intestinal obstruction, hepatic failure, renal failure, abdominal aorta stenosis, and a slow-leaking abdominal aortic aneurysm).

D. Neurologic examination, including evaluation of mental status   ESSENTIAL

As stated earlier, many neurologic conditions can present as acute confusion. Therefore, not only does she require a neurologic examination, but she also needs an evaluation for her mental status changes. The mini mental status examination (MMSE) and the confusion assessment method (CAM) are generally effective tools for evaluating mental status changes and assisting to distinguish between dementia and delirium; however, because of language and cultural barriers, either assessment tool is going to be difficult to perform and interpret.

E. Evaluation for costovertebral angle (CVA) tenderness ESSENTIAL

Because renal abnormalities (including pyelonephritis) can cause acute confusion and her daughter has noticed her rubbing her flank, evaluating for CVA tenderness is indicated.

3. Diagnostic Studies

A. Complete blood count with differential (CBC w/diff) ESSENTIAL

A CBC w/diff is important because it can provide support regarding the presence of nonspecific conditions that could be associated with acute confusional states including leukocytosis (or occasionally a leukopenia) and/or a differential shift indicating the presence of an infectious process; hemoconcentration indicating dehydration; and anemia suggesting a chronic bleed.

B. Blood urea nitrogen (BUN) and creatinine   ESSENTIAL

A BUN and creatinine are important to evaluate renal and hepatic functioning. (For more, please see Case 6-6.)

C. Urinalysis   ESSENTIAL

A urinalysis will provide information regarding whether a urinary tract infection and/or other renal abnormalities are responsible for (or associated with) her acute confusional state. Additionally, the presence of glycosuria and ketonuria could indicate the presence of an impending diabetic ketoacidotic coma in patients who present with confusion, polyuria, polydipsia, nausea, vomiting, and fatigue. However, this is unlikely to be the presentation of diabetes mellitus in a patient of Mrs. Caudwell's age unless a significant infection is present.

D. Urine culture and sensitivity (C&S)   ESSENTIAL

A urine C&S is also indicated for Mrs. Caudwell because she is elderly and there is a concern that she might have a UTI. As stated previously, unless the leukocyte esterase and nitrites are positive on the dipstick and the microscopic examination reveals pyuria and bacteriuria, a urine culture is not indicated. However, because the leukocyte esterase and nitrite test on dipstick examination have a much lower sensitivity and specificity regarding their ability to predict a UTI in the elderly, a culture should automatically be performed if a UTI is suspected.

E. Blood culture and sensitivity (C&S)   ESSENTIAL

Blood cultures are also indicated because Mrs. Caudwell could be septic based on her confusion, fever, and leukocytosis. Septicemia, regardless of the cause (e.g., pneumonia, UTI, cellulitis, bacterial gastroenteritis, and meningitis), can cause an acute confusional state.

4. Diagnosis

A. Alzheimer disease   INCORRECT

Alzheimer disease is a form of dementia (not delirium) associated with degeneration of the brain cells. Because of its chronic nature and gradual onset, it can be ruled out as Mrs. Caudwell's most likely diagnosis. Furthermore, it is not

associated with a fever, CVA tenderness, leukocytosis, pyuria, bacteriuria, or urine abnormalities.

B. Pneumonia   INCORRECT

Pneumonia can present as acute confusion, fever, an elevated WBC count, and even CVA tenderness (in rare cases). However, it can be eliminated as Mrs. Caudwell's most likely diagnosis because of the absence of signs (abnormal breath sounds, dullness to percussion over the affected lung field, and some degree of hypoxemia) and symptoms (e.g., cough, dyspnea, chest discomfort, and intermittent diaphoresis) of pneumonia on her history and physical examination plus the presence of abnormal findings on her urinalysis.

C. Pyelonephritis   CORRECT

Pyelonephritis is an inflammatory process involving the renal pelvis, calyces, and parenchyma of the kidney; the majority of the time, it is caused by an infectious process. The diagnosis is based on a high index of suspicion from the information obtained on the patient's history and physical examination; it is confirmed by the presence of a positive bacterial culture and resolution of symptoms with appropriate antibiotics. It is very suggestive if the patient's urinalysis contains the same findings as a lower urinary tract infection (i.e., positive test for leukocyte esterase and nitrites, bacteriuria, and pyuria) plus WBC casts. RBC casts are occasionally identified as well. In addition to fever and CVA tenderness on the physical examination, nausea, vomiting, myalgias, and malaise are present. Other presentations of pyelonephritis in the elderly include confusion, unstable gait, new onset of falling, suprapubic pain, back pain, and septicemia. A CBC w/diff generally reveals a leukocytosis and a predominate neutrophilia. Although irritative urinary symptoms can be present, they are not necessary to make the diagnosis. Thus, pyelonephritis is Mrs. Caudwell's most likely diagnosis.

D. Interstitial cystitis   INCORRECT

Interstitial cystitis is a marked inflammatory condition of the bladder wall. It is typically associated with severe irritative urinary symptoms (and decreased bladder capacity when severe). It is associated with pyuria without significant bacteriuria (causing some experts to speculate that it might be viral in nature). It is not associated with fever, CVA tenderness, leukocytosis, or WBC (or RBC) casts in the urine. Thus, this is not Mrs. Caudwell's most likely diagnosis.

E. Heart failure   INCORRECT

Heart failure can essentially be ruled out as Mrs. Caudwell's most likely diagnosis based on her history and physical examination. She is not experiencing any of the characteristic symptoms (e.g., dyspnea, orthopnea, paroxysmal nocturnal dyspnea, or cough) nor exhibiting any of the classic physical findings (e.g., cardiomegaly, distant heart sounds, basilar rales, pedal edema, or jugular venous distension) that are the hallmark features of this disorder. Plus, it fails to account for her findings of fever, CVA tenderness, leukocytosis, bacteriuria, and pyuria.

5. Treatment Plan

A. Trial donepezil 5 mg once a day   INCORRECT

Donepezil is a reversible acetylcholinesterase inhibitor that is indicated for the treatment of Alzheimer dementia. Because Mrs. Caudwell's mental status changes appear to be caused by delirium secondary to pyelonephritis, not to Alzheimer dementia, donepezil is unlikely to have any significant effect on her mental status changes. Its most likely outcome for Mrs. Caudwell would be to provide her with unwanted adverse effects.

B. Hospitalization   CORRECT

Because of her moderately elevated WBC count, fever, and confusion, Mrs. Caudwell should be admitted for IV antibodies and fluids as well as close observation.

C. IV ampicillin and gentamicin until C&S results available, then continue or change based on her response and C&S findings   CORRECT

IV antibiotics should be instituted that cover not only *Escherichia coli,* which is responsible for the majority of UTIs, including pyelonephritis, but also other potential pathogens (e.g., *Pseudomonas aeruginosa, Enterococcus faecalis, Staphylococcus aureus, Citrobacter* sp., *Klebsiella* sp., *Proteus* sp., and *Providencia* sp.), because with age, *Escherichia coli* becomes less likely to cause pyelonephritis while these other pathogens become more likely. IV ampicillin and gentamicin is an appropriate first-line choice for pyelonephritis in the elderly.

D. Stat intravenous pyelogram (IVP)   INCORRECT

An IVP is not indicated at this time. With pyelonephritis, an imaging study is not indicated unless the patient is not responding to antibiotic therapy within 72 hours to rule out complications such as calculi, nephrolithiasis, abscesses, and/or obstructions. Then, a spiral CT of the abdomen and pelvis (not an IVP) is most likely to be the imaging study of choice.

E. Promethazine suppositories 12.5 mg every 8 to 12 hours as needed for nausea   INCORRECT

Promethazine suppositories are only FDA approved for use in motion sickness and perioperative nausea and vomiting. However, they are frequently used off-label for significant nausea and vomiting, especially when patients experience vomiting that is so severe they cannot effectively use oral medications. Promethazine oral tablets are indicated for severe nausea and vomiting.

However, because Mrs. Caudwell's nausea and vomiting would not be considered severe at this time, promethazine is not indicated because the potential risks could outweigh the potential benefits that she would derive from this medication. Promethazine and similar drugs can produce drowsiness, confusion, and central nervous system depression; therefore, it could further complicate the ability to accurately evaluate and monitor Mrs. Caudwell's mental status abnormality. Furthermore, these medications should be used with extreme caution in the elderly because of their potential adverse effects, including the potential for an increase in the incidence of falls and their associated consequences.

Epidemiologic and Other Data

The lifetime incidence of pyelonephritis for females in the United States is unknown. The incidence of pyelonephritis among women between the ages of 18 and 49 years old is estimated to be approximately 0.3 per 1000 women. Estimates on the lifetime incidence of an infection anywhere in the female urinary tract vary dramatically between sources, resulting in a range from 133 to 600 per 1000 women. The number of cases per year also varies significantly by source, starting at approximately 7 million and going to over 11 million pathogens involved.

Regardless of the discrepancies in the incidence of female urinary tract infections, there is consensus on the pathogens involved. Approximately 80% are caused by the gram-negative bacilli *Escherichia coli*. The remaining 20% are generally composed of *Enterobacter* sp., *Klebsiella* sp., *Proteus* sp., *Pseudomonas* sp., *Serratia* sp., and *Staphylococcus* sp. Women who require chronic catheterization, have a history of genitourinary instrumentation and/or surgery, and/or have urinary tract abnormalities tend to have urinary infections with a much higher incidence of atypical organisms.

REFERENCES/ADDITIONAL READING

Aghababian RV, ed. *Essentials of Emergency Medicine.* Sudbury, MA: Jones & Bartlett Publishers; 2006.
    Brinsfield K. Female genital tract. 1–94.
    Brown J. Pyelonephritis. 655–659.
    DiBella MD. Male genital tract. 723–727.
    Gomella LG, Letko J. Structural renal disorders. 651–654.
    Igoe G. Glomerular disorders. 660–663.
American Cancer Society. American Cancer Society guidelines for the early detection of cancer. http://www.cancer.org/docroot/PED/content/ PED_2_3X_ACS_Cancer_Detection_Guidelines_36.asp. Accessed October 25, 2008.
American Urological Association. Diagnosis of BPH. http://www.urologyhealth.org/adult/index.cfm?cat=09&topic=173. Accessed October 25, 2008.
American Urological Association. Management of BPH. http://www.auanet.org/guidelines/bph/cfm. Accessed October 25, 2008.
Centers for Disease Control and Prevention. Cancer—prostate cancer screening. http://www.cdc.gov/cancer/prostate/basic_info/screening.htm. (Last updated October 16, 2006.) Accessed October 25, 2008.
Centers for Disease Control and Prevention. Sexually transmitted diseases treatment guidelines, 2006. *MMWR.* 2006;55 (No. RR-11):1–94.
Fauci AS, Kasper DL, Longo DL, et al., eds. *Harrison's Principles of Internal Medicine.* 17th ed. New York: McGraw-Hill Medical; 2008.
    Asplin JR, Coe FL, Favus MJ. Nephrolithiasis. 1815–1820.
    Austen KF. Allergies, anaphylaxis, and systemic mastocytosis. 2061–2070.
    Bhasin S, Jameson JL. Disorders of the testes and male reproductive system. 2310–2324.
    Holmes K. Sexually transmitted infections: overview and clinical approach. 821–835.
    Josephson SA, Miller BL. Confusion and delirium. 158–162.
    Lewis JB. Glomerular diseases. 1782–1797.
    McVary K. Sexual dysfunction. 296–300.
    Scher HI. Benign and malignant diseases of the prostate. 593–600.
    Scher HI. Motzer RJ. Bladder and renal cell carcinomas. 589–593.
    Stamm WE. Chlamydial infections. 1070–1078.
    Stamm WE. Urinary tract infections, pyelonephritis, and prostatitis. 1820–1827.

Gershman K. Common geriatric problems. 1.13 Male sexual dysfunction (impotence). In: Gershman K. Onion DK, series eds. *The Little Black Book of Geriatrics*. 3rd ed. Sudbury, MA: Jones & Bartlett Publishers; 2006:50–51.

Gilbert ND, Moellering RC Jr, Eliopoulos GM, and Sande MA. (eds.) Clinical approach to initial choice of antimicrobial therapy. In: Gilbert ND, Moellering Jr. RC, Eliopoulos GM, and Sande MA.(eds.) *The Sanford Guide to Antimicrobial Therapy 2008*, 38th ed. Sperryville, VA: Antimicrobial Therapy, Inc. 2008:4–58.

Gonzales R, Kutner J. Disease screening, cancer, prostate. In: Gonzales R, Kutner J. eds. *Current Practice Guidelines in Primary Care 2009*. New York: McGraw-Hill Medical; 2009: 32–33.

Krieger JN. The problem with prostatitis. What do we know? What do we need to know? *J Urol*. 2004;172(2):432–433.

Lalani A, Schneeweiss, S. *The Hospital for Sick Children: Handbook of Pediatric Emergency Medicine*. Boston: Jones & Bartlett Publishers; 2008.
  Harrington L. Urological emergencies. 236–245.
  Thull-Freedman J. Renal emergencies. 228–235.

Litwin MS, Saigal CS, eds. *Urologic Diseases in America*. (NIH Publication No. 07-5512). Washington, DC: US Government Printing Office, US Department of Health and Human Services, Public Health Service, National Institutes of Health, National Institute of Diabetes and Digestive and Kidney Diseases; 2007:42–69. http://kidney.niddk.nih.gov/statistics/ uda/Urologic_Diseases_in_America.pdf. Accessed July 16, 2009.
  Griebling TL. Urinary tract infection in men. 587–619.
  McNaughton-Collins M, Joyce GF, Wise M, and Pontari MA. Prostatitis. 8–41.
  Wei JT, Calhoun E, Jacobson SJ. Benign prostatic hyperplasia. 42–69.

Lue TF, Giuliano F, Montorsi F, Rosen RC, Andersson KE, Althof S, et al. Summary of recommendations on sexual dysfunctions in men. *J Sex Med*. 2004;1(1):6–23.

MacLennon WJ. Urinary tract infections in the older patient. *Rev Clin Geront*. 2003;12:119–127.

Mengel MP, Schwiebert LP. *Family Medicine: Ambulatory Care and Prevention*. 5th ed. New York: McGraw-Hill Medical; 2009.
  Halvorsen JG. Sexual dysfunction. 744–759.
  Heydt FA, Epperly TD. Scrotal complaints. 384–389.
  Schwiebert LP. Dysuria in women. 140–145
  Schwiebert LP. Vaginal discharge. 430–434.
  Truong TT. Renal failure. 610–619.
  Waickus CM. Hematuria. 243–255.
  Walker L. Urinary symptoms in men. 413–420.

National High Blood Pressure Education Program. Special situations in hypertension management. *The Seventh Report of the Joint National Committee on Prevention, Detection, Evaluation, and Treatment of High Blood Pressure*. (NIH Publication No. 04-5230). Washington, DC: US Department of Health and Human Services, National Institutes of Health, National Heart, Lung, and Blood Institute; 2004: 33–58.http://www.nhlbi.nih.gov/guidelines/hypertension/jnc7full.pdf Accessed November 17, 2008.

National High Blood Pressure Education Program Working Group on High Blood Pressure in Children and Adolescents. Blood pressure tables. *The Fourth Report on the Diagnosis, Evaluation, and Treatment of High Blood Pressure in Children and Adolescents*. (NIH Publication No. 05-5267). Washington, DC: US Department of Health and Human Services, National Institutes of Health, National Heart, Lung, and Blood Institute; 2005:8–15. http://www.nhlbi.nih.gov/health/prof/heart/hbp/hbp_ped.pdf Accessed November 17, 2008.

Onion DK, series ed. *The Little Black Book of Primary Care*. 5th ed. Sudbury, MA: Jones & Bartlett Publishers; 2006.
  Onion DK, Sears S. Infectious disease. 9.4 Flagellate protozoans. 640–646.
  Onion DK, Sears S. Infectious disease. 9.7 Mycoplasma/Chlamydia. 596–601.
  Onion DK, Sears S. Renal/Urology. 17.9 Acquired renal diseases. 1021–1036.
  Onion DK. Renal/Urology. 17.11 Infections. 1042–1049.
  Onion DK. Renal/Urology. 17.12 Tumors/Cancers. 1049–1061.
  Onion DK, Sears S. Renal/Urology. 17.7 Miscellaneous. 1061–1065.

Pagana KD, Pagana TJ. *Mosby's Diagnostic and Laboratory Test Reference*. 8th ed. St. Louis: Mosby Elsevier; 2007 (multiple pages utilized to provide normal reference values for laboratory tests).

Pak CY. Medical management of urinary stone disease. *Nephron Clin Pract*. 2004;98(2):49–53.

Ronald A. The etiology of urinary tract infections: traditional and emerging pathogens. *Dis Mon*. 2003;49(2):71–82.

Shortliffe LM, McCue JD. Urinary tract infection at the age extremes: pediatric and geriatrics. *Am J Med*. 2002;113(Supp 1A): S55–S66.

US Preventive Services Task Force. Screening for prostate cancer: US Preventive Services Task Force recommendation statement. *Ann Intern Med*. 2008;149:185–191.

Vranken MV. Prevention and treatment of sexually transmitted diseases: an update. *Am Fam Physician*. 2007;76 (12): 1827–1832.

CHAPTER 7

CASES IN REPRODUCTIVE MEDICINE*

CASE 7-1

Cathy Dennison

Mrs. Dennison is a 48-year-old Asian American female who presents for a refill of her oral contraceptives (ethinyl estradiol 35 µg and norethindrone 1 mg daily for 21 days, then off for 7 days). She has been on the same oral contraceptives (OCs) for approximately 16 years without any problems. However, 2 months ago she did not experience any withdrawal bleeding while on her inactive pills. In fact, she has not experienced any visible bleeding or spotting since her last menstrual period (LMP) nearly 3 months ago. Until then, her periods have always been regular, but light, on the OCs. She has not missed any pills nor taken any other medications.

She denies ever experiencing chest pain/pressure, dyspnea, orthopnea, edema, lightheadedness, vertigo, presyncope, headache, abdominal pain, or localized weakness.

She has a history of hyperlipidemia, which is controlled with rosuvastatin 20 mg once a day, and hypertension, which is treated with triamterene 37.5 mg with hydrochlorothiazide 25 mg once a day. She is on no other prescription medications. She does not take any over-the-counter medications, vitamins, supplements, or herbal preparations. Her only surgery was a cesarean section 17 years ago because she was unable to deliver naturally due to the infant's size (10 lb 3oz). That was her only pregnancy, surgery, and hospitalization. She is sexually active with her husband of 25 years. To her knowledge, their relationship is mutually monogamous.

She has undergone annual Papanicolaou (Pap) tests every year for the past 20 years (the last one 1 year ago), and they have always been normal. She has never had a mammogram. Her last lipid panel was done 6 weeks ago and was normal. Her family history is positive for hypertension (mother, father, and older sister), hyperlipidemia (mother, father, and older sister), and nonfatal premature myocardial infarction (MI) (father at 47 years old).

1. Based on this information, which of the following questions are essential to ask Mrs. Dennison and why?

   A. Did she have gestational diabetes mellitus (GDM) with her pregnancy?

   B. Is she experiencing vaginal dryness, hot flashes, or night sweats?

   C. Is she experiencing any fatigue, nausea, vomiting, or breast tenderness?

   D. How old were her paternal grandmother, maternal grandmother, mother, and aunts when they went through menopause?

   E. What is her smoking history?

Patient Responses

Mrs. Dennison had gestational diabetes with her pregnancy, which was controlled with diet alone. Her last fasting plasma glucose (FPG) was 6 months ago and it was normal.

She is not experiencing any signs or symptoms of menopause, including hot flashes, night sweats, or vaginal dryness, or any symptoms of pregnancy, including nausea, vomiting, fatigue, or breast tenderness. She does not know the ages of menopause for her female family members.

She has smoked one pack of cigarettes per day since she was 18 years old (and therefore has a ~30 pack-year history).

2. Based on this information, which of the following components of a physical examination are essential to conduct on Mrs. Dennison and why?

   A. Oropharyngeal examination

   B. Breast examination

   C. Abdominal examination

   D. Pelvic examination

   E. Rectal examination with occult blood testing of any stool obtained

---

*Remember, for each question, none to all of the answers could be correct/essential or incorrect/nonessential. See page 264 for Chapter 7 answers.

Physical Examination Findings

Mrs. Dennison is 5'4" tall and weighs 195 lb (body mass index [BMI] = 33.5). Other vital signs are blood pressure (BP), 140/92 mm Hg; pulse, 88 beats per minute (BPM) and regular; respiratory rate, 12/min and regular; and oral temperature, 98.6°F.

Her oropharyngeal examination is unremarkable.

Her breasts are without visible lesions, retraction, or other abnormalities. They are normal in consistency and without masses. There is no nipple discharge. Axillary, infraclavicular, and supraclavicular lymph nodes are nonpalpable.

Her abdomen has normoactive and equal bowel sounds in all four quadrants. It is soft, nontender, and without masses or organomegaly. Her rectal examination is unremarkable.

Her external genital examination reveals no discolorations, lesions, excoriation, or other skin changes. Her vaginal mucosa is normal in color and without lesions or discharge. Her cervix is normal in appearance with a parous os, without lesions, and without discharge. Her uterus is normal size and shape without any tenderness. Her adnexal areas are without masses or tenderness; however, her ovaries are not palpable (probably because of her truncal obesity).

She does not have any external rectal lesions or fissures. Her internal rectal examination reveals no lesions, masses, or tenderness. Her stool tests negative for blood.

3. Based on this information, which of the following diagnostic studies are essential to perform on Mrs. Dennison and why?

   A. Pap smear
   B. Mammogram
   C. DNA probe testing for chlamydia and gonorrhea
   D. Urinary human chorionic gonadotropin (HCG) test
   E. Screening colonoscopy

Diagnostic Results

Mrs. Dennison's Pap smear, mammogram, DNA probe, urinary HCG, and colonoscopy were negative.

4. Based on this information, which one of the following is Mrs. Dennison's most likely diagnosis and why?

   A. Routine oral contraceptive refill
   B. Oral contraceptive refill for patient with multiple risk factors
   C. Contraceptive counseling for a patient with hyperlipidemia, obesity, and type 2 diabetes mellitus
   D. Contraception counseling for a patient with multiple risk factors for oral contraceptive usage
   E. Class II obesity, hypertension, and hyperlipidemia

5. Based on this diagnosis, which ONE of the following is the most appropriate treatment plan for Mrs. Dennison at this time and why?

   A. Refill combination oral contraceptives for 1 year
   B. Decrease estrogen component of OCs to 20 µg
   C. Advise her that she has too many risk factors (and what they are) to safely continue taking a combination OC;

however, prescribe her current combination OC for 6 months if she promises to modify her risk factors by quitting smoking and losing weight

   D. Advise her that she has too many risk factors (and what they are) to safely continue combination OCs, provide her with information on alternative methods (including mechanism of action, efficacy rates, possible adverse effects, advantages, and disadvantages), and assist her in determining which one she would like to try with assurance that she can switch to another method if she is not satisfied with her initial choice
   E. Refuse to provide oral contraceptives until she gets an electrocardiogram (ECG) and treadmill stress test (TST)

CASE 7-2
Dianne Edwards

Ms. Edwards is a 36-year-old white female who presents complaining of a "female infection." She has been experiencing a slight to moderate amount of a clear, slightly malodorous vaginal discharge for 1 week. She denies dysuria, urinary urgency, urinary frequency, abdominal pain, bowel changes, vomiting, fever, chills, or rash. However, since starting the contraceptive ring ~4 months ago, she sometimes feels nauseous in the morning; however, it resolves when she eats her breakfast.

Her only medication is the etonogestrel/ethinyl estradiol vaginal ring for 21 days every 28 days. She placed her fourth contraceptive ring 18 days ago. However, she removed it yesterday because she was concerned that the discharge could indicate early toxic shock syndrome (TSS). She has been sexually active in what she assumes to be a monogamous relationship for approximately 5 years. She has not had intercourse since removing the ring. She is on no other prescription or over-the-counter medications, vitamins, supplements, or herbal preparations. She does not have any medical problems, has never had surgery, and has never been hospitalized. Her last menstrual period was approximately 3.5 weeks ago and was normal. She has never been pregnant. Her last pelvic examination, Pap smear, and clinical breast examination (CBE) were 4 months ago and reported as normal. Her family history is noncontributory.

1. Based on this information, which of the following questions are essential to ask Ms. Edwards and why?

   A. Why doesn't she have any children?
   B. Is the discharge associated with vulvovaginal itching?
   C. What is her smoking history?
   D. Is she allergic to latex?
   E. What is her douching history?

Patient Responses

Ms. Edwards and her partner have never desired to have children. Her vaginal discharge is not associated with vulvovaginal itching. She has never smoked. To her knowledge she is not allergic to latex. She does not douche.

2. Based on this information, which of the following components of a physical examination are essential to conduct on Ms. Edwards and why?

    A. Palpation of the cervical lymph nodes
    B. Breast examination
    C. Abdominal examination
    D. Rectal examination
    E. Pelvic examination

Physical Examination Findings

Ms. Edwards is 5'4" tall and weighs 125 lb (BMI = 21.5). Other vital signs are BP, 116/62 mm Hg; pulse, 76 BPM and regular; respiratory rate, 10/min and regular; and oral temperature, 98.3°F.

Her cervical lymph nodes are not palpable.

Her breasts are without visible skin changes, retraction, or other abnormalities. They are normal in consistency and without masses. There is no nipple discharge. Axillary lymph nodes are nonpalpable.

Her abdomen has normoactive and equal bowel sounds in all four quadrants. It is soft, nontender, and without masses or organomegaly. Her rectal examination is unremarkable.

Her external genital examination reveals no discolorations, erythema, lesions, excoriation, or other abnormalities. Her vaginal mucosa is slightly erythematous in color and without abnormal lesions. She has a small amount of clear discharge in the posterior fornix of her vagina. Her cervix is normal in appearance with a normal-appearing os and no lesions, discharge, or tenderness. Her uterus is normal in size and shape without any tenderness. Her ovaries are normal size, smooth, and without masses or tenderness.

3. Based on this information, which of the following diagnostic studies are essential to perform on Ms. Edwards and why?

    A. Urinary human chorionic gonadotropin (HCG) test
    B. Pap smear
    C. Wet-mount microscopy of vaginal secretions with or without vaginal pH, "whiff" test for amine odor, and point-of-care testing for vaginal pathogens
    D. DNA testing for *Chlamydia trachomatis* and *Neisseria gonorrhoeae*
    E. Mammogram

Diagnostic Results

Ms. Edwards' urinary HCG test was negative. Her wet-mount microscopy of her vaginal secretions revealed 10 to 15 white blood cells per high-powered field (WBCs/HPF, normal: < 5), a trace bacteria (normal: trace to 1+), 2+ epithelial cells (normal: 1–4+) that are normal in appearance (no clue cells), no trichomonads (normal: none), and no budding yeast or hyphae (normal: none to rare). Her vaginal pH was 4.2 (normal: ≤ 4.5) and her whiff amine test was negative (normal: negative). Her point-of-care test results were also negative (normal: negative). Her Pap smear, mammogram, and DNA testing for chlamydia and gonorrhea are pending.

4. Based on this information, which one of the following is Ms. Edwards' most likely diagnosis and why?

    A. Vulvovaginitis/vaginitis caused by bacterial vaginosis
    B. Vulvovaginitis/vaginitis caused by gonorrhea
    C. Vulvovaginitis/vaginitis caused by trichomoniasis
    D. Early pelvic inflammatory disease (PID)
    E. Adverse effect of the contraceptive ring

5. Based on this diagnosis, which of the following are appropriate components of a treatment plan for Ms. Edwards and why?

    A. Advise her she has a sexually transmitted infection (STI) and to abstain from intercourse until after her partner has been evaluated and treated
    B. Provide appropriate anti-infective therapy
    C. Advise her that the discharge is secondary to her contraceptive ring and her contraception method can be changed if she desires
    D. Advise her that if she desires to continue with the vaginal ring, she should rinse it off with cold to lukewarm water and reinsert it for the remainder of the 21 days for this ring's cycle, then stop for 1 week (as usual) for withdrawal bleeding as scheduled
    E. Advise her that if she wants to continue with her contraceptive ring, she should properly dispose of the ring she removed yesterday and insert a new ring as soon as possible, then wear it for 3 weeks as usual

CASE 7-3
Ernsteine Fickelstein

Ernsteine is a 16-year-old African American female who is accompanied by her mother for evaluation of not reaching menarche. Ernsteine is "embarrassed" because all of her friends have been menstruating for several years now. She has had breast development, pubic hair, and axillary hair since she was 11 years old.

She experiences two types of abdominal pain about the same time every month. The first, she describes as a mild (1 out of 10 on the pain scale) ache in either her right or left lower quadrant for 1 to 2 days. Approximately 2 weeks after this mild pain ceases, she experiences a more severe (4 out of 10 on the pain scale) suprapubic cramping-type pain of 2 to 3 days' duration. She is unaware of any precipitating, aggravating, or alleviating factors for either type of pain. Neither are associated with vaginal bleeding, spotting, or any type of discharge; nor does she experience nausea, vomiting, bowel changes, rectal bleeding, hematuria, dysuria, frequency, fever, chills, or back pain with or without the aforementioned abdominal pain. She denies any trauma or sexual abuse.

She has no known medical conditions. She has never had any surgery nor been hospitalized. She is not taking prescription or over-the-counter medications, vitamins, supplements, or herbal preparations. She denies ever being sexually active, smoking, drinking alcohol, or using illicit drugs. Her mother is concerned her problem stems from a vegetarian diet.

1. Based on this information, which of the following questions are essential to ask Ernsteine and why?

    A. What are her dietary and exercise habits?
    B. Why is she a vegetarian?
    C. Does she experience headaches, visual disturbances, or abnormalities of smell?
    D. What does she think of her body's appearance and size?
    E. Is she experiencing excess emotional stress with family, school, or friends?

Patient Responses

Ernsteine is a vegetarian but she does consume dairy products and eggs. She ensures that she gets adequate protein and calcium in her diet. She's a vegetarian because she is opposed to eating animals. She does aerobic exercises for one-half hour a day at least 5 days per week. Plus, she is currently practicing ballet for 1 to 1.5 hours per day, 7 days a week because she has a recital next week; however, her normal practice routine is 1 hour three times per week.

She denies having headaches, visual disturbances, or abnormalities of smell. She feels that she is "too thin" and her nose is "too big." Other than her ballet recital next week, she claims she is not under any increased stress. Her mother agrees with all of Ernsteine's responses.

2. Based on this information, which of the following components of a physical examination are essential to perform on Ernsteine and why?

    A. Breast examination
    B. Abdominal examination
    C. Pelvic examination
    D. Cranial nerve testing
    E. Skin examination

Physical Findings

Ernsteine is 5'7" tall and weighs 118 lb (BMI = 18.5). Other vital signs are BP, 92/56 mm Hg; pulse, 68 BPM and regular; respirations, 8/min and regular; and oral temperature, 97.7°F.

She has normal breast development for age (Tanner stage 5). They are without masses, tenderness, color changes, skin changes, lesions, or nipple discharge. Her axillary, infraclavicular, and supraclavicular lymph nodes are not enlarged or tender.

Her abdominal examination reveals normoactive bowel sounds in all four quadrants. There are no masses, organomegaly, or tenderness.

Her pubic hair is normal in texture and distribution. Her external genitalia is without abnormalities except for a hymen that is closed, is bulging, and appears to have old blood behind it. Because of this finding, the remainder of her pelvic examination could not be performed. However, a rectal examination confirms the presence of a uterus.

Her skin is normal in temperature but dry and without scaling, excoriations, lesions, abnormalities of color, or increased lanugo.

Her cranial nerves are grossly intact.

3. Based on this information, which of the following diagnostic studies are essential to conduct on Ernsteine and why?

    A. Follicle-stimulating hormone (FSH) level
    B. Prolactin level
    C. Testosterone level
    D. Estradiol level
    E. Urinary human chorionic gonadotropin (HCG)

Diagnostic Test Results

Ernsteine's FSH level was 7.5 IU/L (normal follicular: 1.37–9.9) and her luteinizing hormone (LH) level was 10.5 IU/L (normal follicular: 1.68–15). Her prolactin level was 22 ng/ml (normal nonpregnant adult females: 0–25). Her testosterone was 35 pg/ml (normal 16- to 19-year-old females: < 70). Her estradiol was 175 pg/ml (normal follicular, adult female: 20–350). Her HCG was negative (normal: negative).

4. Based on this information, which one of the following is Ernsteine's most likely diagnosis and why?

    A. Secondary amenorrhea caused by a local genital abnormality
    B. Primary amenorrhea secondary to imperforated hymen
    C. Primary amenorrhea secondary to müllerian agenesis
    D. Primary amenorrhea caused by anorexia nervosa
    E. Secondary amenorrhea caused by polycystic ovarian syndrome

5. Based on this diagnosis, which of the following are appropriate components of a treatment plan for Ernsteine and why?

    A. Refer to gynecologist
    B. Start metformin
    C. Start estrogen therapy
    D. Psychiatric referral for eating disorder
    E. Brain magnetic resonance imaging (MRI) with emphasis on pituitary/hypothalamus

CASE 7-4
Felicia Goldstein

Felicia is a 16-year-old white female who is brought in by her paternal grandmother (and legal guardian) with the chief complaint of very heavy menstrual bleeding. She achieved menarche approximately 1 year ago and this is her fourth menstrual period. In her opinion, her menses have always been much heavier than her friends, and they appear to be getting heavier. Her flow with her last menstrual period (3 months ago) required two super-tampons and an overnight pad every 2 hours at its maximum intensity. Her menses generally last from 7 to 9 days and is most severe on days 3 to 5. She started her current one yesterday and is already requiring two super-tampons and an overnight pad every hour. Her cycles appear to be irregularly irregular. She experiences nausea, hot flashes, sweating, lightheadedness, generalized weakness, and marked fatigue with her menses. Although she has never had a syncopal episode, she felt like she was going to "pass out" earlier today. This is what prompted her visit.

She does not have vomiting, back/flank pain, dysuria, urinary urgency, urinary frequency, bowel changes, fever, chills, palpations, dyspnea, edema, cyanosis, headaches, visual changes, abnormalities of smell, or galactorrhea. Between menses, she is essentially asymptomatic except for moderate fatigue, which her grandmother attributes to being a "teenager."

She is not taking any prescription or over-the-counter medications, vitamins, supplements, or herbal products. She does not have any known medical problems, has not been hospitalized, has not had any surgeries, and has not experienced any major trauma. She denies ever being sexually active, smoking cigarettes, drinking alcohol, or using illicit substances. Her mother is deceased from hemorrhaging while giving birth to Felicia. Otherwise, her family history is unremarkable, including for any known bleeding disorders.

1. Based on this information, which of the following questions are essential to ask Felicia and why?

   A. Does she bruise easily, bleed when she brushes her teeth, take a long time to cease bleeding after a laceration/abrasion, or experience frequent nosebleeds?
   B. Does she experience dysmenorrhea? If yes, what is its severity?
   C. When are she and her boyfriend planning on becoming sexually active?
   D. Does she experience premenstrual symptoms?
   E. Has she recently had any unintentional weight loss, polydipsia, or polyuria?

Patient Responses

Felicia has noticed that she bruises easily and "thinks" she might take longer than "normal" to stop bleeding following minor trauma. She does not have any gingival bleeding with brushing her teeth and has never experienced epistaxis.

She only experiences very mild lower abdominal cramping at the onset of her menses; otherwise, she does not have any abdominal pain or discomfort. Felicia has never experienced any premenstrual symptoms, weight loss, polydipsia, or polyuria. She does not have a boyfriend.

2. Based on this information, which of the following components of the physical examination are essential to perform on Felicia and why?

   A. Heart examination
   B. Breast examination
   C. Abdominal examination
   D. Pelvic examination
   E. Skin and conjunctival examination

Physical Examination Findings

Felicia is 5'5" tall and weighs 125 lb (BMI = 20.9). Other vital signs include BP lying down, 100/64 mm Hg; BP sitting, 88/60 mm Hg; BP standing, 60/40 mm Hg; pulse, 120 BPM and regular; respiratory rate, 12/min and regular; and oral temperature, 98.6°F.

Her heart appears to be regular in rhythm but reveals a tachycardia of 124 BPM. There is no evidence of a murmur, gallop, or rub. Her apical impulse is normal and nondisplaced. Her lungs are clear to auscultation.

Her breasts are normal in contour and consistency. She does not have any skin changes or masses. Her nipples are normal in appearance and do not exhibit any spontaneous or induced discharge.

Her abdomen reveals normoactive and equal bowel sounds in all four quadrants. It is soft and without masses or organomegaly. She does have some mild suprapubic tenderness without rebound or guarding.

Her external genitalia, vaginal mucosa, and cervix are covered with bright red blood, but no lesions or other mucosal abnormalities are apparent. Her posterior fornix is filled with blood and contains a large blood clot. The bleeding is coming from her cervical os, which has another large clot protruding from it. Her uterus is normal size and shape and slightly tender. Her chandelier sign is negative. Her ovaries are normal in size, nontender, and without masses.

Her skin is pale appearing but does not exhibit any evidence of jaundice. It is of normal temperature but slightly diaphoretic; no rashes, lesions, or other abnormalities are identified. Other than slightly pale palpebral conjunctivae, her eye examination is normal.

3. Based on this information, which of the following diagnostic studies are essential to perform on Felicia and why?

   A. Pap test
   B. Urinary human chorionic gonadotropin (HCG) test
   C. Total testosterone level
   D. Complete blood count with differential (CBC w/diff) and actual platelet count
   E. Prothrombin time (PT) and partial thromboplastin time (PTT)

Diagnostic Results

Felicia's urinary HCG was negative. Her testosterone level was 35 ng/dl (normal female ages 16–19 years old with a Tanner stage 4 or 5: < 70 ng/dl). Her Pap smear results are pending.

Her CBC revealed a red blood cell (RBC) count of $3.6 \times 10^6/\mu l$ (normal female: 4.2–5.4) with a mean corpuscular volume (MCV) of 79 μm^3 (normal adult: 80–95), a mean corpuscular hemoglobin (MCH) of 24 pg (normal adult: 27–31), a mean corpuscular hemoglobin concentration (MCHC) of 33 g/dl (normal adult: 32–36), and a red blood cell distribution width (RDW) of 12.5% (normal adult: 11–14.5). Her white blood cell (WBC) count was 8500/mm³ (normal adult: 5000–10,000) with 65% neutrophils (normal: 55–70), 26% lymphocytes (normal: 20–40), 4% monocytes (normal: 2–8), 4% eosinophils (normal: 1–4), and 1% basophils (normal: 0.5–1). Her hemoglobin (Hgb) was 8.8 g/dl (normal female: 12–16) and her hematocrit (HCT) was 27% (normal female: 37–47). Her platelet (thrombocyte) count was 160,000/mm³ (normal adult: 150,000–400,000) and her mean platelet volume (MPV) was 10.3 fl (normal: 7.4–10.4). Her smear was consistent with these results.

Her PT was 11.5 seconds (normal: 11–12.5) and her PTT was 85 seconds (normal: 60–70).

4. Based on this information, which one of the following is Felicia's most likely diagnosis and why?

A. Normal menstruation

B. Ovulatory abnormal vaginal bleeding (AVB)

C. Anovulatory abnormal vaginal bleeding (AVB) caused by a coagulopathy

D. Endometrial carcinoma

E. Spontaneous abortion

5. Based on this diagnosis, which of the following are appropriate components of a treatment plan for Felicia and why?

A. Start two large-bore IV lines of normal saline solution (NSS)

B. Hospitalize and obtain an immediate consultation with a gynecologist

C. Coagulation factor concentrations

D. Administer conjugated estrogens 25 mg IV stat

E. Administer methylergonovine maleate 0.2 mg IM; repeat every 2 to 4 hours as needed

CASE 7-5

Ginger Halstead

Mrs. Halstead is a 41-year-old African American female who presents with the chief complaint of "a strange feeling in my belly." The best she can describe the feeling is an "uncomfortable" (but not really painful) suprapubic sensation that has been present, without change, for approximately 2 to 3 months. It never varies in intensity nor does it fluctuate with her menstrual cycle. She knows of no aggravating or alleviating factors. She has not been experiencing any nausea, vomiting, bowel changes, abdominal pain in other locations, dysuria, urinary urgency, urinary frequency, hematuria, vaginal discharge, fever, chills, or headaches.

Her last menstrual period was 3.5 weeks ago and essentially normal. For the past year, her menses have been slightly heavier than usual; still, she only requires approximately 20 regular tampons per cycle. She has not experienced a change in the type, degree, or duration of her dysmenorrhea. Her menstrual periods continue to be of the same duration (5 days). She still menstruates every 30 days as she has done since her bilateral tubal ligation (BTL) 5 years ago.

She has been married for 15 years and is in what she assumes to be a mutually monogamous relationship. She has three normal children who were all delivered vaginally without any pregnancy, delivery, or postpartum complications. She never had a spontaneous or induced abortion. Besides childbirth, her only other hospitalization was 6 years ago for a nontraumatic deep vein thrombosis. She has no known medical problems. She does not take any prescription or over-the-counter medications, vitamins, supplements, or herbal preparations. She does not drink alcohol. She continues to smoke one pack per day (PPD) as she has done since the age of 16 years. Her last pelvic examination, clinical breast examination (CBE), Pap smear, and mammogram were 9 months ago and reported as normal by her. Her family history is unremarkable.

1. Based on this information, which of the following questions are essential to ask Mrs. Halstead and why?

A. Is her abdominal discomfort associated with intermenstrual vaginal bleeding?

B. Is she experiencing dyspareunia?

C. Has she noticed visual abnormalities or changes in her sense of smell?

D. Has she had any weight gain, cold intolerance, or dryness of her skin?

E. Does she have any other concerns she would like to address?

Patient Responses

Mrs. Halstead is not experiencing any intermenstrual vaginal bleeding, dyspareunia, visual changes, alterations in her sense of smell, weight loss, cold intolerance, or skin dryness. She denies having any other concerns that she wants to address today.

2. Based on this information, which of the following components of a physical examination are essential to conduct on Mrs. Halstead and why?

A. Thyroid palpation

B. Breast examination

C. Heart and lung examination

D. Abdominal examination

E. Pelvic examination

Physical Examination Findings

Mrs. Halstead is 5'5" tall and weighs 120 lb (BMI = 20). Other vital signs include BP, 100/66 mm Hg; pulse, 68 BPM and regular; respiratory rate, 10/min and regular; and oral temperature, 98.8°F.

Her thyroid is not enlarged or tender to palpate; additionally, there are no masses present.

Her heart is regular in rate and rhythm. There are no murmurs, gallops, or rubs. Her lungs are clear to auscultation.

Mrs. Halstead's abdominal examination reveals normoactive and equal bowel sounds in all four quadrants. She has a smooth, slightly firm, symmetric, suprapubic mass that extends approximately 2 cm above her pubic bone at its greatest height. It is not tender to palpate. The remainder of her abdomen is unremarkable.

Her external genital examination reveals no discolorations, erythema, lesions, excoriation, or other abnormalities. She does have two well-healed episiotomy scars at 3 and 9 o'clock. Her vaginal mucosa is normal in color and without lesions or discharge. Her cervix is normal in appearance without lesions or discharge. Her uterus is enlarged to approximately 14 weeks' gestational size; however, it is smooth in contour, normal in consistency, and nontender. Her ovaries are normal sized and without masses or tenderness.

3. Based on this information, which of the following diagnostic studies are essential to perform on Mrs. Halstead and why?

A. Hematocrit and hemoglobin (H&H)

B. Endometrial biopsy

C. Urinary human chorionic gonadotropin (HCG) test

D. Pelvic ultrasound

E. Urinalysis

Diagnostic Results

Mrs. Halstead's hemoglobin was 13.8 g/dl (normal female: 12–16) and her hematocrit was 42% (normal female: 37–47).

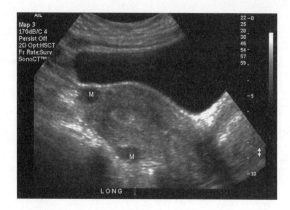

Figure 7-1 Ultrasound revealing multiple discrete solid masses in the uterine wall.

Her urinary HCG was negative. Her urinalysis was within normal limits.

Her pelvic ultrasound revealed an enlarged (~14-week gestational size), slightly asymmetric uterus with multiple discrete, solid masses throughout the uterine wall (the largest being 2 cm); the outer surface of the uterus was smooth; and the uterine cavity was empty and had a relatively smooth mucosal surface. The ovaries were normal sized and without masses. No other abnormalities were identified. Please see **Figure 7-1** for her ultrasound findings. Her Pap smear is pending.

4. Based on this information, which one of the following is Mrs. Halstead's most likely diagnosis and why?

    A. Adenomyosis
    B. Endometriosis
    C. Intramural uterine leiomyomas
    D. Subserosal leiomyomas of the uterus
    E. Submucosal uterine fibroids

5. Based on this diagnosis, which of the following are appropriate components of a treatment plan for Mrs. Halstead and why?

    A. Advise her of the diagnosis, its significance, potential complications, actions required if her symptoms increase, and treatment options
    B. Start her on low-dose combination oral contraceptives to decrease her menstrual flow and alleviate the dysmenorrhea
    C. Insert progesterone intrauterine device (IUD) to decrease her menstrual flow and alleviate the dysmenorrhea
    D. Refer to gynecologist for uterine fibroid embolization
    E. Obtain abdominal computed tomography (CT) scan

CASE 7-6

Hillary Indigo

Mrs. Indigo is a 26-year-old white female who presents with lower abdominal pain. It is a severe (8 out of 10 on the pain scale at its maximum), intermittent, crampy, left lower quadrant to suprapubic pain that radiates into her sacrum. It is associated with minimal vaginal "spotting" but no other vaginal discharge. Her pain began "all the sudden" while she was in the shower this morning and is increasing slightly in intensity and frequency. She is unaware of any aggravating or alleviating factors.

She has been experiencing some early morning nausea for the past 3 to 4 weeks. Although it is unaffected by the pain, it is worsened by smelling and/or drinking coffee. It appears to be alleviated by eating something "bland" for breakfast such as dry cereal, toast, crackers, or oatmeal. She has not experienced any vomiting. She denies bowel changes, fever, chills, myalgias, arthralgias, urinary urgency, urinary frequency, dysuria, and hematuria.

Her LMP was 3.5 weeks ago; however, it was "lighter" than usual in both quantity of flow and duration. She normally has regular menstrual periods at 30-day intervals. She and her husband of 2 years have been attempting to conceive since she discontinued oral contraceptives 4 months ago. She took the same low-dose combination oral contraceptive for approximately 8 years without difficulty. As near as she knows her relationship with her husband is mutually monogamous.

Mrs. Indigo has no known medical problems and has never been pregnant. She has never had any surgeries nor been hospitalized. She is taking folic acid to prevent neural tube defects should she become pregnant. She is on no other prescription or over-the-counter medications, vitamins, supplements, or herbal preparations. She is not allergic to any medications. She does not smoke, drink alcohol, or use drugs. Her family history is negative.

1. Based on this information, which of the following questions are essential to ask Mrs. Indigo and why?

    A. What does she mean by "spotting"?
    B. Has she recently consumed any unwashed fruits or vegetables?
    C. Does she have a history of recent trauma?
    D. Has she ever had pelvic inflammatory disease (PID)?
    E. Has she experienced any lightheadedness, vertigo, presyncope, syncope, tachycardia, or diaphoresis, especially with standing?

Patient Responses

Mrs. Indigo further defines vaginal "spotting" as a small amount of bright red blood on her underwear and on the toilet tissue when she wipes after urinating.

She has not consumed any unwashed fruits or vegetables. She has never had PID.

She denies urinary urgency, urinary frequency, dysuria, hematuria, lightheadedness, vertigo, presyncope, syncope, tachycardia, diaphoresis, or trauma.

2. Based on this information, which of the following components of a physical examination are essential to conduct on Mrs. Indigo and why?

    A. Oral mucosa examination
    B. Examination of the conjunctivae of the eyes
    C. Palpation of the thyroid
    D. Abdominal examination
    E. Pelvic examination

Physical Examination Findings

Mrs. Indigo is 5'5" tall and weighs 140 lb (BMI = 23.3). Other vital signs include BP, and pulse lying down, 106/66 mm Hg and 72 BPM; BP and pulse sitting, 110/68 mm Hg and 76 BPM; BP and pulse standing, 114/70 mm Hg and 84 BPM; respiratory rate, 12/min and regular; and oral temperature, 98.7°F.

Her conjunctivae and oral mucosa are normal in color and without any lesions or other abnormalities. Her thyroid is palpable, smooth, nontender, and normal in size.

Her abdominal examination reveals normoactive bowel sounds in all four quadrants. It is soft but associated with moderate left lower quadrant and suprapubic tenderness without rebound or guarding. She does not have any palpable masses or organomegaly.

Her external genitalia and vaginal mucosa are normal. She does have a small amount of bleeding coming from her cervical os, which appears to be closed and normal in size. The cervix itself is normal in appearance. The uterus is normal in size, shape, and consistency. It is slightly tender to palpate but her chandelier sign is negative. Her right adnexal area reveals a nontender normal-sized ovary. Her left adnexal area is very tender to palpate. Because of this marked tenderness, the size and consistency of her left ovary cannot be adequately assessed.

A urinary HCG test is performed and is positive.

3. Based on this information, which of the following diagnostic studies are essential to perform on Mrs. Indigo and why?

  A. Qualitative serum human chorionic gonadotropin (HCG)
  B. Quantitative serum human chorionic gonadotropin (HCG)
  C. Pelvic ultrasound, preferably with vaginal probe
  D. Hematocrit and hemoglobin (H&H)
  E. Serum progesterone level

Diagnostic Tests Results

Mrs. Indigo's qualitative serum HCG was positive. Her quantitative serum HCG was 7000 mIU/ml (normal nonpregnant: < 5; normal pregnant [depends on gestational week]: < 1 week: 5–50; 2 weeks: 50–500; 3 weeks: 100–10,000; 4 weeks: 1000–30,000; 5 weeks: 3500–115,000; 6–8 weeks: 12,000–270,000; 12 weeks: 15,000–220,000).

Her pelvic ultrasound was normal except for a very small amount of fluid in her cul-de-sac; no uterine sac was identified in her uterine cavity with either the abdominal or vaginal approach. Please see **Figure 7-2** for her ultrasonic findings.

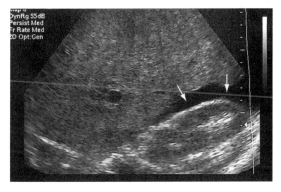

Figure 7-2 Ultrasound revealing empty uterus and edema of lining of fallopian tube.

Her Hgb was 14.4 g/dl (normal adult female: 12–16) and her HCT was 44% (normal adult female: 37–47). Her serum progesterone level was 4 ng/ml (normal pregnancy [varies by trimester]: first trimester: 725–4400; second trimester: 1950–8250; and third trimester: 6500–22,900).

4. Based on this information, which one of the following is Mrs. Indigo's most likely diagnosis and why?

  A. Normal pregnancy
  B. Spontaneous abortion
  C. Threatened abortion
  D. Ectopic pregnancy
  E. Early menstruation caused by an anovulatory cycle

5. Based on this diagnosis, which of the following are appropriate components of a treatment plan for Mrs. Indigo and why?

  A. Hysterosalpingography to evaluate tubal patency
  B. Hospitalization for immediate surgery
  C. Immediate gynecologic consultation
  D. Blood typing
  E. Methotrexate 50 mg/m^2 IM

CASE 7-7

Irene Jackson

Ms. Jackson is a 19-year-old African American female who presents with the chief complaint of abdominal pain. It is located in her right lower quadrant and suprapubic area. It has been present for 2 days and appears to be getting worse. She describes it as a constant dull ache (1 out of 10 on the pain scale) with intermittent severe (10 out of 10 on the pain scale) sharp cramps that appear to be precipitated if she walks fast, rides on rough roads, or jumps. She can generally prevent the cramps by lying still. She knows of no other aggravating or alleviating factors. She denies trauma as the source of her pain.

It is associated with marked nausea and vomiting that has prevented her from being able to "keep anything down" except for cola for the past 24 hours. Her emesis consists of "stomach acid and bile"; however, it does not contain any gross blood, "coffee grounds"-appearing substances, or other abnormalities. She also states she has had a "high fever" but has not checked it with a thermometer. Additionally, she is experiencing chills, shakes, malaise, fatigue, and dyspareunia. She denies bowel changes, headache, myalgias, arthralgias, rhinorrhea, nasal congestion, throat pain, ear pain, cough, wheezing, shortness of breath, chest pain/pressure, urinary urgency, urinary frequency, dysuria, hematuria, vaginal discharge/bleeding, palpitations, lightheadedness, vertigo, presyncope, syncope, or anxiety.

She has no known medical problems. She has never had surgery nor been hospitalized. She does not take any prescription or over-the-counter medications, vitamins, supplements, or herbal preparations (including for her pain). She is not allergic to any medications. She was prescribed oral contraceptives 6 months ago; however, she stopped taking them after 2 months because of a weight gain, which she did not report to the prescriber. Currently she is sexually active with men only and is not using any regular contraceptive method.

She only utilizes male condoms if her partner insists on it and has never used a female condom or dental dam. She participates in oral–anal and receptive anal intercourse. She admits to having multiple partners, many of whom are "one-night stands." She estimates her number of lifetime partners to be over 100, including 15 to 20 new ones in the past month. As near as she knows she nor any of her previous or current partners has ever had a sexually transmitted disease.

Her last Pap smear was 6 months ago and reported to be normal. She is unsure when her LMP occurred, when her next one is expected, or if she has missed one. She denies smoking cigarettes or utilizing illicit substances. She drinks one to two beers two to three per week. She denies any other alcohol consumption. Her family history is noncontributory.

1. Based on this information, which of the following questions are essential to ask Ms. Jackson and why?

 A. Does she have a vaginal discharge?
 B. Is she experiencing any anorexia?
 C. Did her pain begin elsewhere in her abdomen and then migrate to its current location?
 D. Is she experiencing any rectal pressure?
 E. Did her nausea begin before or after the onset of pain?

Patient Responses

She does not have a vaginal discharge, anorexia, or rectal pressure. Her pain has remained in the same location. Her nausea and vomiting began before the onset of her pain.

2. Based on this information, which of the following components of a physical examination are essential to conduct on Ms. Jackson and why?

 A. Oropharyngeal examination
 B. Abdominal examination
 C. Pelvic examination
 D. Rectal examination
 E. Neurologic examination

Physical Examination Findings

Ms. Jackson is 5'7" tall and weighs 157 lb (BMI = 24.6). Other vital signs are BP, 126/64 mm Hg; pulse, 92 BPM and regular; respirations, 14/min and regular; and oral temperature, 102.6°F. She is toxic appearing.

Her oropharyngeal examination reveals no discolorations, lesions, exudates, or structural enlargement/edema.

Her abdominal examination reveals normoactive and equal bowel sounds in all four quadrants. It is soft but with marked right lower quadrant and suprapubic tenderness without rebound or guarding. She has a smooth, firm, round, tender mass that protrudes above her pubic bone and extends to midway between her pubic bone and umbilicus. Doppler confirms the presence of a normal fetal heart rate within the mass. There are no other abnormalities.

Her external genitalia and vaginal mucosa are normal. Her cervix is erythematous, is friable, and has a large amount of a purulent yellowish discharge coming from the os. Her uterus is enlarged to approximately 16 weeks' gestational size (midway between pubic bone and umbilicus) and is

smooth but tender to palpate. She has marked cervical motion tenderness (positive chandelier sign). Her ovaries are normal size, smooth, and tender bilaterally (slightly worse on the right). There are no adnexal masses.

Her neurologic examination is unremarkable.

3. Based on this information, which of the following diagnostic studies are essential to perform on Ms. Jackson and why?

 A. Urinary human chorionic gonadotropin (HCG)
 B. Complete blood count with differential (CBC w/diff)
 C. Erythrocyte sedimentation rate (ESR)
 D. Abdominal MRI
 E. Nucleic acid amplification test of cervical discharge for gonorrhea and chlamydia

Diagnostic Test Results

Ms. Jackson's urinary HCG was positive.

Her CBC revealed an RBC count of $5.2 \times 10^6/\mu l$ (normal female: 4.2–5.4) with an MCV of 89 μm^3 (normal adult: 80–95), an MCH of 30 pg (normal adult: 27–31), an MCHC of 35 g/dl (normal adult: 32–36), and an RDW of 12.5% (normal adult: 11–14.5). Her WBC count was 28,500/mm³ (normal adult: 5000–10,000) with 86% neutrophils (normal: 55–70), 9% lymphocytes (normal: 20–40), 3% monocytes (normal: 2–8), 1% eosinophils (normal: 1–4), and 1% basophils (normal: 0.5–1). Her Hgb was 13.8 g/dl (normal female: 12–16) and her HCT was 43% (normal female: 37–47). Her platelet (thrombocyte) count was 255,000/mm³ (normal adult: 150,000–400,000) and her MPV was 7.9 fl (normal: 7.4–10.4). Her smear was consistent with these results and revealed no cellular abnormalities except for moderate bands.

Her ESR was 55 mm/hr (normal adult female: 0–20).

The MRI scanner was broken; so, the radiologist performed a pelvic ultrasound instead. It was normal except for the presence of a slightly enlarged (approximately the equivalent of 16 weeks' gestational age) uterus with endometrial edema and a viable fetus of 16 weeks' gestational age (GA). The fallopian tubes (right greater than left) were also edematous and filled with fluid. Please see **Figure 7-3** for her ultrasonic findings of her tubes. Her nucleic amplification tests for chlamydia and gonorrhea are pending.

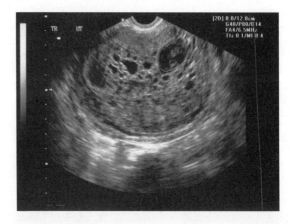

Figure 7-3 Ultrasound revealing edematous fallopian tubes with intraluminal fluid. (Note: Fetus is not visible.)

4. Based on this information, which one of the following is Ms. Jackson's most likely diagnosis and why?

    A. Pelvic inflammatory disease (PID) with pregnancy
    B. Cervicitis with pregnancy
    C. Uterine leiomyoma with pregnancy
    D. Ectopic pregnancy
    E. Appendicitis

5. Which of the following are essential components of Ms. Jackson's treatment plan and why?

    A. Hospitalization
    B. Obstetrical ultrasound
    C. Cefoxitin 2 g IV every 6 hours plus doxycycline 100 mg orally or IV every 12 hours
    D. Levofloxacin 500 mg IV once daily plus metronidazole 500 mg IV every 8 hours
    E. Cefotetan 2 g IV every 12 hours

CASE 7-8

Jackie Khan

Mrs. Khan is a 34-year-old Asian American female who presents to the emergency department (ED) with the chief complaint of severe nausea and vomiting. She is 14 weeks pregnant and has had significant problems with nausea and vomiting since conception. Initially it just occurred in the mornings. However, it progressively worsened in frequency and severity and now her symptoms are present throughout the day and occasionally (one to two times per week) awaken her at night.

She has tried eating small, frequent meals; eating dry meals followed by clear liquid an hour later; munching on crackers; and taking vitamin B$_6$ (pyridoxine), ginger, doxylamine, promethazine, diphenhydramine, and metoclopramide on the advice of her obstetrician without any improvement of her symptoms. She is unaware of any aggravating or alleviating factors.

Mrs. Khan has been experiencing varying degrees of fatigue; however, she attributes this to being pregnant. She cannot remember urinating since this morning (approximately 9 hours ago).

She has not experienced any abdominal pain, bowel changes, fever, chills, malaise, vertigo, presyncopal episodes, syncope, lightheadedness, dysuria, hematuria, or urinary urgency/frequency.

This is her third trip to the ED for this problem. The first one occurred approximately 10 days ago and the second one was 3 days ago. She states that on both occasions, the only diagnostic study performed was a urinalysis. Both visits resulted in the administration of IV fluids and her being discharged home on bed rest and dietary restrictions.

Her LMP was 12 weeks ago and normal. This is her second pregnancy. Her first pregnancy occurred at the age of 20 years and concluded with an elective abortion at 6 weeks. She had no known problems with that pregnancy; however, she remembers the physician who performed the abortion advising her there was "something wrong" with the fetus; however, she didn't go back for follow-up as advised. She is having regular prenatal check-ups with her obstetrician. Her last visit was yesterday. According to Mrs. Khan, her obstetrician has

not conducted nor recommended any special diagnostic studies for her severe nausea and vomiting. However, she is scheduled for an ultrasound to ensure her gestational age is correct and to rule out a multiple gestation because her uterus is "a little bigger than it should be."

Her only current medication is prenatal vitamins; however, she frequently regurgitates them whole. She is not taking any other prescription or over-the-counter medications, vitamins, supplements, or herbal preparations. She is not allergic to any medications. She does not have any known medical problems. Her only surgery was her induced abortion. She has never been hospitalized. She does not smoke cigarettes, drink alcohol, or use illicit substances. Her family history is unremarkable.

1. Based on this information, which of the following questions are essential to ask Mrs. Khan and why?

    A. Has she had any vaginal bleeding/spotting or cramping?
    B. What was her pre-pregnancy weight and how does it compare to her current weight?
    C. Has she ever experienced motion sickness?
    D. Why did she have an abortion?
    E. Has she been experiencing intense pruritus, with or without a rash?

Patient Responses

Mrs. Khan has experienced two separate episodes of light vaginal bleeding that lasted approximately 1 day each since becoming pregnant. Neither was associated with cramping or abdominal pain. The first episode was approximately 2 weeks ago and the second episode was 2 days ago. She states that her obstetrician advised her they were "nothing to be concerned with" but did suggest that she avoid being on her feet for prolonged periods of time and avoid heaving lifting.

She has never experienced any motion sickness or pruritus. She had the abortion following her first pregnancy because it resulted from her being sexually assaulted. She now weighs 2 lb less than her normal pre-pregnancy weight.

2. Based on this information, which of the following components of a physical examination are essential to perform on Mrs. Khan and why?

    A. Thyroid examination
    B. Heart examination
    C. Abdominal examination
    D. Pelvic examination
    E. Lower extremity evaluation for edema

Physical Examination Findings

Mrs. Khan is 5'0" tall and weighs 101 lb (BMI = 19.7). Other vital signs are BP and pulse, 120/60 mm Hg and 96 BPM and regular while supine, 112/56 mm Hg and 100 BPM and regular while sitting, and 96/48 mm Hg and 112 BPM and regular while standing; respirations, 12/min and regular; and oral temperature, 98.9°F.

Her thyroid is mildly enlarged bilaterally but without masses or tenderness. A thyroid bruit is not heard.

Her heart is slightly tachycardic but with a regular rhythm. No murmur, gallop, or rub is noted. Her apical impulse is nondisplaced and without a thrill. Her lungs are clear to auscultation. She does not have any pedal or pretibial edema.

Her abdominal examination reveals normoactive and equal bowel sounds in all four quadrants. Her abdomen is soft and nontender to palpate. Her uterus is palpable at the level of her umbilicus; it is smooth, nontender, and normal in consistency. Fetal heart tones cannot be detected with Doppler. She has no other masses or organomegaly.

External genitalia are normal and without discoloration, lesions, or masses. Her vaginal mucosa and cervix have a slight bluish-purple discoloration (positive Chadwick sign) but are without lesions or discharge. Her cervical os is closed and without any evidence of bleeding. Her cervical isthmus and cervicovaginal junctions are soft (positive Hegar sign). Her uterus is palpable to approximately 20 weeks' gestational size and is smooth and nontender. Adnexal examination reveals normal-sized ovaries without masses or tenderness.

3. Based on this information, which of the following diagnostic studies are essential to perform on Mrs. Khan and why?

 A. Dipstick urinalysis
 B. Blood urea nitrogen (BUN), creatinine, and electrolytes
 C. Quantitative serum human chorionic gonadotropin (HCG)
 D. Obstetric ultrasound
 E. Hematocrit and hemoglobin (H&H)
 F. Thyroid-stimulating hormone (TSH), free thyroxine (FT$_4$), and triiodothyronine by radioimmune assay (T$_3$ by RIA)

Diagnostic Test Results

Mrs. Khan's urine was dark yellow in color, clear, and with a strong odor. Her urinary pH was 4.0 (normal: 4.6–8.0) and her specific gravity was 1.035 (normal: 1.005–1.030). Her dipstick was positive for 1+ ketones and negative for glucose, protein, nitrites, and leukocyte esterase (normal: all negative).

Her BUN was 35 mg/dl (normal adult: 10–20) and her creatinine was 0.8 mg/dl (normal adult female: 0.5–1.1). Her electrolytes revealed a carbon dioxide (CO$_2$) of 26 mEq/L (normal: 23–30), a chloride (Cl) of 102 mEq/L (normal: 98–106), a potassium (K) of 2.8 mEq/L (normal adult: 3.5–5.0), and a sodium (Na) of 134 mEq/L (normal adult: 136–145).

Her quantitative HCG was 300,000 mIU/ml (nonpregnant females: < 5; pregnant females [depends on gestational week]: < 1 week: 5–50; 2 weeks: 50–500; 3 weeks: 100–10,000; 4 weeks: 1000–30,000; 5 weeks: 3500–115,000; 6–8 weeks: 12,000–270,000; 12 weeks: 15,000–200,000; no reference range provided beyond 12 weeks because in a normal pregnancy serum HCG levels peak toward the end of the first trimester, then gradually decline until they plateau near the end of the second trimester).

Pelvic ultrasound did not reveal a heartbeat with Doppler. Uterus was enlarged to approximately 20 weeks' GA size with "snowstorm"-appearing contents. Ovaries were normal. No free fluid was noted.

Her Hgb was 14.0 g/dl (normal adult female: 12–16) and her HCT 42% (normal adult female: 37–47). Her TSH was 7 µU/ml (normal adult: 2–10) and her T$_3$ by RIA was 215 ng/dl (normal 20- to 50-year-old: 70–205); however, instead of performing

an FT$_4$, the laboratory staff performed a total thyroxine (T$_4$), which was 15 µg/dl (normal adult female: 5–12).

4. Based on this information, which one of the following is Mrs. Khan's most likely diagnosis and why?

 A. Pregnancy-induced hyperemesis gravidarum secondary to hyperthyroidism
 B. Multiple gestations with intrahepatic cholestasis
 C. Normal pregnancy with hyperthyroidism
 D. Hyperemesis gravidarum
 E. Hydatidiform mole with hyperemesis gravidarum and dehydration

5. Based on this diagnosis, which of the following are appropriate components of a treatment plan and why?

 A. Admit to hospital for normal saline solution (NSS) IV with potassium chloride (KCl)
 B. Refer to regular obstetrician for continued prenatal care
 C. Refer to regular obstetrician (or gynecologist/obstetrician of the patient's choice) for surgical evacuation of uterine contents and subsequent quantitative serum HCG measurements
 D. Chest x-ray (CXR)
 E. Initiate therapy with propylthiouracil

CASE 7-9

Karen Lane

Ms. Lane is a 25-year-old white female who presents to the ED complaining of dyspnea and palpitations since awakening this morning. Her symptoms vary in intensity; however, they never completely resolve. She is unaware of any aggravating or alleviating factors, including activity. She has also been experiencing myalgias and weakness in her lower extremities as well as fatigue for the past 2 days. She denies any chest pain/pressure, arm/shoulder pain, back pain, cough, wheezing, hemoptysis, fever, chills, malaise, headache, lightheadedness, vertigo, presyncope, syncope, nausea, vomiting, or bowel changes. She also denies any changes in her mood, memory, sleep patterns, appetite, interests, pleasures, or activities.

Her only known medical problem is a compound left mid-tibia/fibula fracture as a result of a motor vehicle accident (MVA) 6 days ago. Her only surgery was the internal fixation of this fracture on the day of injury. Her only hospitalization was the night following the surgery for "observation." She currently is wearing a midthigh to midfoot cast on her left leg and ambulating with crutches (with no weight bearing on the left).

Her current medications consist of celecoxib 200 mg twice a day (prescribed by her orthopedic surgeon), ibuprofen 400 mg four times a day (which she added the day after she was discharged because the celecoxib was not adequately controlling her pain), and a combination oral contraceptive (COC) with ethinyl estradiol (EE) and drospirenone (DRSP). This is her fourth cycle on this COC; she has been taking it regularly and without any difficulties. She is not taking any other prescription or over-the-counter medications, vitamins, supplements, or herbal preparations. Her last menstrual period was 2 weeks ago and normal. She does not currently smoke (however, until her MVA, she smoked one PPD for the previous 10 years). She does not drink alcohol or use illicit substances. Her family history is unremarkable.

1. Based on this information, which of the following questions are essential to ask Ms. Lane and why?

A. How does she define "weakness"?
B. How does she define "fatigue"?
C. Is she experiencing any anxiety or increased stress aside from her tib/fib fracture?
D. Does her cast feel tighter or has she been experiencing paresthesias or discoloration of her toes?
E. Does she have any pedal edema?

Patient Responses

She defines weakness as decreased strength in the muscles of her right leg and foot and her left foot. By fatigue she means tiring easier. When the weakness and fatigue began, she attributed them to walking on crutches and having her sleep interrupted because of leg pain and an inability to "get comfortable" with her cast. Her activity level has decreased since her leg was fractured. She denies anxiety or increased stressors except for her tib/fib fracture. She is not experiencing pedal edema, paresthesias, or discoloration of her toes. Her cast does not feel "tighter" to her.

2. Based on this information, which of the following components of a physical examination are essential to conduct on Ms. Lane and why?

A. Palpation of the thyroid
B. Heart examination
C. Lung auscultation
D. Abdominal examination
E. Evaluation of lower extremities

Physical Examination Findings

Ms. Lane's height and weight cannot be adequately measured as a result of her ambulating with crutches and being instructed not to place weight on her left foot. However, she appears of average height and weight and states she is 5'5" tall and weighs 140 lb which would equate to a BMI of 23.3. Her vital signs are BP, 120/60 mm Hg; pulse, 76 BPM and regular; respiratory rate, 20/min and regular; and oral temperature, 99.8°F. Her oxygen saturation (O_2 sat) by pulse oximetry is 96% on room air. She appears to be in mild distress.

Her thyroid is palpable, smooth, nontender, and equal bilaterally. No bruits are present.

Her heart is regular in rate and rhythm and without murmurs, rubs, or gallops. Her apical impulse is nondisplaced and no thrills are present. Her lungs are clear to auscultation and she has normal and equal breath sounds throughout.

Her abdomen reveals normoactive bowel sounds in all four quadrants. It is soft, nontender, and not associated with masses or organomegaly.

Her toes appear to be normal in color and temperature with normal and equal sensation bilaterally. The fit on her cast appears appropriate. Her entire right leg, left thigh, and left foot are without edema, erythema, or tenderness. Her deep tendon reflexes are normal in her right lower extremity. Her plantar response is normal on the left and equal to her right one. She appears to have very mild quadriceps weakness on the right without evidence of any other muscle weakness or atrophy. It could not be compared to her left because of her cast.

3. Based on this information, which of the following diagnostic studies are essential to perform on Ms. Lane and why?

A. Urinary human chorionic gonadotropin (HCG)
B. Electrocardiogram (ECG)
C. Serum electrolytes
D. D-dimer
E. Chest x-ray (CXR)

Diagnostic Test Results

Her urinary pregnancy test was negative.

Her ECG revealed a first-degree atrioventricular (AV) block with slightly widened QRS waves and flattened P waves. Her T waves were narrow, tall, and peaked in her precordial leads.

Her electrolytes revealed a carbon dioxide (CO_2) of 26 mEq/L (normal: 23–30), a chloride (Cl–) of 102 mEq/L (normal: 98–106), a potassium (K+) of 7.2 mEq/L (normal adult: 3.5–5.0), and a sodium (Na+) of 128 mEq/L (normal adult: 136–145).

Her D-dimer and CXR were normal.

4. Based on this information, which one of the following is Ms. Lane's most likely diagnosis and why?

A. Bradycardia caused by first-degree AV block
B. Pulmonary embolism (PE) secondary to a deep venous thrombosis (DVT)
C. Fibromyalgia syndrome (FMS)
D. Pseudohyperkalemia
E. Severe hyperkalemia secondary to nonsteroidal anti-inflammatory drugs (NSAIDs) and the progestin drospirenone

5. Based on this diagnosis, which of the following are appropriate components of a treatment plan for Ms. Lane and why?

A. Hospitalize and obtain a stat BUN and creatinine level
B. Administer calcium gluconate, glucose, insulin, bicarbonate, and sodium polystyrene sulfonate
C. Start heparin therapy
D. Stop (and avoid in the future) the COC, EE with DRSP, and both of the NSAIDs
E. No treatment is required except to stop the offending agents and monitor serum electrolytes to ensure normalization

CASE 7-1

Cathy Dennison

1. History

A. Did she have gestational diabetes mellitus (GDM) with her pregnancy? NONESSENTIAL

Because of the large size of Mrs. Dennison's baby, there is a concern that she had GDM during her pregnancy. In the past, it was believed that being on oral contraceptives with a history of GDM increased a woman's risk for developing type 2 diabetes mellitus (DM). However, current evidence indicates that the presence of GDM increases the likelihood of a woman acquiring type 2 DM regardless of whether she utilizes a hormonal contraceptive method or not. Hence, the World Health Organization's (WHO) contraindication stratification system does not consider a history of GDM to be a contraindication of any level (e.g. absolute or relative) to low-dose combination oral contraceptive (COC) usage.

Furthermore, despite diabetes mellitus being able to accelerate cardiovascular disease development and its consequences, the WHO still only classifies the presence of DM (regardless of type) as a class 2 contraindication (method is probably safe to use) for oral contraceptive (OC) use. However, if the patient has significant microvascular (e.g., nephropathy and/or retinopathy) or macrovascular (e.g., coronary artery disease and/or peripheral vessel disease) complications or other noteworthy complications (e.g., neuropathy), the WHO acknowledges the risk associated with OC reclassifies it as either a level 3 (relative contraindication) or 4 (absolute contraindication) depending on the severity of the comorbid disease process. (For more information regarding the WHO contraindication stratification, please see the discussion following choice 1 under treatment plan below.)

Regarding screening for the risk of diabetes mellitus, knowing if she has a history of GDM is unnecessary because her obesity already places her in an increased risk category.

B. Is she experiencing vaginal dryness, hot flashes, or night sweats? ESSENTIAL

Although missed menstrual periods can be attributed to the physiologic effects of OCs, they are less likely to be the cause in Mrs. Dennison's case because she has been on the same OC for 16 years without once experiencing this phenomenon. Thus, other possibilities must be explored. Given her age, perimenopause or even menopause could be responsible. The average age of menopause in the United States is slightly older than 51 years, with a range occurring from 41 to 59 years of age.

C. Is she experiencing any fatigue, nausea, vomiting, or breast tenderness? ESSENTIAL

The most common cause for secondary amenorrhea in premenopausal women is pregnancy. Even though Mrs. Dennison is taking her OC regularly, the method is not 100% effective in preventing pregnancy. Thus, because she is sexually active, this possibility must be explored.

D. How old were her paternal grandmother, maternal grandmother, mother, and aunts when they went through menopause? NONESSENTIAL

The age of menopause for these female relatives is inconsequential regarding Mrs. Dennison's complaints. There is some weak observational evidence that the age when a woman's mother and sister(s) underwent menopause is predictive of when she would experience menopause; however, the presence of menopausal symptoms would provide much more useful information.

E. What is her smoking history? ESSENTIAL

Women, especially those age 35 years or older, who smoke and take COCs have an increased risk of cerebral vascular accidents (CVAs). Hence, her smoking history is essential in evaluating the appropriateness of combination oral contraceptives for her. WHO places women who are 35 years of age or older and smoke 15 or more cigarettes per day at a level 3 or 4 risk category, relative or absolute contraindication, respectively.

2. Physical Examination

A. Oropharyngeal examination   NONESSENTIAL

Because Mrs. Dennison is not experiencing any oral or pharyngeal symptoms and her age and sexual history place her in a "low-risk" category for acquiring a sexually transmitted infection (STI), an oropharyngeal examination is not required. The primary reason to perform this exam as part of a routine gynecologic or contraceptive visit is to evaluate for signs of a nongenital STI. The most important would be a human papilloma virus (HPV) infection because approximately 20 to 30% of all oral cancers are related to this virus. HPV is also linked to cervical cancer.

If this were an age-appropriate health maintenance (or cancer screening) visit, an oral examination could be justified based on her age and smoking status. The American Cancer Society recommends all patients over the age of 20 years be screened for an oral cancer with a comprehensive oral examination; however, the National Cancer Institute admits that currently there is insufficient evidence that screening via an oropharyngeal examination (or any method) results in decreased mortality from oral cancer. Nevertheless, tobacco usage is associated with over 90% of all cases. Other risk factors include advancing age, male gender, alcohol use, sunlight exposure, and a diet inadequate in fruits and vegetables.

B. Breast examination   ESSENTIAL

Some organizations (most prominently the US Preventive Services Task Force [USPSTF] and the American Academy of Family Physicians [AAFP]) question the value of a clinical breast examination (CBE) as an early detection method for breast cancer, especially in women older than the age of 40 years, because of the lack of sufficient, good-quality trials demonstrating its usefulness. Thus, some consider it an optional component of the breast cancer screening plan compiled by a woman and her healthcare provider (HCP) based on her known risk factors and the currently available clinical data. However, the American Cancer Society (ACS) still recommends it annually starting at 40 years old (as well as every 2 to 3 years between the ages of 20 and 40 years).

Because there is some evidence to suggest that oral contraceptive usage might be associated with a slightly increased risk of acquiring breast cancer and that if a breast cancer is present, the hormones in the COC might make it enlarge/advance more rapidly, Mrs. Dennison needs a CBE.

C. Abdominal examination   ESSENTIAL

An abdominal examination is an important component of the evaluation for oral contraceptive usage. Although it can determine if there is a suggestion of a large mass, organomegaly, or tenderness over the reproductive organs, this information is more accurately determined via a pelvic examination. Therefore, the greater role of an abdominal examination in a patient taking oral contraceptives is to evaluate for the presence of hepatomegaly, which could be the only sign or symptom of a hepatic adenoma caused by the oral contraceptives. Likewise, it could potentially identify the presence of other hepatic diseases (e.g., cirrhosis or hepatitis) that

could be worsened by oral contraceptive usage and/or cause oral contraceptives to be less effective.

D. Pelvic examination   ESSENTIAL

A pelvic examination is indicated in a contraceptive evaluation to visualize for abnormalities and to assess for the existence, size, shape, and presence of tenderness of the female reproductive organs. Abnormalities could alter the effectiveness of various contraceptive methods (e.g., significant cervical lacerations make it much harder to achieve an effective cervical cap fit, increasing its potential to become dislodged during intercourse, and a substantially abnormal-shaped uterus increases the possibility of expulsion of an intrauterine device [IUD]); could indicate a contraindication to a contraceptive method (e.g., the presence of active pelvic inflammatory disease [PID] is a contraindication to IUD insertion and undiagnosed bleeding and/or cervical abnormalities are a contraindication to prescribing OCs until an evaluation is undertaken and cancer is eliminated as the cause); and/or indicate the presence of an STI or other abnormalities (e.g., ovarian cysts and uterine leiomyomas) that require further evaluation and/or treatment.

E. Rectal examination with occult blood testing of any stool obtained   NONESSENTIAL

3. Diagnostic Studies

A. Pap smear   NONESSENTIAL

The Pap smear is overutilized on many women in the United States. According to the American Cancer Society (ACS), average-risk women older than the age of 30 years who have had three consecutive normal Pap smears only require a Pap smear every 2 to 3 years at the discretion of the HCP. Alternatively, it is appropriate, according to the ACS, for women older than the age of 30 years to be screened every 3 years with a traditional Pap smear or a liquid-based Pap test PLUS DNA testing for HPV. Therefore, because Mrs. Dennison has had multiple normal, consecutive, annual Pap smears, she does not require another one at this time.

Furthermore, the ACS only recommends an annual traditional Pap smear (OR a liquid-based Pap smear every 2 years) for women younger than the age of 30 years starting at age 21 OR within 3 years after becoming sexually active (whichever occurs first). However, recently the findings from three large studies were revealed indicating that liquid-based cytology is not superior to traditional Pap cytology in detecting abnormalities. It is theorized by some that the initial superiority demonstrated with a liquid-based cytology technique had more to do with the adequacy of the specimen, predominately the presence of endocervical cells, than the actual testing procedure; therefore, if an endocervical specimen is obtained with a brush and placed on the slide with the material obtained with a traditional spatula, the difference between these two techniques disappears, thus questioning the recommendation for biannual screening based on the technique utilized to obtain the Pap smear.

The AAFP and USPSTF recommend that any woman with a cervix should have some type of cervical cytologic screening performed at least every 3 years. The USPSTF further states that women can stop having Pap smears at the age of

65 years. The ACS places the upper age limit for screening at 70 years old provided the woman's last three Pap smears were normal AND she has not had an abnormal result in the past 10 years. The ACS, AAFP, and USPSTF all agree that women who do not have a cervix do not require Pap smears if their hysterectomy was for a benign condition and no evidence of a cellular abnormality was identified on the histologic examination of the specimen.

Furthermore, there are some studies currently being published that suggest that screening for the presence of the human papillomavirus (HPV; generally via a modified enzyme-linked immunosorbent assay [ELISA] utilizing an RNA probe to test for the presence of the 13 "high-risk" strains of HPV DNA) is superior to a cytologic approach to prevent invasive cervical cancer (the ultimate goal of a screening Pap smear), especially in women older than the age of 35 years. Because of the higher prevalence rates in younger women, HPV DNA testing is this age group leads to overdiagnosing of spontaneous regressing cervical endoepithelial neoplasm type 2 (CIN2). If these findings are confirmed by additional studies (or preferably in one large clinical trial), then it is possible that HPV DNA testing will replace (or become a recommend adjunctive) to the traditionally cytologic approach followed in cervical cancer screening.

B. Mammogram ESSENTIAL

The decision regarding the need for mammography should occur at all routine gynecologic and contraceptive visits. Many experts would agree that one should be recommended to Mrs. Dennison because she is older than the age of 40 years and has never had one. This recommendation is supported by the ACS and the American College of Obstetrics and Gynecology (ACOG). The ACS recommends annual mammograms for all women beginning at the age of 40 years as long as their life expectancy is greater than 5 years; the ACOG recommends mammograms every 1 to 2 years for women in their 40s.

However, there is even less consensus on this subject by other leading prevention policy makers. The U.S. Preventive Service Task Force (USPSTF) breast screening recommendations, released in 2009, advise against screening average-risk women younger than the age of 50 years by mammography. The rationale is based on the relatively small number of women who develop breast cancer in this age range and its consequences in this "younger" population. However, included in the discussion portion of the recommendation, the task force admits that screening is equivalent in detecting breast cancer in women in their 40s with women in their 50s, and there is moderate certainty that the net benefit of screening women is present, albeit small.

The AAFP, in wake of the updated USPSTF recommendations, reviewed and revised their breast cancer screening recommendations as well. The AAFP now supports holding a discussion with women in their 40s and making the recommendation on an individualized basis that includes the patient's breast cancer risk factors. Because Mrs. Dennison does have some risk factors for breast cancer (e.g., obesity, not breast-feeding, and older age with first child) and has not had a baseline mammogram, in view of these conflicting recommendations, she should still be encouraged to have a mammogram performed at this time.

C. DNA probe testing for chlamydia and gonorrhea NONESSENTIAL

Because Mrs. Dennison is beyond the age where most STIs occur (late teens and early 20s), in an assumed mutually monogamous relationship of 25 years, and lacking signs or symptoms of a sexually transmitted infection, a DNA probe testing for chlamydia and gonorrhea is not indicated.

D. Urinary human chorionic gonadotropin (HCG) test ESSENTIAL

Although Mrs. Dennison's amenorrhea could be related to her long-term COC usage, perimenopause, menopause, obesity, and/or various gynecological, metabolic, or endocrine disorder, pregnancy cannot be ruled out because she is sexually active. Because the presence of a pregnancy needs to be identified as soon as possible to ensure good prenatal care and that timely testing can occur, a urinary HCG is indicated.

E. Screening colonoscopy NONESSENTIAL

A screening colonoscopy is not indicated because Mrs. Dennison is younger than 50 years old and does not have a family history of colorectal cancer (CRC), polyps, or any other conditions that place her in a "high-risk" group for CRC. This is supported by the ACS, AAFP, ACOG, and USPSTF, who all recommend that CRC screening begin at the age of 50 years in average-risk individuals. The screening interval for a normal colonoscopy in an average-risk individual is 10 years.

Other acceptable screening alternatives for average-risk individuals endorsed by the ACS, American College of Radiologists (ACR), and US Multisociety Task Force on Colorectal Cancer (USMTFCC) (composed of the American Geriatrics Society [ACG], the American College of Physicians [ACP], the American Gastroenterological Association [AGA], and the Gastrointestinal Endoscopy American Society [ASGE]) include a flexible sigmoidoscopy (with insertion to at least the splenic flexure), a double-contrast barium enema (DCBE), or a computed tomography colonography (CTC) every 5 years provided that it is normal. These groups also support the annual usage of two to three separate stool samples for fecal occult blood testing (FOBT) using a highly sensitive test for average-risk patients. In average-risk patients, a fecal immunochemical test (FIT) and stool DNA test (sDNA) that are highly sensitive are also acceptable. The FIT should be performed annually. The sDNA interval is uncertain at this time.

The ACOG, AAFP, and USPSTF only support the following alternative to an every 10-year colonoscopy in average-risk individuals: annual FOBT as described previously and/or flexible sigmoidoscopy every 5 years. The ACOG also supports the use of DCBE every 5 years.

4. Diagnosis

A. Routine oral contraceptive refill INCORRECT

Because of Mrs. Dennison's age, smoking status, and comorbid medical conditions, her visit would not be considered "routine." Additionally, instead of an OC prescription, she is going to require significant patient education to ensure that she understands why OCs are not her best contraceptive choice and alternative contraceptive methods are available to her. Thus, this is not her most likely diagnosis.

B. Oral contraceptive refill for patient with multiple risk factors   INCORRECT

Mrs. Dennison certainly has multiple risk factors for OC usage including her age, smoking status, obesity, hypertension, hyperlipidemia, and family history of premature coronary artery disease (CAD). Nevertheless, this is still not her most likely diagnosis because a prudent HCP would not prescribe COCs for her because these risk factors could make OC usage a dangerous option, most notably a significantly increased risk of experiencing a cerebral vascular accident (CVA).

C. Contraceptive counseling for a patient with hyperlipidemia, obesity, and type 2 diabetes mellitus   INCORRECT

Certainly the reason for Mrs. Dennison's visit is contraceptive counseling. Additionally, she has hyperlipidemia and obesity. However, even though Mrs. Dennison had gestational diabetes, she is not currently a diabetic given she reported a normal fasting plasma glucose (FPG) 6 months ago. Thus, this option can be eliminated as her most likely diagnosis.

D. Contraception counseling for a patient with multiple risk factors for oral contraceptive usage   CORRECT

This is the most accurate diagnostic description of Mrs. Dennison's clinical encounter from the choices provided. Contraception counseling is the primary reason for her visit and she does have multiple risk factors (as mentioned previously), making OC usage a less than ideal, and potentially dangerous, contraceptive option for her.

E. Class II obesity, hypertension, and hyperlipidemia INCORRECT

Even though Mrs. Dennison has obesity, hypertension, and hyperlipidemia, her obesity is class I, not class II (please see Case 1-1 for classifications). Furthermore, this diagnosis is not the most accurate description for her visit because it does not address the primary reason for the visit, contraception.

5. Treatment Plan

A. Refill combination oral contraceptives for 1 year INCORRECT

The WHO has compiled a list of signs/symptoms/conditions that could potentially result in adverse events (including death) from utilizing a particular contraceptive method, could interfere with the effectiveness of the method, or could be an unfound concern on the part of the healthcare provider who is advising about and/or prescribing contraceptive methods. Additionally, the WHO rated each of these items with a score from 1 to 4 indicating the appropriateness for utilization of a selected method in a patient with a particular symptom, physical examination finding, or diagnosed condition. A score of 1 means that there are no known reasons not to utilize the selected contraceptive method in a patient with that associated sign, symptom, or condition. A rating of 2 indicates that it is generally safe to utilize the selected method in a person who has a particular sign, symptom, or condition. However, a rating of 3 suggests that the HCP carefully weigh the pros and cons of utilizing a particular method in a selected patient population and only recommend that method if an alternative method is unavailable or unacceptable to the patient; in other

words, a rating of 3 indicates that a relative contraindication exists. A rating of 4 means an absolute contraindication exists between the selected method and the particular patient demographics. However, it is important to remember that these are only recommendations; therefore, all decisions must be made on an individualized basis utilizing sound clinical judgment in conjunction with these evidence-based guidelines.

The broad categories that are considered include age, pregnancy history (including current breast-feeding and future desire), smoking history, body mass index (BMI), blood pressure (BP; according to its severity and level of control), cardiovascular risk factors (including lipids and a history/presence of a vascular disease), venous thromboembolism (VTE) history and risk factors (including valvular heart disease, immobility, planned surgeries, and thrombogenic mutations), neurologic conditions (including headaches, presence of aura with headaches, epilepsy, and depression), reproductive tract disorders (e.g., endometriosis, uterine fibroids, and abnormal vaginal bleeding), history or presence of female carcinomas (including cervical, endometrial, ovarian, and breast), history of typical and atypical sexually transmitted infections, endocrine disorders (e.g., diabetes mellitus and the presence of associated complications and thyroid disease), history or presence of gastrointestinal disorders (including hepatitis, cirrhosis, other liver conditions, cholestasis, and other gallbladder disorders), anemias including the type, and drugs that might increase the possibility of hepatic toxicity and/or affect the effectiveness of the contraceptive method and/or the other medication. Some items are given a range (i.e., 2 or 3) to enable the healthcare provider some degree of flexibility to independently judge the severity of the condition and assign it to the appropriate risk category.

Mrs. Dennison has the following category 3 or 4 items present in her history and physical findings: age 35 years or older plus smoking 15 or more cigarettes per day (4), multiple cardiovascular disease (CVD) risk factors (3 or 4), hyperlipidemia (2 or 3), and a systolic blood pressure of 140 to 150 OR a diastolic blood pressure of 90 to 100 (3). Her category 2 items include age 40 years or older and obesity. She would receive a score of 1 on the remaining items. Nevertheless, she has two to three absolute contraindications (not to mention two to three relative contraindications) to low-dose combination oral contraceptive usage. Therefore, she should not be prescribed oral contraceptives because of the potential for serious cardiovascular disease, including a myocardial infarction (MI) or a CVA.

B. Decrease estrogen component of OCs to 20 μg INCORRECT

Although this option would provide her with less estrogen, it is likely to be associated with frequent breakthrough bleeding, especially because she is obese. Additionally, it could also be a less effective contraceptive choice because of her obesity. Regardless, she still would have the same risk factors and contraindications that were associated with her current OC because both formulations are classified as low-dose pills by the WHO.

C. Advise her that she has too many risk factors (and what they are) to safely continue taking a combination OC; however, prescribe her current combination OC for 6 months if

267

she promises to modify her risk factors by quitting smoking and losing weight   INCORRECT

This would be a potentially viable option if Mrs. Dennison is known by the HCP as a very compliant patient, is prepared and motivated to immediately make these changes, and only had one relative contraindication and no absolute contraindications (because these risk factors are frequently cumulative). However, Mrs. Dennison does not appear to be a highly compliant, motivated patient because she continues to smoke and weighs more than is healthy (despite more than likely being advised to modify these risks in previous years' visits). Regardless, she exceeds the proposed recommendation of one relative contraindication to safely try this option.

Furthermore, as written, this does not address her hyperlipidemia or her hypertension beyond diet and exercise. For this to be a viable treatment option, there must be provisions to ensure that these conditions are in extremely good control to minimize her cardiovascular risks from the COCs. Therefore, this is not an appropriate treatment option for Mrs. Dennison at this time.

D. Advise her that she has too many risk factors (including what they are) to safely continue combination OCs, provide her with information on alternative methods (including mechanism of action, efficacy rates, possible adverse effects, advantages, and disadvantages), and assist her in determining which one she would like to try with assurance that she can switch to another method if she is not satisfied with her initial choice   CORRECT

Because of her age, smoking history, uncontrolled hypertension, cardiovascular risk factors, and hyperlipidemia, this is her best treatment option at this time.

E. Refuse to provide oral contraceptives until she gets an electrocardiogram (ECG) and treadmill stress test (TST) INCORRECT

This is actually a flawed recommendation because having these two tests performed is not going to improve Mrs. Dennison's risk profile for COC use. If they are negative for CAD, there is no assurance that she is disease free because of the potential for false-negative TST results in women, especially when attempting to identify silent ischemia. And, if they are positive for coronary artery disease, her known risk of having a myocardial infarction (MI) from OCs is now higher (and she should definitely not take OCs) because of confirmed CAD.

Additionally, these tests do nothing to address the risk of a CVA, which is probably greater than that of an MI. Thus, this is an inappropriate treatment option.

Epidemiologic and Other Data

The number of sexually active women in the United States is estimated to be approximately 41 million. At least 3 million of these women do not use any form of contraception. Approximately 50% of all pregnancies are unplanned. Of these unplanned pregnancies, ~80 to 85% occur in women who are not utilizing any contraceptive method; the remaining 15 to 20% result from contraception failures.

A disparity exists between the efficacy rates in clinical trials and those found in typical use outside of the "laboratory." Therefore, it is no surprise that the most effective method of contraception in the United States is sterilization, with male rates being slightly higher than female rates. This is followed by other user-independent methods: levonorgestrel implants, IUDs, combination injectables, and progesterone injectables. Other hormonal methods (including pills, patches, and rings) are the next most effective group. Other methods have significantly lower efficacy rates in actual usage situations.

The most commonly utilized method of contraception in the United States is female sterilization.

CASE 7-2
Dianne Edwards
1. History

A. Why doesn't she have any children?   NONESSENTIAL

Whether or not Ms. Edwards has children is irrelevant to her present complaint. Furthermore, the formatting of this question is insensitive. It suggests that there is something "wrong" with her and her partner if they desire to remain childless. Additionally, it lacks the necessary compassion if she is childless as a result of infertility problems.

B. Is the discharge associated with vulvovaginal itching? ESSENTIAL

Vulvovaginal pruritus is frequently associated with vulvovaginitis caused by a yeast infection, most commonly *Candidiasis* sp. The majority of the cases are associated with a thick, white, curd-like discharge. However, early in the course of the infection, the discharge could resemble Ms. Edwards' description. Additionally, an allergic vulvovaginitis can be associated with pruritus. Atrophic vaginitis, which would be highly unlikely to be the cause of Mrs. Edwards' symptoms, can also exhibit pruritus. Lichen simplex chronicus, lichen planus, genital herpes, erythrasma, and, in some cases, vulvular cancer can cause genital pruritus, with or without a vaginal discharge.

C. What is her smoking history?   ESSENTIAL

Smoking status should routinely be sought on all patients. This is even more important for Ms. Edwards because the contraceptive ring is contraindicated in women 35 years of age or older who smoke 15 or more cigarettes per day because of the increased risk of cardiovascular diseases (e.g., MI and CVA).

D. Is she allergic to latex?   NONESSENTIAL

Technically, this is probably a good question to ask every patient before performing a gloved examination regardless of body location (unless a nonlatex glove is being utilized) because of the increasing incidence of latex allergy; however, this information would have hopefully been discovered while questioning the patient regarding medication allergies.

In regard to her current complaint, this question is irrelevant because the only currently available contraceptive ring in the United States is composed of ethylene vinylacetate copolymers; hence, it is latex free.

E. What is her douching history?   ESSENTIAL

Regular douching (defined as greater than once per month) can cause an imbalance of the normal vaginal flora, leading to its overgrowth and subsequent infection, most commonly either bacterial vaginosis or candidiasis. Furthermore, if Ms. Edwards douched in the last 48 hours, it could alter the results of the testing done on her vaginal secretions (i.e., causing changes in the pH and minimizing the presence of leukocytes and bacterial counts), thereby eliminating important diagnostic findings associated with the various causes of vulvovaginitis/vaginitis.

2. Physical Examination

A. Palpation of the cervical lymph nodes   NONESSENTIAL

These would only be positive (enlarged and/or tender) if Ms. Edwards had infection, significant inflammation, or a carcinoma involving her head, eyes, ears, nose, throat, or thyroid gland. If the supraclavicular lymph nodes are also included in the examination of cervical lymph nodes, positive nodes could be caused by these problems of the breasts or lungs.

B. Breast examination   NONESSENTIAL

Ms. Edwards will not require a CBE because she had a normal CBE 4 months ago, does not have any risk factors or previous abnormalities that place her in a greater surveillance pattern, and is not experiencing any current breast complaints.

C. Abdominal examination   NONESSENTIAL

Because Ms. Edwards lacks abdominal pain or gastrointestinal symptoms and the assessment of her reproductive organs (where she is symptomatic) can be much better accomplished by pelvic examination (which will be required with her complaint), an abdominal exam is not essential.

D. Rectal examination   NONESSENTIAL

Without abdominal pain and/or gastrointestinal symptoms, a rectal examination is also unnecessary. However, examination of the pelvic organs rectally is sometimes indicated if after the bimanual examination an enlargement, significant mass, or tenderness appears to exist in a very retroflexed reproductive organ. Still, this would be considered part of the pelvic exam because the rectum (and gastrointestinal tract) is not the focus.

E. Pelvic examination   ESSENTIAL

A pelvic examination is indicated to evaluate for visible abnormalities (e.g., vulvar, vaginal, and cervical erythema; edema; areas of irritation; lacerations; ulcerations; and location of discharge) that could provide important clues as to the cause of Ms. Edwards' vaginal discharge (e.g., cervicitis is generally associated with erythema and discharge limited to the cervix; a discharge from the cervical os is most commonly associated with an upper genital tract infection; vaginitis requires that all the surfaces of the vagina are covered with the discharge; sexually transmitted infections [e.g., genital herpes and syphilis] are suspected by the presence of characteristic lesions; and trauma can be associated with irritations, lacerations, and ulcerations).

Furthermore, a pelvic examination permits the determination of organomegaly, masses, or tenderness affecting Ms. Edwards' reproductive organs that could suggest an upper reproductive tract problem (e.g., endometritis or salpingitis) as the cause of her symptoms.

3. Diagnostic Studies

A. Urinary human chorionic gonadotropin (HCG) test   NONESSENTIAL

A urinary HCG is not indicated because Ms. Edwards has utilized her contraceptive method correctly and consistently (until removing it yesterday) for the past 4 months, has had regular menstrual periods, and has none of the signs and symptoms associated with early pregnancy.

B. Pap smear   NONESSENTIAL

Ms. Edwards does not require a Pap smear at this time because she had a normal one 4 months ago and does not have a history of a previous abnormal smear requiring frequent surveillance. (For more information regarding the frequency of screening Pap smears, please see Case 7-1.)

C. Wet-mount microscopy of vaginal secretions with or without a vaginal pH, "whiff" test for amine odor, and point-of-care testing for vaginal pathogens   ESSENTIAL

Although the distribution of Ms. Edwards' vaginal discharge is not consistent with vaginitis, evaluation of her vaginal secretions, with at least a wet-mount microscopy, is still indicated to rule out a vulvovaginitis and assist in determining the cause of her vaginal discharge.

D. DNA testing for *Chlamydia trachomatis* and *Neisseria gonorrhoeae*   NONESSENTIAL

Because Ms. Edwards is older than the age of 25 years and in an assumed mutually monogamous relationship of 5 years' duration, she is not considered to be at high risk for an infection by either of these organisms. Furthermore, when they do produce symptoms in females, they are generally signs and symptoms of an upper reproductive tract infection (i.e., pelvic inflammatory disease).

E. Mammogram   NONESSENTIAL

A mammogram is not indicated because Ms. Edwards does not have any breast complaints and had a normal CBE 4 months ago. Furthermore, her medical history is negative for risk factors (e.g., being *BRAC1* or *BRAC2* gene positive; having a history of a blood relative who is *BRAC1* or *BRAC2* gene positive; or possessing a family history of any of the following: male breast cancer, bilateral breast cancer, premenopausal breast cancer, breast and ovarian cancer in the same relative, or multiple first-degree relatives with breast cancer) that would indicate that she is at a higher than average risk and requires breast cancer screening younger than the age of 40 years.

4. Diagnosis

A. Vulvovaginitis/vaginitis caused by bacterial vaginosis   INCORRECT

An infectious process is generally considered to be present if there are 5 or more white blood cells (WBCs) per high-power field (HPF) AND a minimum of 2+ bacteria on microscopic examination of the vaginal secretions. In the vast majority of cases, the offending organism is easily identifiable by its presence on a wet-mount microscopy (e.g., mobile trichomonads in trichomoniasis, budding yeast and/or hyphae in candidal infections, and clue cells in bacterial vaginosis). A potassium hydroxide (KOH) mount can enhance the identification of yeast.

The "whiff" test also provides clues regarding the most likely pathogen in vulvovaginitis/vaginitis: candidal infections generally do not have much odor, trichomoniasis is generally malodorous, and bacterial vaginosis has a very malodorous "fishy"-like scent. The vaginal pH provides additional information regarding the most probable pathogen. Candidal infections prefer an acidic to normal environment, whereas trichomoniasis and bacterial vaginosis prefer a more alkaline environment. These organisms can also be identified by point-of-care DNA testing.

Because her discharge was limited to the posterior fornix and her wet-mount microscopy revealed increased leukocytes but normal quantities of bacteria, it is unlikely that she has a vaginal infection. This specific option can be further eliminated as Ms. Edwards' most likely diagnosis because clue cells (which are pathognomonic for bacterial vaginosis) were not identified on her wet-mount microscopy, her whiff amine test was negative, her vaginal pH was normal, and her point-of-care test for bacterial vaginosis was negative.

B. Vulvovaginitis/vaginitis caused by gonorrhea INCORRECT

As previously stated, when gonorrhea is symptomatic in women, it is virtually always a result of any upper reproductive tract infection. Thus, the vaginal discharge would more than likely be of cervical origin; and pain, fever, and other symptoms of PID would be expected. On those extremely rare occasions when gonorrhea is identified as a pathogen in a vulvovaginal or vaginal infection, it is generally associated with a wet-mount microscopy revealing a much higher leukocyte count and significantly more bacteria than were identified on Ms. Edwards' specimen. Thus, vulvovaginitis/vaginitis caused by gonorrhea is not her most likely diagnosis even if she had physical examination findings consistent with vulvovaginitis/vaginitis.

C. Vulvovaginitis/vaginitis caused by trichomoniasis INCORRECT

As stated earlier, vulvovaginitis/vaginitis is characterized by a uniform coating of the vaginal discharge on the vaginal walls; it is not just located in the posterior fornix as is Ms. Edwards'. Additionally, the wet-mount microscopy in trichomoniasis should reveal the presence of mobile protozoans (trichomonads), the whiff amine test should be positive, the vaginal pH should be more alkaline, and the point-of-care test should be positive for this organism. Therefore, vulvovaginitis/vaginitis caused by trichomoniasis is not Ms. Edwards' most likely diagnosis.

D. Early pelvic inflammatory disease (PID) INCORRECT

When a vaginal discharge is caused by PID, it is identifiable as being cervical in origin and revealing a substantial number of leukocytes and bacteria on wet-mount microscopy. Furthermore, the diagnosis of PID cannot be established on a clinical basis without the presence of cervical motion tenderness. Additionally, all women with PID tend to have some degree of pain with palpation of the uterus and/or adnexal areas. Thus, PID is not Ms. Edwards' most likely diagnosis.

E. Adverse effect of the contraceptive ring CORRECT

In view of the minimal number of bacteria on her wet-mount microscopy, the lack of identification of the three major organisms responsible for vulvovaginitis/vaginitis on

both her wet-mount microscopy and point-of-care testing, a normal pH, and a negative "whiff" test, it is extremely unlikely that Ms. Edwards has vulvovaginitis/vaginitis. Thus, the most likely cause of her vaginal discharge would be an inflammatory condition (e.g., an irritant, allergy, or foreign body). Because one of the most frequently reported adverse events in clinical trials involving the vaginal ring was a vaginal discharge (5 to 14%), this is her most likely diagnosis.

Other frequently reported adverse events (also ranging from 5 to 14%) were vaginitis, upper respiratory tract infections, sinusitis, headaches, nausea, and weight gain.

5. Treatment Plan

A. Advise her she has a sexually transmitted infection (STI) and to abstain from intercourse until after her partner has been evaluated and treated INCORRECT

Ms. Edwards' currently available physical and diagnostic findings do not support the assumption that her symptoms are related to an STI; therefore, advising her of such is irresponsible and potentially harmful to her, her partner, their relationship, and the patient–provider relationship.

B. Provide appropriate anti-infective therapy INCORRECT

Because Ms. Edwards does not appear to have an infectious cause for her vaginal discharge, anti-infective therapy is not indicated. Antibiotics should only be utilized when there is sufficient evidence available indicating a bacterial pathogen is responsible for the patient's symptoms. The misuse of antibiotics (prescribing them for nonbacterial infections) only leads to antimicrobial resistance and possible adverse events for the patient.

C. Advise her that the discharge is secondary to her contraceptive ring and her contraception method can be changed if she desires CORRECT

Although Ms. Edwards' vaginal discharge would be considered a "nuisance" adverse effect from her vaginal ring, some women find it intolerable and desire a contraceptive method change. Others are comfortable with continuing the vaginal ring once it is determined that the cause of the vaginal discharge is benign.

However, if the patient does not want a method change at the current time, she should be assured that she can revisit this decision at any time and request an alternative contraceptive method in the future. This will help decrease the incidence of unwanted pregnancies as a result of improperly utilizing or stopping a contraceptive method because of "nuisance" adverse effects.

D. Advise her that if she desires to continue with the vaginal ring, she should rinse it off with cold to lukewarm water and reinsert it for remainder of the 21 days for this ring's cycle, then stop for 1 week (as usual) for withdrawal bleeding as scheduled INCORRECT

This would be an appropriate treatment option for Ms. Edwards if she were on her first or second week of her current ring. However, because she is on her third week, this is incorrect because it could result in an unintended pregnancy.

Additionally, if this incidence had occurred during her first or second week of ring use, she must be advised to use a barrier contraceptive method (e.g., condoms and/or spermicide) for the first 7 days after reinsertion because her ring has been out of her vagina for longer than 3 hours. Having the vaginal ring out of the vagina for longer than 3 hours is associated with a higher method failure rate.

E. Advise her that if she wants to continue with her contraceptive ring, she should properly dispose of the ring she removed yesterday and insert a new ring as soon as possible, then wear it for 3 weeks as usual   CORRECT

If she wants to continue with the contraceptive ring, she should properly dispose of her current ring and insert a new ring as soon as possible. However, she needs to be advised that with this option, she could experience breakthrough bleeding at any time during the next 21 days while using the vaginal ring, and she can expect to have her regular menstrual period once it is removed for the required 7-day time frame. She should also be advised that appropriate tampon usage will not alter the effectiveness of her method. However, she needs to ensure that her ring is not accidentally removed during tampon removal. This option would not require a "back-up" method of contraception.

Another acceptable alternative if she desires to continue on the vaginal ring is to wait until she has withdrawal bleeding; then, insert a new ring no later than 168 hours since the removal of her current one. With this option, she will need to use a "back-up" contraceptive method for the first 7 days postinsertion.

Epidemiologic and Other Data

The hormonal vaginal ring is essentially as effective as other methods of combination hormonal contraceptives that require user participation (i.e., birth control pills and contraceptive patches). The same precautions and contraindications that apply to other hormonal contraceptive methods also apply to women who decide on the vaginal ring for their contraceptive choice.

CASE 7-3
Ernsteine Fickelstein
1. History

A. What are her dietary and exercise habits?   ESSENTIAL

Adolescent girls should be evaluated if menarche has not been reached by 16 years old OR if they lack secondary sexual characteristics (e.g., breast development or pubic hair) by 14 years old.

In addition to knowing if Ernsteine is a vegetarian, it is important to determine what type. The avoidance of eggs and dairy in conjunction with meat makes it more likely for her to develop problems as a result of protein and calcium deficiencies. Even more relevant to her chief complaint is knowing her dietary pattern. Eating disorders (e.g., anorexia nervosa and purging-type bulimia) can be associated with amenorrhea. They consist of abnormal dietary habits including refusing to eat anything, secret eating or purging, or overt binge eating.

Excessive exercise is often a component of eating disorders because the patient attempts to prevent weight gain (or induce weight loss) by expending more calories than consumed.

Plus, adolescent girls who are athletes, dancers, cheerleaders, or involved in other similar activities can have amenorrhea as result of the excessive training without an associated eating disorder. Nevertheless, there is the concern that this could represent the female athlete triad syndrome which consists of amenorrhea, an eating disorder, and osteoporosis.

B. Why is she a vegetarian?   NONESSENTIAL

Although perhaps interesting, her reasoning for selecting a vegetarian diet is not clinically relevant with the exception of her making that decision as a significant weight reduction technique, which should have been identified with the previous question. Furthermore, stated in this manner, it can leave the patient with the impression that a properly done vegetarian diet is not a healthy alternative.

C. Does she experience headaches, visual disturbances, or abnormalities of smell?   ESSENTIAL

Pituitary and hypothalamic abnormalities, especially tumors (both benign and malignant), can produce amenorrhea. The main complaints associated with these tumors are headaches, visual disturbances (especially visual field defects), and decreased olfaction. Additionally, Kallmann syndrome is a rare disorder associated with an intrinsic genetic lack of gonadotropins that can be responsible for primary amenorrhea; its main symptom is a poor sense of smell.

D. What does she think of her body's appearance and size? ESSENTIAL

The majority of adolescents will be able to identify some minor "flaw" in their appearance that they would like to change; this is normal. What is not normal is when a very thin patient describes himself or herself, or a particular body part (e.g., abdomen, thighs, hips, or proximal arms), as "too fat" or too large. This is very suggestive of an eating disorder and requires further evaluation.

E. Is she experiencing excessive emotional stress with family, school, or friends?   ESSENTIAL

Excessive stress, whether positive or negative, can cause amenorrhea. In general, this is a secondary amenorrhea. However, if prolonged and severe, a primary amenorrhea could occur.

2. Physical Examination

A. Breast examination   ESSENTIAL

A breast examination evaluates for development that is appropriate for age and Tanner stage.

The Tanner stage is the most commonly utilized portion of the Tanner growth chart series. It sets forth the parameters for normal growth and development for stages of puberty achieved. The Tanner stages range from 1 (child) to 5 (adult). It is based on breast development (genital development in males) as well as pubic hair growth and distribution. The Tanner stages for females are summarized in **Table 7-1.**

The breast examination should also include visual inspection and palpation for changes in skin color, skin lesions, asymmetry, texture, contour, and masses. Additionally, the nipples need to be evaluated for spontaneous and induced discharge. The majority of nipple discharge is benign; however, it can also be linked with hyperprolactinemia, suggesting

Table 7-1 Tanner Stages for Normal Puberty Development in Females

Stage	Description	Breast Development	Appearance of Pubic Hair
1	Child	None	None
2	Prepubertal	Breast bud present	Minimal, fine, and distributed over the distal mons pubis only
3	Early pubescent	Small amount of subcutaneous growth	Denser, coarser, and with moderate superior distribution
4	Late pubescent	Moderate amount of subcutaneous growth	Midescutcheon
5	Adult	Full amount of subcutaneous growth	Female escutcheon

the possibility of a pituitary problem being responsible for the amenorrhea. Finally, the axillary, infraclavicular, and supra-clavicular lymph nodes need to be palpated for enlargement and/or tenderness.

B. Abdominal examination   ESSENTIAL

An abdominal examination is indicated to evaluate for any organomegaly, masses, or tenderness that could suggest a potential cause (e.g., enlarged uterus or adrenal mass).

C. Pelvic examination   ESSENTIAL

The external examination evaluates pubic hair appearance and distribution for appropriate Tanner stage (as described previously) and gross abnormalities that could be associated with lack of menarche (e.g., congenital defects, enlarged clitoris, small labia, or imperforated hymen). The speculum examination should be able to determine the absence of the uterus or a transverse vaginal septa that could be responsible for the amenorrhea. The bimanual examination further evaluates for the presence and size of the uterus as well as the ovaries for potential conditions that could be causing the amenorrhea (e.g., uterine enlargement with pregnancy and uterine absence with testicular feminization syndrome).

D. Cranial nerve testing   ESSENTIAL

Cranial nerve testing is also indicated, focusing on smell, vision, and visual fields. Abnormalities in these areas can be seen with a pituitary or hypothalamic lesion.

E. Skin examination   ESSENTIAL

A skin examination is indicated to evaluate for signs of a nonreproductive tract cause for her amenorrhea. Examples include hypothyroidism revealing dry skin, myxedema, and/or pallor; Cushing syndrome displaying hyperpigmentation, striae cutis distensae, and/or hirsutism; marked psychological stress showing bitten-down nails, "picked at" skin, and excoriations; and anorexia nervosa revealing loss of body fat, increase of lanugo, and dry, scaly skin.

3. Diagnostic Studies

A. Follicle-stimulating   hormone   (FSH)   level NONESSENTIAL

After ruling out pregnancy, the first step in evaluating a patient who has never menstruated is to evaluate the uterus and/or outflow tract. Because an abnormality was identified,

Ernsteine does not need any further diagnostic evaluation at this time.

However, if treatment of her condition fails to resolve her amenorrhea (or if this abnormality was not present), an FSH level would be indicated. FSH is produced in the anterior pituitary and is responsible for the stimulation of the follicle in the ovary. FSH tends to be elevated (generally twice normal) when ovarian failure is responsible for amenorrhea. However, it is usually decreased (but occasionally normal) in other conditions capable of producing her symptoms (e.g., hypothalamic/pituitary failure, hypothyroidism, or medication adverse effects).

B. Prolactin level   NONESSENTIAL

Again, because a cause for Ernsteine's lack of menarche was identified clinically, further diagnostic evaluation is not necessary at this time. Even without this identifiable cause, a prolactin level would still not be indicated. However, it is the follow-up test of choice if the patient's FSH is low or normal. Because pure ovarian failure is rare, many HCPs order this as an initial diagnostic study assuming the FSH is not going to be elevated.

Prolactin is also released from the anterior pituitary gland and its primary responsibility is lactation. The level tends to decrease with pituitary failure and increase with pituitary tumors, medications, hypothyroidism, or pregnancy as the cause of delayed menarche. The level is generally normal in amenorrhea caused by ovarian problems or short stature.

C. Testosterone level   NONESSENTIAL

Testosterone is considered to be a "male" hormone; however, it is produced in the adrenal glands of both men and women. The level is not routinely checked in the evaluation of lack of menarche unless the presence of ambiguous sexual features was discovered on physical examination, raising the suspicion of hermaphroditism, pseudohermaphroditism, testicular feminization syndrome, or other similar conditions.

D. Estradiol level   NONESSENTIAL

Estradiol is one of the three forms of estrogen produced in the ovaries; because of the extremes of normal throughout the menstrual cycle, it is not useful in evaluating amenorrhea.

E. Urinary   human   chorionic   gonadotropin   (HCG) NONESSENTIAL

Adolescents, especially those who are accompanied by their parent(s) or guardian(s), may not respond honestly to questions regarding sexual activity for fear of disappointment, rejection, or reprisal from these authority figures. Therefore, it is appropriate to perform a pregnancy test despite the teen's denial of sexual activity if appropriate. One is generally indicated in the evaluation of never menstruating because pregnancy can be responsible. However, this is not necessary for Ernsteine because it is virtually impossible for her to have become pregnant with her particular abnormality.

4. Diagnosis

A. Secondary amenorrhea caused by a local genital abnormality   INCORRECT

Secondary amenorrhea is defined as missing three consecutive monthly menstrual periods after attaining menarche and established regular monthly menstrual cycles OR the lack of menses for 6 consecutive months after achieving menarche but with irregular menstrual cycles.

Therefore, regardless of the cause of Ernsteine's amenorrhea, this cannot be her most likely diagnosis because she has never achieved menarche.

B. Primary amenorrhea secondary to imperforated hymen   CORRECT

Primary amenorrhea is defined as not going through thelarche by the age of 14 years or not going through menarche by the age of 16 years. Therefore, Ernsteine's amenorrhea is considered to be primary. The bulging intact hymen on physical examination makes this her most likely diagnosis.

C. Primary amenorrhea secondary to müllerian agenesis   INCORRECT

Müllerian agenesis is a congenital defect consisting of either an absent uterus or a partially formed uterus. Even though Ernsteine has primary amenorrhea, her uterus is palpable on rectal examination and her intact hymen is bulging with what appears to be old blood (indicating that she probably has a working uterus). Thus, primary amenorrhea secondary to müllerian agenesis is not her most likely diagnosis.

A small number of adolescents with what initially appears to be müllerian agenesis actually have testicular feminization syndrome characterized by androgen insensitivity.

D. Primary amenorrhea caused by anorexia nervosa   INCORRECT

Anorexia nervosa can cause both primary and secondary amenorrhea via hypothalamic dysfunction causing a hypogonadotropic amenorrhea. Hypogonadotropic amenorrhea can also be caused by constitutional delays in growth and development (primary cause), endocrine abnormalities (e.g., Cushing syndrome, hypothyroidism, or pituitary tumors), psychological stress, excessive exercise/training, and chronic physiologic stress as a result of medical conditions (e.g., acquired immunodeficiency syndrome [AIDS], cancer, uncontrolled diabetes mellitus, and renal failure). Regardless, anorexia nervosa can essentially be ruled out by Ernsteine's history with her mother's collaboration.

E. Secondary amenorrhea caused by polycystic ovarian syndrome   INCORRECT

Polycystic ovarian syndrome (PCOS) is a complex endocrine disorder that, from a reproductive standpoint, is associated with hyperandrogenism. It is more often associated with oligomenorrhea (less than nine menstrual periods per year) than it is with true secondary amenorrhea (as described earlier). However, some women with PCOS have regular menses. In addition to menstrual abnormalities, the patient often experiences hirsutism, virilization, and/or infertility.

Additionally, it is frequently associated with obesity and abnormal glucose tolerance (and in a few cases overt diabetes mellitus). Furthermore, even when associated with amenorrhea, it is rarely primary amenorrhea. Therefore, PCOS is not Ernsteine's most likely diagnosis.

In the past, to achieve pregnancy, the patient generally had to take a combination of ovulatory-stimulating medications (most frequently clomiphene) and a corticosteroid (most commonly dexamethasone) to suppress adrenocorticotropic hormone (ACTH) and adrenal androgen production. However, pregnancy has been achieved in many women just by treating the insulin resistance and hyperinsulinemia with metformin. Other diabetic medications (e.g., rosiglitazone and pioglitazone) have also been utilized with success. The uses of these diabetic agents to treat PCOS and/or induce pregnancy in patients with PCOS are off-label (not US Food and Drug Administration [FDA]-approved) uses.

5. Treatment Plan

A. Refer to gynecologist   CORRECT

Because Ernsteine has an imperforated hymen, this is an appropriate referral because she will more than likely require some type of surgical correction.

B. Start metformin   INCORRECT

Metformin is used in the treatment of type 2 diabetes mellitus. It is also used off-label in high-risk patients who have abnormal glucose tolerance or metabolic syndrome to prevent (or, more accurately, delay) the onset of type 2 diabetes mellitus and in women with PCOS to treat the disease or induce ovulation. Therefore, it is not indicated for Ernsteine.

C. Start estrogen therapy   INCORRECT

Estrogen therapy is utilized in adolescents only if they have ovarian failure causing amenorrhea. There is no evidence to suspect that Ernsteine has ovarian failure, especially because she is experiencing cyclic monthly pain consistent with Mittelschmerz and she has what appears to be an accumulation of old menstrual blood behind an imperforated hymen.

D. Psychiatric referral for eating disorder   INCORRECT

Although Ernsteine's BMI is at the lower limit of normal and she exercises excessively before upcoming ballet recitals, she does not appear to have an eating disorder based on her history, corroborated by her mother, and the fact that she feels her body is thin, not fat.

E. Brain magnetic resonance imaging (MRI) with emphasis on pituitary/hypothalamus   INCORRECT

There is no reason to suspect that Ernsteine's primary amenorrhea is caused by a pituitary or hypothalamic dysfunction, growth, or tumor; therefore, a brain MRI with emphasis on the pituitary/hypothalamus is not indicated at this time.

Epidemiologic and Other Data

There is a trend in the United States for adolescents to achieve menarche at a much younger age; however, the guidelines for the ages of evaluation have yet to change. African American girls tend to start menses at a younger age compared to any other race.

Primary amenorrhea affects less than 1% of adolescent girls in the United States. Secondary amenorrhea affects between 3 and 5% of women annually.

Menstruation depends on an intact hypothalamic-pituitary-gonadal axis. The hypothalamus must produce gonadotropin-releasing hormone (GnRH) to stimulate the anterior pituitary to produce FSH and luteinizing hormone (LH). The FSH and LH cause the ovaries to produce estrogen and progestin, which serves as a feedback loop to the hypothalamus but also causes proliferation of the endometrium of the uterus in preparation for pregnancy. If implantation of a fertilized egg does not occur, this lining is sloughed off (causing menstruation) as a result of a dramatic drop in the estrogen and progestin levels toward the end of the menstrual cycle.

CASE 7-4

Felicia Goldstein

1. History

A. Does she bruise easily, bleed when she brushes her teeth, take a long time to cease bleeding after a laceration/abrasion, or experience frequent nosebleeds?   ESSENTIAL

Although a significant coagulopathy would more than likely have been diagnosed when Felicia was younger, it is not uncommon for some less severe coagulopathies to only become apparent when a female begins menses. In fact, it is estimated that approximately 50% of all adolescents who present with abnormal vaginal bleeding (AVB) starting at the time of menarche have a bleeding disorder.

B. Does she experience dysmenorrhea? If yes, what is its severity?   ESSENTIAL

The occurrence and severity of dysmenorrhea can provide a clue as to whether a patient with abnormal vaginal bleeding is experiencing ovulatory or anovulatory bleeding. Anovulatory bleeding tends to be associated with mild (if any) dysmenorrhea; conversely, ovulatory bleeding is generally linked to some degree (generally moderate to severe) of dysmenorrhea.

C. When are she and her boyfriend planning on becoming sexually active?   NONESSENTIAL

A very personal question such as this is highly unlikely to be answered honestly by an adolescent, especially in the presence of other significant authority figures (e.g., parents, grandparents, or legal guardians). The only possible relevant piece of information this question could provide is if her final diagnosis were amenable to treatment with COCs, whether she would also be requiring them for contraception. Nevertheless, it would not alter the treatment plan.

Furthermore, this question is inappropriately worded. It makes the assumption that Felicia is in a heterosexual relationship and implies (or certainly can be misconstrued as such) that any other sexual orientation is "wrong," non–mutually exclusive relationships are "wrong," a decision not to be sexually active at her age is "wrong," or something is "wrong" with her because she is not ready for a sexual relationship.

D. Does she experience premenstrual symptoms?   ESSENTIAL

Some women experience a wide array of emotional (e.g., anxiety, crying more easily, mood swings, irritability, and/or insomnia), fluid retentive (e.g., weight gain, edema, bloating, and/or breast tenderness), and pain (headaches, backaches, and generalized myalgias) symptoms before their menses begins. Because these symptoms are related to the luteal phase of the menstrual cycle, their presence also provides clues as to whether Felicia's AVB is ovulatory or nonovulatory. Women who experience premenstrual symptoms are more likely to have ovulatory AVB.

E. Has she recently had any unintentional weight loss, polydipsia, or polyuria?   ESSENTIAL

An infrequent cause of AVB is diabetes mellitus. However, in some women, AVB is the symptom that prompts them to seek medical care. Because Felicia is experiencing intermenstrual fatigue, it is essential to determine whether she has a coexisting condition responsible for it.

2. Physical Examination

A. Heart examination   ESSENTIAL

Because Felicia experienced a presyncopal episode earlier today and now has orthostatic hypotension and tachycardia, a heart examination is essential to evaluate for any signs that could indicate the presence of a congenital or inherited cardiac condition (e.g., aortic stenosis, mitral stenosis, hypertrophic obstructive cardiomyopathy, undiagnosed atrial septal defect with a right-to-left shunt, or a bicuspid aortic valve) that could be responsible for these findings.

B. Breast examination   NONESSENTIAL

With the exception of a hypothalamic or pituitary lesion producing hypo- or hyperthyroidism as the cause of Felicia's AVB (which in some rare cases could be associated with spontaneous galactorrhea), there are essentially no other breast abnormalities that could be associated with AVB. Because this possibility is extremely rare and Felicia lacks symptoms of such (including galactorrhea), a breast examination is unnecessary at this time.

C. Abdominal examination   ESSENTIAL

An abdominal examination is indicated on Felicia to assess for potential causes of a coagulopathy (e.g., splenic enlargement associated with a platelet dysfunction or hepatomegaly caused by a severe hepatic disease) and to determine causes that could be responsible for her orthostatic hypotension and tachycardia (e.g., peritoneal bleeding from an ectopic pregnancy).

D. Pelvic examination   ESSENTIAL

The pelvic examination is essential to determine the source (i.e., vaginal, cervical, or uterine) and extent of Felicia's bleeding. It also permits the pelvic organs to be assessed for abnormalities of size or shape and the presence of tenderness that could represent an alternative diagnosis to a primary menstrual problem as the cause of her AVB (e.g., ectopic pregnancy, spontaneous abortion, or endometritis), because her current menses is more severe than her usual bleeding pattern.

E. Skin and conjunctival examination   ESSENTIAL

Evaluating Felicia's skin and conjunctival mucosa could provide clues suggesting she has an associated anemia (if pallor is present) or a severe liver disease (if jaundice or icterus is present) associated with her AVB. Furthermore, because Felicia has an associated tachycardia (which is most likely related to an acute blood loss and/or anxiety), it is possible that she has a comorbid cardiac (as discussed earlier) or pulmonary condition that could produce cyanosis. As a general rule, central cyanosis is related to pulmonary conditions and peripheral cyanosis is more common in cardiovascular abnormalities.

3. Diagnostic Studies

A. Pap test   NONESSENTIAL

Because of Felicia's age and lack of sexual activity, a screening Pap smear is not indicated. The ACS recommends the first screening Pap smear at the age of 21 years or within the first 3 years after becoming sexually active, whichever comes first. (For more information on screening recommendations for Pap smears, please see Case 7-1.) Nevertheless, if a cervical carcinoma is suspected as the cause of her AVB (which is unlikely because of the quantity of blood present, her endometrium appearing to be its source, her cervix appearing normal, and her never being sexually active), a Pap smear would be indicated. Likewise, if a suspicious cervical lesion is visualized or a cervical lesion persists despite appropriate treatment (i.e., for cervicitis), then a Pap smear and colposcopy are indicated to further evaluate it. Still, even if a Pap smear is indicated for Felicia, it should not be obtained while she is experiencing significant bleeding because the likelihood of it being an adequate specimen is markedly reduced.

B. Urinary human chorionic gonadotropin (HCG) test   ESSENTIAL

Because pregnancy complications (e.g., ectopic pregnancy, placenta previa, placenta abruptio, spontaneous abortion, or adverse effect of an induced abortion) are associated with ~20% of all cases of AVB, a pregnancy test is indicated despite Felicia's claim of never being sexually active. Furthermore, as stated previously, adolescents are not always honest in divulging this type of information, especially in front of authority figures (i.e. her grandmother).

C. Total testosterone level   NONESSENTIAL

The primary indication for a testosterone level in female patients is to diagnose patients who have virilization syndromes, decreased libido, or precocious puberty. It is also utilized in the evaluation of ambiguous sex characteristics, in the evaluation of infertility in men, and as a tumor marker in patients who are status post–ovarian or –testicular malignancies. Because Felicia does not have any signs or symptoms suggestive of any of these conditions and a cause that can produce AVB in an adolescent associated with an abnormal testosterone level is extremely rare, this test is not indicated.

D. Complete blood count with differential (CBC w/diff) and actual platelet count   ESSENTIAL

A CBC w/diff and actual platelet count is an essential component of Felicia's evaluation. The hemoglobin, hematocrit, and red blood cell indices will provide information regarding the presence of an underlying anemia and/or the severity of her acute blood loss. (Remember: The decrease in hemoglobin [Hgb] and hematocrit [HCT] may lag behind the actual blood.)

Her platelet count will determine whether a thrombocytopenia is present, indicating an acquired or inherited bleeding disorder, that can be contributing to her excessive menses. A manual (or actual) platelet count is required because platelet counts obtained via autocounters can have as much as a 10 to 15% error rate as a result of clumping, even in the absence of platelet abnormalities.

E. Prothrombin time (PT) and partial thromboplastin time (PTT)   ESSENTIAL

The severity of Felicia's bleeding, her history of easy bruising (and possibly delayed coagulation), and her AVB commencing at menarche significantly increase the probability that she has an undiagnosed blood dyscrasia. The PT and PTT will assist in determining not only if a coagulopathy is present but also which ones are the most likely. The PT evaluates the extrinsic coagulation pathway. It includes factors II, V, VII, and X. The PTT evaluates the intrinsic pathway and includes factors I, V, VIII, IX, X, XI, and XII.

An elevated PTT in association with a normal PT is consistent with disorders involving factors VIII, IX, XI, and XII; high-molecular-weight kininogen (HK); and prekallikrein. This combination could also represent a deficiency of factors V and X because with these two deficiencies, both the PT and PTT can be either normal or elevated. Factor IX deficiencies are commonly seen in a coagulation abnormality associated with AVB. Other disorders commonly encountered with AVB are von Willebrand disease and symptomatic carriers of hemophilia A.

Fibrinogen and prothrombin abnormalities are associated with an elevation of both the PT and PTT, whereas a factor XIII deficiency can occur in the presence of a normal PT and PTT. Factor VII deficiencies generally have an elevated PT and a normal PTT; other deficiencies associated with this pattern could include those of factors V and X.

4. Diagnosis

A. Normal menstruation   INCORRECT

Normal menses occur at intervals between 21 and 35 days (average 28) and last for 2 to 7 days (average 5). However, it is not uncommon during the first 2 years following menarche for the cycles to be irregular because regular ovulation has not yet been established.

Regardless, the excessive amount of bleeding that Felicia is experiencing and her degree of anemia indicates that she is experiencing significantly more blood loss than the average 25 to 60 ml. Therefore, normal menses is not her most likely diagnosis (even if she were experiencing anovulatory cycles that can frequently be associated with the normal menarche transition).

B. Ovulatory abnormal vaginal bleeding (AVB)   INCORRECT

AVB encompasses a wide array of disorders including hypomenorrhea (menstrual cycles that occur at intervals ≤ 21 days), hypermenorrhea (menstrual cycles that occur at intervals ≥ 35 day), menorrhagia (menstrual blood loss of ≥ 80 ml per menstrual cycle), and metrorrhagia (vaginal bleeding that is irregular and noncyclic). Obviously, these are not exclusive of one another. And, based on these definitions, Felicia certainly has AVB. However, ovulatory bleeding generally is associated with regular and predictable menses. Thus, because of the irregularly irregular pattern of Felicia's menses, this is not her most likely diagnosis.

C. Anovulatory abnormal vaginal bleeding (AVB) caused by a coagulopathy   CORRECT

As previously stated, Felicia can certainly be diagnosed with AVB. In all likelihood, she is experiencing anovulatory cycles because her menses are irregular and unpredictable and not associated with dysmenorrhea or premenstrual symptoms.

Although there is no reported family history of a coagulopathy, it must be considered because of Felicia's elevated PTT and fatal hemorrhage associated with childbirth is extremely rare in the United States. Thus, there is a high index of suspicion that Felicia's mother had some type of a blood dyscrasia that Felicia and her grandmother are not aware. Nevertheless, approximately 25% of all the patients who have AVB secondary to a coagulopathy do not have a positive family history. Thus, anovulatory AVB caused by a coagulopathy is her most likely diagnosis.

D. Endometrial carcinoma   INCORRECT

Cancer of the endometrium often presents as AVB; however, it tends to be much less severe and much more frequent than what Felicia is experiencing. Additionally, it is rare in adolescents and is most frequently in perimenopausal and menopausal women. Furthermore, it is not associated with coagulation abnormalities. Thus, endometrial carcinoma is not Felicia's most likely diagnosis.

E. Spontaneous abortion   INCORRECT

In view of Felicia's history of infrequent episodes of AVB, normal pelvic examination, and negative pregnancy test, a spontaneous abortion can be ruled out as her most likely diagnosis.

5. Treatment Plan

A. Start two large-bore IV lines of normal saline solution (NSS)   CORRECT

Because Felicia has tachycardia and orthostatic hypotension in addition to severe AVB, it is appropriate to institute her treatment with two large-bore IV lines of NSS because she is hypovolemic as a result of her acute blood loss.

B. Hospitalize and obtain an immediate consultation with a gynecologist   CORRECT

Hospitalization is indicated for all women with AVB and a hemoglobin of less than or equal to 7 g/dl OR women whose hemoglobin is between 7 and 10 g/dl if they are tachycardic, hypoxic, or hypotensive (especially if it is orthostatic). Women who are stable and have a hemoglobin greater than or equal to 10 g/dl can generally be safely managed on an outpatient basis. Because Felicia is hemodynamically unstable and has a hemoglobin between 7 and 10 g/dl, hospitalization is indicated for her. Furthermore, she will require a gynecologic consult to help manage her significant AVB.

C. Coagulation factor concentrations   CORRECT

Because of the strong suspicion of a coagulopathy (excessive AVB commencing with the onset of menarche coupled with her elevated PTT), a coagulation factor concentration study should be performed on Felicia to determine the exact nature of her problem. Then, appropriate treatment for it can be instituted into her treatment plan for the AVB.

D. Administer conjugated estrogens 25 mg IV stat   CORRECT

IV conjugated estrogens are the fastest method to stop severe uterine bleeding. The dose is 25 mg IV stat. It is generally repeated every 4 hours for three more doses. At that time, the patient needs to be reevaluated. Ideally, Felicia's coagulation studies would be available and treatment for this underlying abnormality could also be initiated. However, if the gynecologist's consultation is going to take place immediately, it would be appropriate to hold the IV estrogen until the gynecologist has made his or her recommendations regarding appropriate treatment.

Because of IV estrogen's high incidence of nausea and vomiting, some experts recommend providing an antiemetic prior to instituting the estrogen therapy and continuing it for several hours after it is completed in hopes of preventing this adverse effect.

E. Administer methylergonovine maleate 0.2 mg IM; repeat every 2 to 4 hours as needed   INCORRECT

Methylergonovine maleate is a semisynthetic ergot alkaloid that is indicated for the prevention and treatment of postpartum hemorrhage. It is not indicated nor regularly used in AVB.

Epidemiologic and Other Data

The lifetime incidence of AVB is estimated to be nearly 20% of all women. The most common cause is anovulatory bleeding. It is estimated to be responsible for approximately 95% of AVB in women younger than 20 years, approximately 20% in women between the ages of 20 and 40 years, and approximately 90% in women older than 40 years. Ovulatory bleeding represents approximately 10% of all cases of AVB. However, approximately 50% of all women will experience microscopic bleeding or spotting with ovulation. Endometrial hyperplasia and carcinoma account for approximately 10 to 15% in postmenopausal women. Hormonal contraceptives are responsible for an additional 10% in women of reproductive age.

Other less frequent causes include pregnancy complications (including spontaneous abortion and placenta previa), sexually transmitted infections (e.g., gonorrhea, chlamydia, herpes simplex virus, and human papilloma virus), cervicitis, endometritis, benign tumors (e.g., uterine leiomyomas and endometrial polys), trauma (including sexual abuse, assault, and foreign bodies), endocrine abnormalities (e.g., hyperthyroidism, hypothyroidism, and diabetes mellitus), severe liver dysfunction (e.g., cirrhosis and hepatitis), blood dyscrasias, and coagulopathies.

Despite coagulopathies being a rare cause of AVB, they are responsible for approximately half of all cases of AVB that occur at the onset of menses. They are also responsible for approximately 25% of AVB associated with significant blood loss (defined as a hemoglobin of ≤ 10 g/dl) and approximately one third of cases of AVB requiring a transfusion in adolescents.

CASE 7-5

Ginger Halstead

1. History

A. Is her abdominal discomfort associated with intermenstrual vaginal bleeding?   ESSENTIAL

Suprapubic discomfort can result from a variety of urinary, reproductive, and colonic sources. Urinary causes can include cystitis, bladder polyps, bladder cancer, and very distal nephrolithiasis; however, these conditions rarely occur in the absence of irritative urinary symptoms and/or hematuria. Likewise, colonic conditions can produce suprapubic discomfort (e.g., chronic constipation, inflammatory bowel diseases, irritable bowel syndrome, diverticulitis, and/or masses) but rarely occur in the absence of bowel changes (e.g., constipation, diarrhea, mucus, decreased stool diameter, melena, or hematochezia) and/or pain in another abdominal location (i.e., right lower quadrant, left lower quadrant, or periumbilical area).

Because of Mrs. Halstead's lack of urinary and bowel symptoms, there is an increased likelihood that a reproductive tract abnormality is the source of her problem. There exist several uterine abnormalities that can be associated with intermenstrual bleeding and a suprapubic discomfort/fullness including cervicitis, endometritis, leiomyomas, adenomyomas, endometrial hyperplasia, carcinoma, and complications of pregnancy.

B. Is she experiencing dyspareunia?   ESSENTIAL

Enlargement caused by masses (both benign and malignant), prolapse, inflammation, and/or infection of the reproductive organs, bladder, and distal colon can result in dyspareunia. Local physical abnormalities (e.g., atrophic vulvovaginitis and vaginal strictures) and psychological conditions (e.g., anxiety, depression, and posttraumatic stress disorder) can also cause it.

Thus, the presence of dyspareunia is not specific for a particular condition (or even to the reproductive organs). Because of the numerous conditions that can cause dyspareunia, its presence (or absence) does not provide much information on which to reach the patient's correct diagnosis. However, it is still essential to inquire about because its presence can influence the management decisions regarding the condition (e.g., a hysterectomy is considered earlier in the treatment process of uterine leiomyomas if uterine prolapse and/or dyspareunia are present).

C. Has she noticed visual abnormalities or changes in her sense of smell?   NONESSENTIAL

When dealing with a potential reproductive complaint, these symptoms are most often associated with a pituitary abnormality. Because Mrs. Halstead's chief complaint is not consistent with such, inquiring about these symptoms is not going to provide any useful clinical information.

D. Has she had any weight gain, cold intolerance, or dryness of her skin?   NONESSENTIAL

This constellation of symptoms is most frequently inquired about if there is suspicion of hypothyroidism being responsible for the patient's symptoms. However, because Mrs. Halstead lacks symptoms consistent with an endocrinopathy, these questions are not going to be useful.

E. Does she have any other concerns she would like to address?   ESSENTIAL

In individuals with a chronic complaint, something tends to prompt the patient's decision to seek evaluation and treatment of the problem at a particular time. Most frequently it is related to the chief complaint (i.e., condition is worsening or another symptom developed). When that is not the case, it is important to determine what the motivating factor is. Often, it is something unrelated or marginally related that the patient felt was too personal, potentially "embarrassing," "not that important" (but obviously concerning to the patient), or too "stupid" (in the patient's opinion) to make an appointment regarding it.

However, directly inquiring as to why "now is the time" to get this chronic problem evaluated often fails to identify the actual reason for the visit because the patient perceives this wording as confrontational or implying that the HCP is "too busy to be bothered." Thus, providing the patient with a benign open-ended question such as this one often provides him or her with the necessary "permission" to address this underlying concern. However, it is important to remember that occasionally there is no secondary agenda and the patient delayed seeking treatment because he or she had an assumption that the condition would resolve spontaneously, scheduling conflicts, a tendency to procrastinate, fear of a serious or untreatable condition, and/or concerns regarding the cost of having the complaint evaluated or treated.

2. Physical Examination

A. Thyroid palpation   NONESSENTIAL

B. Breast examination   NONESSENTIAL

Mrs. Halstead provides a history of a normal CBE and mammogram 9 months ago. In view of this and her lack of breast complaints, a CBE is not going to assist in her diagnosis and/or treatment.

C. Heart and lung examination   NONESSENTIAL

D. Abdominal examination   ESSENTIAL

Because Mrs. Halstead's discomfort is suprapubic in nature and could represent a wide array of gastrointestinal, genitourinary, and/or reproductive tract conditions, it is essential to perform an abdominal examination on her. While focus should be on the suprapubic area, the entire abdomen should be examined for abnormities of bowel sounds, tender areas, masses, and/or organomegaly in order to correctly diagnose her complaint.

E. Pelvic examination   ESSENTIAL

Because a reproductive tract abnormality is the most likely cause for her suprapubic discomfort, a complete pelvic examination needs to be performed.

3. Diagnostic Studies

A. Hematocrit and hemoglobin (H&H)   NONESSENTIAL

Because Mrs. Halstead does not have any signs or symptoms consistent with anemia, AVB, or other significant bleeding problems, she does not require an H&H at this time.

B. Endometrial biopsy   NONESSENTIAL

Endometrial biopsies are indicated when a sampling of the uterine lining is likely to assist in establishing the diagnosis and treatment plan of the patient. Generally, it is performed when a patient is experiencing AVB that is suspected to be caused by an endometrial hyperplasia but the slight possibility of an endometrial carcinoma needs to be eliminated. Furthermore, it is contraindicated in a pregnant patient. Therefore, in a patient with an enlarged uterus, pregnancy must be satisfactorily eliminated before this procedure can be performed.

C. Urinary human chorionic gonadotropin test (HCG) NONESSENTIAL

Even though Mrs. Halstead is sexually active, it is highly unlikely that pregnancy is the cause of her symptoms because she had a bilateral tubal ligation (BTL) 5 years ago and a normal menses 3.5 weeks ago. Nevertheless, a BTL is not 100% effective. Furthermore, it is not unusual for a woman to have a normal or lighter than normal (but rarely heavier) menses for the first couple of months following conception. Therefore, in view of her enlarged uterus, pregnancy must be eliminated. However, a pregnancy test is not required for this purpose because she will need a pelvic ultrasound to further evaluate her complaints. A pregnancy advanced enough to account for her uterine enlargement will be evident on her ultrasound.

D. Pelvic ultrasound   ESSENTIAL

A pelvic ultrasound is indicated to further assist in identifying the cause of her enlarged uterus.

E. Urinalysis   NONESSENTIAL

Because Mrs. Halstead lacks urinary tract symptoms, a urinalysis is unnecessary at this time.

4. Diagnosis

A. Adenomyosis   INCORRECT

Adenomyosis is a benign invasion of endometrial tissue into the myometrium. Although it can cause an enlarged uterus, it is not Mrs. Halstead's most likely diagnosis because it tends to be associated with moderate to severe tenderness on palpation, AVB, and severe dysmenorrhea.

B. Endometriosis   INCORRECT

Endometriosis occurs when implants consisting of endometrial tissue are located outside of the uterine cavity in abdominal and pelvic sites. These aberrant implants respond to hormonal stimulation in a fashion similar to the endometrial lining of the uterus. It can be eliminated as Mrs. Halstead's most likely diagnosis because it rarely causes uterine enlargement and is generally associated with worsening dysmenorrhea starting several days to a week before the onset of menstruation and lasts until the flow decreases. Eventually, the pain is continuous in the majority of the cases.

Frequently the pelvic examination is normal in endometriosis; however, sometimes tender nodules can be palpable in the rectovaginal wall and/or cul-de-sac. The uterus can be fixed, retroverted, and/or exhibit a positive chandelier sign (in the absence of pelvic inflammatory disease). Additionally, the ovaries can be enlarged because of endometrial implants being located on them, making them palpable and irregular in contour and/or tender to palpation.

C. Intramural uterine leiomyomas   CORRECT

Uterine leiomyomas (also known as uterine fibroids or uterine fibroleiomyomas) are fibrous growths that arise from one of the layers of smooth muscles found in the uterine wall. Classification, or diagnostic type, is based on their physical characteristics as well as in which layer of uterine muscle they arise. Intramural uterine leiomyomas are typically confined to the internal layer of uterine musculature and can cause smooth (symmetric or asymmetric) uterine enlargement. However, they rarely cause a marked irregular (or "bumpy") contour to the uterine fundus on palpation. They are typically not associated with AVB but can cause a mild to moderate increase in the quantity of menstrual flow. From Mrs. Halstead's pelvic ultrasound and physical examination findings, her most likely diagnosis is intramural uterine leiomyomas.

D. Subserosal leiomyomas of the uterus   INCORRECT

Subserosal uterine leiomyomas arise from the outer musculature layer of the uterus; therefore, they tend to produce a markedly irregular shape and contour of the uterus on the bimanual pelvic examination. It is not uncommon, especially in underweight to normal-weight women, to be able to palpate distinct masses on the uterus. Generally, these leiomyomas do not affect the menstrual bleeding pattern. Therefore, based on Mrs. Halstead's physical examination and ultrasound findings, subserosal leiomyomas of the uterus are not her most likely diagnosis.

E. Submucosal uterine fibroids   INCORRECT

Submucosal uterine fibroids are associated with a minimal, if any, enlargement of the uterus and cause a very irregular contour to the uterine cavity. As the leiomyomas protrude into the uterine cavity, excessively heavy menstrual and AVB can occur. Given Mrs. Halstead's clinical picture and ultrasound findings, submucosal uterine fibroids are not her most likely diagnosis.

5. Treatment Plan

A. Advise her of the diagnosis, its significance, potential complications, actions required if her symptoms increase, and treatment options   CORRECT

Patient education regarding the disease, its possible course, and all treatment options is an essential component of any treatment plan. This is especially true in conditions where multiple treatment options are available and there is no clear-cut "best" option. The treatment for each patient must be individualized to her clinical picture, including symptoms, effect on her quality of life, location of the leiomyomas, number and size of the leiomyomas, presence and severity of AVB, presence and severity of menstrual and nonmenstrual pain, associated conditions (including anemia), and existence of comorbid conditions. Treatment options range from observation to complete hysterectomy. Medical approaches include utilizing nonsteroidal anti-inflammatory drugs (NSAIDs) and hormonal manipulation (including combination contraceptives, estrogens, progestins, and GnRH agonists). Surgical options include endometrial ablation, uterine fibroid embolization, myomectomy, and hysterectomy.

B. Start her on low-dose combination oral contraceptives to decrease her menstrual flow and alleviate the dysmenorrhea INCORRECT

This would be an appropriate initial therapy for Mrs. Halstead except she has multiple contraindications to oral contraceptive usage, including a history of a nontraumatic deep vein thrombosis and age older than 35 years with a smoking history of more than 15 cigarettes per day. Furthermore, this option would not serve a dual purpose as a contraceptive method for her because she had a BTL.

C. Insert progesterone intrauterine device (IUD) to decrease her menstrual flow and alleviate the dysmenorrhea INCORRECT

This would also be an appropriate choice for Mrs. Halstead if it were not for her contraindications to utilizing this product (as well as her lack of need for contraception). Her contraindications to the progesterone IUD are the same ones she had to combination oral contraceptives.

Although this treatment option (if not contraindicated for some reason) is appropriate for women with intramural leiomyomas that do not distort the uterine cavity, it is not acceptable for women with intramural (and/or submucosal) leiomyomas that cause distortion of the uterine cavity. The distorted shape of their uterine cavity places them at greater risk of perforation of the uterine wall and expulsion of the device.

D. Refer to gynecologist for uterine fibroid embolization INCORRECT

Referral to a gynecologist for uterine fibroid embolization would be an appropriate treatment option if Mrs. Halstead only had one or two leiomyomas; however, because of the large number that she has, this technique would be impractical for her.

E. Obtain abdominal computed tomography (CT) scan INCORRECT

Mrs. Halstead's pelvic ultrasound clearly identified the abnormal structures as uterine leiomyomas. However, if there is any doubt regarding her diagnosis or concern about the presence of a coexisting condition, then further imaging would be indicated. Still, an abdominal CT would not be the imaging study of choice because it is difficult to distinguish the leiomyomas from the normal myometrium. If an additional imaging study is indicated, an MRI is a much better choice for more precise location of the leiomyomas.

Epidemiologic and Other Data

Uterine leiomyomas (uterine fibroids or uterine fibroleiomyomas) are the most common benign mass responsible for uterine enlargement. They occur most frequently in women between the ages of 25 and 45 years old. They are estimated to be present in 20% of women older than 35 years of age and 40% of women older than 50 years of age. The incidence appears to be even greater in African American women. Additional risk factors for their development include obesity, nulliparity, never smoking, and positive family history of the condition.

Uterine leiomyomas can cause a wide range of symptoms ranging from completely asymptomatic to severe pain and AVB. They are responsible for AVB through two primary pathways. First, intramural (and subserosal) leiomyomas can distort the normal anatomy of the uterine cavity significantly enough to produce AVB. Their second method for producing AVB is when the leiomyoma's needs exceed its own blood supply.

In addition to the three primary types of uterine leiomyomas (intramural, subserosal, and submucosal) defined earlier, there are other types that occur at a much lower incidence. They include external, parasitic, intraligamentous, and cervical. External uterine leiomyomas are considered by some to be a subset of subserosal uterine leiomyomas. They are generally pedunculated and therefore not often palpable unless the mass is large or the woman is thin. Because they are pedunculated, they can be confused for an ovarian mass. External uterine leiomyomas do not affect menstrual flow.

Parasitic uterine leiomyomas are considered by some to be a subcategory of external. They attach to another organ to obtain their required blood supply. Therefore, their pain can be atypical in location and caused by the organ on which they have attached.

Intraligamentous uterine leiomyomas are found affecting the ligaments of the pelvic structures (e.g., suspensory ligaments of the ovary, ovarian ligaments, round ligaments, and medial umbilical ligaments). They generally do not cause uterine enlargement or abnormal menses; however, they can also be mistaken for an ovarian mass on pelvic examination.

Cervical uterine leiomyomas are considered by some to be a form of submucosal uterine leiomyomas. They typically arise from the internal uterine layer in the cervical region and are often pedunculated. Therefore, it is not uncommon for them to protrude through the cervix into the vagina and be mistaken for an endometrial polyp. They are frequently associated with AVB.

CASE 7-6
Hillary Indigo
1. History

A. What does she mean by "spotting"?   ESSENTIAL

The majority of women utilize the term "spotting" to mean some degree of light vaginal bleeding; however, there are some who use this term to refer to minimal urinary incontinence or a small quantity of a nonbloody vaginal discharge. Even when utilized to describe vaginal bleeding, "spotting" can consist of a few drops of bright red blood, a pinkish discharge, or a brownish material noticed on one's underwear or the toilet tissue after wiping, or a menstrual flow that is not quite as severe as a regular menstrual period. Asking for clarification of terms that can have multiple or vague meanings ensures that the HCP clearly understands the patient's complaints, leading to an accurate diagnosis in a timely fashion.

B. Has she recently consumed any unwashed fruits or vegetables?   NONESSENTIAL

The primary concern regarding the consumption of unwashed fruits or vegetables is that her present illness could be an infectious or allergic process resulting from them being contaminated with a bacterium (e.g., *Salmonella*, *Shigella*, or *Escherichia coli*), a pesticide, or a preservative. However, in these illnesses, the patient virtually always has diarrhea, with or without abdominal pain.

C. Does she have a history of recent trauma?   ESSENTIAL

In any painful condition, it is essential to know if trauma was the inciting event because it can dramatically change the differential diagnoses and diagnostic procedures required to assist in confirming the correct diagnosis. This is especially important in women with abdominal pain and "spotting" because this could represent intimate partner violence and/or sexual assault. In both of these conditions, the patient may be reluctant to share this important detail without some prompting.

D. Has she ever had pelvic inflammatory disease (PID)? ESSENTIAL

A history of PID is important to ascertain because it is a risk factor for future episodes of PID as well as an ectopic pregnancy (secondary to scarring and stenosis of the fallopian tubes from the infection). Both of these conditions can present as lower abdominal pain with vaginal bleeding.

E. Has she experienced any lightheadedness, vertigo, presyncope, syncope, tachycardia, or diaphoresis, especially with standing?   ESSENTIAL

The sudden onset of severe abdominal pain can result from the perforation of a hollow viscus and/or hemorrhage into the peritoneal cavity. Therefore, it is important to determine whether there are any signs or symptoms suggestive of hemodynamic instability present.

2. Physical Examination

A. Oral mucosa examination   NONESSENTIAL

An examination of the oral mucosa is indicated if the patient has oropharyngeal and/or dental complaints or if there is a concern regarding his or her hydration status.

B. Examination of the conjunctivae of the eyes NONESSENTIAL

Although pallor of the conjunctivae can be associated with chronic blood loss (i.e., anemia), it is not present with acute blood loss. Likewise, icterus can be seen with severe hepatic, pancreatic, and hepatobiliary diseases; however, these conditions tend to produce upper, not lower, abdominal pain. Furthermore, bleeding disorders caused by severe hepatic disease tend to produce bleeding that is more severe than what Mrs. Indigo is experiencing.

C. Palpation of the thyroid   NONESSENTIAL

D. Abdominal examination   ESSENTIAL

An abdominal examination is essential because Mrs. Indigo is experiencing abdominal pain. Bowel sounds can provide clues to assist in ordering the most appropriate diagnostic studies based on the patient's differential diagnosis list because they are frequently diminished (or absent) in perforation, in constipation, and distal to an obstruction. They tend to be increased in diarrhea, in ileus, or prior to an area of obstructed bowel. Abnormal discoloration of the skin overlying the abdomen, distension, generalized tenderness, and rigidity can be seen in an intraperitoneal hemorrhage. The location and degree of tenderness and masses, as well as the presence of rebound or radiation with palpation, also provide important clues to the patient's most likely diagnosis.

E. Pelvic examination   ESSENTIAL

Because Mrs. Indigo is complaining of lower abdominal pain and slight vaginal bleeding, it is essential to perform a pelvic examination to adequately assess her complaint. Examination of the external genitalia, vaginal mucosa, and cervix

can identify potential sources for her extremely light bleeding (e.g., ulceration caused by genital herpes or syphilis, abrasions and/or lacerations from trauma, or erythema and discharge suspicious for an infectious process). The speculum examination permits visualization of the vaginal mucosa and cervix for these type findings. It also permits the cervical os to be evaluated as the potential source of bleeding and to determine whether it is open or closed and/or contains any foreign bodies or has tissue protruding from it. If the patient's problem was pregnancy related, an opened cervical os is more indicative of a spontaneous abortion, whereas a closed cervical os is more consistent with an ectopic pregnancy. With a spontaneous abortion, it is not uncommon for parts of conception to remain in the cervical os.

Although not pertinent to Mrs. Indigo's evaluation, if the patient is complaining of significant vaginal bleeding and is known to be pregnant, especially if in her third trimester, a speculum (or even a bimanual examination) is contraindicated until an ultrasound examination can be done to rule out the possibility of placenta previa. These maneuvers in the presence of placenta previa can result in hemorrhage, leading to increased fetal and maternal morbidity and mortality.

The size, shape, consistency, and degree of tenderness (if any) of the pelvic organs can also assist in determining the most appropriate diagnostic studies and developing Mrs. Indigo's differential diagnosis list.

3. Diagnostic Studies

A. Qualitative serum human chorionic gonadotropin (HCG) NONESSENTIAL

HCG is released from the placental trophoblasts shortly after fertilization occurs. Urine and serum tests essentially have the same detection threshold (5 to 50 mIU/ml). A qualitative HCG results are reported as either positive (above the threshold) or negative (below the threshold). Therefore, it does not provide any information that could not be obtained from a urine HCG, which does not require a venipuncture.

B. Quantitative serum HCG   ESSENTIAL

The quantitative HCG test provides an actual numerical result for the HCG level as well as references ranges for corresponding weeks of gestation. Thus, it should be relatively simple to determine if the patient is experiencing a "normal" pregnancy because her quantitative HCG result should fall within the corresponding gestational age (GA) range. While theoretically this is true, it is complicated by the tremendous intra-age ranges as well as the wide overlap among age groups. For example, at a gestational age of 6 weeks, the corresponding serum HCG level can range from 12,000 to 270,000 mIU/ml. Likewise, a quantitative HCG result of 15,000 mIU/ml is considered "normal" for gestational ages ranging from 4 to 12 weeks.

This is further complicated in women when an accurate date for their last "true" menstrual period cannot be clearly established. Even in women like Mrs. Indigo who can provide an exact date, determining whether the bleeding experienced at that time represented an actual menstrual period or only a partial shedding of the superficial endometrium lining during an early pregnancy (which is not uncommon) is difficult. For example, Mrs. Indigo reported her last menstrual period

(LMP) as being 3.5 weeks ago. Because it was lighter than her usual menses, it is possible that she was already 1 month pregnant at that time; conversely, it is also possible that it represented an actual menstrual period with a smaller quantity of flow (which is also not uncommon). Thus, if the date provided truly represented the date of her actual LMP, then she is approximately 5.5 weeks pregnant. However, if this menses was "lighter" because she was already pregnant, then her LMP for estimating GA and estimated date of confinement (ECD) would make her previous LMP 7.5 weeks ago, making her fetus' GA 9.5 weeks. From the reference values provided, her level of 5000 mIU/ml is "normal" for either of these dates.

The physical examination can sometimes provide useful information regarding the accuracy of the LMP and the correct fetal GA. For example, Mrs. Indigo's physical examination failed to reveal a Chadwick sign (a bluish discoloration of the cervix and less often the vagina that appears at approximately 7 weeks' gestation) or a Hegar sign (softening of the cervical isthmus that also begins at approximately 7 weeks' gestation). Although the Chadwick sign is not always evident, the Hegar sign is almost always present. This would also indicate that Mrs. Indigo's correct GA is less than 7 weeks pregnant or she has an extrauterine pregnancy.

The bimanual examination is useful in determining GA after 12 weeks, but it is of limited value earlier in a pregnancy because top-normal uterine size is equivalent to a gestational age of approximately 9 weeks. Therefore, if there is still a concern regarding Mrs. Indigo's correct GA, a fetal ultrasound is indicated because it is much more accurate in estimating the actual gestational age. However, it generally takes 4 to 5 weeks after conception for the products of conception to be accurately identified on ultrasound, so it is also not very useful before a GA of 4 to 5 weeks.

Hence, the primary role of the quantitative serum HCG is to assist in determining the viability of the pregnancy. During the first 10 weeks of a normal pregnancy, the HCG level should double every 48 hours. If that fails to occur, then diagnoses such as extrauterine pregnancies, spontaneous abortion, threatened abortion, or inaccurate gestational age must be considered.

After 10 weeks, the serum HCG level continues to rise (just at a slower rate) until the end of the first trimester. Then, it begins to decrease slightly until it plateaus near the end of the second trimester. Still, if toward the end of the first trimester the HCG level fails to increase by at least 66% in 48 hours, a nonviable pregnancy must be considered.

Therefore, repeating Mrs. Indigo's serum HCG level in 48 hours should reveal a doubling of her current serum HCG level if she was pregnant with a viable fetus.

C. Pelvic ultrasound, preferably with vaginal probe ESSENTIAL

A pelvic ultrasound, preferably done vaginally (because structures due to pregnancy can be identified earlier), is essential for Mrs. Indigo's evaluation not so much to determine the true GA but to determine if her pregnancy is intrauterine. Traditional abdominal views are generally able to detect a gestational sac by 5 to 6 weeks' gestation or when the serum HCG level is greater than or equal to 1800 mIU/ml; and, cardiac activity is generally identifiable by 7 to 8 weeks' gestation.

However, with a vaginal probe, a gestational sac can generally be identified by 4 to 5 weeks' gestational age or if the serum HCG level is greater than or equal to 1000 mIU/ml; and, cardiac activity can be identified as early as 5.5 to 6 weeks. The inability to identify at least a gestational sac with a serum HCG level of greater than 6500 mIU/ml is highly suspicious for the presence of an extrauterine pregnancy.

D. Hematocrit and hemoglobin (H&H)   ESSENTIAL

Because Mrs. Indigo is experiencing abdominal pain with vaginal bleeding, an Hgb and HCT are indicated not so much to determine her current blood volume (because her vital signs do not indicate that she hypovolemic) but to establish a baseline to compare future results if needed.

E. Serum progesterone level   ESSENTIAL

In a patient with a positive pregnancy test, abdominal pain, and vaginal bleeding, a serum progesterone level of greater than or equal to 25 ng/ml can almost always exclude the presence of an extrauterine pregnancy despite this value being significantly lower than the levels considered consistent with a first-trimester pregnancy. Furthermore, a serum progesterone level of less than or equal to 5 ng/ml with a positive pregnancy test virtually excludes a viable pregnancy. Levels between 5 and 25 require additional evaluation to determine the pregnancy's viability.

4. Diagnosis

A. Normal pregnancy   INCORRECT

A normal pregnancy can be ruled out as Mrs. Indigo's most likely diagnosis because she has abdominal cramping and very light vaginal bleeding in conjunction with no evidence of a fetal sac on vaginal-probe pelvic ultrasound despite an estimated GA of 5.5 to 9.5 weeks and a serum HCG level of 7000 mIU/ml.

B. Spontaneous abortion   INCORRECT

A spontaneous abortion is not Mrs. Indigo's most likely diagnosis because she is only experiencing minimal vaginal bleeding and has a closed cervical os. In a spontaneous abortion, the bleeding is generally very heavy and the cervical os is generally open. Furthermore, her pelvic ultrasound does not reveal any intrauterine evidence of remaining products of conception.

C. Threatened abortion   INCORRECT

A threatened abortion is a more likely possibility than a spontaneous abortion because Mrs. Indigo is not experiencing heavy bleeding and has no visible products of conception at her cervical os on speculum examination. However, her cervical os is closed and her pelvic ultrasound failed to identify any evidence supporting the presence of an intrauterine pregnancy. Therefore, this is not Mrs. Indigo's most likely diagnosis.

D. Ectopic pregnancy   CORRECT

Despite an ectopic pregnancy not being identified on Mrs. Indigo's ultrasound, this is still her most likely diagnosis because her serum HCG level was 7000 mIU/ml, her serum progesterone level was 4 ng/ml, and her pelvic ultrasound (even with a vaginal probe) failed to identify a gestational sac. Additionally, she did have a mild amount of fluid identified in her cul-de-sac on ultrasound, which is also consistent with an extrauterine pregnancy. The lack of being able to identify an ectopic pregnancy on the ultrasound is not uncommon, especially early in the process.

E. Early menstruation caused by an anovulatory cycle
INCORRECT

Early menstruation caused by an anovulatory cycle is not an unreasonable diagnosis because Mrs. Indigo only discontinued her oral contraceptives 4 months ago after being on them for approximately 8 years. Although OCs do not cause infertility, there is a delay to the return of fertility of several months following discontinuation because of anovulatory cycles. This appears to be greater in women who experienced irregular menses before initiating OCs and in women who utilized them for long durations. However, anovulatory cycles are not associated with an elevated serum HCG level. Thus, this is not Mrs. Indigo's most likely diagnosis.

5. Treatment Plan

A. Hysterosalpingography to evaluate tubal patency
INCORRECT

A hysterosalpingography is a radiologic procedure that involves the instillation of a radiopaque contrast material via the endocervical canal to assess the internal anatomic structure of the intrauterine cavity and, more importantly, the patency of the fallopian tubes. It is most commonly utilized in the evaluation of infertility. It is generally contraindicated in suspected ectopic pregnancies because it could induce or worsen the rupture.

B. Hospitalization for immediate surgery   INCORRECT

The indications for immediate surgery for an ectopic pregnancy include evidence of a definite rupture, hemodynamic instability, inability to comply with outpatient treatment, unwillingness to comply with outpatient treatment, and/or failed medical management.

C. Immediate gynecologic consult   CORRECT

Although Mrs. Indigo is currently hemodynamically stable and has no indication that compliance with outpatient therapy would be problematic, there is a concern that she could have experienced rupturing of an ectopic pregnancy because of the presence of the small amount of fluid in her cul-de-sac on pelvic ultrasound. Even though this could represent a normal finding, it cannot be ignored; therefore, the most prudent treatment option is to obtain an immediate gynecologic consultation to determine whether further diagnostic studies (e.g., paracentesis or culdocentesis) are indicated. Then, the gynecologist can determine if a surgical, medical, or expectant management (including close follow-up, patient education, and repeat serum HCG in 48 hours) is the most appropriate treatment option for Mrs. Indigo at this time.

D. Blood typing   CORRECT

Blood typing is indicated at this time not because surgery is planned but to determine Mrs. Indigo's Rh status. If she is Rh negative, she will require Rho(D) immune globin to prevent Rh incompatibility with future pregnancies.

E. Methotrexate 50 mg/m² IM   INCORRECT

Methotrexate 50 mg/m² IM is an alternative to surgery management that is appropriate for many ectopic pregnancies; however, it is not indicated for Mrs. Indigo primarily because of concern regarding the possibility of a ruptured ectopic

pregnancy. It is only indicated in women who are capable (and willing) to be compliant with outpatient therapy, are hemodynamically stable, lack symptoms suggesting a ruptured ectopic pregnancy and/or an intra-abdominal bleeding, display no evidence of fetal cardiac activity on ultrasound, and have an ectopic pregnancy that is less than or equal to 3.5 to 4.0 cm in diameter. Furthermore, it should not be given until normal results are obtained on a complete blood count (CBC), serum aspartate aminotransferase, and serum creatinine.

Epidemiologic and Other Data

Approximately 2% of all pregnancies in the United States are complicated by an ectopic pregnancy. This translates to nearly 90,000 cases annually. Approximately 95% of all ectopic pregnancies occur in the fallopian tubes; however, other extrauterine sites are possible (e.g., ovary, cervix, or other intra-abdominal site). The highest incidence appears to occur in women in their 20s.

Risk factors include any defect of the fallopian tubes that could affect the progression of the ovum from the ovary to the uterus, including scarring from pelvic inflammatory disease (most frequently caused by chlamydia and/or gonorrhea). Some intrauterine abnormalities can also be associated with an increased risk of ectopic pregnancy (e.g., endometritis, scarring from a prior IUD, or a submucosal leiomyoma that is partially or fully obstructing tubal access to the uterus).

CASE 7-7
Irene Jackson
1. History

A. Does she have a vaginal discharge?   ESSENTIAL

The presence and appearance of a vaginal discharge could provide clues suggestive of potential causes of Ms. Jackson's pain. For example, a clear or mucopurulent discharge could indicate the presence of an infection. The most common would be endometritis; however, it is also possible for her to have a vaginal or cervical infection associated with (or unrelated to) endometritis that could indicate the ascension of normal vaginal flora and atypical organisms instead of an STI. The presence of a bloody discharge as defined in Case 7-6 could indicate a pregnancy complication, trauma, or STI. However, the absence of discharge does not necessarily rule out any of these potential diagnoses.

B. Is she experiencing any anorexia?   ESSENTIAL

Although many medical conditions, including those presenting with acute abdominal pain, can be associated with anorexia, it is much more common in appendicitis, peritonitis, and gastric ulcer disease. Even though its presence (or absence) is not diagnostic, this knowledge can still lend support toward (or against) the patient's various differential diagnoses, assisting in narrowing her list down to the single most likely diagnosis.

C. Did her pain begin elsewhere in her abdomen and then migrate to its current location?   ESSENTIAL

The majority of cases of acute abdominal pain tend to begin and persist in the same approximate location, thereby narrowing the list of potential differential diagnoses to structures located in that particular region (e.g., right lower quadrant abdominal pain is most commonly caused by conditions affecting the appendix, the right side of the colon, the right ovary, the right fallopian tube, and the right ureter). Although abdominal pain can radiate to other locations, it rarely "moves" to another area. The most noteworthy exception is appendicitis. It frequently begins periumbilically and then migrates to the right lower quadrant.

D. Is she experiencing any rectal pressure?   ESSENTIAL

Although rectal pressure is not an uncommon finding in gastrointestinal disorders, it is almost always associated with bowel changes. However, rectal pressure in the absence of bowel changes is frequently associated with a reproductive tract problem. In sexually active young women, the most common is PID. Even though this is not diagnostic for PID, if present, it can provide additional support for the diagnosis.

E. Did her nausea begin before or after the onset of pain? ESSENTIAL

When nausea, with or without vomiting, is present in conditions associated with acute abdominal pain, it almost always precedes the onset of the pain. However, in appendicitis, the nausea typically does not occur until after the pain is present. Although this is not diagnostic for appendicitis, if present, it can provide additional support for the diagnosis.

2. Physical Examination

A. Oropharyngeal examination   ESSENTIAL

The oropharyngeal examination is important to evaluate for signs of nongenital sexually transmitted infections given Ms. Jackson's history. These findings can include pharyngeal erythema with tonsillar enlargements and possibly exudates caused by *Neisseria gonorrhoeae*; a single painless shallow lesion on the pharynx, oral mucosa, tongue, or lips caused by *Treponema pallidum*; multiple painful vesicles or small ulcerations generally on an erythematous base caused by the herpes simplex virus; and wart-like, mucosal-colored growths caused by the human papillomavirus. The identification of any of these findings (or other lesions suggestive of other STIs) increases the probability that a sexually transmitted pathogen is responsible for Ms. Jackson's abdominal pain.

Furthermore, because Ms. Jackson is experiencing vomiting, her oral mucosa should be evaluated for degree of moistness because this will roughly correlate with her hydration status.

B. Abdominal examination   ESSENTIAL

Because Ms. Jackson is complaining of abdominal pain, an abdominal examination is indicated. (For more information regarding an abdominal examination and its implications, please see Case 5-1.)

C. Pelvic examination   ESSENTIAL

Because Ms. Jackson is complaining of right lower quadrant and suprapubic pain accompanied by rectal pressure in the absence of gastrointestinal symptoms, is at risk for an STI, and does not know when her LMP occurred, a pelvic examination is essential to evaluate her complaint. (For more information regarding the pelvic examination and its implications, please see Case 6-7.)

D. Rectal examination   ESSENTIAL

Despite her lack of bowel changes, a rectal examination is indicated because of her complaint of rectal fullness in conjunction with her sexual history. Potential diagnosis could include a forgotten (or unstated) foreign body, proctitis, or PID.

E. Neurologic examination   NONESSENTIAL

Because Ms. Jackson is not complaining of any neurologic abnormalities and does not have any signs or symptoms suspicious for an intracranial cause for her fever, a neurologic examination is unlikely to provide any useful information in formulating her diagnosis or treatment.

3. Diagnostic Studies

A. Urinary human chorionic gonadotropin (HCG) NONESSENTIAL

A urinary HCG is not indicated because an intrauterine pregnancy was confirmed by Doppler during her physical examination.

B. Complete blood count with differential (CBC w/diff) ESSENTIAL

A complete blood count with differential can support the diagnosis of an infectious process (as well as provide an indication of its severity) and/or identify the presence of intra-abdominal hemorrhage. (For more detailed information regarding the CBC w/diff, please refer to Case 1-4.)

C. Erythrocyte sedimentation rate (ESR)   ESSENTIAL

An ESR is a gross determination of the amount of inflammation present in the body; however, it is not specific for any one condition or organ system. Despite it not being a sensitive diagnostic indicator, its result can provide further support toward confirming Ms. Jackson's most likely diagnosis.

It is also one of the additional diagnostic criteria suggested by the Centers for Disease Control and Prevention (CDC) to consider along with the patient's signs, symptoms, and diagnostic test results when the patient meets the minimal accepted diagnostic criteria (adnexal OR uterine OR cervical motion tenderness) for PID. The addition of an elevated ESR provides the much needed supplementary support for the diagnosis of PID because there is high variability among HCPs in diagnosing this condition clinically. Nevertheless, this is not pathognomonic for PID and can occur in other conditions. The other expanded CDC diagnostic criteria can be found in Case 5-9.

Definitive diagnosis of PID requires histopathologic confirmation (via biopsy) of the presence of inflammation and infection of the endometrial or tubal lining. Obviously, this is not feasible. Therefore, the CDC guidelines recommend empiric treatment for all young women presenting with lower abdominal or pelvic pain that cannot be attributed to another cause if they are at risk for an STI and have at least one of the three minimal accepted diagnostic criteria. However, some experts feel all three should be present to make the diagnosis clinically.

D. Abdominal MRI   NONESSENTIAL

MRI is a very effective imaging study for identifying intra-abdominal pathology. However, because Ms. Jackson's diagnosis can be established clinically, this procedure is not necessary.

E. Nucleic acid amplification test of cervical discharge for gonorrhea and chlamydia   ESSENTIAL

These tests are indicated not only because Ms. Jackson has a mucopurulent cervical discharge but also because of her high-risk status for acquiring an STI.

4. Diagnosis

A. Pelvic inflammatory disease (PID) with pregnancy CORRECT

PID is an encompassing term representing any infection of the upper female reproductive tract (i.e., endometritis, salpingitis, and tubo-ovarian abscess). The majority of the cases are a result of ascension of an infection from the cervix or vagina. In rare cases it can occur as a result of direct spread of another intra-abdominal inflammatory process, hematogenous dissemination, complications of an infectious tropical disease, iatrogenic transmission, and parturition. The majority of the cases are caused by a sexually transmitted infection, most notably *Neisseria gonorrhoeae* and *Chlamydia trachomatis*. If untreated, it can spread beyond the reproductive tract and cause peritonitis, pelvic abscesses, perihepatitis, perisplenitis, and/or periappendicitis.

As stated previously, the CDC has established minimal accepted diagnostic criteria for PID that consists of being a patient at risk of an STI with adnexal, uterine, and/or cervical motion tenderness. In addition to satisfying these criteria, Ms. Jackson also meets some of the supplemental diagnostic criteria (fever > 101°F and an elevated ESR) and exhibits other findings strongly supportive of the diagnosis (leukocytosis and mucopurulent cervical discharge).

Because an intrauterine pregnancy was confirmed via fetal heart sounds on Doppler, PID with pregnancy is Ms. Jackson's most likely diagnosis.

B. Cervicitis with pregnancy   INCORRECT

Despite Ms. Jackson having an erythematous, friable cervix on her physical examination and evidence of a viable intrauterine pregnancy, this is still not her most likely diagnosis from the list provided because she has other signs and symptoms that are not accounted for by this diagnosis. Cervicitis is frequently found with PID; thus, in Ms. Jackson's case, it represents a symptom, not an independent diagnosis.

C. Uterine leiomyoma with pregnancy   INCORRECT

Although this choice could account for Ms. Jackson's enlarged uterus with fetal heart sounds, it can be eliminated as her most likely diagnosis because a leiomyoma was not identified on ultra-sound. Furthermore, this diagnosis does not account for the severity of her pain, fever, a positive chandelier sign, adnexal tenderness, and uterine tenderness, cervical edema, erythema, and friability; cervical os discharge; and bilateral adnexal tender-ness or her diagnostic findings of leukocytosis and an elevated ESR.

D. Ectopic pregnancy   INCORRECT

Although an ectopic pregnancy can be responsible for a positive pregnancy test and unilateral adnexal tenderness, it rarely results in bilateral adnexal tenderness. Furthermore, it is not associated with cervical motion tenderness, uterine tenderness, uterine enlargement, fever, or significant leukocytosis.

Finally, Doppler and ultrasound confirmation of a viable intrauterine pregnancy prevents this from being her most likely diagnosis.

E. Appendicitis   INCORRECT

Appendicitis is a possibility because of the elevated white blood cell count along with the abdominal pain, especially in the right lower quadrant, as well as the nausea, vomiting, and fever. However, it alone would not explain her uterine enlargement with Doppler confirmation of a viable intrauterine pregnancy, pelvic organ tenderness, positive chandelier sign, cervical changes, and mucopurulent cervical discharge. Therefore, appendicitis alone is not Ms. Jackson's most likely diagnosis.

5. Treatment Plan

A. Hospitalization   CORRECT

Previous versions of the CDC guidelines for the diagnosis and treatment of PID provided specific circumstances requiring hospitalization of the patient. However, the current edition allows for greater clinical decision making on the part of the HCP and recognizes that the decision to treat a patient as an inpatient or as an outpatient needs to be individualized on a case-by-case basis. However, the CDC does provide "suggestions" of which patient populations might have better outcomes if hospitalized. Ms. Jackson meets at least five of these: severe infection, high fever, pregnancy, vomiting preventing oral medicine administration, and probable poor compliance.

The other indications include lack of definite diagnosis, possible need for a surgical intervention, failure of outpatient therapy, and presence of a tubo-ovarian abscess.

B. Obstetrical ultrasound   INCORRECT

An obstetrical ultrasound would have been indicated for Ms. Jackson to determine an accurate GA because she is unaware of her LMP. However, the radiologist already confirmed this information with the pelvic ultrasound he performed.

Although gestational size can be fairly accurately determined by uterine palpation and measurement, it still needs to be confirmed by ultrasound when the LMP is unknown because of the possibility of multiple gestations, abnormal fetal size, polyhydramnios, and oligohydramnios.

The presence of edematous fluid-filled tubes on ultrasound is considered by some to be equally sensitive as histopathologic confirmation in establishing a definitive diagnosis of PID.

C. Cefoxitin 2 g IV every 6 hours plus doxycycline 100 mg orally or IV every 12 hours   INCORRECT

Although cefoxitin 2 g IV every 6 hours plus doxycycline 100 mg orally or IV every 12 hours is a CDC-recommended regimen A for the parental treatment of PID, it is not indicated for Ms. Jackson because doxycycline has an FDA class D pregnancy rating. (For more information regarding the FDA pregnancy risk categories, please see Case 2-7.)

Clindamycin 900 mg IV every 8 hours plus gentamicin loading dose IV or IM (2 mg/kg of body weight), followed by a maintenance dose (1.5 mg/kg) every 8 hours, is a CDC-recommended regimen B for the parental treatment of PID. However, it would also be contraindicated in Ms. Jackson because gentamicin also has an FDA category D rating.

D. Levofloxacin 500 mg IV once daily plus metronidazole 500 mg IV every 8 hours   INCORRECT

Levofloxacin 500 mg IV once daily plus metronidazole 500 mg IV every 8 hours is a CDC-accepted parental alternative. It would be a better alternative than the previous choice because levofloxacin has a category C and metronidazole a level B rating. However, it is still probably not the best alternative for Ms. Jackson because of the high rate of resistance of gonorrhea to fluoroquinolones as well as potential ligament damage to the unborn fetus and Ms. Jackson herself from these agents.

The other two alternative choices, (1) ofloxacin 400 mg IV every 12 hours with or without metronidazole 500 mg IV every 8 hours (which would have the same concerns as using levofloxacin) or (2) ampicillin/sulbactam 3 g IV every 6 hours with doxycycline 100 mg orally or IV every 12 hours (which, again, doxycycline is a category D drug), are equally as unattractive.

E. Cefotetan 2 g IV every 12 hours   CORRECT

This second-generation cephalosporin is pregnancy category B rated and considered by many experts to be the treatment of choice for pregnant women with PID. The CDC guidelines only state that empiric antibiotics for pregnant patients with PID must cover gonorrhea and chlamydia.

Epidemiologic and Other Data

PID is estimated to affect approximately 0.10 to 0.13 per 100,000 women each year in the United States. However, many experts would argue that this incidence rate is underestimated because a significant number of women with this condition have asymptomatic or subclinical infections. Nevertheless, approximately 1 million women between the ages of 15 and 39 years are diagnosed with PID annually.

The most common pathogens responsible for PID are *Neisseria gonorrhea* and *Chlamydia trachomatis*. These two sexually transmitted infections account for approximately 50% of all cases. Other common causes include ascending and overgrowth of the organisms that are considered to be part of the normal vaginal flora (e.g., *Gardnerella vaginalis*, *Haemophilus influenzae*, *Streptococcus agalactiae*, and assorted gram-negative rods). Much less frequently, PID can result from cytomegalovirus, *Mycoplasma hominis*, *Mycobacterium genitalium*, *Urea urealyticum*, *Escherichia coli*, group B streptococci, and peptostreptococci.

Risks factors for PID include those typically associated with STIs: numerous partners, new partner within the last 3 months, unprotected intercourse, history of PID, history of any STI, history of cervicitis from a sexually transmitted organism, being between the ages of 15 and 29 years, recent IUD placement (generally defined as the first 3 months), and douching.

Common acute complications are tubo-ovarian abscess (estimated to occur in ~15% of all cases) and Fitz-Hugh-Curtis syndrome (estimated to occur in up to 30% of all cases). The most common long-term consequence of the disease is infertility. Women who have had a single episode of PID experience a decrease in their fertility rates of 25%. Subsequent infections are associated with even greater rates of infertility.

CASE 7-8
Jackie Khan
1. History

A. Has she had any vaginal bleeding/spotting or cramping? ESSENTIAL

Some degree of nausea and vomiting is associated with ~90% of all pregnancies. Although mild nausea and vomiting of pregnancy is frequently called "morning sickness," it actually occurs throughout the day in the majority of patients, with a peak of symptoms in the morning and evening. Small frequent feedings, especially of dry food, tend to alleviate the problem for most women. It is theorized to be caused by the rapid elevation of HCG, which is released from the placental trophoblasts. This is supported by the majority of cases occurring in the first trimester, during which the HCG level rises at the fastest rate; and resolving by the end of the first trimester, when the HCG level is not rising nearly as rapidly. During the second trimester, the HCG level decreases slightly until approximately 20 weeks' gestation, when it begins to plateau. This correlates with the resolution of symptoms for nearly all women who experience second-trimester nausea and vomiting.

However, if the nausea and vomiting is severe, is associated with dehydration, accompanied by weight loss, is unresponsive to dietary or medical interventions, or continues beyond the first trimester, it is referred to as hyperemesis gravidarum. The presence of hyperemesis gravidarum requires additional evaluation to determine if there is excessive HCG production. The most common causes of excess HCG production include gestational trophoblastic disease, hyperthyroidism, and multiple gestations. Because molar pregnancies (a form of gestational trophoblastic disease) are almost always associated with some degree of vaginal bleeding, it is imperative to inquire if vaginal bleeding is present when evaluating a patient with hyperemesis gravidarum. Additionally, vaginal bleeding during pregnancy (especially after the first 2 months) is very suspicious for a pregnancy complication.

B. What was her pre-pregnancy weight and how does it compare to her current weight?   ESSENTIAL

In general, the recommended weight gain for a healthy pregnancy is 20 to 40 lb. During the first trimester, the pregnant woman should gain 2 to 5 lb. Afterward, she should not gain any more than 1 lb per week. Women who do not appear to be achieving an adequate weight gain, and especially if they are losing weight, need an evaluation to determine the cause. They can include pregnancy complications (e.g., hyperemesis gravidum, multiple gestations, and gestational trophoblastic disease [i.e., molar pregnancy]), endocrinopathies (e.g., hypothyroidism, hyperthyroidism, adrenal insufficiency, and parathyroid disease), psychological illnesses (e.g., depression, and anorexia nervosa), and renal failure.

It is also important to inquire about comparisons of the weight because minor fluctuations can be accounted for by differences in the facility's scales, patient's clothing, and time of day.

C. Has she ever experienced motion sickness? NONESSENTIAL

Motion sickness is theorized to result from discord between visual and vestibular senses, which is an entirely different mechanism than pregnancy-induced nausea and vomiting. Additionally, there is no evidence to suggest a history of motion sickness is connected to any complications of pregnancy, including nausea and vomiting.

D. Why did she have an abortion?   NONESSENTIAL

Mrs. Khan's decision to electively terminate her first pregnancy was nonmedical in nature. Therefore, her reason will not have any medical consequences on this pregnancy.

Even if there is a legitimate reason for inquiring about the circumstances surrounding her abortion, this request must be worded in a much less judgmental manner.

E. Has she been experiencing intense pruritus, with or without a rash?   ESSENTIAL

Hyperemesis during pregnancy is not restricted to hyperemesis gravidarum or to elevating HCG levels. It is possible that gastrointestinal conditions unrelated to the pregnancy, or resulting from the pregnancy, can be responsible for (or at least contributing to) the severity of the problem. For example, intrahepatic cholestasis can occur with pregnancy probably as a result of pregnancy-related alterations in bile and fatty acid metabolism. It is associated with marked pruritus, generally without a rash; however, excoriations and secondary infections can be present as a result of scratching. Despite this condition being most common during the third trimester, it is possible for it to occur at any time.

2. Physical Examination

A. Thyroid examination   ESSENTIAL

A thyroid examination is indicated for Mrs. Khan because hypothyroidism and hyperthyroidism can be responsible for hyperemesis gravidarum. However, it is important to remember that a benign thyroid enlargement can occur in a very small number (~0.2%) of all pregnancies and a normal thyroid examination does not exclude thyroid dysfunction.

B. Heart examination   ESSENTIAL

Although Mrs. Khan's orthostasis is most likely caused by dehydration secondary to hyperemesis gravidarum, she still should have a heart examination to ensure that there is no evidence of an undiagnosed congenital defect, valvular abnormality, underlying cardiomyopathy, or arrhythmia (which frequently requires cardiac monitoring to detect). This is especially important because the increased blood volume normally seen with pregnancy places additional workload on the heart, which can cause previously unknown cardiac conditions to become evident.

C. Abdominal examination   ESSENTIAL

An abdominal examination is important to measure the fundal height to ensure that it is consistent with patient's gestational age. Furthermore, it is indicated to determine whether there are any abnormalities present that could suggest not only a pregnancy-related complication (e.g., intrahepatic cholestasis of pregnancy) but also a nonpregnancy-related condition (e.g., cholelithiasis, pancreatitis, or bowel obstruction) causing her severe nausea and vomiting.

D. Pelvic examination   ESSENTIAL

A pelvic examination is essential to evaluate for potential complications of pregnancy (e.g., bleeding, cervical os

being partially open, or products of conception evident at the cervical os).

E. Lower extremity evaluation for edema   ESSENTIAL

It is important to evaluate all pregnant women at all visits for pedal edema. The main concern is preeclampsia or eclampsia, which generally isn't a problem until the third trimester. However, in some conditions (e.g., gestational trophoblastic disease [which also can produce hyperemesis gravidarum]), it can occur in the second (and occasionally the first) trimester. Furthermore, hyperthyroidism, which can cause hyperemesis gravidum, can also cause pretibial myxedema.

3. Diagnostic Studies

A. Dipstick urinalysis   ESSENTIAL

All pregnant patients should have a dipstick urinalysis performed at every prenatal visit to evaluate (at minimum) for the presence of protein, ketones, and glucose. The presence of protein can indicate early preeclampsia/eclampsia, ketones can be associated with starvation and/or dehydration, and glucose can indicate the presence of gestational diabetes. Protein can also indicate the presence of renal disease.

Furthermore, dehydration is associated with more concentrated urine (higher specific gravity) and more acidic urine (lower pH). All of these tests are generally performed on a routine urine dipstick. A complete dipstick urinalysis also evaluates for the presence of leukocyte esterase and nitrites, which are frequently found in urinary tract infections.

B. Blood urea nitrogen (BUN), creatinine, and electrolytes   ESSENTIAL

A BUN, creatinine, and electrolytes are indicated to further evaluate Mrs. Khan's renal and hydration status. In renal disease, both the BUN and creatinine are elevated. In dehydration, the BUN is elevated and the creatinine is normal. However, this pattern is not specific for dehydration; gastrointestinal bleeding, hypovolemia, starvation, shock, and sepsis can also produce the same pattern and could potentially be responsible for Mrs. Khan's symptoms. The most common electrolyte abnormality seen from excessive vomiting is hypokalemia; hyponatremia is second.

C. Quantitative serum human chorionic gonadotropin (HCG)   ESSENTIAL

A quantitative serum HCG is indicated because Mrs. Khan has persistent hyperemesis gravidarum and a uterus that is larger than normal for the stated GA. This test could be helpful in screening for potential pregnancy complications; however, it would be much more useful if Mrs. Khan was in her first trimester instead of her second. (For more information regarding quantitative serum HCG testing in determining GA and potential pregnancy complications, please see Case 7-6.)

D. Obstetric ultrasound   ESSENTIAL

An obstetric ultrasound is indicated for Mrs. Khan because there is a discrepancy of approximately 9 weeks between her estimated GA (based on her LMP) and her uterine fundal height, fetal heart tones were not heard with Doppler examination of her uterus (normally, these are evident by 10–12 weeks' gestation), and she is experiencing hyperemesis gravidarum.

E. Hematocrit and hemoglobin (H&H)   ESSENTIAL

An H&H is indicated for Mrs. Khan to ensure that her orthostasis is secondary to dehydration and not blood loss because anemia is common in pregnancy and she had been experiencing some minor vaginal bleeding.

F. Thyroid-stimulating hormone (TSH), free thyroxine (T_4), and triiodothyronine by radioimmune assay (T_3 by RIA)   ESSENTIAL

As stated previously, both hypo- and hyperthyroidism can be associated with hyperemesis gravidarum.

4. Diagnosis

A. Pregnancy-induced hyperemesis gravidarum secondary to hyperthyroidism   INCORRECT

Hyperemesis gravidarum is a complication of pregnancy characterized by severe nausea and vomiting frequently associated with dehydration. Mrs. Khan's clinical picture and diagnostic studies support this diagnosis. However, her elevated total T_4 and T_3 by RIA and normal TSH are not consistent with hyperthyroidism because the elevated thyroid hormone levels must be associated with a suppressed TSH level. Thus, this is not her most likely diagnosis.

However, her thyroid test results are consistent with the normal increase during pregnancy of the total number of thyroxine-binding globulins resulting from the excessive estrogen state associated with pregnancy. This is a result of HCG having a greater affinity for these thyroxine-binding globulin receptor sites than the thyroid hormones do; hence, the thyroid hormones become displaced (resulting in the increase in total hormone serum levels). However, the TSH remains normal. This combination of an elevated total T_4 and T_3 in conjunction with a normal TSH is referred to as pseudohyperthyroidism of pregnancy. If the laboratory had done the FT_4 as ordered, it would likely have been normal.

B. Multiple gestations with intrahepatic cholestasis   INCORRECT

As stated previously, pregnancy causes alterations in bile and fatty acid metabolism. In some women, this can lead to intrahepatic cholestasis, which is a secondary cause for severe nausea and vomiting associated with pregnancy. However, it is not Mrs. Khan's most likely diagnosis because it is generally limited to the third trimester and is associated with severe pruritus.

Furthermore, this diagnosis is incorrect because Mrs. Khan's ultrasound failed to reveal multiple gestations as the cause of her enlarged (for GA) uterus and elevated HCG level.

C. Normal pregnancy with hyperthyroidism   INCORRECT

Based on her diagnostic studies, Mrs. Khan does not have hyperthyroidism (as discussed above) or a "normal" pregnancy. Therefore, this is not her most likely diagnosis.

D. Hyperemesis gravidarum   INCORRECT

As previously stated, hyperemesis gravidarum is a severe, persistent vomiting associated with pregnancy. Some experts feel it cannot be diagnosed unless it results in weight loss, starving ketosis, dehydration, hypochloremic alkalosis, and hypokalemia. Despite Mrs. Khan meeting the basic and expanded definitions, this is still not her most likely diagnosis

from the list provided because it does not account for her other symptoms, abnormal physical examination findings, and diagnostic test results. These indicate that Mrs. Khan has another condition that is causing, or at least contributing to, her hyperemesis gravidarum that must be diagnosed and treated to adequately address her chief complaint.

E. Hydatidiform mole with hyperemesis gravidarum and dehydration   CORRECT

A hydatidiform mole (or molar pregnancy) occurs when the chorionic villi develop into a conglomeration composed of clusters of clear vesicles. It is suspected by the presence of hyperemesis gravidarum (diagnosis confirmed by previous discussion) in her second trimester, her uterus being larger than it should be for her estimated GA based on her LMP, and the absence of fetal heart sounds on Doppler examination. It is confirmed by her characteristic pelvic ultrasound findings and markedly elevated serum HCG level.

Her history of severe emesis and physical examination findings of orthostatic and tachycardia are suggestive of dehydration, which was essentially confirmed by her diagnostic studies (i.e., presence of ketonuria, high urinary specific gravity, low urinary pH, hypokalemia, hypochloremia, and an elevated BUN in the presence of a normal creatinine). Hence, this is Mrs. Khan's most likely diagnosis.

5. Treatment Plan

A. Admit to hospital for normal saline solution (NSS) IV with potassium chloride (KCl)   CORRECT

Because of her dehydration with abnormal electrolyte findings plus her need for surgery for the removal of the hydatidiform mole along with the uterine contents, hospitalization for NSS IV with KCl is indicated. Although serum potassium levels tend to return to normal more quickly with oral potassium, the severity of Mrs. Khan's vomiting eliminates this route at this time.

B. Refer to regular obstetrician for continued prenatal care   INCORRECT

Because the pregnancy needs to be terminated immediately in an attempt to prevent the occurrence of trophoblastic malignancies (primarily a choriocarcinoma or a placental trophoblastic tumor), the conditions that fall at the opposite end of the spectrum of gestational trophoblastic disease from a benign hydatidiform mole, Mrs. Khan does not need further prenatal care at this time.

C. Refer to regular obstetrician (or gynecologist/obstetrician of the patient's choice) for surgical evacuation of uterine contents and subsequent quantitative serum HCG measurements   CORRECT

Once a molar pregnancy is identified, the patient needs the uterine contents evacuated as soon as possible via suction curettage. Histologic examination must be performed on the expelled tissue. If a malignancy is identified, hysterectomy followed by chemotherapy is indicated.

If no evidence of a neoplasm is present, then the patient will require serial quantitative serum HCG levels for 1 year. Initially, they should be performed at 2-week intervals. After two consecutive results are negative (< 5 mU/ml), the measuring interval can be increased to monthly. As long as the results continue to be negative, after six consecutive negative results, the screening interval can be increased to every other month for the remainder of the testing period.

If the HCG levels fail to reach negative, increase from the original level, plateau instead of continuing to decline, or decrease initially and then increase, further evaluation is necessary starting with a repeat ultrasound (to rule out a new pregnancy despite advising patients not to become pregnant for at least 1 year). If it does not appear to be the result of a viable fetus, a repeat chest radiograph and dilation and curettage (D&C) are indicated. Regardless of these findings, the majority of these women are going to be candidates for hysterectomy and chemotherapy.

Hormonal contraceptive methods are not contraindicated and should actually be utilized (unless there is a compelling reason not to) because of their high efficacy rates.

D. Chest x-ray (CXR)   CORRECT

A CXR is also recommended preoperatively to rule out the possibility of pulmonary metastases in case a malignancy is identified on the cytologic examination of the uterine contents.

E. Initiate therapy with propylthiouracil   INCORRECT

Propylthiouracil is the treatment of choice for hyperthyroidism in pregnancy. If ineffective or in cases involving medical urgencies/emergencies from the hyperthyroidism (i.e., thyroid storm), beta-blockers and/or potassium iodine solution may be required. Radioactive iodine is contraindicated in pregnancy because of the adverse effects it has on the developing fetal thyroid. However, because Mrs. Khan has pseudo-hyperthyroidism, she does not require treatment.

However, if she did have actual hyperthyroidism, because her hydatidiform mole will require termination of her pregnancy, radioactive iodine therapy would be the most appropriate treatment option for her. Still, before treatment is initiated, it is essential to determine the cause of her hyperthyroidism. Most likely, it would be secondary to excessive chorionic gonadotropin excretion from her hydatidiform mole. Nevertheless, this cannot just be assumed. Because she does not have signs consistent with Graves disease, multinodular goiter, or a toxic adenoma, she would require a radionuclide thyroid scan to help identify the cause of her hyperthyroidism. Lack of uptake would be consistent with this diagnosis. However, if her scan is positive for uptake, then her more likely diagnoses would include excessive thyroid hormone, excessive iodine, or destructive thyroiditis.

Epidemiologic and Other Data

Hydatidiform moles (or molar pregnancies) represent the benign end of the spectrum of gestational trophoblastic diseases. They are estimated to occur in approximately 1 in 1500 pregnancies in the United States, generally in the first trimester of pregnancy. The incidence rises with increased maternal age. Being older than the age of 45 years at conception is considered to be a risk factor for the development of this complication. The other known risk factor is a history of a previous hydatidiform pregnancy.

The malignant end of the spectrum includes choriocarcinoma and placental-site trophoblastic tumor. These represent less than 1% of all gynecologic carcinomas. The incidence of choriocarcinomas in the United States is approximately 1 in every 25,000 pregnancies (or 1 in every 20,000 live births). Women with a history of a hydatidiform mole are 1000 times more likely to have a choriocarcinoma than women who had previous pregnancies without this complication.

CASE 7-9
Karen Lane
1. History

A. How does she define "weakness"?   ESSENTIAL

Medically, weakness is defined as a decrease in the power than can be produced by muscle(s). However, patients will use this phrase to describe other sensations, such as generalized malaise, the inability to "function normally," weariness, or fatigue (see next choice). In order to establish the correct diagnosis in a timely fashion, it is essential to have a clear understanding of the patient's complaints.

B. How does she define "fatigue"?   ESSENTIAL

Fatigue is another term with various connotations. The actual sensation described as "fatigue" can direct the correct line of questioning necessary to obtain useful clinical information on which to establish the patient's differential diagnoses. For example, if the patient defines "fatigue" as feeling tired or sleepy, it could represent inadequate sleep time, insomnia, or sleep apnea. If the patient defines "fatigue" as a lack of motivation/desire or lassitude, then psychological causes (e.g., depression and/or somatoform disorders) are the most likely culprit. If the patient defines "fatigue" as feeling exhausted with minimal (or at least less than previously required) exertion or tiring more easily, then the most likely cause is an underlying medical condition.

Another generalization that is useful in distinguishing between psychological and physical fatigue is that psychological fatigue tends to be present when the patient awakens (often feeling just as tired as before going to bed), resolves as the day progresses, and decreases (or at least does not worsen) with activity. Conversely, patients who feel "rested" upon arising but whose fatigue returns as the day progresses or with activity generally have a physical illness that is responsible for the fatigue. Although these are important generalizations, it is essential to remember that they are not absolutes.

C. Is she experiencing any anxiety or increased stress aside from her tib/fib fracture?   ESSENTIAL

Anxiety, and in particular, panic attacks can be associated with dyspnea and palpations.

D. Does her cast feel tighter or has she been experiencing paresthesias or discoloration of her toes?   ESSENTIAL

This question addresses two very serious conditions that could be affecting Ms. Lane. First, it determines if there are any signs or symptoms suggestive of a compartment syndrome as a result of the leg swelling in the confining cast.

Second, and more relevant to her chief complaint, it assists in evaluating for the presence of a deep venous thrombosis (DVT). Because Ms. Lane's left leg is essentially immobile and she takes oral contraceptives, she has an increased risk of developing a DVT, which could be responsible for her symptoms (especially if it migrated to her lungs and produced a pulmonary embolism [PE]). Additionally, her risk for a thromboembolic event is also increased by her recent smoking history.

E. Does she have any pedal edema?   ESSENTIAL

Pedal edema can be found in an array of medical conditions; the majority of the time, it represents a cardiovascular, renal, or hepatic condition. Her symptoms could be attributed (partially or completely) to disorders in any of these areas, including tachyarrhythmias, cardiomyopathy, DVT, renal failure, nephrotic syndrome [most likely caused by excessive nonsteroidal anti-inflammatory drug (NSAID) usage in Ms. Lane's case], peptic ulcer disease caused by excessive NSAID usage, and/or hepatic failure.

2. Physical Examination

A. Palpation of the thyroid   ESSENTIAL

Palpitations, tachyarrhythmias, accentuation of the heart sounds, fatigue, myalgias, and dyspnea can be associated with hyperthyroidism. Hypothyroidism can cause fatigue, weakness, myalgias, dyspnea, bradyarrhythmias, and heart failure. Therefore, it is important to check Ms. Lane's thyroid gland for signs of goiter, nodules, other masses, asymmetry, tenderness, consistency changes, and bruits.

B. Heart examination   ESSENTIAL

A heart examination is indicated because Ms. Lane is complaining of palpitations, dyspnea, and fatigue. Possible abnormalities responsible for these symptoms that could be evident on physical examination include structural defects, cardiomyopathy, heart failure, or arrhythmias. (For more details on the complete heart examination, please see Case 1-2.)

C. Lung auscultation   ESSENTIAL

Auscultation of the lungs is essential because Ms. Lane has dyspnea. Abnormalities on this exam could be indicative of either a cardiac or pulmonary condition producing her symptoms. (For more information regarding physical examination of the lungs, please see Case 1-5.)

D. Abdominal examination   NONESSENTIAL

Because Ms. Lane's symptoms do not appear to be gastrointestinal, genitourinary, or gynecologic in origin, an abdominal examination is not necessary at this time.

E. Evaluation of lower extremities   ESSENTIAL

Examination of Ms. Lane's lower legs is essential to evaluate for pedal edema (suggestive of cardiac, hepatic, or renal failure), pretibial myxedema (suggestive of hypothyroidism), calf and thigh tenderness (suggestive of DVT or a myopathy), color or temperature changes (suggestive of a vascular occlusion, dilation, or spasm), presence of true weakness (suggestive of a myopathy or electrolyte abnormality), and abnormal deep tendon reflexes (suggestive of a neuropathy or thyroid condition).

3. Diagnostic Studies

A. Urinary   human   chorionic   gonadotropin   (HCG)   NONESSENTIAL

Ms. Lane is regularly and consistently using a highly effective method of contraception, lacks signs or symptoms of pregnancy (except for fatigue), and had a normal menstrual period 2 weeks ago. Thus, a urinary HCG is not indicated.

B. Electrocardiogram (ECG)   ESSENTIAL

An ECG is indicated because Ms. Lane is complaining of palpitations. Although the ECG only provides a couple of seconds of evaluation of her heart's rate and rhythm, it is possible that an arrhythmia can be identified. (However, longer-term cardiac monitoring is likely going to be necessary to ensure that an arrhythmia is not present.) Furthermore, it permits evaluation of the P, Q, R, S, and T waves; their respective complexes; and associated segments for findings that are suggestive of abnormalities of conduction, cardiac ischemia, myocardial infarction, electrolyte disturbances, cardiomegaly, and areas of hypertrophy that could be causing Ms. Lane's symptoms.

C. Serum electrolytes   ESSENTIAL

Because Ms. Lane's symptoms could be caused by hyperkalemia and she is taking three medications (celecoxib, ibuprofen, and ethinyl estradiol/drospirenone) that could potentially result in this condition, it is important to evaluate her electrolytes for this and other electrolyte disturbances.

D. D-dimer   ESSENTIAL

The signs and symptoms associated with a PE are highly variable and generally nonspecific; thus, additional studies are indicated to rule out this possibility. Therefore, a Wells risk probability assessment was performed on Ms. Lane. A D-dimer is indicated because her Wells score is 4.5 (or intermediate risk).

The Wells scoring system was developed to stratify individuals with signs and symptoms suggestive of a PE into a risk category of either low, intermediate, or high based on their history and physical examination findings. The patient is assigned points for positive results on each of the following items: clinical signs and symptoms suspicious for a PE (3 points), differential diagnoses are less likely to be the patient's correct diagnosis than a PE (3 points), history of a prior VTE (1.5 points), history of cancer (1 point), recent surgery or immobilization (1.5 points), hemoptysis (1 point), and presence of tachycardia on examination (1.5 points). The sum of the items' assigned point value is the patient's score. A patient with a Wells score of 1 or lower is considered to be at low risk for a PE, whereas one with a score of 7 or higher is considered to be at high risk. Patients with a Wells score of 2 to 6 are considered to be at intermediate risk.

E. Chest x-ray (CXR)   ESSENTIAL

Despite clear lung auscultation on her physical examination, Ms. Lane should have a CXR performed because of her dyspnea. It could identify abnormalities that are not yet detectable that may or may not be related to her recent motor vehicle accident (e.g., small pneumothorax, small hemothorax, or a diaphragm tear that is permitting abdominal cavity contents [most commonly the small intestine] to herniate slightly into the chest cavity) and her current symptoms.

4. Diagnosis

A. Bradycardia caused by first-degree AV block   INCORRECT

Despite the presence of a first-degree atrioventricular block (AVB) on her ECG, this is not Ms. Lane's most likely diagnosis because her pulse rate is 76 BPM. Bradycardia is defined as a pulse rate under 60 BPM.

B. Pulmonary embolism (PE) secondary to a deep venous thrombosis (DVT)   INCORRECT

Ms. Lane's medical history (recent compound leg fracture, recent surgery, leg immobilization because of a cast, very recent smoker, and combination oral contraceptive use) is more suspicious for the possibility of a PE causing her chief complaint than all of her clinical signs, symptoms, and diagnostic test results combined.

Aside from her chief complaint, she does not have any other symptoms that are strongly suggestive for this disorder, including chest pain, hemoptysis, and cough. Additionally, her physical examination lacks findings suspicious for both a DVT (e.g., leg edema, erythema, or tenderness) and a PE (e.g., tachycardia, pulmonary friction rub, or rales). A negative D-dimer level in conjunction with her intermediate-risk Wells score significantly decreases the likelihood of this being Ms. Lane's most likely diagnosis.

C. Fibromyalgia syndrome (FMS)   INCORRECT

The American College of Rheumatology's diagnostic criteria for FMS requires the HCP to reproduce the patient's pain by applying moderate pressure over at least 11 of the 18 established trigger points. Because these trigger points were not evaluated on Ms. Lane's physical examination, it would be difficult to conclude that FMS is her most likely diagnosis.

However, irrespective of the trigger-point testing, there is sufficient clinical evidence to accurately conclude that FMS is not Ms. Lane's most likely diagnosis. For example, her muscle pain is acute in nature, only affects her legs, and is associated with true weakness. In contrast, the myalgias associated with FMS tend to be chronic in nature, to involve the whole body (with predominance in the neck, shoulders, hips, and lower back), and to be without identifiable decreased muscle strength. Furthermore, FMS has not been known to cause (or be caused by) an electrolyte abnormality.

D. Pseudohyperkalemia   INCORRECT

Pseudohyperkalemia is a false elevation of the serum potassium level resulting from an influx of potassium out of the intracellular space into the bloodstream immediately prior to or after venipuncture. It is felt to be caused by either hemolysis (caused by a traumatic stick or prolonged tourniquet usage) or clot formation (caused by leukocytosis or thrombocytosis).

This can essentially be eliminated as Ms. Lane's most likely diagnosis because of the associated hyponatremia. The shift caused by potassium exiting the cells is associated with an influx of sodium into the cells. Hence, the serum potassium level elevates while the serum sodium level decreases, or vice versa in the case of hypokalemia and hypernatremia.

E. Severe hyperkalemia secondary to nonsteroidal anti-inflammatory drugs (NSAIDs) and the progestin drospirenone   CORRECT

As stated previously, Ms. Lane has true hyperkalemia because of her associated hyponatremia as well as signs and symptoms consistent with this electrolyte abnormality. Hyperkalemia is considered severe if any of the following conditions are present: (1) a serum potassium level of greater than 8 mEq/L, (2) the presence of ECG findings consistent with hyperkalemia (especially the loss of P waves and the widening of the QRS complex), OR (3) severe neuromuscular symptoms.

Even though Ms. Lane's potassium is still below 8 mEq/L and her neuromuscular symptoms are mild (myalgias, not spasms or flaccid paralysis), she has flattened P waves, a prolonged PR interval, a shortened QRS interval, and T-wave changes on her ECG, which are consistent with hyperkalemia. Therefore, she meets the diagnostic criteria for severe hyperkalemia.

Moderate hyperkalemia is defined as a serum potassium level between 6.5 and 8.0 mEq/L AND no evidence of hyperkalemia-related ECG abnormalities or severe neuromuscular symptoms. Mild hypokalemia is a serum level between 5.5 and 6.5 mEq/L PLUS no evidence of either hyperkalemia-related ECG changes or severe neuromuscular symptoms. It is important to get the patient categorized correctly (mild, moderate, or severe) because treatment decisions are based on the assigned level.

Because Ms. Lane does not have a history of any preexisting renal, hepatic, or adrenal abnormalities and is taking three agents (two NSAIDs and a COC with the progestin drospirenone [DRSP]) that can produce hyperkalemia, in all likelihood it is the combination that caused her potassium to elevate to this significant level. NSAIDs generally cause hyperkalemia as a result of a secondary hypoaldosteronism effect in which impaired sodium reabsorption is responsible for decreased potassium secretion (leading to decreased renal excretion), whereas drospirenone (a spironolactone analog) produces hyperkalemia via the same mechanism except the sodium impairment is caused by a resistance to aldosterone.

Other causes of hyperkalemia include primary hypoaldosteronism causing impaired sodium reabsorption and its associated decreased potassium secretion, enhanced chloride reabsorption resulting in decreased potassium secretion, renal failure, and decreased distal tubular flow.

Unfortunately, there is no simple diagnostic test that can be performed to ensure that Ms. Lane's hyperkalemia is drug related. However, one of the recommended first steps in attempting to determine the cause of hyperkalemia is to eliminate any drugs that could be responsible for the condition. The medications most commonly responsible include heparin, angiotensin-converting enzyme (ACE) inhibitors, angiotensin receptor blockers (ARBs), potassium-sparing diuretics, potassium supplements, and DRSP.

DRSP is a spironolactone analog that has antimineralocorticoid activity. The COC containing ethinyl estradiol (EE) and DRSP has a bolded warning on its packaging label cautioning HCPs not to prescribe this agent to women who have coexisting medical conditions that could cause hyperkalemia. Furthermore, it advises that serum potassium levels be checked during the first cycle of therapy if the patient is on any other medications that could produce an elevated potassium level. Independently, it is estimated that 3 mg of DRSP has an equivalent potential of producing hyperkalemia as 25 mg of spironolactone. Thus, from the choices provided, this is Ms. Lane's most likely diagnosis.

5. Treatment Plan

A. Hospitalize and obtain a stat BUN and creatinine   CORRECT

Because of her palpations, dyspnea, ECG changes, and potassium level, Ms. Lane needs to be admitted to the hospital for cardiac monitoring, further evaluation, and treatment.

Part of her initial assessment should include a measurement of her serum BUN and creatinine to determine if she has any laboratory evidence of renal and/or hepatic insufficiencies. (For more information regarding the interpretation of the BUN and creatinine to evaluate renal and hepatic function, please see Case 6-6.) An impairment of hepatic and/or renal functioning could be responsible for (or contributing to) Ms. Lane's hyperkalemia. Additionally, a drug-related toxicity could be responsible for the hepatic and/or renal impairment (which would further elevate her serum potassium level).

B. Administer calcium gluconate, glucose, insulin, bicarbonate, and sodium polystyrene sulfonate CORRECT

Because of Ms. Lane's symptoms and ECG abnormalities, her potassium excess needs to be corrected as soon as possible to hopefully prevent her from developing a potentially fatal cardiac arrhythmia (most commonly ventricular tachycardia, ventricular fibrillation, or atrial fibrillation) or cardiac ischemia. The calcium chloride (administered IV) will stabilize the cellular membrane (especially of the cardiac muscles) and thereby reduce the possibility of an arrhythmia developing. The combination of insulin and glucose will force the potassium back into the cells (thereby forcing sodium out, resulting in a reduction of the serum potassium level and an increase in the serum sodium level). Bicarbonate (best given as an isotonic solution IV) also promotes the cellular uptake of potassium. Sodium polystyrene sulfonate, a cation exchange resin (given either orally or rectally), works in the gastrointestinal tract to increase the rate of potassium into the cells and the sodium out of the cells.

β_2-Adrenergic agonists are also effective in driving the potassium back into the cells. Hyperkalemia can also be effectively treated using loop diuretics, thiazide diuretics, and hemodialysis to increase the rate of potassium excretion. (Peritoneal dialysis can be used; however, it is significantly less effective than hemodialysis.) Obviously, before any treatment is instituted, the risks versus benefits (including contraindications) need to be carefully considered.

C. Start heparin therapy INCORRECT

At this time, it is unlikely that Ms. Lane has had a thromboembolic phenomenon causing her symptoms; therefore, heparin therapy is not indicated. Furthermore, heparin can produce hyperkalemia and could potentially worsen her condition.

If there are still concerns regarding the presence of a PE, a spiral CT of the lungs should be performed.

D. Stop (and avoid in the future) the COC, EE with DRSP, and both of the NSAIDs CORRECT

As previously stated, the initial approach to managing hyperkalemia includes eliminating any medications suspected of causing the electrolyte disturbance. (It is also important to inquire about herbal preparations and supplements because some of these agents can enhance the potassium shift from the intracellular compartments by the aforementioned methods.)

Furthermore, once this adverse drug effect occurs, it is justified to recommend the patient avoid the agent(s) in the future to prevent a potential recurrence of the hyperkalemia.

E. No treatment is required except to stop the offending agents and monitor serum electrolytes to ensure normalization INCORRECT

Because of Ms. Lane's symptoms, ECG changes, and moderately elevated potassium level, this is not an appropriate treatment option for her. If she had extremely mild hyperkalemia (serum potassium ≤ 6 mEq/L, no ECG or cardiac abnormalities, and no significant neuromuscular abnormalities), this, in conjunction with frequent evaluation, would be appropriate.

Epidemiologic and Other Data

Adverse drug effects are the most common iatrogenic condition in the United States. They are estimated to occur in about 5 to 15% of all patients taking medications. Serious adverse drug effects account for over 100,000 deaths, are responsible for approximately 3 to 6% of all hospitalization admissions, and affect an estimated 6 to 15% of all hospitalized patients annually in the United States.

Approximately 75 to 80% of the all drug reactions are predictable and nonimmunologic mediated. This type of adverse effect includes primary and secondary drug side effects, toxicity, overdosing, and medication interactions. An additional 5 to 10% are considered to be immunologic, or hypersensitive/allergic, in nature. They can occur with all four types of immunologic reactions (acute IgE mediated, delayed cell mediated, formation of immune complex derived, and cytotoxically induced), activation of specific T cells, and other lesser-known (or unknown) mechanisms. The remaining adverse drug effects fall into the category of unpredictable. This group covers drug intolerances, idiosyncratic reactions, and pseudoallergic responses.

REFERENCES/ADDITIONAL READING

Aghababian RV, ed. *Essentials of Emergency Medicine.* Sudbury, MA: Jones & Bartlett Publishers; 2006.
Brinsfield K. Female genital tract. 713–722.
Joyce DM. Fluid and electrolyte disturbances. 189–198.
Michalakes CJ. Contraception, uncomplicated pregnancy, and complicated pregnancy. 461–475.

Alleyassin A, Khademi A, Aghahosseini M, Safdarian L, Badenoosh B, Hamed EA. Comparison of success rates in the medical management of ectopic pregnancy with single-dose and multiple-dose administration of methotrexate: a prospective, randomized clinical trial. *Fertil Steril.* 2006;85(6): 1661–1666.

American Academy of Family Physicians News Staff. Updated AAFP breast cancer screening recommendations stress communication. *AAFP News Now* 2010; Jan. 15. http://www.aafp.org/online/en/home/publications/news/news-now/clinical-care-research/20100115aafp-brca-recs.html. Accessed January 16, 2010.

American Cancer Society. American Cancer Society Guidelines for the Early Detection of Cancer. Revised March 5, 2008. http://www.cancer.org/docroot/PED/content/PED_2_3X_ACS_Cancer_Detection_Guidelines_36.asp. Accessed October 25, 2008.

American Cancer Society. Screening recommendations by age. http://www.cancer.org/Healthy/ToolsandCalculators/Reminders/screening-recommendations-by-age. Accessed September 15, 2010.

Bayer HealthCare Pharmaceuticals Inc. YAZ package insert. Wayne, NJ: Bayer HealthCare Pharmaceuticals Inc; 2007.

Centers for Disease Control and Prevention. Sexually transmitted diseases treatment guidelines, 2006. *MMWR.* 2006; 55(No. RR-11):1–94.

Deutschman M. Advances in the diagnosis of first trimester pregnancy problems. *Am Fam Phys.* 1991;44(suppl 5): S15–S30.

Ehrlich A. Evidence-based medicine: Thinprep cervical cytology does not detect more abnormalities than conventional cytology. *Clin Advisor.* 2009; June:77.

Fauci AS, Kasper DL, Longo DL, et al., eds. *Harrison's Principles of Internal Medicine.* 17th ed. New York: McGraw-Hill Medical; 2008.

Arruda V, High K. Coagulation disorders. 725–731.

Hall J. Menstrual disorders and pelvic pain. 304–307.

Konkle B. Bleeding and thrombosis. 363–369.

Melmed S, Jameson JL. Disorders of the anterior pituitary and hypothalamus. 2195–2216.

Singer GG, Brenner BM. Fluid and electrolyte disturbances. 274–284.

Young R. Gynecological malignancies. 604–610.

Gilbert ND, Moellering RC Jr, Eliopoulos GM, Sande MA, eds. *The Sanford Guide to Antimicrobial Therapy 2008.* 38th ed. Sperryville, VA: Antimicrobial Therapy, Inc; 2008:4–58.

Gilbert ND, Moellering Jr. RC, Eliopoulos GM, and Sande MA. (eds.) Table 1: Clinical approach to initial antimicrobial therapy. 4–58.

Gilbert ND, Moellering Jr. RC, Eliopoulos GM, and Sande MA. (eds.) Table 8: Risk categories of antimicrobics in pregnancy. 74.

Gonzales R, Kutner J. *Current Practice Guidelines in Primary Care 2009.* New York: McGraw-Hill Medical; 2009.

Gonzales R, Kutner J. Disease screening, cancer, breast. 9–14.

Gonzales R, Kutner J. Disease screening, cancer, cervical. 15–19.

Gonzales R, Kutner J. Disease screening, cancer, colorectal. 20–23.

Mengel MP, Schwiebert LP. *Family Medicine: Ambulatory Care and Prevention.* 5th ed. New York: McGraw-Hill Medical; 2009.

Frazier J, Smith C. Vaginal bleeding. 425–429.

Goodwin M. Pelvic pain. 344–352.

Guthrie M. Contraception. 715–721.

Kaufman A. Amenorrhea. 12–18.

Weinstein LC, Altshuler M. Fluid, electrolyte, and acid-base disturbances. 173–181.

National Cancer Institute. Oral cancer. http://www.cancer.org/acs/groups/content/. Accessed September 15, 2010.

National Cancer Institute. Oral cancer screening (PDQ). http://www.cancer.gov/cancertopics/pdq/screening/oral/healthprofessional. Accessed September 15, 2010.

Nelson AL. Menstrual problems and common gynecologic concerns. In: Hatcher RA, Trussell J, Stewart F, et al. eds. *Contraceptive Technology.* 17th ed. New York: Ardent Media; 1998:95–140.

Onion DK, series ed. *The Little Black Book of Primary Care.* 5th ed. Sudbury, MA: Jones & Bartlett Publishers; 2006.

Onion DK, DeJong R. Obstetrics/Gynecology. 11.2 Vaginal/Uterine/Tube disorders. 792–803.

Onion DK, DeJong R. Obstetrics/Gynecology. 11.4 Pregnancy-related conditions. 810–831.

Onion DK, DeJong R. Obstetrics/Gynecology. 11.5 Miscellaneous. 831–849.

Onion DK. Psychiatry. 15.2 Psychiatric diseases. 949–964.

Onion DK. Renal/Urology. 17.6 Hyperkalemia. 1012–1013.

Oral Cancer Foundation. The HPV connection. http://oralcancerfoundation.org/hpv/index.htm. Accessed September 15, 2010.

Organon USA Inc. NuvaRing package insert (NUV-76928). Roswell, NJ: Organon USA Inc; 2008.

Pagana KD, Pagana TJ. *Mosby's Diagnostic and Laboratory Test Reference.* 8th ed. St. Louis: Mosby Elsevier; 2007 (multiple pages utilized to provide normal reference values for laboratory tests).

Riedl MA, Casillas AM. Adverse drug reactions: types and treatment options. *Am Fam Phys.* 2003;68(9):1781–1790.

Ronco G, Gorogi-Rossi P, Carozzi F, et al. Efficacy of human papillomavirus testing for the detection of invasive cervical cancers and cervical intraepithelial neoplasia: a randomised controlled trial. *Lancet Oncol.* 2010;Jan 19 (early online publication) doi:10.1016/S1470–2045(09)70360-2. Accessed January 28, 2010.

Smith HO, Kohorn E, Cole LA. Choriocarcinoma and gestational trophoblastic disease. *Obstet Gynecol Clin North Am.* 2005;32(4):661–684.

Soper JT. Gestational trophoblastic disease. *Obstet Gynecol.* 2006;108(1):176–187.

US Department of Health and Human Services Agency for Healthcare Research and Quality (USDHHS AHRQ). Quality of Health Care. National Healthcare Disparities Report 2007 (Publication No. 08-0041). Rockville, MD: AHRQ; 2008:31–112.

US Preventive Services Task Force. Screening for breast cancer: U.S. Preventive Services Task Force Recommendation Statement. *Ann Intern Med.* 2009;151:716–726.

Wells PS, Anderson DR, Rodger M, et al. Derivation of a simple clinical model to categorize patients probability of pulmonary embolism: increasing the models utility with the SimpliRED D-dimer. *Thromb Haemost.* 2000; 83(3): 416–420.

World Health Organization. Medical eligibility criteria for contraceptive use. 3rd ed. 2004. http://www.who.int.rhl/fertility/contraception/mec_story/en/index.html. Accessed September 6, 2009.

World Health Organization. Selected practice recommendations for contraceptive use. 2nd ed. 2004. http://www.who.int.opics.contraception/en/index.html. Accessed June 6, 2008.

CASES IN MUSCULOSKELETAL DISORDERS*

CASE 8-1

Lillian Myers

Mrs. Myers is a 62-year-old white female who presents complaining of mild (2 out of 10 on the pain scale), aching, bilateral knee pain of 2 years' duration. It is equal bilaterally and is aggravated by walking and standing. Initially, the application of heat effectively alleviated her pain. However, after 1 year, this was no longer effectual. So, she began glucosamine/chondroitin supplements. They provided her with complete relief until 2 months ago. She then added acetaminophen 1000 mg twice a day. This combination has provided her with near-complete resolution of her pain. She came in today for an evaluation of the problem because her daughter felt she might need her "knees replaced" and heard it was better to "have it done early." She denies a history of trauma and/or occupational/recreational activities that involve frequent bending or joint overloading.

Her only known medical problem is hypertension, which is controlled with a diuretic. She has never been hospitalized except for childbirth and has never had any surgery. Her medications consist of triamterene 37.5 mg/hydrochlorothiazide 25 mg once a day, glucosamine 750 mg/chondroitin 400 mg twice daily, and acetaminophen 1000 mg twice a day. She does not take any other prescription or over-the-counter (OTC) medications, vitamins, supplements, or herbal preparations. She is allergic to aspirin, which caused an anaphylactic reaction the last time she took it. She has never smoked and does not drink alcohol. She has regular age-appropriate preventive health examinations with diagnostic testing. Her family history is positive for hypertension and osteoarthritis in both her mother and older sister.

1. Based on this information, which of the following questions are essential to ask Mrs. Myers and why?

   A. How does rest affect her pain?
   B. Does she have stiffness on awakening in the morning or after other periods of inactivity? If yes, how long does it last?

   C. Are any of her other joints affected? If yes, which ones?
   D. What types of limitations are placed upon her because of the pain?
   E. Does she ever have chest pain or pressure?

Patient Responses

Her knee pain is significantly alleviated with rest. She does experience morning stiffness and stiffness after sitting for 1 hour or longer. However, it resolves very quickly (within 5 to 10 minutes). She also has minimal pain (1 out of 10 on the pain scale) and rest-induced stiffness in her hands, especially her fingers. This stiffness also resolves within a few minutes of beginning an activity. She does not experience any functional limitations due to her hand problems. And, the only limitation placed upon her by her knee pain is the necessity to have to stop and rest while doing her grocery shopping. She does not have any chest pain or pressure.

2. Based on this information, which of the following components of the physical examination are essential to conduct on Mrs. Myers and why?

   A. Heart and lung auscultation
   B. Bilateral hip examination
   C. Bilateral ankle examination
   D. Bilateral knee examination
   E. Bilateral hand examination

Physical Examination Findings

Mrs. Myers is 5'2" tall and weighs 225 lb (body mass index [BMI] = 41.1). Other vital signs are blood pressure (BP), 120/66 mm Hg; pulse, 82 beats per minute (BPM) and regular; respiratory rate, 12/min and regular; and oral temperature, 98.4°F.

Her heart is regular in rate and rhythm and does not reveal any murmurs, gallops, or rubs. Her apical impulse is not displaced and without thrills.

---

*Remember, for each question, none to all of the answers could be correct/essential or incorrect/nonessential. See page 306 for Chapter 8 answers.

Her hips do not reveal any gross deformities, bony enlargement, or effusions. They are nontender to palpate but with a slightly decreased range of motion (without pain) in all directions, bilaterally. No crepitus is noted. Her knees reveal a small amount of bony enlargement but no other gross deformities or effusions. They are slightly tender to palpate in the anterior and lateral aspects. The posterior knee is not tender to palpate and does not reveal a mass. She has full extension of her knees but mild to moderate limitation of flexion (only to approximately 90°) with a complaint of mild pain, bilaterally. Mild crepitus is present bilaterally.

Her ankles do not reveal any bony enlargement, gross deformity, effusions, edema, or skin temperature, color, or sensation changes. They are nontender to palpate. She has normal range of motion in all directions that is equal bilaterally and without pain. No crepitus is present.

The skin of her lower extremities does not reveal edema or changes of temperature, color, or sensation. Her lower extremity muscle strength is normal except for a mild, bilateral, and equal quadriceps weakness without obvious atrophy. Her knee, ankle, and plantar reflexes are normal and equal bilaterally. Femoral, popliteal, dorsalis pedis, and posterior tibial pulses are normal and equal bilaterally.

Her hands reveal slight bony enlargement of both her distal interphalangeal (DIP) joints and her proximal interphalangeal (PIP) joints. She also has small bony deposits ~2 to 3 mm in size of her DIP joints (Heberden nodes) and her PIP joints (Bouchard nodes) of all four fingers. There are no effusions, edema, or skin temperature, color, or sensation changes anywhere in her hands. She has a mild decreased range of motion with flexion and a slightly decreased range of motion of extension in all her fingers and thumbs. No crepitus is present. Her hand grip is slightly decreased but equal bilaterally. Her brachial, ulnar, and radial pulses are normal and equal bilaterally. Her triceps, biceps, and brachioradialis reflexes are normal and equal bilaterally.

3. Based on this information, which of the following diagnostic studies are essential to perform on Mrs. Myers and why?

    A. Bilateral knee radiographs
    B. Complete blood count with differential (CBC w/diff)
    C. Serum uric acid level
    D. Synovial fluid analysis from knee
    E. Rheumatoid factor (RF)

Diagnostic Test Results

Her knee radiographs revealed subchondral thickening of the bones, some mild osteophyte formations, and marked joint space narrowing. The left knee was slightly worse than her right.

Her CBC w/diff was normal. Her uric acid level was 3.5 mg/dl (normal adult female: 2.7–7.3). Her RF was negative.

Her synovial fluid analysis revealed a clear, straw-colored aspirate with 100 white blood cells (WBCs), 500 red blood cells (RBCs), and no crystals (normal: appearance: clear and straw colored in appearance with a good mucin clot; cell count: < 200 WBCs/mm³ with normal differential and < 2000 RBCs/µl; polarized light examination: no evidence of any crystals; estimated viscosity test [performed by forcing the synovial fluid out of a syringe]: very viscous or "stringy").

Complement levels, Gram stains, acid-fast stains, and cultures with sensitivities are performed on the synovial fluid as indicated (normal: negative for disease process). Chemical analyses performed on the synovial fluid (e.g., glucose, uric acid, protein, and/or lactate) are normally roughly equivalent to the patient's serum level.

4. Based on this information, which one of the following is Mrs. Myers' most likely diagnosis and why?

    A. Osteoporosis
    B. Osteoarthritis
    C. Rheumatoid arthritis
    D. Gouty arthritis
    E. Lyme disease–associated arthritis

5. Based on this diagnosis, which of the following are appropriate components of a treatment plan for Mrs. Myers and why?

    A. Weight reduction
    B. Physical therapy consultation to develop at-home range-of-motion, strengthening, and aerobic exercise program
    C. Continue acetaminophen
    D. Continue glucosamine/chondroitin supplements if desired
    E. Stop acetaminophen and add naproxen 500 mg twice a day with a proton pump inhibitor (PPI) for gastrointestinal protection

CASE 8-2
Mitchell Nutter

Mr. Nutter is a 26-year-old African American male who works as a block layer. Yesterday at work, while lifting a regular-sized concrete block, he immediately experienced a sharp, crampy pain in the right side of his lower back that was so severe it caused him to drop the block. He finished out the day, but every time he straightened upright after bending forward, he experienced the identical pain. However, if he worked with his back continuously flexed, he could continue to lift and lay blocks with only a mild ache in his lower back. Today his back is essentially the same. It was "stiff" when he got up out of bed this morning; however, that resolved with his shower. Nevertheless, when he stood up after drying his feet, he experienced the identical pain. It recurred again when he assumed an upright position after putting on his underwear, pants, and boots. He rates the baseline achy pain as a 2 out of 10 on the pain scale and the intermittent pain as an 8 out of 10 on the pain scale. He is unaware of any other aggravating or alleviating factors.

He has experienced four or five previous episodes of back pain exactly like this over the past 2 to 3 years. The last episode was approximately 9 months ago. In between these painful events, he is completely asymptomatic. According to Mr. Nutter, the only effective treatment with his previous episodes was a rapid titration of fentanyl patches to 100 µg/hr every 72 hours along with strict bed rest for 6 to 8 weeks, then a slow titration off the fentanyl and bed rest until he could resume his normal activities, which typically takes an additional 6 to 8 weeks. Other treatment modalities including multiple oral analgesics (names unknown by the patient), activities as tolerated, partial bed rest, and physical therapy proved ineffective in the past. Therefore, he would prefer to just start fentanyl and bed rest immediately.

He states that his only known medical problem is his "bad back," for which he cannot provide an actual diagnosis. He has not experienced any additional back injuries nor been involved in a serious accident. He has never had surgery nor been hospitalized. He is taking no prescription or over-the-counter medications, vitamins, supplements, or herbal preparations. He has no known drug allergies (NKDAs). He does not currently smoke; however, up until 5 years ago he smoked one to two packs per day since the age of 16 years. He does not currently drink alcohol. He does not use illicit substances and has never injected any drugs. His family history is negative.

1. Based on this information, which of the following are essential questions to ask Mr. Nutter and why?

- **A.** What, if any, imaging studies has he ever had performed on his back?
- **B.** Does he take potassium supplements?
- **C.** Does he have any urinary incontinence, inability to void, dysuria, urinary urgency, urinary frequency, hematuria, urethral discharge, or impotence?
- **D.** Is he experiencing any radiation of pain, dysesthesias, paresthesias, leg weakness, or other neurologic symptoms?
- **E.** Has he experienced fever, fatigue, weight loss, or a recent bacterial infection?

Patient Responses

With every episode of back pain he has had a plain film radiograph that was reported as "normal" on each occasion. He had a magnetic resonance image (MRI) with his last episode of back pain and it revealed a bulging, but not herniated, disc at L4 to L5. The diagnostic procedures were conducted at the local hospital. As stated in his history, he does not take any supplements, including potassium.

He denies urinary incontinence, inability to void, dysuria, urinary urgency or frequency, hematuria, urethral discharge, impotence, radiation of pain into his buttocks or down his leg, dysesthesias, weakness in his legs, other neurologic symptoms, fever, fatigue, weight loss, or a recent bacterial infection.

2. Based on this information, which of the following components of a physical examination are essential to conduct on Mr. Nutter and why?

- **A.** Heart auscultation
- **B.** Abdominal examination
- **C.** Low back examination with Waddell signs
- **D.** Neurologic evaluation of lower extremities
- **E.** Vascular evaluation of lower extremities

Physical Examination Findings

Mr. Nutter is 6'4" tall and weighs 198 lb (BMI = 23.1). Other vital signs are BP, 126/72 mm Hg; pulse, 88 BPM and regular; respirations, 16/min and regular; and oral temperature, 98.4°F.

Mr. Nutter's heart is regular in rate and rhythm. There are no murmurs, gallops, or rubs. His apical impulse is nondisplaced and without a thrill.

His abdominal examination reveals normal bowel sounds in all four quadrants. It is soft, nontender, nondistended, and without masses or organomegaly. His aorta is palpable, normal size, and without bruit.

His lower back reveals marked decreased range of motion with flexion because of the complaint of pain; however, he does have full extension and lateral movement. It is tender to palpate the paraspinous muscles to the right of L1-L4 and doing so elicited a slight spasm with pain like he had on bending yesterday but not quite as severe. It did not elicit any abnormal facial grimacing or yelling. There is no associated scoliosis. There are no other areas of tenderness or any costovertebral angle (CVA) tenderness. There are no areas of discoloration, temperature change, abnormal sensation, or dermal lesions. He did not experience pain with axial loading or twisting of the body with the spine held in a straight position.

Mr. Nutter's gait is normal. He can squat and get back up without assistance or difficulty. His knee and ankle reflexes are normal bilaterally. He has no areas of abnormal sensation to either sharp or dull touch; furthermore, the sensation was equal bilaterally. His straight-leg-raising test was negative both sitting and lying.

His popliteal, dorsalis pedis, and posterior tibial pulses are normal and equal bilaterally. His legs, including his feet, are normal in color and temperature; they are also equal bilaterally. Capillary refill is normal.

3. Based on this information, which of the following diagnostic studies are essential to perform on Mr. Nutter and why?

- **A.** Lumbosacral (LS) spine radiograph
- **B.** Magnetic resonance imaging (MRI) of LS spine
- **C.** Urinalysis (U/A)
- **D.** Erythrocyte sedimentation rate (ESR)
- **E.** Complete blood count with differential (CBC w/diff)

Diagnostic Testing Results

Mr. Nutter's LS spine radiograph showed a normal curvature of the spine without displacement of the vertebral bodies, obvious bony lesions, fractures, or abnormal disc spaces. His MRI revealed a bulging disc at L4/L5 without evidence of nerve compression. His U/A, ESR, and CBC w/diff were normal.

4. Based on this information, which one of the following is Mr. Nutter's most likely diagnosis and why?

- **A.** Osteoarthritis of the LS spine
- **B.** Osteoporosis of the LS spine
- **C.** Osteomyelitis of the LS spine
- **D.** Lumbar strain with spasm
- **E.** Lumbar disc herniation

5. Based on this diagnosis, which of the following are appropriate components of a treatment plan for Mr. Nutter and why?

- **A.** Rapid titration of fentanyl patches to 100 µg/hr every 72 hours for 6 to 8 weeks, then a slow titration off the fentanyl
- **B.** Cyclobenzaprine 5 mg three times per day with drowsiness and alcohol precautions
- **C.** Bed rest until follow-up appointment in 1 week
- **D.** Referral to physical therapy
- **E.** Referral for laminectomy

CASE 8-3

Natasha O'Hara

Ms. O'Hara is a 33-year-old Asian American female who presents with the chief complaint of "hurting all over." Her pain is achy in nature and she rates it as a 5 out of 10 on the pain scale. It primarily affects the muscles in her neck, shoulders, back, and hips; however, other areas are intermittently symptomatic. It has been present for approximately 2 years without change. It is worsened by almost any activity and only partially alleviated by rest. Acupuncture completely relieves the pain and many of the associated symptoms; however, because it is a "short-lived" therapy, she requires a treatment every 2 to 3 days to maintain relief. Unfortunately, because it is not covered by her insurance, she cannot afford treatment that frequently. Currently, she is receiving a treatment once every 1 to 2 weeks when her symptoms get "real bad." She's requesting "something" that her insurance will cover.

Ms. O'Hara has also been experiencing fatigue and an increased need for sleep for approximately the same time frame. She is generally in bed for 12 hours per night on weekdays; however, she only sleeps approximately 8 of them. She states that it often takes her more than 1 hour to get to sleep because she "just cannot get comfortable." Once she gets to sleep, she is generally awakened every 1 to 2 hours by "a pain somewhere," but not necessarily the same location each time. Then, it takes between 1/2 and 1 hour to get comfortable and back to sleep. On weekends, she remains in bed even longer, sometimes as much as 18 hours per day. Still, she has to force herself out of bed in the morning because she is virtually as tired on arising as she was before retiring. She remains tired throughout the day; however, her fatigue worsens as the day progresses. Before she became ill, she slept 6 to 7 hours per night and awoke refreshed.

Ms. O'Hara has not been experiencing dyspnea, orthopnea, chest pain/pressure, palpitations, vertigo, presyncope, syncope, nausea, vomiting, changes in bowel movements, changes in the texture of her hair or skin, fever, rhinorrhea, nasal congestion, frequent sneezing, itchy or watery eyes, or a rash at any time during her illness. She did not have a viral infection or a known tick or mosquito bite prior to the onset of her illness. She denies being under significant stress. She has not done any foreign travel. She is employed as a sales clerk at a high-end women's boutique where she works 10 hours per day, 5 days a week. When she does not get her acupuncture treatments regularly, she says it is "all I can do to make it through the day." After work, she purchases take-out for dinner, goes home, eats, takes a hot bath, and goes to bed.

Her only medical problem is migraine headaches, which are successfully treated with acupuncture. She experiences one every 4 to 6 months without a known trigger. She has never been hospitalized nor had surgery. She has never been in a serious accident nor had a significant injury. She takes no prescription or over-the-counter medications, vitamins, supplements, or herbal preparations. She is not allergic to any medications. She does not drink alcohol and has never smoked cigarettes. She has not been sexually active in over 1.5 years because of her illness making her "too tired to enjoy it." Her last menses was 3 weeks ago and was normal. She has one regularly every 28 days.

Her family history is positive for a sister with depression and her mother being deceased for 20 years as a result of suicide.

1. Based on this information, which of the following questions are essential to ask Ms. O'Hara and why?

   A. Has she experienced any changes in her appetite, weight, interests, or activities; anhedonia; trouble concentrating; memory difficulties; crying episodes; feeling depressed, blue, sad, or anxious; or suicidal ideations?
   B. Was she sexually molested as a child?
   C. Is she experiencing true weakness of her muscles?
   D. Does she have any joint pain or swelling?
   E. Has anyone ever told her she snores or quits breathing while she is asleep?

Patient Responses

Ms. O'Hara admits her appetite has been decreased; however, she has been "forcing" herself to eat in an attempt to "maintain her strength." Her weight has stayed the same. She is still interested in the same things she was before; however, she rarely participates in them because of her fatigue. When she does participate, she enjoys herself; however, she "has to pay for it" by feeling "even worse" for the next couple of days, especially if the activity has a physical component. She has noticed intermittent problems with concentration, being easily distracted, and forgetfulness. She occasionally has crying episodes or feels "down" when she thinks of how much her life has changed since becoming ill. However, she would not describe it as a true depression. She feels her mood is "upbeat" most of the time. She denies being anxious or having suicidal ideations. She was not sexually molested as a child.

She is not experiencing any muscle weakness, just pain. She has not had any pain, edema, erythema, or other skin changes of her joints; however, her hands feel "swollen" at times.

No one has ever told her that she snores or quits breathing while sleeping. However, she has always slept alone.

2. Based on this information, which of the following components of a physical examination are essential to conduct on Ms. O'Hara and why?

   A. Beck Depression Inventory
   B. Mini-mental status examination (MMSE)
   C. Musculoskeletal examination
   D. Neurologic evaluation of the extremities
   E. Vascular examination of the extremities

Physical Examination Findings

Ms. O'Hara is 4'10" tall and weighs 115 lb (BMI = 24.0). Other vital signs are BP, 106/64 mm Hg; pulse, 80 BPM and regular; respirations, 10/min and regular; and oral temperature, 98.1°F.

Her Beck Depression Inventory is normal as is her MMSE with a score of 30 (maximum score: 30).

She has full range of motion in all her joints without pain except with flexion of her lumbar spine. This maneuver produces generalized low back pain but no loss in range of motion. She has no evidence of scoliosis. None of her joints are erythematous, edematous, or warm to the touch. There are no joint effusions.

She experiences point tenderness when pressure is applied over her occiput where the suboccipital muscle insertions are located, intertransverse processes of her low cervical spine, lateral epicondyles, greater trochanter of hips, and medial aspects of her knees. The tenderness is equal bilaterally. Otherwise, she has no joint or associated structure tenderness.

She also has point muscle tenderness located halfway down the superior border of her trapezius muscles, supraspinatus muscles near the border of the scapula, and superior-lateral quadrant of her gluteal muscles that are equal bilaterally. Otherwise, her muscles are not tender to palpate. Pertinent negative findings include a lack of point tenderness over her second anterior rib near her sternum on either side of her body.

Her biceps, triceps, brachioradialis, knee, ankle, and plantar reflexes are normal and equal bilaterally. She has good and equal muscle strength bilaterally with no evidence of atrophy. Her gait and coordination are normal. Her sensation is intact to both sharp and dull discrimination in both her arms and legs; it is also equal bilaterally.

Her brachial, radial, ulnar, dorsalis pedis, and posterior tibial pulses are normal and equal bilaterally. Her skin is normal in color and temperature and does not blanch. There is no evidence of any dermatologic changes including livido reticularis and Raynaud phenomenon. Her capillary refill is normal bilaterally in her fingers and toes.

3. Based on this information, which of the following diagnostic studies are essential to perform on Ms. O'Hara and why?

    A. Full x-ray series of the spine
    B. Creatine phosphokinase (CPK)
    C. Thyroid-stimulating hormone (TSH)
    D. Liver function testing (LFT)
    E. Cerebral spinal fluid (CSF) analysis for substance P

Diagnostic Test Results

Ms. O'Hara's full spinal x-ray series was reported as negative. Her CPK was 42 units/L (normal adult female: 30–135). Her TSH was 4.5 µU/ml (normal adult: 2–10). Her LFTs were normal as was her CSF analysis for substance P.

4. Based on this information, which one of the following is Ms. O'Hara's most likely diagnosis and why?

    A. Poliomyelitis
    B. Somatoform disorder
    C. Unspecified connective tissue disease
    D. Polymyalgia rheumatica
    E. Fibromyalgia syndrome

5. Based on this diagnosis, which of the following are appropriate components of a treatment plan for Ms. O'Hara and why?

    A. Continue acupuncture as needed
    B. Amitriptyline 25 mg at bedtime, then titrate upward as appropriate
    C. Fluoxetine 20 mg daily
    D. Milnacipran in a tapering dose starting at 12.5 mg once on the first day; twice on days 2 and 3; days 4 through 7, 25 mg twice daily; and after day 7, 50 mg twice a day
    E. Pregabalin 300 mg daily
    F. Naproxen 500 mg twice a day with food

CASE 8-4
Oscar Pence

Mr. Pence is a 72-year-old white male who presents complaining of not being able to fully extend his right ring finger. This condition has been present for several months without any change. He states it does not hurt, interfere with any activities, or cause him any problems. Furthermore, he is not bothered by its appearance. The only reason that he is getting it evaluated is because his daughter insisted. He denies any injury to his hand/finger or any repetitive activities. He has no other musculoskeletal or any type of complaints or concerns.

He has no known medical problems, has never been hospitalized, and has never had any surgery. He does not take any prescription or over-the-counter medications, vitamins, supplements, or herbal preparations. He does not smoke. He admits to drinking a 24 pack of beer (12-oz. cans) per day and has done so since he retired 7 years ago; prior to that, he drank an average of 12 beers per day. He denies drinking any other alcoholic beverages. He does not have regular age-appropriate preventive health evaluations. His family history is unknown.

1. Based on this information, which of the following questions are essential to ask Mr. Pence and why?

    A. What does his wife think about his drinking?
    B. Did he notice any knots, rope-like lesions, or swelling in his palm before this problem began?
    C. Has he noticed any swelling in his neck, crooked penile erections, dyspnea, chronic cough, or wheezing?
    D. Has he had any abdominal pain or swelling, anorexia, nausea, vomiting, constipation, diarrhea, melena, or jaundice?
    E. Has he experienced any change in his weight, malaise, fatigue, chest pain/pressure, or palpitations?

Patient Responses

He doesn't know what his wife thinks of his level of alcohol consumption because he has been divorced for over 10 years.

He did notice some knots in his palms that coalesced together to form a thickened cord before his finger contracted. This had occurred over a multiyear time frame.

He has not noticed/experienced any swelling in his neck, crooked penile erections, dyspnea, chronic cough, wheezing, abdominal pain or swelling, nausea, vomiting, constipation, diarrhea, melena, jaundice, malaise, chest pain/pressure, or palpitations.

He has noticed that his "appetite isn't what it used to be." He has lost approximately 2 lb in the past year and a total of 10 lb in the past 5 years. He admits to some fatigue, which he attributes to "old age."

2. Based on this information, which of the following components of a physical examination are essential to conduct on Mr. Pence and why?

    A. Heart and lung examination
    B. Abdominal examination
    C. Bilateral hand examination
    D. Bilateral foot examination
    E. Skin and sclera examination, especially for jaundice

Physical Examination Findings

Mr. Pence is 5'9" tall and weighs 140 lb (BMI = 20.7). Other vital signs are BP, 124/76 mm Hg; pulse, 78 BPM and regular; respirations, 12/min and regular; and oral temperature, 98.6°F.

His heart is regular in rate and rhythm, without any murmurs, gallops, or rubs. His apical impulse is nondisplaced and without a thrill. His lungs are clear to auscultation.

His abdomen reveals normoactive bowel sounds in all four quadrants and is soft and nondistended. His liver is slightly firm, smooth, nontender, and palpable approximately 5 cm below his right costal margin. There are no other masses or organomegaly.

He has full range of motion of all joints in his hands and wrists except for his right fourth (ring) digit. He cannot fully extend or flex it. It is contracted in a flexed position of ~25° at the metacarpophalangeal (MCP) and ~5° at the PIP joints. He has a palpable, firm, raised, nontender, "cord-like" formation from his midpalm to the base of his fourth digit. Sensation is intact and equal bilaterally in his hands. His ulnar and radial pulses are normal and equal bilaterally and his brachioradialis reflex is normal and equal bilaterally. His grip strength is good and equal bilaterally. His hands are warm to touch, exhibit mild palmar erythema, and have normal capillary refill. No other skin changes were evident including jaundice. He does not have icterus. His foot examination is normal.

3. Based on this information, which of the following diagnostic tests are essential to perform on Mr. Pence at this time and why?

   A. Magnetic resonance imaging (MRI) of his right hand
   B. Radiograph of his right hand
   C. Magnetic resonance imaging (MRI) of his abdomen
   D. Aspartate aminotransferase (AST), alanine aminotransferase (ALT), alkaline phosphatase (ALP), and total bilirubin
   E. Fasting plasma glucose (FPG)

Diagnostic Test Results

Mr. Pence's MRI of his abdomen was reported as normal except for mild hepatomegaly without any intrahepatic lesions. The MRI and radiograph of his right hand were reported as normal except for the flexure contracture of his right fourth MCP and PIP joints.

His AST was 180 units/L (normal adult: 0–35), ALT was 75 units/L (normal adult: 4–36), ALP was 288 units/L (normal adult: 30–120), total bilirubin was 0.8 mg/dl (normal adult: 0.3–1.0), and FPG was 102 mg/dl (normal: 70–110).

4. Based on this information, which one of the following is Mr. Pence's most likely diagnosis and why?

   A. Dupuytren contracture of right fourth digit and alcoholic liver disease
   B. Systemic fibrosing syndrome
   C. Trigger finger and alcoholic cirrhosis
   D. De Quervain tenosynovitis and alcoholic hepatitis
   E. Complex regional pain syndrome

5. Based on this diagnosis, which of the following are appropriate components of a treatment plan for Mr. Pence and why?

   A. Refer to an orthopedic hand surgeon for surgical intervention on right hand
   B. Complete blood count with differential, prothrombin time, and liver ultrasound
   C. Refer for liver biopsy
   D. Provide Mr. Pence with patient education on his condition, advise to cease all alcohol intake, and offer referral to a substance abuse counselor or treatment center
   E. Commit to psychiatric hospital for detoxification and rehabilitation
   F. If patient desires, refer to hand specialist for collagenase *Clostridium histolyticum* injection to his palmar connective tissue excess

CASE 8-5
Paul Quinn

Mr. Quinn is a 25-year-old Pacific Islander male who presents complaining of a very painful (9 out of 10 on the pain scale) swollen right knee. He provides a history of an injury yesterday while working on a home improvement project. While standing upright nailing above his head, he brought the hammer down and accidentally hit himself directly over his right patella. It did not break the skin and was very painful initially. However, the pain gradually subsided without treatment, and by bedtime (approximately 4 hours after the injury) his knee was completely asymptomatic.

However, he awoke at approximately 3:00 a.m. this morning experiencing excruciating (9 out of 10 on the pain scale) right knee pain. It was associated with throbbing, edema, erythema, and calor. His knee was so tender he could not tolerate his pajama pants or the bedcovers touching it. Despite taking 1000 mg of acetaminophen when the pain awoke him, a second dose approximately 4 hours later, and a third dose approximately 4 hours after that (which was approximately 2 hours ago), his knee is just as painful as when it awoke him. The pain worsens if he tries to walk and is alleviated slightly if he sits down and props it up. Heat makes the pain worse and ice does not alter it in any manner. He knows of no other aggravating or alleviating factors. He has never experienced a similar pain in the past.

He has no known medical problems. He has never had surgery nor been hospitalized. His only medication is the acetaminophen. He is not taking any other over-the-counter drugs, prescription medications, vitamins, supplements, or herbal preparations. He is not allergic to any medications. He drinks beer, but no liquor, and averages four to six beers (12-oz. bottles) per month. Normally, he has one or two beers per setting; however, while working on the home improvement project yesterday he drank approximately six bottles over an 8-hour time period. He has never smoked cigarettes nor done illicit drugs. His immunizations are up to date, including a tetanus immunization 2 years ago. His family history is unknown because he is adopted.

1. Based on this information, which of the following questions are essential to ask Mr. Quinn and why?

   A. What type of home improvement project is he performing?
   B. What is his sexual history?

C. Has he been ill or experienced a previous knee injury within the past month?

D. Does he have a fever, fatigue, malaise, or a rash?

E. Are any other joints involved?

Patient Responses

His home improvement project is installing new kitchen cabinets.

He has only been sexually active with women. He has been married and in what he assumes to be a mutually monogamous relationship for the past 5 years. He and his wife have not been using any type of contraception for the past 3 months because they are trying to conceive.

He has not been ill recently nor has he sustained previous trauma to his right knee. He "felt febrile earlier today; however, he did not take his temperature. He has been experiencing some fatigue but denies true malaise. His only skin change is his erythematous knee. No other joints are affected.

2. Based on this information, which of the following components of a physical examination are essential to conduct on Mr. Quinn and why?

A. Bilateral eye examination

B. Bilateral knee examination

C. Bilateral hip and ankle examination

D. Lower extremity pulse and vascular examination

E. Lower extremity reflex and sensation testing

Physical Examination Findings

Mr. Quinn is 5'11" tall and weighs 180 lb (BMI = 25.1). Other vital signs are BP, 126/68 mm Hg; pulse, 92 BPM and regular; respiratory rate, 14/min and regular; and oral temperature, 100.2°F.

His eye examination is unremarkable.

His right knee reveals a hot, extremely tender joint with the overlying skin being a reddish purple in color. There is a moderate-sized prepatellar effusion and a moderately decreased range of motion in both flexion and extension secondary to the complaint of pain. His left knee is normal in appearance, nontender to palpate, and without any effusion or skin changes. It has full range of motion without pain.

His hips and ankles are normal with equal and full range of motion bilaterally. They reveal no evidence of tenderness, edema, effusion, temperature changes, erythema, or other discolorations.

His femoral, popliteal, posterior tibial, and dorsalis pedis pulses are normal and equal bilaterally. His knee jerk is normal on the left but guarded and poorly assessable on the right. His ankle jerks and plantar responses are normal and equal bilaterally.

Sensation is intact and equal bilaterally in his hips, thighs, lower legs, ankles, and feet. However, his right knee appears to be hypersensitive to any sensation compared to his left knee and the rest of his lower extremities.

3. Based on this information, which of the following diagnostic studies are essential to perform on Mr. Quinn and why?

A. Arthrocentesis of right knee with synovial fluid analysis including appearance, viscosity, white blood cell count

with differential, Gram stain, and polarized light examination for crystals

B. Acid-fast stain, Thayer-Martin culture, and fungal cultures of the aspirated fluid

C. Serum and synovial fluid for glucose, uric acid, protein, and lactate levels

D. Thayer-Martin blood culture

E. Radiograph of left knee

Diagnostic Test Results

Mr. Quinn's synovial fluid was slightly cloudy, straw colored, and mildly thin. His WBC count was 1500/mm³ with 80% lymphocytes. No bacteria were identified on microscopic examination or Gram stain. Polarized light examination revealed needle-like crystals with a single refraction (negative birefringent). No cholesterol crystals were identified. Acid-fast stain, cultures, and sensitivities are pending.

His synovial fluid revealed a glucose of 86 mg/dl (normal: ± 10 of serum glucose level), uric acid level of 9.8 mg/dl (normal: essentially same as serum), protein of 7.5 g/dl (normal: essentially same as serum), lactate of 130 units/L (normal: essentially same as serum), and normal complement levels.

His plasma glucose was 95 mg/dl (normal fasting adult: 70–110). His serum uric acid level was 9.7 mg/dl (normal adult male: 4.0–8.5), total serum protein was 7.4 g/dl (normal adult: 6.4–8.3), and serum lactate was 134 units/L (normal adult serum: 100–190).

His right knee radiograph did not reveal any fractures, other bony abnormalities, or foreign bodies. However, a moderate-sized prepatellar effusion was present.

4. Based on this information, which one of the following is Mr. Quinn's most likely diagnosis and why?

A. Acute bacterial arthritis

B. Acute gouty arthritis

C. Pseudogout

D. Rheumatoid arthritis

E. Effusion secondary to trauma

5. Based on this diagnosis, which of the following are appropriate components of a treatment plan for Mr. Quinn and why?

A. Indomethacin 150 mg twice a day for 3 days with food

B. IV colchicine

C. IV antibiotics

D. Tapering dose of methylprednisolone over 1 week

E. Allopurinol 100 mg twice a day; increase by 100 mg/week until desired result is achieved

F. IV Pegloticase and repeat every 2 weeks (after pretreatment prophylaxis with oral prednisone and diphenhydramine)

CASE 8-6

Queenie Rodriquez

Ms. Rodriquez is a 36-year-old Hispanic American female who presents with the chief complaint of "my hands are really bothering me." Her primary concern is her hands have been painful and swollen for approximately 3 months. However, she feels that the problem actually began approximately 6 months ago, when she started experiencing fatigue, mild intermittent hand aching, and morning stiffness. Initially, the fatigue was mild, but it gradually progressed until now it is so severe that "it is all I can do to get up out of bed in the mornings." She defines fatigue as "being totally exhausted." Her fatigue is least during the first couple of hours after awakening, but it gradually worsens until it peaks before bedtime. She has not experienced sleepiness or lack of motivation/desire. The stiffness also began in a much milder form; now, it lasts approximately 2 hours after she arises in the mornings. She also is complaining of numbness of her right thumb and first and second fingers. The numbness appears to be relieved by "shaking my hand a few times." There is no history of trauma or repetitive-use activities.

Hot weather and the application of heat seem to make her hand pain worse. However, the application of ice, a cold environment, and humid days also appear to make her symptoms worse. She has tried over-the-counter acetaminophen, aspirin, ibuprofen, and naproxen for the pain. Acetaminophen did not help with the pain. The other three, especially the aspirin, were helpful; unfortunately, they were all associated with intolerable nausea and heartburn. Her gastrointestinal symptoms resolved immediately upon the cessation of these medications.

She has not had a change in her appetite, interests, or pleasures or felt depressed. She has not experienced a rash, true malaise, cough, dyspnea, or chills. Additionally, she had not been ill, exposed to sick children, or bitten by a tick (to her knowledge) before her symptoms began.

Ms. Rodriquez has no known medical problems, has never been hospitalized, and has never had surgery. She is not taking any prescription or over-the-counter medications, vitamins, supplements, or herbal preparations. She is not allergic to any medicine. She does not drink alcohol and has never smoked. She states that she has not been sexually active for over 1 year now and has no immediate plans to become so in the near future. Her last menstrual period (LMP) was 3 weeks ago and normal. Her cycles occur once every 28 to 30 days. She has never been pregnant. Her family history is unremarkable.

1. Based on this information, which of the following questions are essential to ask Ms. Rodriquez and why?

A. Is she experiencing any myalgias or muscle weakness?
B. When did the numbness begin?
C. What does she mean by the term "numbness"?
D. Which joints are affected?
E. Has she had fever, night sweats, weight loss, or nocturnal symptoms?

Patient Responses

She does not have any myalgias or muscle weakness. She defines numbness as a tingling sensation, which started 1 month ago. She experiences mild erythema, increased warmth, and edema of her affected joints, which are her PIP joints and MCP joints of her second and third (middle and ring, respectively) fingers.

She has felt as though she were running a fever at times. On the rare occasions she checked, it was between 99.5° and 100.0°F. She denies any night sweats, weight loss, and nocturnal symptoms.

2. Based on this information, which of the following components of a physical examination are essential to conduct on Ms. Rodriquez and why?

A. Ear, nose, and throat (ENT) examination
B. Bilateral hand examination
C. Bilateral wrist examination
D. Bilateral shoulder and elbow examination
E. Vascular and neurologic examination of her upper extremities

Physical Examination Findings

Ms. Rodriquez is 5'5" tall and weighs 140 lb (BMI = 23.3). Other vital signs are BP, 110/64 mm Hg; pulse, 88 BPM and regular; respiratory rate, 14/min and regular; and oral temperature, 98.7°F.

Her ENT examination is unremarkable.

Her hands reveal normal and equal range of motion in all joints bilaterally. However, she has mild palmar and affected joint erythema, soft tissue swelling, tenderness, and slightly increased warmth over her second (middle) and third (ring) fingers' PIP and MCP joints, which are bilateral and equal. Additionally, she has a positive squeeze test and some mild ulnar deviation of her MCP joints, which are bilateral and equal.

Her wrists reveal normal range of motion and some mild swelling, tenderness, and increased warmth over the ulnar styloid process, which are bilateral and equal. There is no erythema of her wrists. Pressing the backs of her hands together with her wrists flexed produces the same sensation she has been experiencing in her fingers (positive Phalen test) in her right hand only. Her paresthesias are also reproduced by lightly tapping a couple of times over her right transverse carpal ligament (positive Tinel test). The Tinel test is negative on the left.

Her elbows and shoulders do not reveal any gross deformities, tenderness, effusions, growths, edema, erythema, temperature alterations, or color change.

Her brachial, radial, and ulnar pulses are normal and equal bilaterally. Other than the aforementioned hand abnormalities, there is no edema, effusions, temperature alterations, or color changes noted in her upper extremities. Capillary refill is normal and equal bilaterally.

Her brachioradialis and radial reflexes are normal and equal bilaterally. Sensation appears to be intact and equal in both her upper extremities with the exception of a slight decrease to sharp touch in her right thumb, right first (pointer) finger, second (middle) finger, and medial aspect of her third (ring) finger when compared to her left hand. However, she was able to feel the sensation and discriminate between sharp and dull in these areas. Muscle strength (grip) is slightly decreased in her right hand when compared to the left. The remainder of strength testing of her upper extremities revealed normal and equal findings.

3. Based on this information, which of the following diagnostic studies are essential to perform on Ms. Rodriquez and why?

A. Erythrocyte sedimentation rate (ESR) and C-reactive protein (CRP)
B. Complete blood count with differential (CBC w/diff)
C. Serum uric acid level

D. Rheumatoid factor (RF), anticyclic citrullinated peptide antibody (anti-CCP), and antinuclear antibody (ANA)

E. Nerve conduction study (NCS) of her right upper extremity

Diagnostic Test Results

Ms. Rodriquez's ESR was 62 mm/hr (normal adult female: < 20) and her CRP was 4.0 mg/dl (normal: 1.0). Her CBC w/diff was normal except for a mild thrombocytosis and platelet count of 425,000/mm³ (normal adult: 150,000–400,000).

Her serum uric acid was 3.4 mg/dl (normal adult female: 2.7–7.3).

Her RF was positive at 1:80 (normal: < 1:80) and her anti-CCP was 7.5 units/ml (normal: < 5). Her ANA titer was positive at 1:80 for an immunofluorescent-stained speckled pattern (normal or negative: < 1:40).

Her nerve conduction revealed a mild to moderate sensory conduction delay in the distal medial nerve beginning at the level of the wrist.

4. Based on this information, which one of the following is Ms. Rodriquez's most likely diagnosis and why?

A. Rheumatoid arthritis (RA) with right carpal tunnel syndrome (CTS)

B. Rheumatic fever with right carpal tunnel syndrome (CTS)

C. Osteoarthritis with right wrist involvement and compression of the median nerve

D. Acromegaly-induced arthropathies and right carpal tunnel syndrome (CTS)

E. Lyme disease

5. Based on this diagnosis, which of the following are appropriate components of a treatment plan for Ms. Rodriquez and why?

A. Refer to a rheumatologist

B. Liver function testing (LFT), blood urea nitrogen (BUN), and creatinine

C. Refer to physical therapy for an individualized treatment program

D. Purified protein derivative (PPD) testing

E. Start methotrexate, a tumor necrosis factor (TNF) inhibitor, or other disease-modifying antirheumatic drugs (DMARDs) if the patient's appointment with the rheumatologist is scheduled for more than 1 week away

CASE 8-7

Raquel Summers

Mrs. Summers is a 27-year-old African American female who presents with the chief complaint of "my left knee keeps trying to lock up." This has been an intermittent problem for her for several years. Initially it only occurred once or twice per year. However, it has gradually increased in frequency, and currently she experiences problems once or twice per month. She made today's appointment because her knee became "stuck" in the flexed position yesterday, requiring her to physically "pry" her leg straight. That episode was significantly more painful than when her knee spontaneously "unlocks" and she can feel her patella "going back into place."

These episodes occur primarily when she sits on the floor with her knees bent for a minimum of 30 minutes and goes to straighten out her legs to stand up. As she is attempting to unflex her knee, she experiences a sharp pain in the anterior portion of her knee that quickly resolves when she feels her patella "move back into place." Immediately afterward, her knee is "sore," and occasionally, she has difficulty bearing her full weight on it. The soreness exists for the remainder of the day of the event and occasionally the following day. Her difficulty with full weight bearing on ambulation lasts a maximum of 2 hours.

It is not associated with any edema, effusion, color change, or temperature alteration. She never experiences this problem in her right knee or other joints. She is unaware of any other aggravating factors; however, she does experience left knee pain with jumping. She has not tried anything to alleviate it. She is left-handed. She was not ill prior to the initial onset of symptoms.

She has no known medical problems. She has never had surgery. Her only hospitalizations have been for childbirth, 2 and 4 years ago. Her only medication is a combination oral contraceptive (the name of which she does not remember), which she has taken regularly without difficulty for approximately 2 years. She does not take any other prescription or over-the-counter medications, vitamins, supplements, or herbal preparations. She is not allergic to any medicines. She has regular age-appropriate examinations with diagnostic testing. Her immunizations are up to date. She has never smoked and does not drink alcohol. She does not exercise regularly, which she attributes to her busy lifestyle caring for her family. Her last menstrual period was 1 week ago and normal. Her family history is negative.

1. Based on this information, which of the following questions are essential to ask Mrs. Summers and why?

A. Has she ever experienced a knee injury (especially associated with a "popping sound") or participated in any occupational or recreational repetitive knee activities?

B. Has she felt depressed, sad, or blue or experienced anhedonia lately?

C. Does she experience any difficulty if she remains seated in a chair with her knees flexed at a 90° angle and her feet flat on the floor for over an hour?

D. Does she have any difficulty going up or down stairs?

E. Has she ever experienced her knee "giving away"?

Patient Responses

Mrs. Summers has never had any injury to her knees. Regarding repetitive activities, she states she does a lot of squatting down to pick up her children, their toys, etc. Getting up from the squatting position sometimes causes her some anterior knee pain and occasionally the "catching-like" sensation, especially if she is lifting her oldest child.

She does admit to her knees feeling "stiff" if she sits for long periods of time (positive theater sign) and sometimes has difficulty "getting started" without a slight limp or pain; however, it always occurs in the anterior aspect of her right knee and does not persist for longer than approximately 5 minutes. She occasionally experiences difficulty descending stairs;

however, she feels it occurs less than once per week. She is uncertain if it is associated with her episodes of knee locking and pain. She does not experience a buckling sensation.

She denies feeling depressed, sad, or blue as well as experiencing anhedonia.

2. Based on this information, which of the following components of a physical examination are essential to conduct on Mrs. Summers and why?

A. Bilateral hand examination
B. Bilateral knee examination
C. Bilateral hip and ankle examination
D. Evaluation of the curvature of the lumbar spine
E. Bilateral foot examination

Physical Examination Findings

Mrs. Summers is 5'6" tall and weighs 142 lb (BMI = 22.9). Other vital signs are BP, 120/66 mm Hg; pulse, 82 BPM and regular; respirations, 12/min and regular; and oral temperature, 98.6°F.

Her hands exhibit full range of motion without pain, joint abnormalities, temperature or color changes, or edema bilaterally.

Her knees are normal and equal in color, temperature, and size bilaterally. She has no evidence of masses, effusions (even with milking the suprapatellar pouch), or deformities (including a valgus or varus deformity of her legs) bilaterally. She is experiencing moderate pain when her patella is directly palpated; otherwise, there is no tenderness in her left knee. Her right knee is completely nontender. She appears to have full range of motion that is equal bilaterally and without pain, crepitus, "locking," or a "popping" sound. She does not have either patellar alta or baja with knee flexion.

With her knees fully extended, her "Q" angle is approximately 20° on the right but 30° on the left. Her "J" sign is also positive on the left but not on the right. Her patellar apprehension sign, patellar glide tests, patellar tilt tests, and lateral pull tests are all positive for her left knee but normal for the contralateral knee. She experiences mild to moderate discomfort with the patellofemoral grind test in her left knee only. Her McMurray test, collateral ligament testing, anterior and posterior drawer signs, Lachman maneuver, and pivot shift test are negative bilaterally. Her quadriceps measure 14" on the right and 14.25" on the left. She can ambulate without a limp. She has no abnormal curvature to her spine.

Her hips and ankles reveal normal range of motion without any discomfort bilaterally. There is no edema, erythema, tenderness, or temperature change either.

Her femoral, popliteal, posterior tibial, and dorsalis pedis pulses are all normal and equal bilaterally. Her feet reveal normal color, temperature, and capillary refill.

Her knee reflexes, ankle reflexes, and plantar responses are normal and equal bilaterally. Sensation appears to be intact and equal in her legs and feet bilaterally. Muscle strength is slightly decreased in her left quadriceps compared to her right; however, the remaining muscle testing of her lower extremity muscles appears normal and equal bilaterally.

3. Based on this information, which of the following diagnostic studies are essential to perform on Mrs. Summers and why?

A. Erythrocyte sedimentation rate (ESR) and C-reactive protein (CRP)
B. Complete blood count with differential (CBC w/diff)
C. Patellofemoral degradation antibody (anti-PFD)
D. Radiograph of her left knee in weight bearing, extension, and Merchant view
E. Magnetic resonance imaging (MRI) of her left knee

Diagnostic Test Results

Mrs. Summers' ESR was 8 mm/hr (normal adult female: < 20) and her CPR was 0.5 mg/dl (normal: < 1.0). Her CBC w/diff was normal. Her anti-PDF is pending. Her knee radiographs and MRI revealed no fracture, bony lesions, osteophytes, or joint space narrowing; however, it did reveal that her patella was slightly subluxed and tilted laterally.

4. Based on this information, which one of the following is Mrs. Summers' most likely diagnosis and why?

A. Osteoarthritis of the left knee
B. Patellofemoral syndrome (PFS)
C. Lateral meniscus tear
D. Osgood-Schlatter disease
E. Osteochondritis dissecans (OCD)

5. Based on this diagnosis, which of the following are appropriate components of a treatment plan for Mrs. Summers and why?

A. Nonsteroidal anti-inflammatory drugs (NSAIDs) with food
B. Proton pump inhibitor (PPI)
C. Referral to physical therapy
D. Immediate referral to an orthopedic surgeon
E. Intra-articular hyaluronate injections

CASE 8-8
Sylvia Tincher

Mrs. Tincher is a 72-year-old white female who presents with the chief complaint of "right jaw pain." It began approximately 4 months ago following a dental extraction of a lower right molar, which "broke off and split into pieces" during the procedure. Initially, her pain was achy in nature and estimated to be a 1 or 2 out of 10 on the pain scale. It increased to 4 out of 10 on the pain scale when she chewed, especially if the food was "tough." Currently, she rates her pain as 8 out of 10 on the pain scale, which increases to 10 out of 10 on the pain scale, when she chews. She is not aware of any additional aggravating factors. The pain is alleviated somewhat with acetaminophen; however, it never completely resolves. A couple of days ago, she started experiencing numbness and tingling on the ipsilateral side of her face with mastication, prompting her visit. She has most of her natural teeth but does wear a bridge in place of her upper left premolars. She denies fever, chills, nausea, vomiting, and weight loss.

She saw her dentist approximately 3 months ago for this problem. She states that her dentist advised that the extraction site had healed well; however, she still had a small "pocket" present but it did not contain any purulent material. Her dentist also performed a "full series" of radiographs and advised her they were normal except for mild temporomandibular joint (TMJ) dysfunction. She was fitted with a "mouthpiece" to wear at night, which did nothing for her pain.

Mrs. Tincher reconsulted her dentist approximately 1 month after the final "mouthpiece" fitting because her pain had gradually worsened. She claims the dentist adjusted her "mouthpiece" and advised her to return if her symptoms were not improved after 1 month.

She had that appointment with her dentist 2 weeks ago because her pain has continued to worsen. She states that her dentist obtained jaw radiographs, which were reported as normal except for mild TMJ dysfunction, and he advised her to take acetaminophen regularly before meals and at bedtime. Because it only provides her with partial relief, she just takes it when the pain becomes "intolerable."

Mrs. Tincher's only known medical problem is osteoporosis. Her only hospitalizations were for childbirth three times. She has never had any surgery. Her medications include alendronate 10 mg once a day, calcium 500 mg twice a day, vitamin D 400 IU twice a day, and acetaminophen 1000 mg as needed for pain (currently taking three to four times per day). She has taken the alendronate for approximately 5 years. She is on no other prescription or over-the-counter medications, vitamins, supplements, or herbal preparations. She is not allergic to any medications. She smokes one pack of cigarettes per day and has done so since she was 14 years old. She does not drink alcohol. She has regular preventive health check-ups with diagnostic testing, immunizations, and patient education. Her family history is positive for osteoporosis (mother and two older sisters).

1. Based on this information, which of the following questions are essential to ask Mrs. Tincher and why?

   A. How old were her sisters and mother when they were diagnosed with osteoporosis?
   B. What brand of mouthwash does she use?
   C. Has she had any type of infection (including dental) in the previous 6 months?
   D. Has she ever been diagnosed with cancer?
   E. Has she notice any "grinding" noise or sensation when moving her jaw?

Patient Responses

Her mother and her sisters were all in their early 60s when they were diagnosed with osteoporosis. She has never been diagnosed with cancer. She did not have an infectious process (including dental) within the past 6 months. She has not noticed crepitus or a "grinding" noise/sensation. She does not use mouthwash regularly.

2. Based on this information, which of the following components of a physical examination are essential to conduct on Mrs. Tincher and why?

   A. Ear examination
   B. Oral examination
   C. Heart and lung auscultation
   D. Bilateral TMJ examination
   E. Neurologic examination of the face

Physical Examination Findings

Mrs. Tincher is 5'0" tall and weighs 115 lb (BMI = 22.5). Other vital signs are BP, 136/76 mm Hg; pulse, 84 BPM and regular; respirations, 14/min and regular; and oral temperature, 97.9°F.

Her tympanic membranes are intact and fully mobile bilaterally. They reveal no evidence of erythema, injection, retraction, bulging, middle ear effusions, or middle ear tumors/masses. Her ear canals are clear and without abnormal discharge, discoloration, or lesions, bilaterally.

There is no deviation of her mouth when she opens it. No uvular or palate deviation is present with saying "ah." Her tongue is midline and does not deviate when she extends it out of her mouth. Her vocal cords sound grossly normal when she speaks. Her teeth are in good repair with a bridge present in the space left by the removal of two upper left premolars. The extraction site in her right lower gingiva appears healed; however, there is a small cavity in which a protruding dark, nearly black, object is evident in its lower lateral aspect, which could represent necrotic, exposed bone. There is no associated edema, erythema, discharge, or gingival hypertrophy. Her pharynx, tongue, and oral mucosa are not discolored nor do they reveal any edema, lesions, edema, or exudates.

Her heart is regular in rate and rhythm and without any murmurs, rubs, or gallops. Her apical impulse is nondisplaced and without a thrill. Her lungs are clear to auscultation.

The area over Mrs. Tincher's right TMJ is slightly edematous and slightly warm to the touch when compared to her left. She cannot fully open her mouth. There is no crepitus or other sound/sensation heard or felt when she opens or closes her mouth. There is tenderness to deep palpation of her right anterior/inferior mandible; the remainder of the TMJ is nontender. Her left TMJ is nontender, as is the remainder of her facial bones.

She does have some increased sensation to sharp and dull touch over her right TMJ compared to her left. Discrimination is intact. Otherwise, her sensation is intact and equal bilaterally on the remainder of her face and neck. The remainder of her cranial nerves II through XII are grossly intact.

3. Based on this information, which of the following diagnostic studies are essential to perform on Mrs. Tincher and why?

   A. Radiograph of right TMJ
   B. Magnetic resonance imaging (MRI) of right TMJ
   C. Erythrocyte sedimentation rate (ESR)
   D. White blood cell count with differential (WBC w/diff)
   E. Electromyelogram (EMG) of her right trigeminal nerve

Diagnostic Testing Results

Mrs. Tincher's radiograph of her right TMJ revealed "possible osteoporosis." Her MRI revealed a single, "whitened-out," irregular-shaped area in the lower lateral aspect of her right mandible and generalized mild osteoporosis.

Her ESR was 35 mm/hr (normal adult female: < 20). Her WBC w/diff was normal.

EMG of her right trigeminal nerve was reported as normal.

4. Based on this information, which one of the following is Mrs. Tincher's most likely diagnosis and why?

A. Gingival abscess secondary to dental extraction
B. Osteomyelitis of right TMJ
C. Chondrosarcoma of right TMJ
D. Bisphosphonate-related osteonecrosis of right TMJ
E. Osteoarthritis of right TMJ

5. Based on this diagnosis, which of the following are appropriate components of a treatment plan for Mrs. Tincher and why?

A. Stage Mrs. Tincher's disease
B. Chlorhexidine antiseptic mouthwash
C. Penicillin VK 500 mg four times a day
D. Consultation with an oral surgeon
E. Discontinue bisphosphonate

CASE 8-9
Travis Uno

Mr. Uno is a 27-year-old white male who presents with the chief complaint of "right foot pain." The pain is plantar in location and appears to be greatest over his heel. It is worst when he first attempts to ambulate on arising in the mornings or following periods or inactivity. In fact, he states that it is so severe he "can barely walk" because of the pain. However, after a few steps it is significantly improved, and it resolves completely after a few minutes of ambulation. It worsens if he is not wearing shoes. Occasionally it occurs when he is ascending stairs. He knows of no other aggravating or alleviating factors. It has been present and unchanged for approximately 2 weeks. There is no history of trauma.

He has no known medical problems. However, he does experience chronic low back pain that he has never had evaluated because ibuprofen 200 mg two pills twice per day generally alleviate it. He does not take any other over-the-counter or prescription medications, vitamins, supplements, or herbal preparations. He has never been hospitalized nor had surgery. He is not allergic to any medications. He does not drink or smoke. His family history is negative on his mother's side; however, he has no information concerning his paternal history.

1. Based on this information, which of the following questions are essential to ask Mr. Uno and why?

A. When did his back pain begin, where is it located, and what is its course?
B. Does he experience any nocturnal symptoms?
C. Does he have any problems with diarrhea, constipation, abdominal bloating, abdominal cramping, melena, hematochezia, or rectal discomfort, or urinary symptoms?
D. Has he experienced any fatigue, malaise, fever, visual disturbances, rashes, other musculoskeletal pain, or severe swelling of his fingers?
E. Has he had any dyspnea, cough, chest pain/pressure, or palpitations?

Patient's Responses

Mr. Uno estimates that he has experienced low back pain for approximately 7 to 8 years. It is located beside his lower thoracic and entire lumbar spine and is equal bilaterally. It occasionally radiates into his buttocks and down the back of his legs to midcalf which is also equal bilaterally. It is achy in nature and he rates it as a 3 out of 10 on the pain scale. It is gradually worsening in intensity, and he has recently begun to experience a decrease in flexion. His lumbar pain is aggravated by sitting or lying for extended periods. It is associated with marked morning stiffness requiring several hours to completely resolve; however, if he sits or lies for an extended amount of time, the stiffness returns. "Staying active" seems to make it better, as does a hot shower. He is occasionally awakened by nocturnal lumbar pain; however, this occurs less than once per week. He attributes it to "weak back muscles" secondary to the lack of a regular exercise program.

He has been experiencing some fatigue for approximately 2 to 3 years; however, he attributed this to his demanding work schedule, attending night school, and being a single parent of a second grader. He has experienced tender, migratory, intermittent arthralgias of his fingers, knees, hips, shoulders, and toes for the past year; however, none of these arthralgias has ever been accompanied by edema, erythema, or increased temperature. He denies fever, malaise, weight loss, rash, visual disturbances, gastrointestinal symptoms, abdominal pain/discomfort, dyspnea, cough, chest pain/pressure, or palpitations.

2. Based on this information, which of the following components of a physical examination are essential to conduct on Mr. Uno and why?

A. Heart and lung examination
B. Spine evaluation
C. Bilateral hip examination
D. Bilateral foot and ankle examination
E. Genital and prostate examination

Physical Examination Findings

Mr. Uno is 5'8" tall and weighs 165 lb (BMI = 25). Other vital signs are BP, 130/74 mm Hg; pulse, 76 BMP and regular; respiratory rate, 14/min and regular; and oral temperature, 98.4°F.

His heart is regular in rate and rhythm and without any murmurs, gallops, or rubs. His apical impulse is nondisplaced and without thrills. His lungs are clear to auscultation.

His spine reveals a moderate loss of the normal lumbar lordosis (measured with a modified Schober test), a slight increase in his thoracic curvature, and a slight decrease in the curvature of his cervical spine (with occiput-to-wall testing). He has a markedly decreased range of motion with flexion and a moderate decrease with extension and lateral movements in his entire spine; however, it is most pronounced in this lumbar region. He has tenderness upon palpation of his vertebral prominences in his lumbar spine; otherwise, his back is not tender to palpate. He also has tenderness over his sacroiliac joints and sacral prominence.

A FABERE (**f**lexion, **ab**duction, **e**xternal **r**otation, and **ex**tension) test conducted on his hips is positive for producing sacroiliac pain. His hips exhibit a slightly decreased range of motion in all directions; however, they are not erythematous, edematous, hot, or tender bilaterally.

His feet are normal in appearance except for the presence of significant bilateral pes planus. He has full range of motion of toes, feet, and ankles bilaterally, and the only pain noted was with maximum active flexion of his right ankle and passive inversion of his right midfoot. These maneuvers produce a pain over the medial tuberosity of his right calcaneus that is identical to his presenting complaint. His medial tuberosity of his right calcaneus, at approximately the insertion site of his plantar fascia, is tender to palpate; this finding is absent in his left foot. Otherwise, there is no pain on foot palpation.

He does not have any skin lesions or pedal edema bilaterally.

His knee reflexes, ankle reflexes, and plantar responses are normal bilaterally. Muscle strength of his lower extremities, ankles, and feet are normal and equal bilaterally. Sensation appears to be intact and equal bilaterally in his legs, ankles, and feet.

His femoral, popliteal, posterior tibial, and dorsalis pedis pulses are normal and equal bilaterally. His legs, ankles, and feet are normal in color and temperature bilaterally. There is no change in hair distribution or skin color of his lower extremities. His capillary refill is normal.

His genital and prostate examination is normal.

3. Based on this information, which of the following diagnostic studies are essential to perform on Mr. Uno and why?

  A. Radiograph of his lumbar spine
  B. Erythrocyte sedimentation rate (ESR)
  C. Complete blood count with differential (CBC w/diff)
  D. Radiograph of his right heel
  E. Magnetic resonance imaging (MRI) of his right heel

Diagnostic Test Results

Mr. Uno's lumbar radiograph revealed a loss of the normal curvature of the lumbar spine, bilateral grade 3 sacroiliitis, a slight squaring of lumbar vertebral bodies, and multiple syndesmophytes.

His ESR was 75 mm/hr (normal adult male: < 15). His CBC was normal except for a mild normocytic, normochromic anemia.

The radiograph and MRI of his right heel did not reveal any abnormalities except for a small bone spur on the upper anterior aspect of the calcaneus that did not extend into the tibial/calcaneus junction.

4. Based on this information, which one of the following is Mr. Uno's most likely diagnosis and why?

  A. Osteoarthritis of spine with pes planus
  B. Plantar fasciitis associated with ankylosing spondylitis
  C. Diffuse idiopathic skeletal hyperostosis (DISH) with plantar fasciitis
  D. Ankylosing hyperostosis with right calcaneus fracture
  E. Rheumatoid arthritis of the lumbar spine with a symptomatic posterior calcaneus bone spur

5. Based on this diagnosis, which of the following are appropriate components of a treatment plan for Mr. Uno and why?

  A. Increase his ibuprofen to 800 mg regularly twice a day
  B. Add famotidine 20 to 40 mg once a day
  C. Methotrexate
  D. Infliximab
  E. Calcium with vitamin D

CHAPTER
8

CASES IN MUSCULOSKELETAL DISORDERS

RESPONSES AND DISCUSSION

CASE 8-1
Lillian Myers

1. History

A. How does rest affect her pain? ESSENTIAL

In general, the pain associated with most forms of arthritis, strains, sprains, and overuse syndrome lessens with rest. Conversely, the pain from a bony malignancy actually worsens with rest. Neuropathic joint disease (Charcot joint) may be alleviated or unchanged with rest; however, it rarely worsens. Thus, joint pain that is aggravated by rest is suspicious for a serious underlying abnormality; however, the absence of this finding does not rule these conditions out.

B. Does she have stiffness on awakening in the morning or after other periods of inactivity? If yes, how long does it last? ESSENTIAL

The presence and duration of morning (and prolonged post-inactivity) stiffness are important in distinguishing between the potential causes of joint pain. For example, mild to moderate morning stiffness that resolves fairly quickly (i.e., less than a half hour) is typical of osteoarthritis, whereas moderate to severe morning stiffness taking several hours to resolve is more typical of an inflammatory arthritis.

C. Are any of her other joints affected? If yes, which ones? ESSENTIAL

Monarticular joint pain is most often seen in gouty arthritis, septic arthritis, traumatic injury, or Lyme disease; oligoarticular involvement (two to four joints) is more common in reactive arthritis, Reiter disease, psoriatic arthritis, or arthritis associated with inflammatory bowel disease; and polyarticular involvement (five or more joints) is most commonly seen with the connective tissue diseases, such as rheumatoid arthritis (RA) and systemic lupus erythematosus (SLE).

Regarding hand involvement, osteoarthritis commonly affects the distal interphalangeal (DIP) joints and the proximal interphalangeal (PIP) joints but does not typically affect the

metacarpophalangeal (MCP) joints or the wrists. Conversely, rheumatoid arthritis typically involves the wrists and MCP joints but rarely affects the DIP joints. In regard to other joints, osteoarthritis prefers the knees, hips, cervical spine, lower lumbar spine, and first metatarsophalangeal joints, whereas rheumatoid arthritis affects the knees and feet.

In gouty arthritis, the metatarsophalangeal joint of the first toe is preferred; however, it can also affect the knees, ankles, and tarsal joints. On rare occasions, it can affect a DIP or a PIP joint. The most commonly affected joints in neuropathic joint disease are the tarsals and tarsometatarsal joints; this is followed by the metatarsophalangeal joints and talotibial joints. Although the knees and spine can be affected in neuropathic joint disease, this is rare. Although this list is not all-inclusive and some overlap does exist, the basic patterns of involvement along with the number of joints affected can assist in establishing appropriate differential diagnoses.

D. What types of limitations are placed upon her because of the pain? ESSENTIAL

The treatment goals for joint pain are individualized for both the condition and the patient. For example, in osteoarthritis, the goals of treatment are to alleviate pain, improve joint mobility, and reduce or eliminate functional limitations. In rheumatoid arthritis, the treatment goals include alleviating the pain, reducing associated inflammation, protecting articular structures, maintaining function, and managing systemic symptoms. Therefore, in osteoarthritis, aggressive therapy does not need to be sought if the patient is not having significant pain, severely decreased range of motion, or functional limitations that are important to the patient. Conversely, in RA, early aggressive therapy is necessary to control the underlying disease process.

E. Does she ever have chest pain or pressure? NONESSENTIAL

Although this is an appropriate question to ask an elderly patient, especially one with a history of hypertension like Mrs. Myers, when the patient is seeking health care for an age-appropriate health maintenance visit or other comprehensive physical examination (as part of performing a complete review of systems), a follow-up on hypertension (as part of the screening for cardiovascular complications), or a presenting complaint that is suspicious for cardiac ischemia (as part of the symptom complex). However, it is not a necessary component for the evaluation for her chief complaint.

2. Physical Examination

A. Heart and lung auscultation   NONESSENTIAL

B. Bilateral hip examination   ESSENTIAL

When evaluating a patient with a joint complaint, it is important to evaluate at least the next most proximal joint. Therefore, in the evaluation of Mrs. Myers' knee pain, her hip would also need to be evaluated. The joint examination involves more than just actively or passively putting the joint through its range-of-motion (ROM) evaluation. While performing the ROM evaluation, it is important to listen and feel for crepitus, which is frequently present in osteoarthritis but rare in other forms of arthritis. It is also important to note what maneuvers produce pain, where exactly the pain is located, and whether it is the same pain identified in the chief complaint.

The joint itself needs to be palpated for tenderness and its location noted. For example, generalized pain is common in osteoarthritis, whereas the pain in rheumatoid arthritis is often limited to a bursa. Plus, the joint needs to be palpated and viewed for structural deformities.

The skin overlying the affected joint should also be inspected for edema, warmth, and erythema (suggesting an infectious [e.g., septic arthritis] or inflammatory [e.g., gouty arthritis or rheumatoid arthritis] process). Furthermore, it needs to be evaluated for decreases in temperature and/or pallor (suggesting decreased circulation and/or ischemia involving the joint or causing pain which is referred to the joint). The skin over the area also needs to be evaluated for any other abnormal lesions (e.g., vesicles in a dermatomal distribution suggesting herpes zoster as the cause of the patient's pain or silvery-pink plaques of the flexor surfaces of the joint suggesting the presence of psoriatic arthritis).

Furthermore, it is essential to ensure that the affected area is neurologically intact by checking sensation and reflexes. For example, in diabetic peripheral neuropathy, patients may not notice the decreased sensation in their feet but may notice a deeper pain in their joint from a puncture wound with a foreign body or infection. Finally, the circulation to the area needs to be evaluated to ensure that the pain is not caused by ischemia or claudication by checking the associated pulses and overlying skin as described earlier.

Even if the joint complaint is unilateral, the joint examination must be bilateral. The inclusion of the contralateral joint is not only necessary to provide a comparative "normal" but also to determine if there is evidence of bilateral disease that is asymptomatic or at least not as symptomatic (and hence not as noticeable) as the affected joint(s). This is also a sound medical practice when evaluating joints that are either proximal or distal to the affected one, regardless of whether these other joints are symptomatic or not.

C. Bilatertal ankle examination   ESSENTIAL

Not only does a good orthopedic examination involve the evaluation of at least the next most proximal joint, it also involves the examination of at least one joint distal, to the affected joint. Thus, in the evaluation of Mrs. Myers' knee, her ankle should also be examined.

D. Bilateral knee examination   ESSENTIAL

A knee examination is essential because knee pain is the reason for the patient's visit today.

E. Bilateral hand examination   ESSENTIAL

A hand examination is indicated in the evaluation of Mrs. Myers' knee pain because a history of hand pain was elicited during subsequent questioning. Any changes to the joints of the hands can assist in providing clues to the potential cause of her chief complaint.

3. Diagnostic Studies

A. Bilateral knee radiographs   NONESSENTIAL

Mrs. Myers' diagnosis can be made clinically; therefore, she does not require any diagnostic studies. Knee radiographs are generally only indicated in patients with Mrs. Myers' most likely diagnosis if the pain does not respond to appropriate therapies or if there are atypical signs or symptoms present. This recommendation is based on the fact that typically the knee x-ray findings poorly correlate with the degree of severity of the patient's symptoms.

B. Complete blood count with differential (CBC w/diff) NONESSENTIAL

A CBC w/diff would be indicated if there was a suspicion that Mrs. Myers' problem was caused by an infectious or inflammatory process. Even in that case, a white blood cell count (WBC) with differential is a more appropriate diagnostic option.

C. Serum uric acid level   NONESSENTIAL

An elevated serum uric acid level can add support to suspicion that the patient has a gouty arthritis; however, it is not confirmatory. In order to definitely make the diagnosis of gouty arthritis, the "gold-standard" is synovial fluid analysis. Regardless, it is not indicated in Mrs. Myers' case because her symptoms are not consistent with those typically found in gouty arthritis. Gouty arthritis is generally a monoarticular arthritis, with the affected joint being erythematous, edematous, hot, and tender.

D. Synovial fluid analysis from knee   NONESSENTIAL

Synovial fluid analysis is generally not indicated in the evaluation of joint pain unless there is a suspicion of a condition for which synovial fluid analysis and possibly cultures are likely to assist with the diagnosis and/or treatment plan for the patient (e.g., crystal arthropathy or infectious arthritis) or if a significant effusion is present. It is also indicated if the patient is not responding appropriately to therapy. Nevertheless, in osteoarthritis, some experts feel that synovial fluid analysis is superior to plain film radiographs in evaluating the patient's condition because of the inconsistencies between the radiologic findings and the patient's symptoms.

In evaluating synovial fluid, if the white blood cell count of the synovial fluid is greater than 1000/µL, the patient has an inflammatory process, infectious condition, or crystal-associated arthropathy. Crystal-associated arthropathies can be further distinguished by their characteristic crystals (e.g., gout has monosodium urate [MSU] crystals that are somewhat long, narrow, rod-shaped [also called "needle-shaped"] and negatively birefringent, whereas pseudogout has calcium pyrophosphate dehydrate [CPPD] crystals that are weakly positively birefringent and rod shaped, but rectangular or rhomboid shaped than the "needle-shaped" crystals of true gout). Gram stains and appropriate cultures with sensitivities need to be performed on the fluid if there is a suspicion of an infectious process.

E. Rheumatoid factor (RF)   NONESSENTIAL

RF is not indicated as part of Mrs. Myers' evaluation because she does not have signs or symptoms suspicious for rheumatoid arthritis or any other connective tissue disease. Furthermore, if these findings were present, Mrs. Myers would require a complete evaluation for all connective tissue disease, not just RF. A positive RF is found significantly more frequently in patients with RA than the general population. Nevertheless, an individual can have a positive RF and not have RA. Conversely, he or she can have RA and not have a positive RF.

4. Diagnosis

A. Osteoporosis   INCORRECT

Osteoporosis results from an imbalance in the activity of the osteoclasts and osteoblasts leading to thinner bone that is more susceptibility to fractures, even with no or minimal trauma. Traditionally, it is considered a disease of the trabecular bone because of its role in providing overall strength for the bone. However, cortical bone is also involved as evident by the related fractures. The preponderance of cases occur in women shortly after menopause (explaining why some refer to this condition as "menopausal osteoporosis"). The pain associated with osteoporosis is generally related to a fracture and/or its resultant deformity. The most common sites for osteoporotic fractures are the vertebral bodies, followed by the hip and the distal radius. It is diagnosed by dual-energy x-ray absorptiometry (DEXA) scan.

Osteoporosis can be ruled out as Mrs. Myers' most likely diagnosis because it rarely causes knee pain unless there is an associated lumbar or hip fracture compressing a nerve, or more rarely a blood vessel, causing radiation of pain to the knee, a neuropathic joint, or aseptic (avascular) necrosis. Additionally, Mrs. Myers' pain description and physical examination findings are inconsistent with this diagnosis.

B. Osteoarthritis   CORRECT

Osteoarthritis is a degenerative joint disease that is caused by a defect in the hyaline articular cartilage leading to an irregular pattern of cartilage loss and its resultant consequences of hypertrophy and sclerosis of the subchondral bone plate (and its consequence of osteophyte formation), stretching of the joint capsule, synovitis, and associated muscular atrophy. Because many of these structures have roles in joint protection, their affliction permits further joint damage to occur. Osteoarthritis is characterized by a lack of grossly visible inflammatory changes and predilection for the knee joint. Advanced disease can be associated with internal derangement of the knee. Additionally, it can cause or be caused by

weakness of the supporting muscles surrounding the joint. In patients older than the age of 45 years, it is the most common cause of monoarticular arthritis (however, it frequently affects multiple joints). Based on Mrs. Myers' age, history, and physical examination, osteoarthritis is her most likely diagnosis.

C. Rheumatoid arthritis   INCORRECT

Rheumatoid arthritis (RA) is an autoimmune process that affects the connective tissues of the joints; hence, it is considered to be a connective tissue or autoimmune disease. In the acute phase, the symmetric affected joints are erythematous, edematous, and warm to touch and prodromal symptoms are present. The chronic phase is associated with thickening of the articular soft tissue and a chronic synovitis that can produce articular cartilage, ligament, tendon, and bony erosions with joint space narrowing. Extra-articular manifestations can include subcutaneous (rheumatoid) nodules, Sjögren syndrome, episcleritis, scleritis, small vessel vasculitis, pericarditis, pleural effusions, lymphadenopathy (both localized and generalized), splenomegaly, and leukopenia. RA can be ruled out as Mrs. Myers' most likely diagnosis because her affected joints revealed bony proliferation but no warmth, erythema, or swelling on physical examination. Furthermore, Mrs. Myers did not have any systemic symptoms.

D. Gouty arthritis   INCORRECT

Gouty arthritis (gout) is an inflammatory arthritis that is characterized by the presence of monosodium urate (needle-shaped) crystals in the synovial fluid. Typically, it is monoarticular, unilateral, and infrequently affects the knee (let alone both knees simultaneously). Thus, gouty arthritis can be ruled out as Mrs. Myers' most likely diagnosis.

E. Lyme disease–associated arthritis   INCORRECT

Lyme disease can be ruled out as Mrs. Myers' most likely diagnosis because it is also generally a monoarticular process associated with other systemic symptoms associated with it. Also, her history and clinical findings are inconsistent with a tick-borne infectious process.

5. Treatment Plan

A. Weight reduction   CORRECT

Weight reduction is an essential component of the treatment plan for all individuals who are overweight or obese, especially if they have osteoarthritis of the knee. Essentially, without weight reduction, all other interventions to treat the osteoarthritis are going to be less effective. In cases of extreme obesity, some of the interventions are going to be impossible to perform (e.g., total knee replacement).

B. Physical therapy consultation to develop at-home range-of-motion, strengthening, and aerobic exercise program CORRECT

All of the major organizations dealing with arthritis agree that the nonpharmacologic interventions are the most important aspect of the treatment plan. One component of these nonpharmaceutical interventions includes a physical therapy consultation to develop an at-home range-of-motion, strengthening, and aerobic exercise program. There is some evidence to suggest that physical therapy should be the mainstay of therapy in osteoarthritis because it eliminates the need for medications in many patients.

C. Continue acetaminophen   CORRECT

Currently the acetaminophen appears to be effective in controlling her pain to her satisfaction. If it becomes ineffective, then the next choice would be to have her increase it to its maximum dosage of 1000 mg four times per day. This recommendation is supported by several major medical organizations. The American Geriatric Society's (AGS) guidelines regarding the management of persistent pain in older persons recently reverted to recommending acetaminophen as first-line therapy for older persons with chronic pain. The Osteoarthritis Research Society International (OARSI) also supports acetaminophen as first-line therapy for osteoarthritis.

Additionally, the American Academy of Orthopaedic Surgeons' (AAOS) recently revised guidelines and the most recent American College of Rheumatology (ACR) guidelines for the treatment of osteoarthritis of the knee and hip recommend acetaminophen or a nonsteroidal anti-inflammatory drug (NSAID) as the first-line treatment for osteoarthritis of the knee and hip; however, they recommended adding a gastroprotective agent if utilizing an NSAID. Although NSAIDs appear to be slightly superior to acetaminophen in terms of pain relief, many experts feel the benefit is so slight it doesn't justify the adverse effects of the NSAIDs.

D. Continue glucosamine/chondroitin supplements if desired   CORRECT

To date, there are no good clinical trials supporting that either of these supplements, taken singularly or in combination, offer any significant pain relief for patients with knee or hip osteoarthritis. However, these trials have failed to reveal any evidence to suggest they are harmful. Therefore, if Mrs. Myers feels these supplements are beneficial, she should continue taking them.

However, if the patient has utilized the maximum dosage regularly for 3 months and has not noticed an appreciable improvement, then he or she should stop the supplements because some benefit should be evident in that time frame.

E. Stop acetaminophen and add naproxen 500 mg twice a day with a proton pump inhibitor (PPI) for gastrointestinal protection   INCORRECT

This would be one recommendation for a patient with osteoarthritis if the acetaminophen was not effective in controlling his or her symptoms and is supported by the aforementioned AAOS and ACR guidelines. However, the AGS guidelines recommend that NSAIDs should be used with "extreme caution" because of the gastrointestinal and cardiovascular risks associated with these agents. They recommend usage of opioids as a "safer" alternative for elderly patients who have moderate to severe pain or who are having significant limitations on quality of life because of a painful condition. However, they do recommend that healthcare providers (HCPs) exercise the same precautions, assessments, and responsible prescribing as with any patient placed on a narcotic pain medication. OARSI makes similar recommendations.

Regardless, this would not be an acceptable option for Mrs. Myers because she has had an anaphylactic reaction to aspirin; therefore, technically all NSAIDs would be contraindicated for her, especially those in the same class as aspirin, including naproxen.

If considering a selective cyclooxygenase-2 (COX-2) inhibitor, it is essential to take into account not only the patient's concurrent disease but also his or her risk factors for acquiring diseases that are being associated with these products (e.g., cardiovascular disease, gastrointestinal disease, renal insufficiency, and hepatic toxicity). Currently only one COX-2 inhibitor (celecoxib) is still available in the United States. It is important to remember that selective COX-2 inhibitors have a slightly lower incidence of gastrointestinal (GI) bleeding; however, it is not absent. Consideration should be given to cover these patients with a PPI or misoprostol as well for GI protection.

The AGS and OARSI also mention the benefits of topical agents (e.g., diclofenac sodium 1% gel and capsaicin 0.025% or 0.075%). Diclofenac gel is topical NSAID and is only available by prescription. Even though it is applied topically, there is some systemic absorption. Therefore, it carries the same precautions as oral NSAIDs for serious complications, including gastrointestinal bleeding and thromboembolic cardiovascular diseases. It is unknown at this time if the incidence is lower due to the topical administration and lower dosage of this agent. It is contraindicated in patients who have experienced a serious allergic reaction to other NSAIDs, including aspirin.

Capsaicin is a topical analgesic that is derived from hot peppers. Because it is classified as a dietary supplement, it is not regulated by the US Food and Drug Administration (FDA). Therefore, clinical studies are not required to support claims or test for adverse effects, contraindications with co-existing medical conditions, or drug–drug interactions.

Epidemiologic and Other Data

Osteoarthritis is the most common form of arthritis found in adults residing in the United States. Because the disease is much more common in older individuals and the number of individuals in the United States who are older than 65 years of age continues to increase, it is estimated that the number of Americans affected by the disease could double by 2020. Current estimates in individuals who are 60 years of age or older consist of approximately 12% having symptomatic knee osteoarthritis, 10% having symptomatic hand osteoarthritis, and 4% having symptomatic hip osteoarthritis.

Risk factors for osteoarthritis include older age, female gender, obesity, positive family history, prior joint trauma (including occupational/recreational activities that involved frequent bending or joint overloading), chronic joint misalignment, and associated muscle weakness.

CASE 8-2
Mitchell Nutter
1. History

A. What, if any, imaging studies has he ever had performed on his back?   ESSENTIAL

Knowing the date, location, and results of previously performed diagnostic studies provides some clues as to what was being considered for his differential diagnoses at that time. Plus, it provides the location of these studies in the event they are required for comparison to current ones.

B. Does he take potassium supplements?   NONESSENTIAL

Individuals performing demanding manual labor or athletes participating/practicing sports when ambient temperatures are elevated are at risk for heat-related illnesses, including heat cramps, heat stroke, heat exhaustion, and heat syncope. Heat cramps are severe muscle cramps located in the muscles that the individual utilizes the most, and they almost always occur immediately following the activity. Although heat cramps are theorized to result from an electrolyte imbalance, it is dilutional hyponatremia, not hypokalemia. Some feel that taking salt (sodium chloride) tablets or drinking water containing salt before and during such exposure can prevent heat cramps; however, the literature is conflicting regarding this recommendation.

Although hypokalemia can occur during a heat-related illness, pretreating with potassium supplements has not been shown to have any effect on preventing these conditions. Thus, this question is not going to provide any useful clinical information. Appropriate questions to ask if there is concern that his back pain resulted from heat cramps would include the following: What was the ambient temperature during his shift yesterday? Was he agitated before he began experiencing back pain? Did he experience muscle twitching? Did he experience perspiration with cool-feeling skin? and, Did he have an elevated body temperature?

C. Does he have any urinary incontinence, inability to void, dysuria, urinary urgency, urinary frequency, hematuria, urethral discharge, or impotence?   ESSENTIAL

Previous urinary tract infections, especially in immunocompromised individuals or those who abuse IV drugs, are a significant risk factor for osteomyelitis. Urinary urgency and hematuria can suggest the possibility of pyelonephritis as the cause of his low back pain. Dysuria can indicate the presence of urethritis, cystitis, or prostatitis, which can be associated with low back pain. Urethral discharge is suspicious for urethritis, prostatitis, or epididymitis, which can also produce low back pain. Symptoms of incontinence, inability to void, or impotence could signify a serious neurologic impairment being related to his low back pain.

D. Is he experiencing any radiation of pain, dysesthesias, paresthesias, leg weakness, or other neurologic symptoms?   ESSENTIAL

Pain, especially if burning in nature, and/or paresthesias radiating into the buttocks and down the leg to below the level of the knee (and especially to the foot) are most frequently caused by an irritation of the affected nerve root, most often the sciatic nerve. Potential causes include a herniated nucleus pulposus, spinal stenosis, sacroiliitis, osteoarthritis, or local compression on the nerve by a severe muscle spasm or from external sources (e.g., man's wallet in his back pocket).

Neurologic symptoms, such as bilateral leg weakness and saddle anesthesia, especially in conjunction with urinary tract symptoms (e.g., bladder incontinence, inability to void, or impotence), are very suspicious for cauda equine syndrome, especially if the symptoms are rapidly developing, or evolving, in conjunction with low back pain. It also tends to be characterized by the presence of nocturnal pain as well as pain that is not alleviated (or at least decreased) when in the supine position. The presence of dysesthesias, leg weakness, or other neurologic symptoms requires a more extensive evaluation to ensure that serious conditions are not missed.

E. Has he experienced fever, fatigue, weight loss, or a recent bacterial infection?   ESSENTIAL

The presence of constitutional symptoms (e.g., fever, fatigue, and/or weight loss) as well as a history of a recent bacterial infection also requires a more extensive evaluation to determine if these symptoms represent an infectious, inflammatory, or malignant process, which could result in very grave consequences if not diagnosed and treated in a timely manner.

2. Physical Examination

A. Heart auscultation   ESSENTIAL

Heart auscultation is required because the pain of subacute bacterial endocarditis (SBE) and endocarditis can radiate to the lower back. On auscultation, a regurgitant murmur of the affected valve is frequently audible.

B. Abdominal examination   ESSENTIAL

An abdominal examination is indicated to identify potential intra-abdominal pathology that can radiate to the lower back (e.g., pancreatitis, bleeding or expanding abdominal aortic aneurysm, and penetrating peptic ulcer disease). When intra-abdominal structures are responsible for low back pain, frequently the back pain is reproduced when these structures are palpated.

C. Low back examination with Waddell signs   ESSENTIAL

A low back examination is indicated because Mr. Nutter's presenting complaint is low back pain. However, aside from being able to identify and quantify decreases in range of motion and/or the presence of a muscle spasm, very little clinical information is derived from this exam. Still, there are some rarer conditions that can be identified (or at least suspected) by this examination. For example, point tenderness over a single vertebra, in the absence of trauma, is very suggestive of osteomyelitis. A soft tissue mass could represent a wide array of conditions ranging from a benign lipoma to a neurofibroma. A rash following a dermatome could indicate herpes zoster.

Positive Waddell signs are a nonspecific constellation of inconsistencies in the physical examination that are suggestive, but not absolute, that the patient is not being entirely truthful during the examination for personal gain (e.g., acquiring prescription drugs for abuse/diversion, obtaining a work release, or getting attention from a significant other) or is extremely anxious regarding the examination because of fear it might reproduce (or worsen) the pain, a previous traumatic experience with an HCP, or other cause. These signs include abnormal grimacing or screaming about pain that is out of proportion to the procedure being performed (e.g., lightly touching the skin over the lumbar spine), axial loading producing low back pain, turning the patient's body with his or her spine straight reproducing the pain, or a negative straight-leg-raising test while sitting but a positive test when supine.

D. Neurologic evaluation of lower extremities   ESSENTIAL

A neurologic examination of the lower extremities is essential. The distribution of reflex loss, decreased sensation, and motor function can assist in identifying the site of a disc problem. Significant symptoms (e.g., bilateral leg weakness with saddle anesthesia) are very suspicious for cauda equine abnormalities. Rapidly progressing neurologic deficits can be caused by serious neurologic conditions such as a cauda equine lesion, an epidural abscess, or an extremely large herniated nucleus pulposus.

E. Vascular evaluation of lower extremities   ESSENTIAL

A vascular examination of the lower extremities is also important. It provides clues to conditions such as a ruptured abdominal aortic aneurysm, vascular compression syndrome, compartmental syndrome, or an ischemic event being responsible for, or coexisting with, the low back pain.

3. Diagnostic Studies

A. Lumbosacral (LS) spine radiograph   NONESSENTIAL

In the absence of significant trauma, diagnostic imaging, especially with radiographs of the LS spine, is not indicated because it provides very little useful clinical information unless the patient has "red flags" (alarm or warning signs and symptoms). The presence of these signs or symptoms increases the likelihood that the patient does not have a benign musculoskeletal condition. They include age younger than 20 years or older than 50 years, a history of cancer, pain that worsens with rest or lying down, nocturnal pain, comorbid immunocompromised disease, IV drug abuse, recent bacterial infection, severe or progressing neurologic defects, chronic long-term corticosteroid usage, and osteoporosis. Otherwise, an imaging study is indicated only if the patient's pain persists for longer than 1 month.

B. Magnetic resonance imaging (MRI) of LS spine NONESSENTIAL

An MRI is the diagnostic test of choice to evaluate low back pain in individuals with the aforementioned "red flag" signs and symptoms. Because Mr. Nutter lacks these as well as any evidence to suggest that his bulging disc has herniated, an MRI is not indicated, especially considering an essentially normal study was conducted 9 months ago.

C. Urinalysis (U/A)   NONESSENTIAL

A U/A would only be indicated if Mr. Nutter were exhibiting signs and symptoms suspicious for a genitourinary condition causing (or coexisting with) his low back pain.

D. Erythrocyte sedimentation rate (ESR)   NONESSENTIAL

An ESR would only be indicated if Mr. Nutter's history or physical examination was suspicious for an inflammatory, infectious, or malignant process being responsible for his low back pain.

E. Complete blood count with differential (CBC w/diff) NONESSENTIAL

The same conditions that would necessitate an ESR would also require a CBC w/diff; additionally, the concern of hemorrhage should be added to the list.

4. Diagnosis

A. Osteoarthritis of the LS spine   INCORRECT

Osteoarthritis can cause low back pain if the lumbar spine is affected. However, Mr. Nutter's young age and lack of findings consistent with this condition (please see Case 8-1 for these clinical signs and symptoms) make it unlikely to be his most likely diagnosis.

B. Osteoporosis of the LS spine   INCORRECT

Osteoporosis of the LS spine can essentially be ruled out as Mr. Nutter's most likely diagnosis because of his age and the lack of any comorbid conditions or medications that would be responsible for premature osteoporosis in a male. Furthermore, the back pain from osteoporosis results from the vertebral fractures and their subsequent deformities, which generally are confined to the thoracic spine and are extremely rare in the lumbar spine. Furthermore, the nature of the pain is also different.

C. Osteomyelitis of the LS spine   INCORRECT

Osteomyelitis is an infection of the bone; if lumbar vertebrae are involved, it can produce low back pain. However, this condition can essentially be eliminated as Mr. Nutter's most likely diagnosis because he does not have any constitutional symptoms indicating the presence of a serious infectious process, tenderness to palpation of the spinous processes, or a pain pattern consistent with this diagnosis.

D. Lumbar strain with spasm   CORRECT

Because he provided a history of an acute lumbar injury, has a pain pattern consistent with this diagnosis, and has evidence of a mild muscle spasm on physical examination, Mr. Nutter's most likely diagnosis is lumbar strain with spasm.

E. Lumbar disc herniation   INCORRECT

Lumbar disc herniation can essentially be eliminated as the most likely diagnosis for Mr. Nutter's pain because he is not experiencing a radiculopathy, dysesthesias, or paresthesias suggestive of nerve root compression. With a true herniation, these findings are virtually always present.

5. Treatment Plan

A. Rapid titration of fentanyl patches to 100 µg/hr every 72 hours for 6 to 8 weeks, then a slow titration off the fentanyl INCORRECT

Pain control, improvement of range of motion, and avoiding limitations on functional status are the primary goals for the treatment of acute musculoskeletal pain in the lumbar region. Pain control can generally be partially (if not fully) achieved by topical heat application; however, it typically takes short-term oral analgesics to accomplish this goal. According to the guidelines coproduced by the American College of Physicians (ACP) and the American Pain Society (APS), first-line pharmaceutical therapy should be either acetaminophen, an NSAID, or in rare cases time-limited narcotics.

Fentanyl is an inappropriate choice for Mr. Nutter, regardless of its success in the past, because it should never be used in patients with acute pain, mild to moderate pain, intermittent pain, or postoperative pain unless they are currently taking an opioid and not achieving pain relief. It is indicated for the management of chronic pain in opioid-dependent patients who have failed to obtain relief from lesser agents.

B. Cyclobenzaprine 5 mg three times per day with drowsiness and alcohol precautions   CORRECT

According to the guidelines coproduced by the ACP and APS, there is evidence supporting the use of a muscle relaxant for short-term pain relief. This will be especially helpful for Mr. Nutter because he has a muscle spasm present. When choosing a muscle relaxant, there must be some consideration given to the possibility that Mr. Nutter could have a substance use/abuse problem and agents avoided that could contribute to the condition. Some of these agents are obvious in their abuse potential, such as the benzodiazepines (e.g., diazepam); others are less well known for their abuse potential (e.g., the centrally acting muscle relaxant carisoprodol). Cyclobenzaprine does not have any specifically known abuse potential except that it can potentiate increased central nervous system depression when taken with alcohol. Unfortunately, all of the muscle relaxants have this risk. This must be emphasized to the patient along with the drowsiness precautions upon prescribing.

C. Bed rest until follow-up appointment in 1 week INCORRECT

Even though it has been effective for his pain in the past, bed rest for 1 week is an inappropriate treatment option. Multiple studies have found, and the combined ACP/APS guidelines agree, that individuals who remained as active as possible with an acute lumbar strain had much shorter healing times than those assigned bed rest.

Despite the ACP/APS guidelines recommending the initial follow-up to occur in 4 weeks, it is appropriate to bring Mr. Nutter back in 1 week to ensure he is compliant with not remaining on strict bed rest and to assess his level of pain control. It is essential to remember that evidence-based medical guidelines, such as the ACP/APS's on low back pain management, are just that—guidelines. They are not absolutes; therefore, appropriate clinical judgment has to be part of all evaluation, diagnostic, and treatment plans.

D. Referral to physical therapy   CORRECT

Surprisingly, the ACP/APS guidelines found that an exercise program did little to improve acute musculoskeletal lumbar pain during the first month; however, it was found to be very effective in individuals with persistent pain. Because Mr. Nutter has a history of frequent episodes of LS strain with spasms, he will require education on how to prevent these episodes in the future by learning how to utilize his legs, not his back, to lift; appropriate strengthening exercises for his back and legs; and stretching exercises for his back. Until he is well enough to begin these sessions, the physical therapist can provide pain-reducing modalities (e.g., hot packs, massage, ultrasound, and/or muscle stimulation). This will also hopefully prevent him from remaining on complete bed rest.

E. Referral for laminectomy   INCORRECT

Mr. Nutter provides a history of a prior MRI that revealed a bulging disc, not a herniated disc. In the absence of neurologic symptoms, a surgical procedure is not indicated even with overt herniation. The currently recommended procedure of choice for a herniated nucleus pulposus is a partial hemilaminectomy. Indications for this procedure include the presence of at least ONE of the following: (1) damage to the nerve root resulting in a progressive motor weakness, (2) spinal cord compression, (3) intolerable/incapacitating nerve root pain that is unresponsive to other therapeutic modalities, or (4) recurrent intolerable/incapacitating nerve pain that is unresponsive to nonsurgical approaches.

Caution must be utilized when interpreting a patient's MRI results because it is not uncommon for individuals without any

pain or history of trauma to have one or more bulging, or even herniated, discs. Thus, before instituting a treatment plan for lumbar disc disease, it is essential to ensure that the patient's symptoms are related to the abnormality discovered on MRI.

Epidemiologic and Other Data

It is estimated that approximately 85 to 90% of all low back pain is secondary to a benign musculoskeletal condition. The remainder consists of more serious conditions (e.g., primary bone carcinomas, bony metastatic disease, inflammatory arthropathies, significant neurologic processes, infections, intra-abdominal processes, and pelvic conditions).

The majority of musculoskeletal low back pain resolves without any treatment, or with conservative therapy, within 1 month. However, if the musculoskeletal low back pain involves a worker's compensation claim, the resolution rate at 1 month is significantly lower.

CASE 8-3
Natasha O'Hara
1. History

A. Has she experienced any changes in her appetite, weight, interests, or activities; anhedonia; trouble concentrating; memory difficulties; crying episodes; feeling depressed, blue, sad, or anxious; or suicidal ideations?   ESSENTIAL

With any chronic condition, there are a significant number of individuals who have coexisting depression. In many cases, it is unknown whether the depression predisposed the patient to the condition, the illness caused the depression, or the two are unrelated. Regardless, if not diagnosed or left untreated, it can have a tremendous impact on the outcome of the illness and patient compliance. Therefore, because Ms. O'Hara has hypersomnia, is not engaging in regular pleasurable activities, and has a family history of depression, it is essential to inquire about this possibility.

B. Was she sexually molested as a child?   NONESSENTIAL

Being the victim of sexual molestation as a child is known to result in a variety of psychological, somatic, and physical symptoms. However, it is not uncommon for the victim to successfully repress the memory of the event, so direct questioning might not reveal this information. Furthermore, because this would be a diagnosis of exclusion, it is not necessary to address with Ms. O'Hara at this time.

Approaching very sensitive issues such as this, unless absolutely pertinent to the chief complaint, is best delayed until the patient–provider relationship is better developed. Ideally, it should be broached in the context of a safe, therapeutic environment with a trained mental health professional. Furthermore, other childhood traumas, such as a mother committing suicide, occur much more frequently and can have just as devastating an impact.

C. Is she experiencing true weakness of her muscles? ESSENTIAL

Inquiring about muscle weakness is essential in determining Ms. O'Hara's differential diagnoses. Neuromuscular transmission diseases and myopathies are generally associated with some degree of true muscle weakness. However, polymyositis is associated with muscle weakness without myalgias. Likewise, fibromyalgia is associated with muscle pain but no muscle weakness.

D. Does she have any joint pain or swelling?   ESSENTIAL

The presence or absence of joint pain or swelling is also essential to inquire about. It could provide clues as to whether Ms. O'Hara has an arthritic or autoimmune condition producing her myalgias or coexisting with them. This becomes significant not only in formulating her list of potential differential diagnoses but also in establishing her treatment plan.

The coexistence of arthralgias and myalgias occurs in many conditions (e.g., systemic lupus erythematosus, polymyalgia rheumatica, rheumatoid arthritis with mononuclear cell infiltration of skeletal muscle or joint instability, overlap [mixed] connective tissue disease, osteoarthritis, poor physical conditioning, obesity, and depression). However, the presence of both symptoms could also represent two separate clinical conditions; for example, approximately 20 to 30% of all patients with rheumatoid arthritis also have fibromyalgia.

E. Has anyone ever told her she snores or quits breathing while she is asleep?   ESSENTIAL

Not only can myalgias cause sleep disturbances because of an inability to maintain a comfortable position, but also poor sleep quality can cause severe fatigue and myalgias. One of the most common conditions responsible for the latter is sleep apnea. Although it occurs more frequently in obese individuals, it can occur in individuals with a normal weight, neck size, and uvula.

If a diagnosis cannot be determined or she does not respond appropriately to treatment, it might be beneficial to obtain polysomnography to rule out sleep apnea as the cause of, or at least a contributing factor to, Ms. O'Hara's symptoms.

2. Physical Examination

A. Beck Depression Inventory   NONESSENTIAL

The Beck Depression Inventory is a standardized questionnaire that requires the patient to rate symptoms from 0 (not present) to 3 (severe). It is utilized to establish the presence and severity of depression if there is any question regarding its presence or if the patient does not respond to adequate trials of antidepressant therapy to ensure that the diagnosis is correct. Because depression can essentially be eliminated based on Ms. O'Hara's clinical interview, this test is not currently necessary.

B. Mini-mental status examination (MMSE)   ESSENTIAL

The MMSE is a screening tool designed to evaluate for the presence of dementia. However, it has also been utilized to screen for specific defects in the various components of the test (orientation, registration, recall, attention/calculation, language, and construct). The specific tasks required for each component are scored based on the patient's performance on each of the tasks. The maximum score is 30. A score of less than 27 indicates that an organic process is possible. However, at 33 years of age, it would be unlikely for a dementia to be detected in Ms. O'Hara. Nevertheless, due to her complaints, the test should be performed to evaluate for the presence of defects in cognitive function and mental impairment that would indicate additional testing is warranted.

C. Musculoskeletal examination   ESSENTIAL

Because Ms. O'Hara's chief complaint is generalized myalgias, a musculoskeletal examination is essential. Focus should be on range of motion and areas of tenderness to palpation because she is not experiencing arthralgias. Because her myalgias are generalized, her examination should also include checking the fibromyalgia trigger point locations for tenderness. (Please see response section for their location.)

D. Neurologic examination of the extremities   ESSENTIAL

A brief neurologic examination focusing on muscle strength, sensation, and reflexes is indicated as a component of a musculoskeletal evaluation to determine whether there are any defects that would require further evaluation for a potential neurologic or neuromuscular condition.

E. Vascular examination of the extremities   ESSENTIAL

A vascular examination of the extremities is also an essential component of a properly performed musculoskeletal evaluation. It is indicated to ensure that Ms. O'Hara's symptoms are not caused by a vascular problem, such as vasculitis, claudication, compartmental syndrome, or reflex sympathetic dystrophy.

3. Diagnostic Studies

A. Full x-ray series of the spine   NONESSENTIAL

A full spine x-ray series is not indicated because Ms. O'Hara does not provide a history of back trauma nor any of the "red flag" signs or symptoms indicating immediate radiographic studies are indicated. (To review this list, please see Case 8-2).

B. Creatine phosphokinase (CPK)   NONESSENTIAL

The majority of CPK is found in skeletal muscles, the myocardium, and the brain; however, there is a small quantity in the lungs as well. An injury to any of these structures can cause the total CPK to elevate. To distinguish which area is responsible, CPK isoenzymes (MB [predominately cardiac], MM [predominately muscle], and BB [predominately brain or rarely lungs]) should be performed and the results compared to the information that has been obtained on the patient's history and physical examination. Therefore, if there was concern that Ms. O'Hara was experiencing actual muscle damage, a CPK with isoenzymes should be performed.

However, because Ms. O'Hara's symptoms have been present and unchanged for 2 years, it is unlikely that her CPK is going to be elevated unless caused by a recent acupuncture treatment. Conditions associated with a chronically elevated CPK-MM (e.g., muscular dystrophy, rhabdomyolysis, and hypothyroidism) should worsen over time. Many of the conditions that are responsible for short-term elevations in CPK-MM (e.g., trauma, strenuous exercise, electroconvulsive therapy, seizures, delirium tremens, IM injection, recent surgery, and/or adverse effects caused by medications) can be eliminated based on her history. Other conditions that result in acute, short-term elevations of the CPK-MM (e.g., shock, serotonin syndrome, neuroleptic malignant syndrome, and hyperthermia) can essentially be eliminated by the presence of normal vital signs on her physical examination. Thus, a CPK is unnecessary.

C. Thyroid-stimulating hormone (TSH)   NONESSENTIAL

Hypothyroidism can cause severe fatigue and occasionally myalgias. However, Ms. O'Hara does not exhibit other symptoms that are commonly associated with the condition (e.g., weight increase, dryness of the skin, coarseness of the hair, constipation, or menstrual irregularities).

However, thyroid function studies might be considered if she fails to respond to appropriate therapy or develops some of these other symptoms. Regardless, to adequately assess thyroid function, a minimum of a TSH and a free thyroxine (FT_4) should be performed to ensure a subclinical or secondary hypothyroidism is not missed. However, most HCPs tend to order a thyroid panel that contains a measurement of the triiodothyronine (T_3) in addition to the TSH and FT_4 because it is generally less expensive than ordering these two tests separately.

D. Liver function testing (LFT)   NONESSENTIAL

Some hepatic conditions can also cause fatigue and myalgias (e.g., cirrhosis and hepatitis). Nevertheless, over a 2-year time period, the condition should have spontaneously resolved or significantly worsened. However, if therapy was being considered with hepatotoxic drugs for her condition, a baseline LFT measurement would be appropriate.

E. Cerebral spinal fluid (CSF) analysis for substance P NONESSENTIAL

One of many conditions that can reveal substance P in the CSF analysis is fibromyalgia, which could certainly be responsible for Ms. O'Hara's symptoms. However, it is not pathognomonic for the condition and lacks both sensitivity and specificity significant enough to justify obtaining it.

4. Diagnosis

A. Poliomyelitis   INCORRECT

Poliomyelitis is a viral infection that causes inflammation of the gray matter of the spinal cord. In the acute phase, it can cause muscle weakness; however, this is also associated with other signs and symptoms of an infectious process (e.g., fever, nausea, vomiting, headache, stiff neck, and sore throat, but no myalgias). Later in the course of the illness, the patient can present with signs of a lower motor neuron lesion (e.g., flaccid paralysis, decreased deep tendon reflexes, and muscle atrophy). Because this is not consistent with Ms. O'Hara's symptoms and she should have received vaccinations against the poliomyelitis virus as a child, this is not her most likely diagnosis. The extremely small possibility of a vaccine-induced case is also unlikely considering her symptoms.

B. Somatoform disorder   INCORRECT

A somatoform disorder is basically the manifestation of psychiatric distress as physical symptoms. Patients with this condition have a long-standing history of multiple complaints that are not explainable by any known medical conditions, including substance abuse disorders. The actual diagnostic criteria established by the American Psychiatric Association in the *Diagnostic and Statistical Manual of Mental Disorders,* fourth edition, text revision (DSM-IV-TR) are much more stringent. The DSM-IV-TR requires that the condition be present

before the age of 30 years old and consist of a series of multiple complaints occurring over a several-year period for which the patient has sought treatment or experienced a significant impairment in functioning. Furthermore, it requires that at some time during the course of the illness, the patient experienced at least four separate problems associated with pain, with at least two being gastrointestinal, one sexual, and one pseudoneurotic. Furthermore, the evaluation of these multiple complaints must fail to reveal any known medical condition, medication adverse effect, or substance abuse disorder. And, if there is a coexisting medical condition present, the severity of the symptoms and/or lack of functioning are excessive for that condition. Finally, the symptoms cannot have been intentionally manufactured by the patient.

Therefore, because Ms. O'Hara's symptoms began after the age of 30 years; she does not have a history of multiple complaints in the aforementioned areas (with the exception of her migraine headaches); and a physical condition can account for her symptoms, which are not out of proportion to her level of functioning, a somatoform disorder is not her most likely diagnosis.

C. Unspecified connective tissue disease   INCORRECT

An unspecified connective tissue disease is not Ms. O'Hara's most likely diagnosis because the pain tends to be distributed more in the joints than in the muscles. Additionally, other constitutional symptoms besides fatigue are generally associated with unspecified connective tissue diseases.

D. Polymyalgia rheumatica   INCORRECT

Polymyalgia rheumatica is a vasculitis syndrome that affects the medium-sized blood vessels with the characteristic symptoms of pain and stiffness of the hips and shoulders of several weeks' duration without another diagnosis to account for these symptoms. Although polymyalgia rheumatica can produce back pain, especially in the shoulders and pelvic girdle, it generally is not as widespread as Ms. O'Hara's. Furthermore, it is rare in individuals younger than the age of 50 years. Therefore, it is not Ms. O'Hara's most likely diagnosis.

E. Fibromyalgia syndrome   CORRECT

Fibromyalgia syndrome (FMS) is a chronic widespread pain disorder that predominately affects the muscles and soft tissues. In contradiction to wide-held beliefs, FMS is not a diagnosis of exclusion, but one that is made entirely on the basis of history and physical examination.

The diagnostic criteria for FMS devised by the ACR include 11 of the 18 fibromyalgia pressure points (one on each side of the body in the following areas: occiput where the suboccipital muscle insertions are located, intertransverse processes of the low cervical spine, second intracostal space near the sternum, halfway down the supraspinatus muscle near the border of the scapula, superior lateral quadrant of the gluteal muscle, greater trochanter of the hip, superior border of the trapezius muscle, medial aspect of the knee, and lateral epicondyle) being tender to palpation with a single digit. It ALSO requires that a minimum of one of the tender pressure points be located in the spine AND at least one be located in at least three of the four quadrants of the body. Furthermore, the symptoms must be present for a minimum of 3 months. Ms. O'Hara's history and physical findings are consistent with this, and therefore, fibromyalgia syndrome is Ms. O'Hara's most likely diagnosis.

Because the ACR criteria were technically established as a research tool to ensure all participants in clinical trials had a similar, quantifiable disease, there are some experts in the field who criticize these criteria as too stringent in establishing FMS in the clinical setting. They feel that if the patient has chronic (≥ 3 months) widespread pain, sleep disturbances, mood alterations, and cognitive decline that affects their functional status; a negative musculoskeletal and neurologic examination except for the presence of some, but not 11, positive FMS trigger points; and a normal complete blood count with differential, erythrocyte sedimentation rate, thyroid studies, liver function testing, and muscle enzymes, then it would be appropriate to diagnose the patient as having FMS. Conversely, there are those who feel the ACR guidelines are too vague and lead to the overdiagnosis, not underdiagnosis, of the condition.

5. Treatment Plan

A. Continue acupuncture as needed   CORRECT

As with other chronic pain conditions, the goals of treating FMS include reducing pain, improving function, and decreasing limitations/disabilities.

There is still a significant amount of knowledge that needs to be discovered regarding alternative therapies. Nevertheless, multiple studies indicate that acupuncture does not provide effective relief from fibromyalgia symptoms; however, this could be because of the short-term benefit of acupuncture and the longer treatment intervals and/or duration of the studies. However, many patients, like Ms. O'Hara, feel it is effective for them. Therefore, if the patient feels the treatment is providing benefit and there are no known significant harms, then it is a beneficial therapy, at least for that particular patient, and can be continued, if desired.

B. Amitriptyline 25 mg at bedtime, then titrate upward as appropriate   INCORRECT

Off-label use of tricyclic antidepressants (TCAs) was considered to be the mainstay of FMS therapy several years ago. Despite the fact that multiple studies revealed TCAs to be effective in alleviating the pain of FMS, it was very difficult to achieve doses high enough to determine whether they offered any improvement on the patient's mood and daily functioning because of the intolerability of their adverse effects.

C. Fluoxetine 20 mg daily   INCORRECT

Because of the high intolerability rates and high potential for fatalities in cases of accidental or intentional overdoses with TCAs, they quickly fell out of favor as a preferred antidepressant when the selective serotonin reuptake inhibitors (SSRIs), such as fluoxetine, were introduced to the US marketplace. At that time, many still considered FMS to be a "psychiatric" condition and assumed that the improvement in symptoms from the TCAs was purely from the antidepressant effects. Therefore, many medical practitioners automatically changed FMS treatment from off-label TCA usage to off-label SSRI usage, without any real data to support this change.

After being on the market for a few years, a study was done that found fluoxetine 20 qd was not superior to placebo in the treatment of FMS. Later studies using higher doses found SSRIs to be better than placebo, but still not as effective as TCAs, in managing the pain of FMS. However, they had minimal effects on the other symptoms of the illness, with the exception of mood.

D. Milnacipran in a tapering dose starting at 12.5 mg once on the first day; twice on days 2 and 3; days 4 through 7, 25 mg twice daily; and after day 7, 50 mg twice a day   CORRECT

The introduction of the serotonin-norepinephrine reuptake inhibitors (SNRIs) has significantly impacted the treatment of FMS. Good quality, clinical studies have shown that at least some of these agents, particularly duloxetine and milnacipran, are effective in not only decreasing the pain associated with the disease but also in improving the patient's mood, memory, fatigue, overall physical functioning, and global impression of change (PGIC). Furthermore, these changes appear to persist over time. Duloxetine and milnacipran have FDA approval for the treatment of FMS. There are some smaller studies that suggest the off-label use of other SNRIs are capable of producing similar results. However, larger scale, double-blinded, placebo-controlled randomized trials are indicated to further study their benefits in FMS.

E. Pregabalin 300 mg daily   CORRECT

Pregabalin, an α_2–δ ligand anticonvulsant, at 300 mg daily is also FDA approved for the first-line treatment of FMS. Additionally, it is FDA approved for diabetic neuropathy, postherpetic neuralgia, and some seizure disorders. Clinical trials with pregabalin have shown reductions in pain scores, improvements in global impression, enhancements in functioning, better sleep quality, less fatigue, and improvements in overall quality of life in patients with FMS.

However, it should not be initiated simultaneously with milnacipran. The decision regarding which one of these agents (if either) is best for a patient with FMS includes correlating the patient's signs and symptoms with the mechanism of action, benefits versus risks of each agent (including over-the-counter products and pharmaceuticals with and without FDA approval), comorbid medical conditions, current medications, and other patient factors (e.g., cost, insurance status, medication formularies' preferences, and/or frequency of dosage) and recommending appropriate treatment plans; then, in conjunction with the patient, a course of action is established.

Currently, there are no other FDA-approved medications for the treatment of FMS. Another drug, commonly used off-label, is tramadol. It is often utilized if the patient is experiencing significant pain unalleviated with over-the-counter agents because it is not only an opioid μ-agonist but also an SNRI. Pramipexole, a dopamine agonist approved for Parkinson disease and restless leg syndrome but not specifically for FMS, provides effective relief for patients with restless leg syndrome associated with their FMS.

F. Naproxen 500 mg twice a day with food   INCORRECT

Naproxen is not indicated for Ms. O'Hara because clinical trials failed to reveal any significant improvement, even in pain, when used alone and only a slight reduction in pain when added to a TCA. Additionally, a PPI would need to be added to provide gastroprotection because Ms. O'Hara will require the medication long term. Several adverse effects have been associated with PPI (e.g., increased incidence of osteoporosis at specific sites, *Clostridium difficile* infections, and pernicious anemia) and NSAID (e.g. GI bleed and cardiovascular disease) usage, these potential problems must be considered in prescribing long-term NSAID therapy for any reason.

Epidemiological and Other Data

Utilizing the 1990 ACR criteria for diagnosing fibromyalgia, the incidence of FMS is estimated to be approximately 3.4% of the female population and 0.5% of the male population in the United States. However, some rheumatologic practices cite the rate of fibromyalgia to be as high as 20%.

The incidence actually increases with age. The group with the highest incidence is women 50 years of age or older. Furthermore, it is estimated to affect approximately 7.4% of all US women in their 70s. Still, most patients who present with symptoms are between the ages of 30 and 50 years. Although rare, it does occur in children.

The precise cause of fibromyalgia is unknown. It is theorized that it results from abnormal perceptions of pain. Many differences have been found between control groups and individuals with fibromyalgia; however, none of these differences met adequate sensitivity and specificity to be considered pathognomonic for fibromyalgia. Some of these include disturbances in stage 4 sleep by frequent interruptions of alpha waves; reduced serotonin levels in cerebrospinal fluid; increased levels of substrate P in cerebrospinal fluid; low serum levels of growth hormone; low levels of free cortisol in the urine; decreased serum cortisol levels in response to stress; decreased serum cortisol levels in response to a corticotrophin-releasing hormone; dysfunction of the autonomic nervous system; and decreased blood flow to the thymus, caudate nucleus, and pontine tectum (via single photon emission computed tomography [SPET] scanning).

Patients with fibromyalgia have a much greater incidence (approximately 30%) of psychological comorbidity (e.g., depression, anxiety, hypochondriasis, and somatization disorders) when compared to healthy controls. However, it is uncertain whether the chronic pain and disability from the fibromyalgia produce the psychological comorbidity or the psychological condition predisposes the patient to the development of fibromyalgia.

CASE 8-4
Oscar Pence
1. History

A. What does his wife think about his drinking? NONESSENTIAL

Before inquiring about spouses' impressions/concerns, it is essential to determine if he has a spouse and, if so, the status of their current relationship. If there is concern regarding his alcohol consumption, a CAGE screen would be a more appropriate approach to utilize. It is a screening tool for possible alcohol abuse and consists of four questions. One or more positive responses indicate a potential problem with alcohol abuse requiring further evaluation. These questions are as follows: (1)Have you ever tried to **c**ut down on the amount of alcohol that you consume? (2)Have you ever become **a**ngry

when others suggest you reduce your intake or have a problem with alcohol? (3)Have you ever felt **g**uilty about your drinking? and (4)Have you ever needed an "**e**ye opener" to get started the next morning following an episode of drinking?

B. Did he notice any knots, rope-like lesions, or swelling in his palm before this problem began?   ESSENTIAL

Knots, rope-like lesions, or swelling in the palm, with or without pain, before the development of a flexure contracture of the finger(s) are consistent with. Mr. Pence's most likely diagnosis. Generally, the progression of these changes and the development of a flexure contracture take years.

C. Has he noticed any swelling in his neck, crooked penile erections, dyspnea, chronic cough, or wheezing?   ESSENTIAL

If signs and swelling are present which suggest other areas of the body are affected by fibrosis, (e.g. neck swelling [Riedel struma]; crooked penile erections [Peyronie disease]; or, dyspnea, chronic cough, and wheezing [mediastinal fibrosis]), it raises the suspicion that Mr. Pence's problem represents a systemic process, such as systemic fibrosing syndrome, instead of a localized process.

D. Has he had any abdominal pain or swelling, anorexia, nausea, vomiting, constipation, diarrhea, melena, or jaundice? ESSENTIAL

Because Mr. Pence's condition has a much higher incidence in alcoholic patients, especially those with cirrhosis, hepatitis, or fatty liver disease, it is especially important to inquire about symptoms not only of hepatic diseases but also of upper gastrointestinal bleeding. These symptoms need to be sought because he is at risk for upper gastrointestinal bleeding from the effects of alcohol on the mucosa (e.g., gastritis and peptic ulcer disease), esophageal varices caused by portal hypertension from an underlying hepatic disease, and Mallory-Weiss tears if he is experiencing significant vomiting because of his alcohol consumption.

E. Has he experienced any change in his weight, malaise, fatigue, chest pain/pressure, or palpitations?   ESSENTIAL

Because Mr. Pence's diagnosis can be associated with other chronic diseases (e.g., diabetes mellitus, thyroiditis, seizures disorders, and coronary artery disease), inquiring about the presence of symptoms that could be related to these comorbid conditions is also important. Furthermore, excessive alcohol consumption can result in cardiomyopathies and Mallory-Weiss syndrome, which could also present as chest pain, palpitations, dyspnea, cough, and/or wheezing.

2. Physical Examination

A. Heart and lung examination   NONESSENTIAL

Because his history did not elicit any information suspicious for a cardiac or pulmonary condition, including an alcoholic cardiomyopathy, a heart and lung exam is not indicated.

B. Abdominal examination   ESSENTIAL

Because of the possibility of an associated alcohol-related hepatic disease caused by his regular, heavy alcohol consumption (and its association with his diagnosis), an abdominal examination is indicated to evaluate for hepatomegaly, liver edge irregularities, tenderness, splenomegaly, ascites, or other signs of hepatic disease (e.g., abdominal spider nevi and jaundice).

C. Bilateral hand examination   ESSENTIAL

Obviously, because Mr. Pence has a hand complaint, a hand examination is indicated. It should be bilateral because it provides a "normal" for comparison and permits the unaffected hand to be evaluated for subtle changes.

D. Bilateral foot examination   NONESSENTIAL

There are no foot problems equivalent to his chief complaint nor is he complaining of a foot malady.

E. Skin and sclera examination, especially for jaundice ESSENTIAL

Because of the possibility of an associated alcohol-related hepatic disease, examination of the skin and sclera are indicated to evaluate for jaundice, icterus, and spider nevi. If not performed during the hand evaluation, it is important to examine the skin of the the hand for abnormalities. Palmar erythema is another finding suggestive of alcoholic liver disease or cirrhosis.

3. Diagnostic Studies

A. Magnetic resonance imaging (MRI) of his right hand NONESSENTIAL

The diagnosis of Mr. Pence's chief complaint can be made by history and physical examination. Early in the course of the illness, when just a "knot" is present on the palmar surface, occasionally a biopsy is indicated to rule out a carcinoma.

B. Radiograph of his right hand   NONESSENTIAL

The diagnosis of his chief complaint can be made clinically by history and physical examination findings.

C. Magnetic resonance imaging (MRI) of his abdomen NONESSENTIAL

Even though he had hepatomegaly on his abdominal examination, an MRI of Mr. Pence's abdomen is not indicated at this time. MRIs of the abdomen are generally reserved for cases of hepatomegaly where there is concern about lesions (both benign and malignant) in the liver and/or pancreas or to evaluate the associated vasculature.

If any imaging study was required at this time, it would be an abdominal ultrasound to obtain a measurement of the exact size of the hepatomegaly. Additionally, it would provide information regarding the texture and uniformity of the organ.

D. Aspartate aminotransferase (AST), alanine aminotransferase (ALT), alkaline phosphatase (ALP), and total bilirubin ESSENTIAL

An appropriate first-line diagnostic procedure to evaluate a patient with asymptomatic hepatomegaly is the assessment of the liver function via measurement of the primary liver enzymes—AST, ALT, ALP, and total bilirubin. All four are generally elevated in hepatic problems.

Depending on the degree of elevation and their relationship/ratio to one another, these enzyme values can provide essential information that will assist in establishing the correct diagnosis. For example, with the exception of viral hepatitis, hepatocellular disease is indicated by an ALT:AST ratio (also known as the DeRitis ratio) of less than 1. If the AST is elevated more than the ALT, especially by a factor of two or more, then

it is almost always indicative of an alcohol-related disease. However, in alcohol-induced liver disease, the AST is rarely over 300. In viral hepatitis, the AST and ALT are extremely elevated initially; then, ALP and bilirubin elevations follow. If the bilirubin is elevated, then further breakdown into percentage of direct (conjugated) and indirect (unconjugated) provides additional information regarding the cause. In general, if the major elevation is indirect bilirubin, then the problem is usually caused by some type of hepatocellular dysfunction; however, if direct bilirubin is the fraction that is grossly elevated, then an extrahepatic obstruction is generally the problem.

Alcoholic cirrhosis often has normal laboratory values at first; however, as the disease progresses, there are moderate elevations of the AST and ALP. This is followed by a gradual elevation of the bilirubin as the disease progresses. It is rare for a patient to be jaundiced when the total bilirubin is less than 3.

E. Fasting plasma glucose (FPG)   ESSENTIAL

An FPG is indicated in Mr. Pence because he is experiencing symptoms consistent with type 2 diabetes mellitus (e.g., gradual weight loss and fatigue). Additionally, his diagnosis is found more often in individuals with diabetes mellitus. Chronic pancreatitis, which can result from alcohol abuse, is also frequently associated with diabetes mellitus.

4. Diagnosis

A. Dupuytren contracture of right fourth finger with alcoholic liver disease   CORRECT

A Dupuytren contracture is a chronic flexion deformity of the fourth and/or fifth digits(s) resulting from the thickening and shortness of the fascial bands on the palmar surface of the hand. It is associated with alcoholic liver disease, type 2 diabetes mellitus, thyroiditis, and coronary artery disease. The diagnosis of Dupuytren contracture is generally made clinically.

Alcoholic liver disease, presumably steatosis, is characterized by a nontender, smooth-bordered hepatomegaly without jaundice in conjunction with an AST elevated by a factor of more than 2 compared to an ALT elevation, a normal bilirubin, and an ALP that is elevated less than three times the upper limit of normal. Thus, this is Mr. Pence's most likely diagnosis.

B. Systemic fibrosing syndrome   INCORRECT

Systemic fibrosing syndrome can be ruled out as Mr. Pence's most likely diagnosis because he has no evidence of an additional fibrosing disease (e.g., Riedel struma, Peyronie disease, retroperitoneal fibrosis, and/or mediastinal fibrosis).

C. Trigger finger and alcoholic cirrhosis   INCORRECT

A trigger finger, or stenosing tenosynovitis, involves inflammation of the fibrous sheath at the metacarpophalangeal joint resulting in a nodular constriction of the flexor tendon. It generally involves the second (index) digit, not the fourth digit. It is frequently found in individuals who frequently play tennis, golf, baseball, or racquetball.

Alcoholic cirrhosis must be considered a potential diagnosis because of Mr. Pence's history of alcohol consumption, hepatomegaly, and elevated liver function tests and the overlap between alcoholic liver disease, alcoholic hepatitis, and alcoholic cirrhosis. However, in its pure form as a single diagnosis, alcoholic cirrhosis is much less likely to be the cause of his hepatic abnormalities than alcoholic liver disease because he does not have abdominal pain, ascites, jaundice, tender hepatomegaly, a nodular texture to his palpable liver border, splenomegaly, nausea, and/or vomiting. Although it is possible for a patient to be completely asymptomatic or to have normal liver function testing early in the course of compensated alcoholic cirrhosis, the majority of patients present with findings similar to nonalcoholic cirrhosis. A liver biopsy could provide a definitive diagnosis; however, it is frequently deferred for a minimum of 6 months of abstinence in patients who are currently drinking alcohol because of the possibility of associated bleeding that is frequently unresponsive to vitamin K as well as concerns regarding proper care of the biopsy site following the procedure. Regardless of which alcohol-related hepatic condition Mr. Pence has, this is still not his most likely diagnosis because he does not have a trigger finger.

D. De Quervain tenosynovitis and alcoholic hepatitis INCORRECT

De Quervain tenosynovitis is an inflammation of the abductor pollicis longus and/or the extensor pollicis brevis tendons where they go through a fibrous sheath at the level of the styloid process of the radius. It is generally caused by an overuse syndrome involving repetitive wrist twisting. It is characterized on physical examination by tenderness to palpate the tendon(s) at the styloid process of the radius and a positive Finkelstein sign (the patient's pain is reproducible by moving the wrist laterally with the patient's hand forming a fist with the thumb in the center).

As previously stated, there is an overlay in the signs, symptoms, and diagnostic test results between the hepatic condition of steatosis, hepatitis, and cirrhosis caused by alcoholic liver disease. Hepatic injury caused by ethanol begins as alcoholic fatty liver disease (steatosis), which is present in over 90% of all chronic and binge (defined as more than five alcoholic beverages per setting for men and more than four for women) drinkers. A small percentage of these individuals go on to develop alcoholic hepatitis, which is considered to be a precursor to alcoholic cirrhosis. Therefore, it could be expected that the symptoms experienced by the patient with alcoholic hepatitis would fall somewhere in between these two conditions. However, that is not always the case. The symptoms of alcoholic hepatitis can range from asymptomatic to those seen in severe hepatic failure (e.g., jaundice, ascites, tender hepatomegaly, and the presence of portal hypertension). A liver biopsy is generally required to make an absolute distinction between these conditions. Still, regardless of exactly which alcoholic liver disease Mr. Pence has, this still cannot be his most likely diagnosis because he does not have de Quervain tendosynovitis.

E. Complex regional pain syndrome INCORRECT

Complex regional pain syndrome (formerly known as reflex sympathetic dystrophy) is a painful condition of the affected extremity that is associated with autonomic and vasomotor instability generally following minor trauma. Because of Mr. Pence's palmar erythema, it would be essential to include this in his differential diagnosis because it can cause alterations in the color of the skin in the affected extremity. However, this can be eliminated as his most likely diagnosis because he is not experiencing pain with his chief complaint.

Other characteristic features include edema, temperature changes, and (over time) some degree of dystrophic alterations of the skin and nails of the affected extremity only.

5. Treatment Plan

A. Refer to an orthopedic hand surgeon for surgical intervention on right hand INCORRECT

Referral to an orthopedic hand surgeon for surgical intervention is not an appropriate choice at this time. Surgery is only indicated if the degree of flexure contracture at the MPC is greater than or equal to 30° and/or the PIP is greater than or equal to 10 to 15°. The only indication for surgery when the deformity is less than these values is if it is functionally or cosmetically bothersome for the patient.

B. Complete blood count with differential, prothrombin time, and liver ultrasound CORRECT

These tests are indicated to assess the degree of Mr. Pence's hepatic dysfunction. Anemia, thrombocytopenia, and an elevated PT are associated with a more severe hepatic dysfunction and a poorer outcome. The ultrasound will provide a baseline measurement of his liver's size, texture, and uniformity as well as evaluate for masses and intra-abdominal effusion.

C. Refer for liver biopsy INCORRECT

A liver biopsy is not indicated for Mr. Pence at this time. However, if at follow-up his liver functions fail to improve after ceasing alcohol consumption or continue to worsen (regardless of abstinence status), a liver biopsy will be indicated at that time provided his PT is normal. An abnormal PT significantly increases the risk of hemorrhage from the procedure.

D. Provide Mr. Pence with patient education on his condition, advise to cease all alcohol intake, and offer referral to a substance abuse counselor or treatment center CORRECT

Patient education regarding his liver function tests and their significance, the importance of alcohol cessation, the potential consequences if he continues to drink alcohol, and the importance of proper nutrition are important components of his treatment plan. Direct advice to stop all beer and alcohol consumption is essential because a significant motivator is being advised to cease by a HCP. Furthermore, this prevents any misunderstanding of what action is required on the part of the patient. Finally, a referral to an in- or out-patient treatment facility for substance abuse and proper nutrition are essential components of a treatment plan for Mr. Pence.

E. Commit to psychiatric hospital for detoxification and rehabilitation INCORRECT

Involuntary commitment to a psychiatric hospital is a complex legal process that varies from state to state. Generally, the HCP has to make a case to the local mental hygiene commissioner (or other individual with commitment authority) that the individual is a danger to himself or others. If the mental hygiene commissioner agrees, then the patient can be placed in the facility for an observation period (typically 48 to 72 hours). At the end of the observational period, the facility then makes the determination as to whether the patient is a danger to himself or others. If he is found to be a danger to himself or others, then he can be forced to remain hospitalized for another observational period. If he is found not to be a danger to himself and others, then he is free to leave or has the choice of a voluntary hospitalization. Many facilities do not continue involuntary commitment on individuals with substance abuse problems unless they are extremely severe (or associated with a significant psychological illness) because it is nearly impossible to help individuals with a substance abuse problem until they are willing to admit the problem exists and possess a desire to obtain help in addressing it. Because of the mildness of Mr. Pence's symptoms at this time, it is unlikely that a commitment hearing will result in an involuntary commitment; thus, this action at this time is only going to serve to damage the patient–provider relationship.

F. If patient desires, refer to hand specialist for collagenase *Clostridium histolyticum* injection to his palmar connective tissue excess   CORRECT

Collagenase *Clostridium histolyticum* was approved by the FDA in February 2010 for injection into the palmar connective tissue excess associated with a Dupuytren contracture. It is classified as a biologic agent because it contains a living organism's protein product. It must be injected by an HCP who has the necessary expertise to perform hand injection because of the risk of tendon rupture. Additionally, a small study accompanying the FDA news release only showed a 44% success rate (compared to 5% for placebo). Therefore, it is important to advise patients of this potential for treatment failure when counseling them on their treatment options.

Epidemiologic and Other Data

The exact incidence of Dupuytren contracture/disease is not known; however, it is a commonly encountered disorder. It is most commonly seen in white males older than the age of 50 years. Risk factors include male gender, age older than 50 years, white race, history of alcoholism or alcohol abuse, history of diabetes mellitus, or presence of any chronic systemic medical condition.

CASE 8-5
Paul Quinn
1. History

A. What type of home improvement project is he performing? NONESSENTIAL

The time, date, type, and mechanism of injury have already been determined. Exactly what he was "improving" would add little pertinent information to assist in determining his diagnosis and treatment plan. However, if time permits, such questions are important in establishing good patient–provider rapport and alleviating patient anxiety.

B. What is his sexual history?   ESSENTIAL

Because of the high incidence of morbidity and mortality from septic arthritis (especially when treatment is delayed), all hot, erythematous, edematous painful joints must be considered infectious in nature until proven otherwise. Overall, the most common organism for septic (infectious) arthritis is *Staphylococcus aureus*. However, in healthy, sexually active young adults, *Neisseria gonorrhoeae* is more common. Therefore, it is important to know Mr. Quinn's sexual history to evaluate his risk potential for a sexually transmitted infection (STI) being responsible for his monoarticular arthritis.

Staphylococcus epidermis is also frequently encountered in septic arthritis; however, it is more common in patients with prosthetic joints. In children younger than the age of 5 years, *Haemophilus influenzae* and gram-negative bacillus are the most common pathogens.

C. Has he been ill or experienced a previous knee injury within the past month?   ESSENTIAL

Septic arthritis can result directly from a puncture wound, foreign body, or other joint trauma. However, it can also result indirectly via disseminated hematologic or lymphatic spread from an infection located elsewhere in the body, directly from infected adjacent structures, or nosocomially (e.g., during or immediately following surgery). Even though Mr. Quinn provides a history of trauma, it is unlikely that trauma yesterday could result in a septic joint by today. Therefore, it is essential to determine the existence of any previous, recent injury to his knee or any recent (or current) infection.

D. Does he have a fever, fatigue, malaise, or a rash? ESSENTIAL

Infectious and inflammatory processes can account for all of these symptoms. The location, characteristics, duration, and symptom pattern associated with a rash can not only assist in distinguishing infectious from inflammatory causes but also provide clues to the most likely diagnosis. For example, jaundice would most likely be associated with an acute hepatitis B infection; erythema chronicum migrans is seen with Lyme disease; a maculopapular rash that begins on the face and descends centripetally is fairly characteristic of rubella; and papules, vesicopustules, and petechial lesions, especially with central eschar or necrosis and especially on the distal extremities, are found in disseminated gonococcal infection (DGI). Inflammatory conditions such as SLE are associated with a malar erythema that is frequently sudden in onset and associated with edema, and rheumatoid nodules and vasculitis are found in RA.

E. Are any other joints involved?   ESSENTIAL

Monoarticular arthritis is most frequently caused by trauma, infection, crystal-induced arthropathies, and osteoarthritis (although it is not uncommon for osteoarthritis to be present in other joints and for crystal-induced arthropathies to occasionally be oligoarticular). Therefore, it is important to determine whether this is a true monoarticular arthritis or part of an oligoarticular or polyarticular process in which this one joint is significantly more symptomatic.

2. Physical Examination

A. Bilateral eye examination   NONESSENTIAL

Because of the rarity of conditions presenting with a monoarticular arthropathy and abnormal ocular findings and Mr. Quinn's lack of eye or visual symptoms, an eye examination is not indicated.

B. Bilateral knee examination   ESSENTIAL

Because Mr. Quinn's chief complaint is knee pain, a bilateral knee examination is indicated.

C. Bilateral hip and ankle examination   ESSENTIAL

As stated previously, a properly conducted orthopedic examination of a painful joint always includes the evaluation of the next most proximal and distal joints.

D. Lower extremity pulse and vascular examination ESSENTIAL

As stated previously, a properly conducted orthopedic examination also involves determining the vascular status of the affected area and ensuring that the pain is truly musculoskeletal in nature and not secondary to a vascular phenomenon.

E. Lower extremity reflex and sensation testing ESSENTIAL

Likewise, as previously stated, a properly conducted orthopedic examination involves ensuring that the affected area is neurologically intact and a neurologic or neuromuscular process is not responsible for the patient's pain.

3. Diagnostic Studies

A. Arthrocentesis of right knee with synovial fluid analysis including appearance, viscosity, white blood cell count with differential, Gram stain, and polarized light examination for crystals ESSENTIAL

An erythematous, hot, swollen joint is virtually impossible to diagnose without the benefit of a synovial fluid analysis. Therefore, an arthrocentesis should be performed to obtain synovial fluid to analyze for gross color, clarity, and viscosity; white blood cell (WBC) count with differential; red blood cell (RBC) count; Gram stain; and crystals (via polarized light examination). Normal synovial fluid is straw colored, clear, and of high viscosity with a WBC count of less than $200/mm^3$, an RBC count of less than 2000 μU, a negative Gram stain, and no crystals.

An abnormality in these findings can suggest potential causes for the joint pain. For example, if the synovial fluid is grossly bloody appearing, it is most likely caused by a traumatic process, including a traumatic tap. An RBC count greater than 2000 μU provides confirmation.

If the synovial fluid is yellow and turbid appearing, the pathology could be an infection, inflammation, or crystal-induced process. Likewise, these same three conditions can cause an elevated WBC count in the synovial fluid. However, the degree of WBC elevation and its differential provide clues regarding the most likely source. Infectious causes are generally associated with the greatest levels of leukocytosis ($> 2000/mm^3$); nevertheless, it is possible for inflammatory and crystal-inducing processes to have this significant WBC elevation (although they tend to be in the range of 200 to $2000/mm^3$). However, if the elevated WBC count is predominately neutrophils (especially $> 75\%$), there is an extremely high potential for the cause to be an infectious process. A preponderance of either lymphocytes or monocytes is generally associated with an inflammatory or crystal-inducing process. Furthermore, viscosity is decreased in an inflammatory process. In severe cases, it can be so thin it drips.

The identification of crystal during the polarized light examination is associated with crystal-induced arthropathies. They can be further distinguished by the type of crystal identified (e.g., MSU crystals that are somewhat long, narrow, rod-shaped [also called "needle-shaped"] and negatively birefringent are generally found in gouty arthritis; and CPPD crystals are weakly positively birefringent, rod shaped, but are more rectangular or rhomboid in shape than needle-shaped crystals, and are generally identified in pseudogout). Although cholesterol crystals are sometimes identified, they do not represent a true crystal-induced arthropathy; they are most frequently associated with rheumatoid arthritis.

A positive Gram stain generally provides confirmation of an infectious process; however, it can result from contamination of skin flora during the arthrocentesis. Therefore, it is essential that any positive Gram stain be followed up with appropriate bacterial cultures (including sensitivities). Once the organism is isolated, the patient's symptoms and response to therapy assist in determining whether the culture results represent an actual joint infection or a containment.

B. Acid-fast stain, Thayer-Martin culture, and fungal cultures of the aspirated fluid   NONESSENTIAL

These tests are only indicated if there is a suspicion based on the patient's history, physical examination findings, and initial synovial fluid analysis of a condition that could be identified through one of these methods. Additionally, they are sometimes employed when the initial evaluation failed to identify the cause of the problem or if the patient did not respond to therapy as anticipated. The acid-fast stain is required when there is a concern that a joint infection could be caused by *Mycobacterium tuberculosis*, which accounts for virtually all the human cases of tuberculosis (TB) in the United States. Because musculoskeletal involvement is caused by hematogenous spread from primary pulmonary tuberculosis, the patient generally has a history of current or previous TB or a cough and constitutional symptoms caused by an undiagnosed case.

Thayer-Martin media is utilized almost exclusively to grow the *Neisseriae gonorrhoeae* and *Neisseriae meningitidis* bacteria. Septic arthritis caused by either of these organisms is hematologically spread. Thus, if septic arthritis results from *Neisseriae meningitidis*, the patient should possess a history of a recent infection caused by this organism (i.e., meningococcal meningitis). However, if the joint infection is caused by *Neisseriae gonorrhoeae*, the patient may or may not have a history of a genitourinary or reproductive tract infection, proctitis, and pharyngitis. In fact, the more likely presentation is a history of a recent episode, or current symptoms, of a DGI because gonococcal arthritis occurs more frequently as a complication of this disease. Nevertheless, these organisms should be suspected in young adults who are considered high risk for the acquisition of a sexually transmitted infection and by the presence of gram-negative cocci on the Gram stain. *Neisseriae gonorrhoeae* are intracellular diplococci, whereas *Neisseriae meningitidis* can occur either singly or in pairs; as diplococci they are elongated and paired along their long axis with their adjacent sides kidney shaped.

C. Serum and synovial fluid for glucose, uric acid, protein, and lactate levels   ESSENTIAL

The chemistry analysis of synovial fluid can provide additional clues to the cause of the arthropathy. However, they are most useful when timed matched serum samples are also obtained because the level in the synovial fluid should be essentially equivalent with those in the serum. For example, if the glucose is significantly lower in the synovial fluid than it is in the blood (especially if it is approaching the 50% mark), the most likely cause is a bacterial process. However, this is not an absolute.

The uric acid is generally only elevated in both the synovial fluid and the serum when dealing with gouty arthritis.

However, gouty arthritis can occur with a normal serum uric acid level, especially in the early stages of an acute attack. A synovial fluid uric acid level is unnecessary if the defining crystals are present. Bacterial infections tend to have elevated protein and lactate levels in the synovial fluid, whereas crystal-induced arthritis has normal protein and lactate levels.

Complement levels can also be performed on the aspirated synovial fluid if there is a strong suspicion for the presence of a systemic inflammatory process affecting the joints. The complement is decreased in the synovial fluid of most of the connective tissue diseases (e.g., RA and SLE), but also with immunologic processes (e.g., prosthetic joint rejection). However, the absence of this finding does not rule out any of these conditions.

D. Thayer-Martin blood culture   NONESSENTIAL

If a true septic monoarticular arthropathy is caused by gonorrhea, the likelihood of growing the organism, even on Thayer-Martin culture media, is less than 40% from synovial fluid and virtually nonexistent (0%) from a blood culture. However, if the patient appears ill, has a history of migrating polyarthralgia, or has lesions consistent with DGI (as described earlier), blood cultures on Thayer-Martin media should be considered in an attempt to diagnose DGI, especially if the patient's sexual history places him in an "at-risk" category. Even with DGI, the yield rate for a positive culture, even on Thayer-Martin media, is less than 45% for blood and synovial fluid cultures.

E. Radiograph of left knee   NONESSENTIAL

A radiograph of his left knee is unlikely to provide any useful information because it is his right knee that is affected. However, given his history of trauma and marked physical findings, a right knee radiograph would probably not be considered incorrect for Mr. Quinn.

It is very important to ensure that the correct anatomic site and special views (if indicated, e.g., "sunset" view of Mr. Quinn's patella for easier identification of a patellar fracture) are listed on the diagnostic request slip AND the correct test was performed. Otherwise, this could lead to a misdiagnosis that could result in extensive morbidity and even mortality for the patient.

4. Diagnosis

A. Acute bacterial arthritis   INCORRECT

Despite his elevated temperature and single hot, red, swollen joint, an acute bacterial (septic) arthritis can essentially be eliminated as Mr. Quinn's most likely diagnosis because his synovial fluid analysis revealed a moderate leukocytosis of predominately lymphocytes and a Gram stain without significant bacteria. Furthermore, "needle-shaped" crystals were present. It is important to remember that in addition to infection, significant inflammation can produce fever.

B. Acute gouty arthritis   CORRECT

Acute gouty arthritis is an inflammatory monoarticular arthritis (although rarely it can be oligoarticular) caused by a metabolic defect that results in either the overproduction or undersecretion of uric acid leading to the deposition of monosodium urate crystals in the synovium of the joint. The most commonly affected joints (in order of descending involvement) are the metatarsophalangeal joints of the great toe, the knees, the ankles, and the tarsal joints.

Although only 10% of gouty arthritis occurs in men younger than the age of 30 years, this is Mr. Quinn's most likely diagnosis. This diagnosis is based on his history (e.g., increased alcohol intake, pain awakening him at night, joint intolerant of light touch, acute onset of symptoms, and monoarticular involvement) and physical examination (e.g., a single significantly inflamed joint and fever) findings in conjunction with his synovial fluid analysis (presence of the needle-shaped nonbirefringent crystals and moderate leukocytosis with predominately lymphocytosis).

C. Pseudogout   INCORRECT

Pseudogout is another crystal-induced arthropathy with symptoms very similar to gout. However, on synovial fluid analysis the typical crystals identified are CPPD crystals, which are positively birefringent ones with a more rectangular and rhomboidal shape than the needle-shaped negatively birefringent ones seen in "true" gouty arthritis. Because Mr. Quinn had crystals consistent with MSU, this is not his most likely diagnosis.

D. Rheumatoid arthritis   INCORRECT

RA is a systemic, inflammatory connective tissue disease that is generally characterized by polyarticular arthritis. Although the synovial fluid analysis is consistent with inflammation, the synovial fluid analysis in patients with RA does not reveal MSU crystals; however, cholesterol crystals may be present. Thus, RA is not Mr. Quinn's most likely diagnosis.

E. Effusion secondary to trauma   INCORRECT

An effusion secondary to trauma needs to be considered as a potential diagnosis for Mr. Quinn given his history; however, his physical examination findings (e.g., fever and a severely inflamed joint) are inconsistent with this diagnosis. Furthermore, unless a coexisting disease was present, the synovial fluid should not reveal MSU crystals and a leukocytosis with a predominance of lymphocytosis but, instead, an erythrocytosis. Thus, this is not Mr. Quinn's most likely diagnosis.

5. Treatment Plan

A. Indomethacin 150 mg twice a day for 3 days with food   CORRECT

Indomethacin, or similar NSAIDs, is indicated for the initial treatment of acute gouty arthritis. However, with this medication it is essential to take the extra time to explain possible adverse events and what to do if they occur. Furthermore, in individuals who are at risk of a gastrointestinal bleed or are going be on the medication for more than 1 week, a PPI should be considered along with the drug for gastrointestinal bleeding protection.

B. IV colchicine   INCORRECT

IV colchicine is not a potential treatment for acute gouty arthritis because of the significant incidence of myelosuppression associated with the administration of this drug via this route.

Even oral colchicine is no longer considered to be an acceptable first-line agent for acute gouty arthritis. It should only be utilized in this manner after careful consideration of all other available options, with significant caution, and only if the patient is intolerant of all the recommended treatment options as outlined by the task force report by the Standing Committee for International Clinical Studies Including Therapeutics (ESCISIT). Additionally, it is no longer acceptable medical practice to determine the drug's dosage by continued administration until the patient becomes asymptomatic or develops GI toxicity.

Essentially, oral colchicine is limited in current practice to two main uses. First, it can be used as a once- or twice-daily, long-term treatment option for patients who experience infrequent episodes of acute gouty arthritis and continue to have a slight elevation of their serum uric acid levels despite lifestyle modifications (e.g., weight reduction, avoiding foods with high purine, avoiding alcohol, and changing medicines that could increase the serum uric acid level [such as diuretics and niacin]), after the patient and provider have discussed all the potential treatment options and determined that the patient's hyperuricemia requires treatment and this is the best individual agent for the patient in terms of risks versus benefits. If therapy is undertaken to treat hyperuricemia, then the goal of treatment is to maintain the serum uric acid level at less than 5 mg/dl.

The second recommendation is utilizing colchicine in conjunction with the initiation of a uricosuric agent or a xanthine oxidase inhibitor for the treatment of chronic hyperuricemia to prevent an exacerbation of gouty arthritis caused by the rapid reduction in the uric acid level.

C. IV antibiotics   INCORRECT

IV antibiotics have no role in the treatment of acute gouty arthritis.

D. Tapering dose of methylprednisolone over 1 week CORRECT

Tapering the dose of methylprednisolone over 1 week is one of the ESCISIT task force's recommendations for the treatment of acute gouty arthritis. It has essentially replaced the usage of colchicine in acute gouty arthritis.

E. Allopurinol 100 mg twice a day; increase by 100 mg a week until desired result is achieved   INCORRECT

Using a xanthine oxidase inhibitor while the patient is having an acute episode of gouty arthritis is contraindicated. If it results in a rapid reduction in the serum uric acid levels, there is the potential for it to worsen the patient's pain.

Furthermore, it has yet to be determined if his problem is from excess production of uric acid or decreased secretion. Xanthine oxidase inhibitors will only be effective if Mr. Quinn's problem is caused by an overproduction of uric acid. That information will need to be determined after the acute episode is resolved by performing a 24-hour urine collection for uric acid. If the result is greater than 800 mg/day, then the patient is an overproducer of uric acid and allopurinol would be an acceptable treatment option. However, if the result is less than 800 mg/day, then the patient is an undersecretor of uric acid and would require a uricosuric agent.

However, there exists a minority of patients that never have more than one acute attack or have very infrequent attacks. For these individuals, the risks of using a xanthine oxidase inhibitor (or a uricosuric agent or colchicine, for that matter) probably outweigh the benefits. In general, the risk of

experiencing future episodes of acute gouty arthritis is directly correlated with the patient's serum uric acid level when he is asymptomatic. Thus, he will also require this measurement after his acute episode resolves.

However, if Mr. Quinn begins to experience frequent attacks, forms tophaceous deposits, or develops renal insufficiency because of the gout, then, he will require either a uricosuric drug to block tubular reabsorption or a xanthine oxidase inhibitor to prevent the overproduction of uric acid, depending on the cause of his uric acid elevation.

The other currently available xanthine oxidase inhibitor that is available in the United States for the chronic treatment of hyperuricemia associated with gouty arthritis is febuxostat. Despite being found to be superior to allopurinol in terms of the overall number of individuals able to reach target uric acid levels in some clinical trials, it is generally reserved for use as a second-line agent because it was associated with a high rate of liver function abnormalities. Furthermore, in the aforementioned clinical trials, there was a higher rate of cardiovascular deaths, nonfatal myocardial infarctions (MIs), and nonfatal cerebral vascular accidents (CVAs) in the treatment group receiving the febuxostat compared to the allopurinol group. Although a causal relationship could not be established, the FDA required the drug manufacturer to conduct on-going clinical trials regarding its cardiovascular safety when it was approved in February 2009 and recommends all patients on this agent be monitored for signs and symptoms of angina, TIAs, MIs, and CVAs. Since its approval, there has also been a high incidence of hypersensitivity reactions reported with its usage.

F. IV Pegloticase and repeat every 2 weeks (after pretreatment prophylaxis with oral prednisone and diphenhydramine)   INCORRECT

Pegloticase is a pegylated uricase that was approved by the FDA in September 2010 for the treatment of gouty arthritis in patients who are nonresponders or intolerant of conventional therapy. Therefore, it is not an appropriate initial treatment for Mr. Quinn. However, pre-treatment with a corticosteroid and an antihistamine is recommended because approximately 25% of all the patients in the clinical trials for this medication experienced a hypersensitivity reaction.

Epidemiologic and Other Data

Eighty to 95% of all cases of acute gouty arthritis affect middle-aged and elderly men. The majority of the remaining cases are composed of postmenopausal women who often have hypertension and mild renal insufficiency and are on diuretic therapy. Rarely is gout seen in a premenopausal female. There appears to be a familial association with the condition. Individuals who are native or descendants of the Pacific Islands appear to be at an increased risk.

Foods that are high in purine have been suggested to cause/exacerbate gouty arthritis. These foods include all meats, meat extracts, and gravies; seafood; alcoholic beverages, especially beer; oatmeal; beans and lentils; and a few vegetables (e.g., asparagus, cauliflower, mushrooms, peas, and spinach). Alcohol intake also appears to be a risk factor for the development of the condition.

CASE 8-6
Queenie Rodriquez
1. History

A. Is she experiencing any myalgias or muscle weakness? ESSENTIAL

The presence of myalgias or muscle weakness expands the list of differential diagnoses to not only include intra-articular diseases but also conditions that affect the muscles and other extra-articular structures that can cause perceived joint pain (e.g., tendonitis, bursitis, polymyalgia rheumatica, fibromyalgia, complex regional pain syndrome, and somatization disorders).

B. When did the numbness begin? ESSENTIAL

This question is important because it attempts to determine whether her numbness is part of the same condition, an unrelated problem, or a disorder caused by her initial condition. In general, if all the symptoms began simultaneously, there is a greater probability that they are related. However, if the onset is earlier or later, it is more likely to represent an unrelated ailment. Later could also represent a complication.

C. What does she mean by the term "numbness"? ESSENTIAL

Numbness is a vague term used to describe several sensations (e.g., entire lack of sensation, reduced sensation, paresthesias, and dysesthesias). Additionally, some patients will utilize this term to mean that they are having difficulty using the affected part. Thus, it is essential to understand exactly what Ms. Rodriquez is experiencing in order to establish her most likely diagnosis.

D. Which joints are affected? ESSENTIAL

When evaluating a patient with a complaint of joint pain, it is essential to discern the number of joints affected, which joints are involved, whether inflammation is present, and whether extra-articular manifestations exist. While one entity alone will not provide much assistance in determining the cause of the patient's problem, the combination will assist in narrowing the differential diagnoses significantly. For example, polyarticular arthritis, which Ms. Rodriquez is complaining, is generally caused by a systemic process (e.g., rheumatoid arthritis, SLE, or psoriatic arthritis); rarely do these present as monoarticular arthritis. Conversely, as previously stated, monoarticular arthritis is most frequently caused by trauma, infection, crystal-induced arthropathies, and osteoarthritis; however, these can present with more than one joint involved, especially osteoarthritis. Oligoarticular involvement is more common in reactive arthritis, Reiter disease, and psoriatic arthritis.

Regarding which joints are involved, there are only two conditions that frequently affect the DIP joints: osteoarthritis and psoriatic arthritis. As previously stated, rheumatoid arthritis has a predilection for diarthrodial joints; the main ones that are affected are the PIP joints and MCP joints of the hands, wrists, and knees. Osteoarthritis prefers the knees, hips, lumbar spine, cervical spine, metatarsophalangeal (MTP) joint of the great toes, and DIP and PIP joints of the hands.

Inflammation is more common with connective tissue/autoimmune diseases that produce arthritis (e.g., RA, SLE, and polyarteritis nodosa), crystal-induced arthropathies (gouty arthritis and pseudogout), and septic arthritis.

Extra-articular manifestations tend to occur much more frequently in systemic disease processes (e.g., RA and SLE) as opposed to localized disease processes (e.g., fracture or osteoarthritis). However, extra-articular manifestations can also indicate a disease process that arises outside of the articular structure, as previously discussed.

E. Has she had fever, night sweats, weight loss, or nocturnal symptoms? ESSENTIAL

As previously stated, the presence of a fever is generally seen in an infectious or inflammatory process. However, if Ms. Rodriquez has been febrile for the entire 6-month duration of her illness, it is highly unlikely that an infection is responsible. Although an inflammatory process is most likely, other conditions must be considered. For example, if it is also associated with night sweats, it could indicate that a primary or secondary bone cancer, a *Mycobacterium* infection, or a metabolic condition such as hyperthyroidism is producing her symptoms.

Unintentional weight loss, especially in conjunction with night sweats and/or fever, is highly suspicious for a primary bone cancer or metastasis to the bone from a yet-to-be-identified primary carcinoma. Nocturnal symptoms are also suspicious for a bony malignancy; however, they can occur in other conditions as well (e.g., severe osteoarthritis). Also, the initial painful episode of gouty arthritis tends to occur in the middle of the night.

2. Physical Examination

A. Ear, nose, and throat (ENT) examination NONESSENTIAL

Because Ms. Rodriquez has not experienced an illness involving her upper respiratory tract either before or since the onset of her symptoms, an ENT examination is not necessary.

B. Bilateral hand examination ESSENTIAL

Because she is complaining of hand pain, swelling, and numbness, a hand examination is indicated. However, the benefit of a "normal" comparison is not going to be available because she is complaining of bilateral symptoms. Nevertheless, both hands need to be evaluated carefully to identify any abnormalities and ensure that the changes are symmetric.

C. Bilateral wrist examination ESSENTIAL

Because a properly conducted orthopedic examination includes the next joint distally and proximally, a wrist examination is indicated. Furthermore, because Ms. Rodriquez is experiencing finger paresthesias, it is necessary to evaluate for evidence of a possible nerve entrapment.

D. Bilateral shoulder and elbow examination ESSENTIAL

This examination is indicated to attempt to identify any pathology that could be causing compression or entrapment of a nerve capable of producing her hand paresthesias (e.g., thoracic outlet syndrome, osteoarthritis of either the shoulder or the elbow, or poorly healed fractures at either site). The elbow also needs examined as her next most proximal joint.

E. Vascular and neurologic examination of her upper extremities ESSENTIAL

As previously stated, a vascular and neurologic examination of the affected areas is essential to prevent overlooking

323

an alternative or additional diagnosis besides an intra-articular problem. This is essential in Ms. Rodriquez's case because she is experiencing finger paresthesias, which could be caused by compression/entrapment of a nerve or vascular structure anywhere from the neck to the wrist.

3. Diagnostic Studies

A. Erythrocyte sedimentation rate (ESR) and C-reactive protein (CRP)   ESSENTIAL

The ESR and CRP are both measurements of nonspecific inflammation and are indicated for Ms. Rodriquez. Elevations are not specific for a particular disease entity; however, they can provide additional support toward certain conditions contained in her differential diagnosis list.

Additionally, these tests are utilized to monitor progress during medical therapy and to assist in determining if medication dosage adjustments, combination therapy, or substitution of the drug is required. Therefore, it is important to have a baseline measurement for comparison of response (or lack of response) to the specific treatment(s) instituted.

The ESR is determined by the rate of fall of RBCs in either plasma or saline over a period of 1 hour. The agglutination of red blood cells causes them to be heavier and therefore fall faster, thus causing the ESR to be elevated. Conditions capable of this include infections (both acute and chronic), connective tissue (collagen vascular or autoimmune) diseases, malignancies, tissue infarction, and tissue necrosis.

The CRP is a hepatic protein produced in response to an acute inflammatory process. It is elevated in collagen vascular diseases, bacterial (but not necessarily viral) infections, tissue infarction, and tissue necrosis. It can also be utilized postoperatively to monitor for wound infections and as a predictor of cardiovascular events when utilizing the high-sensitivity assay. The CRP tends to respond faster than the ESR and is also considered to be more sensitive.

B. Complete blood count with differential (CBC w/diff)   ESSENTIAL

A CBC w/diff is indicated to rule out the rare possibility that Ms. Rodriquez's polyarticular arthritis is caused by an infectious process. It is also useful to evaluate for anemia, thrombocytosis, and thrombocytopenia, which can accompany an inflammatory, malignant, or metastatic process.

C. Serum uric acid level   NONESSENTIAL

Elevated serum uric acid levels are often associated with, but are not pathognomonic for, gouty arthritis. Therefore, a serum uric acid level is not indicated for Ms. Rodriquez because it is highly unlikely that she has gouty arthritis because of the number of joints affected, the location of joints involved, and the lack of a significant effusion, erythema, edema, and temperature change of the involved joints. (For more information on gouty arthritis, please see Case 8-5.) Furthermore, if gouty arthritis was strongly suspected to be her most likely diagnosis, then a synovial fluid specimen should be obtained for analysis.

D. Rheumatoid factor (RF), anticyclic citrullinated peptide antibody (anti-CCP), and antinuclear antibody (ANA)   ESSENTIAL

An RF is indicated because one of the primary causes of an inflammatory polyarthritis is RA. A positive RF (defined as 1:80 or greater) and the appropriate arthritis symptoms (such as

those Ms. Rodriquez has) are highly specific, but not absolute for the diagnosis of rheumatoid arthritis. False-positive RFs can occur as a result of other connective tissue diseases, other autoimmune conditions, other inflammatory arthropathies, sarcoidosis, syphilis, positive family history of RA, and even elderly age. Likewise, only 75 to 80% of all patients with RA have a positive RF. Thus, this is just one of the seven factors that the ACR utilizes to establish the diagnosis of RA in a patient.

The CCP antibody results from the conversion of ornithine to arginine. Because this amino acid process can occur early in the disease course of RA (often before the RF is elevated), a positive anti-CCP can lend significant support to a diagnosis of RA. Some experts feel it can replace the ACR's criteria of a positive RF because it actually has greater sensitivity and specificity in diagnosing early RA when compared to the RF.

An ANA is indicated to determine whether SLE is the cause of Ms. Rodriquez's symptoms because many of the inflammatory arthropathies have very similar symptoms. A positive ANA is estimated to be found in over 95% of all patients with SLE. However, depending on the pattern of ANA that is responsible for the test being positive, other autoimmune conditions can be responsible for the elevation.

The four primary patterns and their most commonly associated conditions are (1) outline pattern (or peripheral pattern), which is almost exclusively identified in SLE; (2) homogeneous pattern (or diffuse pattern), which can be associated with not only SLE but also any mixed connective tissue disease; (3) speckled pattern, which can be associated with not only SLE but also RA, mixed connective tissue disease, scleroderma, Sjögren syndrome, and polymyositis; and (4) nuclear pattern, which is typically not seen with SLE but with scleroderma or polymyositis.

ANA tests also have false-negative and false-positive results. Medications are the most commonly interfering factor, with the most significant being corticosteroids associated with false-negatives and aminosalicylic acid with false-positives. Interestingly, both agents are commonly utilized to treat many of these autoimmune inflammatory diseases that the ANA helps to diagnose.

E. Nerve conduction study (NCS) of her right upper extremity   ESSENTIAL

Nerve conduction studies, or electromyography, can detect subtle defects of the motor and sensory portions of the nerves of the arm from their origins. As stated previously, hand paresthesias following the distribution of the median nerve (seen in Ms. Rodriquez's case) can result from nerve compression or entrapment at the wrist, elbow, or shoulder.

Although this compression or entrapment is generally caused by a musculoskeletal abnormality, it can also be seen as a feature of systemic conditions (e.g., rheumatoid arthritis, inflammatory tenosynovitis, and other connective tissue disease; myxedema; hyperparathyroidism; sarcoidosis; leukemia; and pregnancy).

4. Diagnosis

A. Rheumatoid arthritis (RA) with right carpal tunnel syndrome (CTS)   CORRECT

The ACR has established diagnostic criteria for RA consisting of the presence of a minimum of four of the following seven symptoms: (1) morning stiffness of a minimum of 1 hour's duration daily for a minimum of 6 weeks; (2) arthritis of three or more joints for a minimum of 6 weeks with swelling detected by a healthcare provider; (3) involvement of either the PIP, MCP, or wrist joints for a minimum of 6 weeks; (4) symmetric involvement that has been present for a minimum of 6 weeks; (5) presence of rheumatoid nodules; (6) positive RF; and (7) evidence consistent with RA on radiographs of the hands and/or wrists (e.g., erosions or extra-articular osteopenia). Because Ms. Rodriquez's clinical picture is consistent with five of these (given that her previous 6 weeks of physical findings were consistent with today's findings) and her anti-CPP is elevated, she can be diagnosed with RA with a fair degree of certainty.

Regarding right carpal tunnel syndrome, this diagnosis can essentially be established on the characteristic findings in her history and physical examination as well as their correlation to the results of her NCS. Thus, RA with right CTS is her most likely diagnosis.

B. Rheumatic fever (RF) with right carpal tunnel syndrome (CTS)   INCORRECT

Rheumatic fever is a systemic infectious condition that results from pharyngitis caused by group A β-hemolytic *Streptococcus*. It is theorized to be an autoimmune reaction. Rheumatic fever is diagnosed based on the modified Jones criteria. In order to establish the diagnosis, the patient must have a confirmed diagnosis of a preceding group A β-hemolytic *Streptococcus* infection PLUS EITHER two major OR one major and two minor criteria. The major Jones criteria are polyarthritis, subcutaneous nodules, erythema marginatum, chorea, and carditis. The minor criteria include arthralgias, fever, elevated ESR or CRP, and prolonged PR interval on electrocardiogram (ECG).

Based on the information that is available, Ms. Rodriguez does not meet the Jones criteria because she never had a documented streptococcal infection and she only has one of the major criteria (polyarthritis) and one of the minor criteria (elevated ESR or CRP; arthralgias do not count because she was credited with polyarthritis as her major criteria). Thus, rheumatic fever with right carpal tunnel syndrome is not Ms. Rodriquez's most likely diagnosis despite having electromyelographic documented right CTS.

C. Osteoarthritis with right wrist involvement and compression of the median nerve   INCORRECT

Although Ms. Rodriquez's paresthesias could result from compression of her right median nerve at the wrist, she does not have evidence of osteoarthritis in her right wrist. The most obvious distinction between osteoarthritis and her symptoms include the specific joints that are affected in her hands (please see previous discussion for the joints most commonly involved in these two conditions), the presence of joint inflammation (almost always absent in osteoarthritis), the presence of systemic symptoms (rare in osteoarthritis), and her positive diagnostic studies (inconsistent with osteoarthritis). Thus, this is not her most likely diagnosis.

D. Acromegaly-induced arthropathies and right carpal tunnel syndrome (CTS)   INCORRECT

Acromegaly is an endocrine disorder that is virtually always caused by a pituitary adenoma resulting in the hypersecretion of growth hormone and somatotropin. Although it can be associated with arthralgias and right carpal tunnel syndrome, the associated arthritis generally involves the spine, hips, and knees. Despite Ms. Rodriquez not having any lab tests to evaluate for this condition, it can be ruled out as her most likely diagnosis because she lacks the characteristic skeletal abnormalities (e.g. large hands with broadened digits, wide feet, enlarged skull, protrusion of the mandible with prognathism, and dental malocclusion) seen in acromegaly.

E. Lyme disease   INCORRECT

Lyme disease is a systemic inflammatory condition caused by an infection with the spirochete *Borrelia burgdorferi*, which is primarily transmitted by the Ixodes scapularis and the Ixodes pacificus ticks in the United States. The systemic symptoms are generally preceded (or at least accompanied) by the characteristic rash, erythema chronicum migrans. Musculoskeletal, neurologic, and cardiac manifestations are possible. The arthritis associated with Lyme disease is almost always monoarticular and prefers the knee. Although it would be possible for her to have been bitten by a tick without her knowledge, it is unusual for one to be attached for a sufficient enough time frame to cause Lyme disease without the patient's knowledge. Nevertheless, even if she did experience an unnoticed tick bite and attachment, it would be highly unlikely that she also missed the characteristic target lesion. Thus, Lyme disease is not Ms. Rodriquez's most likely diagnosis.

5. Treatment Plan

A. Refer to a rheumatologist   CORRECT

The primary treatment goals in RA consist of (1) alleviating pain, (2) diminishing inflammation, (3) preserving articular structures, (4) maintaining function, and (5) managing systemic manifestations. Involving a rheumatologist early in the treatment process is essential because several well-done studies have documented that patients with RA who are managed by a rheumatologist have better outcomes than those treated by other specialists. Ideally, her initial appointment should occur within 6 weeks of her diagnosis.

B. Liver function testing (LFT), blood urea nitrogen (BUN), and creatinine   CORRECT

The initial therapy must be individualized and is generally based on the patient's current symptomatology and potential for disease progression. In the majority of cases, the pharmacologic approach is likely to involve analgesics, glucocorticoids, and disease-modifying antirheumatic drugs (DMARDs). Baseline LFT, BUN, and creatinine are essential before initiating any of the DMARDs, including traditional (e.g., hydroxychloroquine, methotrexate, and sulfasalazine), biologic (e.g., adalimumab, anakinra, etanercept, infliximab, and rituximab), and immunologic (e.g., azathioprine, cyclophosphamide, cyclosporine, and leflunomide), because of their potential adverse effects on hepatic and/or renal functioning. These results should be sent to the consulting rheumatologist to expedite the patient's treatment program and permit the rheumatologist to focus on more important issues with the patient. Furthermore, this ensures that a baseline study is available for future reference.

C. Refer to physical therapy for an individualized treatment program   CORRECT

In addition to pharmacologic modalities, other treatments are essential if the goals of therapy are going to be met. Therefore, physical therapy is an excellent adjunct. Examples of potential treatments that could be provided include hot packs, cold therapy, hydrotherapy, massage, and passive ROM when the patient is significantly symptomatic; stretching exercises for contracture prevention as tolerated; exercise recommendations to maintain core muscles and stamina; education on how to properly complete tasks with less effort and pain; and training on the usage of assistive devices (if indicated).

D. Purified protein derivative (PPD) testing   CORRECT

Having the patient present to the rheumatologist with results of a recent appropriately performed and interpreted PPD test also enables any therapies deemed necessary to be initiated without further delays. PPD testing should be done prior to initiating any of the immunologic and biologic DMARDs because of their high risk of infections, especially the tumor necrosis factor (TNF) inhibitors (e.g., adalimumab, etanercept, and infliximab). The development of opportunistic infections, such as TB, presents significant morbidity and occasionally mortality for individuals being treated with TNF inhibitors.

Patients who are at high risk of acquiring TB and especially individuals with a positive PPD test pose treatment challenges. It is essential to consider the risks versus benefits of utilizing many of the DMARDs in this patient, even with accompanying rifampin therapy. Such decisions must be made by the rheumatologist, taking the patient's symptoms, predicted disease course, concerns, and preferences into consideration.

E. Start methotrexate, a tumor necrosis factor (TNF) inhibitor, or other disease-modifying antirheumatic drugs (DMARDs) if the patient's appointment with the rheumatologist is scheduled for more than 1 week away   INCORRECT

As stated previously, most experts agree that it is acceptable for the initial rheumatologic consultation to occur within 6 weeks from the time of diagnosis of the patient. Therefore, there is no reason for a primary care provider to initiate treatment with any of the DMARDs if the rheumatology consultation is going to occur during this time frame.

However, it would be considered appropriate in the interim to begin a course of NSAIDs with close observation for GI toxicity. However, because Ms. Rodriquez has already experienced GI symptoms related to the lower, over-the-counter dosages, she should begin her NSAID dose low and gradually increase it. Additionally, a PPI or misoprostol should be utilized for GI protection in conjunction with her NSAID, and she should be observed closely for any signs or symptoms suspicious of GI bleeding.

The NSAID trial would hopefully provide the patient with some symptomatic relief while waiting for the rheumatology appointment. Additionally, it should be helpful to the rheumatologist at the time of the initial consult because it would enable him or her to assess Ms. Rodriquez's response for pain control and tolerability from the NSAID at that visit. The response to NSAID therapy is still utilized by some rheumatologists in determining whether a DMARD is indicated. They feel that if the patient is pain free with this therapy, further medication is not necessary. In a few cases, this is still considered appropriate.

However, the current consensus is to consider adding a DMARD early in the treatment program to prevent further intra-articular damage. However, it is a decision that must be made on an individualized basis taking into account many factors including the severity of the patient's symptoms, coexisting medical conditions, potential for drug interactions, potential for adverse drug effects, potential for acquiring a significant infection, benefits versus risks of each of the medications (alone and in combination), and patient preferences.

If it will be several months before the patient is able to obtain a rheumatology consult and maximum-dose NSAIDs are not alleviating the patient's symptoms, then it would be appropriate to initiate a trial of glucocorticoids and/or a less toxic DMARD (e.g., methotrexate) provided that the patient's hepatic and renal functions are normal. Ideally, biologic and immunologic agents should never be utilized without first obtaining a rheumatology consult unless the HCP is very familiar with utilizing this particular group of drugs.

Epidemiologic and Other Data

RA is considered to be one of the autoimmune inflammatory systemic conditions that have joint involvement. In the case of RA, the major area of joint involvement is the patient's synovial membranes.

It is estimated that the incidence of RA is approximately 1 to 2% of all the individuals residing in the United States. It tends to affect females at three times the rate of males. The average age of onset is in the third through fifth decades of life. A positive family history increases the patient's potential for acquiring the disease.

CASE 8-7
Raquel Summers
1. History

A. Has she ever experienced a knee injury (especially associated with a "popping sound") or participated in any occupational or recreational repetitive knee activities?   ESSENTIAL

Unilateral, single-joint pain can result from several sources (e.g., trauma, osteoarthritis, infection, cancer, and crystal-induced arthropathies). Because trauma is the most common cause of monoarticular joint problems in Mrs. Summers' age group, it is essential to inquire if any has occurred, including repetitive knee activities. Because Mrs. Summers experienced a recent change in her symptomatology, acute trauma is just as important to inquire about as old trauma occurring before her symptoms began.

The association of a "popping" sound, especially followed by an unstable knee joint, could be indicative of a complete ligament (especially the cruciate) tear with or without an associated rupture of the patellar or quadriceps tendon. Likewise, a popping sensation following a tearing sensation in an acute knee injury (especially one that involves a twisting movement of the knee in conjunction with weight bearing) most often represents a meniscal injury. Ligament injuries can generally be differentiated from meniscal injuries by the occurrence of immediate swelling, effusion development, and early ecchymosis compared to meniscal injuries, in which these findings occur much later.

B. Has she felt depressed, sad, or blue or experienced anhedonia lately?   NONESSENTIAL

Although depression can present as a pain syndrome or vague joint symptoms, Mrs. Summers' complaint is relatively specific. Furthermore, pain associated with depression tends to be constant, and patients with depression presenting as a painful condition generally seek medical treatment much sooner than several years after its onset.

C. Does she experience any difficulty if she remains seated with her knees flexed at a 90° angle and her feet flat on the floor for over an hour?   ESSENTIAL

This is known as the theater sign. If present, this is extremely useful information to narrow Mrs. Summers' differential diagnosis list because only a small percentage of all possible causes of monoarticular joint pain are associated with a positive theater sign (e.g., old fractures, osteoarthritis, and patellofemoral syndrome [PFS]). Further delineation among these various conditions can be accomplished by determining exactly what symptom the patient experiences and how long it persists. For example, the stiffness associated with osteoarthritis is short-lived but can be accompanied by increased pain and difficulty in fully using the affected joint for the first few steps.

D. Does she have any difficulty going up or down stairs?   ESSENTIAL

Knee pain can occur from bony conditions, other intra-articular structure abnormalities, supporting structure defects, extra-articular processes, problems involving the adjacent joints and structures, neurologic conditions, and/or vascular abnormalities. Although patients with knee pain frequently experience difficulty ambulating steps, the type of difficulty, the direction associated with the difficulty, and the onset of the difficulty can provide clues to the potential types of conditions involved. For example, patients with proximal muscle weakness have more difficulty ascending stairs, whereas individuals with distal muscle weakness problems have more difficulty descending stairs. Individuals with claudication causing knee pain have pain more frequently ascending stairs; furthermore, it occurs at approximately the same distance on the same flight of steps and resolves almost instantaneously with stopping to rest.

There are some conditions that can be associated with both types of weakness. In pure musculoskeletal conditions, the type of weakness is frequently associated with the duration/severity of the symptoms. For example, weakness of the associated musculature is common in osteoarthritis and patellofemoral syndrome. Although the most common muscle affected is the quadriceps, early in the course of the disease the distal muscles are generally more symptomatic; this is theorized to be related to their overall smaller muscle mass/size.

E. Has she ever experienced her knee "giving away"?   ESSENTIAL

The sensation that the knee "gives away" is essentially always associated with some type of internal derangement. The most common causes include meniscal tears and osteoarthritis. The sensation of "buckling" in conjunction with a history of "locking" of the knee is virtually pathognomonic for a bucket handle tear of the meniscus. However, "locking" alone can be seen in a variety of other conditions (e.g., other meniscal injuries, a foreign body, PFS, osteoarthritis, or chondromalacia patellae).

2. Physical Examination

A. Bilateral hand examination   NONESSENTIAL

Mrs. Summers' symptoms are limited to a single joint and she is not experiencing any other arthralgias, myalgias, systemic symptoms, or upper extremity problems indicating the need for a hand examination.

B. Bilateral knee examination   ESSENTIAL

Obviously, because Mrs. Summers is complaining of left knee pain, she needs to have it examined. However, it is equally important to also examine the contralateral knee as a basis of "normal" for comparison and to evaluate it for subtle abnormalities that could suggest that the patient's condition is not a true monoarticular arthropathy. Observation and palpation of the knees should be performed in the standing, sitting, and lying (both supine and prone) positions. The standing position is best for determining if a malalignment exists as a result of leg length discrepancy and for determining genu varum ("bow legged") or genu valgum ("knocked kneed"), which can represent congenital abnormalities, nutritional deficiencies, growth problems, and an increased risk of chronic patellar subluxation. This position also permits visualization of the posterior knee for edema or a mass, which almost always represents a Baker cyst. However, the best position to palpate a Baker cyst or examine the knee for a smaller cyst is with the knee flexed and the patient in the prone position. The circumference of the thigh should be measured at an equal distance superior to the knee for a size discrepancy, which could represent quadriceps atrophy. However, it is essential to remember that the dominant leg (which is generally associated with ipsilateral hand dominance) can have a slightly greater measurement compared to the contralateral thigh. Obviously, gait must be observed with the patient in an upright position.

Evaluating for the presence of patellar alta (the patella sits superiorly to the anticipated site) or patellar baja (the patella sits inferiorly to its expected position) should be performed while the patient is both standing and supine. If present, they generally represent an ipsilateral rupture of the patellar tendon or the quadriceps tendon, respectively. The supine position is best for evaluating for soft tissue swelling and effusion; effusions are most frequently identified in the suprapatellar pouch; however, they can also exist in the lateral and medial aspects of the knee. They are generally caused by synovium hypertrophy or a frank synovial effusion, and they are typically identifiable on physical examination by visualizing the edema and by balloting the patella inferiorly. Small effusions can be diagnosed with the bulge sign (manually milking the superior and lateral aspects of the knee inferiorly forces the effusion from its preferred site in the suprapatellar pouch, thus producing a visible "bulge" on the medial aspect of the knee). If there is a concern regarding a leg length discrepancy, supine is the best position to measure leg length. The measurement is taken from the medial malleolus to the anterior superior iliac spine.

A complete orthopedic examination not only includes visualizing the affected area for gross deformities, adjacent muscle atrophy, edema, erythema, other color alterations, rashes, and other skin changes and palpating the joint for tenderness, warmth, and crepitus but also evaluating range of motion for abnormalities with flexion, extension, and lateral movement. Additionally, a neurologic and vascular examination should be performed to detect abnormalities that could be causing or contributing to the joint complaint.

In regard to the knee, several special maneuvers can be employed to assist in determining the patient's most likely diagnosis. Anterior and posterior cruciate ligament instability, tears, or ruptures can generally be identified by detecting positive anterior and posterior drawer signs, respectively. These maneuvers are conducted with the patient in a sitting position with the knees flexed 90° and feet supported; the HCP stabilizes the ankle with one hand while applying pressure in a forward motion (anterior) and then in a backward (posterior) motion to the superior position of the lower leg with the other hand. The Lachman maneuver is performed identically to the anterior drawer sign except the patient's knee is in 30° flexion; when positive, it reveals a "stepping up" from the lower aspect of the patella to the tibial tuberosity and represents an anterior cruciate abnormality.

The pivot shift test is performed with the patient supine and hips flexed to 30° with the HCP holding the leg at the ankle with one hand to maintain 20° of internal tibial rotation; with the other hand, the HCP increases the force of internal rotation by grabbing and pulling on the lateral aspect of the lower leg over the superior tibiofibular joint. Then, the HCP applies a valgus force to the knee while slowly flexing and then extending the patient's knee. If a "clunk" is heard during the maneuver, it almost always indicates a rupture of a cruciate ligament. Less significant findings can also be associated with a positive test. For example, a sensation of anterior subluxation with extension can be caused by an anterior cruciate ligament, posterolateral joint capsule, or arcuate ligament tear.

Collateral ligament testing looks for lateral movement of the femur when the HCP stabilizes the patient's fully extended knee with one hand while grasping the lower leg slightly superior to the ankle joint and moving it in lateral and medial directions with the other hand; any laxity detected can indicate an injury to both the collateral and cruciate ligaments. However, if the maneuver is performed with the patient's knee in 30° of flexion, laxity becomes much more specific for a collateral ligament tear. Laxity that occurs when the leg is moved in the lateral direction generally indicates a laxity or tear of the medial collateral ligament; however, if it occurs on medial movement, generally the lateral collateral ligament is affected.

Meniscal injuries can generally be identified by the McMurray test; it consists of palpation of the patella (generally by covering it with a palm) while the patient's knee is being fully extended and the tibia is being rotated internally; then, the maneuver is repeated, except the tibial rotation is externally. A "popping" sound or sensation, a "locking up" of the knee, and/or the reproduction of the patient's symptoms by the maneuver constitutes a positive test. If any of these findings occur during medial rotation, it suggests an injury or a tear to the lateral meniscus, whereas the presence of these findings with lateral rotation suggests an injury or tear to the medical meniscus.

Tests that are fairly specific for patellar dysfunction include the measurement of the "Q" angle, identification of the "J" sign, the patellar apprehension sign, evaluation for patellar irritability, the patellar glide test, the patellar tilt test, the lateral pull sign, and the patellofemoral grind test. In general, the more dramatic the findings are on these tests, the greater the likelihood that a complication exists. The "Q" angle is the angle of the patellar tendon off the patella; it is determined by the HCP viewing the patella as the oval-shaped portion of the letter "Q" and the tail portion as the patellar tendon. Normally, it should be less than or equal to 15%. The "J" sign is visible movement of the patella with flexion of the knee at the end of extension in a path that resembles the letter "J." The patellar glide test involves moving the patella medially and laterally with the patient seated and the knee flexed to approximately 30°. The medial glide test is positive when the patella can be moved in the medial direction, whereas a lateral glide test is positive if the patella can be moved laterally. The patellar apprehension sign is positive if this maneuver produces anxiety and resistance to movement on the part of the patient generally as a result of fear of pain and in patients with a history of lateral patellar instability.

The patellar tilt test is performed by the HCP attempting to lift up the edges of the patella with the patient supine and relaxing his or her quadriceps; a positive sign occurs if the HCP has any degree of success. A lateral pull test is performed in the same manner (and has the same findings for a positive test) as the patellar tilt test except the patient actively contracts his or her quadriceps muscle. The patellofemoral grind test is performed in the same manner as a lateral pull test; however, instead of attempting to lift up the edges of the patella, the HCP applies gentle downward pressure directly over the patella. The test is considered to be positive if the patient experiences pain with the maneuver.

C. Bilateral hip and ankle examination   ESSENTIAL

As stated previously, a good orthopedic examination evaluates not only the affected joint and its contralateral mate but also the next most proximal and distal joints. Additionally, if a patient complaining of knee pain is walking with limp, special attention to the hips is essential because a significant number of knee complaints associated with limping are caused by hip abnormalities.

D. Evaluation of the curvature of the lumbar spine NONESSENTIAL

Although there are a few conditions that can be associated with both lumbar lordosis and knee pain (e.g., decreased joint spaces or osteophyte formation resulting in nerve root irritation or compression causing radiation of pain to the knee, or lordosis causing PFS), it is highly unlikely for them to present without some degree of low back pain. Additionally, the neurologic component of the orthopedic examination should be able to identify the former and tests for patellar stability the latter.

E. Bilateral foot examination   NONESSENTIAL

Although severe talipes planus ("flatfoot") could potentially cause knee pain as a result of structural malalignment, a foot examination would not be indicated unless genu valgum was identified on the standing portion of the knee examination.

3. Diagnostic Studies

A. Erythrocyte sedimentation rate (ESR) and C-reactive protein (CRP)   NONESSENTIAL

An ESR and CRP are not indicated for Mrs. Summers because her history and physical examination findings do not support the suspicion of an inflammatory, infectious, necrotic, cancerous, or metastatic cause to her knee pain. In the first three examples, both tests would prove useful. For the latter two conditions, the ESR would be more likely to be elevated than the CRP.

B. Complete blood count with differential (CBC w/diff)   NONESSENTIAL

A complete blood count with differential is also not indicated because Mrs. Summers' signs and symptoms are not suspicious for an infectious, inflammatory, or malignant condition or one that might be associated with a leukocytosis, thrombocytopenia, or anemia.

C. Patellofemoral degradation antibody (anti-PFD)   NONESSENTIAL

Nice try, but this test doesn't exist.

D. Radiograph of her left knee in weight bearing, extension, and Merchant view   ESSENTIAL

A radiograph of Mrs. Summers' left knee is indicated because of the chronicity of her symptoms. The special views are indicated because she has signs and symptoms of patellar tenderness and patellar dysfunction; these additional views will provide better visualization of her patella.

Some would argue that a radiographic study is not indicated, citing that she does not have a chronic condition but experienced an acute injury. This opinion would be based on the infrequent occurrences and rapid resolution of her symptoms in the past and that, despite a similar mechanism of injury, a different outcome occurred, therefore meaning she has an acute injury with a low risk of fracture and would not require a radiograph.

Nevertheless, even if Mrs. Summers' knee pain represented an acute injury to her left knee, the evidence-based guidelines regarding the ordering of knee radiographs in acute injuries, the Ottawa knee rules, support performing a radiographic study because she has patellar tenderness. The other indications these guidelines cite as reasons for an x-ray study to be performed in an acute knee injury are (1) age 55 years or older, (2) fibular head tenderness, (3) knee flexion of less than or equal to 90°, and (4) limp occurring with a minimum of four steps with weight bearing.

E. Magnetic resonance imaging (MRI) of her left knee   NONESSENTIAL

An MRI of the knees is not currently indicated for Mrs. Summers. It would be considered appropriate if she was being evaluated for a surgical procedure or if there was a strong suspicion of a cartilage, ligament, or meniscus abnormality or a carcinoma being responsible for her symptoms.

4. Diagnosis

A. Osteoarthritis of the left knee   INCORRECT

Osteoarthritis is a degenerative process with a propensity for the knees (for more information, please see Case 8-1). Technically, osteoarthritis is classified as a monoarticular arthritis;

however, with the exception of those cases attributable to trauma, it frequently involves more than one joint (although one joint can be more symptomatic than the rest). Despite similarities to Mrs. Summers' main complaint, osteoarthritis can be ruled out as her most likely diagnosis based on her findings on history and physical examination. Furthermore, her radiographs do not reveal any degenerative changes. Although the radiographic findings do not necessarily correlate with the degree of pain, for osteoarthritis to be the culprit, there should at least be some minimal evidence of the disease present. Furthermore, it is uncommon for the disease, especially the primary form, to occur in individuals younger than the age of 40 years, especially in the absence of prior trauma.

B. Patellofemoral syndrome (PFS)   CORRECT

PFS is a degenerative condition involving the articular cartilage of the patella most frequently caused by atypical knee compression and/or shearing forces that can result in patellalgia and/or patellar dysfunction. Based on the information obtained through Mrs. Summers' history, physical, and diagnostic studies, this is her most likely diagnosis.

She has the typical complaints of a "catch" in her knee associated with difficulty standing from a squatting position, and a positive theater sign. Her findings on her physical examination further support this diagnosis by a "Q" angle of greater than 15 to 20°, a positive "J" sign, a patellar glide test and patellar tilt test suggestive of a rigid lateral retinaculum, and pain with the patellofemoral grind test. Additionally, these suspicions were confirmed on her radiograph by findings of a slightly subluxed and laterally tilted patella.

However, it is important to note that if she exhibited signs and symptoms suggestive of joint inflammation, even with all of these findings consistent with the diagnosis of FPS, an inflammatory condition would more than likely be responsible for her symptoms. If left untreated, FPS can lead to chronic subluxation of the patella, patellofemoral arthritis, or chondromalacia patellae (chronic degeneration of the cartilage of the patella).

C. Lateral meniscus tear   INCORRECT

A tear to the lateral meniscus almost always occurs as a result of trauma; the most common injury is a medial twisting motion of the knee while the foot is in a position of weight bearing. Characteristic physical examination findings include a positive McMurray test on medial rotation of the tibia and evidence of internal derangement of the affected knee joint. Because Mrs. Summers lacks all of these characterizing features but does have patellar pain, tenderness, and instability, a lateral meniscus tear is not her most likely diagnosis. Furthermore, because of the anatomic structure of the knee joint, the medial meniscus is more tightly tethered to the tibia, making it approximately 10 times more likely to be injured than the lateral meniscus.

D. Osgood-Schlatter disease   INCORRECT

Osgood-Schlatter disease, also known as Schlatter disease or Schlatter-Osgood disease, typically presents as pain and point tenderness over the tibial tuberosity caused by inflammation and/or partial avulsion of the apophysis caused by two opposing forces. The vast majority of individuals with this condition present between the ages of 10 and 15 years; however, there have been few cases of it not being identified until later. Nevertheless, this is not Mrs. Summers' most likely diagnosis because she was not complaining of tibial pain, she did not exhibit any tenderness on palpation of her tibial tuberosity, and her radiograph did not reveal any enlargement, fragmentation, or avulsion off the tibial tuberosity.

E. Osteochondritis dissecans (OCD)   INCORRECT

OCD is an inflammation of not only the bone but also its overlying cartilage that generally results in an actual separation of the bone from the cartilage. Frequently it is associated with epiphyseal aseptic necrosis. Although it most frequently involves the knee joint, it can also be eliminated as Mrs. Summers' most likely diagnosis primarily based on the absence of inflammation on her physical examination and her radiographic findings being inconsistent with this diagnosis.

5. Treatment Plan

A. Nonsteroidal anti-inflammatory drugs (NSAIDs) with food   CORRECT

NSAIDs are the mainstay of pain management for PFS. Generally, they are effective; however, occasionally a patient will require a short course of a narcotic analgesic to control pain.

B. Proton pump inhibitor (PPI)   INCORRECT

A PPI or misoprostol is indicated for all patients who are going to be on long-term treatment with NSAIDs or those patients who are at "high risk" for a gastrointestinal bleed from NSAIDs. However, NSAIDs are generally only required for a short period of time in FPS and Mrs. Summers does not have any co-morbid conditions that would increase her risk of this serious complication. Therefore, a PPI is not indicated at this time for her. However, it is appropriate to consider misoprostol or enteric or time-released forumlations to miminize GI risks.

C. Referral to physical therapy   CORRECT

Physical therapy is the mainstay of treatment for PFS.

D. Immediate referral to an orthopedic surgeon   INCORRECT

Surgery for PFS is considered to be a "last resort" treatment option. It is indicated if chronic subluxation exists, recurrences occur with great frequency after relocating the patella, significant complications are rapidly developing, or other treatment modalities have failed.

E. Intra-articular hyaluronate injections   INCORRECT

Intra-articular high-molecular weight sodium hyaluronate injections are only indicated after an intense trial of physical therapy and NSAIDs has proven to be ineffective in managing the condition. It appears to be most effective if complications, especially patellofemoral arthritis, have already occurred. This medication is currently only FDA approved for the treatment of osteoarthritis of the knee.

Epidemiologic and Other Data

PFS affects females at a significantly higher rate than their male counterparts. It is found primarily in two main groups. The first cluster is found in adolescent females who are generally tall, have an abnormal "Q" angle, and participate in sports/activities that involve frequent jumping (e.g., basketball or cheerleading). The second group consists of early-middle-aged females who have abnormal patellar tracking in the patellar groove as a result of poor conditioning, quadriceps weakness, or laxity of the ligaments of the knee that results in subluxation of the patella.

CASE 8-8
Sylvia Tincher
1. History

A. How old were her sisters and mother when they were diagnosed with osteoporosis?   NONESSENTIAL

The age of her relatives when diagnosed with osteoporosis is unimportant because it is not reflective of the actual onset of the disease process nor is it predictive of what age Mrs. Tincher might acquire the condition. Furthermore, Mrs. Tincher already has osteoporosis, so knowing she has a positive family history is irrelevant, regardless of their ages at time of diagnosis.

A positive family history of a first-degree relative with osteoporosis is significant when evaluating a (generally younger) patient's risks for acquiring the disease. Other nonmodifiable risk factors for osteoporosis include advancing age, female gender, white race, personal history of an adult fracture, and presence of dementia. Theoretically, modifiable risk factors include weight under 127 lb, inadequate calcium intake, dietary deficiency of vitamin D, smoking, excessive alcohol consumption, early menopause, prolonged amenorrhea, sedentary lifestyle, poor general health, impaired vision despite corrective lenses, and recurrent falls.

B. What brand of mouthwash does she use?   NONESSENTIAL

Her brand of mouthwash is not going to have any relevance on her pain because it is not aggravated by mouthwash exposure. If it was, this could become significant as its ingredients would need to be determined because alcohol (which is contained in the majority of the products made for adult usage) could be the culprit. Still, there exists the possibility that the symptoms are due to an allergic or more likely an irritative, reaction to another component of the mouthwash.

C. Has she had any type of infection (including dental) in the previous 6 months?   ESSENTIAL

One condition that has to be on her list of differential diagnoses is osteomyelitis. Because it results from the spread of an infection via a hematogenous dissemination or directly from an adjacent structure (including skin), it is essential to know whether Mrs. Tincher has experienced any type of an infectious process at any time during the previous 6 months that could be responsible.

D. Has she ever been diagnosed with cancer?   ESSENTIAL

Osteonecrosis of the tympanomandibular joint (TMJ) has been reported in individuals taking bisphosphonate therapy. A significant risk factor for this condition appears to be taking high-dose aminobisphosphonate therapy for multiple myeloma or metastatic breast cancer and undergoing dental surgery, including an extraction. Furthermore, radiation therapy to the jaw also appears to significantly increase the incidence of this complication. However, cases do exist in patients without any previous carcinoma who have exposed mandibular or maxillary bone.

E. Has she notice any "grinding" noise or sensation when moving her jaw?   ESSENTIAL

The presence of crepitus or a "grinding-like" sensation or sound is an important distinguishing feature. It is usually associated with a loss of articular cartilage and/or degeneration of the joint (e.g., osteoarthritis and true TMJ syndrome).

2. Physical Examination

A. Ear examination   ESSENTIAL

Mrs. Tincher requires an ear examination because it is not uncommon for otic problems to cause pain to radiate into the jaw. This is especially important because she has been diagnosed with TMJ dysfunction and has failed to respond to appropriate treatment.

B. Oral examination   ESSENTIAL

An oral examination is also an essential component of the evaluation of a patient with tympanomandibular joint pain. Dental malocclusions, poor dentition, oral lesions, pharyngeal problems, tongue abnormalities, and gingival conditions can be associated with, present as, or cause an exacerbation of an unrelated condition. An oral examination is especially important for Mrs. Tincher because she is currently on bisphosphonate therapy and recently had a dental procedure performed; therefore, careful evaluation of her oral mucosa and gingival surfaces for any evidence of an area of exposed bone that could be necrotic is essential.

C. Heart and lung auscultation   NONESSENTIAL

D. Bilateral TMJ examination   ESSENTIAL

Because Mrs. Tincher is complaining of tympanomandibular pain, this area must be examined. Even though her symptoms are unilateral, evaluation of her contralateral tympanomandibular joint is essential. Evidence of contralateral disease can alter the patient's potential differential diagnosis list.

E. Neurologic examination of the face   ESSENTIAL

Because Mrs. Tincher is experiencing paresthesias and difficulty with mastication, a neurologic examination of her face, including both sensory and motor function of her cranial nerves, is necessary.

3. Diagnostic Studies

A. Radiograph of right TMJ   NONESSENTIAL

From Mrs. Tincher's history, it appears that a panoramic radiograph and a plain radiograph of her right TMJ have already been performed for this complaint and did not identify any abnormalities. Therefore, in all likelihood, all an additional TMJ radiograph is going to provide is unnecessary radiation exposure for Mrs. Tincher.

B. Magnetic resonance imaging (MRI) of right TMJ ESSENTIAL

Because her radiographic studies were unremarkable despite her having a very symptomatic TMJ, an MRI is indicated because it tends to be more sensitive than radiography in detecting subtle bony abnormalities.

C. Erythrocyte sedimentation rate (ESR)   ESSENTIAL

An ESR will be not only reflective of the degree of inflammation associated with her right TMJ but also indicative

of any inflammation she might have elsewhere. Additionally, it may or may not be elevated with bony necrosis. However, it will be elevated with an infectious, inflammatory, or malignant process; thus, it needs to be performed.

D. White blood cell count with differential (WBC w/diff) ESSENTIAL

A WBC w/diff is indicated because it will provide information regarding the presence (and seriousness) of an infectious, and in many cases an inflammatory, process.

E. Electromyelogram (EMG) of her right trigeminal nerve NONESSENTIAL

An EMG of her right trigeminal nerve is not indicated at this time because her facial motor function is normal and her abnormal sensation does not follow its distribution.

4. Diagnosis

A. Gingival abscess secondary to dental extraction INCORRECT

Because Mrs. Tincher's oral examination failed to reveal any gingival edema, tenderness, erythema, or discharge, even in the gingival cavity remaining after her recent tooth extraction, gingival abscess secondary to dental extraction is not her most likely diagnosis.

B. Osteomyelitis of right TMJ   INCORRECT

Osteomyelitis is an infection of the bone that is acquired directly from adjacent structures, including the skin, or indirectly via hematogenous dissemination. Early in the course of this condition, plain film radiography can be normal; however, it generally reveals some nonspecific signs such as tissue edema, loss of tissue plains, or periarticular loss of bone. Bony erosions, abnormal-appearing callous bone, and periostitis are almost always evident on a plain film radiograph any time after approximately 2 weeks of symptom duration.

Additionally, an MRI scan is considered to be equally as sensitive as a bone scan in making this diagnosis. It can actually detect bone marrow water content changes before cortical disruption occurs. However, at this point in time, her MRI scan should reveal evidence of cortical destruction. In view of her MRI scan not revealing any findings consistent with osteomyelitis, her not experiencing an infection in the previous 6 months, her not having any obvious signs or symptoms of a current infection, and her not having a significant leukocytosis or ESR elevation on her blood work, osteomyelitis is not Mrs. Tincher's most likely diagnosis.

C. Chondrosarcoma of right TMJ   INCORRECT

Chondrosarcoma is a malignancy that arises from cartilage. Because it tends to be associated with "punched out"–appearing lesions on radiography and MRI, this is not her most likely diagnosis.

D. Bisphosphonate-related osteonecrosis of right TMJ CORRECT

Osteonecrosis is death of bone cells. When it affects the tympanomandibular joint as a result of an adverse effect of bisphosphonate therapy, it is known as bisphosphonate-related osteonecrosis of the jaw (BRONJ). Mrs. Tincher has a typical presentation for BRONJ, a vague, mild discomfort that progressively gets worse; increased pain with mastication; a slightly elevated ESR; nonspecific radiographic findings; and a whitened-out area of bone on the mandible on MRI.

According to the American Association of Oral and Maxillofacial Surgeons (AAOMS) position paper, the diagnosis of BRONJ can be made if ALL of the following criteria are met: the patient is currently (or was recently) taking a bisphosphonate, maxillofacial bone has been exposed for at least 8 weeks, and the patient has not received radiation therapy to the area.

Her history definitively establishes that Mrs. Tincher meets the first and third criteria (current bisphosphonate therapy and never receiving radiation therapy). Additionally, she had a difficult dental extraction approximately 4 months ago and necrotic bone is evident in the gingival cavity produced by the procedure. Thus, it is a relatively safe assumption that she meets this criterion as well. Thus, BRONJ is Mrs. Tincher's most likely diagnosis.

Other drugs that have been implicated as capable of producing osteonecrosis are glucocorticoids and alcohol.

E. Osteoarthritis of right TMJ   INCORRECT

Osteoarthritis of the right TMJ can be eliminated as Mrs. Tincher's most likely diagnosis by the lack of audible or palpable crepitus on her history and physical examination as well as evidence of any degree of bony degeneration on her previous radiographs and MRI.

5. Treatment Plan

A. Stage Mrs. Tincher's disease   CORRECT

The primary goals of treatment for Mrs. Tincher are to control any infection that is present, alleviate any pain, and prevent further bone destruction/necrosis. To achieve these goals, the first step is to stage her disease so appropriate treatment can be instituted. The staging system runs from stage 0 to stage 3 in order of worsening severity. Patients who are "at risk" for BRONJ are classified as stage 1. Stage 0 patients have nonspecific symptoms (e.g., tooth pain without a dental cause, sinus pain, dull jaw pain, mild facial paresthesias, and/or another mild cranial nerve dysfunction), nonspecific periodontal disease associated with an unrelated loosening of teeth but no evidence of any necrotic bone, and imaging studies that are negative or reveal nonspecific findings (e.g., thickening of the periodontal ligament, narrowing of the inferior alveolar canal, alveolar bone loss without a clear cause, and/or a trabecular bony pattern).

Patients with stage 1 or stage 2 BRONJ have exposed necrotic bone. However, individuals with stage 1 BRONJ are asymptomatic and infection free, whereas patients with stage 2 BRONJ experience pain and have evidence of an infectious process being present.

Stage 3 BRONJ patients have all the signs and symptoms that are associated with stage 2, plus some type of complication (e.g., bony necrosis or osteolysis that goes beyond region of the alveolar bone, a nontraumatic fracture, and/or fistula formations). Although Mrs. Tincher lacks evidence of a gross infection, she is experiencing pain and her MRI lesion is beyond the alveolar process (superior ridge) of the mandible; thus, she has stage 3 disease.

B. Chlorhexidine antiseptic mouthwash   CORRECT

Patients with stage 1, 2, or 3 BRONJ should be using chlorhexidine (or some other type of antimicrobial) mouthwash on a regular basis.

C. Penicillin VK 500 mg four times a day   CORRECT

Patients who are classified as having either stage 2 or stage 3 disease need to be on regular, systemic antibiotic therapy. Oral penicillin VK is usually sufficient because the majority of the bacteria identified in BRONJ are normal oral flora; thus, it would be unusual to identify one that was resistant to penicillin. However, if there is significant extra-alveolar involvement, IV antibiotics may be required, at least initially.

Short courses of penicillin are useful in stage 0 patients who get an occasional mild infection. Penicillin does not play a role in the treatment of stage 1 BRONJ patients because by definition, they are asymptotic and without a related infection.

If the infection does not seem to be responding to penicillin, then appropriate cultures and sensitivities should be employed to attempt to identify the organism and to which antibiotics it is sensitive. In the interim, empiric therapy with erythromycin, clindamycin, metronidazole, doxycycline, or a quinolone is an appropriate choice as these have proven successful in treating this condition in the past. This approach is also appropriate for individuals who are allergic to or intolerant of penicillin.

D. Consultation with an oral surgeon   CORRECT

A consultation with an oral surgeon is also indicated for Mrs. Tincher because she is being considered as a stage 3 BRONJ patient. Patients in this stage often benefit from surgical débridement, resection, and correction of anatomic defects (e.g., fistulas) to achieve better relief from both the pain and the associated infection.

However, many oral surgeons prefer to delay surgery, when possible, until the involved area is well sequestered. This makes it easier to remove the damaged bone and decreases the potential of leaving noninvolved areas of bone exposed, which often will lead to necrosis of that bony segment as well.

Stage 2 BRONJ patients also require minor surgical débridement to provide pain relief if soft tissue irritation is a significant problem.

E. Discontinue bisphosphonate   CORRECT

Because her bisphosphonate therapy appears to have contributed to her condition, it is reasonable to discontinue it. The AAOMS guidelines recommend discontinuation for a minimum of 6 to 12 months.

Although not listed as one of the treatment options for Mrs. Tincher, analgesics are indicated for the control of pain as needed in stage 0 patients and regularly in stage 2 and 3 BRONJ patients. The lowest effective dose of the least addictive/sedating medication is indicated. However, when prescribing analgesics, one must be careful to consider the patient's other comorbid conditions and allergies, drug adverse effects, and drug-to-drug interactions to prevent further problems. For example, high-dose morphine would be contraindicated in a patient with chronic obstructive pulmonary disease to prevent respiratory depression; oxycodone should be avoided in individuals with a substance abuse problem because it is often difficult to wean them off the product as their pain improves; meperidine should be avoided in patients who are taking serotonergic agents (especially monoamine oxidase inhibitors [MAOIs]) because of the risk of serotonin syndrome; and NSAIDs need to be avoided or utilized with extreme caution with a cytoprotective agent in a patient with a history of a bleeding peptic ulcer disease.

Because of the association between bisphosphonate therapy and osteonecrosis of the jaw, it is accepted practice to have the patient examined by a dentist for any evidence of exposed bone or dental abnormalities prior to the initiation of bisphosphonate therapy. If dental problems requiring treatment are identified, they should be treated and healed before commencing bisphosphonate therapy.

Epidemiologic and Other Data

Despite a black-box label warning by the FDA, the currently available medical evidence suggests a causal relationship between osteonecrosis of the jaw and bisphosphonate usage. Hence, the most correct name for the condition is bisphosphonate-related osteonecrosis of the jaw.

It appears to be greater in women who take IV bisphosphonates compared to those who take them orally. Individuals on IV bisphosphonates with an associated malignancy, particularly bony metastasis, are at the greatest risk; studies place this risk between 0.8 and 12%. For women on oral therapy without an associated malignancy, studies place this risk between 0.00038 and 0.06%. It is further estimated that patients with cancer who are taking IV bisphosphonates have between a 2.7- and 4.2-fold increase compared to patients without cancer who are utilizing IV bisphosphonates. The presence of inflammatory dental disease in these patients with cancer further increases their risk to approximately sevenfold.

Currently, other risk factors appear to include longer duration of therapy, recent dentoalveolar surgery (especially if it involves the lower teeth, gingival area, or deeper structures), abnormalities of the mandible, advanced age, genetic defects, comorbid medical conditions (obesity, diabetes mellitus, renal failure requiring dialysis, and anemia), concurrent corticosteroid usage, exposure to chemotherapeutic agents, and tobacco usage.

Because the bisphosphonates inhibit osteoclastic activity in all the bones of the body, osteonecrosis can occur at any site. However, it is theorized that the majority of the cases affect the jaw because of its extremely high bony turnover and excellent vascular supply.

CASE 8-9

Travis Uno

1. History

A. When did his back pain begin, where is it located, and what is its course?   ESSENTIAL

Mr. Uno's foot pain is a classic presentation and the diagnosis can be made clinically. However, because this enthesopathy is associated with some of the inflammatory seronegative spondyloarthropathies (e.g., ankylosing spondylitis, reactive arthritis, psoriatic arthritis, arthritis of inflammatory bowel disease [IBD], and undifferentiated spondyloarthropathy) and he is complaining of long-standing back pain, it is important to explore this problem.

B. Does he experience any nocturnal symptoms?   ESSENTIAL

In the vast majority of musculoskeletal conditions, the pain is improved when the patient assumes the supine position and sleeps at night. However, as stated previously, with bone cancer or metastatic bone disease, the pain frequently worsens at night. Additionally, the spondyloarthropathies are associated with increased nocturnal pain.

C. Does he have any problems with diarrhea, constipation, abdominal bloating, abdominal cramping, melena, hematochezia, or rectal discomfort, or urinary symptoms?   ESSENTIAL

Because his differential diagnoses include inflammatory seronegative spondyloarthropathies (e.g., arthritis of IBD, reactive arthritis, and ankylosing spondylitis), it is essential to determine if he has been experiencing any symptoms suggestive of colonic and/or ileum inflammation, an enteric infection, or IBD.

D. Has he experienced any fatigue, malaise, fever, visual disturbances, rashes, other musculoskeletal pain, or severe swelling of his fingers?   ESSENTIAL

Because the seronegative spondyloarthropathies are inflammatory in nature, they can share some of the symptoms of the inflammatory seropositive arthropathies (e.g., RA and SLE), including fatigue, malaise, fever, and other constitutional symptoms. Additionally, the seronegative spondyloarthropathies can be associated with other symptoms (e.g., visual disturbances, rashes, enthesitis, or severe swelling of the fingers [also known as "sausage fingers"]). For example, up to 40% of patients with ankylosing spondylitis will experience acute anterior uveitis, and patients with psoriatic arthritis tend to have the typical skin plaquing and nail pitting that is consistent with nonsystemic, dermatologic psoriasis.

E. Has he had any dyspnea, cough, chest pain/pressure, or palpitations?   ESSENTIAL

Some of these inflammatory seronegative spondyloarthropathies, especially ankylosing spondylitis, can be associated with Tietze syndrome, aortic insufficiency, atrioventricular conduction defects, pulmonary fibrosis of the upper lobes, and bronchiectasis. Therefore, it is essential to inquire about symptoms that could represent one of these conditions.

2. Physical Examination

A. Heart and lung examination   ESSENTIAL

A heart and lung examination is necessary because of potential cardiac or pulmonary complications if his low back pain is caused by an inflammatory seronegative spondyloarthropathy.

B. Spine evaluation   ESSENTIAL

Because of the chronic, atypical nature of Mr. Uno's back pain, he requires a thorough assessment of his entire spine to help determine the cause of his back pain and whether it is caused by, related to, or a separate problem from his enthesis.

C. Bilateral hip examination   ESSENTIAL

A bilateral hip examination is indicated for Mr. Uno because of the intimate relationship shared between the spine, pelvis, and hips. Additionally, the hips are commonly affected in some of the inflammatory seronegative spondyloarthropathies, most notably ankylosing spondylitis.

D. Bilateral foot and ankle examination   ESSENTIAL

Because Mr. Uno's presenting complaint is foot pain, he requires a bilateral foot examination. As previously stated, a good orthopedic examination includes not only the affected joint but also the next most proximal and distal joints; thus, an ankle examination is indicated for Mr. Uno.

E. Genital and prostate examination   NONESSENTIAL

Although some of the inflammatory seronegative spondyloarthropathies (e.g., reactive arthritis and ankylosing spondylitis) are associated with urethritis and prostatitis, a genital and prostate examination are not indicated because he is not experiencing any genitourinary symptoms.

3. Diagnostic Studies

A. Radiograph of his lumbar spine   ESSENTIAL

Because of the chronicity of Mr. Uno's low back pain and the possibility of an inflammatory seronegative spondyloarthropathy, a lumbar spine radiograph is indicated. Sometimes early in the disease course of the spondyloarthropathies, joint involvement is not visible on plain film radiographs. Therefore, in patients who have negative lumbar spine radiographs but a high index of suspicion for a spondyloarthropathy, an MRI is indicated. However, because Mr. Uno has been experiencing low back pain for 7 to 8 years and has an abnormal lumbar spine evaluation, if this condition is present, he should have some evidence of it present on his radiographs.

B. Erythrocyte sedimentation rate (ESR)   ESSENTIAL

As stated previously, the ESR is a measurement of nonspecific inflammation. If it is moderately to significantly elevated, it provides additional support that Mr. Uno has a coexisting inflammatory seronegative spondyloarthropathy. His chief complaint independently should not have a significant impact on his ESR.

C. Complete blood count with differential (CBC w/diff) ESSENTIAL

Because Mr. Uno's differential diagnoses include an inflammatory arthritis, regardless of whether it is a seronegative or a seropositive autoimmune condition, he requires a CBC w/diff to evaluate for the common findings of coexisting anemia and/or platelet dysfunction. Because of the chronicity of his back pain, an infection is not a likely possibility.

D. Radiograph of his right heel   NONESSENTIAL

The cause of Mr. Uno's foot pain can be established based on his history and physical examination. A radiograph is not going to provide any useful information but has the potential to complicate the clinical picture. The most common radiographic finding associated with his diagnosis is bone spurs of the calcaneus; however, their presence is not pathognomonic for his condition. Furthermore, it is unlikely that a bone spur is producing any of his symptoms.

It is important to remember that when evaluating any diagnostic abnormality, the patient's history and physical examination should be consistent with the findings to ensure that the "abnormality" represents the true pathology and is not an incidental finding.

E. Magnetic resonance imaging (MRI) of his right heel NONESSENTIAL

If there is significant doubt regarding the patient's diagnosis, concern of a coexisting stress fracture, or unresponsiveness of the patient to appropriate treatment, an imaging study would be indicated. However, this is not Mr. Uno's case.

Because plain film radiographs are generally ineffective in establishing the diagnosis of heal pain in the absence of trauma, another imaging modality is required. However, the diagnostic study of choice would be a bone scan, not an MRI.

4. Diagnosis

A. Osteoarthritis of spine with pes planus   INCORRECT

Although Mr. Uno does have pes planus evident on his physical examination as well as osteophytes and other degenerative changes on his lumbar radiograph, which can be seen with osteoarthritis, this is not his most likely diagnosis. Osteoarthritis generally does not cause a true sacroiliitis, a significant elevation of the ESR, or a normocytic normochromic anemia. Additionally, osteoarthritis tends to be alleviated with rest, aggravated by activity, and associated with morning and inactivity stiffness of a short duration, which is the opposite of what Mr. Uno is experiencing.

B. Plantar fasciitis associated with ankylosing spondylitis CORRECT

Plantar fasciitis is an inflammation of the plantar fascia that occurs most frequently at the insertion of the fascia on the calcaneus. Mr. Uno's history and physical examination findings are a classic presentation of this condition.

Ankylosing spondylitis (AS) is an inflammatory arthropathy that is characterized by vertebral inflammation and degeneration that leads to bony stiffening and later fixation (as a result of a fibrous or bony union) of the vertebral joints, spondylolisthesis (forward slipping of one or more lumbar vertebrae), and syndesmophytes (bony protrusions from the vertebrae that are smaller and more posteriorly located than osteophytes). The classic radiographic finding in advanced disease is the "bamboo spine," which is caused by vertebral slippage, fusion, and consequential straightening of the spine, giving it the appearance of bamboo.

It is currently diagnosed utilizing the modified New York classification criteria, which were originally developed for research and later adapted to the clinical setting. For the diagnosis of definite ankylosing spondylitis, the patient must have at least one of the radiographic criteria (bilateral grade 2 [or higher] sacroiliitis OR grade 3 [or higher] unilateral sacroiliitis) AND one of the following clinical findings: low back pain for a minimum of 3 months associated with stiffness, alleviated with activity, and aggravated by rest; decreased range of motion of the spine in the frontal and sagittal planes; or decreased lung expansion when compared to individuals of the same gender and age. Based on his history, physical examination, and diagnostic studies, Mr. Uno meets the diagnostic criteria for AS. Thus, his most likely diagnosis is plantar fasciitis associated with ankylosing spondylitis. As stated previously, it is not uncommon for patients with ankylosing spondylitis to be afflicted with plantar fascitis.

Incidentally, the diagnosis of probable ankylosing spondylitis via the modified New York classification criteria is defined as having ALL THREE of the aforementioned clinical symptoms OR one of the aforementioned radiologic findings.

C. Diffuse idiopathic skeletal hyperostosis (DISH) with plantar fasciitis   INCORRECT

Diffuse idiopathic skeletal hyperostosis (Forestier disease) is primarily an articular disease that is characterized by calcification and ossification of the paraspinal ligaments. Bony involvement is generally limited to the development of osteophyte formation. Invertebral disc spaces, the sacroiliac joint, and the apophyses are generally spared. The characteristic radiographic finding generally occurs in the late stages of the disease when the ossification of the paraspinous ligaments (especially the anterior longitudinal ligament) is extensive and provides the impression that white wax is flowing over the anterior portion of the vertebral bodies, lending to the descriptive term "flowing wax" appearance.

Because the signs, symptoms, and radiographic features of DISH are inconsistent with Mr. Uno's clinical picture, this cannot be his most correct diagnosis. Additionally, DISH tends to present in a much older age-based population as compared to AS, which generally presents itself in patients in their teens or early 20s. Therefore, even though Mr. Uno has plantar fasciitis based on his history and physical examination findings, DISH with plantar fasciitis is not his most likely diagnosis.

D. Ankylosing hyperostosis with right calcaneus fracture INCORRECT

Ankylosing hyperostosis is another term for DISH; therefore, it can be ruled out based on the aforementioned information. Additionally, a right calcaneus fracture is inconsistent with his diagnosis primarily because calcaneus fractures are unusual without a history of trauma; furthermore, the pain associated with fractures tends to increase with ambulation and be alleviated with rest. Therefore, this is not Mr. Uno's most likely diagnosis.

E. Rheumatoid arthritis of the lumbar spine with a symptomatic posterior calcaneus bone spur   INCORRECT

Even though RA is generally associated with a prolonged period of morning and/or postinactivity stiffness, an elevated ESR, and sometimes a normochromic normocytic anemia, it can be eliminated as a possible cause of Mr. Uno's back pain because RA rarely affects the spine. If there is spinal involvement with RA, it is essentially limited to C1 and C2. Furthermore, RA virtually never involves the sacroiliac joints.

A symptomatic posterior calcaneus bone spur can also be ruled out primarily because his calcaneus tenderness is over the insertion of the plantar fascia, not in the posterior aspect of his heel. Thus, RA of the lumbar spine with a symptomatic posterior calcaneus bone spur can be eliminated as Mr. Uno's most likely diagnosis.

5. Treatment Plan

A. Increase his ibuprofen to 800 mg regularly twice a day CORRECT

NSAIDs on a regular dosing interval are the first-line therapy for the pain of AS. Recent studies indicated that NSAIDs are not only effective in alleviating the pain of sacroiliitis but can also stabilize, and in some cases improve, the radiographic evidence of sacroiliitis. Because there is not one NSAID considered superior to the others nor is there one that works for all patients, if the first medication tried is ineffective, the next most appropriate step is to change to a different NSAID in another NSAID class.

Although virtually all of the NSAIDs are utilized in the treatment of both acute and chronic pain, the majority do not have FDA approval for such. The majority of NSAIDs have an FDA indication for rheumatoid arthritis and/or osteoarthritis. Although ibuprofen does not have an FDA indication for ankylosing spondylitis, some of the other NSAIDs do (e.g., celecoxib, diclofenac, indomethacin, naproxen, and sulindac).

B. Add famotidine 20 to 40 mg once a day   CORRECT

Chronic long-term usage of NSAIDs has been associated with GI complications (e.g., gastritis, peptic ulcer disease, bleeding ulcers, and severe hemorrhage). Multiple studies show that adding a PPI, such as famotidine, significantly reduces the incidence of these complications. However, this is an off-label indication for famotidine. The only PPI that currently has FDA approval for the prevention of NSAID-induced gastric ulcers is lansoprazole.

C. Methotrexate   INCORRECT

Methotrexate, as well as other traditional DMARDs (e.g., sulfasalazine and leflunomide), has not been shown to be effective in the treatment of AS. Therefore, it is not only a poor first-line agent but also a poor choice altogether, except possibly for a patient with significant peripheral joint involvement. However, none of the traditional DMARDs have an FDA indication for ankylosing spondylitis.

D. Infliximab   INCORRECT

Infliximab and other TNF-α inhibitors (e.g., adalimumab and etanercept) have been proven to be very effective in the treatment of patients with AS. However, currently they are only recommended in patients who have failed conventional therapy, but they are FDA approved for this usage. Etanercept and infliximab also carry an FDA indication for psoriatic arthritis.

E. Calcium with vitamin D   CORRECT

Calcium with vitamin D is essential in the treatment of AS because of its association with osteopenia.

Epidemiologic and Other Data

AS, previously known as either Marie-Strümpell disease or Bechterew disease, is an inflammatory arthritis of unknown cause. It is classified as an inflammatory seronegative spondyloarthropathy. Although it is predominately a disease of the spine, peripheral joints and/or extra-articular structures can become involved. Symptoms tend to become apparent in the second or third decades of life. It affects males at a rate that is two to three times that of females.

AS is strongly linked with human leukocyte antigen (HLA)-B27 (one of the histocompatibility antigens), which is found in over 90% of the individuals with this disease. There is a genetic component to the disease. It is much stronger for individuals who have a first-degree relative who is HLA-B27 positive and exhibits AS probands (AS incidence is approximately 10–30%) as compared to individuals who inherit HLA-B27 (AS incidence is approximately 1–6%).

REFERENCES/ADDITIONAL READING

Aghababian RV, ed. *Essentials of Emergency Medicine*. Sudbury, MA: Jones & Bartlett Publishers; 2006:386–390.

Anderson III H. Upper and lower extremity injuries. 940–944.

Habal R. Bony abnormalities. 375–381.

Pierce DL, Jehle DVK. Autoimmune diseases. 291–297.

Pipas L. Overuse syndromes. 391–392.

Roach CN, Bensinger G. Disorders of the Spine. 386–390.

Sloan B. Joint disorders. 382–385.

American Association of Oral and Maxillofacial Surgeons Task Force on Bisphosphonate-Related Osteonecrosis of the Jaws. American Association of Oral and Maxillofacial Surgeons Position paper on bisphosphonate-related osteonecrosis of the jaw—2009 update. *AAOMS*. 2009; 1–23.

American College of Physicians and American Pain Society. Diagnosis and treatment of low back pain: a joint clinical practice guideline from the American College of Physicians and the American Pain Society. *Ann Intern Med*. 2007;147: 478–491.

American College of Physicians and American Pain Society. Reviews of evidence for medications for low back pain. *Ann Intern Med*. 2007;147:505–514.

American College of Physicians and American Pain Society. Reviews of evidence for nonpharmacologic therapies for low back pain. *Ann Intern Med*. 2007;147:492–504.

American College of Rheumatology Subcommittee on Osteoarthritis Guidelines. Recommendations for the medical management of osteoarthritis of the hip and knee. *Arthritis Rheum*. 2000;43:1905–1915.

American College of Rheumatology Committee to Reevaluate Improvement Criteria. A proposed revision to the ACR20: the hybrid measure of the American College of Rheumatology. *Arthritis Rheum*. 2007;57(2):193–202.

American Geriatrics Society Panel on the Pharmacological Management of Persistent Pain in Older Persons. Pharmacological management of persistent pain in older persons *J Am Geriatr Soc*. 2009;57:1331–1346.

American Psychiatric Association. Somatoform disorders. In: American Psychiatric Association. *Diagnostic and Statistical Manual of Mental Disorders*. 4th ed., text revision. Washington, DC: American Psychiatric Association; 2000:485–511.

Arnett FC, Edworthy SM, Bolch DA, et al. The American Rheumatism Association 1987 revised criteria for the classification of rheumatoid arthritis. *Arthritis Rheum*. 1988;31(3): 315–324.

Arnold LM, Clauw DJ, Wohlreich MM, et al. Efficacy of duloxetine in patients with fibromyalgia: pooled analysis of 4 placebo-controlled clinical trials. *Prim Care Companion J Clin Psychiatry*. 2009;11(5):237–244.

Arnold LM, Gendreau RM, Spera, et al. Milnacipran 100 m/day in the management of fibromyalgia: a randomized, double-blind placebo-controlled trial. *AAPM*. 2010; Abstract 109.

Arnold LM, Hess EV, Hudson JI, et al. A randomized, placebo-controlled, double-blind, flexible-dose study of fluoxetine in the treatment of women with fibromyalgia. *Am J Med*. 2002;112:191–197.

Arthritis Foundation. Supplementation guide. http://www.arthritis.org/glucosamine.php. Accessed December 11, 2008.

Assefi NP, Sherman KJ, Jacobsen C, et al. A randomized clinical trial of acupuncture compared with sham acupuncture in fibromyalgia. *Ann Intern Med*. 2005;143(1):10–19.

Atlas SJ. Nonpharmacological treatment for low back pain. *J Musculoskel Med*. 2009;27:1–7.

Bachman LM, Haberzeth S, Steurer J, et al. The accuracy of the Ottawa knee rule to rule out knee fractures: a systemic review. *Ann Inn Med*. 2004;140(2):121–124.

Braun J, Baraliakos X. Treatment of ankylosing spondylitis and other spondyloarthritides. *Curr Opin Rheumatol*. 2009;21 (4):324–334.

Braun J, Sieper J. Ankylosing spondylitis. *Lancet*. 2007;369: 1379–1390.

Burns CM, Wortmann RL. Gout therapeutics: new drugs for an old disease. *Lancet*;2010; doi:10.1016/S0140-6736(10) 60665-4.

Bykerek VP, Keystone EC. What are the goals and principles of management in the early treatment of rheumatoid arthritis? *Best Pract Res Clin Rheumatol* 2005;19:147–155.

Carette S, Bell MJ, Reynolds WJ, et al. Comparison of amitriptyline, cyclobenzaprine, and placebo in the treatment of fibromyalgia. A randomized, double-blind clinical trial. *Arthritis Rheum*. 1994;37:32–40.

Carville SF, Arendt-Nielsen S, Biddal H, et al. EULAR evidence-based recommendations for the management of fibromyalgia syndrome. *Ann Rheum Dis*. 2008;67(4): 536–541.

Centers for Disease Control and Prevention. Targeting arthritis: improving quality of life for more than 46 million Americans. At a Glance 2008. http://www.cdc.gov/nccdphp/publications/AAG/arthritis.htm. Accessed December 11, 2008.

Christian SR, Anderson MB, Workman R, et al. Imaging of anterior knee pain. *Clin Sports Med*. 2006;25(4):681–702.

Dalton BR, Lye-Maccannell T, Henderson EA, Maccannell DR, Louie TJ. Proton pump inhibitors increase significantly the risk of *Clostridium difficile* infection in a low-endemicity, non-outbreak hospital setting. *Aliment Pharmacol Ther*. 2009;29:626–634.

EULAR Standing Committee for International Clinical Studies Including Therapeutics. EULAR evidence based recommendations for gout. Part I: diagnosis. Report of a taskforce of the Standing Committee for International Clinical Studies Including Therapeutics (ESCISIT). *Ann Rheum Dis*. 2006;65 (10):1301–1311.

EULAR Standing Committee for International Clinical Studies Including Therapeutics. EULAR evidence based recommendations for gout. Part II: Management. Report of a taskforce of the Standing Committee for International Clinical Studies Including Therapeutics (ESCISIT). *Ann Rheum Dis*. 2006;65(10):1312–1324.

Fauci AS, Kasper DL, Longo DL, et al., eds. *Harrison's Principles of Internal Medicine*. 17th ed. New York: McGraw-Hill Medical; 2008.

Bacon B. Cirrhosis and its complications. 1971–1980.

Cush JJ, Lipsky PE. Approaches to articular and musculoskeletal disorders. 2149–2158.

Engstrom JW. Back and neck pain. 107–113.

Felson DT. Osteoarthritis. 2158–2165.

Langford CA, Gilliland BC. Fibromyalgia. 2175–2177.

Langford C, Gilliland BC. Arthritis associated with systemic disease and other arthritides. 2177–2186.

Lipsky P. Rheumatoid arthritis. 2083–2094.

Mailliard ME, Sorrell MF. Alcoholic liver disease. 1969–1971.

Parsonnet J. Osteomyelitis. 803–807.

Schumacher HR, Chen LX. Gout and other crystal-associated arthropathies. 2165–2168.

Taurog JD. The spondyloarthritides. 2109–2119.

Fredericson M, Yoon K. Physical examination and patellofemoral pain syndrome. *Am J Phys Med Rehabil.* 2006; 85(3):234–243.

Glodenbery DL, Felson DT, Dinerman H. A randomized, controlled trial of amitriptyline and naproxen in the treatment of patients with fibromyalgia. *Arthritis Rheum.* 1986;29 (11):1371–1377.

Goodwin DL, Clauw DJ, Palmer RH, Mease P, Chen W, and Gendreau RM. Durability of Therapeutic Response to Milnacipran Treatment for Fibromyalgia. Results of a Randomized, Double-Blind, Monotherapy 6-Month Extension Study. *Pain Medicine* 2010;11(2):180–194.

Gramenzi A, Caputo F, Bisselli M, et al. Review article: alcoholic liver disease—pathophysiological aspects and risk factors. *Aliment Pharmacol Ther.* 2006;24(8): 1151–1161.

Katz P, Lee F. Racial/ethnic differences in the use of complementary and alternative medicine in patients with arthritis. *J Clin Rheumatol.* 2007;13:3–11.

Khan MA, Clegg DO, Deodhar AA, et al. 2006 annual research and educational meeting of the Spondyloarthritis Research and Therapy Network (SPARTAN). *J Rheumatol.* 2007;34:1118–1124.

Lafforgue P. Pathophysiology and natural history of avascular necrosis of bone. *Joint Bone Spine.* 2006;73(5):500–507.

Mease PJ, Clauw DJ, Gendreau RM, et al. The efficacy and safety of milnacipran for treatment of fibromyalgia. A randomized, double-blind, placebo-controlled trial. *J Rheumatol.* 2009;36(2):398–409.

Mease PJ, Russell IJ, Arnold LM, et al. A randomized, double-blind, placebo-controlled, phase III trial of pregabalin in the treatment of patients with fibromyalgia. *J Rheumatol.* 2008;35 (3):502–513.

Mease PJ. Fibromyalgia syndrome: a review of clinical presentation, pathogenesis, outcome measures, and treatment. *J Rheumatol Suppl.* 2005;75:S6–S21.

Mengel MP, Schwiebert LP. *Family Medicine: Ambulatory Care and Prevention.* 5th ed. New York: McGraw-Hill Medical; 2009.

Kaminski MA. Knee Complaints. 271–278.

Schwiebert LP. Joint pain. 263–271.

Mikuls TR, Saag KG. Gout treatment: what is evidence-based and how do we determine and promote optimized clinical care? *Curr Rheum Rep.* 2005;7:242–248.

Novartis Consumer Health Inc. Voltaren gel package insert (42035D). Parsippany, NJ: Novartis Consumer Health, Inc. 2009.

Onion DK, series ed. *The Little Black Book of Primary Care.* 5th ed. Sudbury, MA: Jones & Bartlett Publishers; 2006.

Onion DK. Rheumatology/Orthopedics. 18.5 Collagen vascular diseases. 1074–1100.

Onion DK. Rheumatology/Orthopedics. 18.6 Crystal diseases. 1100–1103.

Onion DK. Rheumatology/Orthopedics. 18.7 Inherited and other rheumatologic diseases. 1104–1118.

Onion DK. Rheumatology/Orthopedics. 18.8 Entrapment syndromes. 1118–1130.

Onion DK. Rheumatology/Orthopedics. 18.10 Miscellaneous. 1134–1145.

Pae CU, Marks DM, Shah M, et al. Milnacipran: beyond a role of antidepressant. *Clin Neuropharmacol.* 2009;32(6): 355–363.

Pagana KD, Pagana TJ. *Mosby's Diagnostic and Laboratory Test Reference.* 8th ed. St. Louis: Mosby Elsevier; 2007 (multiple pages utilized to provide normal reference values for laboratory tests).

Pascual E, Sivea F. Why is gout so poorly managed? *Ann Rheum Dis.* 2007;66:1269–1270.

Phillips C, Brasington Jr. RD. Osteoarthritis treatment update: are NSAIDs still in the picture? *J Musculoskel Med.* 2010;27(2): 65–71.

Rayan GM. Dupuytren disease: anatomy, pathology, presentation, and treatment. *J Bone Joint Surg Am.* 2007;89(1): 189–198.

Rudwaleit M, Khan MA, Sieper J. The challenge of diagnosis and classification in early ankylosing spondylitis: do we need new criteria? *Arthritis Rheum.* 2005;52:1000–1008.

Russell IJ, Mease PH, Smith TR, et al. Efficacy and safety of duloxetine for treatment in patients with or without major depressive disorder: results from a 6-month, randomized, double-blind, placebo-controlled, fixed-dose trial. *Pain.* 2008;136(3):432–444.

Saag KG, Teng GG, Patkar NM, et al. American College of Rheumatology 2008 recommendations for the use of nonbiological and biologic disease-modifying antirheumatic drugs in rheumatoid arthritis. *Arthritis Rheum.* 2008;59(6):762–784.

Sarac AJ, Gur A. Complementary and alternative medical therapies in fibromyalgia. *Curr Pharm Des.* 2006;12(1):47–57.

Singh JA, Hodges JS, Toscano JP, Asch SM. Quality of care for gout in the US needs improvement. *Arthritis Rheum.* 2007;57:822–829.

Townley WA, Baker R, Sheppard N, Grobbelaar AO. Dupuytren's contracture unfolded. *BMJ.* 2006;332(7538): 397–400.

Turk DC, Wilson HD. Managing fibromyalgia: an update on diagnosis and treatment. *J Musculoskel Med.* 2009;10:1–8.

US Food and Drug Administration. FDA approves new drug for gout. FDA News Release 2009: February 13. http://www.fda.gov/NewsEvents/Newsroom/PressAnnouncements/2009/ucm149534.htm. Accessed February 13, 2009.

US Food and Drug Administration. FDA approves new drug for gout. FDA News Release 2010: September 14. http://www.fda.gov/NewsEvents/Newsroom/PressAnnouncements/ucm225810.htm. Accessed August 18, 2010.

US Food and Drug Administration. FDA approves Xiaflex for debilitating hand condition. FDA News Release 2010: February 2. http://www.fda.gov/NewsEvents/Newsroom/PressAnnouncements/ucm199736.htm. Accessed February 4, 2010.

US Food and Drug Administration. Potential Signals of Serious Risks/New Safety Information Identified from the Adverse Event Reporting System (AERS) between April - June 2010. http://www.fda.gov/Drugs/GuidanceComplianceRegulatoryInformation/Surveillance/AdverseDrugEffects/ucm223734.htm. Accessed September 18, 2010.

Van Linschoten R, van Middelkoop M, Berger MY, et al. Supervised exercise therapy versus usual care for patellofemoral pain syndrome: an open label randomised controlled trial. *BMJ*. 2009;339:b4074.

Voelker R, for the American Academy of Orthopaedic Surgeons (AAOS). Guideline provides evidence-based advice for treating osteoarthritis of the knee. *JAMA*. 2009; 301(5):475–476.

Wandel S, Jüni P, Tendal B, et al. Effects of glucosamine, chondroitin, or placebo in patients with osteoarthritis of hip or knee: network meta-analysis. *BMJ* 2010;341: c4675.

Wolfe F, Cathey MA, Hawley DJ. A double-blind placebo controlled trial of fluoxetine in fibromyalgia. *Scand J Rheumatol*. 1994;23:255–259.

Woo SB, Hellstein JW, and Kalmar JR. Narrative review: bisphosphonates and osteonecrosis of the jaws. *Ann Intern Med*. 2006;144(10):753–761.

Zhang W, Moskowitz RW, Nuki G, et al. OARSI recommendations for the management of hip and knee osteoarthritis, part I: critical appraisal of existing treatment guidelines and systematic review of current research evidence. *Osteoarthritis Cartilage*. 2007;15(9):981–1000.

Zhang W, Moskowitz RW, Nuki G, et al. OARSI recommendations for the management of hip and knee osteoarthritis, part II: IARSI evidence-based, expert consensus guidelines. *Osteoarthritis Cartilage*. 2007;16(2):137–162.

Zochling J, van der Heijde D, Burgos-Vagas R, et al. ASAS/ EULAR recommendations for the management of ankylosing spondylitis. *Ann Rheum Dis*. 2006;65:442–452.

CASES IN NEUROLOGIC CONDITIONS*

CASE 9-1

Unger Valley

Mr. Valley is a 25-year-old white male who presents with the chief complaint of "headaches." They are located in and around his left eye. He has experienced them intermittently for approximately 4 months. The headaches occur "all the sudden" without warning or provocation. They are sharp in nature and associated with "horrendous" pain ("15" out of 10 on the pain scale). They will last approximately a half hour; then, they resolve just "as quickly as they came." When his headaches occur, he experiences three or four per day for 3 to 4 consecutive days; then, he is essentially asymptomatic for approximately 1.5 months when he experiences that same headache pattern.

Yesterday, he began experiencing headaches again. They are identical to those he previously had. He experienced four seemingly unrelated headaches yesterday, and he has suffered with two thus far today; however, he is not currently experiencing one. He has tried over-the-counter acetaminophen, ibuprofen, and naproxen for them; however, none of these medications were effective in decreasing the length or lessening the severity of the pain.

He did not experience a head injury prior to the onset of his headaches. He's unsure if his headaches are associated with photophobia, phonophobia, diplopia, or other visual disturbances, because they are so severe he "doesn't notice anything else." However, he is certain that they are not associated with nausea, vomiting, lightheadedness, vertigo, presyncope, syncope, problems with ambulation, gait abnormalities, difficulty using his extremities, paresthesias, dysesthesias, aphasia, or other focal neurologic deficits.

He has no known medical problems, never had surgery, and never been hospitalized. He is currently not taking any prescription or over-the-counter medications, vitamins, supplements, or herbal preparations. He is not allergic to any medications. He does not smoke, and he drinks alcohol rarely (approximately one or two drinks per month). The headaches are not related to the consumption of alcohol. His family history is negative, including headaches.

1. Based on this information, which of the following questions are essential to ask Mr. Valley and why?

   A. Are his headaches associated with redness of his eyes, changes in his pupils, lacrimation, edema of his eyelids, drooping of his eyelids, sweating of his forehead or face, nasal congestion, or rhinorrhea?
   B. Does lying down affect his headaches?
   C. Does he experience any bowel changes with the headaches?
   D. Does he experience nocturnal symptoms?
   E. Has he had any changes in his appetite, sleep, mood, interest, activities, or pleasures?

Patient Responses

Mr. Valley has noticed his left eyelid looking swollen and droopy, his left conjunctivae being injected, and his left pupil being very small during the episodes. He has also noticed sweating on his left forehead only. He has not noticed any nasal symptoms. He cannot lie down and rest during the episodes because they seem to make him "agitated and anxious." Therefore, he tends to pace when he gets them. He has never had any bowel changes associated with them.

He has been awakened at night by a headache requiring him to walk around his apartment until it resolved; however, this only occurred once during his initial episode of headaches approximately 3 months prior. He states that he is "anxious" when he experiences the headaches; however, this symptom is completely resolved when he is not experiencing a headache. He denies any other mood disturbances, changes in his appetite, sleeping difficulties, anhedonia, constipation, diarrhea, or other bowel changes.

---

*Remember, for each question, none to all of the answers could be correct/essential or incorrect/nonessential. See page 353 for Chapter 9 answers.

2. Based on this information, which of the following components of a physical examination are essential to perform on Mr. Valley and why?

    A. Palpation of the head
    B. Palpation of the thyroid
    C. Abdominal examination
    D. Cranial nerve evaluation
    E. Cursory neurologic examination, with further evaluation of any abnormalities identified

Physical Examination Findings

Mr. Valley is 5'9" tall and weighs 162 lb (BMI = 23.9). Other vital signs are blood pressure (BP), 124/68 mm Hg; pulse, 78 beats per minute (BPM) and regular; respiratory rate, 14/min and regular; and oral temperature, 98.3°F.

His head is normocephalic, symmetric, and without gross defects, discoloration, or rash. It is not tender to palpate over his cervical, cranial, and facial muscles and arteries. His cranial nerves are grossly intact.

His heart is regular in rate and rhythm and without any murmurs, gallops, or rubs. His thyroid is not palpable or tender, bilaterally. His abdomen is unremarkable.

He has good and equal strength and sensation (to sharp and dull) in his extremities. His gait is normal. His Romberg is negative. Finger to nose, heel to shin, and finger to examiner's finger are all intact and normal.

3. Based on this information, which of the following diagnostic tests are essential to perform on Mr. Valley at this time and why?

    A. Computed tomography (CT) of the brain
    B. Magnetic resonance imaging (MRI) of the brain
    C. Thyroid scintiscan
    D. Erythrocyte sedimentation rate (ESR)
    E. Complete blood count with differential (CBC w/diff)

Diagnostic Test Results

Mr. Valley's CT, MRI, and thyroid scintiscan were all reported as normal. His ESR was 2 mm/hr (normal adult male: < 15). His CBC was within normal limits.

4. Based on this information, which one of the following is Mr. Valley's most likely diagnosis and why?

    A. Migraine headaches without aura
    B. Episodic cluster headaches
    C. Migraine headaches with aura
    D. Paroxysmal hemicrania
    E. Chronic cluster headaches

5. Which of the following are essential components of Mr. Valley's treatment plan and why?

    A. Trial sumatriptan (6 mg SQ or 20 mg intranasally) at onset of headache
    B. Look for triggers of headaches
    C. Discuss possibility of prophylaxis treatment with patient, including potential adverse effects of medications, advantages, and disadvantages

    D. Oxygen therapy
    E. If headache persists beyond a half hour, increases in frequency, increases in intensity, becomes associated with focal neurologic defects, or changes in any way, return to clinic or go to emergency department (ED) immediately

CASE 9-2
Vinnie Winchester

Mr. Winchester is a 39-year-old African American male who presents with the chief complaint of "hands shaking." It has been present for approximately 1 year and appears to be getting worse. It affects both hands equally. He notices that it is most prevalent when he attempts to write, eat soup, or drink from a full cup or glass. It varies in intensity; in fact, he states that it gets so severe that "sometimes I can't even read my own handwriting." The problem worsens with stress and consuming caffeine; however, drinking alcohol appears to temporarily alleviate it. He knows of no other aggravating or alleviating factors. He works as a salesman and is required to frequently entertain clients; therefore, this problem is very embarrassing for him.

He denies any seizurelike activity. He does not have any tremor at rest, in his head, or in his legs, nor does he have any difficulty with gait, tics, speech, jerks, or movement disorders. He denies any significant stressors; an increased stress level; any major life changes (negative or positive); problems with his mood; anhedonia; or changes in sleep, appetite, weight, or activities.

He has no known medical problems. He has never had surgery nor been hospitalized. He does not take any prescription or over-the-counter medications, vitamins, supplements, or herbal preparations. He is not allergic to any medications. He has never smoked nor used illicit substances. He drinks alcohol occasionally (averages one to two drinks two to three times per week). His family history is positive for his father having "senile tremors."

1. Based on this information, which of the following questions are essential to ask Mr. Winchester and why?

    A. Has he experienced any problems with memory or confusion?
    B. Has he had abdominal pain, nausea, vomiting, bowel changes, jaundice, or icterus?
    C. How old was his father when he was first diagnosed with senile tremors?
    D. Has he had palpitations, dyspnea, fever, heat or cold intolerance, changes in perspiration, polydipsia, polyuria, vertigo, lightheadedness, presyncope, or syncope?
    E. Does he experience any problems with balance and/or coordination?

Patient Responses

Mr. Winchester denies problems with memory, confusion, abdominal pain, nausea, vomiting, bowel changes, jaundice, icterus, vertigo, lightheadedness, presyncope, syncope, palpitations, dyspnea, fever, heat or cold intolerance, changes in perspiration, polydipsia, polyuria, gait, balance, or coordination.

His father was 70 years when he was first diagnosed with senile tremors.

2. Based on this information, which of the following components of a physical examination are essential to perform on Mr. Winchester and why?

- **A.** Cornea examination
- **B.** Thyroid examination
- **C.** Cervical spine examination
- **D.** Abdominal examination
- **E.** Cursory neurologic examination, with extended exam if problems are identified

Physical Examination Findings

Mr. Winchester is 5'8" tall and weighs 152 lb (BMI = 23.1). Other vital signs are BP, 122/68 mm Hg; pulse, 76 BPM and regular; respirations, 14/min and regular; and oral temperature, 98.8°F.

His corneas are clear and without any discoloration.

His thyroid is smooth, nontender, palpable, and normal and equal in size bilaterally. His cervical spine exhibits full range of motion and no muscle tenderness or muscle spasms.

Mr. Winchester's abdomen reveals normoactive and equal bowel sounds in all four quadrants. It is soft, nontender, and without masses or organomegaly.

His facial expressions and affect are appropriate. His cranial nerves are grossly intact. His gait and ambulatory coordination are normal with appropriate use of his arms. There is no evidence of bradykinesia. Holding his arms outstretched reveals no arm drift, but does reveal a very mild flexion/extension tremor of hands and arms. The tremor is equal bilaterally and does not vary with distraction. Finger to nose, finger to examiner's finger, and drinking from a cup produces an intention tremor that is slightly less than when he holds his arms in the outstretched position. No tremor is elicited in his legs. Muscle strength in his hands, arms, legs, and feet is normal and equal bilaterally, with no evidence of atrophy. His biceps, triceps, brachioradialis, knee, ankle, and plantar reflexes are normal bilaterally. His sensation is intact to both sharp and dull stimulation in both his arms and legs and is equal bilaterally.

3. Based on this information, which of the following diagnostic tests are essential to perform on Mr. Winchester at this time and why?

- **A.** Thyroid-stimulating hormone (TSH)
- **B.** Liver functioning tests (LFTs)
- **C.** Serum copper (Cu) and ceruloplasmin levels
- **D.** Electroencephalography (EEG)
- **E.** Computed tomography (CT) of the brain

Diagnostic Test Results

Mr. Winchester's TSH was 3.4 µU/ml (normal adult: 2–10). His liver functioning testing consisted of an alkaline phosphatase (ALP) of 50 units/L (normal adult: 30–120), aspartate aminotransferase (AST) of 12 units/L (normal adult: 0–35), and alanine aminotransferase (ALT) of 2 units/L (normal adult: 4–36). His serum copper (Cu) level and ceruloplasmin levels were also normal. The EEG and CT of his brain did not reveal any abnormalities.

4. Based on this information, which of the following is Mr. Winchester's most likely diagnosis and why?

- **A.** Parkinson disease
- **B.** Psychogenic tremor
- **C.** Wilson disease
- **D.** Benign essential tremor
- **E.** Multiple system atrophy

5. Which of the following components are essential parts of Mr. Winchester's treatment plan and why?

- **A.** Primidone 12.5 mg once daily, then gradually increase the dose until symptoms resolve or a maximum dose of 1000 mg is attained, if tolerated
- **B.** Long-acting propranolol 20 mg once a day
- **C.** Relaxation therapy course
- **D.** Liver biopsy
- **E.** Botulinum toxin type A injections

CASE 9-3
Willamette Xandier

Mrs. Xandier is a 76-year-old African American female who presents to the ED complaining of right-sided weakness and difficulty with speech. Her symptoms began approximately 30 minutes ago while she was preparing her breakfast. The weakness affects her right arm, leg, and face. She denies any symptoms on the left side of her body. Her dysarthria involves poorly formed sounds, making it difficult for others to understand her. Her son, who was visiting her when the symptoms began, insisted on bringing her to the ED.

She is experiencing some difficulty with gait as a result of the weakness in her right leg, but she can walk unassisted. She denies headaches, nausea, vomiting, lightheadedness, vertigo, presyncope, syncope, altered level of consciousness, difficulty remembering words, other memory problems, visual abnormalities, chest pain/pressure, pyrosis, dyspnea, wheezing, fever, chills, or any recent/present infections within the previous 6 months. Her son confirms these responses.

She has experienced identical symptoms on approximately five or six occasions during the previous 3 to 4 months. According to Mrs. Xandier, each of the previous episodes resolved just as abruptly as it began, approximately 20 to 30 minutes from its onset. The last episode was 4 to 5 days ago while she was preparing breakfast.

Her past medical history is positive for hypertension; however, she has never been diagnosed as having a transient ischemic attack (TIA) or a cerebrovascular accident (CVA). She has been hospitalized for childbirth three times and has never had any surgeries. Her only medication is triamterene/hydrochlorothiazide 37.5/25 mg once daily. She is on no other prescription or over-the-counter medications, vitamins, supplements, or herbal preparations. She was on hormone replacement for approximately 2 years when she went through menopause (at 52 years old); however, she has not been on it since. She is allergic to aspirin, which caused severe swelling of her face, near closure of her eyelids, inversion of her lips, and marked dyspnea. She has never smoked nor drank alcohol. She lives alone since her husband died

3 years ago. Her son lives "nearby" and "checks on her" as frequently as possible. Her other two children reside out of state. Her family history is positive for fatal myocardial infarction (mother at the age of 76 years) and ischemic cerebral vascular disease (father had multiple CVAs starting at the age of 65 years until a fatal one occurred at the age of 70 years).

1. Based on this information, which of the following questions are essential to ask Mrs. Xandier and why?

   A. What was she preparing for breakfast this morning and the last time she experienced these symptoms?
   B. Is she experiencing any paresthesias or dysesthesias?
   C. Is she experiencing any dysphagia?
   D. Is she experiencing any palpitations?
   E. Were any of these episodes associated with a fall, loss of consciousness, seizurelike activity, or incontinence of her bladder and/or bowels?

Patient Responses

She was preparing oatmeal on both occasions; however, she has oatmeal for breakfast every day.

She is experiencing some "numbness" (described as "feeling funny") and "tingling" around the right side of her mouth. She denies any paresthesias/dysesthesias elsewhere. She denies dysphagia, palpitations, falls, loss of consciousness, seizurelike activity, or incontinence of her bladder and/or bowels with any of the episodes.

2. Based on this information, which components of a physical examination are essential to perform on Mrs. Xandier and why?

   A. BP in all four extremities (in addition to regular vital sign assessment)
   B. Evaluation of all pulses
   C. Heart and lung examination
   D. Neurologic examination
   E. HINTS (**H**ead **I**mpulse/**N**ystagmus/**T**est of **S**kew) testing

Physical Examination Findings

Mrs. Xandier is 5'3" tall and weighs 180 lb (BMI = 31.9). Other vital signs are BP, 176/98 in her right arm and 174/92 in her left arm; pulse, 90 BPM and regular; respirations, 12/min and regular; and oral temperature, 98.7°F. Her systolic BP in her ankles is 180 mm Hg on the left and 182 mm Hg on the right (ankle-brachial index [ABI] ≥ 1).

Her heart is regular in rate and rhythm and without murmur, gallop, or rub. Her apical impulse is nondisplaced and without a thrill. Her lungs are clear to auscultation.

Her carotid, subclavian, and renal arteries are normal and equal bilaterally and without bruits. Her aorta is normal size, nonpulsatile, and without a bruit. Brachial, ulnar, radial, femoral, popiteal, dorsalis pedis, and posterior tibial pulses are normal and equal bilaterally. There is no abnormal discoloration, temperature changes, or lesions on her feet. Her capillary refill is normal bilaterally. She does not have any pedal edema.

Her cranial nerves are intact except she cannot raise her right eyebrow, has slight weakness of her right eyelid, cannot fully smile on the right side of her mouth, and cannot puff out and hold her cheeks. There is no deviation of her tongue,

palate, or uvula. She does not have any evidence of a nystagmus of abnormal skew.

Her right hand and forearm are weaker than her left. Holding her arms outstretched reveals a slight arm drift with ulnar deviation on the right and no arm drift on the left. No tremor is present. Finger to nose, finger to examiner's finger, and drinking from a cup are normal but done slower than average. Her right thigh, lower leg, and foot are weaker than her left. She has mild difficulty in walking as she appears to be slightly dragging her right leg. She cannot do heel-to-toe walking, walk on her heels, or walk on her toes without losing her balance. She can walk in a circle but does it very slowly with many extra steps. There is no evidence of muscle atrophy.

Her biceps, triceps, brachioradialis, knee, ankle, and plantar reflexes are normal and equal bilaterally.

Her sensation is intact to both sharp and dull stimulation in both her arms and legs and is equal bilaterally. She has some decreased sensation to light touch around the right perioral area only. The remainder of her face reveals normal discrimination to sharp and dull stimulation with equal subjective sensation bilaterally.

3. Based on this information, which of the following diagnostic studies are essential to perform on Mrs. Xandier and why?

   A. Computed tomography (CT) of the brain with and without contrast
   B. Electrocardiogram (ECG)
   C. Random plasma glucose (RPG)
   D. Lipid profile
   E. Serial cardiac troponin I and T

Diagnostic Test Findings

Mrs. Xandier's CT of her brain was normal and did not reveal any evidence of either a hemorrhagic or ischemic CVA.

Her ECG showed normal sinus rhythm at a rate of 90 BPM. No abnormalities were seen.

Although a random plasma glucose was ordered, Mrs. Xandier's test was actually a fasting plasma glucose because she didn't eat breakfast; it was 86 mg/dl (normal adult, fasting: 70–110).

Her total cholesterol was 250 mg/dl (normal average-risk adult: < 200), with a high-density lipoprotein (HDL) of 30 mg/dl (normal average-risk adult female: > 55), a low-density lipoprotein (LDL) of 184 mg/dl (normal average-risk adult: 60–180), and a very-low-density lipoprotein (VLDL) of 36 mg/dl (normal average-risk adult: 7–32). Her triglycerides (TGs) were 180 mg/dl (normal average-risk adult female: 35–135).

Her cardiac troponin I was 0.01 ng/ml (normal: < 0.03) and her cardiac troponin T was 0.08 ng/ml (normal: < 0.2).

While these tests were being performed, Mrs. Xandier's symptoms completely resolved subjectively and objectively.

4. Based on this information, in addition to obesity and hypertension, which of the following is Mrs. Xandier's most likely diagnosis and why?

   A. Transient ischemic attack (TIA)
   B. Cerebrovascular accident (CVA) affecting the right anterior cerebral artery
   C. Migraine headache with transient neurologic symptoms

D. Amaurosis fugax

E. Cerebrovascular accident (CVA) affecting the right posterior cerebral artery

5. Which of the following are appropriate components of the treatment plan for Mrs. Xandier and why?

A. Hospitalization

B. Echocardiogram, carotid ultrasound, and lipid panel

C. Aspirin plus dipyridamole 25/200 mg twice a day

D. Clopidogrel 75 mg daily

E. Atorvastatin 80 mg daily

F. Referral for carotid endarterectomy

CASE 9-4

Xeb Yellowstone

Xeb is a 4-year-old Native American male who is accompanied by his parents because his pre-K teacher advised them to have Xeb "evaluated for ADHD" (attention-deficit/hyperactivity disorder). His parents state that his teacher has noticed intermittent episodes of Xeb "refusing to pay attention." The teacher estimates that this behavior persists for "a minute or two at the most" but recurs several times daily. She has tried various techniques in an attempt to obtain his attention, including shaking him, patting his face, snapping her fingers in front of his eyes, and clapping her hands beside his ear; however, none of these have proven successful. She advised his parents that despite any attempt to stimulate him he just "sits and stares." These episodes are associated with him constantly "picking at his shirt tail" with both of his hands. When she does finally get his "attention," he appears to be "normal" but he denies any knowledge of the preceding event. Furthermore, his parents state that his teacher is also concerned because he occasionally appears to "get lost" when he is speaking. According to the account reported to his parents, he will be talking and abruptly ceases for a few seconds. During these episodes, his behavior is virtually identical to that displayed when he "decides not to pay attention." Afterward, he frequently "picks up where he left off." With the exception of these concerns, his teacher told his parents that he is a "delightful boy who is eager to learn." He completes his assignments on time, does not make careless mistakes, and overall does "pretty good" with his work.

Xeb's parents have noticed similar episodes occurring at home during the previous 2 to 3 months. His mother estimates that on the days he does not go to school, they can occur as frequently as five to six times per hour, but they do not appear to be escalating in terms of frequency, intensity, or severity. They did not appear to interfere with Xeb's activity and they were not "too concerned" until yesterday evening. According to Xeb's father, who witnessed the event, Xeb was crossing the street to retrieve their mail (which he has done independently without difficulty on numerous previous occasions) and "just stopped" in the middle of the road. His father yelled for him to move, but Xeb didn't respond. His father began running toward Xeb while continuing to scream for him to move. He managed to grab Xeb and get him to safety "just seconds" before an approaching car reached the location where Xeb was previously standing. Despite appearing "frozen in place," Xeb

felt "normal" to his father when he grabbed him, except he failed to encircle his father's neck with his arms as he normally does when his father picks him up. In fact, his only movement initially was "picking at" the hem of his shirt. However, this quickly resolved and he was interacting normally by the time they got to the curb. Xeb's only memory of the event is starting across the street and ending up in his father's arms.

Neither his parents nor his teacher have noticed any other symptoms related or unrelated to these episodes. Additionally, they are unaware of any aggravating or alleviating factors. He was not ill prior to the onset of his symptoms.

Xeb has no known medical problems. His was a full-term infant who was delivered vaginally without complications. There were no problems prenatally, antenatally, or postnatally. He has never had a serious injury or illness, been hospitalized, or had surgery. His parents and pediatrician (who does regular preventive health check-ups on him) feel he is developing normally. His immunizations are up to date. He does not take any prescription or over-the-counter medications, vitamins, supplements, or herbal preparations. He is not allergic to any medications. His family history is negative.

1. Based on this information, which of the following questions are essential to ask Xeb's parents regarding his symptoms and why?

A. Do they have any pets or does Xeb frequently visit where pets reside?

B. Have they noticed any problems or have any concerns with any of the following: speech, behavior, anger, impulsiveness, frustration, purposeless activities, inability to sit still, inability to concentrate on TV shows or whatever activity he is engaged in, inability to complete tasks, frequently losing things, talking excessively, interrupting others, fidgeting, "always being on the go," or poor self-esteem?

C. Has he ever lost control of his bladder or bowels during the episodes or has he experienced any nausea, sweating, dysphagia, vertigo, presyncope, syncope, loss of consciousness, hallucinations, or inappropriate affect/behavior?

D. Has he been complaining of or have his parents noticed any signs of headaches, stiff neck, fever, chills, malaise, fatigue, cough, wheezing, vomiting, changes in bowel movements, dysuria, hematuria, or urinary frequency?

E. Have they noticed him experiencing polyuria, polydipsia, a weight change, or an abnormal smell to his breath?

Patient Responses

They do not have any pets in the home; however, they do have two cats that they keep outdoors. He does not visit regularly where there are animals. Other than the aforementioned problems, his parents have not noticed any difficulties with Xeb's speech.

They do not feel he has any behavioral problems including problems with anger, impulsiveness, frustration, purposeless activities, inability to sit still, inability to concentrate on TV shows or whatever activity he is involved in, frequently losing things, talking excessively, interrupting others, fidgeting, "always being on the go," or poor self-esteem.

He has not lost control of his bladder or bowels during the episodes. Additionally, they have not noticed nor has he complained of nausea, diaphoresis, dysphagia, vertigo, presyncope, syncope, loss of consciousness, hallucinations, inappropriate affect/behavior, headaches, stiff neck, fever, chills, malaise, fatigue, cough, wheezing, vomiting, bowel changes, dysuria, hematuria, urinary frequency, polyuria, polydipsia, weight change, or an abnormal smell to his breath.

2. Based on this information, which of the following components of a physical examination are essential to perform on Xeb and why?

    A. Ear, nose, and throat (ENT) examination
    B. Palpation of thyroid
    C. Heart and lung examination
    D. Neurologic examination
    E. Assessment of behavior during the examination

Physical Examination Findings

Xeb is 42" tall and weighs 32 lb. Other vital signs are BP, 80/46 mm Hg; pulse, 110 BPM and regular; respirations, 20 and regular; and oral temperature, 98.6°F.

His auditory canals are clear, nonerythematous, and without abnormal discharge, bilaterally. His tympanic membranes are nonerythematous, not injected, and display normal movement, bilaterally. He exhibits no evidence of an effusion/mass in either of his middle ears.

His nasal mucosa, pharynx, and oral mucosa are normal in color and without edema, lesions, or discharge. His tonsils are normal in size and without exudates, bilaterally.

Cervical lymph nodes are not palpable. His thyroid is normal in size, nontender, and without masses, bilaterally.

His heart is regular in rate and rhythm and without murmurs, gallops, or rubs. His apical impulse is nondisplaced and without a thrill. His lungs are clear to auscultation.

His cranial nerves are intact and equal bilaterally. His fundi are normal and without any evidence of papilledema. His meningeal signs are negative. His hands, arms, feet, and legs are of normal strength and equal bilaterally. There is no evidence of muscle atrophy. He has no difficulty with gait. He can walk in a circle, do heel-to-toe walking, walk on his heels, and walk on his toes without difficulty. Finger to nose with eyes open and closed as well as finger to examiner's finger is normal. His biceps, triceps, brachioradialis, knee, ankle, and plantar reflexes are normal and equal bilaterally. Sharp and dull sensation is intact and equal bilaterally.

He sits still on his mother's lap the entire time his history is being taken. He speaks only when questions are addressed to him. His answers are appropriate for age. During the physical examination, he sits on the examination table alone and he only moves when requested to do so. There is no evidence of fidgeting, hyperactivity, or other abnormalities of behavior.

3. Based on this information, which of the following diagnostic studies are indicated at this time for Xeb and why?

    A. Electroencephalogram (EEG)
    B. Echocardiogram
    C. Electrocardiogram (ECG)
    D. Complete blood count with differential (CBC w/diff)
    E. Computed tomography (CT) of the brain

Diagnostic Test Results

His EEG revealed intermittent, very brief, symmetric, 3-Hz spike-and-wave activity.

His echocardiogram, ECG, CBC w/diff, and CT were all reported as normal.

4. Based on this information, which one of the following is Xeb's most likely diagnosis and why?

    A. Absent seizures
    B. Simple partial seizures
    C. Landau-Kleffner syndrome
    D. Psychogenic nonepileptic seizures (PNESs)
    E. Attention-deficit/hyperactivity disorder (ADHD)

5. Which of the following are appropriate components of Xeb's treatment plan and why?

    A. ADHD evaluation
    B. Complete blood count with differential (CBC w/diff)
    C. Trial of valproic acid
    D. Trial of clonazepam
    E. Trial of carbamazepine

CASE 9-5

Yule Zeus

Ms. Zeus is a 38-year-old white female who presents with the chief complaint of "difficulty going to sleep." Her symptoms have occurred nightly for approximately 2 months. She feels tired and sleepy before going to bed; however, once she lies down, she cannot get to sleep because she experiences a "crawling-like" sensation in her lower legs associated with an urge to move them. Moving her legs temporarily alleviates her discomfort. However, approximately once or twice a night, the sensation becomes so intense she is required "to get up and walk around the house" in order to obtain any sustained relief; even with this, she is lucky if the absence of sensation persists for greater than 30 minutes. She is unaware of any other aggravating or alleviating factors.

On average, it takes her approximately 2 hours to achieve sleep. Most nights, once she finally falls asleep, she sleeps throughout the night until her alarm awakens her. However, she is tired the next day. She further defines tired as being "sleepy"; its maximum peak occurs shortly after lunch. She is uncertain if the leg movement persists throughout the night because she is single and sleeps alone. When she awakens her blankets are in disarray; however, she is uncertain whether this results from continued symptoms or her movements while trying to fall to sleep.

Her only known medical problem is depression, which was diagnosed and treatment initiated approximately 4 months ago. She was started on fluoxetine 20 mg/day; it was gradually increased by 20 mg every other week to her current dosage of 80 mg. She feels her depression has completely resolved since the last titration of her medication. She is not taking any other prescription (including oral contraceptives) or over-the-counter medications, vitamins, supplements, or herbal preparations. She has never had any surgeries nor been hospitalized. She does not drink alcohol, smoke cigarettes, or use any illicit substances. Her last menstrual period was 2 weeks ago and normal. Her menses have been regular since menarche at the age of 12 years. Her family history is positive for depression (mother and two sisters).

1. Based on this information, which of the following questions are essential to ask Ms. Zeus and why?

  A. Is she experiencing increased stress, suffering from excessive "worry," having "lots of thoughts running through her head" while attempting to initiate sleep, experiencing difficulty with completing tasks she has initiated, attempting to multitask more than normal for her, or suffering from "hyperactivity"?
  B. Is she experiencing "hot flashes" and "night sweats"?
  C. Are her leg symptoms unilateral or bilateral, associated with paresthesias or dysesthesias besides the "crawling" sensation, or present at other times during the day?
  D. Has she had any pallor, fatigue out of proportion to sleep loss, lightheadedness, vertigo, presyncope, syncope, palpitations, tachycardia, or dyspnea on exertion?
  E. Has she experienced any polydipsias or polyuria?

Patient Responses

Ms. Zeus readily admits to having a very stressful job; however, the amount of stress has not increased and she has been performing the same job for the past 5 years. She feels the fluoxetine also controls her "stress"-related symptoms. She looks forward to going to work.

She denies suffering from excessive "worry," having "lots of thoughts running through her head" while attempting to initiate sleep, experiencing difficulty with completing tasks she has initiated, attempting to multitask more than normal for her, suffering from "hyperactivity," experiencing "hot flashes" or "night sweats," and having polydipsia or polyuria. Furthermore, she has not experienced any pallor, fatigue out of proportion to sleep loss, lightheadedness, vertigo, presyncope, syncope, palpitations, tachycardia, or dyspnea on exertion.

Her leg symptoms are bilateral and equal. She does not experience other paresthesias/dysesthesias. She does have similar symptoms when sitting and watching TV or reading before going to bed.

2. Based on this information, which of the following components of a physical examination are essential to perform on Ms. Zeus and why?

  A. Cranial nerve examination
  B. Thyroid palpation
  C. Auscultation of carotids
  D. Pelvic examination
  F. Vascular and neurologic examination of her lower legs

Physical Examination Findings

Ms. Zeus is 5'5" tall and weighs 142 lb (BMI = 23.6). Other vital signs are BP, 106/68 mm Hg lying, 110/70 mm Hg sitting, and 112/72 mm Hg standing; pulse, 76 BPM and regular lying, 78 BPM and regular sitting, and 83 BPM and regular sitting; respirations, 12/min and regular; and oral temperature, 97.9°F.

Her cranial nerves are grossly intact.

Her thyroid is within normal limits. Her carotids are normal and equal bilaterally without bruit. Her pelvic examination is unremarkable.

She has full range of motion of her hips, knees, ankles, and toes that is equal bilaterally, without pain, and without reproduction of her symptoms. She has a negative straight leg raising test. She does not experience difficulty with gait, heel-to-toe walking, heel walking, or toe walking. She can make a circle in an appropriate number of steps at a rapid pace without difficulty. Her coordination appears normal. Her knee and ankle jerks as well as her plantar responses are normal and equal bilaterally. Muscle strength is normal and equal bilaterally without any evidence of atrophy. Sensation is intact to sharp and dull and is equal bilaterally.

Her skin is normal in temperature and without discoloration or lesions. Capillary refill is normal. Her femoral, popiteal, posterior tibial, and dorsalis pedis pulses are normal and equal bilaterally. There is no thigh or calf swelling or tenderness. She does not have any pedal edema.

3. Based on this information, which of the following diagnostic tests are important to order on Ms. Zeus at this time and why?

  A. Bilateral electromyogram (EMG) of her lower extremities
  B. Glucose tolerance test (GTT)
  C. Iron level, total iron-binding capacity (TIBC), and ferritin levels
  D. Blood urea nitrogen (BUN) and creatinine
  E. Urinary human chorionic gonadotropin (HCG) test

Diagnostic Test Results

Ms. Zeus' bilateral nerve conduction study of her lower extremities showed no abnormalities. Her glucose tolerance test was within normal limits.

Her iron level was 140 µg/dl (normal adult female: 60–160). Her TIBC was 380 µg/dl (normal: 250–460). Her calculated transferrin saturation (TS, transferrin and other mobile iron-binding proteins saturated with iron) was 36.8% (normal female: 15–50). (TS is calculated by dividing the serum level by the TIBC and multiplying the result by 100.) Her ferritin was 100 ng/ml (normal adult female: 10–150).

Her BUN was 11 mg/dl (normal adult: 10–20) and her creatinine was 0.6 mg/dl (normal adult female: 0.5–1.1).

Her urinary HCG test was negative (normal: negative).

4. Based on this information, which one of the following is Ms. Zeus' most likely diagnosis and why?

  A. Peripheral neuropathy
  B. Primary restless leg syndrome
  C. Secondary restless leg syndrome caused by fluoxetine
  D. Pregnancy
  E. Pain secondary to unresolved depression

5. Which of the following are appropriate components of Ms. Zeus' treatment plan and why?

  A. Stretching exercises or a hot bath before bed
  B. Immediately stop fluoxetine
  C. Immediately start sertraline
  D. Start bupropion in 2 weeks
  E. Start pramipexole

CASE 9-6

Zachary Adkins

Zachary is a 17-year-old African American male who is brought to the ED by rescue squad following an episode of unconsciousness after being tackled during a high school football game. The paramedic who was on stand-by at the game states that Zachary was hit on the right side of his rib cage with the helmet of the defensive tackle, which caused him to fall backward. His initial impact with the ground occurred with his left shoulder and was immediately followed by his left posterolateral head. The impact caused Zachary's head to bounce up approximately 6" and hit the ground again. When Zachary did not immediately get up the trainers, coach, and emergency medical services (EMS) staff ran to him. The paramedic estimates he was by Zachary's side in 3 to 4 minutes. His initial assessment revealed that Zachary had a respiratory rate of 6/min and regular, pulse of 50 BPM and regular, and a palpable systolic BP of 88 mm Hg; he was unconscious and unresponsive to painful stimuli.

The EMS team carefully removed his helmet, secured his neck, placed him on a backboard, loaded him onto a stretcher, and transported him to the ED with oxygen at 2 L/min by nasal canula. A 16-gauge IV line with normal saline solution (NSS) running "wide open" was started during transport. Shortly after the IV line was started, the paramedic reported that Zachary regained consciousness; however, Zachary could not remember the incident, his name, where he was (or had been), or the date. Reevaluation of Zachary's vital signs at that time revealed that his pulse was 72 BPM and regular, his respiratory rate was 12/min and regular, and his BP was 90/56 mm Hg.

The paramedic estimates that the time from injury to consciousness was approximately 20 minutes and the time from injury to arriving at the ED was about 25 minutes. According to the paramedic and the EMS squad, the other player sustained no injuries or loss of consciousness at that time or since. Zachary's parents, who were at the game, arrived at the ED almost simultaneously with the ambulance. They confirmed the paramedic's description of the injury.

Zachary is currently conscious; however, he only opens his eyes to verbal or physical stimulation. He is complaining of a severe, generalized headache; however, he cannot quantify or describe it. He is nauseated but has not vomited. He denies diplopia, complete or partial visual field loss, any other visual abnormalities, neck pain, paresthesias, and/or dysesthesias. However, he states he "cannot move his arms or legs" but can wiggle his fingers and toes (however, he is currently strapped to the backboard and stretcher). He is also complaining of right lateral rib pain in his midaxillary line from approximately T5 to T10. It is dull in nature and increases with inspiration. He denies dyspnea, chest pressure, chest pain, lightheadedness, vertigo, abdominal pain, or any other problems. He has no recollection of his injury or being transported to the ED. He is cognizant of being in the ED, but initially he had to be told.

His has no known medical problems. He has never had surgery nor been hospitalized. He takes no prescription or over-the-counter medications, vitamins, supplements, or herbal preparations. He denies smoking cigarettes, drinking alcohol, or using illicit substances. His family history is unremarkable.

1. Based on this information, which of the following questions are essential to ask the paramedics, his parents, or Zachary and why?

   A. Was his helmet broken or dented?
   B. Has he experienced a previous head injury? If yes, when and how severe was it?
   C. Who was the other player?
   D. Has he ever experienced dehydration during or following a game or practice?
   E. How was he feeling before the game?

Patient Responses

According to the paramedic, his helmet was not broken or dented. According to his parents, he has never had a previous head injury, has never experienced a problem with dehydration during (or after) a practice session and/or a game, and was not ill or experiencing any symptoms before the game. No one knew the name of the defensive tackle.

2. Based on this information, which of the following components of a physical examination are essential to perform on Zachary and why?

   A. Heart, lung, and chest wall examination
   B. Abdominal examination
   C. Rectal examination to obtain stool sample to test for occult blood
   D. Glasgow coma scale score
   E. Cursory neurologic examination with abbreviated mental status evaluation, and a more comprehensive examination to follow after imaging studies are completed

Physical Examination Findings

Zachary's height and weight are deferred because he is restrained on a stretcher with a backboard and hard cervical collar in place. Other vital signs are BP, 100/70 mm Hg; pulse, 92 BPM and regular; respirations, 12/min and regular; and tympanic temperature, 97.9°F.

His heart is regular in rate and rhythm without murmurs, gallops, or rubs. His apical impulse is nondisplaced and without a thrill. His lungs are clear to auscultation. His chest wall reveals no gross deformities, swelling, erythema, or contusions; however, he is tender from the posterior axillary line to the anterior axillary line over his ribs extending from T5 to T10.

His abdominal exam reveals normoactive and equal bowel sounds in all four quadrants without tenderness, distension, or ascites. There is no organomegaly or abnormal masses. His aorta is normal in size and pulsation. His aorta and renal arteries are without bruits.

His rectal examination reveals no external lesions or tears, good muscle tone, no internal rectal abnormalities, and a small amount of brown stool that tested negative for occult blood.

He opens his eyes to verbal stimuli (3 points), talks but is confused and occasionally uses inappropriate words

(3 points), and follows commands (6 points), giving him a Glasgow coma score of 12.

He has no gross head deformities or areas of tenderness. His pupils are equal, round, and regular in size and respond to light and accommodation, bilaterally. His funduscopic examination is normal. Within his ability to cooperate, his other cranial nerves are normal. There is no abnormal fluid/blood in his ears, behind his tympanic membranes, or in his nostrils. His cervical spine is nontender. He has normal and equal sensation to sharp and dull stimulation all over the anterior and lateral portions of his body. He has normal and equal hand and foot strength. His plantar response is normal and equal bilaterally.

On his Mini-Mental Status Examination (MMSE), he is able to provide his name and year but not the month, date, or day of the week. (This is an apparent improvement over the initial EMS assessment.) He knows he is in an ED; however, he does not know which one, how he got there, or what happened to cause him to be transported there. He can only remember one out of three objects immediately, and none of them at 5 minutes. He cannot spell "world" backwards. He responds to simple commands. However, the remainder of the MMSE is unable to be performed as a result of his being restrained on the backboard with a hard cervical collar in place.

3. Based on this information, which of the following diagnostic tests are essential to perform on Zachary and why?

A. Cervical spine (C-spine) radiograph
B. Skull series radiograph
C. Right ribs radiograph
D. Chest x-ray (CXR)
E. Computed tomography (CT) of the head

Diagnostic Study Findings

Zachary's C-spine revealed no evidence of fracture or dislocation. His skull series was negative for fracture. His right ribs were negative for fracture. His CXR was normal. The CT of his brain revealed a very small area of homogenous hyperdensities in the superficial posterolateral parietal lobe and a much smaller area located in the superficial anterolateral aspect of the right temporal lobe. There was no evidence of significant edema or gross hemorrhage.

4. Based on this information, which one of the following is Zachary's most likely diagnosis and why?

A. Grade 2 concussion with coup injury
B. Grade 2 concussion with contrecoup injury
C. Grade 3 concussion with coup injury
D. Grade 3 concussion with coup and contrecoup injury
E. Subdural hematoma

5. Based on this information, which of the following are the most appropriate components of Zachary's treatment plan and why?

A. Hospitalize for observation and frequent neurologic and vital sign assessments
B. Discharge to parents' care but advise them to awaken him every 2 hours to check for confusion, drowsiness, increasing symptoms, or other neurologic deficits
C. Neurosurgical consultation

D. Start midodrine to normalize BP
E. Start promethazine for nausea

CASE 9-7
Alec Bradford

Alec is a 12-year-old Hispanic American male who presents, accompanied by his mother, with the chief complaint of "a very sore lump on my head." It is located in his right temporal and periorbital areas; he describes it as crampy in nature and moderate (6 out of 10 on the pain scale) in intensity. His only other symptom is a "migraine headache," which he describes as a moderate (6 out of 10 on the pain scale), constant, throbbing, pressure-type pain located on the right side of his head. It has been present constantly and unchanged for 2 weeks. His symptoms do not affect his sleep; however, he has been sleeping more in the past 2 weeks. Coughing or sneezing, which rarely (twice or less a day) occurs, increases the severity of his headache. Although he denies any visual disturbances, attempting to read or watch TV increases the intensity of his headache. Lying supine with his eyes closed seems to minimally alleviate his headache. Neither ice nor heat impacts on his headache. He is not cognizant of any other aggravating or alleviating factors. However, he has been running a fever intermittently. According to his mother, it has been as high as 102.8°F orally.

His mother took him to the ED for his headache 1 week ago, where he was given the diagnosis of migraine headache and advised to take over-the-counter ibuprofen 200 mg every 6 to 8 hours as needed for pain. The following day, his pain was unaffected by this medication, so his mother took him back to the ED. He was reevaluated by the same physician, who prescribed ibuprofen 800 mg three times a day. Alec feels the higher dose of ibuprofen "might" have had a minimal, if any, impact on alleviating his pain.

His only known medical problem is the "migraine headaches." He has never had any surgeries nor been hospitalized. His only medication is the ibuprofen 800 mg three times a day. He takes no other prescription or over-the-counter medications, vitamins, supplements, or herbal preparations. He is not allergic to any drugs. He denies smoking cigarettes, drinking alcohol, or using illicit substances. He has regular age-appropriate health examinations that have always been reported as normal. His immunizations are up to date. His last purified protein derivative (PPD) test was 1 month ago and showed no reaction. His family history is unremarkable, including being negative for migraines.

1. Based on this information, which of the following questions are essential to ask Alec and why?

A. Has he had any photophobia, phonophobia, nausea, or vomiting?
B. Has he experienced any seizures, signs of meningeal irritation, confusion, weakness, speech problems, gait difficulties, coordination abnormalities, lightheadedness, vertigo, presyncope, syncope, or other neurologic deficits?
C. Is he currently experiencing (or did he experience before getting ill) any of the following symptoms: chills,

eye discharge, otalgia, rhinorrhea, nasal congestion, sore throat, postnasal discharge, cough, or neck pain?

D. Has he been experiencing a depressed or sad mood, irritability, anhedonia, decreased time spent with friends, increased time spent alone, declining grades, sleep changes, appetite changes, or weight changes?

E. Has he experienced any recent head injury or trauma?

Patient Responses

Alec has been experiencing mild photophobia, phonophobia, and nausea since the headache began. He started vomiting 1 week ago (precipitating the ED visit) and has vomited once or twice per day since. There is no blood or "coffee grounds"–appearing materials in his emesis.

He has not had any seizures, neck stiffness, confusion, problems with speech, vertigo, lightheadedness, presyncope, syncope, or eye discharge. However, he has noticed some weakness in his right arm and leg. He is unsure if it affects his gait because he walks slowly and "lightly" because walking at his normal pace causes his headache to increase. This is especially true with "bouncing"-type activities (e.g., walking up stairs).

He and his mother both deny any signs or symptoms of depression, any head injury or trauma, or an upper respiratory tract symptoms of any type. However, his mother states he had a "cold" approximately 1 month ago.

2. Based on this information, which of the following components of a physical examination are essential to perform on Alec and why?

A. Head, eyes, ears, nose, and throat (HEENT) examination

B. Palpation of cervical lymph nodes

C. Meningeal signs

D. Thoracic and lumbar spine examination

E. Neurologic examination

Physical Examination Findings

Alec is 5'0" tall and weighs 105 lb. Other vital signs are BP, 106/62 mm Hg; pulse, 100 BPM and regular; respiratory rate, 15/min and regular; and oral temperature, 102.2°F. He is toxic appearing.

He has marked edema, erythema, and warmth circumorbitally on the right, including his upper and lower eyelids. It extends across his forehead and his temple to just inside his hairline. There is mild pitting of the edema over bony surfaces. There appears to be a well-delineated mass in the area; however, it is difficult to fully evaluate secondary to the marked tenderness. It does not extend below or behind the ear. His mastoid processes do not exhibit dolor, rubor, calor, or tumor. His preauricular lymph nodes are negative.

His auditory canals are clear, nonerythematous, and without abnormal discharge, bilaterally. His tympanic membranes are nonerythematous, not injected, normal in movement, and without any evidence of effusion/mass behind them.

His nasal mucosa, pharynx, and oral mucosa are normal in color and without edema, lesions, or discharge. His tonsils are normal in size and without exudates or other lesions. Cervical lymph nodes, both anterior and posterior chains, are slightly enlarged and tender on the right. The left ones are not palpable.

His Kernig sign and Brudzinski sign are positive for mild to moderate resistance only.

He has full range of motion of his thoracic and lumbar spine without the complaint of back pain. However, full flexion of his lumbar spine does cause his headache to increase in intensity. His thoracolumbar spine and associated muscles are nontender to palpate. The overlying skin reveals no calor, dolor, rubor, tumor, or other lesions.

His cranial nerves appear grossly intact; however, he does have pain in his right eye with medial gaze when testing his extraocular movements (EOMs). He cannot fully open his right eye or completely wrinkle up his right forehead; however, this probably results from his periorbital and facial edema. His funduscopic examination is normal bilaterally.

Muscle strength testing of his right hand, arm, leg, and foot reveals a slight weakness compared to his left. Although he does have a minor right arm drift, there is no deviation of his hand with holding his arms outstretched. Finger-to-nose testing with his eyes open and closed as well as finger-to-examiner's finger testing is normal. His gait is slow and deliberate. He can perform tandem, toe, and heel walking but does it slowly and cautiously. Completing a circle takes a little longer and a few more steps but is without coordination problems, probably secondary to his slow, deliberate gait.

His biceps, triceps, brachioradialis, knee, ankle, and plantar reflexes are normal and equal bilaterally. Sensation is intact to both sharp and dull stimulation in his arms, legs, and face; it is equal bilaterally, except for the swollen area where he states sharp sensations are not as pronounced as the rest of his face.

3. Based on this information, which of the following diagnostic studies are indicated at this time for Alec and why?

A. Blood culture and sensitivity with Gram stain × 2

B. Complete blood count with differential (CBC w/diff)

C. Magnetic resonance imaging (MRI) of the head, with and without contrast

D. Ultrasound of the head mass

E. Computed tomography (CT) of the head without contrast

Diagnostic Test Results

Alec's Gram stain showed mixed flora. His cultures are pending.

His CBC was normal except for a total leukocyte count of 27,500 mm^3 (normal for those older than 2 years of age: 5000–10,000) with 90% neutrophils (normal: 55–70), 7% lymphocytes (normal: 20–40), 1% monocytes (normal: 2–8), 2% eosinophils (normal: 1–4), and 0% basophils (normal: 0.5–1).

His MRI revealed soft tissue edema over his right forehead and around his right eye with a subperiosteal abscess and complete opacification of his frontal sinuses. There was a moderate-sized crescent-shaped hyperintense (compared to cerebrospinal fluid) accumulation of fluid between his inner skull table and dura mater is located under his subcutaneous mass. Additionally, his MRI revealed some abnormalities of his bone marrow as well as disruption of his cortical bone in the associated area of the skull and a small subperiosteal abscess formation.

The ultrasound of the mass was too painful to be performed. His CT revealed the complete opacification of his frontal sinuses and a questionable epidural mass.

4. Based on this information, which one of the following best defines Alec's diagnosis at this time and why?

  A. Pott disease
  B. Pott disease, frontal bone osteomyelitis, and cranial epidural abscess
  C. Pansinusitis
  D. Cranial epidural abscess with frontal bone osteomyelitis and Pott puffy tumor
  E. Migraine headaches

5. Based on this information, which of the following are appropriate components to Alec's treatment plan and why?

  A. Hospitalize
  B. IV cefotaxime, metronidazole, and vancomycin until culture results are available
  C. Stop ibuprofen and start sumatriptan
  D. Amoxicillin plus clavulanic acid orally
  E. Neurosurgical consultation for possible drainage of abscess

CASE 9-8
Bella Chang

Ms. Chang is a 42-year-old Japanese American female who presents with the chief complaint of "something weird is going on with my body." This complaint is further defined as involuntary, irregular, jerking movements of her arms and face of approximately 6 months' duration. Initially, these abnormal movements were rare and infrequent; however, they gradually increased until she is currently experiencing them several times per day. Each episode lasts a maximum of "a couple of minutes." She has no warning to their onset, and they stop just as rapidly as they start. They can occur at rest or with purposeful activities (e.g., eating, pouring beverages, or reaching for objects). She is unaware of any aggravating or alleviating factors. She does not feel they are stress related. She admits to being "embarrassed" by these episodes. She has cut down on social obligations/situations because she's "worried" that one "might happen."

Her past medical history is positive for myoclonic seizures. They were diagnosed approximately 5 years ago via EEG. A follow-up EEG conducted 2 months ago on medication did not reveal any evidence of seizure activity. Her clonazepam level at the same time was 60 ng/ml (optimal drug level: 20–80). Although her seizures lasted only a few minutes, beginning rapidly without provocation or warning and ending "just as quickly," they are otherwise dissimilar to her chief complaint. Her seizures occurred much less frequently and consisted of a series of multiple myoclonic jerks involving her head and trunk. She is conscious and aware during her seizures and not postictal afterward. She never experienced incontinence with them. Her last seizure was at least 3 years ago.

Her seizure disorder was initially treated with phenytoin, which controlled the seizures; however, shortly after initiating the medication, she began experiencing difficulty with memory, problems with completing simple mathematical tasks, and

irritability. This was attributed to an adverse effect of the phenytoin and valproic acid was substituted. The valproic acid also controlled her seizures; however, the change did not remedy her cognitive and emotional symptoms. Thus, the valproic acid was discontinued and clonazepam was initiated. The clonazepam also controlled her seizures but did not alter her cognitive or mood symptoms. At that point, her healthcare provider (HCP) decided her cognitive and mood symptoms were secondary to depression and started her on fluoxetine; however, it did not have any effect on her symptoms. Since then, she has been tried on citalopram, venlafaxine, duloxetine, mirtazapine, and olanzapine/fluoxetine without any improvement.

Examples of her memory problems consist of forgetting where she placed objects (e.g., car keys, purse, or shoes), going into another room to retrieve a needed item but then forgetting what it was, or being unable to recall the "right" word when speaking. Examples of types of mathematical tasks she experiences difficulty with include balancing her checkbook, calculating tips, or determining savings at percentage-off sales. She further defines irritable as being "short with others when I am frustrated"; this primarily occurs when she is experiencing the aforementioned difficulties. She denies feeling depressed, sad, or blue. She is not experiencing any degree of anhedonia. She has not experienced any changes in sleep, appetite, weight, or libido, nor has she exhibited any signs of mania, excessive worry, anxiety, or suicidal thoughts/ideations.

The myoclonic seizure disorder and depression are Ms. Chang's only known medical problems. Her current medications are clonazepam 1 mg twice a day and olanzapine/fluoxetine 12 mg/50 mg once daily which she has been on for approximately 6 months. She is on no other prescription or over-the-counter medications, vitamins, supplements, or herbal preparations. She has never had any surgeries nor been hospitalized. She does not drink alcohol, smoke cigarettes, or use illicit substances. Her last menstrual period was 2 weeks ago and normal. She has regular menstrual cycles. She uses condoms and is sexually active with two current male partners. She has never been sexually active with female partners. She estimates her number of lifetime partners to be greater than 100. Her family history is noncontributory.

1. Based on this information, which of the following questions are essential to ask Ms. Chang and why?

  A. Did she experience any other symptoms before the "jerking movements" began?
  B. Does she have any problem with ambulation?
  C. Does she have a tremor or weakness?
  D. Has she ever had a positive culture for syphilis?
  E. Does she have a family history of anyone with a similar condition?

Patient Responses

Before the actual "jerks" started, Ms. Chang noticed that her limbs were "restless" and she would sometimes have difficulty getting "comfortable." Also, she noticed that she became a "fidgeter." Those symptoms essentially resolved as the myoclonic jerks became more regular. She has noticed some "unsteadiness" to her gait at times, especially when trying to turn around quickly. She denies having a tremor or any muscle weakness.

She has never been tested for syphilis. To her knowledge, no one in her family has similar symptoms or an associated condition.

2. Based on this information, which of the following components of a physical examination are essential to perform on Ms. Chang and why?

    A. Ear, nose, and throat examination
    B. Cardiac examination
    C. Examination of pulses
    D. Neurologic examination
    E. Mini-mental status examination

Physical Examination Findings

Ms. Chang is 4'10" tall and weighs 100 lb (BMI = 21). Other vital signs are BP, 102/62 mm Hg; pulse, 76 BPM and regular; respirations, 13/min and regular; and oral temperature, 98.4°F.

Her auditory canals are clear, nonerythematous, and without lesions or abnormal discharge bilaterally. Her tympanic membranes are nonerythematous, not injected, and fully mobile bilaterally.

Her nasal mucosa, pharynx, and oral mucosa are normal in color and without edema, lesions, or abnormal discharge. Her tonsils are normal size and without lesions or exudates bilaterally. Cervical lymph nodes are nonpalpable.

Her heart is regular in rate and rhythm and without murmurs, gallops, or rubs. Her apical impulse is nondisplaced and without a thrill.

Her carotid and renal arteries are normal, equal, and without bruits bilaterally. Her aorta is normal size and without a mass or bruit. Brachial, ulnar, radial, femoral, popiteal, dorsalis pedis, and posterior tibial pulses are normal and equal bilaterally. Her feet are warm, without discoloration or lesions, and with normal capillary refill. She has no pedal edema.

Her cranial nerves are grossly intact. She can perform finger to nose with eyes open and closed as well as finger to examiner's finger.

Her hands, arms, legs, and feet have normal and equal muscle strength. There is no evidence of a tremor or muscle atrophy. Her gait is wide based, slightly staggering-like, and slightly unsteady. Her turns are exaggerated. She cannot perform tandem walking, and toe and heel walking reveal the same abnormalities as her regular gait. She cannot stand with her feet together with her eyes open or closed.

Her biceps, triceps, brachioradialis, knee, ankle, and plantar reflexes are normal and equal bilaterally. Her sensation is intact to both sharp and dull stimulation in her arms, legs, and face bilaterally; the sensations appear equal bilaterally to the patient.

Her total MMSE score is 21 out of a maximum of 30. Further breakdown reveals that under orientation, she cannot name the facility or what county she is currently located in, or the correct date (7 of 10); under registration, she can immediately recall all three items named to her (3 of 3); under attention and calculation, she misses three of the serial 7's (2 of 5); under recall, she can only recall one of the three objects (1 of 3); under language, she can perform all tasks except write a sentence (hers contains no subject; 7 of 8); under construction, she is able to reproduce the interlocking pentagons (1 of 1).

3. Based on this information, which of the following diagnostic studies are indicated for Ms. Chang and why?

    A. Computed tomography (CT) scan of the brain
    B. Repetitive stimulation testing via electromyography (EMG) of her arms
    C. Lipid panel
    D. White blood cell count with differential (WBC w/diff)
    E. Human immunodeficiency virus (HIV) antibody test

Diagnostic Test Findings

Ms. Chang's CT of her brain revealed mild cerebral atrophy and atrophy of the caudate nucleus. No other abnormalities were noted. Her repetitive stimulation EMG studies were normal.

Her total cholesterol was 150 mg/dl (normal average-risk adult: < 200), with an HDL of 70 mg/dl (normal average-risk adult female: > 55), an LDL of 60 (normal average-risk adult female: 60–180), and a VLDL of 20 mg/dl (normal average-risk adult female: 7–32). Her TGs were 120 mg/dl (normal average-risk adult female: 35–135).

Her WBC w/diff revealed a total white blood cell count of 7250/mm³ (normal adult: 5000–10,000) with 65% neutrophils (normal: 55–70), 25% lymphocytes (normal: 20–40), 5% monocytes (normal: 2–8), 4% eosinophils (normal: 1–4), and 1% basophils (normal: 0.5–1).

Her HIV antibody test was negative (normal: negative).

4. Based on this information, which one of the following is Ms. Chang's most likely diagnosis and why?

    A. Treatment-resistant atypical depression
    B. Parkinson disease
    C. Mild exacerbations of myoclonic seizures
    D. Dentatorubral-pallidoluysian atrophy (DRPLA)
    E. Huntington disease

5. Which of the following treatment possibilities are appropriate components of Ms. Chang's treatment plan and why?

    A. Increase clonazepam 1 mg to three times a day
    B. Recheck clonazepam serum level in 1 month
    C. Reserpine gradually titrated to a total daily dose of 2 to 5 mg depending on response and adverse effects
    D. Donepezil 5 mg a day initially, increasing to 10 mg daily if necessary and tolerated
    E. Refer to psychiatrist for possible electroconvulsive therapy (ECT)

CASE 9-9

Clarence Deets

Mr. Deets is a 19-year-old white male who presents with his fraternity house's residence director (RD), who states that "Clarence is really sick." According to his RD, Mr. Deets' behavior has deteriorated dramatically within the past couple of weeks. He reported that Mr. Deets has essentially remained in his bed asleep for the past week. He did not attend classes, bathe, or go to the cafeteria during this time frame. He refused to eat; however, his friends managed to get him to drink "a little bit" of bottled sports drinks. For the past 2 days he appeared to be confused, forgetful, irritable, and exhibiting slurred speech. The frat brothers who initially witnessed this behavior did not report it until this morning because they assumed he was drunk. According to the RD, they have also noticed Mr. Deets exhibiting inappropriate anger outbursts, confusion, memory loss, lethargy, and fatigue for approximately 1 month. This morning, when the RD noticed Mr. Deets walking "funny," he insisted he "go to the hospital" and immediately drove him here.

When asked about his illness, Mr. Deets states that he does not understand "what all the fuss is about" because he "just has a flu bug." He admits to being fatigued for approximately 1 month; however, he attributes it to the demands of his class schedule. He denies being irritable, forgetful, or confused. He admits to experiencing a generalized headache that is aching in nature and a 2 out of a 10 on the pain scale in severity for the past week. It is associated with anorexia and nausea, and he vomited two times earlier in the week. This is why he is consuming sports drinks instead of eating food. He is unaware of any aggravating or alleviating factors.

He denies diarrhea, melena, hematochezia, mucus in his bowel, other bowel changes, abdominal pain, previous or current upper or lower respiratory tract infection, wheezing, dyspnea, chest pain, palpitations, lightheadedness, vertigo, presyncope, syncope, seizures, visual abnormalities, other cranial nerve abnormalities, dysuria, urinary urgency or frequency, penile discharge, groin pain, or rectal pain. The RD is unaware of any frat brothers or frequent visitors being ill or exhibiting symptoms similar to Mr. Deets' at any time during the past month. As near as he knows, Mr. Deets has not been in close contact with anyone who has been ill. He has not traveled out of the state or country recently.

His only known medical problem is being infected with HIV for approximately 2 years. Thus far, he has not achieved diagnostic criteria for acquired immunodeficiency syndrome (AIDS) or even AIDS-related complex (ARC). He did opt to initiate prophylactic azidothymidine (AZT), lamivudine, and indinavir immediately upon being identified as HIV positive. He took these medications regularly until approximately 3 months ago when he sought prescription refills from the university's health center. He claims that the nurse manning the health center advised him that the prophylactic medications were ineffective for prevention of AIDS and his "counts looked good" so he could discontinue his drugs. Unable to obtain refills and assuming new studies had negated the benefits of prophylaxis, he terminated his medications as advised.

He is not on any prescription or over-the-counter medications, vitamins, supplements, or herbal preparations. He has never been hospitalized nor had surgery. Currently, he is abstinent; however, in the past he has been sexually active with both women and men. He denies drinking alcohol, smoking cigarettes, or using illicit substances. His family history is noncontributory.

1. Based on this information, which of the following questions are essential to ask Mr. Deets and why?

   A. Is he experiencing any constitutional symptoms?
   B. Before becoming ill this week, had he experienced a change in his appetite and/or sleep pattern; anhedonia; feeling depressed, anxious, overwhelmed, sad, and/or worthless; and/or suicidal ideations?
   C. Do they eat at the frat house, in the cafeteria, or at restaurants? Does he eat undercooked or raw meat?
   D. Do they have a cat? If yes, what is his exposure to its litter box?
   E. Do they have a dog? If yes, is it kept indoors or outdoors?

Patient Responses

Mr. Deets has been febrile and experiencing chills since becoming ill with the "flu"; however, he does not know the exact degree of temperature elevation because he does not possess a thermometer. He denies night sweats, lymphadenopathy, and other constitutional symptoms; change in his appetite, weight, and sleep patterns prior to becoming ill; anhedonia; feeling depressed, anxious, overwhelmed, sad, and worthless; or suicidal ideations.

They do not eat meals at the frat house. They either eat in the cafeteria or at a local pizzeria. His RD is unaware of anyone else eating at these establishments becoming ill or a known pathogen "outbreak" associated with them. Mr. Deets does not consume undercooked or raw meat.

They do not have a cat; however, there are several that "roam around" campus with which he interacts. However, he denies any contact with their feces. They do not have a dog.

2. Based on this information, which of the following components of a physical examination are essential to perform on Mr. Deets and why?

   A. Ear, nose, and throat (ENT) examination
   B. Heart and lung examination
   C. Examination of all his pulses
   D. Neurologic examination, including a mini-mental status (MMSE) and meningeal signs
   E. Examination of all his lymph nodes

Physical Examination Findings

Mr. Deets is 5'11" tall and weighs 169 lb (BMI = 23.6). Other vital signs are BP, 112/72 mm Hg; pulse, 98 BPM and regular; respiratory rate, 16/min and regular; and oral temperature, 101.4°F.

He is unkempt and toxic appearing. He maintains his right arm in a flexed posture held against his chest except when he is asked to perform a task requiring him to move it.

His heart is regular in rate and rhythm and without murmurs, gallops, or rubs. His apical impulse is nondisplaced and without a thrill. His lungs are clear to auscultation.

His auditory canals are clear, nonerythematous, and without abnormal discharge, bilaterally. His tympanic membranes are nonerythematous, noninjected, and fully mobile without evidence of an effusion/mass behind them, bilaterally. His nasal mucosa, oral mucosa, and pharynx are normal in color and without edema, lesions, or discharge. His tonsils are normal size and without exudates, bilaterally.

His cranial nerves are grossly intact except for a partial paralysis of the area around his right nasolabial area, ipsilateral forehead, and ipsilateral eyebrow when he attempts to raise his eyebrows; a flattening of his right nasolabial fold with closing of his eyes (this latter maneuver also revealed weakness of the ipsilateral upper eyelid [but it still fully closed]); and a weakness to the right corner of his mouth when asked to smile. He also exhibits some difficulty producing his labial and lingual consonants. However, he does not have deviation of his tongue.

He can perform finger to nose with eyes open and closed as well as finger to examiner's finger without difficulty. His right hand, arm, leg, and foot are slightly weaker than his left. He has a slight arm drift with ulnar rotation of the arm on the right; the left was normal. He has no evidence of a tremor. His gait reveals a slightly circumducted right leg with occasional dragging of the toe with walking. He cannot perform tandem, toe, or heel walking. He cannot stand with his feet together with his eyes open or closed. His biceps, triceps, brachioradialis, knee, ankle, and plantar reflexes are normal and equal bilaterally. His sensation is intact and equal to both sharp and dull stimulation in his arms, legs, and face, bilaterally.

After supplying his name, he refuses to perform any other components of the MMSE. His meningeal signs are negative.

His cervical, axillary, and inguinal lymph nodes are slightly enlarged and tender to palpate, bilaterally. All his pulses were normal.

3. Based on this information, which of the following diagnostic tests are essential to perform on Mr. Deets and why?

A. Computed tomography (CT) of the head, with and without contrast
B. Complete blood count with differential (CBC w/diff)
C. $CD4^+$ lymphocyte cell count and HIV RNA level
D. Polymerase chain reaction (PCR) testing for *Toxoplasma*, *Coccidioides*, cytomegalovirus (CMV), and Epstein-Barr virus (EBV) antibodies; serum cryptococcal antigen; rapid plasma reagin (RPR); and PPD
E. Urine drug screen

Diagnostic Test Results

Mr. Deets' CT revealed a single, 3.5-cm, round, thin-walled lesion in the white matter near the right lateral ventricle. Contrast induced a ringlike enhancement around the lesion.

His CBC w/diff was normal except a mild leukopenia (leukocyte count of 4250 mm^3 [normal adult: 5000–10,000]) with 80% neutrophils (normal: 55–70), 12% lymphocytes (normal: 20–40), 6% monocytes (normal: 2–8), 1% eosinophils (normal: 1–4), and 1% basophils (normal: 0.5–1).

His $CD4^+$ lymphocyte cell count was 110 cells/µl (normal: 600–1500). His HIV RNA viral load was level was 31,000 copies/ml (normal: none detected).

His PCR testing for *Toxoplasma, Coccidioides*, CMV, and EBV were all negative (normal: negative). His serum cryptococcal antigen was not detected (normal: negative). His RPR was negative (normal: < 1:4). His PPD is pending.

His urine drug screen was also negative (normal: negative).

4. Based on this information, what is Mr. Deets' most likely diagnosis and why?

A. Advanced AIDS with *Toxoplasma* abscess
B. AIDS with tuberculoma
C. AIDS with coccidioidoma
D. AIDS with a non-Hodgkin central nervous system (CNS) lymphoma
E. Bell palsy in an HIV-positive patient

5. Which of the following are appropriate components of Mr. Deets' treatment plan and why?

A. Hospitalize in isolation
B. Consult with an infectious disease specialist, a neurosurgeon, and an oncologist
C. Restart triple antiretroviral therapy unless specialist recommends alternative
D. Four- to 6-week trial of sulfadiazine and pyrimethamine unless specialist recommends alternative
E. Start radiation therapy

CASES IN NEUROLOGIC CONDITIONS

RESPONSES AND DISCUSSION

CASE 9-1
Unger Valley

1. History

A. Are his headaches associated with redness of his eyes, changes in his pupils, lacrimation, edema of his eyelids, drooping of his eyelids, sweating of his forehead or face, nasal congestion, or rhinorrhea? ESSENTIAL

One of the conditions that must be included in Mr. Valley's differential diagnosis list is cluster headaches. True cluster headaches, according to the International Headache Society (IHS), must be associated with at least one of the following symptoms on the ipsilateral side of the face as the headache: conjunctival injection, pupillary constriction, epiphora, eyelid edema, eyelid ptosis, lacrimation, forehead sweating, facial perspiration, nasal congestion, nasal discharge, or a sense of agitation or restlessness. However, these findings are far from specific for cluster headaches.

They can present with headaches from numerous causes. For example, brain tumors and other intracranial masses can cause constriction of the pupil; nasal congestion and discharge can be caused by a sinus infection, other upper respiratory infections, or allergic rhinitis; and nasal congestion and lacrimation can be present in migraines, trigeminal autonomic cephalalgias, or paroxysmal hemicranias. Abuse of substances can also produce similar findings depending on the substance being abused (e.g. nasal congestion with cocaine, mydriasis with cocaine or amphetamines, and myosis with heroin).

B. Does lying down affect his headaches? ESSENTIAL

The majority of headaches tend to improve when the patient assumes a supine position; however, there are a few types of headaches that are worsened by or prevent the patient from being able to do such. They include cluster headaches and headaches caused by elevated intracranial pressure (e.g., brain malignancies, metastatic intracranial lesions, meningoma, acoustic neuroma, brain abscess, and pseudotumor cerebri).

Migraines and new daily persistent headache (NDPH) can infrequently be associated with this pattern.

C. Does he experience any bowel changes with the headaches? NONESSENTIAL

Bowel changes are generally not associated with any type of chronic headaches.

D. Does he experience nocturnal symptoms? ESSENTIAL

Difficulty falling asleep would not be an unusual finding in a patient with an acute headache, nor would difficulty lying down in bed be unusual in individuals who are experiencing headaches caused by one of the aforementioned conditions associated with worsening symptoms when supine; however, very few headaches (or associated symptoms) actually awaken the patient from sleep. Headaches with true nocturnal symptoms can include those caused by brain tumors, cluster headaches, paroxysmal hemicrania, temporal arteritis, hypnic headaches, or a major mood disorder. Thus, if a patient is experiencing true nocturnal symptoms, his or her list of differential diagnoses can potentially be significantly reduced. However, it is important to remember that conditions generally cannot be diagnosed based on the presence of one particular symptom, nor can a potential diagnosis be excluded based on the absence of a single symptom.

E. Has he had any changes in his appetite, sleep, mood, interest, activities, or pleasures? ESSENTIAL

Headaches can be caused by stress, anxiety, and depression. In fact, headaches are one of the more common presentations of depression in the primary care setting. Therefore, it is essential not to overlook a major mood disorder as the cause of a headache.

2. Physical Examination

A. Palpation of the head ESSENTIAL

Palpation of the head is unlikely to assist in making the diagnosis of a headache caused by an intracranial process.

However, it can be useful in determining those caused by extracranial causes, including muscle contracture headaches, tension-type headaches (TTHs), temporal arteritis, tympanomandibular syndrome, and occasionally migraines (especially if tenderness is located in the scalp).

B. Palpation of the thyroid   NONESSENTIAL

Hypothyroidism, hyperthyroidism, thyroid masses, thyroid cancers, and other conditions potentially associated with palpable thyroid abnormalities are highly unlikely to produce a headache.

C. Abdominal examination   NONESSENTIAL

Although there are a few conditions that could potentially produce both a headache and intra-abdominal pathology, they tend to be acute (and often infectious) in nature. The likelihood that a patient would have a chronic medical condition associated with a headache and an intra-abdominal process, without any significant gastrointestinal, genitourinary, or reproductive symptoms, is very small.

D. Cranial nerve evaluation   ESSENTIAL

Any patient complaining of a headache should have his or her cranial nerves evaluated. The examination could potentially identify numerous findings (e.g., facial weakness, ptosis, abnormal pupillary response, pain with extraocular movements [EOMs], visual field defects, photophobia, or phonophobia) that could assist in determining the patient's correct diagnosis.

E. Cursory neurologic examination, with further evaluation of any abnormalities identified   ESSENTIAL

Focal neurologic deficits are occasionally seen with headaches. Because some of these are potentially life-threatening (e.g., intracranial hemorrhage, cerebrovascular accident [CVA], benign or malignant space-occupying lesions, and meningitis), an abbreviated neurologic examination must be performed as a routine component of the physical examination of a patient presenting with a headache. Obviously, if any abnormal findings are identified, a more comprehensive neurologic examination is mandatory.

However, not all abnormal neurologic findings identified on the physical examination of a patient complaining of headaches are going to represent a potentially life-threatening condition. There are a few headache syndromes in which patients can develop focal neurologic defects associated with their headache. The most common is probably migraine headache with aura. Conversely, not all abnormal neurologic findings identified on the physical examination of a patient complaining of a headache are necessarily related to the headache.

3. Diagnostic Studies

A. Computed tomography (CT) of the brain   NONESSENTIAL

Because Mr. Valley's history and physical examination are sufficient to establish the cause of his headaches and he did not have any headache "red flags" (alarm or warning symptoms), he does not need an imaging study at this time. However, headaches that are associated with "red flags" require prompt evaluation because their presence significantly increases the probability that the patient's headache does not have a benign cause. Although a significant intracranial

pathology only accounts for an estimated 5 to 10% of all headaches, it is responsible for the vast majority all the morbidity and virtually all the mortality associated with headaches. Thus, the presence of even one of these "red flag" symptoms is justification for a CT scan.

These "red flag" symptoms include headaches that are described by the patient as the "worst" of his or her life; severe and unlike any previously experienced; progressively worsened over days (or even weeks); preceded by vomiting; intensified by bending, lifting, coughing, or sneezing; sleep interrupters; present upon awakening; or associated with a known systemic disease, a fever or other constitutional symptoms, an abnormal neurologic examination, age older than 55 years, or localized tenderness on palpation of the skull/face.

B. Magnetic resonance imaging (MRI) of the brain NONESSENTIAL

An MRI of the brain is not required on Mr. Valley for the same reasons he does not require a CT scan. Unless there is a suspicion of an intracranial bleed (e.g., acute CVA, intracranial hemorrhage, or leaking arteriovenous [AV] malformation or aneurysm), either a contrast-enhanced MRI or CT is essentially equivalent in diagnosing intracranial pathology, with the exception of abnormalities located in the posterior fossa or when there is a suspicion of an early abscess formation; then, an MRI might be slightly better at identifying the abnormality, especially if it is early in the disease process or the abnormality is small. However, when an intracranial hemorrhage is suspected, a noncontrast CT is the imaging study of choice because during the first 24 to 48 hours following a bleed, it is often not evident on MRI.

C. Thyroid scintiscan   NONESSENTIAL

A thyroid scintiscan is indicated when more information is required regarding the location, size, shape, and function of the thyroid gland. Because Mr. Valley has a normal thyroid gland on palpation, lacks symptoms suspicious for a thyroid condition, and has not had any serum thyroid function testing, he does not require a thyroid scintiscan. Furthermore, it would be extremely rare for a thyroid condition to be associated with a headache, especially in the absence of ischemic or other neurologic symptoms. Thus, the most probable outcome of a thyroid scintiscan for Mr. Valley would be unnecessary radiation exposure.

D. Erythrocyte sedimentation rate (ESR)   NONESSENTIAL

Because of Mr. Valley's history and physical examination findings, there is no reason to suspect an inflammatory, infectious, or malignant cause for his headaches, which are the primary indications for an ESR.

E. Complete blood count with differential (CBC w/diff) NONESSENTIAL

Because Mr. Valley's headaches do not appear to have an infectious, inflammatory, or malignant cause, a CBC w/diff is highly unlikely to provide any useful clinical information.

4. Diagnosis

A. Migraine headaches without aura   INCORRECT

Until recently, migraine headaches were assumed to be caused by a vascular phenomenon. However, recent research in this area indicates that migraine headaches are probably caused by an abnormality of serotonin.

According to the IHS second edition of diagnostic criteria for the evaluation of headaches (developed in 1994), in order to establish the diagnosis of a migraine headache WITHOUT aura, ALL of the following criteria must be present: (1) the headache must last a minimum of 4 but no longer than 72 hours, with or without treatment; (2) it must possess a minimum of TWO of the following qualities: unilateral, pulsating, moderate to severe in intensity, or aggravated by normal physical activity (such as walking or climbing stairs); (3) it must be associated with nausea and/or vomiting AND/OR phonophobia and photophobia; and (4) it cannot be attributable to any other condition.

Although migraine headaches are typically unilateral in location, they differ from Mr. Valley's headaches in length of duration, associated symptoms, and descriptive qualities. Therefore, migraine headache without aura is not Mr. Valley's most likely diagnosis.

B. Episodic cluster headaches   CORRECT

Originally, cluster headaches were considered to be a migraine variant, hence the older term of "migrainous neuralgia." However, currently they are considered to be a distinct entity, despite their mechanism of occurrence being unknown. They are characterized by "clusters" of headache episodes in a very similar distribution to what Mr. Valley is experiencing. The IHS defines episodic cluster headache as experiencing a minimum of five headaches that meet ALL four of the following characteristics: (1) it has to be severe to excruciating in nature AND be unilateral AND be located orbitally, supraorbitally, or temporally AND last a minimum of 15 minutes and a maximum of 180 minutes if untreated; (2) the ipsilateral side of the head must have at least ONE of the following: conjunctival injection, constriction of the pupil, tearing, eyelid edema, eyelid ptosis, forehead sweating, facial perspiration, nasal congestion, or nasal discharge, OR a sense of agitation or restlessness; (3) the patient must experience the headache in clusters consisting of no less than one every other day AND no more than eight times per day; (4) there is not a secondary cause for the headache. Thus, episodic cluster headache is Mr. Valley's most likely diagnosis.

C. Migraine headaches with aura   INCORRECT

Migraine headaches with aura are distinguished from other forms of migraines because they are associated with an aura (prodromal symptoms) with photophobia or other visual disturbances, in which patterns of intermittent bright lights being the most common. In order to establish the diagnosis of migraine WITH aura, all the aforementioned criteria for a migraine headache must be met PLUS an aura must be present. Because Mr. Valley does not have any warning of when his headaches are going to occur nor do his headaches meet the diagnostic criteria for migraine headaches, migraine headache with aura is not his most likely diagnosis.

D. Paroxysmal hemicrania   INCORRECT

Paroxysmal hemicrania shares many of the symptoms commonly attributed to cluster headaches. They are located in the same areas and must be associated with at least ONE of the following on the ipsilateral side as the headache: conjunctival injection, constriction of the pupil, epiphora, eyelid edema, eyelid ptosis, forehead sweating, facial perspiration, rhinorrhea, nasal congestion, or a sense of agitation or restlessness. Additionally, they cannot be caused by another condition.

However, paroxysmal hemicrania differs from cluster headaches in regards to their remaining IHS criteria for the condition. These are a minimum of 20 headaches that last from 2 to 30 minutes with or without treatment AND a minimum of five distinct episodes per day at least 50% of the time AND capable of being aborted or prevented with indomethacin. Thus, this is not Mr. Valley's most likely diagnosis.

E. Chronic cluster headaches   INCORRECT

According to the IHS, the diagnostic criteria for chronic and episodic cluster headaches are identical except that chronic cluster headaches must be present at least every other day for a minimum of 1 year OR have remission periods that are shorter than 1 month in duration. Therefore, chronic cluster headaches are not Mr. Valley's most likely diagnosis.

5. Treatment Plan

A. Trial sumatriptan (6 mg SQ or 20 mg intranasally) at onset of headache   CORRECT

Sumatriptan is a selective 5-HT agonist. Although the intranasal formulation does not have a US Food and Drug Administration (FDA) indication for cluster headaches, it has been utilized with some success in patients with this condition. However, the injectable formulation is FDA approved for both migraine and cluster headaches, whereas the tablets are only approved for migraines. The other 5-HT agonists (e.g., almotriptan, eletriptan, frovatriptan, and rizatriptan) only have FDA-approved indications for the treatment of migraines; however, they are probably effective in cluster headaches as well.

B. Look for triggers of headaches   CORRECT

Triggers (e.g., alcohol, spicy foods, and stress) can induce a cluster headache. Therefore, it is important to attempt to identify individual triggers for each patient. If found, they can be eliminated, when possible, to prevent the occurrence of all, or at least some, of his headaches.

C. Discuss possibility of prophylaxis treatment with patient, including potential adverse effects of medications, advantages, and disadvantages   CORRECT

Depending on the severity and frequency of his symptoms, his response to abortive therapy, and the effect of his headaches on his lifestyle (e.g., employment, interpersonal relationships, and recreational activities), he might want to consider utilizing prophylactic medication to prevent, or at least reduce, the frequency and severity of his episodes.

There are three off-label medications that have been proven to be effective for the chronic prevention of cluster headaches: methysergide, lithium, and verapamil. Additionally, off-label use of the prescription drugs gabapentin and topiramate, as well as usage of the over-the-counter product melatonin, has not been proven to be effective in clinical trials; however, they have been reported in the literature as effective for select patients. They would certainly be worth considering in individuals who have medical contraindications to the other agents or are unresponsive or intolerant of them.

Some experts feel that the prophylactic use of verapamil is the safest option. However, before selecting a therapy, it is essential to consider not only the individual medications and their contraindications, drug interactions, and potential adverse effects but also how they impact on the patient's other medical conditions, medications, and drug allergies. This information needs to be shared with Mr. Valley, as well as the fact that these medications do not have FDA approval for this usage. It is also appropriate to inform him that even though the selected medication is not approved for this usage in his condition, there is some evidence to support the usage; explain the cumbersome process of getting new indications for drugs already on the market; and explain the difficulties associated with getting medications to the market for orphan diseases.

Individuals who are resistant to therapy can be considered for radiofrequency therapy to the ganglion pterygopalatinum. Additionally, occipital nerve stimulation is a potential last-resort therapy.

D. Oxygen therapy   CORRECT

Fifteen to 20 minutes of high-dose oxygen therapy (100% at 10 to 12 L/min) has been shown to be very effective in aborting an acute cluster headache, especially if started immediately after the onset of the headache. This therapy should not be utilized in individuals with chronic obstructive pulmonary disease (COPD) because this high flow of oxygen could suppress their respirations as their respiratory drive is based on carbon dioxide, not oxygen.

E. If headache persists beyond a half hour, increases in frequency, increases in intensity, becomes associated with focal neurologic defects, or changes in any way, return to clinic or go to emergency department (ED) immediately   CORRECT

Advising the patient what to do if his symptoms change or persist is also a crucial element of any treatment plan. The aforementioned conditions are not generally associated with cluster headaches and are not typical for Mr. Valley; therefore, they could represent a new-onset headache of a different cause that needs to be promptly evaluated in hopes of preventing serious morbidity and mortality depending on the cause.

Epidemiologic and Other Data

Cluster headaches affect ~0.1% of the US population. The male-to-female ratio is 3:1. There does not appear to be any relevant family clustering of the condition. The onset of the headache occurs at night in approximately 50% of the patients.

The exact mechanism of cluster headaches is unknown. Some support the theory that they occur in posterior hypothalamic regions as a result of abnormalities of the central pacemaker neurons. However, other experts feel they are related to either an abnormality of the vasculature or the neurotransmitter serotonin.

In general, 90 to 95% of all headaches have a benign cause.

CASE 9-2

Vinnie Winchester

1. History

A. Has he experienced any problems with his memory or confusion?   ESSENTIAL

Mr. Winchester appears to be describing an involuntary hyperkinetic movement problem, the most common of which is a tremor. Tremors can be divided into four basic categories (parkinsonian, exaggerated physiologic, essential, and cerebellar) depending on their coarseness, presence at rest, postural component, intentional component, and location. Because only mild distinctions exist between these various categories, atypical presentations occur frequently, they can be associated with certain medical conditions, and they can result from adverse medication effects, it is essential to inquire about symptoms related to these entities in order make the correct diagnosis. For example, the chorea associated with early Huntington disease resembles the tremor of Parkinson disease; however, Parkinson disease is associated with a mild cognitive decline, whereas Huntington disease is associated with a true dementia. Depression can also present with a tremor similar to a parkinsonian type tremor; and, a predominant feature of depression is a memory loss. Partial seizures can also exhibit involuntary movements, especially of the hands; they can be associated with a sense of detached confusion.

B. Has he had abdominal pain, nausea, vomiting, bowel changes, jaundice, or icterus?   ESSENTIAL

Hepatic diseases can cause a wide array of nongastrointestinal manifestations, including neurologic abnormalities (primarily movement, mood, and memory disorders). Involuntary movement disorders are not uncommon in the latter stages of Wilson disease, cirrhosis, and hepatitis.

C. How old was his father when he was first diagnosed with senile tremors?   NONESSENTIAL

Senile tremors are considered to be a subtype of benign essential tremors that are not apparent until the patient is elderly. Benign essential tremors can become apparent at any age, including childhood. However, they become worse and more noticeable as the patient ages. Furthermore, they can vary not only in severity but also in how they impact a patient's life. Therefore, Mr. Winchester's father's age at diagnosis probably correlates poorly with his age when he actually started experiencing symptoms. Thus, his father's age at diagnosis is unrelated to Mr. Winchester's risk of acquiring the condition and is not predictive of the age that he might develop the condition. Nevertheless, because benign essential tremors are an autosomal dominant inherited disorder, Mr. Winchester's father having this condition increases Mr. Winchester's risk of acquiring it.

D. Has he had palpitations, dyspnea, fever, heat or cold intolerance, changes in perspiration, polydipsia, polyuria, vertigo, lightheadedness, presyncope, or syncope?   ESSENTIAL

Metabolic alterations (e.g., hypoxia and hypothalamic conditions), endocrinopathies (e.g., hyperthyroidism, hypothyroidism, and diabetes mellitus), autonomic dysfunction (e.g., dysautonomia, multiple system atrophy, and Shy-Drager syndrome), and adverse effects caused by medications (e.g., amlodipine, propranolol, hydrochlorothiazide, prazosin, clonidine, citalopram, tricyclic antidepressants, and morphine/opioids) can produce involuntary movement disorders. However, with the exception of drug adverse effects, it is highly improbable that any of these conditions would manifest without some other sign or symptom indicating the presence of the causative condition.

E. Does he experience any problems with balance and/or co-ordination?   ESSENTIAL

In regards to attempting to establish the diagnosis of tremors, if the patient reports difficulties with balance and/or coordination, cerebellar tremors must be included among the differential diagnoses. Likewise, if the patient is not experiencing any problems in these areas, it is extremely unlikely that cerebellar tremors are the cause of the patient's symptoms.

2. Physical Examination

A. Cornea examination   ESSENTIAL

The sensory and motor components of the eyes will be evaluated during the cranial nerve examination. However, the cornea itself needs to be examined in patients presenting with tremors for the presence of a Kayser-Fletcher ring (a green-gray or brownish discoloration of the cornea secondary to granular copper deposits). If present, this finding is pathognomonic for Wilson disease. However, the absence of a Kayser-Fechner ring does eliminate Wilson disease from the list of potential diagnoses, especially if other signs and symptoms of the condition are present. In general, if the patient has primarily neuropsychological symptoms, the rings are more likely to be seen than if the patient has predominately hepatic involvement.

B. Thyroid examination   ESSENTIAL

Because tremors are frequently associated with primary and secondary hyperthyroidism and occasionally seen in primary and secondary hypothyroidism, it is essential to palpate the thyroid.

C. Cervical spine examination   NONESSENTIAL

Although the cervical spine can be affected by an involuntary hyperkinetic movement problem, it is generally a cervical dystonia causing contractures of the related spinal musculature resulting in abnormal neck and head postures, not a hand tremor.

D. Abdominal examination   ESSENTIAL

As previously stated, some tremors are associated with conditions that can affect the liver (e.g., Wilson disease and alcoholic cirrhosis). Thus, it is important to perform an abdominal examination on all patients with the complaint of tremor for the presence of hepatomegaly or other abnormalities.

E. Cursory neurologic examination, with extended exam if problems are identified   ESSENTIAL

Because a tremor is a neurologic complaint, a cursory neurologic examination is essential; obviously, a comprehensive neurologic examination is required if any abnormality is identified.

3. Diagnostic Studies

A. Thyroid-stimulating hormone (TSH)   ESSENTIAL

There are very few diagnostic tests that are indicated in the evaluation of a tremor unless a secondary cause is suspected based on the findings of the patient's history and physical examination. Despite Mr. Winchester's clinical picture not being typical for hyperthyroidism, most experts will still agree that a screening TSH is indicated to evaluate for this condition because tremor can be the presenting (and only) symptom.

B. Liver functioning tests (LFTs)   NONESSENTIAL

LFTs are not indicated for the routine evaluation of patients who present with tremor. However, they are indicated if the patient has signs or symptoms that are suspicious for a hepatic cause.

C. Serum copper (Cu) and ceruloplasmin levels   NONESSENTIAL

These tests are only indicated in patients presenting with tremor when their history and physical examination are suspicious for Wilson disease. Although both hepatic and neuropsychiatric symptoms can be the presenting symptoms for patients with Wilson disease, it is highly unlikely that tremors are the only neuropsychiatric symptom upon presentation because the tremors related to Wilson disease result directly from the copper depositing in the basial ganglia of the brain; thus, more evidence of basial ganglia dysfunction should be evident.

D. Electroencephalography (EEG)   NONESSENTIAL

Although simple partial seizures can be associated with focal involuntary muscle movements without a loss of consciousness, they are rarely present and equal in a bilateral distribution. Furthermore, they tend to be more clonic in appearance than a tremor.

E. Computed tomography (CT) of the brain   NONESSENTIAL

CT of the brain is not a usual component of the initial evaluation of a patient with an involuntary movement disorder unless there is some evidence to suggest an intracranial pathology (e.g., intracranial hemorrhage, vascular abnormality, or space-occupying lesion) is present.

4. Diagnosis

A. Parkinson disease   INCORRECT

Parkinson disease (also known as shaking palsy, trembling palsy, or parkinsonism) is a neurodegenerative disorder believed to result from a dopamine deficiency. It is characterized by involuntary muscle tremors that are rhythmic in nature, rigidity of joints, bradykinesis, micrographia, masklike facies, autonomic dysfunction, and depression. Because Mr. Winchester does not have any of these symptoms, Parkinson disease is not his most likely diagnosis.

B. Psychogenic tremor   INCORRECT

Psychogenic tremor, as the name implies, has its cause rooted in a psychopathy. With some effort, mood symptoms can generally be elicited from the patient. Furthermore, distraction frequently alleviates the tremor on physical examination. Thus, this is not Mr. Winchester's most likely diagnosis.

C. Wilson disease   INCORRECT

Although Wilson disease (Westphal-Strümpell disease or hepatolenticular degeneration) is a form of hereditary hemochromatosis in which copper is deposited in the liver, brain, corneas, and kidneys of affected individuals, it is classified as a hepatic condition because its primary physiologic pathology is increased small bowel absorption of copper in conjunction with decreased hepatic elimination of copper. As previously stated, it generally manifests with hepatic and neuropsychological symptoms; one of these symptoms is often an involuntary movement disorder. This abnormality can be either intermittent, regular, fine oscillatory movements (as seen with a tremor) or intermittent or sustained, gross muscle movement frequently associated with abnormal posturing (as seen with a dystonia). The associated dystonia can also produce dysarthria and dysphagia. The tremor can be resting, positional, or intentional. However, as stated previously, it is highly unlikely that a purely neuropsychiatric disease is going to occur in the absence of any other neuropsychiatric symptoms because of the biochemical alterations producing these symptoms. Thus, Wilson disease is not Mr. Winchester's most likely diagnosis.

D. Benign essential tremor   CORRECT

Benign essential tremor is a high-frequency tremor of unknown cause that appears to be autosomal dominant. It primarily affects the upper extremities (but occasionally can involve the head and voice) in an equal, bilateral distribution and has both a postural and kinetic tremor. Plus, it is very frequently aggravated by caffeine consumption and alleviated by drinking alcohol.

To establish the diagnosis of benign essential tremor, the condition must be distinguished from the other primary tremor types. As previously stated, this is complicated by the lack of diagnostic studies to assist with the diagnosis, the majority of signs and symptoms not being pathognomic for any one particular tremor type, and atypical presentations often occurring. Therefore, small, subtle differences assist in establishing the diagnosis of a patient presenting with a tremor. For example, parkinsonian tremors are typically more coarse and "stiffer" than essential tremors. Unlike essential tremors, they tend to be worse at rest; however, they also can have a moderate postural or intentional component. It is not uncommon for the jaw and tongue to be affected by parkinsonian tremors; however, this is rare in other tremors, even those affecting the head. Although parkinsonian tremors resemble those tremors associated with Parkinson disease, if the other defining criteria for Parkinson disease (see earlier) are not present, then the patient does not have the disease.

The head is frequently involved in cerebellar tremors; however, this is not exclusive for this type of tremors. They also tend to be associated with difficulties with balance and coordination. Generally, they are variable in amplitude, rarely occur at rest, and have both postural and intentional components. In contrast, essential tremors (which tend to be uniform in amplitude) generally have a postural component that is slightly more prominent and/or frequent than the intentional component. With cerebellar tremors, the opposite is generally true.

Exaggerated physiologic tremors are fine, rarely occur at rest, and are more postural than intentional, making them the most difficult to distinguish from essential tremors. Nevertheless, from the choices provided, Mr. Winchester's most likely diagnosis is benign essential tremor. This diagnosis is based on his positive family history, his tremor being aggravated by stress and caffeine, alcohol alleviating his tremor temporarily, only his upper extremities being affected, and his postural component being slightly worse than the intentional component.

E. Multiple system atrophy   INCORRECT

Multiple system atrophy (MSA) is the new term for Shy-Drager syndrome. It is a neurodegenerative condition of unknown cause that is progressive and fatal. Its main symptoms are a primary physiologic defect of autonomic nervous system dysfunction. It is generally associated with parkinsonism characteristics and/or ataxia. When the parkinsonism symptoms predominate, it is called MSA-P; it is known as MSA-C when the cerebellar symptoms (e.g., ataxia) predominate. It can also be eliminated as Mr. Winchester's most likely diagnosis because he does not have symptoms consistent with autonomic dysfunction.

5. Treatment Plan

A. Primidone 12.5 mg once daily, then gradually increase the dose until symptoms resolve or a maximum dose of 1000 mg is attained, if tolerated   CORRECT

Primidone is an antiseizure medication that has been proven to be effective in the off-label treatment of benign essential tremor. It is considered to be a first-line medication. Approximately 50% of patients with essential tremor have some response to it. It should be given at night because of its sedation properties; furthermore, the patient must be appropriately warned to take the necessary precautions because of this known adverse effect. Additionally, the patient needs to be apprised that this is an off-label indication and the significance of such.

B. Long-acting propranolol 20 mg once a day   CORRECT

The beta-blocking antihypertensive propranolol, has also been proven to provide some benefit to approximately 50% of patients with benign essential tremor. This is considered to be a first-line agent, and is also an off-label usage. Beta-blockers should be avoided in individuals with a history of cardiac arrhythmias and pulmonary disease. Patients who are intolerant of propranolol should be tried on another beta-blocker because the majority of drugs in this class of medications appear to be nearly as effective in treating essential tremor as propranolol. The patient should be made aware of the potential adverse effects, how to prevent them, and to return to the clinic (or to the nearest emergency department) if problematic. The usual starting dose is 20 mg once daily. It can gradually be increased as tolerated until the patient achieves a symptomatic response or a maximum dose of 320 mg/day. Initial drug therapy should consist of a single first-line medication.

Second-line medications include the off-label use of antiseizure drugs (gabapentin and topiramate), benzodiazepines (clonazepam and alprazolam), and antipsychotic medications (clozapine and olanzapine). Currently, there are no medications approved by the FDA for use in the treatment of benign essential tremor.

C. Relaxation therapy course   CORRECT

Relaxation therapy is also considered to be an acceptable first-line therapy for benign essential tremor, especially if it is mild to moderate in severity and aggravated by stress or anxiety. With appropriate relaxation techniques, the symptoms can be significantly reduced, if not completely eliminated. However, successful therapy does not mean that the patient's condition was psychological (i.e., psychogenic tremor) and was misdiagnosed as benign essential tremor.

D. Liver biopsy   INCORRECT

A liver biopsy is not indicated for Mr. Winchester because he does not have any signs, symptoms, or laboratory findings to indicate that a hepatic problem (e.g., Wilson disease, hepatitis, or cirrhosis) can be implicated as the possible cause of his tremor. The most common signs and symptoms associated with a hepatic cause include right upper quadrant pain, jaundice, icterus, constitutional symptoms, a palpable tender liver, and ascites. Laboratory abnormalities would include abnormal LFTs and disease-specific tests (e.g., elevated serum copper and ceruloplasmin in Wilson disease and hepatitis antibodies and antigen in acute and chronic hepatitis).

E. Botulinum toxin type A injections   INCORRECT

Botulinum toxin type A injections should only be used if medical therapy has failed and the symptoms are causing the patient significant distress and/or disability. They offer some improvement in symptoms, especially in regards to upper extremity and vocal symptoms. However, the procedure is associated with a high rate of muscle weakness, especially if the hand is treated. Additionally there is the rare possibility that the patient can acquire botulism from the injections.

The last-resort effort in treating very symptomatic patients who are experiencing major disruption of their lives secondary to the benign essential tremor include thalamotomy, long-term thalamic deep unilateral brain stimulation, or bilateral thalamic deep brain stimulation. Studies indicate that bilateral thalamic deep brain stimulation is the most effective of the three options, especially if the disease is bilateral. Additionally, studies appear to indicate that either type of stimulation has better success rates than surgery.

Epidemiologic and Other Data

As the most common involuntary hyperkinetic movement disorder, benign essential tremor is estimated to affect approximately 5 to 10 million people in the United States. It is also known as familial tremor or heredofamilial tremor, because over half of the individuals with this condition have a positive family history. It appears to be autosomal dominant inherited. It gradually worsens with age and affects males more often than females.

CASE 9-3
Willamette Xandier
1. History

A. What was she preparing for breakfast this morning and the last time she experienced these symptoms?   NONESSENTIAL

Although this is a terrific question to establish rapport with the patient, possibly put her "more at ease," and assist in determining her preillness level of functioning, it is not essential at this time because it fails to provide any useful clinical information to assist in determining which diagnostic tests should be performed, her most likely diagnosis, and her treatment plan. Furthermore, even if the healthcare provider (HCP) had the time to ask questions, the patient may not. This type of question is best left until all the pertinent information is obtained because Mrs. Xandier's symptoms mandate that her initial evaluation be performed as rapidly, yet thoroughly, as possible because she could have a potentially life-threatening condition.

B. Is she experiencing any paresthesias or dysesthesias?   ESSENTIAL

Unilateral weakness, dysarthria, and paresthesias/dysesthesias can be the presenting features of a multitude of medical conditions including central neurologic conditions involving the upper or lower motor neurons; cerebrovascular ischemia or hemorrhage; peripheral neurologic problems involving the nerves, their plexuses, or their roots; disorders affecting the neuromuscular junction; emboli phenomena from cardiac diseases and/or endothelium dysfunction; infectious diseases; inflammatory conditions; hematologic abnormalities; hypercoagulable disorders; and hypoxia. Nevertheless, it is still important to know if she is experiencing these symptoms, and if so, their location, description, course, duration, and other associated features. This descriptive information is what will be useful in attempting to clarify the exact location of Mrs. Xandier's presenting symptoms as well as in assisting in the development of her differential diagnoses.

It is important to note that the occurrence of intermittent paresthesia/dysesthesia in the absence of any other symptoms could represent ischemic vascular disease of the carotid arteries.

C. Is she experiencing any dysphagia?   ESSENTIAL

Dysphagia, unilateral weakness, and dysarthria can also occur in a wide variety of medical conditions. The most common include transient ischemic attacks (TIAs), CVAs, multiple sclerosis, myasthenia gravis, dysautonomias, somatic disorders, and dysphagia lusoria. Thus, the relevant information obtained from this question has more to do with the actual description of the symptoms as opposed to their presence. For example, an acute onset of dysphagia is highly unlikely to be caused by a mechanical obstruction or a motility disorder (unless this represents the initial episode) because the dysphagia in these disorders tends to be intermittent and/or progressive; however, a CVA or TIA would be associated with an acute onset of dysphagia. Oropharyngeal dysphagia (swallowing difficulty located in the throat) can be caused by either a mechanical obstruction or a motility disorder; the primary distinguishing feature is that motility disorders also exhibit other neuromuscular findings, which would be inconsistent with a mechanical obstruction unless a coexisting condition was present.

Esophageal dysphagia (swallowing difficulty located in either the chest or the pharynx) can also result from mechanical obstructions and motility disorders. With esophageal dysphagia, the most likely cause is determined by whether the problem occurs with solids or with solids and liquids; solids only tend to have an obstructive cause, whereas solids and liquids appear to be related to a motor disorder and are frequently associated with heartburn, except with achalasia. The presence of both pharyngeal and esophageal dysphagia is almost always caused by a neurologic or neuromuscular condition. Psychogenic dysphagia is much rarer than previously assumed and commonly limited to globus hystericus, which is pharyngeal in location and accompanied by the sensation of "a ball in the throat."

D. Is she experiencing any palpitations?   ESSENTIAL

Palpitations can represent an underlying cardiac arrhythmia (which can be independent of or associated with a valvular abnormality) producing decreased perfusion and hypoxia that could account for her presenting symptoms. Additionally, anemia, fever, endocrinopathies (e.g., diabetes mellitus, hyperthyroidism, and/or pheochromocytoma), and psychopathies (e.g., predominately anxiety disorders) can occasionally be the underlying pathology of an arrhythmia (most frequently sinus arrhythmia) that is responsible for the palpitations and their related symptoms.

E. Were any of these episodes associated with a fall, loss of consciousness, seizurelike activity, or incontinence of her bladder and/or bowels?   ESSENTIAL

A history of a fall in conjunction with a loss of consciousness could represent an intracranial hemorrhage, contusion, or edema causing Mrs. Xandier's symptoms. If not witnessed, the occurrence of a tonic-clonic seizure might not be known to the patient; however, he or she should be able to relay a history consistent with postictal symptoms, loss of consciousness, a fall, and urinary (and occasionally bowel) incontinence. Furthermore, the postictal phase following a seizure can cause neurologic defects, including unilateral weakness and dysarthria.

Secondary seizures (as a result of another cause including TIAs, CVAs, hypoglycemia, electrolyte imbalances, hepatic failure, renal insufficiency, meningitis, brain tumors, and other space-occupying brain lesions) can also present as unilateral weakness, dysarthria, or other focal neurologic deficits.

2. Physical Examination

A. BP in all four extremities (in addition to regular vital sign assessment)   ESSENTIAL

Comparisons should be made between the contralateral arms, contralateral ankles, and ipsilateral arm and ankle. When comparing brachial systolic BP between the arms, a difference of greater than 20 mm Hg could indicate an intermittent vertebrobasilar ischemia caused by subclavian steal syndrome.

Comparing the measurements of the BP in the ankle and ipsilateral arm establishes the patient's ankle-brachial index (ABI). The ABI provides an objective measurement that assists in establishing the presence of arterial insufficiency of the lower extremities. The ABI is determined by dividing the systolic BP at the ankle by the systolic BP measured in the brachial artery. A normal ABI is greater than or equal to 1.0. If the ABI is less than 1.0, then arterial insufficiency is present in the lower extremities. If it is less than 0.5, then severe arterial insufficiency of the lower extremities is present.

B. Evaluation of all pulses   ESSENTIAL

Evaluation of all pulses is essential to determine if any are diminished and/or with a bruit, which can indicate the presence of atherosclerosis, subclavian steal syndrome, and/or carotid stenosis that could result in an ischemic or thromboembolic event producing Mrs. Xandier's symptoms.

C. Heart and lung examination   ESSENTIAL

A heart and lung examination is important to evaluate for signs of valvular heart disease that could produce an embolic phenomenon, arrhythmias that could result in poor cerebral perfusion and hypoxia, pulmonary conditions (e.g., chronic obstructive pulmonary disease, asthma, and pneumonia) that could cause central hypoxia, and cardiopulmonary conditions

(e.g., heart failure) that could decrease perfusion. Any of these conditions alone or in combination could be responsible for Mrs. Xandier's symptoms.

The heart and lung examination should include an evaluation for the presence of pedal edema. Bilateral, equal pitting lower extremity edema is commonly seen, but not exclusively, in heart failure (HF). Unilateral lower extremity edema is suspicious for a deep vein thrombosis (DVT); however, other conditions can cause this. HF or a DVT can be responsible for Mrs. Xandier's symptoms: HF via inadequate perfusion and DVT via an embolic phenomenon.

D. Neurologic examination   ESSENTIAL

The neurologic examination is critical in the formation of Mrs. Xandier's differential diagnoses. It evaluates for potential defects and assists in determining which areas of the brain are most likely to be involved; the HCP can then apply these findings to knowledge regarding the innervations of the affected area's sensory and motor components. Additionally, it can be useful in differentiating between upper versus lower motor neuron conditions, central versus peripheral neuropathies, and myopathies that could be responsible for her hemiparesis.

Upper motor neuron conditions typically involve select muscle groups and are associated with spasticity of the affected muscles, but no true atrophy; additionally, they are characterized by increased deep tendon reflexes and an increased plantar response. In contrast, lower neuron diseases are typically associated with muscle atrophy, flaccidity, fasciculations, and decreased (or absent) deep tendon reflexes, and generally no change in the plantar reflex.

Peripheral neuropathies can often be distinguished from one another by the location and extent of the motor and sensory loss in combination with a good working knowledge of the anatomy of nerves, their distribution, and their individual motor and sensory functions. For example, sensory symptoms of the lateral aspect of the thumb are generally caused by radial nerve involvement, whereas sensory symptoms involving the medial aspect of the thumb are generally caused by median nerve involvement, especially if the symptoms also involve the second, third, and half of the fourth digits. However, most of the motor control of the thumb is via the median nerve.

Neuromuscular disorders can often be distinguished from central and peripheral neuropathies by their erratic distribution of weakness, lack of sensory changes, and fluctuations of symptoms over short time spans, at least initially. Myopathies involve the muscles themselves; therefore, initially, weakness is the predominate finding. Later on, atrophy and loss of deep tendon reflexes occur. Additionally, they lack sensory changes.

E. HINTS (**H**ead **I**mpulse/**N**ystagmus/**T**est of **S**kew) testing   NONESSENTIAL

The HINTS test involves checking for evidence of eye instability when rapidly moving the patient's head in alternating lateral directions (head impulse), evaluating for a "jerking" movement when testing the extraocular muscles' movement in the lateral direction (nystagmus), and testing for evidence of eye malalignment in the horizontal position (test of skew). Although certainly not specific for CVA, these abnormalities have been found to be present in individuals who are experiencing marked vertigo in the hours preceding their presentation if a CVA was the cause of their problem. In fact, in the first clinical trial on the concept, the 1-minute eye examination was superior to MRI as it correctly identified 100% of the subset of patients with CVA who presented with acute vestibular syndrome.

Even though testing for skew and nystagmus is a component of any neurologic examination, head-impulse testing generally only is routinely employed when evaluating patients with vertigo. Thus, Mrs. Xandier does not require the full HINTS testing. Because the only study evaluating patients for CVA utilizing this technique was in patients presenting with acute vestibular syndrome, it is inappropriate to extrapolate these finds as indicators of CVAs in patients without this specific syndrome. Furthermore, until larger studies are performed to determine whether this finding is indeed present in 100% (or at least a very significant majority) of patients with CVAs presenting as acute vestibular syndrome and the results are correlated with noncontrast CT (which is the imaging study of choice in patients suspected of having an acute stroke because of MRI's difficulty in identifying CVAs less than 48 hours old), testing for HINTS is probably not beneficial beyond the HCP's own curiosity.

3. Diagnostic Studies

A. Computed tomography (CT) of the brain with and without contrast   NONESSENTIAL

When ordering the initial imaging study for patients with a possible CVA, it is essential to remember that only 85% of CVAs are ischemic and the remaining 15% are caused by hemorrhagic events. Contrast is contraindicated in the case of a potential hemorrhage to prevent the contrast media from adding additional pressure and/or local damage to structures in the affected area of the brain. Thus, the initial imaging study would be a noncontrast CT alone. It evaluates not only for areas of ischemia and/or hemorrhage indicating a possible CVA but also for the presence of other intracranial abnormalities that could be responsible for the patient's symptoms.

B. Electrocardiogram (ECG)   ESSENTIAL

The ECG is important to evaluate for the presence of a cardiac arrhythmia, atrial enlargement, and/or ventricular enlargement that could be causing the patient's symptoms via poor perifusion.

C. Random plasma glucose (RPG)   ESSENTIAL

Hyper- or hypo-glycemia can produce symptoms similar to what Mrs. Xandier is experiencing; therefore, an RPG is essential to determine whether either of these conditions is present. An alteration of blood sugar could also be caused by diabetes mellitus (which increases risk of atherosclerotic and ischemic CVAs), infection, and/or other metabolic conditions.

D. Lipid profile   NONESSENTIAL

Although hyperlipidemia is associated with endothelium dysfunction, which can cause cardiac vessel disease, CVAs, or TIAs, it is not indicated during this diagnostic phase of her evaluation. However, in the near future, she will need to be evaluated for this condition (if it had not recently been done) because if present, it would represent a potentially preventable risk factor for Mrs. Xandier in regards to acquiring the aforementioned conditions that could hopefully be controlled with diet, exercise, and medication.

E. Serial cardiac troponin I and T   NONESSENTIAL

Because Mrs. Xandier is not complaining of any symptoms that could be suggestive of a myocardial infarction (MI) and her ECG failed to identify abnormalities consistent with a MI, serum cardiac troponin levels are not necessary.

4. Diagnosis

A. Transient ischemic attack (TIA)   CORRECT

Because Mrs. Xandier's symptoms are consistent with a CVA; resolved completely during her evaluation process, which was less than 1 hour since the onset of her symptoms; and are associated with virtually identical episodes in the past, which also resolved within 30 minutes from their presentation, a TIA is Mrs. Xandier's most likely diagnosis at time.

By definition, TIAs are transient neurologic symptoms that start and resolve suddenly and are both subjectively and objectively resolved within a maximum of 24 hours from the onset of the patient's symptom(s). However, because the majority of TIAs last less than 30 minutes, a new definition might be forthcoming from the American Heart Association (AHA) limiting the patient's symptoms to a maximum 1 hour time frame.

B. Cerebrovascular accident (CVA) affecting the right anterior cerebral artery   INCORRECT

CVAs and TIAs produce almost identical symptoms, but unlike TIAs, the neurologic symptoms produced by a CVA are not transient. In fact, the current AHA definition requires that the neurologic deficits must persist for greater than 24 hours, regardless of the imaging studies' results. Therefore, for this reason alone, it is unlikely that Mrs. Xandier's most like diagnosis is CVA affecting her right anterior cerebral artery (ACA).

Even though ACA ischemia could account for Mrs. Xandier's dysarthria, it is unlikely to be producing her right-sided arm, leg, and facial weakness as well as her right facial dysesthesias because ACA ischemia generally affects the sensory and motor aspects of the contralateral side of the body. However, symptoms can be bilateral if both postcommunicating segments are occluded. Furthermore, if the occlusion is proximal, it is unlikely to produce significant symptoms because of the excellent collateral circulation to the structures supplied by the ACA.

C. Migraine headache with transient neurologic symptoms   INCORRECT

Migraine headaches with transient neurologic symptoms could potentially present as Mrs. Xandier's did; however, in general, the neurologic deficits associated with migraine headaches are more focal in nature. Likewise, the symptoms tend not to be resolved completely in less than 1 hour from their onset. Despite the fact that rare cases of migraine headaches can occur without a headache, it is highly improbable that they occur without at least one of the other symptoms characterizing a migraine headache (e.g., nausea, vomiting, photophobia, phonophobia, and the desire to lie still in a dark room). Furthermore, because this would represent a new onset of migraine headaches for Mrs. Xandier, it makes this an even less likely possibility of being her most likely diagnosis because the onset of migraine headaches typically occurs when the patient is an older adolescent or young adult.

D. Amaurosis fugax   INCORRECT

Amaurosis fugax is characterized by a unilateral visual loss that lasts from a few seconds to a couple of hours but resolves completely following that time interval. Furthermore, it rarely is associated with other neurologic symptoms. Thus, because of Mrs. Xandier's lack of visual complaints and abnormalities but the presence of other neurologic symptoms, it is extremely improbable that amaurosis fugax is her most likely diagnosis.

E. Cerebrovascular accident (CVA) affecting the right posterior cerebral artery   INCORRECT

Proximal posterior cerebral artery (PCA) lesions generally produce symptoms from ischemia to structures located in the midbrain, thalamus, or subthalamus; whereas distal lesions tend to affect structures located in the medial temporal and occipital lobes. However, the resultant symptoms are located on the contralateral aspect of the body. This in conjunction with the complete resolution of her symptoms during her evaluation being inconsistent with the diagnosis of a CVA (as discussed previously) makes CVA affecting her PCA not her most likely diagnosis.

E. Treatment Plan

A. Hospitalization   CORRECT

Traditionally, even though her symptoms completely resolved, hospitalization would have been indicated because of the high risk of a CVA in the 48 hours following a TIA. However, because the vast majority of these individuals do not develop a CVA before hospital discharge, this practice has come into question. Many experts are now advocating for stratifying individuals into a high-, intermediate-, or low-risk category based on their ABCD2 score. The ABCD2 score represents the sum of all the points (maximum of 9) awarded on certain components of the patient's history and physical examination. These consist of **a**ge at presentation (0 points if younger than 60 years old and 1 point if 60 years of age or older), **b**lood pressure on presentation (1 point if ≥ 140 /90 mm Hg and 0 points if less), **c**linical manifestations (2 points for unilateral weakness, 1 point for speech difficulties, and 0 points for any other symptom[s]), **d**uration of time since symptom onset (2 points if ≥ 60 minutes, 1 point if 10–59 minutes, and 0 points if < 10 minutes), and **di**abetes mellitus as a comorbid condition (1 point if present, 0 points if absent). Interpretation of the findings consists of low risk, 1 to 3; moderate risk, 4 to 6; and high risk, 7 or 8.

Patients who are considered to be low risk and did not experience a crescendo TIA can generally be safely managed as an outpatient, unless a contraindicating comorbid condition exists (e.g., severe atherosclerosis, carotid stenosis, or carotid spasm), provided they are compliant, understand that they should come back immediately if symptoms return, and have an appropriate evaluation of their symptoms within the subsequent 48 hours.

High-risk patients should be hospitalized for observation and to ensure an appropriate diagnostic evaluation is conducted within the next 24 hours. In moderate-risk patients, the treatment setting is left to the discretion of the provider, who bases this decision on patient compliance, time required to obtain necessary diagnostic procedures, and presence of comorbid conditions.

Mrs. Xandier's ABCD2 score is 5 (2 points for unilateral weakness and 1 each for her age, presenting BP, and duration of symptoms), or moderate risk. Hospitalization is indicated for her because this represents her sixth or seventh TIA over a 3- to 4-month period without an evaluation. Furthermore, this episode likely represents an increase in frequency of her symptoms (because this is at least her second TIA this week), plus there are concerns regarding her compliance (i.e., only seeking care despite being symptomatic for over 3 months because her son insisted) in keeping scheduled testing appointments and returning if symptoms recur and for follow-up.

B. Echocardiogram, carotid ultrasound, and lipid panel   CORRECT

During the hospital stay, not only will Mrs. Xandier be closely monitored for any signs of recurring symptoms but also an appropriate evaluation of her symptoms will be completed. Furthermore, another goal is to achieve good blood pressure control to prevent complications from her high blood pressure. These three diagnostic studies are an excellent beginning toward achieving these goals.

An echocardiogram will evaluate for potential sources of emboli, valvular abnormalities, atrial myxoma, cardiomegaly, and hypertrophy (especially of the left ventricle given her long-standing hypertension that appears to be poorly controlled). The carotid ultrasound will determine the presence of plaque, potential thrombus formation, and stenosis in the carotid arteries. The lipid panel will determine whether Mrs. Xandier has hyperlipidemia.

C. Aspirin plus dipyridamole 25/200 mg twice a day   INCORRECT

Aspirin plus dipyridamole 25/200 mg twice a day, aspirin less than or equal to 81 mg once per day, or clopidogrel alone is recommended by the AHA/acetylsalicylic acid (ASA) updated CVA prevention guidelines for women with TIAs as a first-line preventive strategy provided they are older than the age of 65 years; have an ischemic stroke risk that is significantly greater than the possibility of bleeding complications; and have a risk for hemorrhagic CVA, other adverse drug effects, and consequences of a drug–drug interaction (e.g., the coadministration with a nonsteroidal anti-inflammatory drug can increase the risk of gastrointestinal bleeds and abnormal renal function, an oral hypoglycemic may be associated with an increased risk/incidence of hypoglycemia, and a diuretic or a beta-blocker can be less effective in controlling the patient's hypertension that is low.). The primary prevention of CVA following TIAs and the secondary prevention of CVA in patients with a history of an ischemic CVA are FDA-approved indications for aspirin plus dipyridamole. Nevertheless, this medication should not be prescribed for Mrs. Xandier because she has a history of experiencing angioneurotic episodes with aspirin in the past.

D. Clopidogrel 75 mg daily   CORRECT

The platelet aggregation inhibitor clopidogrel is not FDA approved for primary prevention of strokes caused by TIAs; however, it is recommended for this use in the AHA stroke prevention guidelines. Given Mrs. Xandier's history of angioedema secondary to aspirin, this is an appropriate medication choice for her.

E. Atorvastatin 80 mg daily   CORRECT

The new National Cholesterol Education Panel (NCEP) guidelines recommend the use of an HMG-CoA reductase inhibitor (or statin) in any patient who has experienced a TIA, even without a history of coronary heart disease (CHD) or hyperlipidemia, to reduce the risk of a CVA and/or other cardiovascular event. Atorvastatin has an FDA-approved indication for CVA risk reduction.

In theory, any of the other statins (e.g., fluvastatin, lovastatin, pravastatin, rosuvastatin, and simvastatin) should be effective in this capacity; however, only pravastatin and simvastatin have an FDA indication for CVA reduction. The others are approved to treat various forms of hyperlipoproteinemias; to slow the progression of atherosclerotic plaques in patients with an elevated total and/or low-density lipoprotein (LDL) cholesterol; and/or to reduce the risk of myocardial infarction, angina, or a revascularization procedure in patients with symptomatic and/or asymptomatic cardiovascular disease.

F. Referral for carotid endarterectomy   INCORRECT

Carotid endarterectomy is only indicated if the patient has greater than or equal to 70% stenosis of the carotid artery. Thus, Mrs. Xandier would need evidence of a significant stenosis on an imaging study before this would be an appropriate option for her.

Interestingly, a recent study from the United Kingdom suggests that in symptomatic carotid stenosis of greater than or equal to 50%, patients who were managed medically had a better outcome (in terms of lack of an ischemic event) than patients who were surgically managed. However, in patients younger than 75 years of age with asymptomatic carotid artery narrowing, the Asymptomatic carotid Surgery Trial 1 revealed that carotid endarterectomy reduces the 10-year mortality by approximately 46%.

Epidemiologic and Other Data

The incidence of individuals with TIAs is unknown in the United States. However, TIAs significantly increase the risk of the patient having an ischemic CVA. Approximately 15 to 30% of patients with TIAs will have a CVA within the next 3 months, and the majority of those occur within the next 48 hours post-TIA. CVAs account for approximately 200,000 deaths annually in the United States. Additionally, they are responsible for significant morbidity. Eighty-five percent of CVAs are ischemic in nature; the other 15% are hemorrhagic.

Risk factors for both TIAs and CVAs include advancing age, male gender, African American ethnicity, hyperlipidemia, hypertension, diabetes mellitus, smoking, obesity, sedentary lifestyle, excessive alcohol consumption, sympathomimetic use/abuse, established cerebrovascular disease, atherosclerosis, carotid stenosis, coronary artery disease, cardiac arrhythmias (especially atrial fibrillation), peripheral vascular disease, syncope, hypoxemia, fibromuscular dysplasia, migraine headaches, sickle cell disease, and positive family history of cerebrovascular and/or cardiovascular disease.

In the past, a TIA was distinguished from an ischemic CVA based on the time the neurologic defect persisted, regardless of imaging study findings. However, anywhere from 15 to 50% of all TIAs are associated with brain infarcts, despite the symptoms resolving in 24 hours (or being completely asymptomatic). Nevertheless, if the event lasted less than 24 hours, it was considered to be a TIA. If symptoms persisted beyond 24 hours, it was considered to be a CVA. Hence, a proposed updated definition would include TIAs with acute ischemic CVAs, regardless of the duration of symptoms.

CASE 9-4
Xeb Yellowstone
1. History

A. Do they have any pets or does Xeb frequently visit where pets reside?   NONESSENTIAL

Xeb's history is inconsistent with an allergic condition, a zoonosis, or a vector-borne illness; thus, it is irrelevant whether Xeb is exposed to pets and where they are primarily kept. However, asking about pets and other personal issues often assists in establishing good rapport and reducing anxiety for pediatric patients; thus, if time permits, questions regarding pets, activities, school, family, etc. are encouraged.

B. Have they noticed any problems or have any concerns with any of the following: speech, behavior, anger, impulsiveness, frustration, purposeless activities, inability to sit still, inability to concentrate on TV shows or whatever activity he is engaged in, inability to complete tasks, frequently losing things, talking excessively, interrupting others, fidgeting, "always being on the go," or poor self-esteem?   ESSENTIAL

The items listed in this question represent many of the primary symptoms associated with attention-deficit/hyperactivity disorder (ADHD). Because the reason for Xeb's visit is for an evaluation for this condition, these questions are essential to ask his parents. More formalized testing can be conducted if there is a suspicion that the patient does have ADHD based on these screening questions.

C. Has he ever lost control of his bladder or bowels during the episodes or has he experienced any nausea, sweating, dysphagia, vertigo, presyncope, syncope, loss of consciousness, hallucinations, or inappropriate affect/behavior? ESSENTIAL

Given Xeb's age and symptomatology, a seizure disorder must be included in his differential diagnoses. The majority of seizure disorders fall into one of two primary categories: partial seizures and generalized seizures; this grouping is based on whether the brain involvement is localized or generalized, respectively. Partial seizures include simple partial seizures and complex partial seizures. However, occasionally partial seizures can expand their focus and produce generalized brain involvement; when this occurs, the condition is then called partial seizures with secondary generalization. Generalized seizures include absent (formerly called petit mal), tonic-clonic (formerly called grand mal), tonic, atonic, and myoclonic seizure disorders. However, there exist a few seizure disorders that are not readily classified into either of these primary types. The majority of these are seen in the pediatric population, and they can include febrile seizures, neonatal seizures, and infantile spasms.

This particular subset of questions assists in determining whether the patient is suffering from a seizure disorder, a seizure mimic, or an unrelated abnormality, although many of these symptoms would be more pertinent in an adult presenting with "drop attacks" because the potential for cardiac, psychological, musculoskeletal, and other neurologic causes occurs much more frequently in this age group. Nevertheless, the pattern and characteristics of these symptoms can provide some useful clinical information for Xeb and should be asked. For example, incontinence is most commonly associated with generalized, especially tonic-clonic, seizure disorder.

Additionally, these questions can assist in differentiating among the various seizure disorders. For example, symptoms produced by autonomic dysfunction occur at a much higher frequency in patients whose seizure disorder doesn't involve significant myoclonic activity; however, syncopal episodes caused by orthostatic hypotension must be distinguished from a true lack of consciousness, which is a hallmark feature of tonic-clonic seizures. Although definite alterations (but rarely a complete loss) of consciousness occur with complex partial seizures, simple partial seizures are characterized by no alterations of consciousness.

Finally, it is essential to remember that seizures can be either idiopathic (also known as constitutional) or secondary (also known as symptomatic). Idiopathic seizures do not have an identifiable causative agent, whereas secondary seizures result from another cause (e.g., trauma, metabolic alternations, endocrinopathies, vascular diseases, infectious diseases, degenerative disorders, space-occupying brain lesions, and congenital anomalies). Thus, a high index of suspicion and attentiveness for the existence of signs and symptoms suggestive of these coexisting conditions are crucial.

D. Has he been complaining of or have his parents noticed any signs of headaches, stiff neck, fever, chills, malaise, fatigue, cough, wheezing, vomiting, changes in bowel movements, dysuria, hematuria, or urinary frequency?   NONESSENTIAL

Infections can be a secondary cause of seizure activity as a result of fever and/or a central nervous system infection, which incidentally are the most common causes of secondary seizures in his age group. However, the majority of the time, it is an acute process and a tonic-clonic (or some other generalized type of) seizure. Thus, these questions are not extremely important from this aspect.

The other most common causes of secondary seizures in children of this age group are trauma, congenital conditions, and developmental disorders. However, these symptoms are unlikely to reveal a strong suspicion for any of these, with the exception of a headache and trauma, which were previously denied. Although these questions do not need to be asked, a high index of suspicion for trauma must always be maintained in evaluating children with unusual or unexplained symptoms. Idiopathic seizures are also frequently seen in this age group.

E. Have they noticed him experiencing polyuria, polydipsia, a weight change, or an abnormal smell to his breath?   ESSENTIAL

Metabolic derangements secondary to diabetes mellitus can produce symptoms similar to Xeb's; therefore, it is essential to ask questions to evaluate for this endocrinopathy.

2. Physical Examination

A. Ear, nose, and throat (ENT) examination   NONESSENTIAL

If Xeb's symptoms were acute in nature, it would be appropriate to conduct an ENT examination to evaluate for the presence of an infection because an infectious process could be responsible for his symptoms and these locations are involved in the majority of infections in Xeb's age group. However, a central nervous system infection is much more likely to be responsible for his symptoms than an ENT infection. Although central nervous infections in his age group are most frequently caused by hematogenous, lymphatic, or direct extension spread of the pathogen from an ENT infection, it is still generally an acute process.

There is always a remote possibility that a chronic central nervous system infection (i.e., chronic meningitis) could be responsible for his symptoms. However, there would not be any remaining ENT findings to visualize, even if this was the initial focus of infection.

B. Palpation of thyroid   NONESSENTIAL

Xeb's symptoms are highly unlikely to be related to a palpable thyroid abnormality.

C. Heart and lung examination   ESSENTIAL

The cardiac and pulmonary examinations are critical to look for any evidence to suggest that a cardiac (e.g., arrhythmia, valvular abnormality, or structural defect) or pulmonary condition (e.g., asthma or chronic hypoxia) is present that could account for Xeb's symptoms.

D. Neurologic examination   ESSENTIAL

Because Xeb's primary symptom appears to be neurologic in nature, a complete neurologic examination is indicated to evaluate for a primary and/or secondary cause for them.

E. Assessment of behavior during the examination   ESSENTIAL

In every clinical encounter, the HCP makes some assessment regarding the patient's behavior, mood, affect, and appearance and obtains nonverbal cues and information regarding the patient's condition. However, unless an abnormality is detected or the presenting complaint mandates an observational period, these findings rarely are documented in the patient's chart.

This observational assessment is especially important and requires closer attention when evaluating a patient with a suspected psychological or neurologic condition. When patients present with specific behavioral concerns, the presenting condition is likely to manifest itself at some time during the clinical encounter. For example, in patients with true ADHD, "fidgeting," moving freely around the examination room, exploring drawers and cabinets, interrupting the conversation frequently, exhibiting poor impulse control, getting easily frustrated, and being unable to "focus" on a sustained activity can be observed. In both primary and secondary neurologic conditions, the motor complaint can occasionally be visualized. Therefore, this observation should be an integral and documented component of Xeb's physical examination.

3. Diagnostic Studies

A. Electroencephalogram (EEG)   ESSENTIAL

Because a seizure disorder is included on Xeb's differential diagnosis list, an EEG is indicated. It is considered to be the "gold standard" for making the diagnosis of a seizure disorder. Nevertheless, only 7 to 34% of patients presenting with their first seizure will have an abnormal EEG. However, if this test is conducted within the first 24 hours following a seizure, the incidence of identifying underlying seizure activity is slightly greater than 50%. If altered consciousness is associated with the seizure, the incidence of an abnormal EEG increases significantly to nearly 100%. Regardless, if the affected area is small, a significant distance from the corresponding electrodes, or responsible for a simple partial seizure, the spikes may not be visualized, may be obscured by artifact, or may be absent; slowing of the brain waves might be the only abnormality exhibited in these circumstances.

Therefore, patients with seizure disorders can have normal EEGs. Conversely, there are individuals who have epileptiform spike discharges on EEGs who never have a single seizure. Hence, long-term in- and out-patient EEG monitoring in conjunction with video surveillance is being used to increase the probability of discovering and identifying seizure activity.

B. Echocardiogram   NONESSENTIAL

An echocardiogram is indicated if there are signs and symptoms to suggest the presence of a cardiac condition (most commonly a valvular, structural, or congenital anomaly) is responsible for a seizure mimic and/or untreated cardiovascular disease. The most common mechanism for a cardiac abnormality to produce seizurelike activity is via inducing cerebral hypoxia. Because Xeb's history and physical examination failed to reveal findings consistent with an underlying cardiac abnormality or hypoxia, an echocardiogram is not indicated at this time.

C. Electrocardiogram (ECG)   NONESSENTIAL

An ECG is not indicated for Xeb because his history and physical examination were not suggestive of a cardiac rhythm disturbance producing seizurelike activity. With a cardiac arrhythmia, the seizurelike activity is most likely caused by brain hypoxia.

D. Complete blood count with differential (CBC w/diff)   NONESSENTIAL

A CBC w/diff would only be indicated if his history and physical examination findings were suspicious for an infectious, inflammatory, malignant, or other hematologic abnormality causing a seizure mimic.

E. Computed tomography (CT) of the brain   NONESSENTIAL

An imaging study of the brain is indicated in patients with known (or suspected) seizure disorders who have clinical findings consistent with an intracranial lesion, an EEG revealing a focal process, progressing symptoms, and/or an onset of symptoms after the age of 20 years. However, even if Xeb did have one of these conditions, a CT is still not indicated because MRI is generally a superior imaging technique.

4. Diagnosis

A. Absent seizures   CORRECT

Absent seizures are classified as a generalized seizure disorder characterized by extremely brief (generally only seconds) alterations of consciousness with staring but no loss of postural position. Other distinguishing features include a very sharp demarcation between the levels of consciousness; the patient's unawareness of the event; the association of a barely perceptible movement disorder (including automatisms), which is typically bilateral; and signs of autonomic dysfunction. The patient appears to be "daydreaming" by those witnessing the event because he or she tends to be "staring off into space" and is unresponsive to external stimuli.

In addition to the presence of these characteristic symptoms, Xeb's EEG reveals the typical pattern seen in absent seizures (intermittent, very brief, symmetric, 3-Hz spike-and-wave activity). Therefore, absent seizures are his most likely diagnosis.

B. Simple partial seizures   INCORRECT

Simple partial seizures are classified as a partial seizure disorder. Depending on the specific area of the cerebral hemisphere involved, patients can experience varying degrees of sensory, motor, autonomic, or (less commonly) psychic symptoms. The motor symptoms are more noticeable than those seen in absent seizures and are generally clonic in nature. However, tonic symptoms can occur independently of or in conjunction with the clonic movements. A rare movement disorder can sometimes be seen with this condition that consists of a very localized area of clonic activity that gradually "marches" over a period of a few minutes to involve a larger adjacent muscle group (e.g., finger to forearm or toes to lower legs [sometimes referred to as a jacksonian march]).

The sensorial component can consist of paresthesias, dysesthesia, and Todd paralysis; however, it can also present with signs and symptoms of autonomic dysfunction (e.g., orthostatic hypotension, tachycardia, hyperhidrosis, anhydrosis, flushing, and mydriasis) or flashes of light. Psychiatric symptoms can include auditory, visual, olfactory, and gustatory hallucinations.

They are distinguished from complex partial seizures by preservation of consciousness during the seizure. An EEG performed when the patient is asymptomatic is unlikely to reveal any significant abnormalities; however, if performed during the seizure, small spikes in a limited region correlate with the area of cerebral involvement. Nevertheless, simple partial seizures are not Xeb's most likely diagnosis.

C. Landau-Kleffner syndrome   INCORRECT

Landau-Kleffner syndrome, or acquired epileptic aphasia, is a generalized seizure disorder of childhood characterized by not only seizure activity but also psychomotor components, with the most characteristic one being a deterioration of language skills until aphasia is achieved. There also tends to be cognitive decline, behavioral problems, and a greater motor component to the seizure activity than is seen in absent seizures. Thus, this is not Xeb's most likely diagnosis.

D. Psychogenic nonepileptic seizures (PNESs)   INCORRECT

PNESs are a seizure mimic that is theorized to be a conversion disorder related to a current or previous severely stressful life event. However, they can be seen in association with other psychiatric conditions. The major differences between PNESs and true tonic-clonic seizures are that with PNESs, the eyes are generally closed, movements of the limbs are flailing instead of rhythmic in pattern, thrusting of the hips is common, lateral rolling of the head occurs, and *la belle indifference* regarding the symptoms is present. Nocturnal seizures and incontinence are rare with PNESs but common with tonic-clonic seizures. Nevertheless, PNESs can be eliminated as Xeb's most likely diagnosis.

E. Attention-deficit/hyperactivity   disorder   (ADHD) INCORRECT

ADHD is a psychological disorder that can be a seizure mimic. It is characterized by the inability to sustain attention, easy distractibility, difficulty in completing tasks, impulsivity, and often learning disabilities. It can occur with or without the motor/physical hyperactivity. Because of its characteristic symptoms and the lack of the "daydreaming"-like component, it can essentially be ruled out as Xeb's most likely diagnosis.

5. Treatment Plan

A. ADHD evaluation   INCORRECT

There are no diagnostic tests to establish the diagnosis of ADHD; however, there are some tools that can assist in this task. Because it is diagnosed primarily by the presence of core symptoms, the evaluation process frequently begins with a questionnaire for the teacher, the parents, and other significant caregivers to complete regarding their observations for the presence and severity of many of the characteristic symptoms of this condition. These symptom questionnaires are utilized along with the observation of the patient during the clinical visit to diagnose this condition. If the primary care provider is uncertain as to whether the condition is present, a psychiatric consult for more comprehensive testing is appropriate.

However, because the symptomatology provided by Xeb's parents is inconsistent with the diagnosis of ADHD but consistent with the diagnosis of absent seizure disorder, further evaluation for ADHD is not currently required. If there is still a concern regarding the possibility of ADHD after his seizure disorder is adequately controlled, symptom questionnaires might be indicated at that time.

B. Complete blood count with differential (CBC w/diff) CORRECT

A baseline CBC w/diff should be performed at this time because the first-line medications utilized to treat absent seizures have the rare potential to cause blood dyscrasias, platelet abnormalities, and anemia. Most experts recommend baseline and routine monitoring for these conditions by repeating the CBC w/diff every 6 to 12 months (provided it is normal) while the patient is on the medication. Any abnormality discovered must be thoroughly evaluated to determine its cause, significance, and impact on current therapy.

C. Trial of valproic acid   CORRECT

Valproic acid is considered a first-line treatment for absent seizures and the one with the least adverse events. The other first-line agent is ethosuximide. Both of these drugs have FDA approval for use in absent seizures.

D. Trial of clonazepam   INCORRECT

Clonazepam is considered to be a second-line drug for absent seizures in those patients who fail to respond to the succinimides. This benzodiazepine can either be tried in place of one of the first-line agents or in addition to that medication. This medication is FDA approved as a second-line agent for absent seizures.

E. Trial of carbamazepine   INCORRECT

Carbamazepine should not be considered as part of Xeb's treatment plan because it has not been shown to be effective in treating absent seizures. Its FDA-approved indications include generalized tonic-clonic seizures, partial seizure disorders, and mixed-type seizure disorders.

Epidemiologic and Other Data

Absent seizures (formerly called petite mal seizures) are considered to be the most common type of childhood seizures. They are estimated to account for approximately 15 to 20% of all childhood seizure disorders. The age of onset is typically between 4 and 8 years. However, in adolescence, spontaneous resolution occurs in approximately 60 to 70% of the individuals affected with the condition.

CASE 9-5
Yule Zeus
1. History

A. Is she experiencing increased stress, suffering from excessive "worry," having "lots of thoughts running through her head" while attempting to initiate sleep, experiencing difficulty with completing tasks she has initiated, attempting to multitask more than normal for her, or suffering from "hyperactivity"?   ESSENTIAL

Insomnia associated with depression tends to be terminal (awakening early and unable to return to sleep), whereas that associated with anxiety tends to occur while attempting to initiate sleep. However, it is not uncommon for major mood disorders (MMDs) to coexist and/or have some overlapping of symptoms. Therefore, even though her depression appears to be in remission, she could still experience atypical symptoms and/or have a coexisting MMD (e.g., anxiety or bipolar disorder).

Additionally, bipolar disorder, especially type II, is sometimes not apparent until the patient's depression (assumed to be a unilateral depression) is treated and the manic (or hypomanic) symptoms manifest, including decreased need for sleep and insomnia. Patients suffering from hypomanic symptoms can experience daytime fatigue.

B. Is she experiencing "hot flashes" and "night sweats"? NONESSENTIAL

Although "hot flashes" or "night sweats" can be related to other conditions capable of producing vasomotor instability (e.g., carcinomas, carcinoid syndromes, and hyperthyroidism), they are typically considered to be signs of the menopausal transition. "Night sweats" tend to interrupt sleep because the patient becomes uncomfortably warm and/or her bed clothing becomes saturated with perspiration, arousing her from sleep. "Hot flashes" tend to be a nonnocturnal complaint. Nevertheless, if a "hot flash" or "night sweat" would occur while Ms. Zeus was attempting to initiate sleep, the period of discomfort would be very short lived (generally a few minutes) and would not cause a 2-hour delay in sleep onset. Furthermore, it is unlikely that perimenopause/menopause is responsible for Ms. Zeus' symptoms because of her age and lack of experiencing the main symptom associated with this condition—menstrual irregularities.

C. Are her leg symptoms unilateral or bilateral, associated with paresthesias or dysesthesias besides the "crawling" sensation, or present at other times during the day? ESSENTIAL

Paresthesias and dysesthesias in the legs can occur in a variety of conditions (e.g., herniated lumbar nucleus pulposus, sciatica, peripheral neuropathies, restless leg syndrome [RLS], periodic limb movements of sleep [PLMS], periodic limb movement disorder [PLMD], diabetes mellitus, anemias, and akathisias) and as a result of adverse effects of medications. The location, associated symptoms, and timing of the sensation are essential to establish the correct diagnosis and treatment plan for the patient. For example, the paresthesias/dysesthesias caused by a herniated lumbar nucleus pulposus, sciatica, or peripheral neuropathy can be described as a "crawling" sensation; however, it is much more frequently described as a pain or burning-type sensation.

Paresthesias and dysesthesias associated with a herniated lumbar nucleus pulposus and sciatica tend to be unilateral, whereas peripheral neuropathies can be either bilateral or unilateral depending on the nerve(s) involved. The other conditions listed previously tend to be bilateral in distribution. The abnormal sensations associated with a herniated lumbar nucleus pulposus, sciatica, and peripheral neuropathies are present during the day; however, they can be exacerbated by postural changes that increase compression of the affected nerves. This includes lying down in bed at night. RLS and PLMS are generally restricted to when the patient is tired, required to maintain the same position for an extended period of time (e.g., sitting in a meeting), enjoying periods of inactivity late in the evening (e.g., watching television), or recumbent in bed prior to the onset of sleep. PLMD is the term utilized to describe PLMS that results in disturbed sleep.

D. Has she had any pallor, fatigue out of proportion to sleep loss, lightheadedness, vertigo, presyncope, syncope, palpitations, tachycardia, or dyspnea on exertion? ESSENTIAL

RLS and PLMS can be primary (idiopathic) or secondary (related to another condition or medication adverse effect). One of the major secondary causes is iron deficiency anemia. In rare cases, other types of anemia can also be responsible for the conditions. Additionally, peripheral neuropathies can be seen in late vitamin B_{12} deficiency anemia. The initial symptoms associated with anemia are related to the decreased blood volume and include those in this question. Later in the course, deficient specific symptoms (e.g., glossitis, cheilosis, and brittle nails with iron deficiency and paresthesias, balance difficulties, and cerebral dysfunction with B_{12} deficiency) occur.

E. Has she experienced any polydipsia or polyuria? ESSENTIAL

RLS, PLMS, and peripheral neuropathies can occur as a complication of diabetes mellitus; therefore, it is important to know whether Ms. Zeus is experiencing any symptoms that could indicate that she has undiagnosed disease.

2. Physical Examination

A. Cranial nerve examination NONESSENTIAL

Evaluating for signs of a motor or sensory deficit of Ms. Zeus' cranial nerves is unlikely to be useful because she is not complaining of facial weakness, abnormal facial sensations,

visual abnormalities, hearing problems, alterations in her sense of smell, mastication difficulties, or dysphagia.

B. Thyroid palpation NONESSENTIAL

Because Ms. Zeus is experiencing sleepiness, not true fatigue, and does not have any symptoms to indicate the presence of a thyroid abnormality, a thyroid examination is unnecessary.

C. Auscultation of carotids NONESSENTIAL

Carotid auscultation is performed when the patient's symptoms indicate that carotid stenosis might be present and account for her symptoms or in evaluating the radiation of a heart murmur.

D. Pelvic examination NONESSENTIAL

E. Vascular and neurologic examination of her lower legs ESSENTIAL

A complete examination of her legs, including musculoskeletal, neurologic, and vascular examinations, is essential to assist in establishing Ms. Zeus' most likely diagnosis.

3. Diagnostic Studies

A. Bilateral electromyogram (EMG) of her lower extremities NONESSENTIAL

Indications for an EMG include motor weakness, atrophy, and sensory defects on the physical examination in conjunction with a strong suspicion of a muscular disorder, neuromuscular condition, or peripheral neuropathy being responsible for the patient's chief complaint.

B. Glucose tolerance test (GTT) NONESSENTIAL

A glucose tolerance test is unnecessary unless Ms. Zeus has a fasting plasma glucose which falls between the upper end of normal (100 mg/dl) and the lowest level used to diagnose diabetes mellitus (126 mg/dl).

C. Iron level, total iron-binding capacity (TIBC), and ferritin levels NONESSENTIAL

As stated previously, a potential secondary cause for Ms. Zeus' symptoms could be iron deficiency anemia, which she is at risk for because she is a menstruating female. Iron stores are generally significantly depleted before changes occur in hemoglobin and hematocrit levels. Nevertheless, there are subtle changes detectable in the red blood cell (RBC) indices much sooner. Additionally, other anemias (albeit less commonly) can also be responsible for her symptoms. Thus, a better approach to determine if vitamin and/or mineral deficiencies are responsible for Ms. Zeus' symptoms is to order a complete blood count with differential. Testing for specific deficiencies can then be conducted based on the RBC morphology. (For more information on utilizing the RBC morphology to characterize anemias, please see Case 1-4.)

D. Blood urea nitrogen (BUN) and creatinine ESSENTIAL

A BUN and creatinine are typically indicated to evaluate for possible uremia or renal failure because this can also be responsible for RLS and/or RMLS.

E. Urinary human chorionic gonadotropin (HCG) test NONESSENTIAL

Although pregnancy is a secondary cause of RLS and some peripheral neuropathies, Ms. Zeus does not require a urinary HCG test. This is because she is not currently sexually active, has not missed a menstrual period, and has not experienced any menstrual irregularities.

4. Diagnosis

A. Peripheral neuropathy   INCORRECT

The discomfort associated with a peripheral neuropathy follows the distribution of the damaged or compressed nerve(s) from the site of involvement distally. The description of the abnormal sensation experienced is generally determined by the type of nerve fiber involved in the neuropathy. Small-fiber sensory disturbances are frequently described as a sharp, stabbing, burning, and/or lancing pain or allodynia, whereas large-fiber sensory disturbances are typically a dysesthesia described as being "dead," "numb," "pins and needles," or "tingling" in sensation. If the motor component is also affected, the patient can experience weakness, cramps, myoclonus, and/or foot drop (if the distal extremity is involved). Autonomic involvement is also possible and consists of signs of dysautonomia (e.g., peripheral vasoconstriction and hypohidrosis) in conjunction with the sensory symptoms.

The clinical presentation can also provide clues as to whether the underlying cause is axonal, demyelinating, or affecting the dorsal root ganglion. Axonal neuropathies are typically intermittent initially and may gradually progress to a more continuous pain pattern. They tend to follow a stocking-glove distribution, affect small fibers more frequently than large fibers, and cause distal weakness when the motor portion of the nerve is involved; the sensory component is more pronounced than the motor component, areflexia is distal only, and sensations of pain and temperature are more frequently affected than vibration and proprioception. In contrast, a demyelinating neuropathy is associated with a more discriminating onset, equal proximal and distal segment involvement, and generalized areflexia; the sensory component reveals large fibers being affected more frequently than small fibers, sensory and motor components are affected equally, and abnormal sensations of vibration and proprioception occur at a greater incidence than alterations in pain and temperature. Neuronal neuropathies are associated with a rapid onset, non–length-dependent involvement, motor component greater than sensory, proprioceptive motor involvement, and vibration and proprioception more frequently affected than pain and temperature sensations. Obviously, these distinctions are not as dramatic in the clinical setting, but the preponderance of characteristics consistent with one of these groups is still frequently useful in narrowing the list of potential diagnoses. Still, this is not Ms. Zeus' most likely diagnosis.

B. Primary restless leg syndrome   INCORRECT

Restless leg syndrome is characterized by an abnormal sensation in the legs, especially the distal portions, that is associated with an irresistible urge to move the legs. The sensation primarily occurs in the evenings at rest and is especially apparent when the patient lies down in bed to go to sleep. It is alleviated by moving the legs. The sensation often prevents one from going to sleep and getting restful sleep; hence, it is associated with daytime sleepiness. It can be primary (idiopathic) or secondary to another medical condition or a medication side effect.

Even though this description matches Ms. Zeus' symptoms, primary restless leg syndrome can be ruled out as her most likely diagnosis because a secondary cause can be identified.

C. Secondary restless leg syndrome caused by fluoxetine   CORRECT

As previously alluded, Ms. Zeus' history and physical are consistent with the diagnosis of RLS. Because her symptoms became apparent within 2 weeks of increasing her to high-dose fluoxetine and selective serotonin reuptake inhibitors (SSRIs) can cause RLS, her most likely diagnosis is secondary restless leg syndrome caused by fluoxetine.

In addition to the SSRIs, other neuropsychiatric medications that can cause secondary RLS include tricyclic antidepressants and lithium.

D. Pregnancy   INCORRECT

Despite pregnancy being a secondary cause for RLS, it can be ruled out as Ms. Zeus' most likely diagnosis because she is not experiencing menstrual irregularities and is not sexually active.

Other medical conditions that can be responsible for secondary RLS include diabetes mellitus, peripheral neuropathies, spinal cord abnormalities, iron deficiency anemia, other anemias, uremia, renal failure, and being on dialysis.

E. Pain secondary to unresolved depression   INCORRECT

Depression can manifest as several physical symptoms, including pain. However, this is unlikely to be Ms. Zeus' most likely diagnosis because her symptoms are not described as painful but as dysesthesias. Furthermore, her psychological symptoms of depression have been responsive to pharmacologic interventions; hence, physical symptoms caused by the disease should also be resolved, or at least improving.

5. Treatment Plan

A. Stretching exercises or a hot bath before bed   CORRECT

Some studies have found that stretching or a hot bath before bed is useful in relaxing the muscles and preventing RLS symptoms; however, this is not consistent in the literature. Nevertheless, these are relatively harmless activities (unless the bath water is too hot and it causes a burn or produces other symptoms [e.g., weakness, lightheadedness, presyncope, or syncope] that might provide Ms. Zeus with relief. Other complementary treatments that have been found helpful in smaller studies (or less consistently in the literature) include cool water baths, walking before bed, massage, and acupuncture.

B. Immediately stop fluoxetine   INCORRECT

Because fluoxetine can cause RLS and Ms. Zeus' symptoms began at approximately the same time it was increased to her current dose, it makes sense to stop the medication. However, in order to avoid SSRI withdrawal symptoms (e.g., flulike illness, agitation, and dysphoria), Ms. Zeus' fluoxetine needs to be gradually tapered instead of abruptly ceased.

C. Immediately start sertraline   INCORRECT

Despite Ms. Zeus' depressive symptoms currently being resolved, she should be placed on another agent to prevent them from recurring. It is recommended that initial antidepressant therapy be continued for a minimum of one year. At that time, a reevaluation of the patient's symptoms, life stressors, concurrent medical conditions, number of previous episodes of depression (if any), adverse medication effects, and other relevant data must be considered before a decision is made to stop, decrease, or continue the antidepressant therapy.

Because of the concern that RLS could be class specific, it is probably advisable to avoid utilizing another SSRI, unless she appears to be treatment resistant to other options. Furthermore, it would also be advisable to wait until her dose is tapered somewhat before instituting another antidepressant because her high dose of fluoxetine combined with a new agent has the potential of inducing a serotonin syndrome. Therefore, starting sertraline is not a good treatment option at this time.

D. Start bupropion in 2 weeks   CORRECT

Bupropion is an antidepressant in another class (aminoketone) that has not been linked with RLS. Thus, it is an appropriate medication for Ms. Zeus' depression. Waiting for Ms. Zeus' fluoxetine level to decrease before instituting this agent is important to prevent the possibility of serotonin syndrome.

E. Start pramipexole   INCORRECT

If changing Ms. Zeus' antidepressant is ineffective in resolving her symptoms, then her symptoms must be reevaluated to ensure that RLS is still her most likely diagnosis. If she stills appears to have RLS and no causative condition or medication is identified, it would be appropriate to institute therapy with pramipexole. Pramipexole is classified as a nicergoline dopamine agonist and has a high selectivity for D_2 and D_3 receptors. It holds an FDA indication for RLS.

The only other medication that has FDA approval for RLS is ropinirole, which is a nonergot dopamine agonist. However, other dopaminergic agents (e.g., L-dopa/benserazide, or L-dopa/carbidopa), the benzodiazepines, gabapentin, and opioids have been shown to be effective as off-label treatment; thus, they are considered to be part of the "standard of care" for RLS.

Epidemiologic and Other Data

RLS can either be primary (idiopathic) or secondary to a medical condition or an adverse reaction to a medication. Primary RLS is a chronic disorder that actually varies in intensity throughout the course of the illness. Symptoms appear to be worsened with inadequate amounts of sleep (which could result in a vicious cycle), caffeine intake, and alcohol consumption.

It is estimated to affect 1 to 5% of adults younger than the age of 60 years and 10 to 20% of individuals older than the age of 60 years in the United States. Nevertheless, its onset is typically before the age of 40 years, but in rare cases, it can present during childhood. There appears to be a family history of the condition present in approximately 33% of the cases. This familial association is greatest in those who are diagnosed with the condition at a younger age. It occurs at a much greater incidence in non-Hispanic Caucasians compared to other racial groups.

The majority of patients with RLS also have PLMS; however, the majority of patients with PLMS do not have RLS.

CASE 9-6
Zachary Adkins
1. History

A. Was his helmet broken or dented?   ESSENTIAL

Any major damage to protective equipment utilized during an injury is suggestive of a more serious condition. Conversely, it is possible that the protective gear reveals significant damage yet the patient's injury is minor because the protective gear absorbed the impact of the injury.

B. Has he experienced a previous head injury? If yes, when and how severe was it?   ESSENTIAL

It is extremely important to be cognizant of previous head injuries and their severity because of the cumulative "stacking" effect that results from the occurrence of a second injury before the first one is completely resolved, which can result in "second impact syndrome." In this resultant condition, a relative minor head injury can result in significant edema, contusion, hemorrhage, and in some cases death.

This is especially important when dealing with athletes who want to "get back into the game." In making this determination, the American Academy of Neurology's Quality Standards Subcommittee established evidence-based guidelines. Their criteria include the severity (grade) of the concussion, history of previous head injuries, and neurologic findings.

If on the field, the patient is found to have a grade 1 concussion (grades are defined below under diagnosis), he should be "benched" immediately and an initial assessment should be undertaken. If this is his first head injury of the season, then he should be evaluated at 5-minute intervals to ensure that he is oriented to person, place, and time can perform finger-to-nose testing with his eyes open and closed; can do tandem walking; exhibits a negative Romberg test; and has normal pupillary reactions. Finally, a postexertion evaluation needs to be performed, paying particular attention to subjective symptoms and signs for headache, vertigo, presyncope, syncope, and/or other neurologic findings is/are present. The most common exertion techniques include having the patient to perform five push-ups, sits-ups, or knee bends. Occasionally, a 40-yard dash is utilized, especially in players whose position requires them to be able to regularly perform this activity.

If this is the athlete's initial head injury of the season and he is completely asymptomatic after 15 minutes of observation and testing, it is probably safe for him to return to the game. However, if this is his second (or greater) grade 1 concussion, he should be restricted from play for a minimum of 1 week, including practices. Furthermore, he should not be permitted to return to participation until he obtains neurologic clearance from an HCP. If any subsequent evaluation reveals any suggestion of deterioration from his initial assessment, he should immediately be transported to the nearest emergency department for evaluation.

A grade 2 concussion also requires that the patient be "benched" on the sidelines immediately, observed frequently, and not permitted to return to this game. He should have an evaluation by an HCP no later than 24 hours postinjury or sooner if his condition worsens. If the HCP's initial evaluation is normal, the patient should be reevaluated in 1 week following the resolution of all his symptoms (or immediately if his condition deteriorates) for a neurologic evaluation, including postexertional testing as discussed previously. However, the guidelines state that it is permissible for the HCP, at his or her discretion, to reevaluate the patient sooner. If the patient's postconcussion evaluation is normal and this is his initial head injury of the season, then he can return to full participation at that time. However, if this is his second (or higher) grade 2 concussion, he should be eliminated from play for a minimum of 2 weeks. If his symptoms worsen at any time, he needs to be reevaluated immediately.

A player with a grade 3 concussion should not be removed from the field except by EMS personnel, and he should be immediately transported to a hospital for evaluation and treatment. If the initial evaluation is normal, then treatment is very similar to a grade 2 concussion. If the patient's loss of consciousness (LOC) was present for a few seconds and this was his first head injury of the season, then his return to participation should not be any sooner than a minimum of 1 week; furthermore, he should be required to have HCP clearance. If the patient's LOC lasted for a few minutes or longer, then he cannot participate for a minimum of 2 weeks, and he requires an HCP's clearance to return to participation. If this is his second (or greater) grade 3 concussion, he should not participate for a minimum of 1 month. Again, return to participation should be accompanied by an HCP's clearance.

C. Who was the other player?   NONESSENTIAL

The only purpose this question might serve is to satisfy the ED staff's curiosity.

D. Has he ever experienced dehydration during or following a game or practice?   ESSENTIAL

A history of dehydration related to exertion could indicate that Zachary experiences difficulty in maintaining his body's delicate balance between preventing hypovolemia and fluid overload, either of which could worsen intracranial damage from sustaining a head injury. If the response is positive, the patient will likely require immediate electrolyte testing and more vigilant observation/testing for potential electrolyte abnormalities. If not diagnosed and treated in a timely manner, this could place him at risk for further complications, including cardiac arrhythmias, alkalosis, and seizures.

A heat stroke (or severe heat exhaustion) could be partially or completely responsible for Zachary's altered level of consciousness, nausea, and headache. A clue to either of these conditions collectively is an elevated core body temperature. A heat stroke is characterized by anhydrosis, whereas a patient experiencing heat exhaustion maintains moist skin. Rhabdomyolysis (more common in heat stroke), myalgias, and/or muscle cramping are generally present.

E. How was he feeling before the game?   ESSENTIAL

His state of health preceding the game can potentially affect his list of differential diagnoses. For example, if he was already febrile, complaining of a headache, experiencing myalgias, or vomiting (with or without nausea), a coexisting condition could be responsible for some (if not all) of Zachary's symptoms assumed to have resulted from his head injury.

2. Physical Examination

A. Heart, lung, and chest wall examination   ESSENTIAL

A heart, lung, and chest examination is mandatory as part of Zachary's physical examination because he experienced a direct-impact injury to his right lateral chest wall followed immediately by blunt trauma to his contralateral shoulder. This could result in musculoskeletal abnormalities (e.g., contusions or fractures), pulmonary problems (e.g., pneumothorax or hemothorax), or cardiac complications (e.g., pericardial effusion or cardiac tamponade).

B. Abdominal examination   ESSENTIAL

Despite Zachary's denial of abdominal pain, an abdominal examination is indicated to ensure there are no signs of an intra-abdominal hemorrhage or free air under his diaphragm. This is important because his altered level of consciousness may prevent him from being aware of or able to adequately communicate symptoms related to either of these conditions; furthermore, it provides a baseline for comparison in case symptoms occur later.

C. Rectal examination to obtain stool sample to test for occult blood   NONESSENTIAL

If Zachary has intra-abdominal bleeding caused by his injury, it is much more likely to be found in his peritoneum than in his gastrointestinal lumen. Thus, this test will not detect the bleeding.

However, depending on the findings on his neurologic assessments, a rectal examination might be indicated as part of Zachary's more comprehensive neurologic examination to evaluate his rectal muscle strength, sphincter tone, and "wink" reflex.

D. Glasgow coma scale score   ESSENTIAL

A Glasgow coma scale (GCS) score provides an objective measurement of the patient's level of consciousness based on eye opening (point range: 1 [none] to 4 [spontaneous]), motor activity (point range: 1 [none] to 6 [obeys commands]), and verbal response (point range: 1 [none] to 5 [oriented]). The resultant score (total: 3–15 points) is important for subsequent evaluation to detect improvement and/or deterioration based on a quantitative measurable tool.

Additionally, the score has some predictive value in terms of overall survival for the patient. For example, the overall survival rate for the first 24 hours is estimated to be less than 15% if the GCS score is less than 5. In contrast, the overall survival rate is estimated to be greater than 90 to 95% if the GCS is greater than 11. Scores between these extremes are directly proportional to the likelihood of survival.

Other criteria for a poorer outcome independent of the GCS score include advanced age, lack of pupillary response, hypoxia, hypotension, brain stem compression, midline shift, increased intracranial pressure, and/or delay in evacuation of hematomas.

E. Cursory neurologic examination with abbreviated mental status evaluation, and a more comprehensive examination to follow after imaging studies are completed   ESSENTIAL

When a patient presents to the ED with a potentially serious injury, the first step in the evaluation and treatment process is to attend to the patient's ABCs (airway, breathing, and circulation). While the patient is being stabilized, the history and physical examination should be conducted simultaneously, if possible, to evaluate for signs of other potentially life-threatening conditions that also need to be addressed.

In a patient with a head and/or neck injury, a cursory neurologic examination must be performed to evaluate for signs and/or defects that could indicate a serious problem that has not yet been identified in the patient's differential diagnoses. However, a more comprehensive examination cannot be conducted until the cervical spine is "cleared" of any fractures to prevent complications (including death) from spinal cord injuries. If the imaging studies are negative, the patient can be removed from the neck brace and backboard and a complete neurologic assessment can be performed. If hemiparesis, gaze preference, and/or miosis are present on the initial physical assessment, typically at least a moderate-sized intracerebral contusion is present.

The site of involvement frequently produces additional symptoms consistent with the area of the brain that is involved. For example, a temporal lobe injury is associated with personality changes, the most common being combative and aggressive behavior; however, delirium is possible. Diabetes insipidus can result from a contusion involving the pituitary stalk or the median eminence. Frontal lobe involvement can produce a taciturn state.

Because memory and confusion are defining symptoms for a concussion, it is essential to perform an abbreviated mental status examination during this cursory neurologic examination. Its main purpose is to establish a baseline for further serial comparisons. The mini-mental status examination (MMSE) was initially developed as a screen for dementia; however, its application has been extended to evaluate cognitive function in a wide array of conditions. Obviously, this test is going to require some modification for Zachary because he is strapped to a stretcher and cannot accomplish some of the tasks (e.g., copying a figure, folding the paper, and placing the paper on the floor). However, it will still provide a baseline of his orientation, registration, attention and calculation, recall, language, and construction within these expected limitations.

Orientation (maximum 10 points) is an expanded technique to check orientation to person, place, and time. Registration (maximum 3 points) involves providing the patient three unrelated objects to memorize; it checks for instant recall. Recall (maximum 3 points) involves asking the patient to name those objects after approximately 5 minutes. Attention and calculation (maximum 5 points) is generally assessed by having the patient count backward by 7s from 100 to 65; alternatively, the patient counts backward by 3s from 20 or spells the word "world" backward. Language (maximum 8 points) determines whether the patient comprehends both written and spoken language as well as being able to write a sentence. Construction (maximum 1 point) involves the patient reproducing a drawing of two interlocking pentagons.

In screening for dementia, a score less than 27 is suggestive for its presence. However, it is important to note that in educated adults, the MMSE could be normal despite the existence of mild organic pathology. Likewise, individuals with very low educational levels, English as a second language, significant visual impairments, or other physical impairments may have false-positive test results. Therefore, if there is a strong suspicion of a physiologic cause, comprehensive neuropsychological testing might be indicated. In acute brain trauma, the total score possesses much less significance.

3. Diagnostic Studies

A. Cervical spine (C-spine) radiograph   ESSENTIAL

Because Zachary suffered a significant head injury, it is possible that he also has an associated cervical spine abnormality, the most common being a fracture or dislocation (which can compromise the spinal cord). If a spinal cord injury is present and goes undiagnosed, it can result in further damage to the spinal cord, including paralysis or even death.

The most accepted method of determining cervical spine (C-spine) involvement is via C-spine radiographs. The first films should be cross-table lateral views (with the cervical collar still in place if possible); if these are normal, then the remainder of the C-spine series can be completed. However, it is essential to ensure all views include the entire cervical spine from the odontoid process to C7.

If the radiographs have questionable results, a CT or MRI of the C-spine may be required to clarify the finding.

B. Skull series radiograph   NONESSENTIAL

Skull radiographs are not necessary because Zachary's injuries are severe enough to require a CT scan. Therefore, if a skull fracture is present, it would be discovered via that procedure.

Skull fractures generally follow a linear course extending from the site of impact to the base of the skull and may be associated with a basilar skull fracture. Basilar skull fractures have characteristic, but not pathognomic, clinical features; however, some of these are not evident on the initial assessment of the patient, especially the battle sign (postauricular ecchymosis). Other findings can include hemotympanum (collection of blood in the middle ear visible by viewing the patient's tympanic membrane) and "raccoon sign or raccoon eyes" (periorbital ecchymosis).

The presence of a skull fracture generally indicates a more serious injury. Approximately 66% are associated with an intracranial lesion. Furthermore, there is an increased risk of a subdural and/or an epidural hematoma. Because the brain is exposed to air "outside" the skull, skull fractures are also associated with a significantly greater risk of meningitis, pneumocephalus, cerebrospinal fluid (CSF) leakage, and/or cavernous-carotid fistulas.

C. Right ribs radiograph   ESSENTIAL

Right ribs radiographs are indicated not only because they represent the location of Zachary's primary injury (a direct-impact blow that resulted in his fall) but also because he is complaining of pain in that area. It is important to differentiate between rib contusions and fractures before manipulating the patient through the remainder of the physical examination to avoid an unwanted complication (e.g., hemothorax, pneumothorax, penetration of the renal capsules, and splenic rupture) caused by displacement of one (or more) of the sharp surfaces of comminuted or oblique rib fractures.

D. Chest x-ray (CXR)   ESSENTIAL

Along the same lines, a CXR is indicated to identify whether a pulmonary complication (e.g., pneumothorax or hemothorax) is present.

E. Computed tomography (CT) of the head   ESSENTIAL

A CT of the head is indicated for Zachary because of his prolonged loss of consciousness, posttraumatic amnesia, complaints of a severe headache, and initial GCS score of less than 13. Any significant loss of consciousness results in, some degree of brain contusion, petechial hemorrhage, edema, and tissue destruction. The CT scan can quantify these findings. If the impact was significant, the deeper structures, including the blood vessels, are displaced via mechanical forces, leading to the potential for a deeper hemorrhage, contusion secondary to the brain impacting the skull at the site of injury (coup injury), and/or contusion of the contralateral area of the brain where it impacted the skull (contrecoup injury).

Other indications for CT scanning with an acute head injury include obvious bony deformities of the skull, known or suspected basilar skull fracture, posttraumatic seizures, focal neurologic deficiency, history of a blood dyscrasia, current or recent anticoagulation therapy, and/or previous craniotomy with shunt.

Contusions are evident as homogenous hyperdensities on a CT scan. They are identified by hyperintensities on MRI scanning.

4. Diagnosis

A. Grade 2 concussion with coup injury   INCORRECT

A concussion is a brain injury that results from head trauma and is characterized by an alteration in the level of consciousness (from "dazed" to complete loss of consciousness) even if only present for a few seconds, some degree of confusion, and a brief period of both retrograde and anterograde amnesia. Histologically, there does not appear to be any specific gross or microscopic abnormalities identifiable from the condition; however, new research suggests that certain biochemical changes occur at the cellular level. As stated previously, when a head injury is severe enough to produce a loss of consciousness, there is some degree of petechial bleeding, contusion formation, edema, and tissue destruction. Although these findings are not pathognomic for a concussion, in conjunction with a history of a head injury, they are extremely suspicious for the process. Nevertheless, some consider these abnormal imaging findings not to represent a concussion but an associated intracranial process that resulted from the same injury that produced the concussion, with the two coexisting as separate entities. For the most part, the diagnosis of concussion is made clinically, explaining why imaging studies are only indicated for a small portion of patients with head injuries.

The terminology used to quantify the severity of a concussion is not consistent. Some HCPs use the newer grade classification of a 1, 2, or 3. Others use the older terminology of mild, moderate, or severe. Unfortunately, the defining criteria of a grade 1 and a mild concussion; a grade 2 and a moderate concussion; and a grade 3 and a severe concussion are not equivalent. In the numerical grading system, a grade 1 concussion is defined as confusion that is resolved within 15 minutes AND is not associated with amnesia surrounding the event; a grade 2 concussion is EITHER confusion that persists for 15 minutes or longer without amnesia OR the presence of any posttrauma amnesia; and a grade 3 concussion is characterized by any loss of consciousness.

Therefore, even though Zachary has a concussion, it is not a grade 2; thus, this is not his most likely diagnosis.

B. Grade 2 concussion with contrecoup injury   INCORRECT

Grade 2 concussion with contrecoup injury can also be eliminated as Zachary's most likely diagnosis because he experienced a loss of consciousness. Therefore, utilizing the aforementioned diagnostic criteria, his concussion would be considered a grade 3, not a grade 2.

Furthermore, a coup injury is associated with some degree of bruising or swelling of the brain on the ipsilateral side of the injury, whereas a contrecoup injury is ultramicroscopic bruising or swelling of the brain on the contralateral side of the brain. From the description of the head injury provided (i.e., an initial impact followed by a "bounce"), he is much more likely to have sustained both a coup and contrecoup injury along with his concussion. Additionally, his CT scan is consistent with this injury pattern.

C. Grade 3 concussion with coup injury   INCORRECT

Although Zachary has a grade 3 concussion and a coup injury (as defined above), he also has evidence of a hyperdense area in the superficial anterolateral aspect of his right temporal lobe. Therefore, this diagnosis alone would not account for all his physical and diagnostic findings. Thus, this is not his most likely diagnosis.

D. Grade 3 concussion with coup and contrecoup injury   CORRECT

Zachary's most likely diagnosis is a grade 3 concussion with coup and countrecoup for the aforementioned reasons.

E. Subdural hematoma   INCORRECT

A subdural hematoma can present with symptoms similar to Zachary's and can even coexist with a concussion. However, it can be eliminated as Zachary's most likely diagnosis at this time because of his negative CT scan for evidence of this condition. However, if his condition deteriorates, he will need a repeat CT scan to rule out this potential complication as they are not always evident on the initial imaging study. In fact, they can evolve in a subacute fashion, not appearing clinically for days or even weeks post-injury.

5. Treatment Plan

A. Hospitalize for observation and frequent neurologic and vital sign assessments   CORRECT

Zachary's head injury is severe enough to require hospitalization to ensure immediate and appropriate interventions are initiated to prevent further morbidity, and even mortality, if necessary.

In general, indications for hospitalization following a head injury include (1) a loss of consciousness of greater than 2 minutes, (2) the presence of any type of skull fracture, (3) the association of any type of focal neurologic deficit, or (4) the occurrence of lethargy.

B. Discharge to parents' care but advise them to awaken him every 2 hours to check for confusion, drowsiness, increasing symptoms, or other neurologic deficits   INCORRECT

Because of Zachary's prolonged loss of consciousness, he is not a candidate for outpatient therapy.

C. Neurosurgical consultation   CORRECT

A neurosurgical consultation is indicated for Zachary because of his extensive period of loss of consciousness (a neurosurgical consult is generally indicated with a loss of consciousness of > 5 minutes), abnormal physical examination, severe headache, posttrauma amnesia, and CT results.

Other indications for a neurosurgical consult in a patient with a head injury include a GCS score of less than 12, worsening headache, the development of nausea and vomiting with a headache, a posttraumatic seizure, a focal neurologic deficit, the presence of a skull fracture, a history of a bleeding disorder, a history of anticoagulant usage, a history of previous brain surgery (especially if a shunt is present), and/or a suspicion of child abuse.

D. Start midodrine to normalize BP   INCORRECT

Midodrine is an α_1-agonist that is indicated for the treatment of orthostatic hypotension. It is not indicated to treat generalized hypotension, especially when it is associated with a headache, because it can cause not only hypertension but also hypoxia of the brain because of its vasoconstrictive properties. Even if it was an acceptable treatment for hypotension, it would not be indicated for Zachary because his latest set of vital signs was within the range of normal.

It should be noted that in August of 2010, the FDA issued a "Proposal to Withdraw Marketing Approval and Notice of Opportunity for a Hearing" to the manufacturers of this drug because it was approved under an accelerated program using a surrogate endpoint and the required clinical studies to confirm the proposed clinical benefits were never conducted or submitted to the FDA for review. Currently, the future availability of this product is questionable.

E. Start promethazine for nausea   INCORRECT

The phenothiazine, promethazine, is indicated for motion sickness and perioperative nausea and vomiting. However, it is frequently used off-label for the treatment of severe nausea with or without vomiting. Despite Zachary's complaint of nausea, it is not indicated as part of his treatment plan primarily because of its likelihood of producing drowsiness; therefore, it would be difficult to distinguish increasing drowsiness as a result of his head injury or an adverse drug effect.

Furthermore, promethazine has been associated with the adverse effects of hypertension, hypotension, respiratory depression, lowered seizure threshold, and worsening of nausea. These problems could result in additional complications of Zachary's head injury and/or "mask" deterioration of his condition as the changes could be assumed to be caused by the medication.

Epidemiologic and Other Data

Head injuries are a significant cause of morbidity and mortality in the United States. It is estimated that each year there are approximately 10 million head injuries with approximately 2 million resulting in some degree of brain damage. In many cases, the severity of the brain damage is directly correlated with the length of time the patient has retrograde amnesia.

Unless previous psychological or substance abuse conditions (diagnosed or undiagnosed at the time of injury) are present, it is rare for a single, uncomplicated concussion to result in any sustained significant neurobehavioral symptoms except for minimal memory loss and difficulty with concentration.

CASE 9-7
Alec Bradford
1. History

A. Has he had any photophobia, phonophobia, nausea, or vomiting?   ESSENTIAL

The presence of a mass, edema, and fever in conjunction with the continuous and chronic nature of Alec's headache makes the diagnosis of migraine headache suspect. As previously stated, the IHS criteria to establish the diagnosis of migraine headache requires the patient to experience a minimum of five distinct episodes of headache that are extremely similar in location, nature of pain, intensity of pain, and associated symptoms and that occur for at least 4 but no longer than 72 hours, regardless of treatment.

Because there is a concern about the accuracy of his diagnosis of migraine headache based on this, it is worthwhile to pursue whether he has other symptoms typically associated with this condition. According to the IHS criteria, at least one of the following symptom combinations must exist in order to make the diagnosis with any degree of certainty: nausea and/or vomiting AND/OR phonophobia and photophobia. The other criteria are outlined in Case 9-1.

B. Has he experienced any seizures, signs of meningeal irritation, confusion, weakness, speech problems, gait difficulties, coordination abnormalities, lightheadedness, vertigo, presyncope, syncope, or other neurologic deficits?   ESSENTIAL

Because of the aforementioned inconsistencies with his diagnosis of migraine as outlined by the IHS criteria, it is imperative to question the patient regarding symptoms related to other conditions that could be responsible for the headache.

C. Is he currently experiencing (or did he experience before getting ill) any of the following symptoms: chills, eye discharge, otalgia, rhinorrhea, nasal congestion, sore throat, postnasal discharge, cough, or neck pain?   ESSENTIAL

The presence of meningeal signs, eye discharge, and/or symptoms of an upper respiratory tract infection, in conjunction with a headache, fever, and an erythematous, edematous, hot mass, increases the potential of an infectious process (e.g., meningitis, encephalitis, abscess, osteomyelitis, or periorbital cellulitis) being responsible for Alec's chief complaint.

D. Has he been experiencing a depressed or sad mood, irritability, anhedonia, decreased time spent with friends, increased time spent alone, declining grades, sleep changes, appetite changes, or weight changes?   NONESSENTIAL

Although headaches can be linked with major mood disorders, this tends to be more common in adults compared to preadolescents. Additionally, the associated symptoms and headache pattern being experienced by Alec are inconsistent with this diagnosis.

E. Has he experienced any recent head injury or trauma? ESSENTIAL

The presence of a head injury or trauma in conjunction with a headache is suspicious for an intracranial process. Furthermore, the presence of a "lump" makes it even more important to explore this potential cause.

2. Physical Examination

A. Head, eyes, ears, nose, and throat (HEENT) examination ESSENTIAL

Alec's head needs to be visualized and palpated to better assess his "lump" in regards to exact location, size, shape, and consistency as well as the presence of edema, skin discoloration, ulceration, other skin abnormalities, temperature alterations, and tenderness. Furthermore, the remainder of his head needs to be visualized and palpated to determine whether similar (or different) lesions are present. A localized lesion is much more likely to represent an isolated problem in contrast to a systemic illness (e.g., neurofibromatosis, amyloidosis, sarcoidosis, Sweet syndrome, or dysthyroid eye disease). However, localized infectious processes of the skin can progress to serious infections (e.g., osteomyelitis, mastoiditis, or meningitis).

Because Alec is complaining of periorbital edema and pain, it is essential to ensure that there is no eye involvement or visual defects present. Likewise, it is important to examine the ears, nose, throat, and other oral structures for the presence of any signs of an infectious process that could be responsible for Alec's chief complaint (e.g., ethmoid sinusitis or a dental abscess producing periorbital cellulitis).

B. Palpation of cervical lymph nodes ESSENTIAL

Enlarged and/or tender cervical lymph nodes increase the potential that an infectious, auto-immune, or malignant process is producing Alec's symptoms. However, it is important to note that cervical lymphadenopathy is not specific for ocular, periorbital, or even temporal processes. Any structure that lymphatics drain into the cervical chain could be involved.

C. Meningeal signs ESSENTIAL

Because of the potential for a central nervous system infection being responsible for Alec's symptoms, it is important to check for signs of meningeal irritation, which are suspicious for meningitis. The two most commonly performed meningeal signs are Kernig sign (with the patient supine and hip and knee flexed to 90°, straighten knee while checking for resistance and/or pain) and Brudzinski sign (with patient supine, flex the neck while watching for flexion of knees and hip). However, these are not specific for meningitis; the Kernig sign can be positive with disc disease (especially a herniated nucleus pulposus), and the Brudzinski sign can be present with arthritis, muscle strain/sprain, and other musculoskeletal abnormalities of the cervical spine.

D. Thoracic and lumbar spine examination NONESSENTIAL

E. Neurologic examination ESSENTIAL

A neurologic examination is indicated because Alec has been having a continuous headache for approximately 2 weeks plus signs and symptoms that could represent increased intracranial pressure, meningitis, a space-occupying mass, or a subdural hematoma (or less likely an intracranial hemorrhage).

3. Diagnostic Studies

A. Blood culture and sensitivity with Gram stain × 2 ESSENTIAL

Because Alec is toxic appearing, blood cultures are necessary in an attempt to isolate the organism(s) involved in case an infectious process is responsible. A minimum of 2 specimens from different sites is required. The bacteria's characteristics on Gram stain can aid in the initial antibiotic selection.

B. Complete blood count with differential (CBC w/diff) ESSENTIAL

A CBC w/diff is indicated to add additional support for or against a diagnosis of an infectious cause being responsible for Alec's symptoms as well as an estimation of its severity.

C. Magnetic resonance imaging (MRI) of the head, with and without contrast ESSENTIAL

An MRI, with and without contrast, is the best imaging test to evaluate for pathology not only in his intracranial structures but also in his sinuses, bony structures, and subcutaneous areas. Furthermore, it is the best imaging technique to assess his mass.

D. Ultrasound of the head mass NONESSENTIAL

An ultrasound would provide good information regarding the nature of the mass (i.e., cystic vs solid). However, it cannot evaluate the bony and intracranial structures for abnormalities, which are crucial given Alec's symptoms.

Additionally, it would be a technically difficult procedure to do without sedation because of the severity of the tenderness experienced by Alec when the mass was palpated. Adequate sedation would more than likely produce drowsiness, which would make it difficult to evaluate for deterioration of Alec's condition in terms of level of consciousness, drowsiness, and confusion. Because there are imaging studies without these limitations, they should be performed instead.

E. Computed tomography (CT) of the head without contrast NONESSENTIAL

Although CT is a good diagnostic study to evaluate for the presence of sinusitis as well as cerebral hemorrhage, ischemia, or infarction, it is inferior to MRI for evaluating bone and skin. Without contrast, it is also inferior to MRI in evaluating for intracranial abnormalities. To adequately evaluate the necessary structures, an MRI is still going to be required. Thus, it would be redundant to perform a CT that is unlikely to add anything but unnecessary radiation.

4. Diagnosis

A. Pott disease INCORRECT

Pott disease is a *Mycobacterium tuberculosis* infection involving the lumbar and/or thoracic spine without extraspinal involvement. Because of Alec's facial mass, headache, lack of back pain, and negative purified protein derivative (PPD) test 1 month ago, Pott disease is not Alec's most likely diagnosis.

B. Pott disease, frontal bone osteomyelitis, and cranial epidural abscess INCORRECT

A cranial epidural abscess most commonly occurs as a rare complication of an upper respiratory tract infection (e.g., sinusitis [most commonly the frontal and/or the ethmoid], otitis media, or mastoiditis). However, it can occur from other sources (please see Epidemiologic and Other Data to follow). It generally develops slowly over an extensive period of time because of its marked adherence to the dura. Thus, the patient generally does not have any upper respiratory tract symptoms at the time of presentation and frequently cannot remember experiencing one in the preceding months.

In patients with consistent history and physical examination findings, a cranial epidural abscess can generally be confirmed by the presence of a lentiform or crescent-shaped fluid-filled lesion in the epidural space.

Osteomyelitis is an inflammation of the bone marrow and adjacent bone. It is most commonly due to an infectious process, most commonly a bacteria or mycobacteria. Despite Alec having signs, symptoms, and diagnostic imaging evidence of a cranial epidural abscess and frontal bone osteomyelitis, this is not his most likely diagnosis because he does not have Pott disease, as previously discussed.

C. Pansinusitis   INCORRECT

Although Alec has pansinusitis, it alone is not going to produce a significant facial mass, marked facial edema and inflammation, focal neurologic deficits, or the other changes exhibited on his MRI scan. Therefore, pansinusitis is not his most likely diagnosis.

D. Cranial epidural abscess with frontal bone osteomyelitis and Pott puffy tumor   CORRECT

Although Pott puffy tumor sounds like it would be related to Pott disease, they are distinct entities. A Pott puffy tumor is formed via a fistula from a subperiosteal abscess and is characterized by varying degrees of pitting, pedal edema over the frontal bone. It would be exceedingly rare for a Pott puffy tumor to be related to a tuberculosis infection of the spine, especially in the absence of back pain. Because Alec's history, physical examination, and diagnostic imaging studies are consistent with the diagnosis of Pott puffy tumor, a cranial epidural abscess (as discussed earlier), and frontal bone osteomyelitis (as previously discussed), this is Alec's most likely diagnosis.

E. Migraine headaches   INCORRECT

Migraine headaches can be ruled out as Alec's most likely diagnosis because he failed to meet the IHS's criteria for the diagnosis of this condition as previously discussed.

5. Treatment Plan

A. Hospitalize   CORRECT

Because of Alec's fever, elevated leukocyte count, toxic appearance, and MRI findings, he cannot be managed as an outpatient. He is going to require hospitalization with IV antibiotics to cover potential pathogens until the blood cultures (which are unfortunately negative in the vast majority of patients) are available.

However, if the abscess is drained by a neurosurgeon, the cultures obtained on that purulent material is much more likely to grow true pathogens. Nevertheless, blood cultures are an essential element of Alec's evaluation process.

B. IV cefotaxime, metronidazole, and vancomycin until culture results are available   INCORRECT

Because approximately 50% of patients with an epidural abscess are infected with α- or β-hemolytic *Streptococcus* and other common pathogens (*Staphylococcus aureus*, *Haemophilus influenzae*, and *Enterobacteriaceae*), it is essential that these common as well as other respiratory pathogens are adequately covered by the empiric antibiotic selection. Because of the possibility of methicillin resistant *S. aureus* (MRSA) as well as gram-negative organisms, a third-generation cephalosporin, metronidazole, and vancomycin are an

appropriate combination until culture results are available, then they can be adjusted accordingly. However, because Alec is going to require neurosurgery to drain his abscess, it is recommended to only use the third-generation cephalosporin, ceftazidime, or the broad-spectrum antibiotic, meropenem.

C. Stop ibuprofen and start sumatriptan   INCORRECT

Sumatriptan is a selective 5-HT receptor agonist that is indicated to treat migraine and cluster headaches. Because migraine headache has been eliminated as Alec's most likely diagnosis, it is unlikely that this disease-specific analgesic will be effective in alleviating his headache.

Nevertheless, his ibuprofen needs to be discontinued and a more potent analgesic instituted because the ibuprofen is not adequately controlling Alec's pain and may be contributing to his nausea. Narcotic analgesics are indicated at this time to alleviate his pain. Acetaminophen can be utilized for fever reduction when necessary without the concern of gastrointestinal toxicity. However, if the chosen narcotic analgesic also contains acetaminophen, it is essential to remember to maintain the total daily dosage of acetaminophen under the recommended limit of 4 g/day to prevent liver toxicity.

D. Amoxicillin plus clavulanic acid orally   INCORRECT

Amoxicillin plus clavulanic acid will not adequately cover all the potential pathogens associated with Alec's condition, making it a poor first-line agent. Furthermore, it is an inappropriate choice because of the seriousness of his illness, the importance of good brain tissue penetration, and the need to achieve a therapeutic level quickly. Hence, at this time all of Alec's antibiotics should be given intravenously.

E. Neurosurgical consultation for possible drainage of abscess   CORRECT

A neurosurgical consultation is indicated because of the severity and extent of Alec's infection. Studies exist showing that long-term antibiotics (without abscess drainage) have been sufficient in resolving small abscesses; however, these studies also show a greater number of deaths than in those who were treated surgically. Nevertheless, Alec's MRI scan revealed a moderate-sized cranial epidural abscess and bone involvement. Therefore, Alec should have the benefit of a neurosurgical consult to determine the most appropriate course of action, which will likely, at minimum, require surgical drainage of his abscess.

Epidemiologic and Other Data

A cranial epidural abscess is an infection located between the dura of the brain and interior of the skull. It is responsible for approximately 2% of all localized suppurative infections of the central nervous system in the United States. The two most frequently encountered central nervous system focal infectious processes are brain abscess (approximately 80%) and subdural empyema (approximately 15–25%). Other rare conditions occur at a rate even smaller than those seen with a cranial epidural abscess.

A cranial epidural abscess can result from the bacterial infection entering the brain directly from a skull fracture; a complication of a craniotomy, with or without osteomyelitis; reflux spreading from upper respiratory tract infections (e.g., otitis media, sinusitis, and mastoiditis); or retrograde infection from either orbit. Rarely are they the result of hematologic spread or from sites that are not adjacent to the affected area.

CASE 9-8

Bella Chang

1. History

A. Did she experience any other symptoms before the "jerking movements" began? ESSENTIAL

Ms. Chang appears to be describing chorea, which consists of involuntary, rapid, and jerky movements that are irregular and unpredictable. They can occur at rest or with purposeful movement. They tend to be more rapid than an athetosis and slower than a myoclonus. In contrast, a tremor (which is also an involuntary movement) is a regular, shaking motion. However, tremors can occur at rest (resting tremor), with purposeful movements (intention tremor), and when attempting to maintain the same position (postural tremor).

She also appears to be describing a mild dementia. The most common disorder affecting middle-aged individuals with the primary symptoms of chorea and dementia is Huntington disease. Because it is gradual in onset, it is important to inquire about other symptoms before onset of the irregular, jerking movements. The typical pattern of the chorea in Huntington disease is for it to begin as a sensation of restlessness and/or fidgetiness that gradually increases until true myoclonus occurs. Then, the myoclonus becomes progressive.

B. Does she have any problem with ambulation? ESSENTIAL

Another feature of Huntington disease as well as other movement disorders is cerebellar ataxia; therefore, if gait problems exist, it is important to know exactly what difficulty the patient is experiencing. Although patients will often experience difficulties in attempting to describe their gait abnormality, the question should still be asked. For diagnostic purposes, it is frequently easier to identify and classify a gait abnormality by observing it during the physical examination or while entering or exiting the examination room. It is never inappropriate to have the patient repeat an abnormal gait to better identify its characteristics.

Cerebellar ataxia is characterized by an unsteady, staggering, wide-based gait associated with difficulty in maneuvering turns. Furthermore, the patient is unable to stand steady with his or her feet together, regardless of whether the eyes are open or closed. Tandem walking is associated with a decompensation of balance. In contrast, a patient with a sensory ataxia also exhibits the wide-based, unsteady gait; however, when standing with feet together, he or she only experiences difficulty when the eyes are closed. Furthermore, a patient with sensory ataxia tends to raise his or her feet higher than normal when ambulating and bring them down with a slap while observing the ground to ensure accurate steps.

A sensory ataxia varies from a steppage gait; with the latter, the knees are lifted higher and are more flexed when walking. A patient with a steppage gait will also not have a positive Romberg sign (not being able to stand with feet close together and eyes closed) and his or her gait is steadier and not as wide based. Whereas a patient with a characteristic parkinsonian gait exhibits short, shuffling steps with ambulation. To maintain balance, the patient with a parkinsonian gait tends to be flexed forward at the waist so the upper trunk is parallel to the front of the feet; additionally, the knees and hips tend to be slightly flexed to maintain this new center of gravity. Furthermore, arm movements are limited and the gait appears "stiff," especially when the patient is completing turns. It is also known as a "freezing" gait.

Gait apraxia, or frontal gait disorder, is characterized by wide, often shuffling, short steps with significant difficulty executing starts and stops. This gait must be distinguished from a stiff-legged (or spastic) gait and a cautious gait. Although the stiff-legged gait is characterized by a shuffling step, the feet are also circumducted and the legs "stiff" appearing because of an inequality of muscle tone. A cautious gait is also associated with short steps, but there tends not to be much shuffling of the feet with movement. Furthermore, patients with a cautious gait tend to have a lower center of gravity. It is theorized to be caused by a fear of falling.

C. Does she have a tremor or weakness? ESSENTIAL

For the most part, Huntington disease can be differentiated from most other movement disorders because it is generally not associated with a tremor or a true muscle weakness.

D. Has she ever had a positive culture for syphilis? NONESSENTIAL

Neurosyphilis occurs when a syphilis infection involves the central nervous system (CNS) of an infected individual. Typically, the involvement is classified into one of four patterns (asymptomatic, meningeal, meningovascular, and parenchymatous); however, mixed patterns are more prevalent than a single entity, with the exception of asymptomatic neurosyphilis. Parenchymatous is generally divided into general paresis and tabes dorsalis. Traditionally, it was believed that neurosyphilis only occurred late in the course of untreated disease (tertiary syphilis); however, it is now known that CNS involvement can occur as early as the first few weeks of the illness. However, the time from infection until symptom development frequently correlates with the type of CNS involvement the patient experiences. For example, meningeal syphilis can become symptomatic in less than 1 year after inoculation. However, meningovascular, general paresis parenchymatous, and tabes dorsalis parenchymatous typically don't occur until 5 to 10 years, 20 years, and 25 to 30 years postinfection, respectively.

Meningeal syphilis frequently presents as meningitis; thus, mental status changes are possible. Meningovascular syphilis' most common presentation is a cerebrovascular accident (frequently in a patient much younger than normally anticipated) and it can have associated psychological abnormalities. General paresis parenchymatous syphilis involves widespread parenchymal damage and can present with abnormalities of personality, affect, sensorium, intellect, and speech. Other findings frequently include Argyll-Robertson pupils (or other ocular changes) and hyperreflexia. The symptoms of tabes dorsalis are related to demyelination of the poster columns, dorsal roots, and dorsal root ganglia.

Therefore, neurosyphilis, irrespective of disease duration, can be associated with a variety of memory, mood, and cognitive changes; thus, it could potentially be responsible for Ms. Chang's nonmyoclonic symptoms. However, syphilis is not diagnosable by any culturing techniques primarily because it is a spirochetal infection. It is primarily diagnosed via serum antibody testing, although properly performed dark-field examination and/or immunofluorescence techniques can identify the organism in "moist" lesions (e.g., primary chancre and condyloma lata); and pleocytosis, increased protein, and reactive Venereal Disease Research Laboratory (VDRL) tests of cerebrospinal fluid. Thus, asking if Ms. Chang had a positive culture for syphilis is unnecessary because the test does not exist.

E. Does she have a family history of anyone with a similar condition?   ESSENTIAL

In evaluating patients with hyperkinetic movement disorders, it is important to inquire about a positive family history of relatives, which could assist in determining her most likely diagnosis because several potential differential diagnoses are inherited conditions (e.g., Huntington disease, Machado-Joseph disease, Friedreich ataxia, McLeod syndrome, and dentatorubral-pallidoluysian atrophy). Others appear in family clusters (e.g., ischemic cerebrovascular accidents, autoimmune disorders, Tourette syndrome, and paraneoplastic syndromes), whereas others appear unrelated (e.g., Sydenham chorea, human immunodeficiency virus [HIV], neurological complications, CNS infections, alcohol/drug intoxication, and medication adverse effects).

2. Physical Examination

A. Ear, nose, and throat examination   NONESSENTIAL

B. Cardiac examination   ESSENTIAL

The discovery of a cardiac murmur or arrhythmia could indicate a potential embolic source causing a CVA, multiple "mini-strokes," or TIAs as the cause of Ms. Chang's symptoms.

C. Examination of pulses   ESSENTIAL

Examination of her pulses for decreased sensation and/or bruits evaluates for probable atherosclerosis. This could also indicate the possibility of an ischemic CVA, multiple "mini-strokes," or TIAs as possible causes of her symptoms.

D. Neurologic examination   ESSENTIAL

Because her presenting symptoms are primarily neurologic in nature, a neurologic examination is indicated to assist in determining Ms. Chang's most likely diagnosis.

E. Mini-mental status examination   ESSENTIAL

Because Ms. Chang is complaining of memory loss, an MMSE is important to conduct. For more information regarding the MMSE, please see Case 9-6.

3. Diagnostic Studies

A. Computed tomography (CT) scan of the brain   ESSENTIAL

A brain CT scan is indicated because of the neurologic deficits identified on Ms. Chang's physical examination. Although a movement disorder could be responsible for those findings, it is essential to rule out intracranial pathology (e.g., ischemic or hemorrhage CVA, other brain hemorrhages, primary or secondary brain tumors, other space-occupying lesions, and/or infection) as the cause because of the potential serious (and even fatal) consequences if they remain undiagnosed and untreated.

B. Repetitive stimulation testing via electromyography (EMG) of her arms   NONESSENTIAL

Repetitive stimulation testing via EMG is generally indicated when a neuromuscular junction disorder (e.g., myasthenia gravis, Lambert-Eaton syndrome, or botulism) is suspected.

The typical presentation is a progressive and/or variable-intensity pattern of actual muscle weakness, with or without atrophy, which is typically exacerbated by activity.

C. Lipid panel   NONESSENTIAL

Although an ischemic vascular process could potentially be responsible for Ms. Chang's symptoms, a lipid panel is not indicated because other signs and symptoms suggesting this possibility are absent.

However, if the purpose of Ms. Chang's visit is for age-appropriate health maintenance instead of a problem-focused evaluation, she would require a screening lipid panel if she never had one or her last one was performed over 5 years ago. The NCEP III recommends this test for all adults every 5 years (provided it is normal) starting at age 20 years. For other organizations' screening recommendations, please see Case 1-3. Regardless of the purpose of the visit, it is important to establish whether the patient has regular age-appropriate health maintenance visits. If not, the patient should be encouraged to have such.

D. White blood cell count with differential (WBC w/diff)   NONESSENTIAL

Although a central nervous system infection or an inflammatory condition could be responsible for Ms. Chang's symptoms, her physical examination findings do not support either of these conditions. Although a leukocytosis can be caused by tissue necrosis, trauma, leukemia, and physiologic stress and a leukopenia can occur in response to bone marrow suppression/failure, possible dietary deficiencies, and some viral illnesses, her history and physical findings are inconsistent with any of these conditions.

E. Human immunodeficiency virus (HIV) antibody test   ESSENTIAL

HIV complications in the central nervous system (e.g., toxoplasmosis, CNS lymphoma, acquired immunodeficiency syndrome [AIDS] dementia complex, HIV myelopathy, and progressive multifocal leukoencephalopathy [PML]) can produce focal neurologic defects, aphasia, seizures, spastic paresis, memory problems, cognitive difficulties, and emotional changes with or without other symptoms (headache, fever, hemiparesis, and visual disturbances, are typically associated with these disorders). Given Ms. Chang's history of more than 100 lifetime sexual partners, she is at risk for acquiring a sexually transmitted infection (STI), including HIV.

4. Diagnosis

A. Treatment-resistant atypical depression   INCORRECT

Up to 66% of all patients with major unilateral depression will not respond to their initial antidepressant. However, if the patient does not respond to the second medication, it is the standard of care to reevaluate the patient to ensure that the diagnosis is correct. Because Ms. Chang is on her sixth medication, it is becoming more and more likely that this is not her correct diagnosis, and a more extensive evaluation is indicated to attempt to identify the cause of her symptoms.

Unfortunately, when patients present with physical complaints, especially those that involve neurologic, musculoskeletal, and gastrointestinal systems, that do not "fit" nicely into easily recognizable conditions, all too often the treating HCP decides the cause of these symptoms is psychological in nature. However, before making such a diagnosis, it is essential to ensure that there is not a rare underlying condition present. Remember that one of the defining criteria for depression is that the patient's symptoms cannot be explained by another condition.

To establish the diagnosis of depression, the patient must be experiencing a persistently depressed mood and/or chronic anhedonia. The term "atypical depression" denotes that the patient's associated disease features do not correspond to those generally anticipated (e.g., hypersomnia, increased weight, increased appetite, "leaden" paralysis [sensation of limbs being weighted down], and mood reactivity [the depressed mood is responsive to external stimuli]). Although depression is the most frequent cause of memory loss in middle-aged individuals, it is far from the only one. Other causes must be pursued with an open mind.

B. Parkinson disease   INCORRECT

Parkinson disease is a neurodegenerative condition of the basal ganglia that typically occurs in late life. It is believed to result from a dopamine deficiency and is characterized by tremor, rigidity, festination, shuffling gait, and a stooping posture. The associated dementia tends to occur later in the course of the illness. Because Ms. Chang does not have a tremor, a shuffling gait, rigidity, or a stooping posture; her dementia occurred early in the course of her illness; and she appears unresponsive to dopamine, Parkinson disease is not her most likely diagnosis.

C. Mild exacerbations of myoclonic seizures   INCORRECT

As stated previously, Ms. Chang's description of her chief complaint more closely resembles a chorea than a myoclonus. Additionally, she states that her current "jerking movements" are different from those experienced with seizure. Based on this alone, an exacerbation of her myoclonic seizure disorder, even a mild one, is not her most likely diagnosis.

Further support for an alternative diagnosis includes a repeat EEG conducted 2 months ago failed to reveal a return of the abnormality initially utilized to establish her diagnosis; her trough medication level performed 2 months ago was therapeutic and her dosage has not been altered since that time; and dementia is generally not a feature of a myoclonic seizure disorder.

D. Dentatorubral-pallidoluysian   atrophy   (DRPLA) CORRECT

DRPLA is an autosomal dominant disease that is almost exclusively found in individuals of Japanese heritage. Its characteristic features include the presence of a myoclonic seizure disorder, chorea, progressive ataxia, and dementia. Thus, dentatorubral-pallidoluysian atrophy is Ms. Chang's most likely diagnosis.

E. Huntington disease   INCORRECT

As stated previously, Huntington disease is the most common disorder presenting with both chorea and dementia in middle-aged patients. This autosomal dominant disorder can also begin as a sensation of restlessness or fidgetiness that gradually increases to a focal chorea. Later in the course of this progressive, fatal illness, the chorea becomes generalized and associated with myoclonus, spasticity, rigidity, bradykinesis, gait disturbances, dystonia, dysarthria, cognitive difficulties, vision problems, memory problems, and mood alterations.

Although Huntington disease is an excellent possibility, it can be eliminated as Ms. Chang's most likely diagnosis because she lacks a family history of the condition (which is almost always present), has a history of myoclonic seizures (which is generally not seen), and another diagnosis is a better possibility.

5. Treatment Plan

A. Increase clonazepam 1 mg to three times a day INCORRECT

Because an exacerbation of her seizure disorder does not appear to be the cause of her symptoms and she is not experiencing anxiety, raising her clonazepam is unlikely to provide her with any symptom relief but could increase the potential for her to develop adverse effects as a result of the medication (e.g., drowsiness, depression, dyspepsia, and hepatic toxicity).

B. Recheck clonazepam serum level in 1 month   INCORRECT

Because her trough level was therapeutic 2 months ago, a medication adjustment has not occurred, another drug was not added that could potentially alter the metabolism of the clonazepam, and she is not experiencing seizures, a repeat level in 1 month is not indicated.

Typically seizure medications do not require regular monitoring of the drug level. Generally, the level is only checked if seizures recur, there is a question of compliance with the therapeutic regimen, adverse effects of the medication are suspected, medications that have the potential to alter the serum level are added, or the patient develops (or already has) hepatic and/or renal (depending on excretion route) insufficiency/failure.

C. Reserpine gradually titrated to a total daily dose of 2 to 5 mg depending on response and adverse effects   CORRECT

A trial of reserpine with gradual titration of dose based on response and/or the development of adverse effects is an appropriate choice. It is one of two medications that are effective in controlling the dyskinesis in patients with DRPLA. The other medication choice is haloperidol.

Although both of these medications tend to be associated with multiple adverse effects, reserpine is generally better tolerated; thus, it is considered to be the first-line treatment drug of choice. However, if there are significant behavioral symptoms associated with the condition, haloperidol is generally utilized as the first-line agent. Haloperidol is also used if the patient is intolerant of reserpine or does not respond to the maximum dose (or highest tolerated dose) of it. Because dentatorubral-pallidoluysian atrophy is a rare condition, neither of these medications has an FDA-approved indication for use in the condition.

D. Donepezil 5 mg a day initially, increasing to 10 mg daily if necessary and tolerated   INCORRECT

Although donepezil 5 to 10 mg/day is somewhat effective in improving the cognitive symptoms associated with Alzheimer disease, it has not been shown effective in treating any of the symptoms associated with dentatorubral-pallidoluysian atrophy.

F. Refer to psychiatrist for possible electroconvulsive therapy (ECT)   INCORRECT

ECT is a proven, effective therapy for treatment-resistant depression. It is generally reserved for those severe cases of acute or treatment-resistant depression in which the patient is at extremely high risk of suicide, unable to provide basic self-care (e.g., bathing, feeding, and/or dressing), and/or exhibiting vegetative symptoms (e.g., not eating, not getting out of bed, and/or not responding to external stimuli).

Nevertheless, it is not indicated for Ms. Chang because she fails to meet the minimum established diagnostic criteria for a major depressive disorder, and her mood symptoms most likely represent a component of her neurologic disease process; however, they could represent her reaction to the illness and its debilitating symptoms. In general, "mood" symptoms caused by neurologic pathology are unresponsive to treatment with medication; however, psychotherapy might provide her some benefit by offering her coping mechanisms to handle her illness, its symptoms, and its impact on her life.

Epidemiologic and Other Data

DRPLA is considered to be one of the autosomal spinocerebellar ataxias (SCAs). Other SCAs include episodic atrophy type 1, episodic atrophy type 2, Machado-Joseph disease (MJD) or SCA type 3, SCA type 1, SCA type 2, and SCA types 4 to 28. Genotyping has become the "gold standard" for differentiating between the various SCAs. The incidence of these conditions, including DRPLA, is unknown; however, they are considered to be extremely rare. DRPLA is almost exclusively found in individuals of Japanese heritage.

CASE 9-9

Clarence Deets

1. History

A. Is he experiencing any constitutional symptoms? ESSENTIAL

Patients who are HIV positive, regardless of their CD4+ lymphocyte cell counts and HIV RNA levels, represent some of the most clinically challenging cases, especially when they present with new symptoms. Not only can the immunodeficiency itself produce a multitude of infectious and/or malignant conditions in virtually every body system, but also the adverse effects of their antiviral therapies can produce similar symptoms. Additionally, these patients can develop other conditions that are unrelated to their HIV status.

Because of the propensity of HIV-positive patients to develop infections and malignancies, it is essential to determine if Mr. Deets is experiencing constitutional symptoms (e.g., unplanned weight loss, fever, chills, night sweats, or generalized lymphadenopathy) that could represent the development of either of these problems. Additionally, these symptoms in conjunction with an opportunistic infection and cytopenia could represent AIDS-related complex (ARC).

B. Before becoming ill this week, had he experienced a change in his appetite or sleep pattern; anhedonia; feeling depressed, anxious, overwhelmed, sad, or worthless; or suicidal ideations?   ESSENTIAL

HIV-infected individuals can have mood symptoms caused by CNS involvement from the virus, mood disorders related to accepting and coping with their HIV status, and mood disorders unrelated to their HIV infection. Major mood disorders can present with physical symptoms (e.g., headache, anorexia, fatigue, and increased need for sleep) as well as

cognitive symptoms (e.g., memory loss and confusion) in addition to the psychological symptoms (e.g., anhedonia, avoiding others, shirking responsibility, and lack of concern with personal hygiene).

C. Do they eat at the frat house, in the cafeteria, or at restaurants? Does he eat undercooked or raw meat?   ESSENTIAL

Because Mr. Deets discontinued his antiretroviral therapy 3 months ago, he must be considered immunosuppressed until proven otherwise. Thus, the same concerns regarding the potential for acquiring infectious and/or malignant conditions that any immunosuppressed HIV-infected patients have must be addressed. This includes being susceptible to common as well as opportunistic infections that can result in marked CNS involvement.

For example, if an immunocompetent individual consumes food tainted with *Salmonella*, the likely result would be a self-limited episode of gastroenteritis with bloody diarrhea; however, if an immunosuppressed patient consumes *Salmonella*-tainted food, it can result in a *Salmonella* septicemia and CNS symptoms. Thus, knowing that their food is prepared on-site should lead to questions regarding consumption of foods recently reported as contaminated with *Salmonella*, their washing process regarding fruits and vegetables, their handling of meat products, and whether others are ill (and what symptoms they are exhibiting). If they eat primarily in the cafeteria, questions regarding other ill students and faculty as well as any known *Salmonella* contamination at the facility should be sought. If they eat primarily in restaurants, knowing which ones, histories of recent *Salmonella* outbreaks related to that particular establishment, and whether there have been other ill patrons become important follow-up questions.

Additionally, questions addressing the hygiene practices of the individuals preparing the food, regardless of the setting, are important because cytomegalovirus and *Mycobacterium tuberculosis* (two of the major CNS pathogens in HIV-infected patients) can be transmitted from an individual who is infected with either of these organisms and practices poor hygiene after defecating, sneezing, coughing, or producing sputum because these diseases can be transmitted by the fecal–oral route, saliva contamination, and/or respiratory droplets. Additionally, there is a slight risk of acquiring *Mycobacterium tuberculosis* from drinking unpasteurized milk. Therefore, the source of some of the ingredients may also need to be sought.

Another serious CNS infection related to food consumption is toxoplasmosis. It is often acquired from eating undercooked or raw meat. Toxoplasmosis has been linked with primary lymphoma of the brain in HIV-infected patients.

D. Do they have a cat? If yes, what is his exposure to its litter box?   ESSENTIAL

Toxoplasmosis is also frequently encountered in the feces of cats. Therefore, the amount of exposure a potentially immunosuppressed patient has to cat feces becomes important not only for toxoplasmosis infection but also for lymphoma.

E. Do they have a dog? If yes, is it kept indoors or outdoors? NONESSENTIAL

There are no known zoonoses transmitted by the canine species that place HIV-positive individuals at increased for acquiring an infection. Thus, this question is not relevant.

However, another relevant question involves the ownership of exposure to birds. *Cryptococcus* is frequently found in bird feces, especially pigeon droppings, and is another important organism in the development of opportunistic CNS infections in HIV-positive patients.

2. Physical Examination

A. Ear, nose, and throat (ENT) examination   ESSENTIAL

An ENT examination will provide information regarding a potential upper respiratory tract infection that could explain some of his symptoms and/or represent a source for CNS pathogens in the event a CNS infection is responsible for his symptoms.

B. Heart and lung examination   ESSENTIAL

The cardiac examination is important to evaluate for a valvular disease or an arrhythmia that could potentially result in vascular embolic phenomena (e.g., TIAs or CVAs) that could explain at least some of his current symptoms. Additionally, by evaluating the valves for a murmur, which could represent a potential bacterial endocarditis, and could also account for many of his symptoms.

The primary function of the lung examination is to evaluate for a potential infectious locus.

C. Examination of all his pulses   NONESSENTIAL

With the possible rare exception of a bruit in his carotid artery representing an atherosclerotic process producing his symptoms via a thromboembolic TIA or CVA, an evaluation of his pulses is extremely unlikely to yield any useful clinical information. Furthermore, the potential of an atherosclerotic process being responsible for Mr. Deets' symptoms is very small given his age.

D. Neurologic examination, including a mini-mental status (MMSE) and meningeal signs   ESSENTIAL

Because of his headache, fever, chills, hypersomnia, confusion, and other neuropsychiatric symptoms, a neurologic examination with an MMSE and meningeal irritation testing is essential. (For additional information regarding the MMSE, please refer to Case 9-6; for further information regarding the meningeal signs, please see Case 9-7.)

E. Examination of all his lymph nodes   ESSENTIAL

Because he is HIV positive, susceptible to a wide array of infections and malignancies, and currently experiencing a fever, it is important to evaluate all his lymph nodes to identify other potential sources of an initial infection that could result in Mr. Deets' current symptoms.

3. Diagnostic Studies

A. Computed tomography (CT) of the head, with and without contrast   ESSENTIAL

A CT scan of Mr. Deets' head, with and without contrast, is essential to identify any potential structural abnormalities that could be consistent with a space-occupying lesion, infection, ischemia, hemorrhage, and/or atrophy that could be responsible for his current condition.

B. Complete blood count with differential (CBC w/diff)   ESSENTIAL

The complete blood count with differential is essential because it can provide information regarding the presence of infection, inflammation, lymphoma, bleeding disorder, anemia, hypovolemia, and other conditions that could be causing and/or exacerbating Mr. Deets' symptoms. (For more information regarding the role of the CBC w/diff, please refer to Case 1-4.)

C. CD4$^+$ lymphocyte cell count and HIV RNA level   ESSENTIAL

These tests are essential because Mr. Deets is HIV positive. The combination of these two levels provides critical information regarding his HIV diagnosis (i.e., HIV infected, ARC, or AIDS) and crucial clinical decisions, including the need to reinstitute antiretroviral therapy for prophylaxis, initiate treatment for ARC or AIDS, evaluate for the need for prophylactic therapy for opportunistic infections, and determine if an opportunistic infection causing Mr. Deets' current symptoms.

D. Polymerase chain reaction (PCR) testing for *Toxoplasma*, *Coccidioides*, cytomegalovirus (CMV), and Epstein-Barr virus (EBV) antibodies; serum cryptococcal antigen; rapid plasma reagin (RPR); and PPD   ESSENTIAL

All of these tests are important to obtain because they are highly sensitive and specific in detecting the major pathogens that are responsible for CNS infections in HIV-positive patients toxoplasmosis, coccidiosis/coccidioidmycosis, CMV infection, EBV infection, cryptococcosis, syphilis, and tuberculosis, respectively. Any of these could present with the signs and symptoms that Mr. Deets is exhibiting if they affect the central nervous system.

E. Urine drug screen   ESSENTIAL

Despite Mr. Deets' denial of illicit substance use/abuse, a urine drug screen should be performed. Positive results could account for some of the behavioral and memory symptoms as well as his lack of personal hygiene, desire for food, and denial of symptoms, especially because some of these problems seemed to have appeared before he became acutely ill.

4. Diagnosis

A. Advanced AIDS with *Toxoplasma* abscess   INCORRECT

Because Mr. Deets is HIV positive and has a CD4$^+$ cell count of less than 200 cells/µl, the diagnosis of AIDS can be established. In order to be diagnosed with advanced AIDS, his CD4$^+$ cell count would need to be less than 50 cells/µl. Nevertheless, with a CD4$^+$ cell count less than 200 cells/µl, he is at risk for acquiring an opportunistic infection and/or malignancy, such as toxoplasmosis.

A *Toxoplasma* abscess could account for his fever and his neurologic symptoms. However, advanced AIDS with *Toxoplasma* abscess is not his most likely diagnosis because his *Toxoplasma* serology is negative (and his CD4+ cell count is greater than 50). Furthermore, despite toxoplasmosis being associated with a thin-walled, round lesion with ringlike enhancement with contrast on CT, it tends to present with multiple lesions.

B. AIDS with tuberculoma   INCORRECT

As stated previously, because Mr. Deets has a CD4$^+$ cell count of less than 200 cells/µl in conjunction with a positive HIV serology, he meets the disease-defining criteria for AIDS and is at risk for acquiring opportunistic infections, including those caused by *Mycoplasma tuberculosis*.

Although a tuberculoma could account for Mr. Deets' clinical picture and his PPD result is unavailable, AIDS with tuberculoma can still be eliminated as his most likely diagnosis because of his CT results and lack of respiratory symptoms. A CNS tuberculoma generally appears as a nodular density on CT scanning and is almost always associated with respiratory tract symptoms.

C. AIDS with coccidioidoma   INCORRECT

As previously stated, Mr. Deets meets the disease-defining criteria for a diagnosis of AIDS and is at risk for subsequent opportunistic infections and malignancies. A central nervous system infection/abscess would certainly account for his history and physical examination findings. Thus, coccidioidoma is a potential differential diagnosis; however, it can be eliminated as his most likely diagnosis because a coccidioidoma appears as a nodular density on imaging studies and is generally associated with a positive serology for *Coccidioides*.

D. AIDS with a non-Hodgkin central nervous system (CNS) lymphoma   CORRECT

As previously stated, Mr. Deets meets the diagnostic criteria for AIDS and is at risk for the development of opportunistic infections and malignancies. A lymphoma of the brain can certainly account for his clinical picture. Furthermore, it is characterized by a single, thin-walled, round lesion with ringlike enhancement with contrast on CT scanning. This can further be confirmed as Mr. Deets' most likely diagnosis because of his negative serology not only for *Toxoplasma* but also for *Coccidioides*, CMV, EBV, *Cryptococcus*, and syphilis. However, definitive diagnosis is going to involve a biopsy of the brain lesion.

E. Bell palsy in an HIV-positive patient   INCORRECT

Although Mr. Deets' cranial nerve testing revealed a lower motor neuron paralysis, which is consistent with Bell palsy, the presence of a mass on CT scanning is not. Additionally, Bell palsy alone, even in an HIV-positive patient, is not going to produce his clinical picture. Thus, this is not his most likely diagnosis.

5. Treatment Plan

A. Hospitalize in isolation   CORRECT

Because of his brain lesion, extremely low CD4+ cell count, high HIV RNA level, and toxic appearance, Mr. Deets needs to be hospitalized in isolation. The purpose of isolation is not to protect the staff and other patients from acquiring an HIV infection, because it is not an air-borne virus, but to protect him from acquiring a nosocomial infection, because he is extremely susceptible to any infection and its complications at this point.

B. Consult with an infectious disease specialist, a neurosurgeon, and an oncologist   CORRECT

Mr. Deets needs the expert input from all three of these specialists. Then infectious disease specialist will need to have experience with AIDS patients, not only because of all the potential complications from the disease itself, the complexity of the medication plans, the potential adverse effects and interactions caused by these medications, the need for prophylaxis from opportunistic infections, and the need for frequent follow-up with extensive patient education and appropriate laboratory testing, but also because of the frequent changes in the recommendations regarding the ultimate management strategies for patients with AIDS. Hence, the best provider to follow Mr. Deets' AIDS is an infectious disease specialist with the necessary experience and expertise to appropriately treat AIDS patients.

A neurosurgeon should be consulted because Mr. Deets has a mass lesion on his CT scan. In conjunction with his other providers, the neurosurgeon will determine whether a stereotactic needle biopsy (or some other diagnostic procedure) is necessary to confirm the diagnosis, and if deemed necessary, the ideal time to perform the procedure. Furthermore, he or she will be required to determine whether the lesion is compressing a vital structure, and if so, whether it will require surgical resection (or some other procedure) immediately or in the near future. Additionally, if the anti-infective agents are not effective in reducing the size of the lesion or the patient cannot tolerate the medication combination, then surgical intervention is probably going to be required at that time.

Additionally, an oncologist should be consulted to work in conjunction with the other specialists to obtain his or her recommendation regarding a trial of anti-infective agents, the need for biopsy (and when), if and when corticosteroids will be required, and whether chemotherapy and/or radiation therapy should be included in Mr. Deets' treatment plan.

C. Restart triple antiretroviral therapy unless specialist recommends alternative   CORRECT

Because Mr. Deets meets the established criteria for AIDS, his need for antiretroviral therapy depends to a great extent on his HIV RNA levels and CD4+ cell counts. If the HIV RNA level is greater than 30,000 copies/ml, therapy is recommended for all patients irrespective of symptoms and CD4+ cell counts. Because Mr. Deets falls into this category, his antiretroviral therapy should be reinstituted. However, the infectious disease (or the oncology and/or neurosurgical) specialist might recommend another combination in view of Mr. Deets' previous course of antiretrovirals and/or current lymphoma. If so, it is prudent to follow his or her advice. If the primary HCP feels the recommendation would be more harmful than helpful, then he or she needs to discuss those concerns with the specialist instead of ignoring or cancelling the recommended course of therapy.

On the other hand, if the HIV RNA level is 5000 to 30,000 copies/ml, therapy is recommended for all symptomatic patients and for those with CD4+ counts of less than 500 cells/µl. Therapy is also considered for patients with an HIV RNA level in this range, even if the CD4+ count is greater than 500 cells/µl. If the HIV RNA level is less than 5000 copies/ml with a CD4+ count of less than 350 cells/µl, antiretroviral therapy should be recommended. However, if the HIV RNA level is less than 5000 copies/ml with a CD4+ count between 350 and 500 cells/µl, therapy should be considered. If the HIV RNA level is less than 5000 copies/ml with a CD4+ count greater than 500 cells/µl, therapy should be deferred.

D. Four- to 6-week trial of sulfadiazine and pyrimethamine unless specialist recommends alternative   CORRECT

Generally, when a single, thin-walled ring-enhanced lesion is identified on an imaging study of the brain, a 4- to 6-week trial of sulfadiazine and pyrimethamine is the treatment of choice. However, if one of the specialists recommends an alternative medical and/or surgical approach, again, the primary HCP should take the advice of the specialist. If the primary HCP has concerns regarding the recommendation, then he or she needs to immediately address these concerns with the specialist.

E. Start radiation therapy INCORRECT

Even though radiation, highly active antiretroviral therapy (HAART), and corticosteroids are the cornerstone of management of a CNS lymphoma in an HIV-positive patient, it is not appropriate to start radiation therapy without the input and recommendation of an oncologist.

Epidemiologic and Other Data

Based on CSF testing, it is estimated that over 90% of all patients with AIDS have some degree of CNS involvement. Complications from CNS involvement are estimated to occur in approximately 33% of all patients with AIDS. This number is significantly lower in patients who are started on appropriate antiretroviral therapy early and take it regularly. Nevertheless, these CNS complications result in significant morbidity and mortality.

The most common CNS problems are damage caused by HIV itself (primary) or an infectious or malignant process (secondary). The most common infectious processes include toxoplasmosis, cryptococcosis, and progressive multifocal leukoencephalopathy. The most common malignancy is CNS lymphoma.

REFERENCES/ADDITIONAL READING

Aboulafia DM. AIDS-related non-Hodgkin lymphoma: evolving clinical issues in the HAART era. *Infect Med.* 2007;24: 445–451.

Adams RJ, Albers G, Alberts MJ, et al. The American Heart Association/American Stroke Association (AHA/ASA) Writing Committee for the Prevention of Stroke in Patients With Stroke and Transient Ischemic Attack (TIA). Update to the AHA/ASA recommendations for the prevention of stroke in patients with stroke and transient ischemic attack. *Stroke.* 2008;39(5):1647–1652.

Aghababian RV, ed. *Essentials of Emergency Medicine.* Sudbury, MA: Jones & Bartlett Publishers; 2006.
Go S. Headache. 444–449.
Nelson D. Seizures. 543–549.
Peralta R, Hirsh M. Pediatric injuries. 970–974.
Pierce DL, Jehle DVK. Autoimmune diseases. 291–297.
Reiser RC. Seizures. 440–443.
Sullivan JM. Cerebrovascular disorders. 403–414.

Amarenco P, Bogousslavsky J, Callahan A 3rd, et al. Stroke Prevention by Aggressive Reduction in Cholesterol Levels (SPARCL) Investigators. High-dose atorvastatin after stroke or transient ischemic attack. *N Engl J Med.* 2006;355:549–559.

American Academy of Neurology Quality Standards Subcommittee. Practice parameter: the management of concussion in sports (summary statement). Report of the Quality Standards Subcommittee. *Neurology.* 1997;48:581–585.

American Psychiatric Association. Mood disorders. In: *American Psychiatric Association, Diagnosis and Statistical Manual of Mental Disorders.* 4th ed., text revision. Washington, DC: American Psychiatric Association; 2000:345–428.

Brathen G, Ben-Menachem E, Brodtkorb E, et al., in conjunction with The EFNS Task Force on Diagnosis and Treatment of Alcohol-Related Seizures Members of the Task Force. EFNS guidelines on the diagnosis and management of alcohol-related seizures: report of the EFNS task force. *Eur J Neurol.* 2005;12(8):575–581.

Brindani F, Vitetta F, Gemignani F. Restless legs syndrome: differential diagnosis and management with pramipexole. *Clin Interv Aging.* 2009;4:305–313.

Cardoso F, Seppi K, Mair KJ, Wenning GK, Poewe W. Seminar on choreas. *Lancet Neurol.* 2006;5(7):589–602.

Chandratheva A, Mehta Z, Geraghty OC, et al. Oxford vascular study: population-based study of risk and predictors of stroke in the first few hours after a TIA. *Neurology.* 2009;72(22):1941–1947.

Department of Health and Human Services, Agency for Healthcare Research and Quality. Quality of health care. In: *Department of Health and Human Services, Agency for Healthcare Research and Quality National Healthcare Disparities Report 2007.* Rockville, MD: Department of Health and Human Services, Agency for Healthcare Research and Quality; 2007:31–112.

Easton JD, Saver JL, Alberts GW, et al. Definition and evaluation of transient ischemic attack. A scientific statement for healthcare professionals from the American Heart Association/American Stroke Association Stroke Council; Council on Cardiovascular Surgery and Anesthesia; Council on Cardiovascular Radiology and Intervention; Council on Cardiovascular Nursing; and the Interdisciplinary Council on Peripheral Vascular Disease. *Stroke.* 2009;40:2276–2293.

Fauci AS, Kasper DL, Longo DL, et al., eds. *Harrison's Principles of Internal Medicine.* 17th ed. New York: McGraw-Hill Medical; 2008.
Chaudhry V. Peripheral neuropathy. 2651–2667.
Czeisler CA, Winkelman JW, and Richardson GS. Sleep disorders. 171–180.
Fauci AS, Lane CL. Human immunodeficiency virus disease: AIDS and related disorders. 1137–1204.
Goadsby PJ, Raskin NH. Headache. 95–107.
Goyal, RK. Dysphagia. 237–240.
Lowenstein DH. Seizures and epilepsy. 2498–2512.
Lukehart SA. Syphilis. 1038–1046.
Olanow CW. Hyperkinetic movement disorders. 2560–2565.
Roos KL, Tyler KL. Meningitis, encephalitis, brain abscess, and emphysema. 2621–2641.
Ropper AH. Concussion and other head injuries. 2596–2601.
Rosenberg R. Ataxic disorders. 2565–2571.
Smith WS, English JD, Johnston SC. Cerebrovascular diseases. 2513–2536.

Flemming KD, Brown RD Jr, Petty GW, et al. Evaluation and management of transient ischemic attack and minor cerebral infarction. *Mayo Clin Proc.* 2004;79(8):1071–1086.

Fothergill A, Christianson TJH, Brown RD Jr, Rabinstein AA. Validation and refinement of the ABCD2 score: a population-based analysis. *Stroke.* 2009;40:2669–2673.

Germiller JA, Monin DL, Sparano AM, Tom LW. Intracranial complications of sinusitis in children and adolescents and their outcomes. *Arch Otolaryngol Head Neck Surg.* 2006;123:969–976.

Gershman K. Onion DK, series ed. *The Little Black Book of Geriatrics*. 3rd ed. Sudbury, MA: Jones & Bartlett Publishers; 2006.

    Gershman K. Neurology. 4.1 Neurology. 117–1263.

    Gershman K. Neurology. 4.2 Parkinson's disease. 126–138.

Giles MF, Rothwell PM. Substantial underestimation of the need for outpatient services for TIA and minor stroke. *Age Ageing*. 2007;36(6):676–680.

Halliday A, Harrison M, Hayter E, et al., on behalf of the Asymptomatic Carotid Surgery Trial (ACST) Collaborative Group. "10-year stroke prevention after successful carotid endarterectomy for asymptomatic stenosis (ACST-1): A multicentre randomised trial" *Lancet*. 2010;376:1074–84.

Headache Classification Subcommittee of the International Headache Society. The international classification of headache disorders, 2nd ed. *Cephalalgia*. 2004;24(Sept 1).

Higgins DS. Huntington's disease. *Curr Treat Opitons Neurol*. 2006;8(3):236–244.

Holmes GL, Zhao Q. Choosing the correct antiepileptic drugs: from animal studies to the clinic. *Pediatr Neurol*. 2008; 38:151–162.

Johnson SC, Rothwell PM, Nguyen-Huynh MN, et al. Validation and refinement of scores to predict very early stroke risk after transient ischaemic attack. *Lancet*. 2007;369:283–292.

Josephson SA, Sidney D, Pham TN, et al. Higher ABCD2 score predicts patients most likely to have true transient ischemic attack. *Stroke*. 2008;39(11):3096–3098.

Kattah JC, Talkad AV, Wang DZ, et al. HINTS to diagnose stroke in the acute vestibular syndrome: three-step bedside oculomotor examination more sensitive than early MRI diffusion-weighted imaging. *Stroke*. 2009;40:3504–3510.

King MA, Newton MR, Jackson GD, et al. Epileptology of the first-seizure presentation: a clinical, electroencephalographic, and magnetic resonance imaging study of 300 consecutive patients. *Lancet*. 1998;352:1007–1011.

Komboriorgas D, Solanki GA. The Pott's puffy tumor revisited: neurosurgical implications of this unforgotten entity. *J Neurosurg*. 2006;105(suppl 2):143–149.

Lalani A, Schneeweiss S, eds. *The Hospital for Sick Children: Handbook of Pediatric Emergency Medicine*. Sudbury, MA: Jones & Bartlett Publishers; 2008.

    Al-Ansari, K. Seizures and status epilepticus. 371–387.

    Jarvis DA. Head injury. 43–49.

    Schneeweiss S. Sinusitis. 119–123.

Levine AM. AIDS-related malignancies. *Curr Opin Oncol*. 1994;6:489–494.

Little A. Treatment-resistant depression. *Am Fam Physician*. 2009;80(2):167–172.

Louis ED. Essential tremor. *Lancet Neurol*. 2004;4(2):100–110.

Manzardo C, Del Mar Ortega M, Sued O, García F, Moreno A, Miró JM. Central nervous system opportunistic infections in developed countries in the highly active antiretroviral therapy era. *J Neurovirol*. 2005;11(suppl 3).72 82.

Marquardt L, Geraghty OC, Mehta Z, Rothwell PM. Low risk of ipsilateral stroke in patients with asymptomatic carotid stenosis on best medical treatment: a prospective, population-based study. *Stroke*. 2010;41:e11–e17.

McArthur JC, Brew B, Nath A. Neurological complications of HIV infections. *Lancet Neurol*. 2005;4(9):543–555.

Ondo WG. Essential tremor: treatment, options. *Curr Treat Options Neurol*. 2006;8(3):256–257.

Onion DK, series ed. *The Little Black Book of Primary Care*. 5th ed. Sudbury, MA: Jones & Bartlett Publishers; 2006.

    Onion DK, Sears S. Infectious disease. 9.21 Viral infections. 666–706.

    Onion DK. Neurology. 10.2 Headache. 718–723.

    Onion DK. Neurology. 10.3 Seizure disorders. 723–730.

    Onion DK. Neurology. 10.4 Sleep disorders. 731–735.

    Onion DK. Neurology. 10.5 Movement disorders. 735–742.

    Onion DK. Neurology. 10.11 Miscellaneous. 772–786.

Pagana KD, Pagana TJ. *Mosby's Diagnostic and Laboratory Test Reference*. 8th ed. St. Louis: Mosby Elsevier; 2007 (multiple pages utilized to provide normal reference values for laboratory tests).

Pandey DK, Gorelick PB. Should statin agents be administered to all patients with ischemic stroke? *Arch Neurol*. 2005; 62:23–24.

Quinn TJ, Cameron AC, Dawson J, Lees KR, Walters MR. ABCD2 scores and prediction of noncerebrovascular diagnoses in an outpatient population: a case-control study. *Stroke*. 2009;40:749–753.

Reeves MJ, Gargano JW, Wehner S, et al. Abstracts from the 2008 International Stroke Conference. 122: Ability of the ABCD2 clinical prediction rule to identify low-risk TIA cases in community-based emergency departments (p. 558). *Stroke*. 2008;39:527–729.

Restless Leg Syndrome Foundation. Restless leg syndrome. www.rls.org. Accessed December 20, 2008.

Ropper AH, Brown RH. Cerebral vascular disease. In: Ropper AH, Brown RH, eds. *Adams and Victor's Principles of Neurology*. 8th ed. New York: McGraw-Hill; 2005:660–746.

Schapira AH. Restless leg syndrome: an update on treatment options. *Drugs*. 2004;64(2):149–158.

Solenski NJ. Transient ischemic attacks: part I. Diagnosis and evaluation. *Am Fam Physician*. 2004;69(7):1665–1680.

Svenson JE, Spurlock JE. Insurance status and admission to hospital for head injuries: are we part of a two-tiered medical system? *Am J Emerg Med*. 2001;19(1):19–24.

US Food and Drug Administration. FDA news release: midodrine hydrochloride: FDA proposes withdrawal of low blood pressure drug. 2010(Aug 16). http://www.fda.gov/NewsEvents/Newsroom/PressAnnouncements/ucm222580.htm

Van Kleff M, Lataster A, Narouze S, et al. Evidence-based medicine; evidence-based interventional pain medicine according to clinical diagnoses: 2. Cluster headache. *Pain Practice*. 2009;9(6):435–442. (Published online 10/27/09. doi: 10.1111/j.1533–2500.2009.00331.x. Accessed October 31, 2009.)

Vincent JL, Berré J. Primer on medical management of severe brain injury. *Crit Care Med*. 2005;33(6):1392–1399.

Winter CD, Adamides AA, Lewis PM, Rosenfeld JV. A review of the current management of severe brain injury. *Surgeon*. 2005;3(5):329–337.

Yogev R. Focal suppurative infections of the central nervous system. In: Long SS, Pickering LK, Prober CG, eds. *Textbook of Principles and Practice of Pediatric Infectious Diseases*. Philadelphia: Churchill Livingstone; 2003:301–312.

CASES IN PSYCHIATRIC ILLNESSES*

CASE 10-1

Debbie Ellison

Mrs. Ellison is a 25-year-old white female who presents with the chief complaint of fatigue and headaches. Her symptoms have been present for approximately 4 to 5 weeks, and they are worsening in severity, frequency, and duration. Her headaches are generalized and nonpulsating. She states it feels "like my skin is too tight for my head." She experiences an average of four to five headaches per week. They are not associated with an aura, nausea, vomiting, photophobia, phonophobia, visual abnormalities, focal neurologic defects, neck pain, irregular eating habits, or skipping meals. There are no precipitating or aggravating factors of which Mrs. Ellison is aware. They are alleviated in less than 1 hour by taking two regular-strength acetaminophen tablets.

She is not experiencing any daytime sleepiness or insomnia, yet she awakens "just as tired" as she was before retiring. In an attempt to alleviate this problem, she adjusted her bedtime several times to "get more sleep"; unfortunately, this was not effective. She is now sleeping approximately 11 to 12 hours per night. She misses approximately 1 day of work per week because she is "just too tired to get up and go." She works as a bank teller and has been reprimanded by her supervisor several times in the past few months not only for her frequent absenteeism but also for taking too long to complete customer transactions, frequent errors (which the patient attributes to being "too tired to think straight"), easy distractibility, difficulty in remembering, and being irritable toward coworkers and customers.

Her headaches and fatigue do not appear to be any different on weekends as they are on weekdays. She denies excessive stress, anxiety, depression, or sadness. However, she does feel "down" because she fears getting fired from her job. She suffers from anhedonia and declines social invitations because "I am just too tired." She is not experiencing any fever; changes in the texture of her hair, oiliness and texture of her skin, or consistency and strength of her fingernails; jaundice; icterus of her sclera; bowel changes; abdominal pain; chest pain/pressure; palpitations; shortness of breath; or pedal edema.

She saw her regular healthcare provider (HCP) approximately 2 weeks ago, who performed serologic and magnetic resonance imaging (MRI) studies. She claims that her HCP advised her that the diagnostic studies were "normal" and her symptoms were caused by "stress." He prescribed lorazepam 0.5 mg at bedtime. However, she did not start this medication because, she emphatically denies this possibility as being her diagnosis because she has not experienced any increase in her stress level.

Her only medication is acetaminophen as needed (maximum of once daily); she is not taking any other over-the-counter or prescription medications, vitamins, supplements, or herbal preparations. She has no known medical problems. She has not had any surgery nor been hospitalized. She does not smoke, drink alcohol, or use any illicit drugs. Her family history is positive for depression in her mother, two maternal aunts, and two sisters.

She has been married for 3 years and has no children by mutual choice. She denies any problems with her marriage or relationship with her husband. She is sexually active and utilizes a copper-containing intrauterine device (IUD) for birth control. It was inserted 3 months ago. Her last menstrual period (LMP) was 2 weeks ago and normal. Her IUD string was palpable after her last menses.

1. Based on this information, which of the following questions are essential to ask Mrs. Ellison and why?

   A. How does she define fatigue and what is its pattern over a typical day?
   B. Has she been experiencing a sore throat, cervical lymphadenopathy, axillary lymphadenopathy, arthralgias, myalgias, or severe postexertional fatigue?
   C. Has she experienced a recent, unintentional weight change?

---

*Remember, for each question, none to all of the answers could be correct/essential or incorrect/nonessential. See page 399 for Chapter 10 answers.

D. Has she ever experienced any episodes of increased activity associated with a decreased need for sleep, grandiosity, enhanced self-esteem, euphoria, behavior unusual or outrageous for her, beginning many projects but not finishing any, or racing thoughts?

E. Has she considered suicide? If yes, does she have a plan?

Patient Responses

Mrs. Ellison describes her fatigue as "no energy" and occasionally as "no desire." It improves as the day progresses. She does not experience weakness. She has not been experiencing a sore throat; cervical or axillary lymphadenopathy; arthralgias; myalgias; severe postexertional fatigue; any episodes of increased activity associated with decreased need for sleep, grandiosity, euphoria, enhanced self-esteem, behavior unusual or outrageous for her, beginning many projects but not finishing any, racing thoughts; or suicidal thought or ideations. She has gained 20 lb the past month without a change in activity or appetite.

2. Based on this information, which of the following components of a physical examination are essential to conduct on Mrs. Ellison and why?

A. Overall appearance and affect
B. Palpation of thyroid
C. Heart examination
D. Abdominal examination
E. Pelvic examination

Physical Examination Findings

Mrs. Ellison is 5'3" tall and weighs 145 lb (body mass index [BMI] = 25.7). Other vital signs are blood pressure (BP), 126/66 mm Hg; pulse, 92 beats per minute (BPM) and regular; respiratory rate, 10/min and regular; and temperature, 97.8°F.

She looks tired. Her hygiene is good. However, her hair appears to only be partially combed. She is not wearing any make-up or earrings in her pierced ears. She is dressed appropriately; however, her pants and blouse have not been pressed. Her affect is somewhat flat and her speech slightly slow despite her appearing "apprehensive."

Her thyroid is normal in size and equal bilaterally. There are no masses or tenderness.

Her heart is regular in rate and rhythm. There are no murmurs, gallops, or rubs. Her apical impulse is nondisplaced and without a thrill.

Her abdominal and pelvic examinations are normal.

3. Based on this information, which of the following diagnostic studies are essential to perform on Mrs. Ellison and why?

A. Urinary human chorionic gonadotropin (HCG)
B. Thyroid function studies
C. Complete blood count with differential (CBC w/diff)
D. Liver function tests (LFTs)
E. Erythrocyte sedimentation rate (ESR)

Diagnostic Test Results

Her urinary HCG was negative. Her thyroid function studies, CBC w/diff, and LFTs were within normal limits. Her ESR was 5 mm/hr (normal adult female: 0–20).

4. Based on this information, which one of the following is Mrs. Ellison's most likely diagnosis and why?

A. Chronic fatigue syndrome
B. Major depressive episode
C. Dysthymic disorder
D. Adverse effect from hormones in contraceptive method
E. Somatization disorder

5. Based on this diagnosis, which of the following are appropriate components of a treatment plan for Mrs. Ellison and why?

A. Lamotrigine 25 mg/day for 2 weeks, then 50 mg/day for 2 weeks, then 100 mg daily
B. Citalopram 20 mg once a day for a minimum of 1 week, then increase to 40 mg daily if required
C. Psychotherapy
D. Tranylcypromine 10 mg three times a day for 2 weeks, then increase by 10 mg/day every 2 to 3 weeks as necessary to a total dose of 60 mg daily
E. Patient education on her disease, medication, potential of suicidal ideations, time before symptom relief, and what to do if adverse effects or concerns develop before follow-up appointment

CASE 10-2
Ellen Franklin

Mrs. Franklin is a 37-year-old African American female who presents for follow-up on her major depressive episode. She has been on her current dosage of medication (sertraline 200 mg once daily) for 5 weeks and states she "feels even worse." She has been experiencing an increase in crying episodes, fatigue, and irritability over minor incidents (e.g., store clerk providing her with incorrect amount of change or waitress getting her order incorrect). Furthermore, she has gained an additional 2 lb (total 5 lb in the past 3 months) despite attempting to lose weight by decreasing calorie consumption and increasing exercise.

She denies feeling depressed, "down," or "blue" or experiencing anhedonia. She has not limited her social activities and continues to enjoy spending time with family and friends. She does not have frequent work absences or complaints on her job performance. She does not experience insomnia and sleeps her usual 8 hours per night. She awakens less tired than before retiring; however, she is not as refreshed as she was before becoming ill. Her fatigue worsens as the day progresses. She didn't have an infectious illness before (or since) her symptoms began.

She first noticed her symptoms approximately 6 months ago. They gradually progressed until she decided to seek medical care approximately 4 months ago. At that time, she was diagnosed with major depressive episode and started on citalopram 10 mg once a day. When she returned for her follow-up appointment 2 weeks later, her symptoms were not improved (and were possibly slightly worse); thus, her citalopram was increased to 20 mg daily. After 1 month on the 20 mg of citalopram, she returned for a follow-up visit and her symptoms were actually worse. Thus, the citalopram was discontinued and she was started on sertraline 50 mg daily for 1 week and advised to increase it to 100 mg daily after one week. When that did not alleviate her symptoms after 2 weeks, it was increased to 150 mg daily for 1 week, followed by 200 mg daily. Two weeks later, her symptoms were definitely not improving (and might have even been slightly worse); however, her HCP advised her to continue it at the same dose to "give the medicine a little more time" and recommended she consider psychotherapy. Because her medical insurance doesn't cover psychotherapy, she scheduled today's appointment in hopes of being prescribed a different drug.

Her only medication is sertraline 200 mg daily. She takes no other prescription or over-the-counter medications, vitamins, supplements, or herbal preparations. She has never had surgery nor been hospitalized. She is not experiencing any marital discord and enjoys a satisfying sex life with her husband of 4 years. For contraception, her husband had a vasectomy 2 years ago when she turned 35 years old and "could no longer take the pill," because they had mutually decided not to have any children. He was azoospermic at his postvasectomy check-up. Her last menstrual period was 6 weeks ago and normal; however, they have been "getting heavier" since she stopped her oral contraceptives. Normally, she experiences menses every 28 to 30 days. She does not smoke cigarettes or do illicit drugs. She used to drink two alcoholic beverages per week; however, she stopped all alcohol when she began her antidepressant. Her family history is noncontributory, including being negative for depression.

1. Based on this information, which of the following questions are essential to ask Mrs. Franklin and why?

  A. What, if anything, provokes her crying episodes?
  B. Is she experiencing a change in appetite; psychomotor slowing or agitation; feelings of worthlessness or inappropriate guilt; problems with thinking processes, concentration, memory, or indecisiveness; or recurrent thoughts of death or suicide?
  C. Has she experienced any recent bowel changes, abdominal pain, fever, chills, night sweats, myalgias, arthralgias, or lymphadenopathy?
  D. Has she experienced any polydipsia, polyuria, or changes in her skin, lips, hair, or fingernails?
  E. Has she experienced any recent changes in her heart rate or breathing?

Patient Responses

Her crying episodes are precipitated by major (e.g., hearing of the death of a friend or of a family member being in a serious accident) and minor (e.g., her husband not liking what she cooked for dinner, a co-worker commenting on her weight gain, or watching a "sad" movie) incidents.

She has not experienced a change in appetite; psychomotor slowing or agitation; feelings of worthlessness or inappropriate guilt; problems with thinking processes, concentration, memory, or indecisiveness; recurrent thoughts of death or suicide; hematochezia; change in the color/consistency of her stool; frequency of bowel movements; abdominal pain; polydipsia; polyuria; fever; chills; night sweats; myalgias; arthralgias; or lymphadenopathy.

She has noticed her skin and lips being drier than usual but no change in color or the appearance of lesions. Additionally,

her hair has become slightly dry and brittle, and her nails are "softer" and breaking more easily. Additionally, she has noticed a slight amount of shortness of breath if she overexerts herself. She denies the episodes being associated with palpitations, tachycardia, bradycardia, wheezing, or coughing. All of these symptoms started at approximately the same time as her fatigue.

2. Based on this information, which of the following components of a physical examination are essential to conduct on Mrs. Franklin and why?

  A. Ear, nose, and throat (ENT) examination
  B. Gross external eye examination
  C. Skin examination
  D. Heart examination
  E. Pelvic examination

Physical Examination Findings

Mrs. Franklin is 5'5" tall and weighs 156 lb (BMI = 26.0). Other vital signs are BP, 120/56 mm Hg; pulse, 64 BPM and regular; respiratory rate, 9/min and regular; and oral temperature, 97.6°F.

Overall, Mrs. Franklin's appearance is normal except she looks a little pale. She is dressed appropriately and is well groomed. She has on nicely done make-up and jewelry, and her shoes and purse match her outfit. Her affect appears normal as do her mannerisms.

Her scleras are normal color without evidence of icterus, erythema, or injection. Her conjunctivae are paler than expected.

Her skin is normal in color without erythema, jaundice, or carotenemia. There is no evidence of a rash; however, her skin does appear to be slightly "dry." Her nails are short but without clubbing, pitting, jagged edges, or other abnormalities.

Her heart is regular in rate and rhythm. There are no murmurs, gallops, or rubs. Her apical impulse is nondisplaced and without a thrill. Her lungs are clear to auscultation.

Her pelvic examination is normal.

3. Based on this information, which of the following diagnostic studies are essential to perform on Mrs. Franklin and why?

  A. Urinary human chorionic gonadotropin (HCG)
  B. Total thyroxine (T$_4$)
  C. Erythrocyte sedimentation rate (ESR)
  D. Complete blood count with differential (CBC w/diff)
  E. Short-form version of Yesavage Depression Scale

Diagnostic Test Results

Mrs. Franklin's urinary HCG was negative.

Her total T$_4$ was 4.8 µg/dl (normal adult female: 5–12). Her ESR was 5 mm/hr (normal female: < 20).

Her CBC w/diff revealed a red blood cell (RBC) count of 4.2×10^6/µl (normal adult female: 4.2–5.4) with a mean corpuscular volume (MCV) of 81 µm^3 (normal adult: 80–95), a mean corpuscular hemoglobin (MCH) of 27.1 pg (normal adult: 27–31), a mean corpuscular hemoglobin concentration (MCHC) of 33.5 g/dl (normal adult: 32–36), and a red blood cell distribution width (RDW) of 11.5% (normal adult: 11–14.5). Her white blood cell (WBC) count was 7500/mm^3

(normal adult: 5,000–10,000) with 64% neutrophils (normal: 55–70), 27% lymphocytes (normal: 20–40), 5% monocytes (normal: 2–8), 3% eosinophils (normal: 1–4), and 1% basophils (normal: 0.5–1). Her hemoglobin (Hgb) was 11.4 g/dl (normal adult female: 12–16) and her hematocrit (HCT) was 34% (normal adult female: 37–47). Her platelet (thrombocyte) count was 225,500/mm³ (normal adult: 150,000–400,000) and her mean platelet volume (MPV) was 8.9 fl (normal: 7.4–10.4). Her smear was consistent with this and revealed rare hypochromic, microcytic cells.

The result of her short-form version of the Yesavage Depression Scale was 4 (normal ≤ 5).

4. Based on this information, which one of the following is Mrs. Franklin's most likely diagnosis and why?

    A. Major depressive episode
    B. Treatment-resistant depression
    C. Pregnancy
    D. Hypothyroidism
    E. Iron deficiency anemia

5. Based on this diagnosis, which of the following are appropriate components of a treatment plan for Mrs. Franklin and why?

    A. Stop sertraline
    B. Start cognitive behavioral therapy (CBT)
    C. Start duloxetine 20 mg twice a day
    D. Start levothyroxine 25 μg once a day
    E. Check serum iron, serum ferritin, total iron-binding capacity, and transferrin saturation

CASE 10-3
Freddie Gleason

Mr. Gleason is a 22-year-old white male who presents accompanied by a police officer for "an evaluation before incarceration." According to the police officer, Mr. Gleason is in the process of being arrested on charges of indecent exposure, grand theft auto, breaking and entering, being a public nuisance, and resisting arrest. Apparently, earlier this evening an individual left her vehicle running while she ran inside a convenience store to make a quick purchase. In the process of checking out, she noticed the patient unzip his pants, urinate on her front tire, get into her vehicle, and drive off.

Later this evening, a man and a woman returned home from dinner and found this stolen vehicle in their driveway, their front door open, what appeared to be urine on their front porch, and the patient sleeping in one of their beds. They phoned the police, who immediately responded to the call. Upon their arrival, they assumed the patient was "probably drunk and just passed out there"; however, when they awoke him to remove him from the premises, the patient immediately commenced barking and growling at them and would not permit them to approach him. While attempting to apprehend the patient, he jumped off the bed, ran down the stairs, and exited out the open front door.

They found him with his pants unzipped, crouched on his hands and knees, urinating on their cruiser's tire. When they approached, he shouted "Ret aray, rit's rine rowl" and reconvened barking and growling at them "like a dog." After several unsuccessful attempts by the accompanying officer's partner to restrain the patient, the officer claims he opened the back door of the cruiser and threw a doughnut inside while shouting, "Here, boy." The patient immediately jumped into the backseat and began eating the doughnut off the seat using his mouth only. They closed the door and took him to the police station for processing without further incident. While searching him for weapons, they discovered an expired out-of-state driver's license without his photo and a few dollars in a wallet in his back pants pocket. However, his front pockets were full of dog biscuits. When asked his name, he responded, "Ruby Doo." When asked where he resides, he stated, "Rhat rever rouse R ree ron." While his partner was requesting permission from their superior officer to obtain a medical/psychological evaluation on the patient, the accompanying officer witnessed him climbing onto the floor on his hands and knees, circling three times in one spot, lying down there, and falling asleep. At this point the booking process was ceased and he was brought in for evaluation.

The officer is asked to wait in the hall and a male nursing assistant replaces him in the examination room. Upon inquiring how he is feeling, the patient responds, "Rine." He confirms that he heard what the officer claimed he did. Then, he spontaneously adds, "Rits rot rue, Raggy rold re ro do rit." He continues to talk spontaneously, going from one unrelated subject to another. Working through the "r's" in his speech, it appears that he believes that he is the cartoon dog Scooby Doo. Furthermore, he believes that if you urinate on an object, it belongs to you. He also explains how his friend, Shaggy, has been attempting to care for him since he was evicted from his apartment an unknown time ago. Apparently, Shaggy advises him on which cars to take, which homes to enter, what to eat, and where to sleep. He cannot see Shaggy when Shaggy talks to him. Shaggy's voice appears to come from "outside" of his head.

He denies any medical or psychiatric conditions. He denies currently or previously being on any prescription medications other than an occasional antibiotic for a "cold." He does not take any over-the counter medications, vitamins, supplements, or herbal preparations. He denies ever being hospitalized or having surgery. He denies smoking cigarettes, drinking alcohol, or doing illicit drugs/substances. His family history is positive for his mother being "razy"; however, he could not provide her diagnosis.

1. Based on this information, which of the following questions are essential to ask the patient and why?

    A. Where is the rest of the "gang"?
    B. Has he recently had any fever, chills, weight changes, fatigue, headaches, arthralgias, myalgias, problems with gait, difficulty with coordination, or visual changes?
    C. Has he experienced any palpitations, dyspnea, weakness, or cold intolerance?
    D. Has he experienced any changes in sleep, appetite, or mood; feelings of depression; anhedonia; or thoughts of harming himself or others?
    E. If he is a dog, where is his tail?

Patient Responses

According to the patient, "Ru rest rof ru rang ris rout runting rhosts." He denies fever, chills, weight changes, fatigue, headaches, arthralgias, myalgias, problems with gait, difficulty with coordination, visual changes, palpitations, dyspnea, weakness, cold intolerance, changes in his appetite, alterations of his mood, or feeling depressed. He has noticed that he tends to sleep more during the day and is awake more at night; however, he sleeps approximately the same total number of hours and awakens refreshed. He is experiencing anhedonia. He denies any suicidal or homicidal ideations. He had his tail "clipped" when he was a pup.

2. Based on this information, which of the following components of a physical examination are essential to conduct on the patient and why?

   A. General appearance, affect, and mannerisms
   B. Examination for minor head/facial deformities
   C. Preauricular lymph node palpation
   D. Neurologic examination, with mini-mental status examination (MMSE)
   E. Skin/nail examination

Physical Examination Findings

Mr. Gleason is 5'11" tall and weighs 172 lb (BMI = 24). Other vital signs are BP, 110/62 mm Hg; pulse, 84 BPM and regular; respiratory rate, 12/min and regular; and tympanic temperature, 97.9°F. The patient appears not to have showered, shaved, or brushed his teeth in several days. His clothing is dirty and unkempt. During the officer's report, the patient lies on the examination table with his arms and legs curled under him and his head resting on his arms. When the officer leaves the room, the patient gets up on his hands and knees and pants when he is acknowledged. He then sits back down on the table with his legs crossed in an "X" and his arms extended straight until the palms of his hands touched the table. Otherwise, he exhibits no unusual behavior or mannerisms. His mood is neither excessively euphoric nor depressed. His affect is normal.

He has a minor, but bilaterally equal, slightly peaked shape to the auricles of his ears. His eyes appear to be set normally. His palate is markedly arched and higher than usual. Otherwise, no head or facial deformities or tenderness is noted. His preauricular lymph nodes are not palpable or tender.

His cranial nerves are grossly intact. He has good and equal muscle strength as well as intact sensation to sharp and dull stimulation in his face, hands, arms, feet, and legs. His coordination is somewhat poor and he walks with his knees flexed, even after the HCP requests that he straighten them. Sitting down, he could fully extend them. He refuses to attempt a Romberg test. His has no arm drift or tremor. Finger-to-nose, finger-to-finger, and rapid alternating motions are intact. His biceps, triceps, brachioradialis, knee, and ankle reflexes are normal and equal bilaterally. His plantar reflexes are normal bilaterally. His Brudzinski and Kernig signs are negative.

He has poor insight and judgment. Other than the "r's," his speech is intact. He frequently changes subjects without an obvious connection from one to the next. His speech is not rapid or pressured. His total mini-mental examination score is 17; however, he refuses to perform tasks requiring reading or writing because "rogs ran't read ror rite." He takes the paper with his left hand instead of his right when instructed. Other language areas are intact. Under orientation, he knows he is located on the first floor of a building; however, he thinks it is a veterinarian's office. Otherwise, he is not oriented to time, place, or person. However, he can remember all three objects immediately and upon recall, and he can perform serial 7's correctly.

Besides being slightly "dry" and dirty, his skin is normal in color and without evidence of pallor, erythema, jaundice, or carotenemia. There is no evidence of a rash or any lesions. His nails are short, dirty, torn, and jagged; however, they are without clubbing, pitting, Beau lines, or other significant abnormalities.

3. Based on this information, which of the following diagnostic studies are essential to perform on this patient and why?

   A. Computed tomography (CT) of brain without contrast
   B. 8 a.m. and 4 p.m. cortisol levels
   C. Thyroid panel with thyroid-stimulating hormone (TSH), free thyroxine (FT$_4$), and triiodothyronine by radioimmunoassay (T$_3$ by RIA)
   D. Complete blood count with differential (CBC w/diff)
   E. Urinary drug screen

Diagnostic Test Results

The CT of his brain with contrast revealed mild atrophy of his left hippocampus-amygdala and left posterior superior temporal gyrus. Otherwise, it was unremarkable.

His 8 a.m. cortisol level was 15 µg/dl (normal adult: 5–23) and his 4 p.m. cortisol level was 8 µg/dl (normal adult: 3–13).

His TSH was 8 µU/ml (normal adult: 2–10), FT$_4$ was 1.9 ng/dl (normal adult: 0.8–2.8), and T$_3$ by RIA was 150 ng/dl (normal adult 20–50 years of age: 70–205).

His CBC w/diff was within normal limits and his urinary drug screen was negative.

4. Based on this information, which one of the following is Mr. Gleason's most likely diagnosis and why?

   A. Schizophrenia, undifferentiated type
   B. Schizophreniform disorder
   C. Schizoaffective disorder
   D. Delusional disorder
   E. Psychotic disorder, not otherwise specified

5. Based on this diagnosis, which of the following are appropriate components of a treatment plan for Mr. Gleason and why?

   A. Hospitalize on psychiatric service
   B. Observe for signs/symptoms/behaviors suggestive of suicidal ideations, especially while his psychosis is resolving
   C. Olanzapine 5 mg once a day, increase to 10 mg once a day after 4 days if tolerating
   D. Haloperidol decanoate 200 mg IM daily
   E. Fasting blood glucose and lipid panel before initiating any atypical neuroleptic

CASE 10-4

Ginger Halstead

Ginger is a 17-year-old white female who is accompanied by her mother who provides the chief complaint of "I'm worried Ginger's bulimic." Her mother saw a movie on television where the main character had bulimia and was astounded when she realized Ginger exhibits several of the same behaviors as the actress. These include spending a lot of time alone in her room, especially if she is "upset over little things" (e.g., fight with her boyfriend; bad grade [defined as a "B"] on a test; or disagreement with her parents over her wardrobe, car privileges, curfew, and friends). Additionally, like the girl in the movie, Ginger appears secretive (e.g., not wanting her parents in her room, cleaning her own room [including emptying the trash directly into and running the trash compactor], and refusing to discuss personal matters with her mother). Also, Ginger was an overweight child who "slimmed down" with puberty. This was followed by a couple of years in which Ginger experienced wide fluctuations in her weight (as much as 10 lb in 1 week). Her mother also notes that Ginger seems excessively concerned regarding her appearance, and in particular her weight, and exercises excessively (e.g., practices kickboxing 2 hours every morning and 2 hours every evening even if ill, tired, or injured).

The day after viewing the movie while Ginger was at school, her mother searched her room and discovered a box on the floor of her closet under a big pile of clothing containing candy bars, snack cakes, cookies, syrup of ipecac, laxatives, and diuretics. Ginger denies owning the box and its contents. She told her mother that she was "keeping it for her friend"; however, she would not reveal which one.

Her mother denies noticing Ginger appearing depressed, taking less time/care with her appearance, having difficulty or a changing pattern with sleep, increasing or decreasing food consumption, being excessively tired, experiencing anhedonia, laughing less, withdrawing from friends, slipping in her grades, having problems with memory or concentration, being "hyper," or talking/reading/obsessing about death.

After having her mother leave the examination room, Ginger admits that she intermittently feels "sad" or "upset" over certain situations (e.g., conflict with her parents, boyfriend, or other friends; not meeting her expectations on a test or a kickboxing match; or when "things just don't go the way I planned"). However, she estimates that this only occurs once or twice a week and lasts for a couple of hours maximum. She states that she resolves these feelings by "being alone in my room" doing "nothing special, just lying on my bed, thinking, listening to music, reading, and stuff like that."

She denies changes in quality or quantity of sleep, amount of energy, appetite, activities, enjoyment derived from previously pleasurable activities, memory, concentration, or thought processes. She also denies experiencing anxiety, suicidal ideations, increased energy, expansive mood, binging, purging, nausea, vomiting, diarrhea, constipation, or changes in stool color or consistency. Even with her mother out of the examination room, Ginger still denies ownership of the box (and its contents) that her mother found in her closet. She spontaneously adds that she didn't even know, until her mother told her, the uses of the medications found in the box, and she is now concerned that her friend might have an eating disorder and plans on talking to her about this possibility.

She doesn't feel like she eats any more than anyone else would in the same time frame. She admits to minor weight fluctuations; however, she attributes them to premenstrual bloating, the frequency of her kickboxing matches, and the duration and intensity of her training. However, she quickly adds that it "can't be more than 2 or 3 pounds." She doesn't feel that her kickboxing training is excessive and adds "it's what you have to do to be the best."

She denies smoking cigarettes, drinking alcohol, using drugs, or being sexually active with males or females. She achieved menarche at the age of 12 years and menstruates every 26 to 28 days. Her LMP was 3 weeks ago and normal. She denies taking any prescription or over-the-counter medications, vitamins, supplements, or herbal products. She denies having health problems, ever being hospitalized, having surgery, or having any health concerns. All her immunizations are up to date. Her family history is negative.

1. Based on this information, which of the following questions are essential to ask Ginger and why?

   A. Why is she lying about the contents of the box not belonging to her?
   B. What kind of grades does she get in school, is she pleased with them, and how difficult is it for her to obtain them?
   C. How good of a kickboxer is she, how much does she enjoy it, and why?
   D. How does she feel about herself overall and especially her appearance?
   E. How often does she weigh herself?

Patient Responses

She still angrily denies the contents of the box being hers. She gets mostly A's, with an occasional B, in school. When she does get a B, she feels she has let her parents down and she could have done better. She has to work "hard" to obtain her grades but feels it is worth the effort to see her parents pleased. She states she is an "OK" kickboxer. She likes it "OK" but thinks her mother likes it better because "she can show off all my trophies to her friends." She does it to "stay healthy" and please her mother. She feels "OK" about herself but would not elaborate further on that or her appearance. She weighs herself every morning before practicing kickboxing, and some days she increases her workout intensity and duration if she has gained weight.

2. Based on this information, which of the following components of a physical examination are essential to conduct on Ginger and why?

   A. Ocular conjunctival examination
   B. Oral mucosa, pharynx, and teeth
   C. Salivary glands
   D. Breast and pelvic examination
   E. Bilateral hands with emphasis on the metacarpophalangeal (MCP) joints

Physical Examination Findings

Ginger is 5'3" tall and weighs 148 lb (BMI = 26.2). Other vital signs are BP, 108/64 mm Hg; pulse, 72 BPM and regular; respiratory rate, 12/min and regular; and oral temperature, 98.1°F.

Her sclerae are normal in color without any evidence of icterus, injection, erythema, or subconjunctival hemorrhages. Her lower palpebral conjunctivae reveal rare pinpoint petechiae ranging from faint pink to bright red in color, bilaterally.

Her oral mucosa and pharynx are normal except she has a few linear-shaped petechiae that are varied in color (from a barely visible pale pink to a bright red) on her soft palate. There is no tonsillar enlargement or exudates. There appears to be a minor dental enamel loss on the lingual surface of her upper incisors and she has had multiple repaired cavities.

Her salivary glands are normal in size and nontender, except her parotid glands that are slightly enlarged, bilaterally. Her cervical lymph nodes are negative.

Her breast and pelvic examinations are normal.

Her hands are normal in color with her nails cut short and painted bright red. There is no evidence of acrocyanosis and her capillary refill is normal. Her left hand is without lesions. Her right hand reveals mild callus formation (Russell sign) and small abrasions over the dorsum of her first and second MCP joint (which she spontaneously attributes to kickboxing).

3. Based on this information, which of the following diagnostic studies are essential to perform on Ginger and why?

   A. Dual energy x-ray absorptiometry (DEXA) scan
   B. Electrolytes and serum magnesium level
   C. Amylase and lipase
   D. Urine toxicology for bisacodyl, emodin, aloe-emodin, and rhein
   E. Electrocardiogram (ECG)

Diagnostic Test Results

Her DEXA scan revealed a T score of –1.0 (normal: T score > –1.0).

Her electrolytes revealed a carbon dioxide (CO_2) of 32 mEq/L (normal: 23–30), a chloride (Cl) of 95 mEq/L (normal: 98–106), a potassium (K) of 3.1 mEq/L (normal adolescent and adult: 3.5–5.0), and a sodium (Na) of 130 mEq/L (normal adolescent and adult: 136–145). Ginger's serum magnesium was 1.0 mEq/L (normal adolescent and adult: 1.3–2.1).

Her amylase was 150 Somogyi units/dl (normal adolescent and adult: 60–120). Her lipase was 180 units/L (normal: 0–160).

Her urine tested positive for bisacodyl, emodin, and aloe-emodin (normal: negative). It was negative for rhein (normal: negative).

Her ECG revealed normal sinus rhythm (NSR) at a rate of 74 BPM without any premature beats, a normal PR interval, a normal QTc interval, and no ST-T changes.

4. Based on this information, which one of the following is Ginger's most likely diagnosis and why?

   A. Anorexia nervosa, purging type
   B. Bulimia nervosa, purging type
   C. Klein-Levin syndrome
   D. Major depressive episode, with atypical features
   E. Bacterial gastroenteritis

5. Based on this diagnosis, which of the following are appropriate components of a treatment plan for Ginger and why?

   A. Urinalysis (U/A), blood urea nitrogen (BUN), and serum creatinine
   B. Hospitalization
   C. Nutritional, personal, and family counseling
   D. Fluoxetine 20 mg once a day to start, increase as tolerated to 60 mg once a day
   E. Desipramine 100 mg once a day, increased to 300 mg once a day by the end of week 1

CASE 10-5

Harriett Iverson

Ms. Iverson is a 32-year-old white female who presents with the chief complaint of "I need help and don't know where else to turn." According to Ms. Iverson, she has just been fired from her third job this year and her parents are refusing to assist her financially. According to her, they told her "It was time to grow up and be responsible your life," that they had "pulled a lot of strings" to help her obtain her real estate agent license, and that "the least you could do was show some gratitude by putting it to proper use." Furthermore, they suggested she "get some help."

According to Ms. Iverson, she was fired from her most recent job as a real estate agent because she missed appointments with clients, became distracted while showing properties, failed to complete the appropriate paperwork on sales, procrastinated on assignments, and was totally unorganized. She admits this is true and adds, "If I were my boss, I would have fired me too." She went on to explain that she didn't intentionally miss appointments with clients; she would just "forget" them. She didn't intentionally not do the paperwork, just found something more "fun" to do like match a potential buyer with "the right house." She tried to "get organized" but despite all her efforts couldn't (e.g., reading books on the subject, making "to do" lists, writing reminders, using a small tape recorder to record reminders, and purchasing an electronic PDA [which, incidentally, she never started using because of its extensive set-up requirements, e.g., reading the instructional manual, entering all the initial data, and "whatever else was involved"]). She further explained, "It's not that I am lazy; in fact, I am always on the go." Then, she added that her boyfriend likes to tease her that she is "like that bunny in the battery commercial."

She has a pattern of not being able to maintain employment longer than 3 or 4 months maximum, and she was fired from her previous positions for the same or similar reasons as this incident. She admits that this has affected her self-esteem, but not her outlook on life. She feels life is worth living and is optimistic about the future despite her unemployed status and difficulty with her parents. She denies feeling depressed, sad, or "blue" and states that she has never had any problems with depression. She is not experiencing any changes in her appetite, weight, or sleep and has never experienced difficulties in these areas. She denies feeling anxious or worried. She continues to do things that she previously enjoyed and still enjoys them. She denies hallucinations, delusions, headaches, myalgias, arthralgias, nausea, vomiting, abdominal pain, changes in her bowel habits or stool appearance, or any physical complaints.

She is not taking any prescription or over-the-counter medications, vitamins, supplements, or herbal preparations. She has no medical problems. She has never been hospitalized nor had surgery. She is not allergic to any medications. Her last menstrual period was 3 weeks ago and normal. She uses condoms regularly for contraception. Her family history is negative.

1. Based on this information, which of the following are essential questions to ask Ms. Iverson and why?

    A. Has she ever experienced episodes of being unusually euphoric, being hyperactive, needing less sleep, having racing thoughts, having increases in goal-directed behavior, starting multiple projects and finishing none, or going on extensive shopping sprees that she could not afford?

    B. Does she make impulsive decisions, take impromptu trips, purchase items "on a whim," or interrupt while others are talking?

    C. Is she a "fidgeter"?

    D. What types of grades did she get in school, was she ever "held back," did she ever get into trouble, or was she ever tested for or diagnosed with "hyperactivity"?

    E. Before starting school, could she sit and finish a game or view an entire TV show without having to "get up," was she able to wait her turn at play, did she often interrupt others, or did she have the urge to get up and move around a lot?

Patient Responses

She denies having episodes of being unusually euphoric, being hyperactive, having a decreased need for sleep, having racing thoughts, having increases in goal-directed behavior, starting multiple projects and finishing none, or going on extensive shopping sprees that she couldn't afford. She admits to being impulsive when making important (or any) decisions, taking impromptu trips, purchasing items "on a whim," interrupting while others are talking, and being a "fidgeter."

She was an average student who made mostly C's with an occasional B or D. She was "held back" in kindergarten because "they didn't think I was ready for first grade." She was also held back in second and third grades because "I was not smart enough." She often got into trouble for not staying in her seat, not waiting to take a turn, blurting out responses to questions, not "listening," not "paying attention," not being able to locate her homework, not being able to find "stuff" when she needed it, not "following directions," and making careless errors.

She cannot remember what she was like before she went to school; however, she remembers having difficulty being able to sit still through an entire TV show or finishing a board game while she was in grade school.

2. Based on this information, which of the following components of a physical examination are essential to conduct on Ms. Iverson and why?

    A. Ear examination
    B. Eye examination
    C. Heart examination
    D. Abdominal examination
    E. Skin examination

Physical Examination Findings

Ms. Iverson is 5'7" tall and weighs 135 lb (BMI = 21). Other vital signs are BP, 114/64 mm Hg; pulse, 84 BPM and regular; respirations, 10/min and regular; and oral temperature, 98.5°F.

Ms. Iverson's ear canals are normal in color and without deformity, edema, or abnormal discharge, bilaterally. Her tympanic membranes are normal in color, noninjected, and freely mobile. Her eyes are normal in appearance. Her pupils are equal and round, and they react to light and accommodation. Her funduscopic examination is normal.

Her heart is normal in rate and rhythm and without any murmurs, gallops, or rubs.

Her abdominal examination is normal.

Her skin is normal in color, nonedematous, and without any lesions.

3. Based on this information, which of the following diagnostic studies are essential to perform on Ms. Iverson and why?

    A. Complete blood count with differential (CBC w/diff)
    B. Thyroid panel (TSH, FT_4, and T_3 by RIA)
    C. Computed tomomgraphy (CT) scan of the brain, with and without contrast
    D. Brown Attention-Deficit Disorder Scale for Adults
    E. Scott Adult Attention-Deficit/Hyperactivity versus Bipolar Disorder Scale

Diagnostic Test Results

Ms. Iverson's CBC w/diff, thyroid panel, and CT of the brain were all within normal limits. Her Brown Attention-Deficit Disorder Scale for Adults was positive. Her Scott Adult Attention-Deficit/Hyperactivity vs Bipolar Disorder Scale results are pending.

4. Based on this information, which one of the following is Ms. Iverson's most likely diagnosis and why?

    A. Major depressive disorder
    B. Bipolar I disorder
    C. Bipolar II disorder
    D. Attention-deficit/hyperactivity disorder, not otherwise specified
    E. Conduct disorder

5. Based on this diagnosis, which of the following are appropriate components of a treatment plan for Ms. Iverson and why?

    A. Atomoxetine 40 mg once in the morning; after 3 days, increase to one in the morning and one midafternoon
    B. Cognitive behavioral therapy

C. Lamotrigine 25 mg/day for 2 weeks, then increase to 50 mg/day

D. Lithium carbonate 300 mg twice a day

E. Check lithium level in 1 week

CASE 10-6

Ivan Jackson

Ivan is a 17-year-old African American male who was involved in a multiple car collision approximately 1 hour ago. He was riding restrained in the middle position of the middle seat of a large SUV when the driver apparently lost control, went into the oncoming lane, and struck a small car head-on. The speed of each vehicle was estimated to be approximately 70 miles per hour. All three individuals in the small car as well as the driver of the SUV were pronounced dead at the scene. The passenger in the front seat of the SUV was taken from the scene via helicopter to the closest trauma center for bilateral compound femur fractures, abdominal injuries, and a head injury. The only other passenger was riding restrained in the passenger-side position of the third-row seat. He appeared "shaken but okay" at the scene; however, he was also transported for evaluation.

According to the emergency medical technician (EMT) who accompanied the patient, Ivan was conscious when they arrived on the scene, buckled in his seat, and mumbling incomprehensible "nonsense." Within a few seconds he appeared more alert but was slurring his speech. He vomited once, claimed he was uninjured, and initially refused transportation to the hospital for evaluation. He confided to the EMT that he drank "a couple of beers" earlier in the evening and was concerned his parents would discover his underage alcohol consumption if he went to the emergency department (ED). The quick-thinking EMT, who was concerned about Ivan not being properly evaluated, advised him that the news cameras were already on the scene filming, so his parents would definitely become cognizant of his drinking if he remained on the scene because they could view his behavior on television. Ivan then agreed to be transported to the ED.

Ivan denies any injuries; however, he states he has a headache from the "stress" of the evening's events. It is generalized in location and feels like a tight band around his head. He rates it as a 4 out of a 10 on the pain scale. He has had similar headaches previously when he was under "stress." They occur approximately once per month and are alleviated with acetaminophen. He denies nausea, vomiting (including at the scene), photophobia, visual abnormalities, difficulty with speech, problems with swallowing, paresthesias, direct head injury, loss of consciousness, vertigo, lightheadedness, presyncope, syncope, chest pain/pressure, shortness of breath, abdominal pain, limb or joint pain, or other symptoms except for a mild phonophobia. He doesn't think that he has any problems using his extremities. However, he is uncertain because he is still strapped to the backboard with a cervical collar awaiting the results of his lateral cervical spine films.

He denies any medical (including psychiatric and substance abuse) problems, hospitalizations, or surgeries. He is not taking any prescription or over-the-counter medications, vitamins, supplements, or herbal preparations. He is not allergic to any medicine. He is up to date on his immunizations, including a tetanus "booster" 2 years ago. He denies smoking cigarettes and illicit drug use. He claims he only drinks "socially." His family history is negative.

His cervical spine radiographs are negative; thus, the restraints, backboard, and cervical collar are removed and he is permitted to sit.

1. Based on this information, which of the following questions are essential to ask Ivan and why?

A. What is his definition of drinking "socially"?

B. Does he currently require greater quantities of alcohol to reach or maintain the same level of euphoria than he previously did? If yes, is this a repetitive pattern?

C. Has alcohol caused him any problems at home, at school, at work, in relationships, or with the law?

D. Has he ever had withdrawal symptoms (e.g., tremors, agitation, headaches, seizures, disorientation, or hallucinations) after not drinking for a couple of days?

E. How intoxicated was the driver of the vehicle?

Patient Responses

He only drinks beer but averages 12 to 18 cans (12 oz.) over a 3- to 4-hour time frame when he drinks. He consumes this amount of beer every Friday, Saturday, and Sunday evening with his friends and has been doing so for approximately 1 year. He does not require any more alcohol than in the past to achieve and/or maintain the same level of euphoria.

He has been suspended from school twice for drinking on campus. Both occasions were on Monday mornings when he required an "eye opener." Now, if he wakes up "hung over" on Monday, he stays home from school (which he estimates occurs two to three times per month). He does not have a job. His parents have been "on his case" about his drinking and school absenteeism. His girlfriend left him several times because of his drinking. The final time he supposedly made a pass at a waitress in a bar while they were out drinking with his friends; however, he claims not to remember the incident. He also admits to "not remembering" other things that allegedly occurred while he has been drinking. He has successfully reduced his alcohol consumption by half on multiple occasions in the past to please others. He, his parents, and some of his friends (including his ex-girlfriend) feel he needs to cut back on his drinking. He has never experienced withdrawal symptoms.

He claims the driver was not drinking before the accident.

2. Based on this information, which of the following components of a physical examination are essential to conduct on Ivan and why?

A. Ear and nose examination

B. Heart and lung examination

C. Abdominal examination

D. Musculoskeletal survey

E. Neurologic examination, including orientation

Physical Examination Findings

Ivan is 5'9" tall and weighs 150 lb (BMI = 22.2). Other vital signs are BP, 130/68 mm Hg; pulse, 86 BPM and regular; respiratory rate, 12/min and regular; and oral temperature, 98.8°F.

His ear canals are normal in color, nonedematous, and without any abnormal discharge, fluid, or blood. His tympanic membranes are intact, nonerythematous, fully mobile, and without any other evidence of middle ear effusion or blood. His nasal mucosa is normal and his nares are without abnormal fluid.

His heart is regular in rate and rhythm. There are no murmurs, gallops, or rubs. The apical impulse is nondisplaced and without a thrill. The lungs are clear to auscultation. His rib cage does not reveal any deformities, abrasions, lacerations, contusions, or tenderness.

His abdomen reveals bowel sounds that are normoactive and equal in all four quadrants. He does not have any ascites, masses, organomegaly, or tenderness. His renal arteries and aorta are without bruits. His aorta is normal size with an abnormal pulsation. His abdominal wall is free of abrasions, lacerations, or contusions.

His shoulders, elbows, wrists, hands, hips, knees, ankles, and feet have equal, full range of motion (ROM) bilaterally. They are nontender and without abrasions, lacerations, or contusions. The long bones of his arm and legs are nontender to palpate and lack abrasions, lacerations, and contusions. His cervical, thoracic, and lumbar spines exhibit full ROM as well as no tenderness, abrasions, lacerations, or contusions. His carotid, brachial, radial, ulnar, femoral, popliteal, posterior tibia, and dorsalis pedis pulses are normal and equal bilaterally.

He is oriented to person, place, and time. Appearance and palpation of his skull reveal no deformities or tenderness. His head, including his face, does not reveal any abrasions, lacerations, or contusions. His cranial nerves are intact except he is still talking with somewhat "slurred" speech; however, it is not as significant as it was during his initial presentation. He cannot perform finger-to-nose, finger-to-finger, rapid alternating movements or Romberg test with eyes open or closed. His gait is normal and he can heel and toe walk; however, he cannot perform tandem walking or walking in a circle without taking extra numbers of large steps. His neck, hands, arms, legs, and feet appear to have normal and equal strength and sensation, bilaterally. His biceps, triceps, brachioradialis, knee, and ankle reflexes are normal and equal bilaterally. His plantar reflexes are normal bilaterally.

3. Based on this information, which of the following diagnostic studies are essential to perform on Ivan and why?

    A. Blood alcohol level (BAL) and toxicology screen
    B. Urinalysis
    C. Computed tomography (CT) of the head, without contrast
    D. Hepatic panel
    E. Complete blood count with differential (CBC w/diff)

Diagnostic Test Results

Ivan's BAL was 150 mg/dl (normal: none), or 0.15% (< 0.05% not under the influence, 0.05% to 0.1% impaired > 0.10% intoxicated). His toxicology screen was positive for alcohol only.

His urinalysis did not reveal any microscopic hematuria or other abnormalities.

His brain CT was normal with and without contrast.

His hepatic panel revealed an alanine aminotransferase (ALT) of 42 units/L (normal: 4–36), an aspartate aminotransferase (AST) of 88 units/L (normal 12–18 years old: 10–40), an alkaline phosphatase (ALP) of 130 units/L (normal 16–21 years old: 30–200), a total bilirubin of 0.9 mg/dl (normal adolescent and adult: 0.3–1.0), a direct (conjugated) bilirubin of 0.1 mg/dl (normal adolescent and adult: 0.1–0.3), an indirect (unconjugated) bilirubin of 0.8 mg/dl (normal adult: 0.2–0.8), a γ-glutamyl (GGT) of 145 units/L (normal adolescent and adult male: 8–38), a total protein of 6.6 g/dl (normal adolescent and adult: 6.4–8.3), an albumin of 3.5 g/dl (normal: 3.5–5), and a prothrombin time (PT) of 11.5 (normal: 11–12.5).

His CBC w/diff revealed an RBC count of $4.9 \times 10^6/\mu l$ (normal males: 4.7–6.1) with an MCV of 102 μm^3 (normal adult: 80–95), an MCH of 35 pg (normal adult: 27–31), an MCHC of 34.4 g/dl (normal adult: 32–36), and an RDW of 12.5% (normal adult: 11–14.5). His WBC count was 9500/mm³ (normal adolescent and adult: 5,000–10,000) with 63% neutrophils (normal: 55–70), 38% lymphocytes (normal: 20–40), 5% monocytes (normal: 2–8), 3% eosinophils (normal: 1–4), and 1% basophils (normal: 0.5–1). His Hgb was 17.2 g/dl (normal male: 14–18) and his HCT was 50% (normal male: 42–52). His platelet (thrombocyte) count was 125,000/mm³ (normal adolescent and adult: 150,000–400,000) and his MPV was 7.9 fl (normal: 7.4–10.4). His smear was consistent with this and revealed no other cellular abnormalities.

4. Based on this information, in addition to being involved in a motor vehicle accident without any serious injuries, which one of the following is Ivan's most likely diagnosis and why?

    A. Alcohol intoxication and abuse
    B. Alcohol intoxication and dependence
    C. Secondary alcoholism
    D. Acute alcoholic hepatitis
    E. Alcohol intoxication and acute alcoholic hepatitis

5. Based on this diagnosis, which of the following are appropriate components of a treatment plan for Ivan and why?

    A. Advise Ivan that he has a major abuse problem with alcohol and it appears to be affecting his liver; that he needs to totally abstain from consuming alcohol of any type and have his LFTs rechecked in 1 month; and that if they are still elevated, he will require further evaluation
    B. Psychological and addiction counseling with Alcoholics' Anonymous meetings to assist in becoming and staying sober
    C. Hospitalize immediately
    D. Advise him to avoid old hangouts, friends, etc., to maintain sobriety
    E. Start disulfiram immediately

CASE 10-7
Jessica Kennedy

Mrs. Kennedy is an 82-year-old white female accompanied by her daughter who supplied the chief complaint of "she seems confused." Her daughter is uncertain of the exact onset of her mother's confusion; however, she knows it started within the last 2 weeks. Her daughter defines her mother's confusion as not being able to sustain a conversation, losing her "train of thought," "rambling" about an unrelated topic, and responding to a question with the answer to the previously asked question. According to her daughter, Mrs. Kennedy's symptoms appeared to be much worse last night than they are today. Furthermore, her daughter is also concerned because she arrived at her mother's home at 10:00 a.m. this morning and discovered her in bed asleep. Her daughter states that she is unaware of her mother ever sleeping past 7:00 a.m.

Mrs. Kennedy denies having any problems with confusion or memory. However, she does admit to being unable to fall asleep until 3 or 4 a.m. for the past week; therefore, she has been sleeping later. Otherwise, her only complaint is "some heartburn" last week that she attributed to her arthritis medication. She began taking cimetidine which completely alleviated her symptoms. She has not had any episodes of hematochezia, dark or "tarry"-appearing stools, diarrhea, constipation, or vomiting.

She has not experienced any recent or remote head injury, headache, loss of consciousness, seizures, tremors, problems with gait, dysphagia, vertigo, dizziness, lightheadedness, presyncope, syncope, palpitations, chest pain/pressure, dyspnea, edema, wheezing, cough, fever, fatigue, rhinorrhea, nasal congestion, sore throat, otalgia, dysuria, urinary urgency, urinary frequency, bladder or bowel incontinence, anxiety, depression, mood changes, appetite alterations, weight changes, decreased energy, decreased activity level, anhedonia, hallucinations, delusions, or thoughts of death.

Her only known medical problem is bilateral knee osteoarthritis, which is well controlled with celecoxib. She has never had surgery. Her only hospitalizations were for childbirth. Her medications consist of celecoxib 200 mg once a day for 6 months and cimetidine 100 mg twice a day for approximately 1 week. She denies taking any other over-the-counter or prescription medications, vitamins, supplements, or herbal preparations. She is not allergic to any medications. She has regular health maintenance check-ups with appropriate patient education and diagnostic studies. She is currently up to date on all age-appropriate immunizations. She has never smoked and does not drink alcohol. Her family history is noncontributory.

1. Based on this information, which of the following questions are essential to ask Mrs. Kennedy and/or her daughter and why?

    A. Is she experiencing any aphasia, agnosia, or apraxia?
    B. Does she have any problems with planning activities, developing her schedule for the day, or initiating either?
    C. Is she easily distracted by "irrelevant stimuli"?
    D. Is she experiencing any misperceptions, illusions, or hallucinations?
    E. When did she last change her hearing aid batteries?

Patient Responses

Neither Mrs. Kennedy nor her daughter has noticed Mrs. Kennedy experiencing aphasia, agnosia, apraxia, or difficulty in executive functioning. Mrs. Kennedy has noticed that she does appear to be distracted by noises that previously did not bother her. In fact, she suspects that her difficulty in falling asleep is because the ticking of her alarm clock is now very apparent to her. She denies having any hallucinations or illusions; however, she has noticed a couple of "incorrect assumptions" regarding sounds during the last couple of nights. For example,

she was awakened by the wind blowing a branch against her bedroom window (as it has done for several years now); however, when she first heard it she feared it was someone breaking into her second-story window.

She does not wear a hearing aid; therefore, she could not change its batteries.

2. Based on this information, which of the following components of a physical examination are essential to conduct on Mrs. Kennedy and why?

    A. Thyroid palpation
    B. Heart and lung examination
    C. Abdominal examination
    D. Evaluate for pedal edema
    E. Neurologic examination with mini-mental status examination

Physical Examination Findings

Mrs. Kennedy is 5'2" tall and weighs 125 lb (BMI = 22.8). Other vital signs are BP, 122/62 mm Hg; pulse, 82 BPM and regular; respiratory rate, 12/min and regular; and oral temperature, 98.2°F. She appears slightly "drowsy." Her affect, dress, and hygiene are appropriate.

Her heart is regular in rate and rhythm. There are no murmurs, gallops, or rubs. The apical impulse is nondisplaced and without a thrill. Her lungs are clear to auscultation. Her carotid, brachial, radial, ulnar, femoral, popliteal, posterior tibial, and dorsalis pedis pulses are normal and equal bilaterally. She has normal capillary refill and no pedal edema.

Her abdomen reveals bowel sounds that are normoactive and equal in all four quadrants. She does not have any masses, organomegaly, or tenderness. Her renal arteries are without bruits. Her aorta is normal size and without abnormal pulsation or bruit.

Her mini-mental status examination reveals a score of 22 (abnormalities include the following: orientation—she is unable to provide name of the facility, what floor she is on, the date, or the day of the week; attention and calculations—she can only perform two of required five correct on serial 7's; and recall—she can only recall two of the three objects). She can pantomime the ability to use a comb, toothbrush, and knife.

Her cranial nerves are intact. She can perform finger-to-nose, finger-to-finger, rapid alternating movements, and a Romberg test with eyes open and closed; however, she does latter slowly and cautiously. Her gait is normal. She can perform heel walking, toe walking, and tandem walking. She can walk in a circle but does it slowly and deliberately with a few extra steps. Her face, neck, shoulders, arms, hands, hips, legs, and feet appear to have normal and equal strength and sensation, bilaterally. Her biceps, triceps, brachioradialis, knee, and ankle reflexes are normal and equal bilaterally. Her plantar reflexes are normal and equal bilaterally.

3. Based on this information, which of the following diagnostic studies are essential to perform on Mrs. Kennedy and why?

    A. Magnetic resonance imaging (MRI) of the brain, with and without contrast
    B. Serum electrolytes and glucose
    C. Complete blood count with differential (CBC w/diff)

D. Blood urea nitrogen (BUN) and creatinine

E. Urinalysis (U/A)

F. Liver function testing (LFT)

Diagnostic Test Results

Mrs. Kennedy's MRI was normal with and without contrast. It did not reveal any areas of ischemia, atrophy, hemorrhage, ventricle defects, or white or gray matter changes.

Her electrolytes revealed a carbon dioxide (CO_2) of 26 mEq/L (normal: 23–30), a chloride (Cl) of 99 mEq/L (normal: 98–106), a potassium (K) of 3.9 mEq/L (normal adult: 3.5–5.0), and a sodium (Na) of 140 mEq/L (normal adult: 136–145). Her fasting serum glucose was 84 mg/dl (normal: 70–126).

Her CBC revealed an RBC count of $5.4 \times 10^6/\mu l$ (normal females: 4.2–6.4) with an MCV of 82 μm^3 (normal adult: 80–95), an MCH of 26 pg (normal adult: 27–31), an MCHC of 32 g/dl (normal adult: 32–36), and an RDW of 12.5% (normal adult: 11–14.5). Her WBC count was 7500/mm³ (normal adult: 5,000–10,000) with 62% neutrophils (normal: 55–70), 24% lymphocytes (normal: 20–40), 2% monocytes (normal: 2–8), 1% eosinophils (normal: 1–4), and 1% basophils (normal: 0.5–1). Her Hgb was 14.2 g/dl (normal female: 12–16; elderly patients can be slightly lower) and her HCT was 45% (normal female: 42–52; elderly patients may be slightly decreased). Her platelet (thrombocyte) count was 225,000/mm³ (normal adult: 150,000–400,000) and her MPV was 8.9 fl (normal: 7.4–10.4). Her smear was consistent with this and revealed no other cellular abnormalities.

Her creatinine was 0.5 mg/dl (normal adult female: 0.5–1.1; may be decreased in elderly patients with decreased muscle mass) and her BUN was 18 mg/dl (normal adult: 10–20; may be slightly elevated in elderly patients).

Her urine was pale yellow in color, clear, and with normal odor. Her pH was 6.5 (normal: 4.6–8.0) and her specific gravity was 1.010 (normal: 1.005–1.030; values can be slightly decreased in elderly patients). Her dipstick was negative for glucose, protein, nitrites, ketones, and leukocyte esterase (normal: negative). Her microscopic examination revealed 2 WBCs per low-power field (normal: 0–4), no WBC casts (normal: 0), 1 RBC per low-power field (normal: ≤ 2), no RBC casts (normal: 0), no crystals per low-power field (normal: no crystals of any type), and no casts (normal: no casts of any type).

Her hepatic panel revealed an ALT of 22 units/L (normal: 4–36), an AST of 28 units/L (normal adult: 0–35), an ALP of 60 units/L (normal adult: 30–120), a total bilirubin of 0.6 mg/dl (normal adult: 0.3–1.0), a direct (conjugated) bilirubin of 0.2 mg/dl (normal adult: 0.1–0.3), an indirect (unconjugated) bilirubin of 0.4 mg/dl (normal adult: 0.2–0.8), a GGT of 24 units/L (normal adult male: 8–38), a total protein of 6.9 g/dl (normal adult: 6.4–8.3), an albumin of 4.5 g/dl (normal: 3.5–5), and a PT of 12.25 (normal: 11–12.5).

4. Based on this information, which one of the following is the most likely diagnosis for Mrs. Kennedy and why?

A. Amnesic disorder

B. Vascular dementia

C. Substance-induced delirium

D. Delirium caused by a general medical condition

E. Dementia caused by Parkinson disease

5. Based on this diagnosis, which of the following are appropriate components of a treatment plan for Mrs. Kennedy and why?

A. Haloperidol 0.5 mg at bedtime, increase to 1 mg if necessary

B. Quetiapine 25 mg once a day, may increase to twice a day if necessary

C. Discontinue celecoxib 200 mg and start acetaminophen

D. Discontinue cimetidine

E. Quadriceps strengthening

CASE 10-8

Kashia Lamont

Ms. Lamont is a 24-year-old African American female who was brought in by emergency medical services (EMS) after her younger sister called 911 because she was "real bad sick and I don't know what was wrong with her." When the EMTs arrived they found a drowsy, confused, agitated, shaking young female with an obvious nystagmus in the lateral gaze. She informed them she "just had the flu" and apologized for her sister bothering them. About that time, her sister emerged from the bathroom with an empty vial of lithium time-release 1200 mg (#30) dated 2 days ago and a bottle of divalproex 300 mg (#90) dated 2 weeks ago with 41 pills in it. They confronted Ms. Lamont and she reluctantly admitted to taking all the lithium last night before going to bed in a suicide attempt. She has today and tomorrow off from her waitressing job and "couldn't stand the thought of being alone that long." She had not anticipated her sister skipping school thinking they could "just hang out" because she knew Ms. Lamont was off.

At the ED, Ms. Lamont denies ever feeling suicidal except for last night. She states that "all the sudden I realized how alone I am and what a mess my life is." She defines a "mess," as she is tired of "making mistakes," does not appear to be responding to the lithium, is only getting 1 or 2 hours of sleep per night, can't stop her brain from "racing" with nonsensical thoughts, is unable to focus on customers' orders and consequently gets them incorrect, is close to getting "fired" from work, can't resist "picking up" customers who are complete strangers and having intercourse with them, and has her credit cards "maxed" out from when she goes on impulsive shopping sprees for "stuff I don't even need." She states that she is "really trying to get better" by taking her medications, keeping her appointments with her counselor, and seeing her psychiatrist as scheduled; however, "nothing works out, no matter how hard I try." She is extremely hopeless about the future; however, she denies any plans to harm herself again.

She has not participated in social activities for at least 1 month because "nothing's fun anymore." She is anorexic and has lost 10 lb in the past month. She provides a history of depression but currently denies feeling depressed. She denies hallucinations and delusions.

She is nauseated but has not vomited. She has not had any diarrhea, abdominal pain, polyuria, polydipsia, palpitations, chest pain/pressure, shortness of breath, weakness, seizures, lightheadedness, vertigo, presyncope, or syncope.

Her only known medical problem is bipolar I disorder. She has never had any surgery. Her only hospitalization occurred when her bipolar illness was first diagnosed approximately 1 year ago. Her family history is positive for bipolar illness (maternal aunt); however, there is no family history of a suicide attempt or successful suicide. Her only medications are lithium time-release 1200 mg at bedtime (current dose for approximately 2 months) and divalproex 300 mg three times a day (added approximately 2 weeks ago because she was unresponsive to lithium and her lithium dose was "as high as it could be"). She is not taking any other prescription or over-the-counter medications, vitamins, supplements, or herbal preparations. She denies drinking alcohol, using illicit substances, or smoking cigarettes. She is sexually active and uses condoms for contraception and "protection." She is unable to estimate her number of lifetime partners. Her LMP was 1 week ago and normal.

1. Based on this information, which of the following questions are essential to ask Ms. Lamont and why?

    A. Approximately how many of the lithium pills did she take and when?

    B. How does she feel about taking the overdose? How does she think others will respond?

    C. Why was she hospitalized when her bipolar illness was initially diagnosed?

    D. What is her religious affiliation and does she attend church regularly?

    E. Does she have a gun in her home?

Patient Responses

Ms. Lamont admits to taking 30 lithium (extended release, 1200 mg) pills at approximately 1 a.m. (8 hours ago). She currently feels embarrassed and confused about taking the overdose. She thinks her family will be disappointed but concerned; however, she feels her "friends" will be even more distant because they will be certain she is "crazy." She was hospitalized upon diagnosis of her bipolar illness because she was experiencing auditory hallucinations; however they have not recurred since she was released from the hospital.

    She is of Catholic faith, but does not attend church regularly. She does not have any guns in her home.

2. Based on this information, which of the following components of a physical examination are essential to conduct on Ms. Lamont and why?

    A. Hearing assessment

    B. Heart examination

    C. Evaluation of pulses

    D. Abdominal examination

    E. Neurologic examination

Physical Examination Findings

Ms. Lamont is 5'5" tall and weighs 130 lb (BMI = 21.6). Other vital signs are BP, 110/62 mm Hg lying and 112/62 mm Hg standing; pulse, 96 BPM and regular lying and 106 BPM and regular standing; respiratory rate, 12/min and regular; oral temperature, 97.3°F.

She is alert, oriented to person and place but not completely to time (she cannot supply the correct date, even after multiple attempts), mildly to moderately drowsy appearing, and dressed in pajamas. Her hearing is grossly normal.

Her heart is regular in rate and rhythm. There are no murmurs, gallops, or rubs. The apical impulse is nondisplaced and without a thrill. Her lungs are clear to auscultation.

Her carotid, renal, and aortic arteries are without bruits. The aorta is normal size and has no abnormal pulsation. Her carotid, brachial, radial, ulnar, femoral, popliteal, posterior tibial, and dorsalis pedis pulses are normal and equal bilaterally.

Her abdomen reveals normoactive bowel sounds that are equal in all four quadrants. She does not have any masses, organomegaly, or tenderness.

Ms. Lamont's mini-mental status score is 28; her only errors include not being able to state the date in orientation or to repeat the sentence in language on the first try. However, at times it took her longer than expected to come up with a response or she self-corrected herself, especially in the areas of registration, attention, calculations, and recall.

Her cranial nerves are grossly intact except for a bilateral lateral nystagmus. She cannot perform finger-to-nose, finger-to-finger or rapid alternating movements possibly because of her moderate, yet significant, tremor or the mild clonus of her arms, both of which are bilateral and essentially equal. There is no evidence of clonus of her legs. However, her gait is moderately ataxic. Her hands, arms, legs, and feet appear to have slightly decreased but equal strength bilaterally. Facial, neck, and shoulder muscles appear normal in strength. Sensation is intact bilaterally. Her biceps, triceps, brachioradialis, knee, and ankle reflexes are normal and equal bilaterally. Her plantar reflexes are normal and equal bilaterally.

3. Based on this information, which of the following diagnostic studies are essential to perform on Ms. Lamont and why?

    A. Lithium level and serum toxicology

    B. Electrocardiogram (ECG)

    C. Blood urea nitrogen (BUN) and creatinine

    D. Electrolytes

    E. Complete blood count with differential (CBC w/diff)

Diagnostic Test Results

Ms. Lamont's lithium level was 2.5 mEq/L (therapeutic range: 0.8–1.2; toxic > 2.0).

Her ECG revealed normal sinus rhythm without any PR segment or QTc prolongation, ST-segment elevation or depression, or T-wave inversion.

Her electrolytes revealed a carbon dioxide (CO_2) of 24 mEq/L (normal: 23–30), a chloride (Cl) of 122 mEq/L (normal: 98–106), a potassium (K) of 3.3 mEq/L (normal adult: 3.5–5.0), and a sodium (Na) of 137 mEq/L (normal adult: 136–145). Her fasting serum glucose was 76 mg/dl (normal: 70–126).

Her BUN was 28 mg/dl (normal adult: 10–20) and her creatinine was 1.5 mg/dl (normal adult female: 0.5–1.1).

Her CBC revealed an RBC count of 5.1 × 10^6/µl (normal females: 4.2–6.4) with an MCV of 90 µm^3 (normal adult: 80–95), an MCH of 28 pg (normal adult: 27–31), an MCHC of 31 g/dl (normal adult: 32–36), and an RDW of 12.5% (normal adult: 11–14.5). Her WBC count was 9750/mm^3 (normal adult:

5,000–10,000) with 55% neutrophils (normal: 55–70), 40% lymphocytes (normal: 20–40), 2% monocytes (normal: 2–8), 2% eosinophils (normal: 1–4), and 1% basophils (normal: 0.5–1). Her Hgb was 14.4 g/dl (normal female: 12–16) and her HCT was 46% (normal female: 42–52). Her platelet (thrombocyte) count was 275,000/mm³ (normal adult: 150,000–400,000) and her MPV was 8.9 fl (normal: 7.4–10.4). Her smear was consistent with this and revealed no other cellular abnormalities.

4. Based on this information, which one of the following is Ms. Lamont's most likely diagnosis and why?

   A. Unsuccessful suicide attempt with lithium toxicity and dehydration, completely or partially exacerbated by divalproex
   B. Aborted suicide attempt with lithium toxicity and dehydration, completely or partially exacerbated by divalproex
   C. Suicidal ideation with lithium toxicity and dehydration, completely or partially exacerbated by divalproex
   D. Deliberate self-harm with lithium toxicity and dehydration, completely or partially exacerbated by divalproex
   E. Deliberate self-harm with lithium, unrelated to divalproex

5. Based on this diagnosis, which of the following are appropriate components of a treatment plan for Ms. Lamont and why?

   A. Hospitalize on telemetry; ensure secure airway; frequent monitoring of mental status, vital signs, electrolytes, and lithium levels; intake and urine output; suicidal precautions; psychiatric consultation; and notify regular counselor and psychiatrist (if not doing consult)
   B. 0.5% normal saline solution (NSS) adjusted to maintain good hydration
   C. Gastric lavage (GL) with large-bore nasogastric (NG) tube and warmed NSS
   D. Hemodialysis
   E. Antiemetic agent and rectal tube, followed by gastrointestinal (GI) decontamination with polyethylene glycol solution at 2L/hr via NG tube until rectal tube is clear

CASE 10-9
Lydia Mortising

Mrs. Mortising is a 45-year-old Asian American female who presents with the chief complaint of "the flu." She woke up at about 4 a.m. today with an oral temperature of 103.9°F, chills, diaphoresis, nausea, vomiting, diarrhea, muscle pains, and objective vertigo. Since awakening, she has experienced a minimum of 10 bowel movements and vomited twice. She is also complaining of intermittent tachycardia and palpitations that do not appear to be related to exertion or standing. She is not experiencing any abdominal pain, hematochezia, steatorrhea, dark "tarry"-appearing stools, rhinorrhea, sneezing, nasal congestion, sore throat, otalgia, cough, wheezing, dyspnea, chest pain/pressure, syncope, presyncope, or headache. She was not constipated before the onset of her symptoms, nor did she consume any food or beverages not eaten by someone else in the household. No one else in the household is ill.

Her known medical problems consist of major depressive disorder and a fractured right index finger (diagnosed yesterday). She denies ever being hospitalized or having any surgeries. Her medications consist of fluoxetine 60 mg once a day for 6 months (which is controlling her depression) and tramadol 100 mg every 4 to 6 hours as needed for pain (which is controlling her finger pain). She has taken three does of the tramadol since it was prescribed (two yesterday and one earlier today). She is not taking any other prescription or over-the-counter medications, vitamins, supplements, or herbal preparations. She is not allergic to any medications. Her health maintenance is up to date including appropriate diagnostic testing and immunizations. Her last menses was 3 weeks ago and normal. Her family history is positive for depression (older sister).

1. Based on this information, which of the following questions are essential to ask Mrs. Mortising and why?

   A. Has she had any confusion, problems staying focused, or memory difficulties?
   B. Has she been unusually aggravated, agitated, or irritated since her symptoms began?
   C. Is she having photophobia, pain with moving her eyes, or burning of her eyes?
   D. Where are her muscle pains located and how would she describe them?
   E. Has she tried an antipyretic for her fever? If yes, what medication and what was the response?

Patient Responses

Mrs. Mortising has noticed feeling "fuzzy" in the head and having problems staying "focused" on tasks this morning; however, she attributes it to the tramadol for her finger fracture. She has been very irritable since she got up this morning and has already apologized to her daughter, granddaughter, and husband regarding it.

She is not experiencing photophobia, pain with moving her eyes, or burning of her eyes. Her muscle pains are located in her upper legs and neck only. She describes this sensation as "jerking," similar to "what your body does right before you fall asleep; it is greatest in her thighs." She has not tried an antipyretic.

2. Based on this information, which of the following components of a physical examination are essential to conduct on Mrs. Mortising and why?

   A. General appearance
   B. Heart and lung examination
   C. Abdominal examination
   D. Pelvic examination
   E. Neurologic examination, including a mini-mental status examination (MMSE)

Physical Examination Findings

Mrs. Mortising is 5'1" tall and weighs 105 lb (BMI = 19.8). Her remaining vital signs are BP, 148/88 mm Hg lying and 154/88 mm Hg standing; pulse, 112 BPM and regular lying and 120 BPM and regular standing; respiratory rate, 12/min and regular; and oral temperature, 104.2°F.

She is a very small woman who obviously doesn't feel well (but is not toxic appearing). She is appropriately and neatly dressed with good hygiene but obviously diaphoretic. Furthermore, she has a generalized tremor and myoclonus of her neck (neck appears to straighten out and then her head jerks to the right) and upper legs (primarily hip flexion) despite trying to sit still. The jerking motions are irregular in interval and intensity; but they are asymmetric.

Her heart is mildly tachycardic (rate 108 BPM and regular) but of regular rhythm and with no murmurs, gallops, or rubs. Her apical impulse is nondisplaced and without a thrill. Her lungs are clear to auscultation.

Her abdominal examination reveals slightly hyperactive but equal bowel sounds in all four quadrants. There is no tenderness, masses, or organomegaly. Her pelvic examination is unremarkable.

She is alert and oriented to person, place, and time. Her MMSE score is 26. (She is able to register all three items; however, it takes three tries for it to occur. In attention and concentration, she cannot perform serial 7's beyond two numbers [similar defects are seen when she attempts to count backward from 20 by 3's or spell the word "world," backward] and she can not remember one of the items in recall.)

Her cranial nerves are intact except for equal mydriasis of her pupils and a lateral nystagmus bilaterally. She cannot perform finger-to-nose, finger-to-finger, or rapid alternating movements bilaterally. However, this is most likely a result of an obvious moderate-intensity tremor of her hands and arms, which is essentially equal bilaterally and worse at rest. Even with her foot held in flexion, there is no evidence of ankle clonus bilaterally. She does not have an asterixis of her wrist. Her gait is ataxic. Her hands, arms, legs, and feet appear to have slightly decreased but equal strength. Facial, neck, and shoulder muscles appear normal in strength. Sensation is intact bilaterally. Her biceps, triceps, brachioradialis, knee, and ankle reflexes are normal and equal bilaterally. Her plantar reflexes are normal. Myoclonus is present as previously described. Kernig and Brudzinski signs are negative.

3. Based on this information, which of the following diagnostic studies are essential to perform on Mrs. Mortising and why?

    A. Serum fluoxetine level
    B. Blood urea nitrogen (BUN) and creatinine

    C. Creatine phosphokinase (CPK)
    D. Electrocardiogram (ECG)
    E. Electrolytes and magnesium level

Diagnostic Test Results

Her fluoxetine level was within therapeutic range.

Her BUN was 12 mg/dl (normal adult: 10–20) and her creatinine was 0.6 mg/dl (normal adult female: 0.5–1.1). Her CPK was 50 units/L (normal adult female: 30–135) and her magnesium level was 1.5 mEq/L (normal adult: 1.3–2.1).

Her ECG revealed a sinus tachycardia with a rate of 112 BPM; there was no PR or QTc interval prolongation, ST-segment elevations or depressions, T-wave changes, P-wave abnormalities, or QRS abnormalities.

Her electrolytes revealed a carbon dioxide (CO_2) of 24 mEq/L (normal: 23–30), a chloride (Cl) of 96 mEq/L (normal: 98–106), a potassium (K) of 3.4 mEq/L (normal adult: 3.5–5.0), and a sodium (Na) of 137 mEq/L (normal adult: 136–145). Her magnesium level was 1.8 mEq/L (normal adult: 1.3–2.1).

4. Based on this information, which one of the following is Mrs. Mortising's most likely diagnosis and why?

    A. Moderate serotonin syndrome
    B. Severe serotonin syndrome
    C. Neuroleptic malignant syndrome
    D. Uremia
    E. Alzheimer disease

5. Based on this diagnosis, which of the following are appropriate components of a treatment plan for Mrs. Mortising and why?

    A. Telemetry monitoring in the ED with frequent vital sign assessment
    B. Discontinue both fluoxetine and tramadol
    C. Cyproheptadine 4 to 8 mg every 2 hours until symptom reversal occurs or a maximum of 32 mg is given
    D. Reduction of body temperature with tepid water spraying and fanning of unclothed patient
    E. Admit to intensive care unit; IV with 0.5 NSS; diazepam for muscle cramping; intubation and mechanic ventilation if necessary

CASES IN PSYCHIATRIC ILLNESSES

RESPONSES AND DISCUSSION

CASE 10-1

Debbie Ellison

1. History

A. How does she define fatigue and what is its pattern over a typical day?   ESSENTIAL

Fatigue is not an exclusive symptom of any particular condition. In fact, it can be present in diseases affecting virtually every body system. Therefore, a clear understanding of exactly what the patient is describing with this complaint is essential in developing an accurate differential diagnosis list. For example, if the patient's definition of fatigue is a weakness or postexertional exhaustion, possible causes can include poor physical conditioning, a musculoskeletal condition, a neurologic problem, a neuromuscular disease, or an anemia. Fatigue defined as sleepiness can be associated with hypoxemia caused by conditions such as sleep apnea, chronic pulmonary diseases, cardiac abnormalities, insomnia, or narcolepsy. Psychological fatigue is generally described as "no energy," "too tired to do anything," or a lack of motivation or desire.

Furthermore, the pattern of the fatigue over the course of a typical day is significant. Patients with fatigue caused by a physical condition tend to awaken feeling more refreshed (although often not completely) than before they retired the previous evening and their fatigue tends to worsen (or at least remains relatively stable) throughout the day. They also experience postexertional fatigue. By contrast, individuals with fatigue caused by a psychological disorder tend to awaken feeling tired. In some cases, their unrefreshed sleep makes them feel equally, if not more, tired than before they went to bed, regardless of the presence of insomnia. They tend to feel the worst first thing in the morning; however, their fatigue tends to lessen as the day progresses. It is not uncommon for the patient to feel less fatigued following exertion.

B. Has she been experiencing a sore throat, cervical lymphadenopathy, axillary lymphadenopathy, arthralgias, myalgias, or severe postexertional fatigue?   ESSENTIAL

Chronic fatigue syndrome is a condition that must be included in the differential diagnosis list for patients complaining of unremitting fatigue. Unrefreshed sleep, new types of headache, impaired concentration, and memory difficulties are some of the defining criteria for the condition. The others include sore throat, cervical or axillary lymphadenopathy, arthralgias, myalgias, and severe postexertional fatigue.

C. Has she experienced a recent, unintentional weight change? ESSENTIAL

Significant weight changes (defined as at least 5% of the patient's previous body weight in 1 month's time) can occur in a wide array of illnesses that are associated with fatigue. For example, fatigue and weight loss can be seen in new-onset diabetes mellitus, hyperthyroidism, cancer, and depression, to name a few. Conditions associated with fatigue and weight gain include hypothyroidism, heart failure, and atypical depression.

D. Has she ever experienced any episodes of increased activity associated with a decreased need for sleep, grandiosity, enhanced self-esteem, euphoria, behavior unusual or outrageous for her, beginning many projects but not finishing any, or racing thoughts?   ESSENTIAL

When a depressive mood disorder is included in the patient's differential diagnosis list, it is imperative to determine whether the symptoms represent a strict unilateral depression or the depressive symptoms found in bipolar I, bipolar II, or cyclothymia. Therefore, the patient must be questioned regarding the potential presence of any symptoms that could represent manic or hypomanic episodes. This is essential not only to establish the correct diagnosis (and subsequent treatment plan) but also to prevent inducing a manic (or hypomanic) episode in a patient with a bipolar illness by initiating antidepressant therapy.

E. Has she considered suicide If yes, does she have a plan? ESSENTIAL

The major cause of death in a patient with a major depressive episode (both unilateral and bilateral) is suicide. Therefore, if a depressive disorder is strongly being considered as the patient's diagnosis, it is important to inquire about the presence of thoughts of suicide. Questioning patients regarding suicidal ideations or plans does not "put the thought in their head." However, it permits this very frightening symptom to be validated as one that is not uncommon in patients with major depressive illnesses.

Furthermore, asking about a plan (and what it is if the patient has one) permits a gross determination of the patient's potential for acting upon such thoughts. If it is a fleeting thought and the patient does not have a history of impulsive behavior, the likelihood is much less than if it the thoughts are persistent and intrusive. The establishment of a plan, especially if the means exist to carry it out, is associated with the greatest risk. Other risk factors for successful suicide include the presence of past attempts (especially if nearly lethal), a positive family history of attempted (and especially completed) suicides, male gender, older age, and the presence of a coexisting chronic medical condition. All of this information must be considered in the development of the treatment plan to ensure that the patient remains "safe."

2. Physical Examination

A. Overall appearance and affect   ESSENTIAL

The patient's general appearance and affect are critical in evaluating a patient with a suspected mood disorder. Areas that need to be considered include personal hygiene, appropriateness of clothing (e.g., fit, coordination, style, consistent with age, suitable for weather, and condition [e.g., wrinkled, dirty, or new]), affect (e.g., flat, normal, or euphoric), mannerisms (e.g., none, flamboyant, or inappropriate), and nonverbal communication (e.g., is body language consistent with spoken words). These observations provide objective data to correlate for consistency with the subjective data gathered from the patient. For example, poor hygiene, unkempt appearance, and dirty clothes can be signs of a more serious depression indicating that the patient "just doesn't care" or is "too tired to make the effort," of a psychotic illness where the disorganization of the thought process can often adversely affect the patient's hygiene and appearance, or of a chronic medical illness when the patient is just too ill or tired to "care" or "bother" about appearance.

B. Palpation of thyroid   ESSENTIAL

Because both hypo- and hyper-thyroidism can be responsible for fatigue, it would be appropriate to palpate Mrs. Ellison's thyroid for abnormalities. However, a normal thyroid gland does not exclude these conditions.

A strong suspicion should be confirmed by serologic testing. More likely than not, Mrs. Ellison's thyroid function was evaluated serologically in the battery of tests performed by her regular healthcare provider (HCP). Therefore, obtaining copies of those records would be important.

C. Heart examination   ESSENTIAL

Although unlikely to occur without any other symptoms, it is possible that a cardiac rhythm abnormality and/or a valvular problem could be causing Mrs. Ellison's fatigue.

D. Abdominal examination   ESSENTIAL

Although gastrointestinal conditions (e.g., carcinoma, inflammatory bowel diseases, and malabsorption syndromes) can cause chronic fatigue, it is highly unlikely for one of these to be causing Mrs. Ellison's complaint in the absence of gastrointestinal symptoms. Still, an abdominal examination needs to be performed to identify other potential intra-abdominal causes. For example, leukemias, myeloproliferative disorders, hemoglobinopathies, other hematologic conditions, and infectious mononucleosis can present as fatigue with splenomegaly. Fatigue and hepatomegaly can be seen in cirrhosis, hepatitis, and liver failure. Ascites can be seen with some intra-abdominal malignancies. Adrenal tumors can produce fatigue and occasionally are palpable if they are large and/or the patient is thin.

E. Pelvic examination   NONESSENTIAL

A pelvic examination is not going to provide any useful information regarding Mrs. Ellison's symptoms unless they are related to a pregnancy in at least the second trimester (which is extremely unlikely because of her normal menstrual period 2 weeks ago, her utilization of an extremely effective method of contraception, and her palpable intrauterine device [IUD] string following her last menstrual period) or a carcinoma (which, with the exception of ovarian carcinoma, is highly unlikely to be of sufficient size to be palpable without other symptoms being present). A weight loss, not a gain, would increase the suspicion that a malignancy was responsible for her symptoms.

3. Diagnostic Testing

A. Urinary human chorionic gonadotropin (HCG) NONESSENTIAL

For the reasons stated previously, it is highly unlikely that Mrs. Ellison is pregnant. Even if she were pregnant (unless she is experiencing normal periods during her pregnancy), sufficient time has not lapsed since her last menstrual period (LMP) for detectable levels of HCG to occur.

B. Thyroid function studies   NONESSENTIAL

Even though hypo- and hyper-thyroidism can cause some of the symptoms Mrs. Ellison is experiencing and some HCPs routinely perform thyroid function testing to rule-out hypothyroidism in patients with what appears to be a major depressive disorder, thyroid testing is still not indicated for Mrs. Ellison because it is highly likely they were performed in the recent battery of tests reported to her as normal. Thus, obtaining these results would be a more appropriate option.

Furthermore, depression is not a diagnosis of exclusion. Therefore, if it appear to be the patient's most likely diagnosis, it is appropriate to initiate antidepressive therapy and only check for thyroid dysfunction at a later time if the patient's symptoms fail to respond to appropriate doses and adequate durations 2 drugs.

C. Complete blood count with differential (CBC w/diff) NONESSENTIAL

Even though many anemias, leukemias, hemoglobinopathies, myeloproliferative disorders, and other hematologic abnormalities can produce fatigue (and in some cases headaches), testing for them at this time is not necessary. Based on Mrs. Ellison's history and physical examination findings, there is a much greater likelihood that she has a mood disorder compared to one of these conditions. Because mood disorders are not considered diagnoses of exclusion (except perhaps when very atypical features are present), Mrs. Ellison does not require a CBC w/diff at this time. Furthermore, in all likelihood, this test was performed as part of the diagnostic evaluation conducted by her regular HCP. Therefore, unless there is some urgency for the test results, reviewing her previously conducted test results is a much more appropriate, and cost-effective, option than repeating the test.

D. Liver function tests (LFTs)   NONESSENTIAL

Hepatic abnormalities (e.g., hepatitis, cirrhosis, hepatocellular dysfunction, and primary or secondary malignancies) can produce fatigue. However, in the absence of any other symptoms to suggest one of these is her most likely diagnosis, performing LFTs is unlikely to produce any useful clinical information and does not need to be performed.

A "shotgun" approach to diagnostic testing is inappropriate, expensive, and unlikely to establish a diagnosis. The purpose of diagnostic testing is to confirm the working diagnosis made on the basis of the history and physical examination or to follow a chronic condition.

E. Erythrocyte sedimentation rate (ESR)   NONESSENTIAL

An ESR is a nonspecific measurement of generalized inflammation, and without a specific inflammatory condition being suspect, it is not going to provide any useful clinical information.

4. Diagnosis

A. Chronic fatigue syndrome   INCORRECT

According to the criteria established by the Centers for Disease Control and Prevention (CDC), chronic fatigue syndrome is defined as severe fatigue that has been present for a minimum of 6 months without a definite diagnosis PLUS the presence of four or more of the following eight criteria: unrefreshed sleep, new type of headaches, impaired concentration or memory, sore throat, cervical and/or axillary lymphadenopathy, arthralgias, myalgias, and severe postexertional fatigue. Because Mrs. Ellison's illness appears to have a cause, has only been present for 4 to 5 weeks, and is only associated with three of the other defining criteria, chronic fatigue syndrome is not her most likely diagnosis.

B. Major depressive episode   CORRECT

The American Psychiatric Association's *Diagnostic and Statistical Manual of Mental Disorders*, 4th edition, text revision (DSM-IV-TR) provides criteria for the diagnosis of virtually every psychological disorder and its subtypes. According to the DSM-IV-TR, in order to establish the diagnosis of major depressive episode, the patient has to have a minimum of five of the following nine symptoms present on more days than not during a consecutive 14-day period, PLUS one of them must be either a depressed mood or anhedonia: (1) a subjectively or objectively evident depressed mood (or an irritable mood, especially in kids or adolescents); (2) subjective or objective reports of significant decreased interest and/or pleasure in almost all previously enjoyable activities; (3) a significant change in appetite or an unintentional weight change of less than or greater than 5% over a period of 1 month; (4) the presence of insomnia or hypersomnia; (5) objective psychomotor slowing or agitation; (6) fatigue and/or decreased energy; (7) feelings of

worthlessness or inappropriate guilt; (8) objectively or subjectively reported problems with thinking processes, concentration, or indecisiveness; and (9) recurrent thoughts (not fear) of death, recurrent suicidal ideations with or without a plan, or a suicide attempt. Additionally, these symptoms cannot be accounted for by another condition (e.g., medical, psychiatric, substance abuse, or bereavement), must interfere with the patient's level of functioning (or be distressing), and must represent a significant change from the patient's previous state.

Although Mrs. Ellison denies a depressed mood, she does have irritability (which is considered by some to be any atypical symptom that is equivalent to depressed mood) as well as anhedonia. Additionally, she has weight gain, hypersomnia, objective psychomotor retardation, fatigue, and problems with thinking. Thus, she meets seven out of the nine of the established diagnostic criteria with anhedonia. Therefore, her most likely diagnosis is a major depressive episode.

C. Dysthymic disorder   INCORRECT

Dysthymia is a chronic, low-grade depressive disorder, in which the patient experiences symptoms on the majority of days in the previous 2-year time frame (and never goes for longer than 60 days without experiencing the symptoms). It consists of a minimum of two of the following six criteria: (1) objectively or subjectively defined depressed or "blue" mood, (2) fatigue (or low energy), (3) difficulty making decisions or concentrating, (4) low self-esteem, (5) feelings of hopelessness, and (6) insomnia or hypersomnia. Also, as with any condition diagnosed by the established DSM-IV-TR criteria, her symptoms cannot be better accounted for by another psychological, substance abuse, or medical disorder. It can be ruled out as Mrs. Ellison's most likely diagnosis because her symptoms have only been present for 4 to 5 weeks plus they interfere with her functional status (whereas those in a dysthymic disorder do not) and are better accounted for by another condition (major depressive episode).

D. Adverse effect from hormones in contraceptive method INCORRECT

Although hormonal contraceptives have been known to produce mood symptoms, this can be ruled out as Mrs. Ellison's most likely diagnosis because her copper-containing IUD does not contain hormones.

E. Somatization disorder   INCORRECT

Somatization disorder can be eliminated as her most likely diagnosis because she lacks a long-standing history of multiple physical complaints in which a definite diagnosis could not be established. Furthermore, she does not meet the DSM-IV-TR diagnostic criteria regarding the number of physical ailments required over the course of the illness to establish the diagnosis (i.e., four pain syndromes in four separate areas of the body; two gastrointestinal symptoms; one sexual symptom; and one pseudoneurologic symptom besides pain).

5. Treatment Plan

A. Lamotrigine 25 mg/day for 2 weeks, then 50 mg/day for 2 weeks, then 100 mg daily if required   INCORRECT

Lamotrigine is approved by the US Food and Drug Administration (FDA) for bipolar illness maintenance and seizure disorders. However, it has been successfully used as an adjunct to unresponsive unipolar depression. Nevertheless, it is not a good first-line drug to treat Mrs. Ellison's major depressive episode.

B. Citalopram 20 mg once a day for a minimum of 1 week, then increase to 40 mg daily if required   CORRECT

A meta-analysis conducted by the American Psychiatric Association (APA) concluded that all the antidepressant medications are essentially equally effective in treating major depressive episode when compared to placebo. However, recent data from Italy indicate that this might not be the case. The authors of this most recent meta-analysis reviewed 117 randomized, controlled trials that were conducted between 1991 and 2007 that involved what they termed to be "new generation" antidepressants—bupropion, citalopram, duloxetine, escitalopram, fluoxetine, fluvoxamine, milnacipran, mirtazapine, paroxetine, reboxetine, sertraline, and venlafaxine. The total number of enrolled patients exceeded 25,000. Their evaluation of the data determined that mirtazapine, escitalopram, venlafaxine, and sertraline were more efficacious than duloxetine, fluoxetine, fluvoxamine, paroxetine, and reboxetine. Furthermore, they determined that escitalopram, sertraline, citalopram, and bupropion were better tolerated than two of the most efficacious agents, mirtazapine and venlafaxine. In conclusion, the authors felt that escitalopram and sertraline are the better first-line agents in the treatment of major depressive disorder.

Regardless, there is not one drug that works well on everyone. Therefore, many other factors go into the decision of choosing the initial medication, if one is going to be utilized, for the treatment of major depressive episode. They include severity of depression, risk of overdosing with the medication, coexisting medical conditions, other medications, drug allergies, the presence of alcohol or substance abuse disorders, adverse effects of the medications, cost of the medications, the patient's ability to follow dietary restrictions, and the patient's previous experiences with antidepressants.

For first-line drug treatment for major depressive episode, the APA recommends a selective serotonin reuptake inhibitor (SSRI); the serotonin-norepinephrine reuptake inhibitor (SNRI), venlafaxine; the tricyclic antidepressants (TCAs), desipramine and nortriptyline; and the aminoketone, bupropion, for patients with mild to moderate depression. For severe depression, they suggest the usage of the monoamine oxidase inhibitors (MAOIs) or nondrug treatment with electroconvulsive therapy (ECT). However, because of potential adverse effects and the possibility of a successful suicide attempt with TCAs, and the dietary restrictions and drug interactions with MAOIs, they state that most psychiatrists go with an SSRI as first-line treatment. However, in their latest update in 2005, they caution against using the new agents because of lack of long-term data regarding their usage.

Regardless, it is accepted practice to utilize either an SSRI or an SNRI as first-line drug therapy for a major depressive episode because they tend to have the best tolerability, safety, and adverse effect profiles. Thus, citalopram, an SSRI, is an appropriate first-line choice for Mrs. Ellison.

C. Psychotherapy   CORRECT

Because of its effectiveness the APA recommends psychotherapy alone for the treatment of a mild to moderate major depressive disorder and in combination with a medication (and possibly ECT) in severe cases. Meta-analysis revealed that, with the exception of traditional psychotherapy, all forms of psychotherapy can be as effective as cognitive behavioral therapy (CBT) in treating patients with a major depressive episode. They recommend attempting to match the type of therapy with the patient's symptoms, goals, and preferences.

Although there are mixed results regarding the use of CBT alone in a severe major depressive episode, a recent meta-analysis revealed that it is equally effective as medication in this setting as well. Furthermore, the combination of CBT and an antidepressant appears to be more effective than either treatment modality alone, especially in elderly patients.

D. Tranylcypromine 10 mg three times a day for 2 weeks, then increase by 10 mg/day every 2 to 3 weeks as necessary to a total dose of 60 mg daily   INCORRECT

Tranylcypromine is an oral MAOI. Therefore, extensive food (predominately tyramine) and medication restrictions are associated with its usage. Furthermore, it is associated with significant adverse events. For these reasons, even though it is recommended as a possible treatment for first-line depression, the APA agrees that MAOIs should probably be reserved for treatment-refractory depression. Additionally, if an MAOI is determined to be appropriate for a patient, it is probably best to go with the transdermal formulation, selegiline. It appears to be better tolerated and the dietary restrictions are not as extensive.

E. Patient education on her disease, medication, potential of suicidal ideations, time before symptom relief, and what to do if adverse effects or concerns develop before follow-up appointment   CORRECT

As with any condition, the patient should be provided with patient education on all of these aspects. Information on her disease process should include an explanation of neurotransmitter deficiencies appearing to be its cause. Anecdotal information indicates that this is associated with better acceptance of the diagnosis and compliance with the medication.

Although the black-box warning issued by the FDA on suicidality and antidepressant medication usage relates to children and adolescents, it is sound medical judgment to make all patients aware of this potential. Whether this represents an actual adverse drug effect, the natural course of the depressive illness (i.e., the medication alleviates the patient's symptoms sufficiently to make him or her capable of attempting suicide; and it is seen more often in children and adolescents because of their limited coping mechanisms and increased impulsivity), or discouragement because the medication is not working as rapidly as the patient desires is unknown. What is known is that suicide is the most common cause of death in patients suffering from major depressive illness. Furthermore, suicidal ideations, and especially plan formulation, are very frightening for patients, especially if this is their first episode and they lack intimate knowledge of the illness. Acknowledging that these feelings could occur, that they are "normal," and that help is available to prevent action on them is beneficial for the patient, regardless of his or her age.

Furthermore, patients should be advised on other common potential adverse effects, what action to take if they occur, and the risks of suddenly discontinuing medication. They should also be advised of the name of the medication being prescribed and its mechanism of action. Furthermore, they should be informed that it generally takes a couple of weeks before much symptom improvement is noticeable and can take as long as 6 to 8 weeks to achieve maximum improvement from the medication.

She should also be encouraged to keep all follow-up appointments and informed of their significance. The frequency of follow-up is determined by a number of factors, including the severity of the symptoms, the likelihood of self-harm, prior suicidal attempts and their severity, the possibility of the patient's noncompliance, concern that medication might be taken incorrectly, the need for encouragement to continue treatment, and history of problems with medications. Therefore, the scheduling for the follow-up appointment can range from the next day to 1 month later.

Epidemiologic and Other Data

The onset of major depressive episode generally occurs during adolescence to the mid-20s. However, it can occur any time from childhood to old age. The incidence of a major depressive disorder is greatest in individuals who are older than the age of 50 years and in postpartum women. In the United States, women are affected at twice the rate as men.

Depression has a recurrence rate of approximately 66%. The lifetime incidence of having a major mood disorder in the United States is estimated to be between 5 and 25%. This extensive span may be explained by the gender, cultural, and ethnic differences in the presentation of this illness; the high index of suspicion by the HCP; and variations in the rate of screening. It is unusual for a major depressive disorder to occur without a positive family history.

CASE 10-2

Ellen Franklin

1. History

A. What, if anything, provokes her crying episodes? ESSENTIAL

In the United States, it is "normal," and in some situations expected, for females to cry upon receiving bad news, being made aware of an extremely sad situation or event, or becoming "upset." Women with fatigue, regardless of the cause, tend to have a lower threshold for crying; however, it is still provoked. With depression, this threshold becomes even lower to the point where minor annoyances and oversensitive perceptions can induce tearful episodes or they can occur without any precipitating event. Therefore, it is important to determine what, if anything, is responsible for her crying episodes in an attempt to determine this "threshold."

B. Is she experiencing a change in appetite; psychomotor slowing or agitation; feelings of worthlessness or inappropriate guilt; problems with thinking processes, concentration, memory, or indecisiveness; or recurrent thoughts of death or suicide?   ESSENTIAL

If a patient is unresponsive to a second therapeutic trial (adequate dose for adequate length) of an antidepressant, the diagnosis must be reevaluated. A diagnosis of a major depressive episode is suspect for Mrs. Franklin because she denies

both feeling depressed and experiencing anhedonia. One or the other of these symptoms is required in order to establish the diagnosis. Nevertheless, it is important to determine how many of the other symptoms are present. If a significant number is present, then it is important to revisit her responses, providing alternative words and examples to determine whether signs and symptoms of a depressed mood and/or anhedonia can be elicited. Currently, it appears that Mrs. Franklin only has one on the defining list (for the complete list, please see Case 10-1); thus, other diagnostic possibilities must be explored.

C. Has she experienced any recent bowel changes, abdominal pain, fever, chills, night sweats, myalgias, arthralgias, or lymphadenopathy?   ESSENTIAL

As stated previously, because Mrs. Franklin has taken maximum doses of two different antidepressants without an improvement, her diagnosis needs to be reevaluated. Basically, her primary complaints are fatigue, mild weight increase despite attempting to lose weight, crying episodes involving major and minor incidences, and being irritable with others. The latter two symptoms could be attributed to her fatigue alone. Furthermore, the weight gain is minimal and could easily be a result of the time of day she was weighed, what she was wearing, when and how much she had last consumed, constipation, premenstrual bloating, unnoticed decreased activity from the fatigue, or the underlying condition responsible for the fatigue. Hence, it would be reasonable to assume that the fatigue is her primary problem.

Unfortunately, virtually every body system has conditions that can cause fatigue. Some examples of fatigue and the associated bowel changes can include the following: diarrhea in inflammatory bowel disease (IBD), irritable bowel syndrome (IBS), or hyperthyroidism; constipation with hypothyroidism, IBS, and multiple neurologic conditions; dark tarry stools and/or frank bleeding from IBD, colon cancer, bleeding ulcers, esophageal varices, or anemia; greasy, malodorous stools with malabsorption syndromes; and any condition that could result in an obstruction in the pancreaticobiliary tree. Therefore, inquiring about any recent bowel changes and what type would be beneficial in determining a list of potential differential diagnoses for Mrs. Franklin.

The presence of abdominal pain (and its description, including location) is important not only to narrow the list of potential differential diagnoses; (e.g. the pain from hepatitis and cholelithiasis is typically found in the right upper quadrant; the pain from IBD as well as diverticulitis is most commonly identified in the left lower quadrant, and epigastric discomfort could indicate peptic ulcer disease) but also to indicate the possibility of intra-abdominal pathology that does not originate in the gastrointestinal (GI) tract (e.g., nephrolithiasis, endometriosis, ovarian cyst, chronic pelvic inflammatory disease).

Bowel changes are also important because certain gastrointestinal and nongastrointestinal conditions could be suggested by such. For example, constipation can be seen in irritable bowel syndrome-constipation predominant, colonic masses, hypothyroidism, multiple sclerosis medication adverse effects, and depression. Whereas, diarrhea is more common in inflammatory bowel diseases, malabsorption syndromes, hyperthyroidism, chronic alcohol ingestion, and medication adverse effects. The timing of symptoms is also important (e.g., nocturnal GI symptoms are more commonly related to a physiologic process than a psychological one).

The other symptoms asked about in this question are also important in evaluating other potential causes of fatigue. For example, lymphadenopathy could be present with chronic fatigue syndrome, infectious processes, and cancer. Night sweats could indicate a carcinoma or premature menopause. Arthralgias could indicate the presence of an inflammatory arthropathy. Myalgias could represent fibromyalgia or myositis.

D. Has she experienced any polydipsia, polyuria, or changes in her skin, lips, hair, or fingernails?   ESSENTIAL

Endocrinopathies, hematologic abnormalities, autoimmune diseases, and hepatic diseases can also produce fatigue. Thus, it is essential to ask some screening questions to potentially identify some of the more common of these conditions. For example, the presence of polydipsia and polyuria is suspicious for diabetes mellitus, whereas changes in the texture, thickness, and color of her skin, lips, hair, or fingernails or the appearance of a rash or skin lesion can be seen with a wide variety of conditions; however, these changes are often indicative of a limited number of conditions, thus narrowing the list of potential diagnoses. For example, a malar rash on the face can be associated with lupus or pregnancy; dry skin, lips, hair, and brittle fingernails can be seen with hypothyroidism and anemia; glossitis can be associated with severe anemia or cirrhosis; pitting of the nails and a silvery plaquelike rash are seen in psoriatic arthritis; palmar erythema can be seen in cirrhosis; spider nevi are present with hepatic conditions, especially cirrhosis; excessive facial hair can be present in a variety of hormonal conditions; spooning of nails and cyanosis can be seen with hypoxia secondary to chronic pulmonary diseases; and Raynaud phenomenon can be seen in a wide array of autoimmune, neurologic, and circulatory conditions (or it can be idiopathic and unrelated).

E. Has she experienced any recent changes in her heart rate or breathing?   ESSENTIAL

Fatigue associated with changes in the cardiac rate, respiratory rate, and respiratory effort can be indicative of several diseases including arrhythmias (e.g., sinus tachycardia, paroxysmal supraventricular tachycardia [PSVT], and atrial fibrillation [AF]), valvular heart problems, anemias, asthma, chronic obstructive pulmonary disease (COPD), primary or secondary pulmonary hypertension, and hyper- and hypothyroidism, as well as poor physical conditioning.

2. Physical Examination

A. Ear, nose, and throat (ENT) examination   NONESSENTIAL

Because Mrs. Franklin was not ill before her fatigue began and has not experienced any symptoms suspicious for an upper respiratory infection (or allergic process), an ENT examination is not needed.

B. Gross external eye examination   ESSENTIAL

Abnormalities visualized during inspection of the external structures of the eyes can indicate the presence of systemic conditions that can produce fatigue (e.g., scleral icterus is seen in severe hepatic disease [e.g., hepatitis and cirrhosis],

conjunctival pallor is found in anemia, and Graves ophthalmopathy is seen in Graves disease).

C. Skin examination   ESSENTIAL

A skin examination is important to evaluate for changes in color, texture, and temperature as well as for lesions or rashes to correlate with the aforementioned conditions and/or make new conditions suspect.

D. Heart examination   ESSENTIAL

A heart examination can confirm the presence of an arrhythmia, valvular disease, or cardiomegaly that can be associated with fatigue caused by some of the aforementioned conditions.

E. Pelvic examination   NONESSENTIAL

A pelvic examination is not necessary to perform on Mrs. Franklin because in view of her symptoms, it is unlikely to yield any useful clinical information. Obviously, with her late menstrual period, there is a concern regarding the potential for pregnancy; however, a pelvic examination is unlikely to provide any insight into the possibility of this condition because the typical signs of pregnancy would not be evident based on the date of her last menstrual period. These include Chadwick sign (a bluish discoloration of the cervix and sometimes the vagina that appears at approximately 7 weeks' gestation), Hegar sign (softening and easy compressibility of the uterine isthmus that occurs at approximately 8 weeks' gestation), and uterine enlargement (generally not significant until at least 12 weeks' gestation). Furthermore, clinical findings suggestive of a pregnancy would be more likely to be confirmed by pregnancy testing than a pelvic examination given the date of her last menses.

3. Diagnostic Testing

A. Urinary human chorionic gonadotropin (HCG)   ESSENTIAL

Although pregnancy is not the only condition associated with fatigue and a late menstrual period, it is essential to rule it out because Mrs. Franklin's stated contraceptive method is partner dependent and she is taking sertraline, which is classified as a pregnancy category C drug. This classification means that animal studies have identified fetal risk(s) and/or there are no adequate human studies performed on the medication to determine its effect on the fetus. Hence, the benefits to the mother may outweigh the risks to the developing fetus. (For more information regarding the current FDA pregnancy categories, please see Case 2-7.)

Nevertheless, the decision to stop her sertraline, change to a medication with a more favorable rating, or continue her current medication if she were pregnant must be made on an individualized basis after conducting a comprehensive review of various factors including her history, physical examination, current level of global functioning (compared to level before medication was initiated), current symptoms, the particular medication and dose, length of therapy, prior episodes of depression and their severity, and prior suicide attempts and their severity.

If a medication must be used during pregnancy, preference would be for a category A drug because these medications failed to demonstrate any fetal risks during human trials in the first trimester of pregnancy and/or have not revealed evidence of any adverse effects attributed to the medication if used during the second or third trimesters. Unfortunately, none of the antidepressants currently on the market in the U.S. fall into this category.

Pregnancy category B drugs are those in which animal studies did not show any harm to the fetus; however, there are no adequate human studies to collaborate these findings in human use. Alternatively, a pregnancy category B rating can mean that fetal harm was identified in an animal study but human studies failed to identify the same problem. Unfortunately, none of the antidepressants have this rating either. The majority of the commonly used antidepressants fall into category C, with the exception of the SSRI paroxetine, which is a category D. Category D drugs have been proven to cause adverse effects in the human fetus; still, the benefits of taking the medication may outweigh the risks.

Pregnancy category X drugs are those in which either human or animal studies have confirmed a definite association between the medication and serious fetal abnormality or toxicity. It is the only category where the risks definitely exceed any benefit that could be derived.

B. Total thyroxine (T_4) to screen for thyroid disease NONESSENTIAL

Although total T_4 is a effective test to screen newborns for hypothyroidism, screening for (or attempting to diagnose) hypothyroidism with a total T_4 in adults is inadequate. It will fail to identify those patients with subclinical hypothyroidism and secondary hypothyroidism. Furthermore, there are several medical conditions (including pregnancy) and drugs (including sertraline) that can cause false-positive or false-negative results of this test because it measures both the bound and unbound T_4, whereas the free thyroxine (FT_4) measures only the unbound, or metabolically active, T_4. Thus, an FT_4 is probably a more accurate measurement of actual thyroid function. However, an FT_4 will still, at minimum, require a thyroid-stimulating hormone (TSH) to adequately screen for thyroid abnormalities.

C. Erythrocyte sedimentation rate (ESR)   NONESSENTIAL

The ESR is a gross indicator of the presence of inflammation anywhere in the body; it is not specific for any particular disorder. Therefore, its primary use is to confirm and quantitate the suspicion of an inflammatory process and to follow disease progression. Nevertheless, without a specific disease process identified on the patient's differential diagnosis list, it is not going to provide much clinically useful information and does not need to be performed.

D. Complete blood count with differential (CBC w/diff) ESSENTIAL

A CBC w/diff is important to evaluate for not only the presence of anemia but also other hematologic disorders that could be associated with fatigue (e.g., leukemias, myeloproliferative disorders, and hemoglobinopathies). It can also provide support for an infectious diagnosis; however, this is unlikely because of the long-standing nature of her symptoms.

E. Short-form version of Yesavage Depression Scale NONESSENTIAL

The short-form version of the Yesavage Depression Scale is a screening, not diagnostic, tool to evaluate for depression in the elderly. It consists of 15 questions regarding mood, satisfaction with life, outlook for the future, and presence of anhedonia.

4. Diagnosis

A. Major depressive episode   INCORRECT

As stated previously, Mrs. Franklin does not meet either of the two major criteria for major depressive episode—depressed mood or anhedonia—and at least one must be present to establish this diagnosis. Furthermore, she is not experiencing any impairment in her ability to function vocationally, socially, or familiarly (which is another criterion that must be met to make the diagnosis of a major depressive disorder). Therefore, major depressive episode is not her most likely diagnosis.

B. Treatment-resistant depression   INCORRECT

As stated previously, Mrs. Franklin does not meet the established diagnostic criteria for a major depressive episode which is the condition referred to by the term, depression. Therefore, treatment-resistant depression cannot be her most likely diagnosis.

C. Pregnancy   INCORRECT

Pregnancy has essentially been eliminated as Mrs. Franklin's most likely diagnosis because she has a negative urinary HCG test, which is highly sensitive.

D. Hypothyroidism   INCORRECT

Although hypothyroidism is a likely potential diagnosis for Mrs. Franklin, it cannot be accurately diagnosed (or eliminated) based on the information obtained thus far, because appropriate thyroid studies have not been performed. Thus, it cannot represent her most likely diagnosis.

However, this potential diagnosis serves as an excellent example of the importance of ensuring that the diagnostic tests ordered are going to provide the desired information. As stated previously, total T_4 levels can be inaccurate because of a variety of conditions that are capable of altering the amount of thyroid-binding globulins (TBGs) present. Generally, an increase in TBGs results in a false elevation of the total T_4. Although it is not clear as to the exact role TBGs play in all cases of factitiously decreased total T_4 levels, there are certainly some conditions capable of inducing this phenomenon, including the antidepressant, sertraline.

Thus, even if erroneously selected, the total T_4, the slightly suppressed total T_4 obtained from that test offers no useful information to support or refute the diagnosis of hypothyroidism. As previously stated, Mrs. Franklin is still going to require a TSH and ideally an FT_4 (although many providers will order a thyroid panel consisting of a TSH, FT_4, and triiodothyronine by radioimmunoassay [T_3 by RIA] because in most labs the panel is actually less expensive than ordering the other two tests individually, plus the T_3 offers additional support regarding the accuracy of the results) to properly assess her thyroid function. In general, obtaining an inappropriate diagnostic test is only going to result in higher healthcare costs, patient stress over having an abnormal test result, patient confusion regarding which test result is correct and why, and increased provider time to explain the actual interpretation of the initial test as well as the need for additional testing.

E. Iron deficiency anemia   CORRECT

From the information thus far obtained and the choices provided, iron deficiency anemia is Mrs. Franklin's most likely diagnosis based on her symptoms, clinical picture, and laboratory testing revealing a normocytic, normochromic anemia. The initial laboratory finding in iron deficiency is actually low iron stores. Once an anemia develops, it is a normocytic, normochromic anemia. Only after it has been present for a while does it become a microcytic, hypochromic condition.

5. Treatment Plan

A. Stop sertraline   CORRECT

Stopping the sertraline is indicated because it appears Mrs. Franklin never met the criteria for a major depressive disorder; therefore, she should not be on an antidepressant. Still, from her current dosage and the fact she has been on it for longer than 6 weeks, her sertraline dose should be tapered before ceasing to hopefully prevent (or at least minimize) any potential withdrawal symptoms (headache, nausea, vertigo, weakness, anxiety, insomnia, decreased concentration, paresthesias, rhinorrhea, and nasal congestion).

Nevertheless, because this assessment is being made with retrospective data provided by the patient, it is essential to observe her for the development of depression symptoms.

B. Start cognitive behavioral therapy (CBT)   INCORRECT

CBT would be indicated if Mrs. Franklin had a major depressive episode. However, current evidence indicates this is not the case.

C. Start duloxetine 20 mg twice a day   INCORRECT

Changing to a different antidepressant in another drug category would be a viable treatment strategy if Mrs. Franklin was experiencing treatment-resistant depression. However, because it appears that she does not meet the APA's criteria for a major depressive episode, it is highly suspected that she has any depressive illness, including treatment-resistant depression. Therefore, she does not require any antidepressant therapy at this time.

D. Start levothyroxine 25 µg once a day   INCORRECT

Levothyroxine is indicated for the treatment of hypothyroidism. It is also utilized off-label, with some degree of success, as an adjunct in treatment-resistant depression. Because Mrs. Franklin does not have evidence of either of these conditions, it is not indicated for her.

E. Check serum iron, serum ferritin, total iron-binding capacity, and transferrin saturation   CORRECT

Checking Mrs. Franklin's serum iron, serum ferritin, total iron-binding capacity, and transferrin saturation is indicated to confirm the diagnosis of iron deficiency anemia.

Epidemiologic and Other Data

The greatest prevalence of iron deficiency anemia in the United States occurs in women of reproductive age generally as a result of heavy menses, pregnancy, childbirth, and nursing. The next most commonly affected group is adolescent females, followed by children between the ages of 1 and 2 years.

CASE 10-3
Freddie Gleason
1. History

A. Where is the rest of the "gang"?   NONESSENTIAL

Although it is unlikely that Mr. Gleason would be offended by this comment at this point in time, hallucinations and delusions are signs of serious conditions and should be afforded the same degree of professionalism as any complaint. It is irresponsible and inappropriate for the HCP to treat the patient with anything other than respect, compassion, and concern. Furthermore, it provides staff with the impression that the HCP doesn't care about the patient and that it is permissible for the staff to treat the patient in a similar, if not worse, manner.

B. Has he recently had any fever, chills, weight changes, fatigue, headaches, arthralgias, myalgias, problems with gait, difficulty with coordination, or visual changes?   ESSENTIAL

Psychotic disorder caused by a general medical condition involves the presence of psychosis symptoms (e.g., hallucinations and delusions) that are not produced or mediated by a psychological cause but are a direct result of the physical condition. This category also includes dementias, delirium, adverse medication effects, and substance-induced psychotic disorder. Some of these general medical conditions can be identified by observing the patient for signs of abnormal movements and/or altered or fluctuating levels of consciousness. For example, choreiform disorders (e.g., Huntington disease or Sydenham chorea) can be identified by their distinctive pattern of movements; interictal, ictal, and postictal psychosis are usually identifiable by the observation of a seizure, the level of consciousness following the seizure, or a gradual improvement of symptoms over a short period of time to a nonpsychotic level of functioning.

However, others are not as easily identifiable and require a high index of suspicion. Hopefully, the patient can answer basic questions to assist in eliminating the majority of these associated conditions so the focus can be placed on the few remaining ones. Alternatively, family members, good friends, and even staff can assist in this process by providing their observations regarding complaints and behavior. A few of these conditions can be made more or less suspect depending on the responses to a few basic screening questions, such as those listed in this question. Possible conditions include subdural hematoma, organic brain syndromes with symptoms besides dementia, meningitis, brain tumors, leukemia, leukodystrophy, multiple sclerosis, autoimmune conditions, or endocrine abnormalities of the thyroid or adrenal glands.

C. Has he experienced any palpitations, dyspnea, weakness, or cold intolerance?   ESSENTIAL

The presence of some of these symptoms suggests an endocrine, metabolic, or hematologic disorder that can produce secondary, nonschizophrenic psychotic symptoms. Examples include hyperthyroidism, hypothyroidism, Cushing syndrome, anemia, and Wilson disease.

D. Has he experienced any changes in sleep, appetite, or mood; feelings of depression; anhedonia; or thoughts of harming himself or others?   ESSENTIAL

Psychosis can result secondarily to severe mood disorders; the most common is psychotic depression. These disorders can be identified not only by directly questioning the patient regarding the presence of these symptoms but also by relying on observations from significant others and staff.

E. If he is a dog, where is his tail?   NONESSENTIAL

Immediate confrontation to any part of the delusional system is not beneficial. Instead of immediately attempting to dismantle delusions, the HCP should work toward establishing a relationship with an appropriate level of rapport so the patient can feel safe and be able to freely discuss any concern without fear of judgment or mockery.

Furthermore, asking this question in this manner at this time could be interpreted as insensitive and rude and lead to the aforementioned problems from such an action.

2. Physical Examination

A. General appearance, affect, and mannerisms   ESSENTIAL

The thoughtful evaluation of general appearance, affect, and mannerisms is just as, if not more, important in evaluating a patient with psychotic symptoms as it is in patients with a mood disorder or medical condition. In addition to the aforementioned information obtainable, clues to previous, older (first-generation or typical) neuroleptic exposure might be indicated by the identification of subtle movement abnormalities suspicious for residual tardive dyskinesia, extrapyramidal symptoms, and/or parkinsonian movements because these neuroleptic-induced adverse effects often never fully resolve. However, these automatisms may also be evident in patients with new-onset schizophrenia. They can include lip licking, tongue smacking, tongue protrusion, mild chewinglike movement of the jaw, grunting, and sniffing.

B. Examination for minor head/facial deformities   ESSENTIAL

Patients with schizophrenia can exhibit minor craniofacial abnormalities that suggest the presence of this congenital condition. These findings include wide-set eyes, close-set eyes, mild deformities of the external ear, and a palate that is markedly arched and high. Additionally, this exam serves as a gross evaluation for potential head trauma, which could indicate the presence of intracranial bleeding and/or edema that could be responsible for Mr. Gleason's symptoms.

C. Preauricular lymph node palpation   NONESSENTIAL

The preauricular lymph nodes are not responsible for drainage from very many structures; they are basically limited to abnormalities of the ipsilateral ear, eye, and lateral aspect of the superficial forehead. Thus, it is highly unlikely that an infectious or malignant process in one of these areas is capable of producing Mr. Gleason's symptoms.

D. Neurologic examination, with mini-mental status examination (MMSE)   ESSENTIAL

A neurologic examination, including a mini-mental status examination (MMSE), is indicated to evaluate for subtle neurologic symptoms that are seen in schizophrenia (e.g., left/right confusion or poor coordination), the differentiation between a dementia and delirium (the first being much more common in primary psychotic conditions but it can also be present in organic brain diseases), clues to other neurologic conditions that

can induce or be associated with psychotic symptoms (e.g., temporal lobe seizures, temporal lobe brain tumor, stroke, multiple sclerosis, peripheral neuropathies caused by leukodystrophy, and tremors or dystonia caused by Wilson disease), and abnormal movements caused by choreiform disorders.

E. Skin/nail examination   ESSENTIAL

A skin and nail examination is indicated to rule out psychotic disorder caused by a general medical condition (e.g., hypothyroidism, anemia, psoriatic arthritis, systemic lupus erythematosus [SLE], Wilson disease, and Cushing syndrome).

3. Diagnostic Testing

A. Computed tomography (CT) of brain without contrast   ESSENTIAL

Although a CT of the brain can detect subtle cortical atrophy of the hippocampus-amygdala and/or posterior superior temporal gyrus, other temporal lobe structural abnormalities, and mild ventricular dilation, which can be seen in schizophrenia, as well as abnormalities that could suggest the presence of a psychotic disorder caused by a general medical condition (e.g., ventricle dilatation suggesting hydrocephalus, mass effect suggesting a brain tumor, areas of ischemia suggesting a cerebrovascular accident, and meningeal inflammation suggesting meningitis), the primary indication for a CT of Mr. Gleason's brain without contrast is to evaluate for the presence of a subdural hematoma or other intracranial hemorrhage. As stated previously, this can produce symptoms similar to Mr. Gleason's. A delay in diagnosis can lead to disastrous consequences; thus, the CT examination should be performed despite minimal other signs and symptoms on his history and physical examination to suggest this possibility.

Interestingly, some evidence exists suggesting that in schizophrenia, the severity of the patient's psychotic symptoms is directly correlated to the degree of temporal cortical atrophy.

B. 8 a.m. and 4 p.m. cortisol levels   NONESSENTIAL

The easiest method to screen for Cushing syndrome is to perform 8 a.m. and 4 p.m. cortisol levels. Because cortisol has a diurnal variation, it tends to be highest between 6 a.m. and 8 a.m. and lowest around midnight. Therefore, a level drawn at 4 p.m., if normal, should be 33 to 66% of the morning value. Although Cushing syndrome is a potential cause for a psychotic disorder caused by a general medical condition, screening for this condition is not indicated in the absence of any other signs and symptoms suggesting it.

C. Thyroid panel with thyroid-stimulating hormone (TSH), free thyroxine (FT$_4$), and triiodothyronine by radioimmunoassay (T$_3$ by RIA)   NONESSENTIAL

Although hypothyroidism and hyperthyroidism (and therefore pituitary and hypothalamic failure and overproduction) can cause a psychotic disorder caused by a general medical condition, these tests do not need to be performed on Mr. Gleason at this time because his history and physical examination failed to identify any signs or symptoms to suggest the presence of these endocrinopathies.

D. Complete blood count with differential (CBC w/diff)   NONESSENTIAL

His most like diagnosis can be made on the basis of history and physical examination. Thus, there are no "routine" tests indicated when a patient presents with psychotic symptoms. However, if there is evidence to suggest the presence of a general medical condition that can produce psychotic disorder, tests directed toward these specific conditions are indicated. Concerns regarding a condition associated with a high incidence of morbidity and mortality also justify the performance of diagnostic studies appropriate to that condition. However, because Mr. Gleason lacks any signs or symptoms to indicate that his symptoms are caused by a significant infectious, inflammatory, or hematologic condition, a CBC w/diff is not indicated at this time.

E. Urinary drug screen   ESSENTIAL

Even though Mr. Gleason denies substance use or abuse, it is still appropriate to screen for this potential cause for his symptoms because this question is not always answered honestly, especially in individuals presenting in the custody of law enforcement. Furthermore, if hospitalization is not indicated and he has a chemical dependency problem, it can go untreated. Furthermore, unmonitored withdrawal from the substance can result in serious medical consequences.

4. Diagnosis

A. Schizophrenia, undifferentiated type   INCORRECT

Although Mr. Gleason exhibits the required minimum of two of the five defining characteristic symptoms for schizophrenia (hallucinations, delusions, disorganized speech, significantly disorganized behavior or catatonia, and negative symptoms [e.g., flat affect, anhedonia, abulia, alogia, absence of thoughts, and loss of function]) as determined by the DSM-IV-TR AND probably a functional impairment (can be either occupational, social, or self-care), the diagnosis cannot be established as Mr. Gleason's most likely diagnosis because it is unknown how long he has been exhibiting symptoms. The DSM-IV-TR diagnostic criteria require that in order to establish the diagnosis of schizophrenia, the patient must be exhibiting these symptoms the majority of the time for a minimum of 1 month and have at least some evidence of the condition for at least 6 months. The exceptions to this time criteria include if the patient is successfully treated within this time frame, the delusions are out of the ordinary, or the hallucinations consist of either a running dialogue between a minimum of two voices or a single voice providing continuous comments regarding the patient's activity and/or ideas.

Furthermore, a schizoaffective or mood disorder, a general medical (or even a substance abuse) disorder, and a pervasive developmental disorder cannot be excluded as the actual cause of his symptoms based on this single brief encounter, which also prevents schizophrenia from being diagnosed at this time. Finally, even though he appears to have some degree of functional difficulty, it is unclear how this compares to his preillness level. Essentially, the functional difficulties must be significantly worse than they were before the onset of this illness in order to establish the diagnosis of schizophrenia.

B. Schizophreniform disorder   INCORRECT

The DSM-IV-TR diagnostic criteria for schizophreniform disorder, as for schizophrenia, require that the symptoms cannot be caused by a medical or substance abuse disorder and that a minimum of two of the aforementioned defining characteristic symptoms must be present almost every day for a minimum of

1 month. However, unlike schizophrenia, the disease does not have to affect social or occupational functioning, but it has to be completely resolved in a maximum of 6 months. Because the length of symptom duration to date, as well as when the illness is anticipated to cease, is unknown, schizophreniform disorder cannot be Mr. Gleason's most likely diagnosis.

C. Schizoaffective disorder   INCORRECT

The DSM-IV-TR diagnostic criteria for schizoaffective disorder require the presence of an underlying major mood disorder (e.g., major depressive episode, bipolar illness, or mixed episode exhibiting depression, mania, or mixed symptoms, respectively), to be present. However, these symptoms must be interrupted by a minimum of a 2-week period during which the patient experiences hallucinations and/or delusions without the mood symptoms. Then, the patient returns to the underlying mood disorder for the duration of the illness. And, like schizophrenia and schizophreniform disorder, a schizoaffective disorder cannot be caused by an underlying substance abuse disorder, medical condition, or medication adverse effects. Thus, schizoaffective disorder can be ruled out as Mr. Gleason's most likely diagnosis because he is unable to provide a history of a previous mood disorder.

D. Delusional disorder   INCORRECT

The DSM-IV-TR diagnostic criteria for delusional disorder require the delusion to be nonbizarre and to not affect function impairment beyond what the delusion itself causes. Additionally, it requires the delusion to be present for a minimum of 1 month. Because it does not appear that Mr. Gleason's symptoms match this description and the length of his illness is unknown, delusional disorder is not his most likely diagnosis.

E. Psychotic disorder, not otherwise specified   CORRECT

Psychotic disorder, not otherwise specified is the only one of the provided diagnoses that does not require a specific time frame for the presence, duration, and/or cessation of the psychotic symptoms. According to the DSM-IV-TR, this diagnosis is utilized in cases where there is inadequate information to make the diagnosis of schizophrenia or one of the other disorders with psychotic features. Thus, from the list provided, this is Mr. Gleason's most likely diagnosis.

If at a later date there is sufficient evidence to establish one of the other disorders associated with psychotic symptoms, his diagnosis can be changed.

5. Treatment Plan

A. Hospitalize on psychiatric service   CORRECT

Hospitalization on psychiatric service is appropriate for Mr. Gleason for observation, his own safety, and medication management because he is experiencing significant hallucinations and delusions.

B. Observe for signs/symptoms/behaviors suggestive of suicidal ideations, especially while his psychosis is resolving   CORRECT

As with depression, the risk of suicide in patients with psychotic symptoms tends to be greatest during the time period when his or her symptoms are beginning to improve. Thus, close observation is mandatory after initiating antipsychotic therapy, especially if there is some response.

Furthermore, it is important to remember that the risk of both suicidal behavior and completed suicides in patients with psychotic illnesses is actually greater in the postpsychotic period than during the psychotic episode itself.

C. Olanzapine 5 mg once a day, increase to 10 mg once a day after 4 days if tolerating   CORRECT

Olanzapine 5 mg once a day, increasing to 10 mg once a day after 4 days, if tolerating, is an appropriate choice for Mr. Gleason's initial neuroleptic therapy. It is classified as an atypical, or second-generation, drug. The atypical neuroleptics tend to be much better tolerated because they possess significantly lower rates of anticholinergic, extrapyramidal, and autonomic side effects when compared to the first-generation, or typical, antipsychotics. Additionally, there is some suggestion that they may be slightly more efficacious than the typical antipsychotics.

D. Haloperidol decanoate 200 mg IM daily   INCORRECT

Haloperidol decanoate is indicated for maintenance of patients with schizophrenia who have been successfully treated with haloperidol orally but are experiencing difficulty in taking their medications as scheduled. Additionally, it is prescribed at dosing intervals of 28 days, not daily.

E. Fasting blood glucose and lipid panel before initiating any atypical neuroleptic   CORRECT

Although the second-generation medications are better tolerated and possibly slightly more efficacious than the first-generation drugs, these benefits do not come without some tradeoffs. The atypical antipsychotics, as a group, are known for their adverse effects of weight gain, lipid abnormalities, and blood sugar elevations. Therefore, a baseline fasting blood glucose and lipid panel before initiating any atypical neuroleptic is essential. Any abnormalities identified must be addressed and the tests repeated at appropriate intervals based on the patient's test results, coexisting medical conditions, and symptoms.

Epidemiologic and Other Data

The lifetime prevalence rate of acquiring schizophrenia in the United States is approximately 1%. The incidence increases by 10-fold if there is a family history of a first-degree relative with the disorder. However, if that first-degree relative happens to be a monozygotic twin, the other twin's lifetime risk of acquiring schizophrenia is approximately 50%.

The disease onset tends to occur in adolescence to the early 30s. The suicide rate in patients with the diagnosis of schizophrenia is approximately 10%. Interestingly, individuals of Asian descent obtain the same symptom relief from approximately half the dose of medication required for individuals who are not of Asian descent.

CASE 10-4
Ginger Halstead
1. History

A. Why is she lying about the contents of the box not belonging to her?   NONESSENTIAL

Immediately confronting the patient is extremely unlikely to change her answer. However, it is extremely likely to adversely affect the patient–provider relationship. This would be unfortunate because if Ginger truly has an eating disorder, trust and rapport must exist between the HCP and Ginger for her treatment program to have its greatest potential for success. Besides, the answer to this question is obvious—to prevent anyone from discovering her "secret" behavior.

B. What kind of grades does she get in school, is she pleased with them, and how difficult is it for her to obtain them?   ESSENTIAL

Inquiring about her grades provides a "soft" measurement of her intelligence level while simultaneously serving as a relatively "neutral" topic to start developing rapport. Furthermore, knowing what her grades are and whether she is pleased with them provides some insight into the patient's expectations of herself and sense of self-worth. Individuals with eating disorders tend to be perfectionists who never quite live up to their own expectations; therefore, they often struggle with poor self-esteem. Knowing what degree of difficulty Ginger is encountering in maintaining her high expectations (if she is currently having such difficulty) provides insight into the potential degree of effort she will likely apply toward correcting any problems identified, once she acknowledges their existence. Furthermore, it provides a gross estimate of the degree of stress she is currently experiencing and whether it can be adversely influencing/producing any psychopathology that might be present.

C. How good of a kickboxer is she, how much does she enjoy it, and why?   ESSENTIAL

Inquiring about her kickboxing not in terms of potentially representing an excessive compensatory mechanism for an eating disorder but as a pleasurable activity makes it another relatively "safe" or "neutral" topic to discuss in hopes of establishing the necessary rapport. Furthermore, inquiring as to her opinion regarding her abilities again provides some insight into her level of self-esteem. Also, knowing if she is motivated by self-improvement, desire for perfectionism, desire to please others, and/or weight maintenance provides some insight as to the presence of inappropriate attitudes that would require addressing in order to achieve optimal mental health, regardless of the presence of an eating disorder.

D. How does she feel about herself overall and especially her appearance?   ESSENTIAL

In many instances the "way" Ginger responds to this question provides more insight regarding her level of self-esteem than the actual spoken words. Refusal to discuss her appearance beyond a vague "OK" is often an indicator that her dissatisfaction goes beyond the normal adolescent concerns regarding a specific aspect of physical appearance. This is important information to obtain because virtually all patients with an eating disorder have a distorted body image.

E. How often does she weigh herself?   ESSENTIAL

This question actually serves to screen for the likelihood of an eating disorder. In general, individuals with eating disorders are obsessed with their body's appearance and weight; thus, they tend to weigh themselves much more frequently (often once or more a day) than individuals without an eating disorder.

2. Physical Examination

A. Ocular conjunctival examination   ESSENTIAL

Vomiting, if forceful enough, can produce subconjunctival hemorrhages and palpebral conjunctival petechiae. Although a recent subconjunctival hemorrhage is hard to miss, the conjunctivae must be specifically evaluated for this abnormality because if resolving, it can be overlooked. Furthermore, the eyelids must be retracted to observe the palpebral conjunctivae.

However, these findings are not specific for an eating disorder; they can occur as a result of other events (e.g., trauma, forceful coughing and sneezing, and blood dyscrasia). Nevertheless, when encountered in a patient who is at risk for an eating disorder, it should not be quickly dismissed. It is important to maintain a high index of suspicion because individuals with eating disorders rarely present complaining of such. If not recognized and addressed early by a concerned family member or friend, the presenting symptoms are frequently caused by late complication(s) from the illness (e.g., cardiac arrhythmia, electrolyte disturbances, malnutrition, fatigue, orthostatic hypotension, syncope, gastrointestinal bleeding, or menstrual irregularities).

Because these diseases are shrouded in secrecy and denial, it often takes an astute HCP with a high index of suspicion to link the subtle early findings (e.g., subconjunctival hemorrhage, palpebral conjunctivae petechiae, facial petechiae, parotid gland hypertrophy, poor dentition, and posterior metacarpophalangeal [MCP] joint callus formation and/or abrasions) together to suspect the diagnosis. Even then, and even if the HCP utilizes a compassionate, nonjudgmental approach, the patient is likely to deny the presence of an eating disorder. In this case, the HCP may elect to elicit the assistance of a qualified mental health specialist with expertise in eating disorders, representatives from a treatment facility, and the patient's family, close friends, minister, and/or significant others to conduct an intervention to get the patient into treatment as soon as possible in hopes of controlling the illness and preventing complications from it.

B. Oral mucosa, pharynx, and teeth   ESSENTIAL

One of the most widely utilized compensatory purging behaviors seen in patients with an eating disorder is self-induced vomiting. The patient often utilizes a finger because it is readily available and easy to "hide" if someone accidentally intrudes while the patient is engaging in this behavior. Still, the use of foreign bodies (e.g., spoons, table knives, toothbrushes, firm straws, or drumsticks) to induce the gag reflex is common. This stimulation can produce small traumatic abrasions, lacerations, or petechiae on the soft palate when the object (or fingernail) isn't removed from the pharynx before the initial upward movement of the reflex occurs.

However, just as the presence of soft palate/pharyngeal abnormalities is not exclusively found in an eating disorder, an eating disorder can be present without these findings. This can result from the patient being able to remove the object quick enough to prevent the trauma; however, it is most frequently found when another method of vomiting induction is utilized. For example, after a while, some patients can vomit "at will." Additionally, others will stimulate vomiting by utilizing syrup of ipecac.

Regardless of how regurgitation is initiated, the resultant stomach acid is generally irritating to the oral mucosa, teeth, gums, and lips. Chronic exposure can result in the formation of small lesions or shallow ulcers on the oral mucosa, minor edema and erythema of the gingival surfaces, and erosion of the tooth enamel. The teeth affected most often by this acidic process, because of their location, are the lingual surfaces of the upper incisors. Therefore, when evaluating a patient for a possible eating disorder, it is essential to look specifically for these changes as they too can often be subtle and easily overlooked or dismissed as a normal variant.

C. Salivary glands   ESSENTIAL

With frequent vomiting, it is not uncommon for the salivary ducts to become obstructed and/or irritated by the retrograde stomach contents, which results in edema of the associated glands. Similarly, vomiting can directly stimulate the salivary glands to produce saliva; over an extended period of time, this can lead to hypertrophy of the affected glands. Unless the purging is severe and long-standing, the changes are likely to be minor and subtle, with the parotid glands being affected most often. Thus, close observation specifically for these changes is essential.

D. Breast and pelvic examination   NONESSENTIAL

This examination is not indicated for Ginger as she is not experiencing any reproductive symptoms.

E. Bilateral hands with emphasis on the metacarpophalangeal (MCP) joints   ESSENTIAL

Individuals with eating disorders who engage in self-induced vomiting as a compensatory mechanism frequently utilize the index finger of their dominant hand for this activity. This can result in abrasions, ulcerations, and eventually calluses of the dorsal aspect of at least the first two MCP joints. Therefore, visually inspecting and palpating these areas are essential. Inspection of the nondominant hand may make subtle changes more obvious.

3. Diagnostic Testing

A. Dual energy x-ray absorptiometry (DEXA) scan   NONESSENTIAL

Screening DEXA scans are not routinely recommended for premenopausal women unless they are taking long-term medications that could increase their risk of osteoporosis (e.g., lithium, glucocorticosteroids, certain anticonvulsants, levothyroxine, and aromatase inhibitors) or have a medical condition that predisposes them to the condition (e.g., hyperparathyroidism, premature ovarian failure, and malabsorption syndrome). In general, patients with a confirmed eating disorder do not require a DEXA scan unless they experience at least 6 months of amenorrhea.

B. Electrolytes and serum magnesium level   ESSENTIAL

If purging behaviors results in vomiting and/or diarrhea that is significant and/or frequent, electrolyte and mineral abnormalities can occur. The first findings are hypokalemia and hypomagnesemia. As the purging behaviors become more chronic, severe, and/or frequent, hyponatremia and hypochloremia are evident. If the primary cause of the electrolyte abnormality is vomiting, hypercarbia and metabolic alkalosis can result. If the electrolyte abnormalities are caused by laxative-induced diarrhea, metabolic acidosis often results. The most serious complications from an electrolyte abnormality occurring in patients with eating disorders is in conjunction with prolongation of the QTc segment on electrocardiogram (ECG), which can result in arrhythmias and even sudden death. If the patient is anorexic and/or dehydrated, oral refeeding may be required to attempt to prevent and correct this cardiac abnormality.

C. Amylase and lipase   ESSENTIAL

Amylase is secreted by the pancreatic acinar cells; therefore, the vast majority of cases of hyperamylasemia result from damage to the pancreatic acinar cells and to the pancreatic duct, which forces the amylase into the intrapancreatic lymphatic system and the peritoneum, where it readily enters circulation. Thus, a gastrointestinal perforation can also result in hyperamylasemia via this same mechanism (i.e., intraluminal amylase being released into the peritoneum). Additionally, amylase is found in small quantities in the salivary glands, the ovaries, and the skeletal muscles; diseases affecting these organs can also result in hyperamylasemia. A few labs have the capabilities to perform fractionation of the isoenzymes to determine the exact source.

In regards to eating disorders, unless another condition is present that is capable of elevating the amylase level (e.g., mumps parotiditis and ectopic pregnancy), hyperamylasemia is caused by one of three complicating conditions: (1) salivary gland inflammation (as discussed previously), (2) gastrointestinal perforation (most frequently an esophageal tear or gastric rupture secondary to intense vomiting), or (3) pancreatitis. In most cases, the patient's history and physical examination findings will be able to distinguish which one of the three is responsible.

Nevertheless, the rate, degree, and pattern of the elevation of the amylase can also provide additional confirmation. In acute pancreatitis, the amylase begins to elevate approximately 12 hours after the onset of the condition and is resolved within 48 to 72 hours; however, the peak elevation is significant, up to three or more times the upper limit of normal. With a bowel perforation or a salivary cause, the elevation is not nearly as dramatic.

The associated degree of lipase elevation will follow a similar but delayed pattern, offering additional confirmation as to the correct source. In acute pancreatitis, the serum amylase will not begin to elevate until approximately 24 to 48 hours after the disease onset and will remain elevated for 5 to 7 days. The degree of elevation will be dramatic, generally greater than three times the upper level of normal and in some cases as high as 5 to 10 times the upper level of normal. In other conditions that can cause a lipase elevation (e.g., salivary gland enlargement, GI perforation, and obstructions), the elevation is not nearly as dramatic. Lipase levels can also be elevated in renal failure, cholecystitis, cholangitis, and intestinal infarction.

Specifically in the diagnosis and treatment of eating disorders, in the absence of an intestinal perforation and overt pancreatic disease, an elevation of these values can serve two purposes. First, it can provide objective evidence of the presence of the condition, which is useful not only in confirming the diagnosis but also in confronting patients and doing interventions. Second, it can provide an indication regarding the frequency of the

patient's purging behavior because it is theorized that the degree of amylase elevation is directly proportional to it.

D. Urine toxicology for bisacodyl, emodin, aloe-emodin, and rhein   ESSENTIAL

Urine screen for bisacodyl, emodin, aloe-emodin, and rhein is useful in patients who are suspected of laxative abuse but are denying it. The presence of any of these four drugs in the urine (or stool) is proof that a laxative has been ingested recently.

E. Electrocardiogram (ECG)   ESSENTIAL

An ECG is important to evaluate the patient for rhythm and conduction defects that can be seen with, but are not specific for, eating disorders. These include QTc prolongations, bradycardia, other arrhythmias, increased PR intervals, first-degree heart block, and ST-T elevations or suppressions. An ECG can also provide clues to the presence of a rare cardiomyopathy that results from the frequent use/abuse of syrup of ipecac.

4. Diagnosis

A. Anorexia nervosa, purging type   INCORRECT

Anorexia nervosa is an eating disorder that is defined by the DSM-IV-TR as requiring ALL four of the following criteria to be satisfied in order to establish the diagnosis: (1) inability to achieve and/or maintain body weight at an acceptable level (defined as ≥ 85% for height and weight in adolescents and a body mass index [BMI] of ≥ 18.5 for adults), (2) unreasonable and intense fear of obesity and/or weight gain despite being underweight, (3) distorted body image and/or refusal to acknowledge the serious nature of current weight, and (4) amenorrhea. Thus, because Ginger technically could only meet the third criterion, this is not her most likely diagnosis.

Furthermore, this can be eliminated as her most likely diagnosis because purging (by itself) is not a recognized subtype of anorexia nervosa in the DSM-IV-TR. The closest diagnosis is anorexia nervosa, binge-eating/purging type. To meet the established criteria for this condition, the patient must meet the diagnostic criteria for anorexia nervosa as defined previously AND participate in binge-eating OR purging activities while the anorexia nervosa is active.

B. Bulimia nervosa, purging type   CORRECT

Bulimia nervosa is an eating disorder defined by the DSM-IV-TR as requiring ALL of the following five criteria be established before the patient can be diagnosed with the condition: (1) experiencing repeated incidents of binge eating defined as either (a) consuming a quantity of food that is significantly larger than most individuals would consume in the same period of time in the same situation or (b) inability to control food intake during the period of time in question; (2) repeat use of inappropriate compensatory mechanisms to attempt to control weight at or below current level; (3) both 1 and 2 occur a minimum of twice a week for a minimum of 3 months; (4) self-worth is disproportionately determined by body size, shape, and weight; and (5) the behavior cannot be accounted for by anorexia nervosa.

Bulimia nervosa, purging type is further characterized by the current inappropriate compensatory mechanisms consisting of inducing vomiting, diarrhea, or diuresis via mechanical, chemical, or pharmacologic means. Although the specific criteria for the condition cannot be definitively established because Ginger is currently denying the existence of most of these defining characteristics, some of them can be inferred by the history provided by her mother and her laboratory test results. For example, her mother's finding of candy, cakes, and cookies in Ginger's closet is suspicious for binge eating. Her electrolyte disturbances, stool toxicology examination for compounds essentially limited to laxatives, and having laxatives discovered in her possession by her mother are suspicious for the inappropriate compensatory mechanism of the purging variety. And her daily weigh-ins, combined with adjusting her training routine based on her weight, offer support of further inappropriate compensatory mechanisms being present. Hence, from the list of diagnoses provided, this is Ginger's most likely diagnosis.

C. Klein-Levin syndrome   INCORRECT

Klein-Levin syndrome is an extremely rare condition consisting of 1- to 2-week episodes of hypersomnia (often > 18 hours/day) with hyperphagia and hypersexuality when awake. Initially, the patient will experience these episodes approximately two to four times per year; then, as the patient ages, the episodes decrease in frequency and virtually disappears by the time the patient enter his or her forties. There are no inappropriate compensatory mechanisms to counteract for the increased caloric intake. Because Ginger is not complaining of any sleep alterations and is not sexually active, Klein-Levin syndrome is not her most likely diagnosis.

D. Major depressive episode, with atypical features   INCORRECT

According to the DSM-IV-TR, an "atypical features" specifier can be added to most of the major mood disorders if ALL three of the following criteria exist: (1) depressed mood is alleviated by real, perceived, or possible positive influences in the patient's environment; (2) at least TWO of the following four symptoms are present: (a) noteworthy increase in appetite and/or weight, (b) hypersomnia, (c) "weighted" sensation in extremities, and (d) history of chronic interpersonal functioning adversely affected by inappropriate response to real or perceived rejection by others; and (3) melancholic and catatonic features specifiers are not satisfied.

Thus, even if Ginger met the diagnostic criteria for a major depressive episode (which can essentially be eliminated by her lack of a depressed mood and anhedonia) as outlined in Case 10-1, her inability to satisfy these qualifiers prevents this from being her most likely diagnosis.

E. Bacterial gastroenteritis   INCORRECT

Bacterial gastroenteritis could account for Ginger's electrolyte abnormality; however, it would not account for her lack of symptoms of this condition (e.g., diarrhea, abdominal pain, fever, and possibly nausea/vomiting), toxicology results, and mother's concerns. Therefore, bacterial gastroenteritis can be eliminated as Ginger's most likely diagnosis.

5. Treatment Plan

A. Urinalysis (U/A), blood urea nitrogen (BUN), and serum creatinine   CORRECT

This testing combination allows a determination to be made whether Ginger's induced vomiting and diarrhea are significant enough to have caused dehydration, which is highly likely given her electrolyte abnormalities. Dehydration produces an elevation in both the BUN and serum creatinine; however, this abnormality is not specific to this condition. Other conditions frequently associated with an elevated BUN and creatinine include glomerulonephritis, renal failure, pyelonephritis, acute tubular necrosis, urinary tract obstructions, and shock. Although the urine specific gravity can be affected by many of these conditions, it is only elevated with dehydration (and renal failure if caused by renal artery stenosis). In general, glomerulonephritis, renal failure, and pyelonephritis are associated with a decreased specific gravity, whereas obstructions, acute tubular necrosis, and shock don't impact the specific gravity significantly. Therefore, the combination of an elevated serum creatinine, an elevated BUN, and a decreased urinary specific gravity is fairly specific for dehydration. Furthermore, it is important to note that if Ginger is dehydrated, her serum potassium level could actually be lower than what's reflected via testing.

B. Hospitalization   CORRECT

Normally hospitalization is not required for patients with bulimia nervosa. However, it is recommended for Ginger because she has hypokalemia, hypomagnesemia, and other metabolic abnormalities. The presence of either hypokalemia or hypomagnesemia in a child or adolescent or the presence of any metabolic abnormality in a patient of any age with bulimia nervosa is an indication for hospitalization. Other admission criteria for patients with bulimia nervosa include bradycardia, orthostatic hypotension, blood pressure (BP) less than 80/50 mm Hg, hypophosphatemia, hematemesis, uncontrolled vomiting, other serious medical conditions, suicidal ideation with plan, failure of outpatient treatment, and coexisting medical, psychological, and/or substance disorders.

C. Nutritional, personal, and family counseling   CORRECT

Nutritional counseling is essential to assist Ginger in determining what an appropriate diet is for her, what a "normal" serving size consists of, and what her nutritional needs are that must be met or supplemented. Personal counseling is crucial to enable Ginger to identify and eliminate binge triggers, deal with interpersonal conflict and stress in an acceptable manner, work on self-esteem issues, set reasonable goals for herself, eliminate the desire to always please others, and address other issues that develop during the course of therapy. Family counseling is necessary to assist her family to understand, deal with, and be able to provide support for Ginger during her recovery and remission; develop techniques of dealing with interpersonal conflict appropriately; identify methods of observing Ginger for signs of recurrence without invading her privacy; and address other issues as they develop.

D. Fluoxetine 20 mg once a day to start, increase as tolerated to 60 mg once a day   CORRECT

Fluoxetine is an SSRI and the only medication currently approved by the FDA for bulimia nervosa. It has been proven effective in treating this disorder in several placebo-controlled clinical trials. Its recommended dosage for bulimia nervosa is 60 mg/day; however, studies indicate that its maximum daily dose of 80 mg may be necessary to achieve the desired results in many patients.

E. Desipramine 100 mg once a day, increased to 300 mg once a day by the end of week 1   INCORRECT

Desipramine is a tricyclic antidepressant that is FDA approved for depression. However, there are some studies suggesting that off-label use of this medication is beneficial in patients with eating disorders. Its recommended starting dose for this use is 100 to 200 mg daily in adults and 25 to 100 mg daily in elderly patients and adolescents. Its maximum recommended daily dose is 300 mg for adults and 150 mg for elderly patients and adolescents. Additionally, because of its significant anticholinergic side effects, even if this were a recommended dose for Ginger, increasing from 100 to 300 mg is likely to be an intolerable dosage escalation. Generally, titration needs to occur at a slower rate to enable the patient sufficient time to "adjust" to these nuisance side effects. However, because it is associated with significantly more side effects than SSRIs (and has a significantly higher lethality rate in an overdose), this drug at this dose is not an appropriate first-line choice for Ginger.

Epidemiologic and Other Data

Bulimia nervosa is predominately a disease of women, beginning in adolescence to early adulthood. The lifetime prevalence incidence for females is approximately 1 to 3%. Only 10% of all cases of bulimia nervosa are found in males, providing men with a lifetime prevalence rate that is approximately one-tenth that of women. It is found at a disproportionally higher rate in non-Hispanic white females in this country. Additionally, the condition is associated with a lifetime prevalence of a substance abuse disorder, particularly stimulant medications or alcohol, of approximately 30%.

CASE 10-5

Harriett Iverson

1. History

A. Has she ever experienced episodes of being unusually euphoric, being hyperactive, needing less sleep, having racing thoughts, having increases in goal-directed behavior, starting multiple projects and finishing none, or going on extensive shopping sprees she could not afford?   ESSENTIAL

With the symptoms that Ms. Iverson is describing, bipolar I and II must be included in her differential diagnosis list. These questions will assist with ruling in (or potentially eliminating) the likelihood of either condition because they represent some of the predominant symptoms.

B. Does she make impulsive decisions, take impromptu trips, purchase items "on a whim," or interrupt while others are talking?   ESSENTIAL

Another condition that must be considered among Ms. Iverson's differential diagnoses is attention-deficit/hyperactivity disorder (ADHD). ADHD involves symptoms in three main areas: inattention, hyperactivity, and impulsivity. These questions are geared toward determining whether impulsivity is present. Impulsivity can also be seen in bipolar illness.

C. Is she a "fidgeter"?   ESSENTIAL

In childhood, one of the main characteristics of the hyperactivity component of ADHD is the inability to sit still for extended periods of time. As the child becomes older, this behavior becomes a "fidgeting" with hands and feet or "squirming" in a chair if forced to remain seated. These latter characteristics remain in adulthood ADHD.

D. What type of grades did she get in school, was she ever "held back," did she ever get into trouble, or was she ever tested for or diagnosed with "hyperactivity"?   ESSENTIAL

Knowledge of school performance, types of difficulties, or previous treatment/testing for ADHD is important in distinguishing between ADHD, conduct disorder, and mental retardation as potential causes of Ms. Iverson's current complaints.

E. Before starting school, could she sit and finish a game or view an entire TV show without having to "get up," was she able to wait her turn at play, did she often interrupt others, or did she have the urge to get up and move around a lot?   ESSENTIAL

Currently, in order to establish the diagnosis of ADHD, the DSM-IV-TR requires that the symptoms began prior to the age of 7 years. Because it is difficult for many adults to distinguish between their preschool and early school years, some experts feel that asking adults to remember preschool behaviors results in the production of "false" memories (and consequently unreliable data). Thus, they suggest this age criteria be revised to "during childhood but before adolescence."

2. Physical Examination

A. Ear examination   NONESSENTIAL

B. Eye examination   NONESSENTIAL

C. Heart examination   NONESSENTIAL

D. Abdominal examination   NONESSENTIAL

E. Skin examination   NONESSENTIAL

3. Diagnostic Testing

A. Complete blood count with differential (CBC w/diff)   NONESSENTIAL

The primary diagnoses that can be supported by a CBC w/diff are infectious diseases, inflammatory conditions, and hematologic malignancies. None of these are currently in Ms. Iverson's differential diagnosis list.

B. Thyroid panel (TSH, FT_4, and T_3 by RIA)   NONESSENTIAL

Hypothyroidism and hyperthyroidism are not potential diagnoses for Ms. Iverson at this time.

C. Computed tomomgraphy (CT) scan of the brain, with and without contrast   NONESSENTIAL

There is no evidence to suggest that an intracranial pathology (e.g., hemorrhage, ischemia, mass, or infection) is producing Ms. Iverson's symptoms.

D. Brown Attention-Deficit Disorder Scale for Adults   ESSENTIAL

The Brown Attention-Deficit Disorder Scale for Adults is a 40-question screening scale designed to evaluate the childhood symptoms of ADHD, as defined by the DSM-IV-TR, as they develop into adulthood. It places more emphasis on the inattention criteria and little to none on the impulsivity and hyperactivity criteria. This instrument is considered by some to be more valid in the establishment of the diagnosis of ADHD in adults than the current DSM-IV-TR diagnostic criteria. Hence, it would be helpful in collaborating the HCP's impression regarding the presence of ADHD.

E. Scott Adult Attention-Deficit/Hyperactivity versus Bipolar Disorder Scale   NONESSENTIAL

Nice try, but this diagnostic scale does not exist.

4. Diagnosis

A. Major depressive disorder   INCORRECT

According to the DSM-IV-TR, in order to establish a diagnosis of depression, one of the symptoms that must be present is either a depressed mood or anhedonia. (For the remaining criteria, please see Case 10-1.) Additionally, a diagnosis of a major depressive disorder requires that the patient experiences one or more major depressive episodes. Because Ms. Iverson is not experiencing a depressed mood or anhedonia and lacks a history of a major depressive episode, major depressive disorder cannot be her most likely diagnosis.

B. Bipolar I disorder   INCORRECT

The DSM-IV-TR diagnostic criteria for bipolar I disorder include an obvious change in personality or mood for a minimum of 1 week (this criterion can be eliminated if the patient is hospitalized for the condition), which generally consists of a constantly expansive, euphoric state with three or more of the defining symptoms OR an atypical, irritable mood with four or more of the defining symptoms. These defining symptoms are (1) greatly enhanced self-esteem or pompous ideations, (2) marked reduction in sleep needs, (3) subjective or objective flight of ideas, (4) subjective or objective pressured speech, (5) more distractible than usual, (6) psychomotor agitation or more "driven" to meet goals, and (7) unrestrained in pleasurable activities that could result in negative consequences (see later). Furthermore, the condition has to be significant enough to interfere with occupational, social, or relationship functioning; not caused by substance abuse, an adverse medication reaction, or a general medical condition; and not diagnosable as a mixed episode.

Hence, bipolar I disorder can also be excluded as Ms. Iverson's most likely diagnosis because she fails to meet the diagnostic criteria established by the DSM-IV-TR for a major manic episode. Furthermore, she has not experienced the associated cyclic depressive symptomatology.

C. Bipolar II disorder   INCORRECT

The DSM-IV-TR diagnostic criteria for bipolar II disorder are very similar to the criteria for bipolar I disorder. The main distinctions are that the symptoms do not have to result in a functional impairment, the symptoms only need to be present for a minimum of 4 days, and the mood/personality changes have to be obvious to another individual. Since Ms. Iverson does not have the correct symptomatology but does has functional impairment, bipolar II is also not her most likely diagnosis.

D. Attention-deficit/hyperactivity disorder, not otherwise specified   CORRECT

The DSM-IV-TR also includes established criteria for the diagnosis of ADHD. The key characteristic is an unrelenting pattern of symptoms that are more prominent and visible more regularly than those exhibited by developmentally comparable

individuals starting before the age of 7 years. And, as with most of the other significant psychopathologies, the symptoms for ADHD, regardless of whether it is the predominately inattentive, predominately hyperactive-impulse, or combined type, cannot be caused by another mental or physical illness and must cause significant functional impairment. However, ADHD's criteria mandate that the functional impairment occurs in a minimum of two spheres (e.g., social, interpersonal, occupational, or educational). Furthermore, the symptoms must be evident in at least two settings (e.g., home and work).

To qualify as inattentive type, a minimum of six of the following nine symptoms must be present in addition to meeting the aforementioned criteria: (1) is inattentive to details; (2) has difficulty maintaining concentration on task at hand; (3) does not appear to hear when addressed directly; (4) displays frequent incompletion of tasks or duties; (5) is disorganized; (6) shows avoidance, procrastination, or dislike of activities that require continuous mental effort; (7) frequently misplaces necessary materials/items; (8) is capable of being easily distracted; and (9) forgets routine day-to-day activities.

For hyperactivity-impulsivity, at least six of the following nine symptoms must be present as well as the aforementioned criteria: (1) is a "fidgeter," especially with hands and/or feet, and/or is "squirmer" if seated; (2) leaves seat frequently despite decorum dictating it improper; (3) displays increased and excessive activity (e.g., running or climbing) in inappropriate settings (in adolescents or adults this criteria can be met by feelings of restless); (4) experiences difficulty participating in "quiet" leisure time activities; (5) is continuously moving, (6) talks excessively; (7) often blurts out responses before question is completed or when it is not addressed to him or her; (8) feels it is virtually impossible to wait for own turn; and (9) interrupts others' conversations and/or activities. The first six are considered to be primarily the hyperactivity symptoms, whereas the last three are predominately impulsivity symptoms.

If the patient meets both sets of symptoms (inattentive and hyperactivity-impulsivity) with an onset before the age of 7, has a functional impairment in at least two spheres, has symptoms in at least two settings, and lacks another psychological or medical condition that could be responsible for the symptoms, then he or she is said to have ADHD, combined type. However, ADHD, not otherwise specified is Ms. Iverson's most likely diagnosis because even though she meets the symptom criteria for ADHD, predominately inattentive type, she cannot be diagnosed as such because her history does not positively reveal the onset of her symptoms prior to the age of 7 years.

E. Conduct disorder   INCORRECT

According to the DSM-IV-TR, conduct disorder is characterized predominately by a persistent and recurring behavioral problem that features being cruel to other individuals and/or animals, destroying property belonging to others, lying, deceiving, stealing, or committing major infractions of rules. Because Ms. Iverson does not exhibit any of these behaviors, conduct disorder is not her most likely diagnosis.

5. Treatment Plan

A. Atomoxetine 40 mg once in the morning; after 3 days, increase to one in the morning and one midafternoon   CORRECT

This is an appropriate initial treatment for Ms. Iverson. Atomoxetine is an SNRI that is FDA approved for use in adults with ADHD. Other medications approved for use in adults with ADHD include mixed amphetamine and dextroamphetamine salts, methylphenidate, dexmethylphenidate, and lisdexamfetamine. However, atomoxetine is frequently considered to be the first-line drug of choice because it does not appear to have a significant abuse potential. The lack of a significant abuse potential is important because substance abuse is a common comorbid problem for many with ADHD.

B. Cognitive behavioral therapy   CORRECT

Cognitive behavioral therapy has recently been proven to enhance effectiveness of medication in the treatment of ADHD.

C. Lamotrigine 25 mg/day for 2 weeks, then increase to 50 mg/day   INCORRECT

Lamotrigine is indicated for bipolar illness and seizure disorders. It has not been used successfully in ADHD.

D. Lithium carbonate 300 mg twice a day   INCORRECT

Lithium carbonate is FDA approved for bipolar disorder. However, it has been used off-label with good results as an alternative treatment option for ADHD when traditional therapies are ineffective.

Other alternative therapies that are not FDA approved for adults but are approved for children include dexmethylphenidate, methamphetamine, and pemoline. However, these agents also appear to be effective in treating adult disease. Pemoline is generally reserved for patients who are unresponsive to the other agents and then only with exceeding caution because it has been associated with rare cases of hepatic toxicity that is sometimes fatal.

Adjunctive medications are sometimes required. Although none are FDA approved for this indication, the following agents have been used with good results: bupropion, modafinil, desipramine, clonidine, risperidone, and haloperidol.

E. Check lithium level in 1 week   INCORRECT

Because Ms. Iverson is not being placed on lithium, checking the level in 1 week is unnecessary.

Epidemiologic and Other Data

To establish the diagnosis of ADHD, the onset of symptoms must occur before the age of 7 years. It is estimated that 3 to 7% of school-aged children are affected. The prevalence rate among all ages of Americans is approximately 3 to 5%. In childhood, males are affected much more frequently than females; estimates range from 2 to 10 times more likely. However, by adolescence, the incidence is relatively equal. In adults, women are affected twice as often as men.

CASE 10-6

Ivan Jackson

1. History

A. What is his definition of drinking "socially"?   ESSENTIAL

Knowing the amount and frequency of alcohol consumption permits a determination to be made regarding the degree of concern that needs to be afforded to Ivan's alcohol intake in addition to the fact that he is underage. Consumption of four or more drinks per day for males (three or more for females) or 14 to 17 or more drinks per week for males (7 to 12 or more for females) is indicative of problem drinking. What the patient is drinking and what he or she considers a serving is also important because drinking the same quantity of beer, wine, or liquor is not equivalent. Twelve ounces of beer is equivalent to 5 oz. of wine or 1.5 oz. of 80-proof liquor. These quantities are considered to be a single serving of the respective substances.

Many HCPs will follow a positive response to quantity with a quick screening tool such as the CAGE (have you ever tried to **c**ut down on your drinking; been **a**nnoyed by someone criticizing your drinking; felt **g**uilty about your drinking; or required an **e**ye-opener the next morning?) or TWEAK (do you have a high **t**olerance, defined as being able to drink six or more drinks or requiring three or more drinks at a time to get an intoxicated feeling; are your friends or family **w**orried about your drinking; do you need an **e**ye-opener the next morning; have you ever had **a**mnesia of events that occurred while you were drinking; or have you ever made plans to **k**ut down on the amount you drink?) to further determine whether the patient has a problem with alcohol. Any positive response is suspicious for alcohol-related problems and mandates additional evaluation. The more positive responses the patient provides, the greater the likelihood of a significant alcohol problem. The TWEAK has been determined to be the more sensitive screening tool; however, the CAGE has been deemed the more specific of the two.

B. Does he currently require greater quantities of alcohol to reach or maintain the same level of euphoria than he previously did? If yes, is this a repetitive pattern?   ESSENTIAL

The development of tolerance, especially when it is repetitive, is associated with a greater potential that the patient is developing (or has developed) an alcohol dependency problem instead of an alcohol abuse problem. This is true for any substance of abuse.

C. Has alcohol caused him any problems at home, at school, at work, in relationships, or with the law?   ESSENTIAL

Alcohol-related interpersonal, social, occupational, or legal problems indicate a more serious alcohol abuse problem and perhaps even a dependency on the substance.

D. Has he ever had withdrawal symptoms (e.g., tremors, agitation, headaches, seizures, disorientation, or hallucinations) after not drinking for a couple of days?   ESSENTIAL

A history of withdrawal is associated with a much greater likelihood that the patient has developed dependency on alcohol and is not just abusing it. Additionally, the type and severity of withdrawal symptoms experienced previously assist with the decision as to whether the patient can safely try outpatient treatment or requires an inpatient setting to cease his alcohol consumption. This also holds true for other substances of abuse.

E. How intoxicated was the driver of the vehicle?   NONESSENTIAL

The level of intoxication of the driver is irrelevant in terms of diagnosing and treating Ivan's injuries as well as whether Ivan has an alcohol-related abuse and/or dependency problem.

2. Physical Examination

A. Ear and nose examination   ESSENTIAL

Ivan requires an ear and nose examination to check for evidence of leaking cerebrospinal fluid (CSF) and hemotympanum, indicating the possibility of a skull fracture.

B. Heart and lung examination   ESSENTIAL

Even though Ivan's vital signs are stable and he denies chest pain/pressure or dyspnea, because of his altered mental status, his heart and lungs require evaluation for signs of trauma (e.g., pericardial tamponade, cardiac valvular rupture, hemothorax, and pneumothorax).

C. Abdominal examination   ESSENTIAL

Despite Ivan's normal vital signs and apparent lack of abdominal pain, his altered mental status necessitates an examination to rule out signs of trauma (e.g., ecchymosis, contusions, and abrasions), distension, tenderness, and other findings suggestive of the presence of a peritoneal hemorrhage or other intra-abdominal pathology caused by the motor vehicle accident (MVA).

D. Musculoskeletal survey   ESSENTIAL

Although Ivan denies any musculoskeletal problems (including pain), he still requires a cursory examination to evaluate for possible musculoskeletal injuries because he has an altered level of awareness.

E. Neurologic examination, including orientation   ESSENTIAL

Ivan requires a complete neurologic examination because he was involved in a serious motor vehicle accident and was initially found to be "confused" and "disoriented" by the emergency medical services (EMS) personnel at the scene. Furthermore, his appearance of "intoxication" could represent the effects of alcohol and/or other substances of abuse. However, it could also represent an intracranial hemorrhage, brain contusion, concussion, or other brain injury, or a combination of both. Additionally, regardless of the cause of his intoxicated-like behavior, Ivan is a poor historian regarding exactly what happened and what injuries he sustained.

3. Diagnostic Testing

A. Blood alcohol level (BAL) and toxicology screen   ESSENTIAL

Because Ivan appears intoxicated, a BAL needs to be performed to confirm that this is indeed the case. The use/abuse of other substances can also present with a similar picture; therefore, a toxicology screen to evaluate for their presence is equally important. If alcohol or another substance is not identified on these tests, an intracranial abnormality must be even more diligently sought.

B. Urinalysis   ESSENTIAL

A urinalysis is essential to evaluate for hematuria, which could indicate genitourinary trauma.

C. Computed tomography (CT) of the head, without contrast   ESSENTIAL

Because Ivan appears intoxicated, the accuracy of his denial of a closed head injury and/or a loss of consciousness associated with the MVA is questionable, especially considering it was reported that he appeared "confused" and incoherent at the scene. Furthermore, he is claiming amnesia of the reported episode of vomiting at the scene, and he is currently complaining of a headache. Thus, a CT of the head, without contrast, is indicated. Once a hemorrhage and hematoma are eliminated, contrast can be utilized if there are suspicious areas that require further evaluation.

Furthermore, if his BAL is elevated (and/or his toxicology screen is positive), it will sufficiently complicate his clinical picture and make it much more difficult to eliminate the possibility of intracranial pathology with any degree of certainty. Likewise, even if his BAL and/or other toxicology screen are positive, there is no guarantee that his poor coordination and slurred speech are solely a result of his being under the influence.

D. Hepatic panel   ESSENTIAL

Because of the excessive amount of alcohol Ivan admits to drinking (which some experts would argue is representative of approximately 50% of the patient's actual consumption), a hepatic panel is indicated to evaluate for hepatocellular damage, especially before any medications that could potentially be hepatotoxic are prescribed for his headache. Additionally, if abnormalities are present and consistent with alcohol damage, this could serve as "sobering" news to the patient regarding the effect his alcohol consumption is having on his body.

E. Complete blood count with differential (CBC w/diff)   ESSENTIAL

Although it is highly unlikely in a hemodynamically stable patient for a significant acute blood loss to be present and identifiable on a CBC w/diff, Ivan still requires one to establish a baseline for comparison in the unlikely event a subtle bleed is present and the symptoms are not evident to him.

Furthermore, a mean corpuscular volume (MCV) measurement is part of the "triple screen" for alcohol abuse. A positive "triple screen" consists of an elevated MCV, elevated γ-glutamyl transpeptidase (GGT), and an aspartate aminotransferase (AST)–to–alanine aminotransferase (ALT) ratio of greater than 2. Studies indicate that having all three of these abnormalities is nearly 100% reliable for alcohol abuse. If two of the three indicators are present, it is still over 90% accurate.

Additionally, a GGT greater than 30 units/L (which is still within "normal" range in many laboratories) is theorized to be associated with alcohol consumption of more than four drinks per day.

A new biomarker, carbohydrate-deficient transferrin (CDT), is very accurate in determining alcohol abuse. Consumption of four to five drinks per day for a minimum of 2 weeks causes this test to be elevated. Furthermore, it is associated with a much lower incidence of false-positive results as the individual tests comprising the "triple screen." For example, the MCV can be elevated with pernicious anemia or folic acid deficiency; the AST-to-ALT ratio can be elevated to at least greater than 1 in liver congestion and metastatic liver cancer. Furthermore, the individual components can produce an inaccurate ratio if either is affected by another condition (e.g., an AST elevation can be found with acute cardiac disease, skeletal muscle trauma, recent seizure activity, hemolytic anemia, and pancreatitis; a low AST can be seen in acute renal disease, pregnancy, and diabetic ketoacidosis; an elevated ALT can occur in myocardial infarction, skeletal muscle trauma, myositis, pancreatis, severe burns, and shock; and a decreased ALT can be caused by hypothyroidism or malnutrition). The GGT can also potentially be elevated with pancreatic abnormalities (e.g., carcinoma and pancreatitis), acute myocardial infarctions, viral infections (e.g., cytomegalovirus and Epstein-Barr virus), and Reye syndrome.

4. Diagnosis

A. Alcohol intoxication and abuse   CORRECT

The established diagnostic criteria for substance, including alcohol, abuse are outlined in the DSM-IV-TR. Substance abuse can be diagnosed if the pattern of usage has caused significant disruption, discord, and/or problems in one or more of the following four areas within the past 12 months: (1) failing to meet expected important obligations at home, work, or school; (2) using substance frequently in situations where it could be physically harmful to oneself or others; (3) having legal difficulties/issues; or (4) continuing to use the substance despite its usage resulting in, or exacerbating, a continued negative impact on relationships. Because Ivan's history indicates difficulties in at least three of these areas and his clinical picture and BAL are consistent with alcohol intoxication, this is his most likely diagnosis.

B. Alcohol intoxication and dependence   INCORRECT

Although Ivan's behavior and BAL meet the diagnostic criteria for alcohol intoxication, he fails to meet the DSM-IV-TR criteria for the diagnosis of substance (including alcohol) dependence. The primary difference between abuse and dependence is that dependence is associated with tolerance and withdrawal symptoms, which Ivan denied.

C. Secondary alcoholism   INCORRECT

Alcoholism is a term (not used by the DSM-IV-TR) that essentially refers to an alcohol dependence disorder (because both tolerance and withdrawal must be present) that has become chronic and is characterized by a strong desire to consume alcohol despite the occurrence of adverse consequences. Secondary alcoholism would then be alcoholism that is caused by another psychological (or in rare cases a physical) disorder. The most commonly identified associated illnesses include depression, bipolar illness, generalized anxiety disorders, and schizophrenia. Because Ivan's history does not supply any known medical (including psychological) illnesses, alcohol tolerance, or withdrawal symptoms during the week when he is not drinking alcohol, he fails to meet the standard definition for alcoholism; thus, secondary alcoholism cannot be his most likely diagnosis.

D. Acute alcoholic hepatitis   INCORRECT

Acute alcoholic hepatitis is an acute form of hepatitis caused by excessive alcohol consumption. Although Ivan does have some evidence of hepatocellular damage, he does not have any findings on his history and physical examination to suggest the presence of hepatitis (e.g., abdominal pain, jaundice, or hepatomegaly). Additionally, his laboratory values are inconsistent with the diagnosis. In acute alcoholic hepatitis the ALT-to-AST (or DeRitis) ratio would be greater than 1; the aminotransferase levels would be markedly elevated (if early in the illness; if later, the bilirubin and ALP would be elevated); and the CBC w/diff would reveal a white

blood cell (WBC) count in the low-normal to low range with a predominance of lymphocytes. Thus, this is not Ivan's most likely diagnosis.

E. Alcohol intoxication and acute alcoholic hepatitis   INCORRECT

Although Ivan's clinical picture and laboratory findings are consistent with alcohol intoxication, they are not consistent with acute alcoholic hepatitis for the reasons described earlier. Thus, alcohol intoxication and acute alcoholic hepatitis is not his most likely diagnosis.

5. Treatment Plan

A. Advise Ivan that he has a major abuse problem with alcohol and it appears to be affecting his liver; that he needs to totally abstain from consuming alcohol of any type and have his LFTs rechecked in 1 month; and that if they are still elevated, he will require further evaluation   CORRECT

It is imperative that Ivan be advised that he has a major abuse problem with alcohol that appears to be impacting him not only emotionally and functionally but also physically. If his liver abnormalities are completely a result of the effects of alcohol, they are potentially reversible if he abstains from any alcohol intake. Thus, when repeated in 1 month, they should be dramatically improved, if not resolved. If they are not, additional evaluation is required to evaluate for the presence of cirrhosis, alcoholic hepatitis, viral hepatitis, or other conditions that could be producing hepatocellular damage.

Furthermore, because he has an alcohol abuse problem, total abstinence is necessary to prevent it from progressing into a dependency problem and the related consequences.

B. Psychological and addiction counseling with Alcoholics' Anonymous meetings to assist in becoming and staying sober   CORRECT

Psychological counseling is an especially important component of his treatment plan because he is still an adolescent and was just involved in an MVA that resulted in the death of four individuals, including a friend. Addiction counseling will assist him in developing coping skills, identifying "high-risk" situations, and providing insight into his excessive alcohol consumption. Alcoholics' Anonymous (AA) will complement his counseling and assist him in becoming and staying sober; additionally, he will receive the benefit of seeing and hearing first-hand accounts of how alcohol has adversely impacted others' lives.

C. Hospitalize immediately   INCORRECT

There is no indication for hospitalization for Ivan at this time. Regarding the MVA, his evaluation and CT were normal. So, even though he will require observation for symptom development and/or condition deterioration, this can safely be accomplished by his parents on an outpatient basis.

Regarding his alcohol abuse, his BAL is not toxic, his liver abnormalities are neither symptomatic nor severe, he has not tried outpatient therapy, he has never experienced withdrawal symptoms (despite consumption being limited to weekends), and he is currently not a danger to himself or others; thus, hospitalization is not indicated at this time for alcohol abuse.

D. Advise him to avoid old hangouts, friends, etc., to maintain sobriety   CORRECT

Avoiding old hangouts, friends, etc., is a hard, yet essential, component of the initial maintenance of sobriety. Therefore, it must be recommended and encouraged.

E. Start disulfiram immediately   INCORRECT

Disulfiram is an aldehyde dehydrogenase inhibitor that significantly increases the serum acetaldehyde concentration (up to 10 times higher than seen with normal alcohol metabolism) when taken in conjunction with alcohol. This significantly elevated acetaldehyde level can produce a variety of autonomic symptoms including flushing, diaphoresis, excessive thirst, orthostatic hypotension, vertigo, tachycardia, chest pain, blurred vision, hypertension, headache, nausea, or vomiting (commonly known as the "disulfiram-alcohol" reaction). Its clinical application is as an adjunct treatment to counseling and Alcoholics' Anonymous in patients who are experiencing (or fear they will experience) difficulty maintaining sobriety.

It should only be utilized in highly motivated individuals without coexisting cardiovascular, pulmonary, or other disease that could potentiate the disulfiram-alcohol reaction and with informed consent because there have been reported fatalities from the resultant reaction. Furthermore, because the half-life of disulfiram is very long (estimated to be up to 120 hours), a reaction could potentially occur with the ingestion of alcohol as long as 2 weeks following the cessation of this medication. Additionally, the patient must be vigilant in his or her quest to identify and avoid "hidden sources" of alcohol in not only foods (e.g., select vinegars, pickles, salad dressings, dips, and sauces) but also hygienic products (e.g., alcohol-based mouthwashes, waterless hand sanitizers, aftershave lotions, colognes, and perfumes) because of the potential of topical absorption of alcohol from even correct usage of these products. Even these minuscule quantities are sufficient to incite a disulfiram-alcohol reaction.

Thus, Ivan's lack of any attempts to maintain sobriety combined with the spontaneous nature of most adolescents make him a less than ideal candidate for disulfiram therapy. However, even if he was committed and well informed, it still could not be instituted immediately because he currently has an elevated blood alcohol level. As long as there is alcohol in the system that requires metabolism, there is the potential of a disulfiram-alcohol reaction. Therefore, in order to safely institute disulfiram therapy, the patient's blood alcohol must be zero.

Epidemiologic and Other Data

The lifetime risk of alcohol dependence in the United States is estimated to be approximately 10 to 15%, with an overall current rate of approximately 5% of the US population. However, alcohol abuse occurs at a much higher rate, with estimates reaching as high as 60% of all males and 30% of all females at some point in their lives. Men are affected at approximately three times the rate of women. The onset of the illness is generally during late adolescence or the 20s; onset after the age of 45 is unusual. The onset in women tends to occur slightly later in life than in men. Approximately 15% of all patients who are alcohol dependent die from completed suicide. Genetic factors appear to be involved in the development of the condition.

CASE 10-7
Jessica Kennedy
1. History

A. Is she experiencing any aphasia, agnosia, or apraxia? ESSENTIAL

Confusional states can be divided into two primary categories: dementias and deliriums. In general, deliriums tend to be acute in nature with fluctuations of symptoms, whereas dementias are chronic and progressive over time. Dementias are characterized by memory impairments, whereas attention difficulties tend to predominate in delirium. Nevertheless, early and subtle dementias can often go undetected until a dramatic change is apparent, often leading to the misperception that the condition is acute in nature. Therefore, it is essential to obtain further information to clarify whether the patient's confusion represents a dementia or delirium to ensure that appropriate conditions are included in the patient's differential diagnosis list.

Aphasia, the deterioration of language abilities that results in being unable to name common objects, having vague speech, or utilizing multiple words and even sentences to describe an object instead of its name; agnosia, an impairment in the ability to recognize or understand sensory stimuli (e.g., objects, words, and/or phrases); and apraxia, the inability to perform certain motor functions despite having the necessary physical ability (e.g., pantomime brushing teeth, using a comb, or slicing bread) are considered to be hallmark cognitive disturbances seen in dementia. Sometimes these changes are not obvious to the patient or he or she will deny their existence out of embarrassment (or some other reason); therefore, whenever possible, it is advisable to obtain this (and similar) information from a reliable observer.

B. Does she have any problems with planning activities, developing her schedule for the day, or initiating either? ESSENTIAL

This question also attempts to distinguish between dementia and delirium. Impairment in executive functioning, such as planning, preparing, arranging, organizing, or carrying out tasks in the proper sequence, is another defining characteristic of dementia.

C. Is she easily distracted by "irrelevant stimuli"?   ESSENTIAL

This question further attempts to distinguish between dementia and delirium. Being easily distracted by "irrelevant stimuli" (e.g., clock chiming on the hour, refrigerator motor engaging, or car door closing down the block) is generally associated with a delirium, not dementia.

D. Is she experiencing any misperceptions, illusions, or hallucinations?   ESSENTIAL

This question further attempts to distinguish dementia from delirium. Perceptual disturbances (e.g., misperceptions, illusions, or hallucinations) are examples of the disorientation that is more commonly found with delirium, especially if acute in onset and exhibiting diurnal fluctuations.

E. When did she last change her hearing aid batteries? NONESSENTIAL

Although a hearing impairment could potentially account for some of Mrs. Kennedy's symptoms (e.g., difficulty in sustaining a conversation or answering the "wrong" question), it cannot account for the presence of others (e.g., change in sleep patterns or "losing train of thought").

Nevertheless, this question is irrelevant because it has not been established that Mrs. Kennedy has any hearing impairment, let alone one that is being treated with hearing amplification devices. Furthermore, many elderly individuals are very sensitive when an assumption (whether correct or not) is made that they are experiencing presbycusis (or some other hearing loss) and would find this question offensive. Therefore, if there was a concern regarding a hearing loss contributing to the patient's chief complaint, a nonjudgmental approach is preferable.

2. Physical Examination

A. Thyroid palpation   ESSENTIAL

Determining whether Mrs. Kennedy's confusion most likely represents a dementia or a delirium is only the initial step toward establishing her diagnosis. The next step involves determining the actual cause for the condition. The primary categories for dementia include dementia of the Alzheimer type, vascular dementia, dementia caused by human immunodeficiency virus (HIV), dementia caused by head trauma, dementia caused by Parkinson disease, dementia caused by Huntington disease, dementia caused by Pick disease, dementia caused by Creutzfeldt-Jakob disease, dementia caused by other general medical conditions (e.g. multiple sclerosis and sarcoidosis), substance-induced persistent dementia, dementia caused by multiple etiologies, and dementia not otherwise specified.

Delirium's primary categories are delirium caused by a general medical condition, substance-induced delirium, delirium caused by multiple etiologies, and delirium not otherwise specified.

Thus, both dementia and delirium can be seen in conjunction with other medical conditions. In general, delirium tends to result from acute processes, whereas dementia tends to result from chronic conditions, most frequently neurodegenerative processes. However, dementia can be caused by hypothyroidism; and endocrinopathies, including both hyperthyroidism and hypothyroidism, can cause delirium.

B. Heart and lung examination   ESSENTIAL

Cardiovascular and pulmonary conditions can also cause dementia and delirium; however, a heart and lung examination is unlikely to identify findings to suggest the cause of a dementia. These typically represent atherosclerotic or necrotic (from infarctions) conditions (e.g., vascular dementia, cerebrovascular accidents, cranial arteritis, and meningovascular syphilis).

However, some of the causes of delirium can be suggested by findings on a heart and lung examination (e.g., cardiac arrhythmia secondary to electrolyte abnormalities, an acute myocardial infarction, or a conduction pathway abnormality, or idiopathic; cardiomegaly secondary to heart failure or cardiomyopathy; pneumonia; hypoxia; or hypercarbia).

C. Abdominal examination   ESSENTIAL

An abdominal examination is necessary to evaluate for signs of conditions that could represent both hepatic disease and those more specifically seen in delirium alone (e.g., renal disease, urinary tract infection, and other systemic infections). It also permits evaluation of the renal arteries and aorta to provide support for a vascular cause (hence, a dementia) if a bruit is discovered.

D. Evaluate for pedal edema   ESSENTIAL

Pedal edema is seen in heart failure, renal failure, hepatic failure, and some autoimmune diseases. All of these can be responsible for delirium, whereas only a hepatic condition can cause dementia (e.g., alcohol-induced cirrhosis, Wilson disease).

E. Neurologic examination with mini-mental status examination   ESSENTIAL

A neurologic examination with MMSE is essential to assist in establishing Mrs. Kennedy's diagnosis. The mini-mental status examination is going to be extremely helpful in evaluating Mrs. Kennedy's confusion and distinguishing between dementia and delirium. For more information regarding the MMSE, please see Case 9-6.

The remainder of the neurologic examination should focus on identifying abnormalities that could suggest the presence of general medical conditions that could be associated with or causing Mrs. Kennedy's confusion. Conditions that could produce either a dementia or a delirium include cerebrovascular accident, anoxia, vascular dementia, Pick disease, other frontotemporal degenerative disorders, central nervous system infections (note that true dementia is generally limited to the aforementioned conditions), space-occupying brain lesion (including cancer), and traumatic brain injuries.

Characteristic dementia is Alzheimer disease. It is the most common cause of dementia in the United States. The other two most common dementias are neurodegenerative dementia (e.g., Parkinson disease, other Lewy body disorders, Pick disease, and other frontotemporal degenerative disorders), and chronic intoxication (e.g. alcohol, prescription drugs, and illicit substances) which, as previously noted, can also cause delirium. Other much rarer neurologic causes include multiple sclerosis, normal-pressure hydrocephalus, and Huntington disease. Neurologic disorders that tend to cause delirium but not dementia include encephalopathies, seizure disorders, and focal lesions located on either the right parietal lobe or the inferomedial surface of the occipital lobe.

3. Diagnostic Testing

A. Magnetic resonance imaging (MRI) of the brain, with and without contrast   ESSENTIAL

An MRI of the brain without contrast is indicated in any patient presenting with confusion without any focal neurologic defects to evaluate for a possible intracranial hemorrhage. Once eliminated, a contrast study should be undertaken to assist in evaluating for some primary causes of dementia (e.g., hippocampal atrophy and/or cortical atrophy in Alzheimer disease, significant white matter abnormalities in vascular dementia, Lewy bodies with Parkinson disease, and frontotemporal degeneration with Pick disease), secondary causes of dementia, and medical causes for delirium as listed previously.

B. Serum electrolytes and glucose   ESSENTIAL

Abnormalities of serum electrolytes and glucose are important indicators of a metabolic disturbance that could be responsible for her cognitive symptoms (e.g., hypocarbia, hypoglycemia, sodium–potassium imbalances, dehydration, and acid–base disturbances).

C. Complete blood count with differential (CBC w/diff)   ESSENTIAL

CBC w/diff is essential to perform because it provides information regarding the presence of an occult infection (e.g., pneumonia, septicemia, meningitis, encephalitis, or pyelonephritis), an anemia (e.g., acute blood loss, iron deficiency anemia, B_{12} deficiency anemia), or alcohol abuse as suggested by an isolated elevation of the MCV (for more information, please see Case 10-6).

D. Blood urea nitrogen (BUN) and creatinine   ESSENTIAL

A BUN and creatinine can provide information regarding the possibility of other medical conditions that could be responsible for Mrs. Kennedy's confusion. These include renal failure, nephrotoxicity as a result of medications, shock, and dehydration (BUN and creatinine elevated); GI bleeding, heart failure, sepsis, and starvation (BUN elevated and creatinine normal); and liver failure, syndrome of inappropriate antidiuretic hormone (SIADH), malnutrition, and malabsorption (BUN decreased and creatinine normal).

E. Urinalysis (U/A)   ESSENTIAL

A urinalysis can also provide information regarding the cause of Mrs. Kennedy's confusion. For example, leukocyte esterase, nitrites, leukocytosis, pyuria, and WBC casts could indicate the presence of pyelonephritis; proteinuria, increased red blood cells, red blood cell casts, WBC casts, hyaline casts, waxy casts, fatty casts, and granular casts could be the result of glomerulonephritis; an elevated specific gravity could indicate dehydration; and a low specific gravity could implicate renal disease, especially if its in conjunction with proteinuria.

F. Liver function testing (LFT)   ESSENTIAL

LFTs, if abnormal, could indicate hepatic failure, hepatotoxicity as a result of medications, cirrhosis, and/or a hepatic encephalopathy as possible medical causes for Mrs. Kennedy's symptoms.

4. Diagnosis

A. Amnesic disorder   INCORRECT

An amnesic disorder can be separated from a dementia and a delirium because the patient is not experiencing true "confusion" but a significant impairment of memory. Additionally, amnesic disorder is not associated with any other signs or symptoms to suggest cognitive impairment. Therefore, amnesic disorder is not Mrs. Kennedy's most likely diagnosis.

B. Vascular dementia   INCORRECT

The DSM-IV-TR defines dementia as a neurodegenerative disorder that involves both memory and cognitive difficulties. Memory problems include not being able to remember previously known information and/or not being able to learn new materials. Cognitive impairments must involve at least one of the following four areas: (1) aphasia, (2) apraxia, (3) agnosia, and (4) abnormalities in executive functioning. Additionally, it involves a significant decrease from a higher level of functioning to one that now causes a functional impairment in some area of the patient's life (e.g., social, personal, or independence).

Furthermore, to diagnose vascular dementia (previously termed multi-infarct dementia), there should be objective evidence of the disease on physical examination (e.g., extremity

weakness, gait abnormalities, hyperactive deep tendon reflexes, extensor plantar response, and/or pseudobulbar palsy) relating to the white matter and cortical infarcts, which are the hallmark of the disease. Finally, it cannot be better attributed to another cause or exclusively caused by an episode of delirium. Because Mrs. Kennedy's symptoms do not meet the diagnostic criteria for dementia nor does she have any of the aforementioned neurologic signs, this is not her most likely diagnosis.

C. Substance-induced delirium   CORRECT

To meet the established DSM-IV-TR diagnostic criteria for delirium, the patient must exhibit an alteration in level of consciousness with impaired inability to concentrate, maintain, and/or reallocate attention. Mild cognitive dysfunctions can occur such as disorientation, reversal of the sleep/wake cycle, and decreased memory. Furthermore, it tends to be acute in onset and fluctuant in symptomatology, with symptoms tending to be worse in the evenings and at night.

Substance-induced delirium and substance intoxication delirium have the same DSM-IV-TR diagnostic criteria. The primary difference between the two is that substance intoxication delirium is generally caused by the abuse of a substance (e.g., alcohol, marijuana, inhalants, cocaine, opioids, benzodiazepines, and/or phencyclidine), whereas substance-induced deliriums are generally limited to adverse effects of medications being utilized for therapeutic benefits.

Both nonsteroidal anti-inflammatory drugs (NSAIDs) and histamine-2 blocking agents can cause problems with orientation and cognitive awareness. Combining two or more of these agents can enhance the effect and cause significant symptoms. Because Mrs. Kennedy had been on the NSAID without difficulty for several months and the cimetidine was just added before the symptoms began, the latter is the more likely culprit. Thus, this is her most likely diagnosis.

Other drugs that can produce problems with orientation and levels of awareness (and meet the diagnostic criteria for delirium) include narcotics, corticosteroids, antidiarrheals, and antihypertensive agents (particularly clonidine). Many other medications can produce cognitive problems (including delirium), especially for the elderly. For example, tricyclic antidepressants, antihistamines, muscle relaxants, and antispasmodics can affect the patient's ability to pay attention, learn new information, and recall previously learned information. Drowsiness and decreased alertness can result from medications such as benzodiazepines, antipsychotics, narcotics, and antiseizure medications.

D. Delirium caused by a general medical condition   INCORRECT

Even though Mrs. Kennedy's clinical picture represents a delirium, delirium caused by a general medical condition is unlikely to be her most likely diagnosis because there is no evidence of a medical condition capable of causing her delirium present. Furthermore, when using this diagnosis for dementia, the name of the medical condition should be included in the diagnosis (e.g., delirium caused by pneumonia, delirium caused by heart failure, or delirium caused by thiamine deficiency).

E. Dementia caused by Parkinson disease   INCORRECT

Dementia caused by Parkinson disease can also be excluded as Mrs. Kennedy's most likely diagnosis because she does not meet the required criteria to make the diagnosis of dementia (see earlier). Furthermore, she does not exhibit any of the characteristic features associated with Parkinson disease (e.g., cog-wheeling, tremor, muscle rigidity, or poverty of movements) and her MRI failed to reveal any of the changes consistent with this diagnosis.

5. Treatment Plan

A. Haloperidol 0.5 mg at bedtime, increase to 1 mg if necessary   INCORRECT

Because Mrs. Kennedy's delirium is likely reversible and not associated with any significant behavioral problems or psychosis, the first-generation neuroleptic haloperidol is not indicated.

B. Quetiapine 25 mg once a day, may increase to twice a day if necessary   INCORRECT

Although FDA approved for use in schizophrenia, this second-generation neuroleptic has been shown to provide similar behavioral effects as haloperidol but with significantly less bothersome adverse effects. Nevertheless, this is not an appropriate choice for Mrs. Kennedy for the same reasons as haloperidol.

C. Discontinue celecoxib 200 mg and start acetaminophen CORRECT

Because the possibility of celecoxib causing, or at least contributing to, Mrs. Kennedy's confusion exists and its usage is being attributed to causing pyrosis, it is best to discontinue the medication to prevent further complications. The recently released guidelines from the American Academy of Orthopedic Surgeons (AAOS) state that NSAIDs and acetaminophen are essentially equivalent in terms of pain relief and are both appropriate first-line agents for osteoarthritis of the knee. Thus, acetaminophen is an appropriate choice.

If the pyrosis alone was the problem, a proton pump inhibitor or other cytoprotective agent could be instituted to prevent GI complications from celecoxib. However, it is essential to remember that the second-generation NSAIDs, or cyclooxygenase-2 (COX-2) inhibitors, decrease, but do not eliminate, the potential for serious gastrointestinal adverse effects, including hemorrhage. Likewise, cytoprotective prophylaxis is not 100% effective.

D. Discontinue cimetidine   CORRECT

Because the problem began shortly after the initiation of the cimetidine, it is definitely appropriate to discontinue it. However, Mrs. Kennedy will need to be followed closely to ensure that her confusion resolves with this action and her pyrosis does not return after stopping this agent and her NSAID. If not, Mrs. Kennedy will require further evaluation for her complaints.

E. Quadriceps strengthening   CORRECT

The recently released AAOS guidelines list quadriceps strengthening as an essential component of the treatment of osteoarthritis of the knee. This is a logical and worthwhile treatment for Mrs. Kennedy. It can be initiated under the guidance of a physical therapist or an HCP with adequate knowledge in such training recommendations, and then transformed into a home program.

Epidemiologic and Other Data

The highest incidence of delirium is found in the elderly. It is estimated to occur in about 50% of patients with hip fractures and approximately 15% of overall elderly surgical patients, regardless of surgical procedure. Dementia's prevalence rate tends to increase as the patient ages. For example, it affects approximately 5% at age 70 years, about 20% at age 80 years, an estimated 40% at age 85 years, and approximately 50% by age 90 years. It is more commonly seen in patients who already have an underlying dementia.

Approximately half of the cases of dementia are caused by Alzheimer disease, a minimum of 25% are vascular multi-infarction type, and approximately 15% are related to Lewy body abnormalities (with approximately 25% of these being caused by Parkinson disease). The incidence appears to be increased in patients with elevated homocysteine levels and decreased in patients who consume alcohol one to six times per week.

It is estimated that approximately 10% of all reversible causes of dementia are a result of medication adverse effects. Furthermore, nearly one quarter of all patients who present for a dementia evaluation or a general medical condition have reversible dementia, most commonly the result of an adverse effect of a medication. Polypharmacy in the elderly makes these statistics even higher.

CASE 10-8
Kashia Lamont
1. History

A. Approximately how many of the lithium pills did she take and when?   ESSENTIAL

Knowing the total dose (number of pills multiplied by strength), the formulation (short- or long-acting), and time since ingestion are crucial elements in establishing an appropriate medical management strategy for Ms. Lamont's overdose.

B. How does she feel about taking the overdose? How does she think others will respond?   ESSENTIAL

This set of questions is important because it provides an indirect assessment of Ms. Lamont's current mood, plans for the future, support system, importance placed on opinion of others, and likelihood of repeat attempts in the near future.

C. Why was she hospitalized when her bipolar illness was initially diagnosed?   ESSENTIAL

Unless there is significant psychopathology, coexisting substance/alcohol abuse/dependency problems, significant suicidal ideations, or another comorbid condition, generally individuals with bipolar illness are not hospitalized after diagnosis. Because prior suicidal activity (even significant ideations) and substance/alcohol use/abuse are associated with an increased risk of future suicide attempts, it is important to ascertain the exact nature of the confounding problem.

D. What is her religious affiliation and does she attend church regularly?   ESSENTIAL

Regular church attendance is generally associated with an additional support system. Furthermore, the denomination of faith that is practiced has been found to be associated with the likelihood of successful completion of a suicide (e.g., Protestants are more likely to successfully complete suicide as compared to individuals of the Catholic or Jewish faith).

Other factors associated with successful suicidal completion are male gender, older age, non-Hispanic white nationality, significant depression, mood swings, hopelessness regarding the future, loss of interest in life, anhedonia, impulsiveness, current hallucinations or delusions, alcohol/substance use/abuse, poor overall heath, poor support system, noteworthy recent loss, humiliating and significant social stressors, unlikely to be discovered following an attempt, prior suicide attempts, high lethality potential with previous attempts, current suicidal ideation (especially if plans involve an extremely lethal or violent method), and a positive family history of successfully completed suicide(s).

E. Does she have a gun in her home?   ESSENTIAL

Guns are the number one method of successful completed suicides. Access to a firearm places the patient at a higher risk of a successfully complete suicide. Therefore, it is important to be aware of whether patients who are potentially suicidal can access firearms and where. Removal of all firearms from the home is critical before permitting a patient with a recent suicide attempt, whether with a firearm or not, to return to that environment.

2. Physical Examination

A. Hearing assessment   NONESSENTIAL

Lithium toxicity is not associated with decreased hearing or even the development of tinnitus.

B. Heart examination   ESSENTIAL

Lithium can be cardiotoxic in overdose situations; therefore, a heart examination is essential to evaluate for any signs of cardiotoxicity (e.g., arrhythmia or cardiomegaly).

C. Evaluation of pulses   NONESSENTIAL

Checking all of Ms. Lamont's pulses will not provide any more information in the treatment of her lithium overdose than checking a single pulse at one site or auscultating her heart because the only piece of useful information that could be obtained is her cardiac rate.

D. Abdominal examination   NONESSENTIAL

Although lithium toxicity is likely to be associated with nausea, vomiting, and/or diarrhea, an abdominal examination is unlikely to provide any additional information in the absence of abdominal pain (which Ms. Lamont denies).

E. Neurologic examination   ESSENTIAL

A neurologic examination, including orientation and an MMSE, is essential in all patients who have taken an overdose of medication (regardless of whether it was intentional or not) to evaluate for confusion and/or indicators of potential toxicities, including lethality. Special emphasis should be placed on attempting to identify subtle neurologic abnormalities associated with the particular drug ingested (if known).

Although not exclusive, neurologic findings associated with early (or mild) lithium toxicity include drowsiness (or occasionally exhilaration), dysarthria, mild ataxia, vertigo, nystagmus, muscle weakness, hyperreflexia, tremor, and myoclonus. Signs seen with moderate to severe (or worsening) lithium toxicity can include not only those found in mild toxicity but also agitated mood, blurred vision, marked muscle fasciculations, clonus, choreoathetoid movements, severe ataxia, syncope, hyperactive deep tendon reflexes, marked confusion, stupor, and coma. Additionally, it is essential to remember that the neurologic findings associated with lithium toxicity can lag behind the actual blood level (sometimes by several days) because of the slow passage of lithium across the blood–brain barrier.

3. Diagnostic Testing

A. Lithium level and serum toxicology   ESSENTIAL

A lithium level is essential because Ms. Lamont took an overdose of lithium. However, because she took a sustained-release formulation and it has been only 8 hours since her ingestion, it is likely that her peak lithium level is not going to be achieved until later. Furthermore, in all probability, it will likely be significantly higher without some type of immediate intervention.

Because of lithium's very narrow therapeutic window, levels must be interpreted in conjunction with the patient's clinical picture. A patient can be toxic with a normal level and nontoxic with a slightly elevated level. Furthermore, a coexisting renal disease and/or dehydration can produce a false elevation of the lithium level. Therefore, in interpreting lithium levels, it is essential to evaluate for the presence of these conditions as well. Hence, the diagnosis of lithium toxicity is technically a clinical one. Nevertheless, Ms. Lamont needs to be monitored by serial serum levels in conjunction with her clinical status.

A serum toxicology is also indicated to evaluate not only for the presence of any additional medications that could have been taken during the suicide attempt but also for any substances that the patient might be using and/or abusing that could exacerbate her response or complications as a result of the lithium toxicity as well as increase her risk of future suicide attempts (including a successful one) if not addressed.

B. Electrocardiogram (ECG)   ESSENTIAL

An ECG is essential in any potential drug overdose to evaluate for signs of cardiac toxicity. Lithium can produce serious and sometimes fatal cardiac abnormalities. The most common are prolongation of the QTc segment, torsades de pointes, complete heart block, diffuse depression of the ST segments, and generalized inversion of the T waves.

C. Blood urea nitrogen (BUN) and creatinine   ESSENTIAL

A BUN and creatinine are essential to look for indications of renal disease (because lithium is totally excreted renally) because an impairment can delay the elimination of lithium from Ms. Lamont's system. It also serves as a good screen for the presence of dehydration, which can produce false elevations of the lithium level and can lead to renal impairment in lithium toxicity.

D. Electrolytes   ESSENTIAL

Electrolytes are indicated because they reveal changes that could indicate dehydration (e.g., hyperchloremia, hypernatremia, and/or hypokalemia) or diabetes insipidus (hypernatremia). This is important because of the aforementioned effects of dehydration on lithium levels and the fact that lithium, in normal doses, can cause nephrogenic diabetes insipidus. Lithium toxicity enhances the possibility of developing this disease.

E. Complete blood count with differential (CBC w/diff) ESSENTIAL

A CBC w/diff is indicated to rule out any associated conditions that could have an adverse outcome on Ms. Lamont's condition (e.g., a low hemoglobin and hematocrit are indicative of an anemia, and an elevated MCV can be seen with alcohol abuse). Furthermore, lithium toxicity can cause a leukocytosis with a predominance of neutrophils and can serve as confirmation of the condition when it is evident clinically but not per diagnostic test levels.

4. Diagnosis

A. Unsuccessful suicide attempt with lithium toxicity and dehydration, completely or partially exacerbated by divalproex CORRECT

To determine if this is Ms. Lamont's most likely diagnosis, the easiest method is to evaluate its individual components for accuracy. An unsuccessful suicide attempt is defined as a suicide attempt that is associated with a high level of lethality and intent to die but that, for whatever reason, results in a nonfatal outcome. This definition correctly describes Ms. Lamont's attempt. Her clinical picture and lithium level are consistent with lithium toxicity and her electrolytes, BUN, and creatitine indicate dehydration, which adds additional support for this being her most likely diagnosis. Finally, the FDA issued an alert in December 2008 cautioning HCPs about an association between suicidality and antiepileptic medications (including divalproex). The fact that Ms. Lamont did not experience any suicidal ideations until beginning divalproex therapy approximately 2 weeks ago makes the association between her attempt and the medication very likely. Therefore, from the choices provided, this is Ms. Lamont's most likely diagnosis.

B. Aborted suicide attempt with lithium toxicity and dehydration, completely or partially exacerbated by divalproex INCORRECT

In an aborted suicide attempt, the individual has plans to die via a method that has a high fatality potential; however, for whatever reason, the individual does not proceed with the endeavor. Because Ms. Lamont actually carried out her suicide plan, this is not her most likely diagnosis, even with clinical and laboratory confirmation of lithium toxicity and dehydration in conjunction with a high index of suspicion between the suicide attempt and the initiation of the divalproex.

C. Suicidal ideation with lithium toxicity and dehydration, completely or partially exacerbated by divalproex   INCORRECT

A suicidal ideation is a thought about killing oneself. It can range from infrequent thoughts of death to a very detailed, very lethal plan. However, it is never carried out for whatever reason. Even though Ms. Lamont's clinical picture and laboratory studies are essentially confirmatory for lithium toxicity and dehydration, plus there exists a high index of suspicion between the suicide attempt and the initiation of the divalproex, this cannot be her most likely diagnosis because she acted upon her thoughts.

D. Deliberate self-harm with lithium toxicity and dehydration, completely or partially exacerbated by divalproex INCORRECT

Deliberate self-harm is the act of injuring oneself but having no intention of it resulting in a fatal outcome. So again, even though Ms. Lamont's clinical picture and laboratory studies are essentially confirmatory for lithium toxicity and dehydration, plus there exists a high index of suspicion between the suicide attempt and the initiation of the divalproex, this cannot be Ms. Lamont's most likely diagnosis because the high fatality rate associated with her chosen method, her plan to not be discovered until missing her next shift at work, her initial circumvention of the possibility, and her symptom severity indicate that she truly had intentions for a fatal outcome.

E. Deliberate self-harm with lithium, unrelated to divalproex INCORRECT

As previously stated, Ms. Lamont's suicide attempt has every indication of being an actual endeavor to end her life, not just a means to self-inflict pain, gain attention, or attempt to make others feel guilty. Furthermore, the timing between the onset of the divalproex and the suicidal behavior is very suspicious for a relationship between the two. Thus, this is not her most likely diagnosis.

5. Treatment Plan

A. Hospitalize on telemetry; ensure secure airway; frequent monitoring of mental status, vital signs, electrolytes, and lithium levels; intake and urine output; suicidal precautions; psychiatric consultation; and notify regular counselor and psychiatrist (if not doing consult)   CORRECT

The decision to hospitalize a patient after a suicide attempt for psychiatric reasons depends on several factors. Unfortunately, there is no "magic formula," screening tool, or other assessment method to accurately determine which patients are at risk for successfully completing a future suicide or even attempting suicide again. Much of the information generated in attempting to make this critical assessment is provided by the patient; unfortunately, this information may not be accurate, especially if the patient is determined to make another attempt in hopes of being successful with this future act. Therefore, as a general rule, hospitalization is indicated when the risk of the individual attempting suicide again outweighs his or her present abilities to cope with whatever events precipitated the current attempt.

Risk factors that indicate that the patient should be hospitalized include the current attempt being of a highly lethal and serious nature, the lack of a strong support network, current suicidal ideations possessing greater lethality or violence than the current attempt, patient possessing the means to carry out the new plan, anhedonia, hopelessness, delusional thinking, impulsivity, significant social/occupational/personal stressors, alcohol/substance use/abuse, previous significant attempts, and a family history of a successful suicide. If there is any doubt, the HCP should obtain a stat psychiatric consult to assist with the determination. If immediate consultation cannot be arranged, the patient should be hospitalized until one can be obtained.

However, in Ms. Lamont's case, hospitalization is also indicated for medical reasons because her lithium toxicity requires detoxification, the time span since taking the overdose is short, dehydration is present, and there is a potential for cardiac problems as a result of either the lithium toxicity or electrolyte disturbance.

Obviously, in treating any patient with a potentially fatal condition, the first step is to follow the ABCs (airway, breathing, and circulation) of medical treatment. Therefore, a secure airway and telemetry are required. Frequent monitoring of mental status will provide information regarding whether or not her toxicity is worsening; her lithium levels will provide some confirmation, but with the aforementioned limitations. Frequent monitoring of vital signs will provide early indications to the potential of a deterioration of Ms. Lamont's respiratory and cardiovascular condition. Intake and output will provide useful information not only on her hydration status but also on the potential development of nephrogenic diabetic insipidus.

Because her admitting medical condition is a direct result of a serious suicide attempt, she should be placed on suicidal precautions and a psychiatric consult obtained as soon as possible. Professionalism and continuity of care demand that her current therapist and psychiatrist be notified unless they are going to be providing/consulting on her inpatient treatment.

B. 0.5% normal saline solution (NSS) adjusted to maintain good hydration   CORRECT

This is essential in Ms. Lamont's case because she is already dehydrated, and the treatment of her lithium toxicity could result in further dehydration. Furthermore, it will help preserve her renal function, which can also be adversely affected by lithium toxicity.

C. Gastric lavage (GL) with large-bore nasogastric (NG) tube and warmed NSS   CORRECT

Despite GL not being proven beneficial except for very ill patients whose ingestion occurred less than 1 hour previously, there are exceptions where it should still be considered. In Ms. Lamont's case, these would include that the ingested medication is a controlled/time-release formulation, the dosage is sufficient to be lethal, and the treatment could be difficult.

Other notable circumstances to consider utilizing GL beyond the 1 hour postingestion rule include overdose occurring less than 2 hours ago, medication known to "clump" together in the stomach when ingested in large quantities, the substance having significant anticholinergic properties that would cause gastric emptying to be delayed, no effective antidote or treatment being available for the agent ingested, and the ingested medication being resistant to activated charcoal.

D. Hemodialysis   INCORRECT

Hemodialysis is indicated in lithium toxicity only if the patient is experiencing severe symptoms (e.g., coma, apnea, marked hypotension, fluid/electrolyte/acid-base imbalances, or hypothermia) AND the serum lithium level is still greater than 4 mEq/L 12 hours after ingestion OR if the patient has an underlying medical condition that would prevent the drug from being removed with traditional techniques. However, if Ms. Lamont's condition deteriorates, her lithium level increases to greater than 4 mEq/L, or one of these other conditions develops, hemodialysis should be considered at that time.

E. Antiemetic agent and rectal tube, followed by gastrointestinal (GI) decontamination with polyethylene glycol solution at 2 L/hr via NG tube until rectal tube is clear   CORRECT

This treatment is generally effective for lithium toxicity. The antiemetic agent is indicated to attempt to prevent vomiting, and subsequent aspiration, of the polyethylene glycol solution.

Epidemiologic and Other Data

In the United States, the lifetime incidence of a suicidal ideation is approximately 10%. The lifetime prevalence of attempting suicide is approximately 0.3%. The lifetime incidence of completing a successful suicide is approximately 0.012%. The majority (approximately 70–90%) of individuals who complete suicide have a coexisting psychiatric condition; the most common are depression and alcoholism. Males are much more likely to complete suicide than females (estimates range from approximately two to seven males per one female); however, females are much more likely to attempt suicide.

Increasing age is associated with an increased likelihood of a successfully completed suicide. Non-Hispanic white females and males younger than the age of 40 years successfully complete suicides at a slightly greater rate than equivalent African American age- and gender-matched patients. However, after the age of 40 years, the rate of successful suicides becomes significantly higher for non-Hispanic white males. Native American males' successful suicide rate is even higher than that of white males.

CASE 10-9
Lydia Mortising
1. History

A. Has she had any confusion, problems staying focused, or memory difficulties?   ESSENTIAL

The vast majority of elevations in body temperature are the result of fever. Nevertheless, in any patient taking a serotonergic drug who develops a significant, sudden elevation in body temperature, the potentially fatal conditions of drug-induced hyperthermia and serotonin syndrome must be considered among the initial differential diagnoses. Hyperthermia as a result of one of the adverse drug reactions tends to be associated with neurologic symptoms not typically seen with fever (unless the source is a central nervous system problem or dementia is also present) including confusion, problems staying focused, and memory difficulties.

B. Has she been unusually aggravated, agitated, or irritated since her symptoms began?   ESSENTIAL

Symptoms that are frequently prominent in patients with serotonin syndrome, and to a lesser degree drug-induced hyperthermia, that are not typically seen with fever include being unusually aggravated, agitated, or irritated. These are especially important to inquire about in Mrs. Mortising's case because she on a higher-dose SSRI, and an analgesic known to potentiate serotonin syndrome (tramadol) was added to it yesterday.

Other medications that have been implicated as capable of causing serotonin syndrome in patients on SSRIs include other SSRIs, SNRIs, TCAs, MAOIs, other antidepressants with serotoninergic properties, lithium, St. John's wort, linezolid, dopamine antagonists, and triptans.

C. Is she having photophobia, pain with moving her eyes, or burning of her eyes?   ESSENTIAL

Patients will utilize the term "flu" to describe several conditions besides a true influenza illness. Some examples include any febrile illness, any infectious illness associated with muscular aches, a severe upper respiratory tract infection, and viral gastroenteritis (i.e, "stomach flu"). Therefore, when a patient complains of "flu" (or presents with symptoms suspicious for influenza), it is important to distinguish these other conditions from true influenza. Although not specific for true influenza, determining whether the patient is experiencing photophobia, pain with eye movement, or ocular burning can be helpful because they occur at a very high rate in true influenza.

D. Where are her muscle pains located and how would she describe them?   ESSENTIAL

Some patients define any abnormal sensation in their muscles as an ache or pain, leading the HCP to (correctly or incorrectly) deduce that the patient is experiencing myalgias. However, true myalgias are an aching sensation in the muscles that are typically generalized and associated with constitutional symptoms. They are common in influenza.

Abnormal muscle sensations that are more localized (e.g., fasciculations, myoclonus, clonus, tremor, and/or stiffness) tend to represent other problems. These generally are not common in influenza; hence, other causes must be sought. Similar confusion can occur when the term "chills" is not clarified because a patient will often use the term to represent any involuntary muscle sensation when actually it could represent an involuntary muscle movement.

E. Has she tried an antipyretic for her fever? If yes, what medication and what was the response?   ESSENTIAL

In general, pyrogenic cytokine-mediated fever (and even hyperpyrexia) is responsive, to some degree, to basic antipyretics (e.g., acetaminophen, aspirin, and ibuprofen), whereas hyperthermia not secondary to fever tends to be unresponsive. Thus, this is another question that can assist in distinguishing the cause of the patient's elevated temperature when more than fever is suspected.

2. Physical Examination

A. General appearance   ESSENTIAL

The general appearance of a patient who has a temperature as high as Mrs. Mortising's is essential because it provides an estimation of the severity of the illness and the degree of toxicity. If the markedly elevated temperature is not secondary to an infectious process, but the result of a hyperthermia from some other cause, the patient will often appear ill or unwell, but not toxic. Causes of hyperthermia include adverse medication effects, serotonin syndrome, neuroleptic malignant syndrome, malignant hyperthermia, heat-induced illnesses, endocrinopathies, damage to the central nervous system, and some malignancies (although the hyperthermia that occurs in the majority of malignancies is cytokine mediated and would technically be classified as "fever").

B. Heart and lung examination   ESSENTIAL

Mrs. Mortising requires a heart and lung examination because she has an elevated body temperature and is complaining of tachycardia, palpitations, and vertigo. Because her tachycardia is not related to activity or position (including standing), it most likely represents a sinus tachycardia as a physiologic response to fever. However, because of the presence of the palpitations (which can be sensed in some patients experiencing sinus tachycardia) and vertigo, it is essential to ensure that she is not experiencing a nonsinus arrhythmia, autonomic dysfunction, or an undiagnosed orthostasis. Additionally, the heart and lungs need to be auscultated for the presence of signs that could represent an infectious process (e.g., acute bacterial endocarditis, subacute bacterial endocarditis [SBE], pneumonia, or bronchitis) as the cause of her elevated temperature.

C. Abdominal examination   ESSENTIAL

Because the patient is experiencing nausea, vomiting, and diarrhea in conjunction with an elevated body temperature, an abdominal examination is indicated primarily to evaluate for an infectious source; however, inflammatory processes are also possible (e.g., inflammatory bowel disease, appendicitis, pancreatitis, and cholelithiasis). Although nongastrointestinal inflammatory and infectious process can also produce fever, nausea, and vomiting, they are unlikely in the presence of diarrhea in the absence of abdominal pain.

D. Pelvic examination   NONESSENTIAL

E. Neurologic examination, including a mini-mental status examination (MMSE)   ESSENTIAL

Neurologic examination, including an MMSE, is essential because Mrs. Mortising's history reveals myoclonus instead of myalgias, tremor instead of chills, hyperpyrexia possibly not caused by fever, autonomic symptoms (e.g., diaphoresis, tachycardia, and vertigo), and subtle mood and cognition symptoms. The MMSE can assist in determining whether the patient's sensation of altered awareness, concentration problems, and irritability are caused by fatigue from her illness, an adverse medication effect, a dementia, or a delirium.

The neurologic examination is also indicated to evaluate for findings that could indicate her symptoms are caused by serotonin syndrome (e.g., uncontrollable shivering, hyperreflexia, tremors, myoclonus, and muscle rigidity [but not as significant as "lead-pipe" rigidity, which is more common in neuroleptic malignant syndrome]). Advanced stages of serotonin syndrome can be characterized by seizures, status epilepticus, coma, cardiovascular collapse, and even death. Additionally, it can evaluate for the presence of a central nervous system infection or other neurologic conditions that could account for her symptoms.

3. Diagnostic Testing

A. Serum fluoxetine level   NONESSENTIAL

A fluoxetine level, even if available on-site and able to provide immediate results, is still not going to provide any clinically useful information. Serum fluoxetine levels measure the amount of medication in the bloodstream; however, they do not measure, nor can they predict, the concentration of the medication at the neurosynaptic junction where it is active.

B. Blood urea nitrogen (BUN) and creatinine   ESSENTIAL

BUN and creatinine are important because they provide useful information regarding the function of the kidneys. Kidney problems (e.g., pyelonephritis, uremic syndrome, and renal encephalopathy) can produce symptoms that are very similar to Mrs. Mortising's present illness.

C. Creatine phosphokinase (CPK)   ESSENTIAL

The CPK elevates in response to tissue and/or nerve damage in skeletal muscles (CPK-MM), heart muscle (CPK-MB), or the brain (CPK-BB). It is indicated on Mrs. Mortising to determine whether any muscle damage has occurred as a result of her myoclonus and tremor. It can also be elevated in other conditions that could be responsible for some, if not all, of Mrs. Mortising's symptoms. These include myositis, rhabdomyolysis, infectious pericarditis, a myocardial infarction, encephalopathy, encephalitis, or meningitis. If positive, isoenzymes might be necessary to confirm a suspicion.

D. Electrocardiogram (ECG)   ESSENTIAL

An ECG is indicated to determine whether Mrs. Mortising's tachycardia is caused by a sinus tachycardia (as would be expected if a result of fever) or some other regular rhythm alteration (e.g., paroxysmal ventricular tachycardia, autonomic tachycardia, ventricular tachycardia, or torsades de pointes).

E. Electrolytes and magnesium level   ESSENTIAL

These tests are indicated because of the severity of Mrs. Mortising's diarrhea. As stated previously, hyperchloremia, hypernatremia, and/or hypokalemia can occur with dehydration. Although hypokalemia and hypomagnesemia are primary electrolyte disturbances seen from acute vomiting and/or diarrhea, they can also be found in chronic renal diseases. Furthermore, hypomagnesemia and/or hyponatremia are other potential causes for patients who present with a delirium and myoclonus. Hypocarbia, potassium–sodium imbalances, severe dehydration, and/or acid–base disturbances could be responsible for her cognitive changes.

4. Diagnosis

A. Moderate serotonin syndrome   CORRECT

Serotonin syndrome results from the overstimulation of serotonin; it can occur as an adverse effect from any serotoninergic medication. However, more commonly the cause is a combination of medications with serotonergic properties (see earlier). It is characterized by hyperpyrexia, abnormal muscle movements, tachycardia, diaphoresis, and uncontrollable shivering. It is further divided into mild, moderate, and severe depending on the symptoms. In general, the treatment is dependent upon the severity of the illness. Mild serotonin syndrome consists of symptoms such as low-grade tachycardia, diaphoresis, shivering, tremors, dilated pupils, myoclonus, and hyperreflexia. Moderate serotonin syndrome is characterized by the symptoms found in mild disease plus hypertension and significant hyperpyrexia that can exceed 40°C. (The formulas for converting temperatures can be found in Case 1-4.) Other symptoms include hyperactive bowel sounds, ankle and neck clonus, agitation, irritability, and pressured speech. Thus, Mrs. Mortising's most likely diagnosis is moderate serotonin syndrome.

When assigning a severity level to serotonin syndrome, it is important to remember that not all the symptoms need to be present to assign the patient to a particular level; however, a majority do. If there is any doubt regarding which level should be assigned to the patient, it is better to err on the side of

overdiagnosis than underdiagnosis and assign him or her the more severe condition because serotonin syndrome can be fatal.

B. Severe serotonin syndrome   INCORRECT

Severe serotonin syndrome consists of the aforementioned symptoms for mild and moderate disease plus malignant hypertension and significant tachycardia that frequently leads to shock. Temperature can be in excess of 41°C. Coma, seizures, and status ellipticus are not uncommon. Muscles change from flaccid to rigid and hypotonia begins to develop, especially in the lower extremities. Metabolic acidosis and rhabdomyolysis are frequently present. Thus, this can be ruled out as Mrs. Mortising's most likely diagnosis.

C. Neuroleptic malignant syndrome   INCORRECT

Neuroleptic malignant syndrome (NMS) is an idiosyncratic reaction to a neuroleptic medication. It is theorized to be caused by excessive dopamine receptor blockade and/or inadequate levels of CNS dopamine. It is similar to serotonin syndrome in that it produces autonomic nervous system dysfunction, is associated with an elevated temperature (although generally not as high), and muscle rigidity (although tends to be more severe and "lead-pipe" like in nature). Hypotonia and altered mental status are also possible in NMS. Clinically, they are very difficult to distinguish without access to a list of current (and recent) medications. Because Mrs. Mortising's was prescribed tramadol while being on an SSRI, and not a neuroleptic, NMS is not her most likely diagnosis.

D. Uremia   INCORRECT

Uremia can present as a peripheral neuropathy, lassitude, anorexia, nausea, vomiting, muscle cramping, and hypertension. However, it is associated with renal failure, anemia, and either hyperkalemia or hypokalemia. The hypertension is generally caused by the sodium overload. Regardless, Mrs. Mortising's diagnostic studies are inconsistent with uremia being her most likely diagnosis.

E. Alzheimer disease   INCORRECT

Alzheimer disease is the prototypical dementia characterized by a gradual onset of decreasing cognitive functioning from a previously higher level. It is further characterized by losses in both memory and cognitive impairment that result in some degree of functional impairment. Furthermore, the cognitive defect cannot be caused by another medical disorder, a psychological illness, a substance abuse problem, or an adverse effect from a medication.

Alzheimer disease alone cannot be Mrs. Mortising's most likely diagnosis because it fails to account for her hyperthermia, gastrointestinal symptoms, neuromuscular abnormalities, hypertension, and sinus tachycardia. Furthermore, her MMSE is more consistent with a delirium, not a dementia. Incidentally, serotonin syndrome can be associated with delirium.

5. Treatment Plan

A. Telemetry monitoring in the ED with frequent vital sign assessment   CORRECT

In treating a mild to moderate serotonin syndrome, monitoring in the ED with telemetry, 0.5% NSS for hydration, and frequent vital sign assessment are generally adequate as long as the patient responds to therapy.

B. Discontinue both fluoxetine and tramadol   CORRECT

It is essential to discontinue both the fluoxetine and tramadol because Mrs. Mortising's serotonin syndrome is caused by serotonin stimulation from this combination of medications. Ideally, it would be best to avoid both of these agents because they could precipitate serotonin syndrome in the future at much lower doses. Other serotoninergic drugs should be utilized only with extreme caution to ensure that serotonin syndrome does not develop from their usage.

C. Cyproheptadine 4 to 8 mg every 2 hours until symptom reversal occurs or a maximum of 32 mg is given   CORRECT

Cyproheptadine is classified as an antihistamine; however, it has significant serotonin 5-HT$_2$ receptor properties, making it very effective as an off-label treatment for serotonin syndrome. The usual dosage is 4 to 8 mg every 2 hours until symptom reversal occurs or a maximum of 32 mg is reached. This is considered to be the treatment of choice for moderate serotonin syndrome.

D. Reduction of body temperature with tepid water spraying and fanning of unclothed patient   CORRECT

This is considered to be the standard of care as the first-line treatment for hyperthermia reduction in serotonin syndrome regardless of its severity level. If the hyperthermia is unresponsive, the patient may require general anesthesia to accomplish temperature reduction. Antipyretics have no role in the reduction of hyperthermia caused by serotonin syndrome because they have been proven ineffective; however, they are recommended if the hyperthermia is caused by fever.

E. Admit to intensive care unit; IV with 0.5 NSS; diazepam 10 mg IV for muscle cramping; intubation and mechanic ventilation if necessary   INCORRECT

In moderate serotonin syndrome, this intensive of treatment is generally unnecessary unless the patient's condition deteriorates. However, this is the treatment of choice for severe serotonin syndrome.

Epidemiologic and Other Data

The actual incidence of serotonin syndrome in the United States is unknown, primarily because many of the cases are extremely mild and resolve without sequelae within 24 hours of discontinuing the medication. However, estimates are in the thousands of cases annually.

The rate is increasing because of the increased incidence of individuals being prescribed SSRIs and other medications with serotoninergic properties. Additionally, it is estimated to occur in approximately 15% of all overdoses caused by SSRIs. It is estimated that nearly 60% of all patients who are going to develop serotonin syndrome do so within 6 hours of initiating a serotoninergic drug, having a dosage increased or another drug added, or taking an unintentional or accidental overdose. It is theorized that the condition results from the excessive stimulation of the 5-hydroxytryptamine receptors.

REFERENCES/ADDITIONAL READING

Aghababian RV, ed. *Essentials of Emergency Medicine.* Sudbury, MA: Jones & Bartlett Publishers; 2006.
Heron C, Boyer E. Lithium. 825–826.
Menditto D, Hoffman RJ. Toxidromes: an approach to the poisoned patient. 785–788.
Schier JG. Gastric decontamination. 789–791.
American Psychiatric Association. *Diagnosis and Statistical Manual of Mental Disorders.* 4th ed., text revision (DSM-IV-TR). Washington DC: American Psychiatric Association; 2000.
American Psychiatric Association. Alcohol intoxication and abuse. 191–295.
American Psychiatric Association. Delirium, dementia, and amnesiac and other cognitive disorders. 135–180.
American Psychiatric Association. Disorders usually first diagnosed in infancy, childhood, or adolescence. 39–134.
American Psychiatric Association. Eating disorder. 583–595.
American Psychiatric Association. Mood disorders. 345–428.
American Psychiatric Association. Schizophrenia and other psychotic disorders. 297–343.
American Psychiatric Association. Somatoform disorders. 485–511.
American Psychiatric Association. Practice guideline for the treatment of patients with substance use disorders, 2nd edition. In: *American Psychiatric Association Practice Guidelines for the Treatment of Psychiatric Disorders: Compendium 2006.* Arlington, VA: American Psychiatric Association; 2006:291–563.
Anton RF, O'Malley SS, Ciraulo DA, et al. COMBINE Study Research Group. Combined pharmacotherapies and behavioral interventions for alcohol dependence: the COMBINE study: a randomized controlled trial. *JAMA.* 2006;295(17):2003–2017.
Boyer EW, Shannon M. The serotonin syndrome. *N Engl J Med.* 2005;352(11):1112–1120.
Brown TE. *Brown Attention-Deficit Disorder Scales (Manual).* San Antonio, TX: The Psychological Corporation; 1996.
Cipriani A, Furukawa TA, Salant G, et al. Comparative efficacy and acceptability of 12 new-generation antidepressants: a multiple-treatments meta-analysis. *Lancet.* 2009; 373(9665):746–758.
Connery HS, Kleber MD. Guideline watch: practice guidelines for the treatment of patients with substance use disorders, 2nd ed. *Focus.* 2007;5(2):1–4.
Farone SV, Biderman J, Spencer T, et al. Diagnosing adult attention deficit hyperactivity disorder: are late onset and subthreshold diagnosis valid? *Am J Psychiatry.* 2006;163: 1720–1729.
Fauci AS, Kasper DL, Longo DL, et al., eds. *Harrison's Principles of Internal Medicine.* 17th ed. New York: McGraw-Hill Medical; 2008.
Bird TD, Miller BL. Dementia. 2536–2564.
Dinarello CA, Porat R. Fever and hyperthermia. 117–121.
Josephson SA, Miller BL. Confusion and delirium. 158–162.
Reus VI. Mental disorders. 2710–2723.
Schuckit MA. Alcohol and Alcoholism. 2724–2729.
Walsh BT. Eating disorders. 473–477.
Feldman HH, Jacova C, Robiliard A, et al. Diagnosis and treatment of dementia. *CMAJ.* 2008;178(7):825–836.

Fennell J, Husssain M. Serotonin syndrome: case report and current concepts. *Ir Med J.* 2005;18(2):143–144.

Fick DM, Cooper JW, Wade WE, et al. Updating the Beers criteria for potentially inappropriate medication use in older adults: results of a US consensus panel of experts. *Arch Intern Med.* 2003;163(22):2716–2724. (Correction appeared in *Arch Intern Med.* 2004;164[3]:298.)

Fochtmann LJ, Gelenberg AJ. *Guideline Watch: Practice Guidelines for the Treatment of Major Depressive Disorder.* 2nd ed. Arlington, VA: American Psychiatric Association; 2005. http://www.psych.org/psych_pract/treatg/pg/prac_guide.cfm. Accessed December 20, 2008.

Green M, Wong M, Atkins D, et al. *Diagnosis of Attention Deficit/Hyperactivity Disorder: Technical Review 3* (Publication 99-0050). Rockville, MD: US Department of Health and Human Services, Agency for Health Care Policy and Research; 1999.

Iwuagwu CU, Steiner V, Raji MA. Medical-related cognitive impairments in the elderly. *Clin Geriatr.* 2008;16(8):11–14.

Jacobs DG, Baldessarini RJ, Yeates C, et al. Workgroup on Suicidal Behaviors. *Practice Guidelines for the Assessment and Treatment of Patients with Suicidal Behavior.* Washington, DC: American Psychiatric Association; 2003.

Karasu TB, Gelenberg A, Merriam A, Wang P. American Psychiatric Association's Workgroup on Major Depressive Disorder. *Practice Guidelines for the Treatment of Major Depressive Disorder.* 2nd ed. Washington, DC: American Psychiatric Association; 2000: April.

Keegan MT, Brown DR, Rabinstein AA. Serotonin syndrome from the interaction of cyclobenzaprine and other serotonergic drugs. *Anesth Analg.* 2006;103(6):1466–1468.

Kooij JJ, Boonstra A, Swindles SH, et al. Reliability, validity, and utility of instruments for self-report and informant report concerning symptoms of ADHD in adults. *J Atten Disord.* 2008;11(4):445–458.

Larson EB, Reifier, BV, Sumi SM, et al. Feature of potentially reversible dementia in elderly outpatients. *West J Med.* 1986;145(4):488–492.

Lieberman JA. The Clinical Antipsychotic Trials of Intervention Effectiveness (CATIE) Investigators. Effectiveness of antipsychotic drugs in patients with chronic schizophrenia. *N Engl J Med.* 2005;353(12):1209–1223.

Mason PJ, Morris VA, Balcezak TJ. Serotonin syndrome: presentation of 2 cases and review of the literature. *Medicine.* 2000;79(4):201–209.

Moraga AV, Rodriquez-Pascual C. Accurate diagnosis of delirium in elderly patients. *Curr Opin Psychiatry.* 2007;20(3):262–267.

National Institute on Alcohol Abuse and Alcoholism. *Helping Patients Who Drink Too Much: A Clinician's Guide.* 2005 ed. (updated). http://pubs.niaaa.nih.gov/publications/Practitioner/CliniciansGulide2005/clinicians_guide.htm. Accessed December 16, 2008.

Newcomer JW. Second-generation (atypical) antipsychotics and metabolic effects: a comprehensive literature review. *CNS Drugs.* 2005;19(suppl 1):1–93.

Onion DK, series ed. *The Little Black Book of Psychiatry.* 3rd ed. Sudbury, MA: Jones & Bartlett Publishers; 2006.
Moore DP. Delirium, dementia, and related disorders. 67–112.

Moore DP. Early onset disorders. 22–67.
Moore DP. Eating disorders. 259–264.
Moore DP. Mood disorders. 175–202.
Moore DP. Other conditions. 15.8 Serotonin syndrome. 329–331
Moore DP. Other conditions. 15.12 Suicidal behavior. 336–341.
Moore DP. Schizophrenia and other psychosis. 147–173.
Moore DP. Substance-related disorders. 113–145.

Onion DK, series ed. *The Little Black Book of Primary Care.* 5th ed. Sudbury, MA: Jones & Bartlett Publishers; 2006.
Onion DK. Emergencies. 1.2 Emergency protocols. 2–25.
Onion DK. Emergencies. 1.3 Overdoses/poisonings. 25–48.
Onion DK. Endocrine/metabolism. 5.7 Thyroid diseases. 247–323.
Onion DK. Hematology/oncology. 8.2 Vitamin deficiency anemias. 349–418.
Onion DK, Gershman K. Geriatrics.7.4 Dementia. 422–433.
Onion DK, Neurology. 10.11 Miscellaneous. 772–786.
Onion DK. Pediatrics. 13.4 Infectious/acquired diseases. 882–890.
Onion DK. Psychiatry. 15.1 Medications. 937–949.
Onion DK. Psychiatry. 15.2 Psychiatric diseases. 949–964.

Pagana KD, Pagana TJ. *Mosby's Diagnostic and Laboratory Test Reference.* 8th ed. St. Louis: Mosby Elsevier; 2007 (multiple pages utilized to provide normal reference values for laboratory tests).

Rabins PV, Blacker D, Rovner BW, et al. American Psychiatric Association Work Group on Alzheimer's Disease and other Dementias. American Psychiatric Association practice guidelines for the treatment of Alzheimer's disease and other dementias, 2nd ed. *Am J Psychiatry.* 2007;164 (suppl 12):5–56.

Ramsay JR, Rostain AL. *Cognitive-Behavioral Therapy for Adult ADHS: An Integrative Psychological and Medical Approach.* New York: Routledge; 2007.

Sadock BJ, Saddock VA, Sussman N. *Kaplan & Sadock's Pocket Handbook of Psychiatric Drug Treatment.* 4th ed. Philadelphia: Lippincott Williams & Wilkins; 2006.
Sadock BJ, Saddock VA, Sussman N. Disulfiram and acamprosate. 112–116.
Sadock BJ, Saddock VA, Sussman N. Lithium. 143–156.
Sadock BJ, Saddock VA, Sussman N. Selective serotonin reuptake inhibitors. 193–207.
Sadock BJ, Saddock VA, Sussman N. Sympathomimetics and related drugs. 221–230.

Safren SA, Otto MW, Sprich S, et al. Cognitive-behavioral therapy for ADHD in medication-treated adults with continued symptoms. *Behav Res Ther.* 2005;43:831–842.

Spiegel DR, Dhadwal N, Gill R. "I'm sober, Doctor, really": best biomarkers for underreported alcohol use: when and how to use highly specific combinations to access withdrawal risk. *Curr Psychiatry.* 2008;7(9):15–27.

Terao T, Hikichi T. Serotonin syndrome in a case of depression with various somatic symptoms: the difficulty in differential diagnosis. *Prog Neruopsychopharmacol Biol Psychiatry.* 2007;31(1):295–296.

US Food and Drug Administration. FDA requires warnings about risk of suicidal thoughts and behaviors for antiepileptic medications. *FDA News.* 2008; Dec. 16.

http://www.fda.gov/bbs/topics/NEWS/2008/NEW01927.html. Accessed December 16, 2008.

US Food and Drug Administration. *Labeling Change Request Letter for Antidepressant Medications*. Rockville, MD: Food and Drug Administration; 2004: Oct. 28. http://www.fda.gov/cder/drug/antidepressants/SSRIlabelChange.htm. Accessed December 20, 2008.

Vergare MJ, Binder RL, Cook IA, Galanter M, Lu F. American Psychiatric Association's Workgroup on Psychiatric Evaluation. *Practice Guidelines for the Psychiatric Evaluation of Adults*. 2nd ed. Washington, DC: American Psychiatric Association; 2006: June.

Voelker R. Guideline provides evidence-based advice for treating osteoarthritis of the knee. *JAMA*. 2009;301(5):475–476.

Weiss MD, Weiss JR. A guide to the clinical treatment of adults with ADHD. *J Clin Psychiatry*. 2004;65(suppl 3):27–37.

Williams SH. Medications for treating alcohol dependency. *Am Fam Physician*. 2005;72(9):1775–1780.

Yager J, Halmi KA, Herzog DB, Mitchell JE III, Powers P, Zerbe KJ. American Psychiatric Association's Workgroup on Major Eating Disorders. *Practice Guidelines for the Treatment of Patients with Eating Disorders*. 3rd ed. Washington, DC: American Psychiatric Association; 2006: June.

CHAPTER 11

MISCELLANEOUS CASES IN HEMATOLOGY, DERMATOLOGY, AND INFECTIOUS DISEASES*

CASE 11-1

Monty Nutter

Mr. Nutter is a 62-year-old white male who presents with the chief complaint of "my side hurts." Further clarification revealed that he is experiencing left lateral chest pain, which is sharp in nature, tender to touch, very painful (7–8 out of 10 on the pain scale), and of 2 days' duration. His pain intensifies slightly with deep inspiration, any touch (including shirt and sheet on bed), and heat. Otherwise, he is unaware of any aggravating or alleviating factors. There is no history of trauma. He denies chest pressure, left arm/shoulder pain, diaphoresis, nausea, vomiting, pyrosis, fever, signs of a respiratory infection (including sputum production), dyspnea, wheezing, or pedal edema.

Mr. Nutter's only known medical problem is emphysema. He has never been hospitalized nor had any surgeries. His only medication is an albuterol metered-dose inhaler (MDI) as needed (estimates usage at once per week). He does not take any other prescription or over-the-counter medications, vitamins, supplements, or herbal preparations. He has regular age-appropriate preventive health maintenance check-ups with diagnostic studies and immunizations. He smoked two packs of cigarettes per day for 40 years but quit 5 years ago secondary to the cost of cigarettes.

1. Based on this information, which of the following questions are essential to ask Mr. Nutter and why?

    A. Has he experienced any episodes of strenuous or forceful coughing recently?
    B. Does he have a rash or skin lesion(s) in the area?
    C. Did he have any paresthesias before the onset of the pain?
    D. Did he have varicella as a child?
    E. Has he received the vaccination for herpes zoster?

Patient Responses

He has not experienced any forceful or strenuous coughing episodes recently. He noticed a few erythematous papules yesterday; however, he attributed them to the heating pad he used to try to alleviate the pain. The area did appear to "sting and burn" for a couple of days before it became painful; he is unsure whether the paresthesias are still there because of the intensity of the pain.

He did have varicella when he was in the first grade. He deferred the zoster vaccination.

2. Based on this information, which of the following components of a physical examination are essential to conduct on Mr. Nutter and why?

    A. Eye examination
    B. Heart examination
    C. Lung auscultation
    D. Chest wall examination
    E. Lower leg examination for edema

Physical Examination Findings

Mr. Nutter is 6'0" tall and weighs 180 lb (body mass index [BMI] = 24.4). Other vital signs are blood pressure (BP), 140/76 mm Hg; pulse, 96 beats per minute (BPM) and regular; respiratory rate, 14/min and regular; and oral temperature, 97.6°F.

His conjunctivae are clear. His extraocular motions are normal. His pupils are equal and round and respond to light and accommodation. His funduscopic examination is unremarkable.

His heart is regular in rate and rhythm. There is no murmur, gallops, or rubs. His apical impulse is nondisplaced and without a thrill. His lungs are clear to auscultation.

---

*Remember, for each question, none to all of the answers could be correct/essential or incorrect/nonessential. *See* page 445 for Chapter 11 answers.

He has rare papular lesions, multiple vesicles, a few ulcerations, and minimal crusting on an erythematous base extending from just medial to his spine to his left anterior axillary line between his seventh and eighth ribs. There is no purulent discharge or discoloration to the crusting. (Please see **Figure 11-1**.) Palpation of the lesions elicits tenderness, but the underlying bony structure is not tender.

He does not have any pedal edema.

3. Based on this information, which of the following diagnostic studies are essential to perform on Mr. Nutter and why?

A. Skin biopsy of lesions
B. Chest x-ray (CXR)
C. Radiograph of left ribs
D. Electrocardiograph (ECG)
E. Complete blood count with differential (CBC w/diff)

Diagnostic Test Results

His skin biopsy is pending.

His CXR revealed normally inflated lungs and no acute changes. His left rib radiographs were negative for fracture. His ECG revealed normal sinus rhythm (NSR) at a rate of 95 BPM and no abnormalities. His CBC w/diff was unremarkable.

4. Based on this information, which one of the following is Mr. Nutter's most likely diagnosis and why?

A. Herpes simplex dermatitis
B. Herpes zoster
C. Angina
D. Left rib contusion
E. Contact dermatitis

5. Based on this diagnosis, which of the following are appropriate components of a treatment plan for Mr. Nutter and why?

A. Valacyclovir 1000 mg three times a day for 7 days
B. Prednisolone starting at 60 mg daily, then gradually tapering-off over 3 weeks
C. Acetaminophen with codeine #3 four times a day on a regular basis for 1 week
D. Triple antibiotic ointment twice a day to lesions

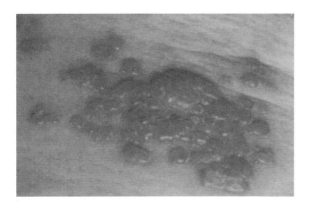

Figure 11-1 Vesiclular lesions characterizing his rash.

E. Advise him to discuss with household members and persons with whom he has had close or intimate contact their risk of acquiring a varicella-zoster virus (VZV) infection from him

CASE 11-2
Nina Olive

Nina is a 14-year-old Hispanic American female who presents crying because "my skin is peeling off." She is accompanied by her mother. Although her chief complaint only started this morning, Nina's illness actually began approximately 5 days ago. At that time she was completely asymptomatic until she awoke with marked fatigue, anorexia, nausea, vomiting, fever of 101.2°F (taken orally), chills, generalized headache, generalized arthralgias, and a sore throat. She did not experience diarrhea, constipation, other bowel changes, abdominal pain, vaginal discharge, or vaginal odor.

The following morning, Nina awoke with a fine, rough, moderately erythematous rash on her neck and in her axillae. By the subsequent morning, it had spread to encompass her entire body and had turned bright red in color. By the fourth day of her illness, she was feeling somewhat better. She was afebrile and no longer experiencing chills, arthralgias, headache, nausea, and vomiting; however, she was still somewhat anorexic, slightly fatigued with a mild sore throat. Not only did the rash persist, but also it now appeared to be increasing in the intensity of the erythema in her axillae, groin, and extensor surfaces of her elbows and knees.

Today, when she awoke, she was no longer anorexic or as fatigued. Her sore throat had further lessened in severity; however, it is still not completely resolved. However, her primary concern is that the skin on her face was "peeling." A couple of hours later, she noticed that the desquamation had expanded to involve her neck and anterior chest. She is frightened that "all my skin is going to come off."

Her mother is wondering if the rash and desquamation could be the result of an allergic reaction to a strawberry-scented bubble bath that Nina initially used a few days before becoming ill. Otherwise, there have not been any changes in soaps, deodorants, detergents, fabric softeners, linens, clothing, or other articles that might have come in contact with Nina's skin.

Her mother states that Nina has no known medical problems, has never had surgery, and has never been hospitalized. Nina was taking acetaminophen for the fever and arthralgias; however, she discontinued it when her symptoms resolved. Currently, she is not taking any prescription or over-the-counter medications, vitamins, supplements, or herbal preparations. She is not allergic to any medications. She is currently finishing a normal menstrual period. She denies being sexually active, smoking cigarettes, drinking alcohol, or using illicit substances. She is not aware of anyone else with similar symptoms. Her family history is noncontributory.

1. Based on this information, which of the following questions are essential to ask Nina and why?

A. Does she use pads, tampons, or both?
B. Did the rash involve the palms of her hands or the soles of her feet?

    C. Has she experienced any otalgia, rhinorrhea, nasal congestion, sinus pressure, postnasal discharge, eye discharge, cough, wheezing, or dyspnea?

    D. Has she experienced any pruritus with her rash?

    E. Which joints were affected by the arthralgias and were they erythematous, edematous, or hot to the touch?

Patient Responses

Nina states that she uses pads only during her menstrual periods. The rash did not involve the soles of her feet or the palms of her hands. It was slightly pruritic at the onset and again now in the areas of desquamation. She has not experienced otalgia, rhinorrhea, nasal congestion, sinus pressure, postnasal discharge, eye discharge, cough, wheezing, or dyspnea with her current illness. All of her joints were involved with the arthralgias; however, none of them were red, hot, or swollen.

2. Based on this information, which of the following components of a physical examination are essential to conduct on Nina and why?

    A. Ears, nose, and throat examination

    B. Lymph node examination

    C. Heart examination

    D. Pelvic examination

    E. Skin examination

Physical Examination Findings

Nina is 5'1" tall and weighs 101 lb. Other vital signs are BP, 96/58 mm Hg; pulse, 92 BPM and regular; respiratory rate, 12/min and regular; and oral temperature, 99.1°F.

Her external auditory canals are brightly erythematous but not edematous or associated with any discharge. Her tympanic membranes are nonerythematous, not injected, in normal position, and fully mobile. Her nasal mucosa is slightly erythematous, but not edematous, and does not reveal any discharge. Her oral mucosa and hard palate are moderately erythematous but without edema, lesions, or discharge. Her pharynx is very erythematous and her soft palate has small petechiae on an erythematous base. Her tonsils are enlarged, erythematous, and with a small amount of whitish exudates. Her tongue is bright red and papillae more visible ("strawberry tongue").

Her cervical lymph nodes are slightly enlarged and slightly tender in her anterior and posterior chains. Her preauricular, supraclavicular, infraclavicular, axillary, and inguinal lymph nodes are not palpable.

Her heart is regular in rate and rhythm, without any murmurs, rubs, or gallops. Her apical impulse is nondisplaced and without a thrill. Her lungs are clear to auscultation.

Her pelvic examination is normal.

Her entire body, except the soles of her feet, the palms of her hands, and her perioral area, is covered with a bright erythematous, "sunburn"-appearing rash (see **Figure 11-2**) with a darker erythema in her axillary area, groin area, flexure surface of her elbows, flexure aspects of her knees, and waistline (Pastia lines). It is composed of discrete papules that are rough and "sandpaper"-like in texture; the papules blanch except in the Pastia lines. There is mild desquamation of the skin at the corners of her mouth, nose, and eyes as well as across her forehead and in a patchy distribution on her neck and anterior chest. A Nikolsky sign is negative.

3. Based on this information, which of the following diagnostic studies are essential to perform on Nina and why?

    A. Rapid strep screen of the throat

    B. Throat culture, if rapid strep screen is negative

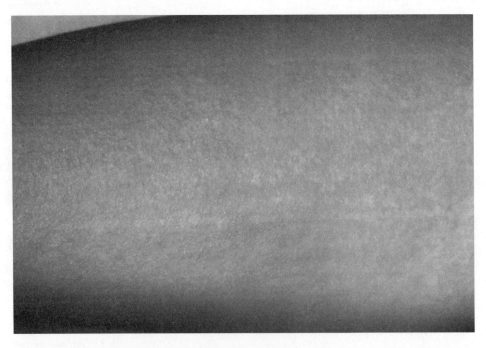

Figure 11-2 Characteristic fine, erythematous, papules of Nina's most likely diagnosis.
Source: Courtesy of CDC.

C. Skin culture
D. Immunofluorescence skin biopsy
E. Complete blood count with differential (CBC w/diff)

Diagnostic Test Results

Her rapid strep screen was negative. Her CBC was normal except for a mild leukocytosis of 15,250 mm³ (normal adult and children older than 2 years: 5,000–10,000) with 83% neutrophils (normal: 55–70), 11% lymphocytes (normal: 20–40), 2% monocytes (normal: 2–8), 3% eosinophils (normal: 1–4), and 1% basophils (normal: 0.5–1).

Her throat culture, skin culture, and skin biopsy results are pending.

4. Based on this information, which one of the following is Nina's most likely diagnosis and why?

A. Scarlet fever
B. Staphylococcal scalded skin syndrome
C. Erythema infectiosum
D. Toxic shock syndrome
E. Contact dermatitis caused by bubble bath

5. Based on this diagnosis, which of the following are appropriate components of a treatment plan for Nina and why?

A. Penicillin 500 mg four times a day for 10 days
B. Advise her not to use any more of the strawberry bubble bath
C. Advise her that only the very top layer of her skin will "peel" off; however, it will likely occur all over her body and can take up to 6 weeks before completed
D. Encourage her not to "pick, scratch, or peel" the skin because of the risk of secondary infection
E. Advise her of the signs and symptoms of secondary infection and to return to clinic immediately if they occur

CASE 11-3
Owen Pickens

Mr. Pickens is a 25-year-old white male who presents with the chief complaint of "a spot on my leg." It is painless, blackish-brown in color, and located on the posterior aspect of his right calf. He first noticed it yesterday. Today, it is much larger (estimated at approximately 150% of yesterday's size).

Mr. Pickens denies any trauma to the area; however, he does note that the lesion appears to be located in the same area in which he experienced some pain approximately 5 days ago while on a hiking trip. At that time, he attributed the discomfort to the elastic in his higher-topped socks that he wore for the first time that day. In fact, wearing his socks "rolled down" significantly decreased his pain almost immediately, and within a couple of hours, the pain was completely resolved. However, the area was still "achy" feeling, slightly itchy, and "a little" swollen. By the next morning, his leg was completely asymptomatic. Thinking about it now, he remembers experiencing some mild intermittent itching of the area since his hiking trip. To his knowledge he was not bitten/stung by an insect nor did he experience trauma to the area.

He has no known medical problems, has never had any surgeries, and has never been hospitalized. He is not taking any prescription or over-the-counter medications, vitamins, supplements, or herbal preparations. He is not allergic to any medications. He has never been married and is sexually active with women only. He does not have a current partner and has not had intercourse in approximately 4 months. He does not smoke cigarettes, drink alcohol, or use illicit drugs. His family history is negative.

1. Based on this information, which of the following questions are essential to ask Mr. Pickens and why?

A. Following the initial pain, swelling, and itchiness that occurred on his camping trip, did he develop "flulike" symptoms, a rash, or other skin lesion(s)?
B. Where did he go on his camping trip?
C. Has he experienced hematuria, bleeding of his gums when flossing or brushing his teeth, bruising more easily, taking longer to stop bleeding, or other signs of a bleeding diathesis since he first experienced his leg symptoms?
D. Did the leg pain or swelling that he experienced on his camping trip return?
E. Has he experienced restlessness, myoclonus, uncontrollable shaking, blurred vision, marked lacrimation, excessive salivation, profuse rhinorrhea, diaphoresis, tachycardia, palpitations, slurred speech, or high fever associated with the enlarging lesion?

Patient Responses

The day following his initial leg symptoms, he awoke feeling nauseated and feverish (but did not have access to a thermometer) and experiencing chills, generalized arthralgias, and myalgias. He vomited once only following breakfast. He did not have diarrhea. He attributed these symptoms to "a touch of food poisoning" from fish they had caught in a nearby stream.

By evening he was feeling somewhat better but noticed he had an asymptomatic, "weird-looking," "target-like" lesion on the posterior aspect of his right calf. He further described the lesion as being raised and purplish in the center, surrounded by a ring of "whiter than usual" looking skin, and surrounded by another, larger "reddish" ring. The following day, it did not look as "bright"; however, it appeared that a vesicle was starting to develop in the middle of the central purplish-colored area. Because it was asymptomatic, he really didn't "give it much more thought." However, while he was showering last night, he remembered the lesion and "decided to see what it looked like"; that was when he discovered the painless, blackish-brown lesion. He and his friends went hiking in the Mississippi valley.

He has not experienced hematuria, bleeding of his gums when brushing/flossing his teeth, bruising more easily, or being slower to stop bleeding since the onset of symptoms. The leg pain and swelling have not returned. Furthermore, he has not experienced any restlessness, myoclonus, uncontrollable shaking, blurred vision, marked lacrimation, excessive salivation, profuse rhinorrhea, diaphoresis, tachycardia, palpitations, slurred speech, or high fever since his leg symptoms began, let alone within the past 24 hours.

2. Based on this information, which of the following components of the physical examination are essential to conduct on Mr. Pickens and why?

    A. Heart examination
    B. Lung examination
    C. Skin examination
    D. Genital examination
    E. Inguinal lymph node examination

Physical Examination Findings

Mr. Pickens is 6'3" tall and weighs 175 lb (BMI = 21.9). Other vital signs are BP, 108/68 mm Hg; pulse, 68 BPM and regular; respiratory rate, 12/min and regular; and oral temperature, 99.2°F.

His heart is regular in rate and rhythm without murmurs, gallops, or rubs. His lungs are clear to auscultation bilaterally.

His skin is without lesions except for a slightly irregular, necrotic-appearing, blackish-brown circular 3-cm superficial ulcer on the medial/posterior aspect of his right calf approximately 10 cm above his medial malleolus. There appears to be mild to moderate eschar formation in the center. It is not tender to palpate, but it is slightly cooler than the surrounding skin. However, the surrounding skin is slightly erythematous, but not edematous, to approximately 2 cm beyond the edges of this lesion. His calves are not tender to palpate bilaterally. His calf circumferences, measured at three equivalent locations, are equal in size. There is no pitting edema bilaterally. His feet are warm to touch and with good capillary refill.

His genitalia are without any gross abnormalities/deformities. His testicles are descended bilaterally and are smooth, without masses, and nontender. There is no evidence of a hernia. He does not have any skin discoloration, rash, or lesions. His inguinal lymph nodes are not palpable and nontender, bilaterally.

3. Based on this information, which of the following diagnostic studies are essential to perform on Mr. Pickens and why?

    A. Urinalysis (U/A)
    B. Complete blood count with differential (CBC w/diff)
    C. Prothrombin time (PT) and partial thromboplastin time (PTT)
    D. Renal function studies
    E. Culture and sensitivity (C&S) of the lesion

Diagnostic Test Results

Mr. Pickens' urine was moderate to dark yellow in color, clear, and with normal odor. His pH was 6.5 (normal: 4.6–8.0) and his specific gravity was 1.015 (normal: 1.005–1.030). His dipstick was negative for nitrites, leukocyte esterase, glucose, protein, and ketones (normal: negative). His microscopic examination revealed 1 to 2 white blood cells (WBCs; normal: 0–4), no WBC casts (normal: 0), 2 to 3 red blood cells (RBCs, normal: ≤ 2), no RBC casts (normal: 0), no bacteria (normal: none), and no crystals or casts (normal: none) per low-power field.

His CBC revealed an RBC count of $4.9 \times 10^6/\mu l$ (normal male: 4.7–6.1) with a mean corpuscular volume (MCV) of $83.8 \ \mu m^3$ (normal adult: 80–95), a mean corpuscular hemoglobin (MCH) of 30 pg (normal adult: 27–31), a mean corpuscular hemoglobin concentration (MCHC) of 32.2 g/dl (normal adult: 32–36), and a red blood cell distribution width (RDW) of 12.5% (normal adult: 11–14.5). His WBC count was $5500/mm^3$ (normal adult: 5,000–10,000) with 62% neutrophils (normal: 55–70), 30% lymphocytes (normal: 20–40), 4% monocytes (normal: 2–8), 4% eosinophils (normal: 1–4), and 1% basophils (normal: 0.5–1). His hemoglobin (Hgb) was 14.8 g/dl (normal adult male: 14–18) and his hematocrit (HCT) was 46% (normal male: 42–52). His platelet (thrombocyte) count was $125,000/mm^3$ (normal adult: 150,000–400,000) and his mean platelet volume (MPV) was 7.9 fl (normal: 7.4–10.4). His smear was consistent with these results and revealed no cellular abnormalities.

His PT was 12.0 seconds (normal: 11.0–12.5) and his PTT was 67 seconds (normal: 60–70). His blood urea nitrogen (BUN) was 18 mg/dl (normal adult: 10–20) and his creatinine was 1.0 mg/dl (normal adult male: 0.6–1.2). His C&S of the lesion is pending.

4. Based on this information, which one of the following is Mr. Pickens' most likely diagnosis and why?

    A. Lyme disease
    B. Rocky Mountain spotted fever
    C. Brown recluse spider envenomation with mild loxoscelism
    D. Toxic epidermal necrolysis
    E. Erythema multiforme major

5. Based on this diagnosis, which of the following are appropriate components of a treatment plan for Mr. Pickens and why?

    A. Tetracycline 500 mg four times a day for 7 to 10 days
    B. Surgical consult for débridement and possible excision with skin grafting
    C. Dapsone 50 mg once daily
    D. Diphenhydramine 25 to 50 mg every 4 to 6 hours as needed for itch up to four times per day
    E. Hyperbaric oxygen therapy

CASE 11-4
Paul Queen

Mr. Queen is a 67-year-old white male who presents with the chief complaint of "a rash on my elbows and knees." For approximately 3 months, he has been experiencing itchy, thickened, slightly scaly areas on the extensor surfaces of his knees and elbows. The lesions have gradually increased in size since their onset. He does not know of any skin lesions elsewhere on his body. He has not changed soaps, lotions, laundry detergents, fabric softeners, or any other products that regularly come in contact with these areas. Other than some mild, nonprogressing fatigue, which started at approximately the same time as these skin lesions, he claims he "feels fine."

His only medical problem is hypertension (diagnosed approximately 6 months ago). He has never had any surgeries nor been hospitalized. His only medication is propranolol 50 mg daily (which is effectively controlling his hypertension) which he has taken since he was diagnosed with hypertension.

He does not take any other prescription or over-the-counter medications, vitamins, supplements, or herbal preparations.

He had an age-appropriate preventive health examination with diagnostic testing, immunization, and patient education approximately 6 months ago. He has been married for 49 years and does not have any sexual partners other than his wife. He admits to drinking alcohol "occasionally" (defined as a 12 pack of beer every Friday and Saturday night) and has done so since he was 17 years old. He quit smoking 20 years ago. His family history is noncontributory.

1. Based on this information, which of the following questions are essential to ask Mr. Queen and why?

   A. Does he find himself scratching the affected areas?
   B. Has he ever had this type of skin lesion, or a similar one, in the past?
   C. Does he have any changes of his nails or itching/flaking of his scalp?
   D. Is he experiencing any arthralgias, oral lesions, eye injection/erythema, eye discharge, penile discharge, dysuria, urinary urgency, or urinary frequency?
   E. Has he recently had strep throat?

Patient Responses

Although the rash itches, he rarely scratches it. He has had a similar but much milder form of the rash for most of his adult life. It was predominately located on the extensor surfaces of his knees; however, he did occasionally experience some elbow involvement as well. It seemed to occur if he worked "on his knees" frequently or if he bumped his knee or elbow (Koebner phenomenon). Since he retired from carpentry work, he rarely got the lesions until this current exacerbation. He hasn't noticed any nail changes; however, he states "they've always looked beat up." He has always had problems with "dandruff." He denies any arthritis, arthralgias, mouth lesions, eye injection, eye erythema, eye discharge, penile discharge, dysuria, urinary urgency, or urinary frequency. To his knowledge, he has never had strep throat.

2. Based on this information, which of the following components of a physical examination are essential to conduct on Mr. Queen and why?

   A. CAGE alcohol screen
   B. Oral examination
   C. Skin examination
   D. Scalp examination
   E. Nail examination

Physical Examination Findings

Mr. Queen is 5'11" tall and weighs 180 lb (BMI = 25). Other vital signs are BP, 136/78 mm Hg; pulse, 92 BPM and regular; respirations, 12/min and regular; and oral temperature, 98.7°F.

He responds negatively to all four CAGE questions. His oral examination is negative.

Mr. Queen has extensive scaly, silvery-colored, rough, well-demarked, symmetric plaques on an erythematous base located on the flexure surfaces of both of his elbows and knees.

Scraping of a scale causes bleeding (positive Auspitz sign). No other skin lesions are noted. His scalp is "flaky"; however, no discrete skin lesions are identifiable. His fingernails and toenails are finely stippled (pitted), with the fingernails being much more involved.

3. Based on this information, which of the following diagnostic studies are essential to perform on Mr. Queen and why?

   A. Potassium hydroxide preparation (KOH prep) of skin lesions
   B. Human immunodeficiency virus (HIV) testing
   C. Antistreptolysin O titer (ASO)
   D. Complete blood count with differential (CBC w/diff) and coagulation studies
   E. Skin biopsy

Diagnostic Test Results

The KOH prep of his skin lesions was negative for hyphae and budding yeast (normal: negative). His HIV test, ASO titer, CBC w/diff, and coagulation studies were normal.

His skin biopsy is pending.

4. Based on this information, which one of the following is Mr. Queen's most likely diagnosis and why?

   A. Guttate (eruptive) psoriasis
   B. Plaque-type psoriasis exacerbated by beta-blocker and binge drinking
   C. Erythrodermic psoriasis exacerbated by beta-blocker
   D. Lichen simplex chronicus
   E. Reactive arthritis (Reiter syndrome)

5. Based on this diagnosis, which of the following are appropriate components of a treatment plan for Mr. Queen and why?

   A. High-potency corticosteroid ointment twice a day for 2 weeks, then decrease to once a day if responding
   B. Calcipotriene ointment twice a day for 2 weeks, then decrease to once a day if responding
   C. Clotrimazole ointment twice a day for 2 weeks, then decrease to once a day if responding
   D. Change propranolol to another antihypertensive outside of the beta-blocker class
   E. Encourage him to stop, or at least significantly decrease, his alcohol consumption because of the likely effect it is having on his psoriasis and blood pressure

CASE 11-5
Rachel Smith

Rachel is a 5-year-old white female accompanied by her mother, who provided the chief complaint of "pain under her right arm." It has been present for approximately 3 days and is worsening. It is alleviated with children's acetaminophen. To her mother's knowledge there are no other alleviating or aggravating factors. There is no known history of trauma.

Rachel is also experiencing a fever that has been as high as 101.4°F (orally), sore throat, anorexia, nausea without vomiting, malaise, fatigue, and a mild (2 out of 10 on the pain scale) generalized headache. Acetaminophen is also effective in alleviating her headache and fever. She has not experienced any rhinorrhea, nasal congestion, otalgia, sneezing, stiff/painful neck, diarrhea, constipation, abdominal pain, cough, wheezing, dyspnea, or chest pain.

She has no known medical problems. She has never been hospitalized nor had any surgeries. Her only medication is children's acetaminophen three to four times per day for fever and pain. She does not take any other over-the-counter or prescription medications, vitamins, supplements, or herbal preparations. She is not allergic to any medication.

Her age-appropriate well check-ups, including immunizations, are up to date. Her last purified protein derivative (PPD) test was 1 month ago before she entered school and it was negative (no reaction at all). Her last diphtheria, tetanus, and acellular pertussis (DTaP) was given at the same time. No one else in her family is ill.

1. Based on this information, which of the following questions are essential to ask Rachel and/or her mother and why?

   A. Has Rachel been in contact with a cat or kitten? If yes, could she have been scratched, bitten, or licked by it; where is the animal located; what is its current health; and is it current on its rabies vaccination?
   B. Has Rachel experienced any type of a rash within the past 2 months?
   C. Has she been complaining of arthralgias or bone pain?
   D. Has she experienced any eye discharge, conjunctival injection, eye pain, or photophobia?
   E. Which hand is her dominant one?

Patient Responses

According to her mother, Rachel has a kitten that is "always scratching her." It is kept in their home, current on its rabies immunizations, and not ill. Her mother did notice that approximately 2 weeks ago, one of the kitten's scratches developed into a pustule. It was asymptomatic and resolved spontaneously within a "couple of days." Otherwise, she has not had rash or skin lesions within the past 2 months.

Rachel has not been complaining of (nor has her mother noticed) any arthralgias, bone pain, eye discharge, conjunctival injection, eye pain, or photophobia. Rachel is right-handed.

2. Based on this information, which of the following components of a physical examination are essential to conduct on Rachel and why?

   A. General appearance
   B. Lymph node examination
   C. Heart examination
   D. Abdominal examination
   E. Bilateral hand/arm/shoulder/axilla examination

Physical Examination Results

Rachel is 40" tall and weighs 41 lb. Other vital signs are BP, 80/56 mm Hg; pulse, 110 BPM and regular; respiratory rate, 18/min and regular; and oral temperature, 99.1°F.

She is resting comfortably on her mother's lap. She appears slightly ill, but definitely not toxic.

She has a single, slightly firm, slightly tender, palpable right lateral axillary lymph node of approximately 1.5 cm in size. She also has a single, firm, nontender, palpable right epitrochlear lymph node of approximately 0.5 cm in size. She does not have any additional palpable nodes in her right or left axillary and epitrochlear regions. Her cervical, preauricular, supraclavicular, infraclavicular, and inguinal lymph nodes are not palpable.

Her heart is regular in rate and rhythm. There is no murmur, rub, or gallop. Her apical impulse is not displaced and does not reveal a thrill.

Her bowel sounds are normoactive and equal in all four quadrants. She does not have any masses, organomegaly, or tenderness. Her renal arteries and aorta are without bruits. Her aorta is normal size without an abnormal pulsation or bruit.

The dorsum of both of her hands reveals multiple superficial excoriations. Additionally, she has a scabbed area of approximately 5 mm in size that is healing nicely on the dorsum of her right hand (her mother states this is the location of the pustule). Otherwise, there are no discolorations, rashes, lesions, temperature alterations, edema, or tenderness present on her upper extremities, including shoulders.

The musculoskeletal examination, including long bone palpation, is unremarkable.

3. Based on this information, which of the following diagnostic tests are essential to perform on Rachel and why?

   A. Abdominal ultrasound
   B. Biopsy with Gram stain, culture and sensitivity of the largest affected lymph node
   C. Purified protein derivative (PPD) skin test
   D. Spinal tap for cerebrospinal fluid (CSF) analysis including Gram stain and culture with sensitivity
   E. Serology for *Bartonella henselae* titer

Diagnostic Test Results

Her abdominal ultrasound was normal. Her *Bartonella henselae* titer was 1:256 (negative for acute infection: < 1:64). Her lymph node biopsy, PPD test, and spinal tap analysis are pending.

4. Based on this information, which one of the following is Rachel's most likely diagnosis and why?

   A. Atypical cat-scratch disease
   B. Infectious mononucleosis
   C. Lymphogranuloma venereum
   D. Typical cat-scratch disease
   E. Burkitt lymphoma

5. Based on this diagnosis, which of the following are appropriate components of a treatment plan for Rachel and why?

   A. Continue acetaminophen
   B. Doxycycline 100 mg with rifampin 300 mg twice a day for 4 to 6 weeks
   C. Ciprofloxacin 500 mg twice a day for 2 weeks
   D. Diphtheria, tetanus, and acellular pertussis (DTaP)
   E. Have vet decapitate the cat and send its head to the state health department to be examined for rabies

CASE 11-6

Sabrina Tabatherson

Ms. Tabatherson is an 18-year-old white female who presents with the chief complaint of "a cough." It began approximately 3 weeks ago; and, initially, she thought she just had a "cold." In the beginning, her cough was nonproductive and associated with rhinorrhea, sneezing, nasal congestion, postnasal discharge, epiphora, and anorexia. She did not have any fever, chills, wheezing, dyspnea, or chest pain tightness.

After approximately 5 to 6 days, her symptoms began gradually improving. However, yesterday she began experiencing "spasms" of cough associated with dyspnea and a high-pitched "weird" sound with inspiration that began and ended suddenly without any provocation. These brief episodes leave her feeling "drained" and slightly dyspneic. However, her cough remains nonproductive. This morning she awoke with the lateral aspect of her left eye being "red"; thereby causing her to decide to be evaluated.

Ms. Tabatherson does not have any problems with her vision, eye pain, photophobia, or discharge. She doesn't think she has been running a fever. She has not experienced any nausea, vomiting, pyrosis, reflux of stomach contents, diarrhea, constipation, or any other bowel change. She also denies any dizziness, vertigo, presyncope, syncope, chest pain/pressure/discomfort, or palpitations.

She is not taking any prescription or over-the-counter medications, vitamins, supplements, or herbal preparations. She is not allergic to any medications. She has no known medical problems, has never had surgery, and has never been hospitalized. Her last menstrual period was 1 week ago and normal. She is not sexually active. Her family history is negative.

1. Based on this information, which of the following questions are essential to ask Ms. Tabatherson and why?

   A. What has been the pattern of her cough since becoming ill?
   B. Does she experience dyspnea between coughing episodes?
   C. Are her immunizations up to date, including a recent tetanus toxoid, diphtheria toxoid and acellular pertussis (Tdap) vaccine?
   D. What color is her rhinorrhea?
   E. Has she ever had pertussis, or "whooping cough"?

Patient Responses

Ms. Tabatherson states that her cough is currently worse at night; however, initially, it occurred more during the daytime and only occasionally at night. She does not experience any dyspnea between coughing episodes. Her rhinorrhea is clear. She did not receive a Tdap vaccine as a preteen or as an adolescent. She has never had pertussis.

2. Based on this information, which of the following components of a physical examination are essential to conduct on Ms. Tabatherson and why?

   A. Ear, nose, and throat (ENT) examination
   B. Bilateral eye examination
   C. Heart examination
   D. Lung examination
   E. Abdominal examination

Physical Examination Findings

Ms. Tabatherson is 5'4" tall and weighs 115 lb (BMI = 19.7). Other vital signs are BP, 100/76 mm Hg; pulse, 88 BPM and regular; respiratory rate, 10/min and regular; and oral temperature, 98.6°F.

Her ear canals are normal color without edema or abnormal discharge. Her tympanic membranes are normal color and noninjected and display normal movement. There is no evidence of a middle ear effusion or lesion, bilaterally. Her nasal mucosa is slightly erythematous, is slightly edematous, and has a small amount of clear discharge. Her oral mucosa is normal except for a few isolated petechiae on her hard and soft palate. Her pharynx is slightly erythematous with no tonsillar enlargement, exudates, or postnasal discharge.

Her left sclera reveals a brightly erythematous area in the lateral aspect that is well demarked at its superior and lateral borders but not as distinct at its inferior edge. There is a slightly yellow appearing area below it; however, the remainder of her left sclera is white. The area is not connected to her iris. (Please see **Figure 11-3**.) Her right sclera is unremarkable. Her lower eyelids reveal a moderate amount of petechiae bilaterally. Her pupils are round and equal and react to light and accommodation, bilaterally. Her funduscopic examination is normal.

Her heart is regular in rate and rhythm and without murmurs, gallops, or rubs. Her apical impulse is nondisplaced and without thrills. Her lungs reveal rhonchi in the lower bases, bilaterally. Otherwise, they are unremarkable.

Her abdominal examination is unremarkable.

3. Based on this information, which of the following diagnostic studies are essential to perform on Ms. Tabatherson and why?

   A. White blood cell count with differential (WBC w/diff)
   B. Nasal swab for culture on Bordet-Gengou agar and a DNA polymerase chain reaction (PCR) assay for *Bordetella pertussis*
   C. Enzyme-linked immunosorbent assay (ELISA) IgA and IgG serum antibody titers for pertussis
   D. Chest x-ray (CXR)
   E. Electroencephalogram (EEG)

Diagnostic Findings

Ms. Tabatherson's WBC w/diff revealed a leukocytosis of 29,250 mm^3 (normal adult and children older than 2 years: 5,000–10,000) with 11% neutrophils (normal: 55–70), 78% lymphocytes (normal: 20–40), 5% monocytes (normal: 2–8), 4% eosinophils (normal: 1–4), and 1% basophils (normal: 0.5–1).

Her DNA PCR was positive (normal: negative) and her ELISA IgA and IgG for *Bordetella pertussis* are both positive at 1:64 and 1:32 (normal: negative for both), respectively.

Her CXR and EEG were both normal. Her nasal culture is pending.

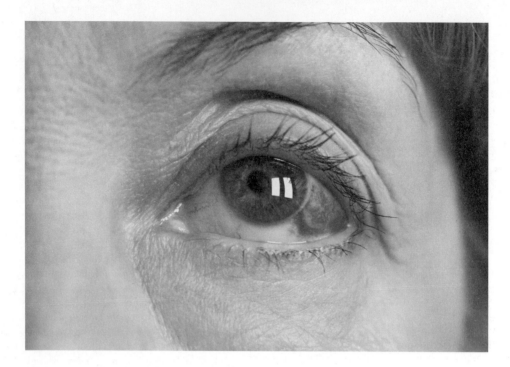

Figure 11-3 Erythematous area of Ms. Tabatherson's sclera.
Source: © Susan Law Cain/ShutterStock, Inc.

4. Based on this information, which one of the following is Ms. Tabatherson's most likely diagnosis and why?

   A. Bronchiolitis
   B. Pertussis with subconjunctival hemorrhage probably secondary to cough
   C. Acute asthma
   D. Gastroesophageal reflux disease (GERD)
   E. Adenovirus infection

5. Based on this diagnosis, which of the following are appropriate components of a treatment plan for Ms. Tabatherson and why?

   A. Azithromycin 250 mg two tablets stat, then one tablet a day for 2 to 5 more days
   B. Erythromycin estolate 500 mg twice a day for 5 days
   C. Prophylaxis of household/dormitory contacts
   D. Esomeprazole 20 mg once a day
   E. Prednisone tapered over 14 days, starting with 60 mg

CASE 11-7
Tami Upjohn

Ms. Upjohn is a 24-year-old white female who presents with the chief complaint of "abdominal pain" for one day. It is located in her right upper quadrant, achy in nature, and moderate (5 out of 10 on the pain scale) in intensity. It does not radiate; however, she is also experiencing a burning epigastric discomfort. It is associated with severe nausea and vomiting. She estimates vomiting a minimum of 20 times since its onset. The emesis did not contain any blood or dark, "coffee

grounds"-appearing material; however, it consisted of bile with undigested food and pill fragments (if occurring shortly after ingesting them). She tried calcium carbonate over-the-counter antacids this morning, and they "might have helped" the epigastric burning slightly. She is not aware of any other aggravating or alleviating factors.

Otherwise, she is asymptomatic, including being afebrile and without lower abdominal pain. She was diagnosed with pelvic inflammatory disease (PID) 4 days ago. At that time, she was given ceftriaxone 250 mg IM and was started on a combination of oral doxycycline 100 mg twice daily and metronidazole 500 mg twice daily for 14 days. She was reevaluated 48 hours later and was much improved.

Her medications consist of oral contraceptives (the name of which she doesn't know) daily for 21 days every 28 days, doxycycline 100 mg twice daily, metronidazole 500 mg twice daily, and the single dose of calcium carbonate antacid earlier today. She is not taking any other prescription or over-the-counter medications, vitamins, supplements, or herbal preparations. She has no known drug allergies. Her partner has not been evaluated or received treatment; however, she has not resumed intercourse. She has not missed any doses of her oral contraceptives or her antibiotics.

On her initial visit, her CBC w/diff was normal except for a leukocytosis of 17,750 mm^3 (normal adult: 5,000–10,000) with 81% neutrophils (normal: 55–70), 12% lymphocytes (normal: 20–40), 2% monocytes (normal: 2–8), 4% eosinophils (normal: 1–4), and 1% basophils (normal: 0.5–1). Her erythrocyte sedimentation rate (ESR) was 55 mm/hr (normal female: < 20), her urinary human chorionic gonadotropin (HCG) test was negative (normal: negative), and her DNA amplification testing for both gonorrhea and chlamydia came back positive (normal: negative).

1. Based on this information, which of the following questions are essential to ask Ms. Upjohn and why?

    A. When was her last menstrual period (LMP) and was it normal?

    B. Has she had any constipation, diarrhea, or color change of her stool?

    C. Has she noticed any changes in her skin or yellowing of her sclera?

    D. Has she had any nasal discharge?

    E. Has she been drinking any alcohol?

Patient Responses

Ms. Upjohn's LMP was 3.5 weeks ago and normal. She denies constipation, diarrhea, color change of her stool, color change of her skin or sclera, a rash, nasal discharge, or drinking any alcohol.

2. Based on this information, which of the following components of a physical examination are essential to conduct on Ms. Upjohn and why?

    A. Ear and nose examination

    B. Sclera and skin examination

    C. Abdominal examination

    D. Pelvic examination

    E. Back examination

Physical Examination Findings

Ms. Upjohn is 5'5" tall and weighs 132 lb (BMI = 22). Other vital signs are BP, 112/72 mm Hg; pulse, 86 BPM and regular; respirations, 13/min and regular; and oral temperature, 98.7°F.

Her ears and nose are unremarkable. Her sclerae do not show any icterus. Her skin does not reveal any rash or jaundice.

Her abdominal examination reveals normoactive bowel sounds that are equal in all four quadrants. She has slight epigastric and right upper quadrant tenderness without rebound. There are no other areas of tenderness. There are no masses or organomegaly.

Her external genitalia and vaginal mucosa are normal in appearance and free from lesions. Her cervix is still slightly erythematous and friable but without any visible discharge. She still has a slight amount of cervical motion tenderness. Her uterus and ovaries are normal size but without any masses, enlargement, or tenderness.

Her back examination is unremarkable.

3. Based on this information, which of the following diagnostic studies are essential to perform on Ms. Upjohn and why?

    A. Abdominal ultrasound

    B. Repeat Complete blood count with differential (CBC w/diff) and erythrocyte sedimentation rate (ESR)

    C. Repeat testing for gonorrhea and chlamydia

    D. Liver function tests (LFTs)

    E. Testing for hepatitis B and C

    F. Electrolytes

Diagnostic Test Results

Ms. Upjohn's abdominal ultrasound did not reveal any abnormalities.

Her repeat CBC w/diff was normal except for a leukocytosis of 12,750 mm³ (normal adult: 5,000–10,000) with 71% neutrophils (normal: 55–70), 22% lymphocytes (normal: 20–40), 3% monocytes (normal: 2–8), 3% eosinophils (normal: 1–4), and 1% basophils (normal: 0.5–1). Her ESR was 32 mm/hr (normal female: < 20).

Her repeat urinary HCG test was negative (normal: negative) and DNA amplification testing for both gonorrhea and chlamydia were positive (normal: negative).

Her LFTs revealed a total protein of 6.8 g/dl (normal: 6.4–8.3), albumin of 3.9 g/dl (normal: 3.5–5.0), total bilirubin of 0.5 mg/dl (normal: 0.3–1.0), alkaline phosphatase (ALP) of 42 units/L (normal adult: 30–120), alanine aminotransferase (ALT) of 16 units/L (normal: 4–36), aspartate aminotransferase (AST) of 17 units/L (normal: < 35), γ-glutamyl transferase (GGT) of 17 units/L (normal: 8–38), and PT of 11.3 seconds (normal: 1.0–12.5).

Her electrolytes revealed a carbon dioxide (CO_2) of 26 mEq/L (normal: 23–30), a chloride (Cl) of 102 mEq/L (normal: 98–106), a potassium (K) of 3.2 mEq/L (normal adult: 3.5–5.0), and a sodium (Na) of 140 mEq/L (normal adult: 136–145). Her testing for hepatitis B and C are pending.

4. Based on this information, which one of the following is Ms. Upjohn's most likely diagnosis and why?

    A. Hyperemesis gravidarum

    B. Acute hepatitis B and/or C

    C. Fitz-Hugh and Curtis syndrome

    D. Hepatoma secondary to oral contraceptives

    E. Gastrointestinal (GI) intolerance of antibiotics causing mild dehydration and hypokalemia

5. Based on this diagnosis, which of the following are appropriate components of a treatment plan for Ms. Upjohn and why?

    A. Change oral doxycycline and metronidazole to ciprofloxacin 500 mg bid for 14 days and continue treatment as an outpatient

    B. Add esomeprazole 20 mg once a day to outpatient regimen

    C. Hospitalize and provide antibiotics by IV and treat hypokalemia

    D. Add potassium chloride orally twice a day

    E. Refer to gastroenterologist for a liver biopsy

CASE 11-8
Ulisa VanDyke

Ulisa is a 4-year-old white female who presented accompanied by her mother, who provided the chief complaint of "a real high fever." According to her mother, Ulisa woke up this morning with a low grade fever (99.9°F orally), rhinorrhea, anorexia, and irritability. Her mother assumed she was getting a "cold" and gave her children's acetaminophen. By noon, her temperature had increased to 100.6°F (orally) and she was more irritable, refused to eat lunch, and was complaining of a sore throat. At this time, her mother gave her another dose of children's acetaminophen, which she has been giving her every 4 hours since.

She appeared to continue to get sicker as the day progressed. By midafternoon, her temperature had increased to 101.2°F (orally), and she began experiencing vomiting and diarrhea. Her mother estimates the quantity to be approximately 10 episodes of each. By this evening (approximately 12 hours after Ulisa's symptoms began), her temperature had increased to 102.8°F (orally) and she started experiencing chills. Approximately 1 hour ago, she began crying inconsolably, appearing "confused," complaining of head and neck pain, experiencing photophobia, and developing a rash on her ankles.

Her only medication is children's acetaminophen as needed (her last dose was approximately 1 hour ago) and a children's chewable vitamin daily. She does not take any other over-the-counter or prescription medications, vitamins, supplements, or herbal preparations. She is not allergic to any medications. She has never had surgery nor been hospitalized. Her well-child visits and immunizations are up to date. She has not experienced any trauma. Her family history is noncontributory.

1. Based on this information, which of the following questions are essential to ask Ulisa's mother and why?

  A. Have there been any recent changes in soaps, shampoos, lotions, detergents, fabric softeners, or other products that come into contact with Ulisa's body?
  B. Has Ulisa been experiencing any myalgias, arthralgias, seizures, lightheadedness, vertigo, presyncope, or syncope?
  C. Has Ulisa's rash changed in any manner since it began?
  D. What does she mean by "confused"?
  E. Has she noticed any changes in Ulisa's urine's frequency or color?

Patient Responses

According to Ulisa's mother, she has not changed soaps, shampoos, lotions, detergents, fabric softeners, or other products that come into contact with Ulisa's skin. Ulisa has been complaining of generalized myalgias; however, she is not complaining of (nor does she appear to be experiencing) arthralgias, seizurelike activity, lightheadedness, vertigo, presyncope, syncopal episodes, pruritus, paresthesias, or dysesthesias. Her rash appears to be unchanged except she has more lesions.

Her mother defines "confused" as Ulisa just "seemed out of it." Examples include "forgetting" how to wash her hands, not being able to put on her clothes correctly, and staring at a glass of electrolyte replacement fluid instead of drinking it.

Ulisa's urine appears to be slightly darker in color and slightly less in quantity than usual; however, she is still urinating every 3 to 4 hours. Also, she has tears when she cries.

2. Based on this information, which of the following components of a physical examination are essential to conduct on Ulisa and why?

  A. General appearance
  B. Skin examination
  C. Eyes, ears, nose, and throat (EENT) examination
  D. Abdominal examination
  E. Neurologic examination

Physical Examination Findings

Ulisa weighs 34 lb and is 35″ tall. Other vital signs are oral temperature, 102.6°F; pulse, 120 BPM and regular; respiratory rate, 20/min and regular; and BP, 82/54 mm Hg.

She is toxic appearing, sitting limply on her mother's lap, and crying tears despite her mother's attempts to comfort her.

She has scattered petechiae of approximately 1 to 3 mm in size around her ankles and wrists and in her axillary areas. The greatest concentration is on her ankles.

Her sclerae are normal in color and noninjected. Her lower eyelids reveal scattered, 1- to 2-mm petechial lesions. The only discharge appears to be tears. Her pupils are equal in size, are round, and react to light and accommodation. Extraocular motions appear to be intact but are difficult to fully assess secondary to the patient's unwillingness to cooperate. For the same reason, her funduscopic examination is limited; however, the presence of papilledema is excluded.

Her ear canals are normal in color and without edema or abnormal discharge bilaterally. Her tympanic membranes are intact, nonerythematous, and moderately injected, but fully mobile, bilaterally. There is no evidence of middle ear effusion or masses.

Her nasal mucosa is slightly erythematous and edematous with a moderate amount of thin, clear discharge, bilaterally.

Her oral mucosa is moist and normal in color, but does exhibit scattered, 1- to 2-mm petechiae on the hard and soft palate. Her pharynx is moderately erythematous and her tonsils are slightly enlarged and erythematous but without exudates. Her lips are also moist appearing.

Her bowel sounds are slightly hyperactive in all four quadrants; however, there does not appear to be any tenderness. No masses or organomegaly are present.

Ulisa appears to be alert but crying inconsolably. Within the limits of her ability to cooperate, cranial nerves II through VII are grossly intact. She appears to have use of all extremities with normal muscle tone; however, she refuses to perform mental status, muscle strength, discrimination, coordination, or gait testing. Her biceps, triceps, brachioradialis, knee, and ankle reflexes are normal and equal, bilaterally. Her plantar reflexes are normal and equal, bilaterally. Her sensation appears to be intact and equal to touch only in both her arms and legs. Her Brudzinski (passive flexion of her neck results in flexion of her knees) and Kernig (passive extension of the knee while holding the hip at a 90° angle produces hamstring pain) signs appear to be positive.

3. Based on this information, which of the following diagnostic studies are essential to perform on Ulisa and why?

  A. Blood culture and sensitivity (C&S) with Gram stain
  B. Lumbar puncture (LP) with Gram stain, culture and sensitivity (C&S), and routine analysis of the cerebrospinal fluid (CSF)
  C. Complete blood count with differential (CBC w/diff)
  D. Electrolytes, serum glucose, blood urea nitrogen (BUN), creatinine, prothrombin time (PT), and partial thromboplastin time (PTT)
  E. Polymerase chain reaction (PCR) testing of blood and cerebrospinal fluid (CSF) for *Neisseria meningitides*

Diagnostic Test Results

Ulisa's blood Gram stain revealed too numerous to count (TNTC) WBCs per high-power field (HPF) and gram-negative diplococci (normal: < 5 WBC/HPF and no organisms).

Her LP revealed an opening pressure of 22 cm H_2O (normal: < 20) and a closing pressure of 22 cm H_2O (normal: < 20 PLUS the opening and the closing pressure should be essentially equal). Her CSF was purulent and yellow in color without any visible blood (normal: clear and colorless). She did not have any red blood cells (normal: none). Her CSF white blood cell count was greater than 1000 cells µg/L (normal for children 1–5 years of age: 0–20) with 80% neutrophils (normal: 0–6), 11% lymphocytes (normal: 40–80), and 9% monocytes (normal: 15–45). Her CSF Gram stain revealed TNTC WBC/HPF and gram-negative diplococci (normal: no organisms). Her CSF total protein was 75 mg/dl (normal in child: 15–70), glucose was 25 mg/dl (normal: 50–75 OR 60–70% of blood glucose level), lactate dehydrogenase (LDH) was 50 units/L (normal: ≤ 40), lactic acid (LA) was 33 mg/dl (normal: 10–25), and glutamine was 7 mg/dl (normal: 6–15).

Ulisa's serum CBC revealed an RBC count of $4.2 \times 10^6/µl$ (normal for children 1–6 years of age: 4.0–5.5) with an MCV of 85 µm^3 (normal: 80–95), an MCH of 31 pg (normal: 27–31), an MCHC of 36 g/dl (normal: 32–36), and an RDW of 12.5% (normal given for adult values only: 11–14.5). Her WBC count was 22,750/mm^3 (normal: 5,000–10,000) with 86% neutrophils (normal: 55–70), 8% lymphocytes (normal: 20–40), 2% monocytes (normal: 2–8), 3% eosinophils (normal: 1–4), and 1% basophils (normal: 0.5–1). Her Hgb was 12.9 g/dl (normal for children 1–6 years of age: 9.5–14) and her HCT was 36% (normal for children 1–6 years of age: 30–40). Her platelet (thrombocyte) count was 150,000/mm^3 (normal child: 150,000–400,000) and her MPV was 7.9 fL (normal: 7.4–10.4). Her smear was consistent with this and revealed no cellular abnormalities except for a moderate amount of bands.

Her PT was 11.6 seconds (normal: 11–12.5) and PTT was 60 seconds (normal: 60–70). Her electrolytes revealed a potassium of 3.3 mEq/L (normal child: 3.4–4.7), chloride of 88 mEq/L (normal child: 90–110), carbon dioxide 30 mEq/L (normal child: 20–28), and sodium of 134 mEq/L (normal child: 136–145). Her glucose was 80 mg/dl (normal for children older than 2 years of age: 70–110), BUN was 17 mg/dl (normal child: 5–18), and creatinine was 0.5 mg/dl (normal child: 0.3–0.7). Her blood and CSF C&S are pending. PCR testing of her blood for *N. meningitides* is also pending.

4. Based on this information, which one of the following is Ulisa's most likely diagnosis and why?

A. Meningococcemia with meningitis
B. Disseminated gonococcal infection (DGI) with meningitis
C. *Haemophilus influenzae* meningitis with disseminated intravascular coagulation (DIC)
D. Pneumococcal meningitis with dehydration
E. Viral encephalitis

5. Based on this diagnosis, which of the following are appropriate components of a treatment plan for Ulisa and why?

A. Hospitalization
B. IV dexamethasone with first dose of IV antibiotics

C. IV ceftriaxone every 12 hours
D. IV vancomycin every 6 hours
E. GI rest and IV fluids to maintain hydration

CASE 11-9

Van Watson

Mr. Watson is a 62-year-old white male who presents with the chief complaint of "headaches." They are generalized in location, aching in nature, moderate (5 out of 10 on the pain scale) in intensity, and gradual in onset. He has been experiencing approximately two headaches per week for approximately 6 months. They have not changed in any manner since their onset.

His headaches are associated with bilateral tinnitus, occasional bilateral blurred vision, and less frequently lightheadedness. They are not associated with true vertigo, presyncope, syncope, palpitations, chest pain/pressure, dyspnea, photophobia, phonophobia, nausea, vomiting, problems using his extremities, difficulties with gait, confusion, abnormalities of speech, dysphagia, nausea, vomiting, bowel changes, rhinorrhea, nasal congestion, or epiphora. The tinnitus is a "ringing" sensation and does not appear to be related to the beating of his heart. It appears to be equal bilaterally. The blurred vision is a slight "fuzziness" of his vision, but no dimness, complete visual loss, or visual field loss is present. It appears to be equal in both eyes.

Furthermore, he has noted that on the day the headaches occur, and sometimes the day before, he will experience episodes of his hands and occasionally his forearms becoming erythematous with a generalized "burning" sensation. These episodes can last from a few minutes to several hours. He is not bothered by any other burning-type sensations or rashes. These hand and forearm symptoms resolve with the headache.

He attributes his headaches to stress. They are alleviated within 1 hour by taking two regular-strength aspirin tablets. Then, he will not experience another one for a couple of days. He has always taken the aspirin at the onset of the headache; therefore, he does not know what his headache pattern would be if left to progress on its own. Otherwise, he knows of no other aggravating or alleviating symptoms.

He does not take any over-the-counter or prescription medications except for the occasional aspirin. He is on no vitamins, supplements, or herbal preparations. He denies any medical problems, previous surgeries, or prior hospitalizations. He smokes 1.5 packs of cigarettes per day (PPD), which is up from one PPD about 1 year ago. He has been smoking since age 15 years. He denies drinking alcohol. His family history is negative.

1. Based on this information, which of the following questions are essential to ask Mr. Watson and why?

A. Has he been bothered by pruritus?
B. Has he experienced any fatigue, night sweats, malaise, unintentional weight loss, fever, or chills?
C. Is he experiencing any insomnia, appetite change, excessive worry, panic attacks, depression, difficulty with memory, anhedonia, or feelings of worthlessness?

D. Has he experienced any abdominal pain, discomfort, or pressure?

E. Has he done any recent traveling or mountain climbing?

Patient Responses

He has noticed experiencing intense generalized pruritus, especially following a hot shower or a trip to his health club's sauna. This has also been occurring for approximately 6 months.

He has been having some fatigue lately, defined as a weakness (not sleepiness, lack of motivation, or exhaustion). The fatigue tends to worsen as the day progresses or with activity. The only difficulty he experiences sleeping is an occasional initial insomnia because of the generalized pruritus and/or the upper extremity dysesthesias if they are occurring when he retires. Once he is asleep, he does not have any difficulty with frequent or early morning awakenings.

He denies night sweats, malaise, unintentional weight loss, fever, chills, appetite change, excessive worry, panic attacks, depression, difficulty with memory, anhedonia, feelings of worthlessness, or any abdominal pain/discomfort/pressure. He has not done any recent travel or mountain climbing.

2. Based on this information, which of the following components of a physical examination are essential to conduct on Mr. Watson and why?

A. Oxygen saturation and evaluation for hypoxia

B. Skin examination

C. Heart, lung, and pulse examination

D. Abdominal examination

E. Neurologic examination

Physical Examination Findings

Mr. Watson is 5'10" tall and weighs 175 lb (BMI = 25.1). Other vital signs are BP, 126/74 mm Hg; pulse, 82 BPM and regular; respiratory rate, 14/min and regular; and oral temperature, 98.2°F.

His oxygen saturation is 97% on room air. He has no central or peripheral cyanosis or pallor. His fingers and toes are warm to the touch, and they have normal and equal sensation. His capillary refill is normal. There is no clubbing of his fingernails. His toes and feet are normal in color; however, his hands are slightly erythematous in comparison to the color of the rest of his skin. There are no other skin lesions or abnormalities noted.

His heart is regular in rate and rhythm without any murmurs, gallops, or rubs. His apical impulse is nondisplaced and without a thrill. His lungs are clear bilaterally.

His carotid pulses are normal and equal bilaterally and without bruits. His brachial, ulnar, radial, femoral, popiteal, dorsalis pedis, and posterior tibial pulses are normal and equal bilaterally. His renal arteries and aorta are without bruits. His aorta is normal in size and pulsation.

His abdomen reveals normoactive bowel sounds in all four quadrants. There is no evidence of any abnormal masses. However, his spleen is palpable and slightly tender. No other organomegaly or tenderness is noted.

Mr. Watson is alert and oriented to person, place, and time. His mini-mental status examination is normal (score: 30 out of 30). His cranial nerves are grossly intact. His pupils are round and equal and react to light and accommodation, bilaterally. He has slight conjunctival injection bilaterally. There is no evidence of sclera or other discolorations. His funduscopic examination is normal except his retinal veins appear to be slightly engorged; this finding is also bilateral and equal.

He can perform finger to nose and finger to examiner's finger without difficulty. He has good and equal strength in his hand, arm, leg, foot, neck, shoulder, and facial muscles. There is no evidence of a tremor. He has no difficulty with coordination or gait. He can perform tandem, heel, and toe walking without difficulty. His Romberg test is normal. He has normal sensation (to sharp and dull stimulation) in his extremities and face. His biceps, triceps, brachioradialis, knee, and ankle reflexes are normal and equal bilaterally. His plantar reflexes are normal and equal bilaterally.

3. Based on this information, which of the following diagnostic studies are essential to perform on Mr. Watson and why?

A. Computed tomography of the head, with and without contrast

B. Complete blood count with differential (CBC w/diff) and absolute reticulated platelet count

C. Erythropoietin (EPO)

D. Carboxyhemoglobin

E. Abdominal ultrasound

Diagnostic Study Findings

Mr. Watson's CT of his head, with and without contrast, was normal.

His CBC revealed an RBC count of $7.2 \times 10^6/\mu l$ (normal adult male: 4.7–6.1) with an MCV of 100 μm^3 (normal adult: 80–95), an MCH of 44.4 pg (normal adult: 27–31), an MCHC of 30.5 g/dl (normal adult: 32–36), and an RDW of 12.8% (normal adult: 11–14.5). His WBC count was 17,500/mm^3 (normal adult: 5000–10,000) with 20% neutrophils (normal: 55–70), 15% lymphocytes (normal: 20–40), 0% monocytes (normal: 2–8), 24% eosinophils (normal: 1–4), and 41% basophils (normal: 0.5–1). His Hgb was 22 g/dl (normal adult male: 14–18) and his HCT was 72% (normal adult male: 42–52). His absolute reticular platelet (thrombocyte) count was 450,000/mm^3 (normal adult: 150,000–400,000) and his MPV was 8.9 fl (normal: 7.4–10.4). His smear was consistent with this and revealed no cellular abnormalities and normal RBC morphology.

His EPO level was 3.8 IU/L (normal: 5–35). His carboxyhemoglobin was 4% (normal in smokers: ≤ 12). His abdominal ultrasound was unremarkable except for mild to moderate splenomegaly.

4. Based on this information, which one of the following is Mr. Watson's most likely diagnosis and why?

A. Chronic myeloid leukemia

B. Myelofibrosis

C. Polycythemia vera

D. Secondary polycythemia

E. Essential thrombocytosis

5. Which of the following treatment options are appropriate components of Mr. Watson's treatment plan and why?

   A. Phlebotomy, 1 unit every 7 days until HCT is less than 45%, then as necessary to maintain his HCT at 45% (but no more frequently than once every 7 days)
   B. Hydroxyurea 500 to 1500 mg/day
   C. Low-dose aspirin 75 to 81 mg/day
   D. Diphenhydramine 25 to 50 mg every 4 to 6 hours as needed up to four times per day
   E. Daily paroxetine if diphenhydramine is ineffective

CASE 11-10

William Xylophone

William is a 7-month-old African American male who is brought in by his foster mother, who supplied the chief complaint, "I think his feet hurt." Yesterday evening he began to experience edema of his hands and feet as well as a low-grade temperature (99.9°F, tympanically). When he awoke this morning, the edema was much worse and he was fussy, anorexic, and not as active as usual. Otherwise, he appears "fine" to his foster mother. His foster mother is unaware of any previous episodes of similar symptoms; however, William has only been living with her for 1 week.

He has not experienced any rhinorrhea, nasal congestion, sneezing, cough, wheezing, dyspnea, cyanosis, pallor, skin lesions, chills, abdominal pain, vomiting, diarrhea, constipation, or changes in the appearance of his bowels.

His only medication is ibuprofen as needed for "fever and pain," which he took two doses of yesterday and one this morning (approximately 2 hours ago). However, his foster mother does not think it is altering any of his symptoms. He takes no other over-the-counter or prescription medications, vitamins, supplements, or herbal preparations. As near as his foster mother knows he does not have any drug allergies.

He saw a pediatrician 4 days ago for a well-child examination, his initial set of immunizations, blood work, and age-appropriate patient education. He is scheduled to return next week for laboratory results and to have his weight rechecked because he appeared underweight for height and head circumference (HC). His foster mother does not have any information regarding William's or his family's medical histories.

1. Based on this information, which of the following questions are essential to ask his foster mother and why?

   A. How much ibuprofen and which formulation has she been giving him?
   B. Has he been experiencing any skin lesions or facial edema?
   C. Has she noticed any changes in his skin color, sclera, or urine?
   D. Which immunizations did he receive at his well-child examination?
   E. Is he being breast- or bottle-fed?

Patient Responses

According to his foster mother, she has been giving him 0.5 ml of the ibuprofen oral drops every 6 to 8 hours as needed.

She has not noticed any rash, skin lesions, skin discoloration, scleral abnormalities, facial edema, or urinary changes. He received his HepB, DTaP, Hib, PCV, and IPV immunizations. He is being bottle-fed.

2. Based on this information, which of the following components of a physical examination are essential to conduct on William and why?

   A. General appearance
   B. Eyes, ears, nose, and throat (EENT) examination
   C. Abdominal examination
   D. Hand and foot examination
   E. Skin examination

Physical Examination Findings

William is 28.3" long and weighs 13.5 lb, and his HC is 17.75". His pulse is 146 BPM and regular and his respirations are 42/min and regular. (For normal values of cardiac and respiratory rates from birth to 36 months, please see Tables 2-1 and 2-2 in Case 2-2.) His rectal temperature is 101.1°F and he is moderately to severely ill appearing.

His sclerae are normal in color; his palpebral conjunctivae appear slightly pale but there is no edema. His pupils are round and equal; they respond to light and accommodation. He can follow a light with his eyes. His red reflex is present in both eyes.

His ear canals are normal in color and without edema or abnormal debris, bilaterally. His tympanic membranes are normal in color, without erythema, and fully mobile. There is no evidence of middle ear effusions or masses in either inner ear.

He has no facial edema. His nasal mucosa is slightly pale bilaterally but with no edema or discharge. His septum is not deviated.

He does not have any perioral or lip edema. His oral mucosa is slightly paler than expected; however, it does not have any lesions or abnormalities. His pharynx is nonerythematous and without tonsillar enlargement or exudates.

His heart is regular in rate and rhythm and without any murmurs, gallops, or rubs. His apical impulse is nondisplaced and without a thrill. His lungs are clear to auscultation.

His abdomen reveals normoactive bowel sounds in all four quadrants and is not tender. His spleen is palpable and slightly tender at the left costal margin; otherwise, there are no masses or organomegaly noted.

His skin does not reveal any evidence of a rash or jaundice. It appears to be normal in color except for his hands and feet, which are slightly erythematous. They are also edematous (fingers and toes greater than hands and feet, providing a "sausage" appearance to them), slightly warm, and tender to the touch. The findings are poorly demarked at the wrists and ankles and equal bilaterally.

3. Based on this information, which of the following diagnostic studies are essential to perform on William and why?

   A. Complete blood count with differential (CBC w/diff) and manual smear
   B. Manual reticulocyte count and level
   C. Blood typing and cross-match
   D. Hemoglobin electrophoresis
   E. Total, conjugated, and unconjugated bilirubin levels

Diagnostic Test Results

William's CBC revealed an RBC count of $3.2 \times 10^6/\mu l$ (normal infant 6–12 months of age: 3.5–5.2) with an MCV of 44.3 μm^3 (normal child: 80–95), an MCH of 9 pg (normal child: 27–31), an MCHC of 36.6 g/dl (normal child: 32–36), and an RDW of 16.8% (normal adult value only: 11–14.5). His WBC count was 17,500/mm^3 (normal child younger than 2 years of age: 6,200–17,000) with 75% neutrophils (normal: 55–70), 15% lymphocytes (normal: 20–40), 6% monocytes (normal: 2–8), 3.5% eosinophils (normal: 1–4), and 0.5% basophils (normal: 0.5–1). His Hgb was 5.2 g/dl (normal child 1–6 years of age: 9.5–14) and his HCT was 14.2% (normal child 1–6 years of age: 30–40). His platelet (thrombocyte) count was 145,000/mm^3 (normal infant: 200,000–445,000) and his MPV was 8.9 fl (normal: 7.4–10.4). His smear was consistent with this but revealed approximately 25% crescent-shaped RBCs and numerous RBCs that were nucleated and contain Howell-Jolly bodies and/or target cells. Additionally, there appeared to be an elevated reticulocyte count which was confirmed by a manual count of 4.1% (normal infant: 0.5–3.1). His reticulocyte index was 1.6 (normal: 1) and manual platelet count was 145,500/mm^3. His blood type was reported as AB positive.

William's hemoglobin electrophoresis revealed 0% of Hgb A$_1$ (normal: 95–98), 2% of Hgb A$_2$ (2–3), 2% of Hgb F (normal child older than 6 months of age: 1–2; normal adult: 0.8–2), 94% Hgb S (normal: 0), 0% of Hgb C (normal: 0), and 0% of Hgb H (normal: 0).

His total bilirubin was 1.2 mg/dl (normal child: 0.3–1); unconjugated, or indirect, bilirubin was 1.0 mg/dl (normal child: 0.2–0.8); and conjugated, or direct, bilirubin was 0.2 mg/dl (normal child: 0.1–0.3).

4. Based on this information, which one of the following is William's most likely diagnosis and why?

    A. Acute gastrointestinal blood loss and cholestasis from ibuprofen

    B. Hand-foot syndrome of sickle cell anemia

    C. Sickle cell trait arthropathy

    D. Thalassemia major

    E. Viral syndrome and iron deficiency anemia

5. Based on this diagnosis, which of the following are appropriate components of a treatment plan for William and why?

    A. Increase ibuprofen oral drops to 1.5 ml every 6 to 8 hours as needed for pain/fever up to four times per day and return if still symptomatic in 2 days

    B. Hospitalize

    C. Provide blood transfusion

    D. Refer for splenectomy

    E. Ensure adequate hydration and pain control

MISCELLANEOUS CASES IN HEMATOLOGY, DERMATOLOGY, AND INFECTIOUS DISEASES

RESPONSES AND DISCUSSION

CASE 11-1
Monty Nutter
1. History

A. Has he experienced any episodes of strenuous or forceful coughing recently? ESSENTIAL

It is possible to cough with sufficient force to produce a rib fracture; however, this information is generally not elicited when questioning the patient regarding trauma. Therefore, it is important to specifically ask this question. In patients with chronic obstructive pulmonary disease, these coughing spasms can occur frequently, making the occurrence less noteworthy to the patient.

B. Does he have a rash or skin lesion(s) in the area? ESSENTIAL

From the description obtained thus far, Mr. Nutter's pain appears to be superficial. Therefore, in order to establish the most accurate differential diagnosis for Mr. Nutter in the most efficient manner, questioning must address superficial causes, predominately limited to musculoskeletal, neurologic, and dermatologic processes. Musculoskeletal causes have been sufficiently addressed currently by questioning the patient regarding trauma and strenuous coughing episodes. The presence of a rash or some other type of skin lesion(s) significantly increases the likelihood that a dermatologic process is responsible for Mr. Nutter's symptoms.

Equally important is a good description of the rash, if present, including its initial appearance, location, distribution, size, characteristics, growth, evolution, and associated symptoms (e.g., pruritus, paresthesias, or dysesthesias). Few dermatologic conditions that can affect the chest wall are described as truly painful, and the vast majority of those are the result of an infectious cause (e.g., herpes zoster, herpes simplex, cellulitis, and/or abscesses).

C. Did he have any paresthesias before the onset of the pain? ESSENTIAL

Chest pain produced by a superficial neurologic condition almost always involves paresthesias, which will frequently precede the pain. If this pain is also accompanied by a rash, the list of differential diagnoses decreases significantly more. For example, a distinguishing characteristic of the herpes viruses is the presence of paresthesias before the onset of the pain or the rash.

D. Did he have varicella as a child? ESSENTIAL

Herpes zoster (or shingles) is a condition that must be included in Mr. Nutter's differential diagnosis list. It is a reactivation of a latent varicella-zoster virus (VZV) from the dorsal root ganglia; therefore, he could not have herpes zoster if he did not have a history of varicella. However, some individuals might have had a mild case or "forgotten" that they had the disease; therefore, a negative response would not completely rule out the possibility. Additionally, individuals who received the immunization for VZV but never had varicella can develop herpes zoster from that exposure.

E. Has he received the vaccination for herpes zoster? ESSENTIAL

A vaccine now exists with a much higher content of the VZV than the pediatric formulation. It is approved for use in and is recommended for all individuals older than the age of 60 years regardless of whether they have a personal history of herpes zoster or varicella unless they have a medical contraindication (i.e., immunocompromising condition except for infection with human immunodeficiency virus [HIV] unless the $CD4^+$ T-lymphocyte count is < 200 cells/μL). This vaccine has been shown in clinical trials to decrease the incidence of acquiring herpes zoster by over 50%. And in those who do acquire the disease despite the vaccine, the severity of the illness is decreased by almost 66% and the incidence of postherpetic neuralgia is decreased by approximately 66%.

2. Physical Examination

A. Eye examination NONESSENTIAL

An eye examination would only be indicated if Mr. Nutter were experiencing ocular symptoms. Even if his truncal rash is caused by herpes zoster, he cannot autoinoculate his eye and acquire herpes zoster ophthalmicus. This condition requires the eruption to be distributed in the ocular area (most commonly affecting the nasociliary or trigeminal nerve). Infection via autoinoculation, however, is a concern with the herpes simplex virus.

B. Heart examination   ESSENTIAL

Even though Mr. Nutter's description of his chest pain makes a cardiac origin unlikely, it is still appropriate to examine his heart because he is complaining of chest pain.

C. Lung auscultation   ESSENTIAL

Likewise, from the information obtained thus far, it does not appear that Mr. Nutter's chest pain is pulmonary in origin; however, it is still appropriate to examine his lungs to ensure that there are no signs to suggest otherwise, especially with his history of emphysema.

Additionally, with severe chest wall pain, especially if associated with pain on deep inspiration or a history of chronic pulmonary disease, special attention needs to be directed to the bases of his lungs to ensure that he has not developed a complication as a result of his chest expansion being limited (e.g., pneumonia or atelectasis).

D. Chest wall examination   ESSENTIAL

Because Mr. Nutter has a rash, a skin examination is essential to assist in establishing the correct diagnosis. Logical analysis of the location, distribution, characteristics, and associated signs and symptoms correlated with the patient's history is essential to accomplish this task. Although not an uncommon occurrence in some clinical settings, it is NEVER appropriate to compare the patient's rash to photos in a dermatology textbook as a method of diagnosis.

Furthermore, patients with chest wall pain should have the affected area palpated to evaluate for areas of tenderness resulting from a musculoskeletal cause.

E. Lower leg examination for edema   NONESSENTIAL

A lower leg examination for pedal edema is only indicated if there exists a suspicion that an illness associated with this condition (e.g., a cardiovascular, renal, hepatic abnormality) is responsible for his symptoms.

3. Diagnostic Studies

A. Skin biopsy of lesions   NONESSENTIAL

A skin biopsy is not indicated because the diagnosis of Mr. Nutter's condition can be made clinically in virtually every case.

B. Chest x-ray (CXR)   NONESSENTIAL

A CXR is not necessary because there are no findings in Mr. Nutter's history or physical examination suggesting a pulmonary cause (or complication) is present.

C. Radiograph of left ribs   NONESSENTIAL

Even though forceful coughing can occasionally result in a spontaneous rib fracture, rib radiographs are not indicated for Mr. Nutter because he does not provide a history of rib trauma (including forceful coughing), nor does he have rib tenderness on the physical examination.

D. Electrocardiograph (ECG)   NONESSENTIAL

Although Mr. Nutter is an elderly male complaining of chest pain, his history and physical findings are inconsistent with a cardiac cause. Thus, an ECG is unnecessary.

E. Complete blood count with differential (CBC w/diff) NONESSENTIAL

4. Diagnosis

A. Herpes simplex dermatitis   INCORRECT

Herpes simplex dermatitis is a possibility because it is typically characterized by all the various lesion stages (papules, vesicles, ulcerations, and crusting) that Mr. Nutter's rash exhibited on physical examination. However, in herpes simplex, the base tends not to be as erythematous, the lesions more superficial appearing, the individual lesions not as large, and the area of involvement not dermatomally distributed, as seen in Mr. Nutter's case.

Furthermore, nongenital herpes simplex infections tend to be more commonly associated with pruritus and/or a stinging sensation instead of frank pain. They can vary from a single lesion to a small patch of a few lesions to a disseminated infection. For these reasons, a nongenital herpes simplex infection can be ruled out as Mr. Nutter's most likely diagnosis.

B. Herpes zoster   CORRECT

Herpes zoster, or shingles, is caused by reactivation of a latent varicella (chicken pox) infection. The typical illness pattern consists of paresthesias and/or pain preceding the onset of a papular rash, which evolves into deep-seated vesicles that ulcerate and crust before healing. Unless the patient is immunocompromised, the rash is always unilateral, never crosses the midline of the body, and is generally limited to a single dermatome.

C. Angina   INCORRECT

Angina can be ruled out as Mr. Nutter's most likely diagnosis based on the lack of typical, or even atypical, anginal symptoms and the presence of a rash consistent with the pain pattern.

D. Left rib contusion   INCORRECT

The lack of a history of trauma and chest wall tenderness make a left rib contusion highly unlikely to be Mr. Nutter's most likely diagnosis.

E. Contact dermatitis   INCORRECT

Contact dermatitis results from a topical exposure to an allergen. It tends to be associated with pruritus, not pain, which occurs with the onset of (or very shortly before or after) the appearance of the lesions. The typical rash consists of small, erythematous papules, although vesicles can sometimes occur. The distribution of the rash follows that of the exposed area, not a dermatome. Thus, contact dermatitis can be eliminated as Mr. Nutter's most likely diagnosis.

5. Treatment Plan

A. Valacyclovir 1000 mg three times a day for 7 days CORRECT

An antiviral agent effective against herpes zoster, such as valacyclovir, is recommended for all patients who have had the rash for less than 72 hours if they are older than the age of 50 years, are at risk for postherpetic neuralgia, and have moderate to severe disease, moderate to severe pain, and/or nontruncal involvement.

After the 72-hour window, antiviral therapy should be considered for individuals who are older and still experiencing new vesicle formation, severe pain, ocular involvement, cutaneous complications, or neurologic symptoms.

The recommended duration of use is 1 week; however, if the patient is still experiencing new lesion formation at the end of 7 days of therapy, a longer course should be considered.

B. Prednisolone starting at 60 mg daily, then gradually tapering-off over 3 weeks   CORRECT

Tapering corticosteroid therapy appears to be effective in assisting with pain reduction; however, an extended course starting with 60 mg daily is recommended. Studies regarding corticosteroids' ability to prevent postherpetic neuralgia (PHN) are currently conflicting.

Pregabalin and gabapentin are approved by the US Food and Drug Administration (FDA) for the prevention of postherpetic neuralgia. They should also offer another pathway of pain reduction. They can be used in conjunction with the antivirals and/or corticosteroids to maximize the patient's therapy.

There are a few studies suggesting that tricyclic antidepressants (TCAs) and other anticonvulsants might be effective as an off-label use in preventing postherpetic neuralgia when given along with an antiviral. These agents are not considered to be part of the standard of care; however, they could be an option in a patient who is unable to take or is intolerant of corticosteroids, gabapentin, and pregabalin.

C. Acetaminophen with codeine #3 four times a day on a regular basis for 1 week   CORRECT

Acetaminophen with codeine #3 four times a day on a regular basis for 1 week is indicated for Mr. Nutter because his pain would be considered moderate to severe. However, it is important to caution him regarding driving, operating equipment, or conducting any other activity requiring alertness and sound reflexes because of its propensity to cause drowsiness.

If his pain was mild to moderate, acetaminophen or nonsteroidal anti-inflammatory drugs (NSAIDs) are likely to be sufficient in controlling his pain. Therefore, they are considered to be the first-line agents of choice. Likewise, if his pain was severe, the first-line agent for pain should be a stronger opioid analgesic (e.g., oxycodone or morphine).

Having Mr. Nutter take his pain medication on a regular schedule, as compared to an as-needed basis, tends to make whatever analgesic prescribed (or recommended) more effective. Obviously, if the medication is not controlling his pain, changing it to a stronger analgesic, adding gabapentin or pregabalin (if not already prescribed), performing a neural block, and referring the patient to a pain management expert are all appropriate treatment options.

D. Triple antibiotic ointment twice a day to lesions   INCORRECT

Over-the-counter triple antibiotic ointment is contraindicated in herpes zoster because it tends to delay healing. Furthermore, many individuals are allergic to neomycin, and the associated drug reaction in combination with the rash from the herpes zoster will only serve to intensify the patient's discomfort and potentially confuse the clinical picture.

E. Advise him to discuss with household members and persons with whom he has had close or intimate contact their risk of acquiring a varicella-zoster virus (VZV) infection from him   CORRECT

Individuals do not contract herpes zoster from another individual with herpes zoster. Instead, if they are not adequately immunized against the VZV, they will contract varicella. Therefore, it is important for him to identify any household members or persons with whom he has had close (defined as being in the same room) or intimate (defined as anyone he has touched in any manner, including hugging) contact to determine whether they are considered "immune" or "nonimmune" to the VZV.

Individuals are assumed to be "immune" if they had a healthcare provider (HCP)-confirmed diagnosis of varicella or herpes zoster, or if they received the childhood vaccine for VZV and are younger than the age of 60 years. However, there is some concern regarding the duration of effect from the childhood vaccine and whether a "booster" dose is indicated. If they are older than 60 years of age and have been immunized with the adult VZV vaccine, they are also considered "immune."

Therefore, if the individual is an adolescent or older and is immunocompromised or has an illness that could be complicated from acquiring varicella, he or she should avoid any contact with Mr. Nutter until he is no longer considered contagious (generally defined as when all the lesions are "crusted" over). If that individual has already had contact with Mr. Nutter, then he or she needs to see his or her HCP so an individualized assessment can be made to determine whether varicella-zoster immune globulin (VZIG) is indicated.

Additionally, individuals who are considered to be "nonimmune" and "at risk" may also be candidates for VZIG. The "at risk" population includes women who are pregnant, newborn infants, premature infants, immunocompromised individuals (regardless of underlying condition), and anyone who would experience significant complications/problems should they acquire varicella. The VZIG works best if given within 72 hours postexposure; however, it can be given up to 96 hours postexposure.

If there is a contraindication to receiving VZIG or if more than 96 hours has passed since exposure, this "at-risk" group might still gain some advantage by taking a full course of antiviral medication effective against VZV (unless there is a contraindication) if less than 1 week has lapsed since exposure. Even if the antiviral medication does not prevent the individual from acquiring the infection, it tends to shorten the course and severity of the illness.

Epidemiologic and Other Data

Although herpes zoster can occur at any age, the incidence of herpes zoster increases with advancing age. In fact, it is estimated that approximately 66% of all cases occur in individuals older than the age of 50 years, with the highest incidence occurring in the sixth decade of life. Furthermore, it is estimated that there are approximately 1,200,000 cases annually in the United States.

Despite the existence of an effective VZV vaccine given in childhood, the incidence of this disease is increasing in the United States. Epidemiologists feel this increase is a result of the increasing number of older adults who are living with immunocompromising conditions.

Because of the significant complications and sequelae, especially PHN, that can result from a herpes zoster infection, the aforementioned adult VZV vaccine was recently developed for usage in individuals older than the age of 60 years. All patients older than the age of 60 years, unless there is a contraindication, should be given the vaccine.

CASE 11-2
Nina Olive
1. History

A. Does she use pads, tampons, or both?   ESSENTIAL

If considering all the potential exanthemas the number of conditions characterized by a brightly erythematous rash with subsequent desquamation is limited. One such condition is toxic shock syndrome (TSS). Any foreign body that comes in prolonged contact with any mucous membrane has the potential to cause TSS. Therefore, because Nina is currently menstruating, it is important to know whether she uses tampons.

B. Did the rash involve the palms of her hands or the soles of her feet?   ESSENTIAL

Very few dermatologic manifestations involve the palms of the hands and soles of the feet; however, if they are affected, the number of potential diagnoses is significantly decreased. Examples include toxic shock syndrome, Rocky Mountain spotted fever, syphilis, contact dermatitis, erythema multiforme, urticaria, and hand-foot-mouth disease.

C. Has she experienced any otalgia, rhinorrhea, nasal congestion, sinus pressure, postnasal discharge, eye discharge, cough, wheezing, or dyspnea?   ESSENTIAL

Several viral exanthems, as well a few bacterial illnesses, that are associated with a sore throat also have other symptoms indicating the presence of an upper respiratory tract infection. This knowledge can dramatically alter the list of potential differential diagnoses for Nina.

D. Has she experienced any pruritus with her rash?   ESSENTIAL

Rashes can be asymptomatic or associated with pain (e.g., cellulitis, abscess, and herpes zoster), paresthesias (e.g., herpes zoster and herpes simplex), or pruritus (e.g., scarlet fever, contact dermatitis, and urticaria).

E. Which joints were affected by the arthralgias and were they erythematous, edematous, or hot to the touch?   ESSENTIAL

Serious systemic conditions (e.g., rheumatic fever, rheumatoid arthritis, systemic lupus erythematosus, Still disease, and infectious arthritis) are associated with a true arthritis (joint pain associated with erythema, warmth, and edema), whereas arthralgias (joint aches and pains) can occur in a wide array of musculoskeletal, infectious, neurologic, and psychological conditions. This distinction also assists in developing an appropriate differential diagnosis list.

Furthermore, which joints and the number affected are also important because specific conditions are frequently characterized by the number and location of joints involved. (For more information please see Cases 5-4 and 8-1).

2. Physical Examination

A. Ears, nose, and throat examination   ESSENTIAL

Because Nina's illness involved a sore throat that has still not completely resolved, an ear, nose, and throat (ENT) examination is required to determine whether there are any signs indicative of an acute, chronic, or resolving upper respiratory tract infection.

B. Lymph node examination   ESSENTIAL

Because an infectious cause must be high on Nina's list of differential diagnoses, an examination of her lymph nodes is indicated.

C. Heart examination   ESSENTIAL

A heart examination is indicated because there are some organisms (e.g., *Staphylococcus aureus*, *Streptococcus viridans*, group A β-hemolytic *Streptococcus,* or *Neisseria gonorrhoeae*) that can produce a rash and infective endocarditis, which could present as a cardiac murmur of the affected valve.

D. Pelvic examination   NONESSENTIAL

If toxic shock syndrome from tampon usage remains high on Nina's final differential diagnosis list, a pelvic examination would be indicated to evaluate for a retained tampon, a purulent discharge, and/or evidence of a coexisting pelvic inflammatory disease. Additionally, it would be indicated to obtain appropriate cultures.

E. Skin examination   ESSENTIAL

Because her primary complaint is a rash, a skin examination is necessary. It enables the characteristics, variability, and distribution to be studied carefully and considered in conjunction with the patient's history. Furthermore, it permits special maneuvers to be performed (e.g., testing for Nikolsky sign [gentle rubbing of the skin results in separation of the epidermis from the basal layer, which can be seen in pemphigus vulgaris, Stevens-Johnson syndrome, and toxic epidermal necrolysis] and diascopy [compression of an erythematous lesion with a glass plate causes blanching if it is a true purpuric lesion]). The unaffected skin, especially surrounding the lesion, also needs to be examined for the presence of associated findings (e.g., secondary infection, excoriation, petechiae, ecchymosis, bruising, or subcutaneous nodules). Gloved palpation confirms texture, nodularity, confinement to the epidermis or dermis, mobility, and other palpable features.

3. Diagnostic Studies

A. Rapid strep screen of the throat   ESSENTIAL

A rapid strep screen of the throat is indicated because it would be the quickest method to confirm the presence of group A β-hemolytic *Streptococcus* infection because she has pharyngitis as part of her illness complex. This is especially important because her other symptoms could be consistent with an endotoxin-producing streptococcal infection.

The rapid strep screen is considered to be more than 95% specific for the diagnosis of group A β-hemolytic *Streptococcus*. Therefore, if it is positive, it can be assumed with a high degree of accuracy that a streptococcal infection is present.

B. Throat culture, if rapid strep screen is negative   ESSENTIAL

However, a negative rapid strep screen is not nearly as indicative of the absence of group A β-hemolytic *Streptococcus*. In fact, there is much controversy regarding the sensitivity of the rapid strep screen. Compared to throat cultures, strep screens' sensitivity ranges from 55 to 90% in studies; hence, a negative strep screen should be followed up by throat culture. Thus, a throat culture will either confirm or refute the rapid strep screen's negative result. It is important to note that acquiring an appropriate specimen, correctly performing the rapid strep screen, and appropriately processing the culture can all affect the reliability of the respective tests. Thus, it is remotely possible to have both a negative rapid strep test and bacterial culture despite a group A β-hemolytic *Streptococcus* infection being present.

C. Skin culture   NONESSENTIAL

Because Nina's rash is not associated with any exudative material, it is highly unlikely that a skin culture is going to grow anything besides normal skin flora. This would only serve to complicate the clinical picture.

D. Immunofluorescence skin biopsy   NONESSENTIAL

An immunofluorescence skin biopsy is not indicated because the information thus far obtained is not consistent with an immune-mediated rash. Thus, attempting to identify immunoglobulin and complement deposits in the tissue is not going to be useful.

E. Complete blood count with differential (CBC w/diff)   ESSENTIAL

The primary purpose of a CBC w/diff for Nina is to provide confirmatory information regarding the presence and severity of the infection as well as clues as to whether it is more likely to be viral or bacterial in origin.

4. Diagnosis

A. Scarlet fever   CORRECT

Scarlet fever, or scarlatina, is an acute infectious process caused by erythrogenic toxin-producing streptococcal organisms; the most common is group A β-hemolytic *Streptococcus*. The typical clinical course consists of the rapid onset of a sore throat and constitutional symptoms, without any additional symptoms to indicate the presence of upper respiratory tract infection. The sore throat is generally followed by a fine sandpaper-like rash 12 to 48 hours later, which most commonly begins on the neck and trunk and then spreads distally, creating Pastia lines in the prominent skin creases and sparing the palms of the hands and soles of the feet. Desquamation frequently occurs approximately 1 week later. Another nearly pathognomonic feature is a "strawberry tongue." Despite the negative strep screen, scarlet fever is Nina's most likely diagnosis from the choices provided.

B. Staphylococcal scalded skin syndrome   INCORRECT

Staphylococcal scalded skin syndrome is primarily seen in children younger than the age of 5 years. The rash is generally described as painful, not pruritic. The spread and desquamation occur much more quickly and extensively than the description provided by Nina. Additionally, the desquamation is severe, with the skin coming off in "sheets." A positive Nikolsky sign is also present. Thus, staphylococcal scalded skin syndrome is not Nina's most likely diagnosis.

C. Erythema infectiosum   INCORRECT

Erythema infectiosum, also known as fifth disease, is characterized by prodromal viremic symptoms for approximately 1 week before the development of the rash. The rash is typically bright red on the cheeks (hence the term "slapped cheeks") and has a fine, lacy, reticular-type pattern on the body. It does not desquamate, but fades and recurs over a period of several months. Based on this description, and because the majority of cases are generally seen in children who are slightly younger than Nina, erythema infectiosum is not her most likely diagnosis.

D. Toxic shock syndrome   INCORRECT

TSS is a systemic infectious illness caused by the endotoxin toxic shock syndrome toxin 1 (TSST-1), which is most generally produced by either group A *Streptococcus* or *Staphylococcus aureus*. Diagnostic criteria have been established by the Centers for Disease Control and Prevention (CDC) for the condition. In addition to the characteristic bright erythematous sunburnlike rash, which typically involves the face, chest, trunk, and extremities, including the palms of the hands and soles of the feet, at least four of the following five established criteria must be met: (1) the rash does not desquamate until 1 to 2 weeks following the onset of the illness; (2) hypotension is present; (3) the patient has a fever of 39.8°C or higher; (4) there is evidence of involvement in three or more body areas not counting the skin—the mucous membranes, gastrointestinal (GI) system, kidneys, liver, musculoskeletal system, central nervous system, or blood; and (5) serologic testing is negative for other possible pathogens (e.g., rubeola, Rocky Mountain spotted fever, and leptospirosis). Although TSS tends to commence as a "flulike" illness, diarrhea is virtually always present at the time of onset. Because of these disease features, TSS is not Nina's most likely diagnosis.

E. Contact dermatitis caused by bubble bath   INCORRECT

Contact dermatitis is an inflammatory reaction that develops in response to an allergic or irritative reaction to a substance that has come in direct contact with the skin. Because Nina's rash began on her neck and axillae (areas that generally do not receive significant, and definitely not maximum, exposure from utilizing bubble bath) and spread distally affecting all her body, including her face (which should only be minimally exposed, if at all, to a product contained in bath water), contact dermatitis to bubble bath is not her most likely diagnosis. Additionally, the prodromal symptoms are inconsistent with this diagnosis.

5. Treatment Plan

A. Penicillin 500 mg four times a day for 10 days   CORRECT

The drug of choice for scarlet fever is penicillin. In mild to moderate infections, oral antibiotics are appropriate. However, in the presence of a severe infection, parental penicillin may be necessary. If the patient is penicillin allergic, then the first-line agent would be erythromycin.

B. Advise her not to use any more of the strawberry bubble bath   INCORRECT

Advising her to avoid her strawberry bubble bath would not be of any benefit in treating her illness because her problem is not contact dermatitis caused by the bubble bath.

C. Advise her that only the very top layer of her skin will "peel" off; however, it will likely occur all over her body and can take up to 6 weeks before completed   CORRECT

Although this might be disappointing news for Nina, it is important to address her concerns openly and honestly. Thus, advising her of the anticipated course of her disease is a very essential and appropriate component of her treatment plan.

D. Encourage her not to "pick, scratch, or peel" the skin because of risk of secondary infection   CORRECT

Advising a patient with a rash, especially one in which the epidermis is broken, not to manipulate the skin or the lesions in hopes of preventing a coinfection is also an essential component of the treatment plan.

E. Advise her of the signs and symptoms of secondary infection and to return to clinic immediately if they occur   CORRECT

Providing the patient with information regarding the signs and symptoms of a coinfection is essential, as is advising the patient of the appropriate course of action to take should this complication occur.

Epidemiologic and Other Data

Scarlet fever is almost always caused by the production of enterotoxin A, B, or C by group A β-hemolytic *Streptococcus* or *Streptococcus pyogenes*. It is a gram-positive coccus, which is often found in chains. However, in extremely rare cases, if scarlet fever is present without a sore throat, the causative agent could be *Staphylococcus aureus*.

The incidence of acquiring scarlet fever is very low. There is estimated to be less than 1 case of scarlet fever per 100,000 cases of group A β-hemolytic *Streptococcus* pharyngitis when the pharyngitis is appropriately treated. Untreated, there is estimated to be approximately 1 case of scarlet fever per 10,000 cases of pharyngitis.

CASE 11-3
Owen Pickens
1. History

A. Following the initial pain, swelling, and itchiness that occurred on his camping trip, did he develop "flulike" symptoms, a rash, or other skin lesion(s)?   ESSENTIAL

The development of "flulike" symptoms following the occurrence of localized pain, pruritus, or paresthesias but preceding the development of an unusual-appearing skin lesion is highly suspicious for an envenomation reaction, regardless of whether the individual remembers being bitten or stung. Common vectors include black widow spiders, brown recluse spiders, most thin-tailed scorpions (i.e., Scorpionidea and

Ischnuridae families), ticks, and fire ants. Recent sea water exposure can expand the list of potential creatures to include Portuguese man-o-war, jellyfish, and stingray bites or stings; however, the patient is generally aware of these envenomizations unless the situation was associated with decreased sensation (e.g., prolonged cold water exposure, substance [including alcohol] intoxication, and coexisting peripheral neuropathies).

The list of potential differential diagnoses is further reduced if the subsequently developed rash or skin lesion is ischemic, hemorrhagic, necrotic, or ulcerative in nature. Of the potential culprits, the most likely would then include brown recluse spider bite, Lyme disease, and secondary cellulitis. However, because of their frequent outdoor acquisition, other diseases that result in similar types of skin lesions can be blamed on a bite or sting. Therefore, a high index of suspicion must be maintained for these conditions (e.g., tularemia, sporotrichosis, cutaneous anthrax, necrotizing fasciitis, and chemical burns).

A good description, if known, of what a lesion looked like before it became necrotic is extremely important in determining the culprit because of the atypical lesions seen with many of the aforementioned bites and stings. For example, a "whiplike" pattern can be seen following contact by a jellyfish tentacle, a large puncture or jagged-edged wound with inconsistent severity of pain (especially located on a lower extremity) is suspicious for a stingray envenomization, and diffuse urticaria on exposed skin only following natural sea water exposure is suspicious for larval anemone exposure.

B. Where did he go on his camping trip?   ESSENTIAL

Because many of the aforementioned vectors are endemic to certain areas, both inside and outside of the United States (depending on the species), it is imperative when considering a particular reptile, marine inhabitant, insect, arachnid, or other ectoparasites as the culprit that the creature is endemic to where the patient resides or has recently traveled. For example, naturally residing aquatic leeches are limited to Africa, Asia, and southern Europe; in the United States, black widow spiders are most abundant in the southeastern portion, whereas tarantulas are found primarily in the southwestern United States.

C. Has he experienced hematuria, bleeding of his gums when flossing or brushing his teeth, bruising more easily, taking longer to stop bleeding, or other signs of a bleeding diathesis since he first experienced his leg symptoms?   ESSENTIAL

Envenomizations from many of these creatures can lead to hemolytic anemia, platelet dysfunction, and even frank disseminated intravascular coagulation (DIC); therefore, it is important to determine whether the patient has had any signs or symptoms of abnormal platelet function/bleeding when considering such a diagnosis.

D. Did the leg pain or swelling that he experienced on his camping trip return?   ESSENTIAL

Although the pain and swelling that Mr. Pickens experienced most likely represented a local inflammatory reaction related to his chief complaint, there is always the rare possibility that it represented an unrelated pathology (e.g., muscle strain or sprain, overuse syndrome, or, significantly more serious, a deep venous thrombus [DVT]). Therefore, it is essential to know if, and when, these symptoms returned and their subsequent course to ensure that a potentially life-threatening condition is not overlooked because of the unusual findings associated with his chief complaint. Furthermore, the return of these symptoms could also represent a complication as a result of his present illness (e.g., necrosis, cellulitis, and hematoma development).

E. Has he experienced restlessness, myoclonus, uncontrollable shaking, blurred vision, marked lacrimation, excessive salivation, profuse rhinorrhea, diaphoresis, tachycardia, palpitations, slurred speech, or high fever associated with the enlarging lesion?   NONESSENTIAL

These symptoms are most consistent with neurotoxic envenomization caused by a venomous (or poisonous) host (e.g., broad-tailed scorpions or snakes). However, because of the larger size of these creatures as well as the significant pain associated with their "bite," it is rare to have an unknown exposure. Nevertheless, rare cases have been reported to occur in sleeping and/or intoxicated individuals. Regardless, these symptoms occur shortly after envenomization and tend to peak in a few hours postexposure. Even if delayed, it is extremely unlikely that this neurotoxic reaction is not going to manifest itself after five days or the development of localized tissue necrosis.

2. Physical Examination

A. Heart examination   ESSENTIAL

Infectious endocarditis would be the most likely cardiac abnormality associated with fever and vague "flulike" symptoms followed by a skin lesion. Despite his initial lesion description being very atypical for the dermatologic manifestations that can be visualized with infective endocarditis (e.g., septic arterial emboli, petechiae subungual hemorrhages, Janeway lesions, Roth spots, and Osler nodes), his current description of a painless, dark lesion is more consistent despite it appearing to be singular in number.

B. Lung examination   ESSENTIAL

Although Mr. Pickens does not have any symptoms that are highly suggestive of a pulmonary problem, he does have a history of several vague complaints (e.g., unilateral leg edema, fever, and "flulike" symptoms) that are likely attributable to his lower leg lesion but nevertheless could represent a coexisting pulmonary abnormality (e.g., early pneumonia or pulmonary embolism), which could be potentially serious, if not life-threatening. Additionally, in rare cases pulmonary edema can be associated with his most likely diagnosis.

C. Skin examination   ESSENTIAL

Because Mr. Pickens' chief complaint is a skin lesion of his lower leg, a skin examination is indicated not only to evaluate this lesion but also to evaluate for the presence of additional skin abnormalities.

D. Genital examination   NONESSENTIAL

E. Inguinal lymph node examination   ESSENTIAL

Because the inguinal lymph nodes are also responsible for the lymphatic drainage from the lower extremities and Mr. Pickens is experiencing an atypical-patterned, dark skin lesion (which could be hyperpigmented until it is examined), his inguinal lymph nodes should be evaluated.

3. Diagnostic Studies

A. Urinalysis (U/A)   ESSENTIAL

Because of the potential for fatal complications including hemolytic anemia, renal failure, and hemoglobinuria with Mr. Pickens' most likely diagnosis, a urinalysis is necessary to evaluate for the presence of gross hematuria, microscopic hematuria, red blood cells, blood cell casts, hemoglobinuria, proteinuria, decreased specific gravity, hyaline casts, fatty casts, and waxy casts, which could suggest the presence of one or more of these complications. Additionally, a urinalysis done at this time can serve as a baseline for future studies.

B. Complete blood count with differential (CBC w/diff) ESSENTIAL

Because of the concern for hemolytic anemia, hemolysis, and platelet dysfunction associated with Mr. Pickens' most likely diagnosis, a CBC w/diff is also indicated not only to look for signs of these conditions but also to serve as a baseline for comparison of future repeat studies. Furthermore, it can provide clues regarding the presence or absence of a primary or secondary bacterial infection.

C. Prothrombin time (PT) and partial thromboplastin time (PTT)   ESSENTIAL

A PT and a PTT are also indicated because they provide more conclusive information regarding the potential of a bleeding disorder. These too can serve as baseline studies.

D. Renal function studies   ESSENTIAL

Renal function studies are indicated because, along with Mr. Pickens' urinalysis results, they can not only evaluate for early signs of uremia/renal failure but also allow appropriate treatment to be instituted if necessary. Furthermore, they can also serve as a baseline for future comparison.

E. Culture and sensitivity (C&S) of the lesion   ESSENTIAL

A culture and sensitivity of the wound is indicated to determine whether a secondary bacterial infection (and hopefully which one, if present) is associated with the lesion.

4. Diagnosis

A. Lyme disease   INCORRECT

Lyme disease (Lyme borreliosis) is caused by the spirochete *Borreliosis burgdorferi* and transmitted by the *Ixodes scapularis* tick in the United States. It is associated with pain at the site of envenomization, "flulike" symptoms, and a "target" lesion (erythema migrans). It begins as an erythematous lesion that expands outward, leaving an area of central clearing.

Therefore, the characteristic "target" lesion is white in the center and surrounded by erythema, in contrast to Mr. Pickens' lesion, which was violaceous in the center with an inner white ring and a concentric outer erythematous ring. Furthermore, the appearance of erythema migrans does not occur until approximately 1 week after being "bitten" by the *Ixodes scapularis* tick. Thus, Lyme disease can be ruled out as Mr. Pickens' most likely diagnosis.

B. Rocky Mountain spotted fever   INCORRECT

Rocky Mountain spotted fever is caused by infection with the bacteria *Rickettsia rickettsii*, which is also transmitted by

Ixodid ticks (*Dermacentor variabilis* [American dog tick] in the eastern United States, *Dermacentor andersoni* [Rocky Mountain wood tick] in the western half of the country, and *Rhipicephalus sanguineus* [brown dog tick] in some areas of eastern Arizona). It is another tick-borne infection that is associated with what could be classified as "target" lesions ("doughnut" lesions) consisting of much smaller lesions composed of an area of central clearing with an erythematous "ring" surrounding it as well as the presence of constitutional symptoms. However, it can be eliminated as Mr. Pickens' most likely diagnosis because the "flulike" syndrome and the rash do not appear until an average of 1 week postexposure. Furthermore, the rash consists of multiple, smaller, maculopapular lesions that begin on the wrist and ankles and spread centrally. One of the hallmark signs of this condition is that the lesions can appear on the palms of the hands and the soles of the feet.

C. Brown recluse spider envenomation with mild loxoscelism CORRECT

Mr. Pickens' description of his initial lesion as a raised "target" lesion that was purplish in the center and surrounded by a ring of extremely white skin, surrounded by another, larger erythematous ring that all became duller and vesicular appearing in the center within 24 hours, is characteristic of the lesion associated with envenomation of a brown recluse spider.

Furthermore, the sequence of symptoms, the "flulike" syndrome, the present necrotic lesion, and a visit to an endemic area make a brown recluse spider envenomation with mild loxoscelism Mr. Pickens' most likely diagnosis.

D. Toxic epidermal necrolysis   INCORRECT

Toxic epidermal necrolysis (Lyell syndrome) does not consist of a single, localized area of necrotic tissue. It involves a markedly erythematous generalized skin involvement with associated flaccid bullae in which desquamation of the skin occurs in large sheets. It is most commonly attributed to an adverse drug reaction; however, there are other cases not pharmacologically induced and of unknown cause. Therefore, toxic epidermal necrolysis can be eliminated as Mr. Pickens' most likely diagnosis.

E. Erythema multiforme major   INCORRECT

Erythema multiforme major also presents with "target" lesions. However, these are numerous small lesions known as "iris lesions" that typically involve all the dermal surfaces, including the palms of the hands and the soles of the feet. Furthermore, it is almost always associated with some degree of mucous membrane involvement. Most cases are caused by an adverse drug reaction/sensitivity or an allergic process. Thus, erythema multiforme major is not Mr. Pickens' most likely diagnosis.

5. Treatment Plan

A. Tetracycline 500 mg four times a day for 7 to 10 days INCORRECT

There is no role for antibiotic therapies, such as tetracycline, in the treatment of a brown recluse spider bite unless a secondary bacterial infection is present. Then, the medication decision would be made empirically based on the most likely organism and confirmed by culture and sensitivity.

B. Surgical consult for débridement and possible excision with skin grafting   CORRECT

The treatment of envenomation from a brown recluse spider depends on the severity of the disease. Much more aggressive treatment is required if renal and/or hematologic abnormalities are present. However, the severity of the skin lesion itself also determines the extent of the treatment of the skin. It can range from simple cleansing and débridement for superficial lesions to removal and full-thickness skin grafts when deeper structures are involved. Therefore, an early surgical consult is imperative for Mr. Pickens, especially given the results of his diagnostic studies.

C. Dapsone 50 mg once daily   INCORRECT

If started within the first 72 hours of a brown recluse spider bite, dapsone has been shown in some animal studies to be beneficial in stopping, or at least slowing down, the progression of the necrosis. Unfortunately, human studies have yielded less impressive results. Therefore, because it has been longer than 72 hours since Mr. Pickens was bitten, dapsone would not be indicated.

D. Diphenhydramine 25 to 50 mg every 4 to 6 hours as needed for itch up to four times per day   CORRECT

Over-the-counter diphenhydramine is indicated for Mr. Pickens to use on an as-needed basis for the mild itching. Its primary mechanism of action is via the blocking of histamine-1 (H_1). Its most common adverse effect is drowsiness. If this occurs, he can substitute it for one of the over-the-counter nonsedating antihistamines. However, if either (or both) fails to alleviate his pruritus, a prescription nonsedating antihistamine can be tried. Alternatively, over-the-counter ranitidine can be used off-label in combination with an antihistamine for its histamine-2 (H_2)-blocking ability.

E. Hyperbaric oxygen therapy   INCORRECT

The results of animal studies utilizing hyperbaric oxygen (HBO) for brown recluse spider envenomation have also been disappointing. Therefore, HBO is not indicated.

Epidemiologic and Other Data

The brown recluse spider, *Loxosceles reclusa*, is endemic to the southeastern portion of the United States. This area is often defined as the western edge being southeastern Nebraska, the northern demarcation being southern Ohio, the eastern boundary being Georgia, and the southern border being the Gulf of Mexico. The southwest and lower Mississippi River Valley tends to be the area of greatest concentration. Therefore, a high index of suspicion for envenomation reactions must be considered in individuals residing in or recently vacationing in these areas.

CASE 11-4
Paul Queen
1. History

A. Does he find himself scratching the affected areas? ESSENTIAL

There are a limited number of conditions that cause skin plaquing, especially on the extensor surfaces of the joints. The most common one is psoriasis; however, another possible condition is lichen simplex chronicus. The hallmark of this latter condition is that the skin lesions are a result of a chronic itch-and-scratch cycle.

Other common conditions characterized by papulosquamous lesions, albeit typically with less predilection for the extensor surfaces and a more generalized distribution, include lichen planus, pityriasis rosea, dermatophytosis, seborrheic dermatitis, sebopsoriasis, and atypical urticaria.

B. Has he ever had this type of skin lesion, or a similar one, in the past?   ESSENTIAL

Although psoriasis is the most common cause of plaques on the extensor surfaces of the knees and elbows, it is unusual for it to begin in individuals who are younger than the age of 30 years or older than the age of 60 years. Therefore, it is important to inquire if he has experienced the same, or similar, lesions in the past. Furthermore, knowing whether this episode represents a worsening of a long-standing dermatologic condition, an intermittent exacerbation of the chronic process, or a new entity also assists in establishing an accurate differential diagnosis list.

C. Does he have any changes of his nails or itching/flaking of his scalp?   ESSENTIAL

Psoriasis can be associated with a fine stippling, or pitting, of the nails as well as scaling scalp lesions; however, the presence of these nail changes or scaling scalp is not pathognomonic for this condition. For example, nail pitting can also be seen with hand eczema and alopecia areata. Onychomycosis is another common condition that can cause abnormal-looking nails and a scaly rash. However, the nail changes are usually more dystrophic and the skin lesions on the flexure surfaces have more erythema and less plaquing than seen with psoriasis. Seborrheic dermatitis and sebopsoriasis are characterized by papulosquamous dermatologic manifestations and scaling scalp lesions; however, they rarely have significant nail involvement. Hand eczema and alopecia areata tend to be associated with nail lesions but minimal scalp scaling.

D. Is he experiencing any arthralgias, oral lesions, eye injection/erythema, eye discharge, penile discharge, dysuria, urinary urgency, or urinary frequency?   ESSENTIAL

Papulosquamous skin lesions can also be representative of an underlying systemic process. For example, psoriatic arthritis is an inflammatory arthritis that predominately affects the hands (in a distribution similar to that of rheumatoid arthritis) and the sacroiliac joint. It is associated with the characteristic skin and nail changes seen in cutaneous psoriasis. Likewise, reactive arthritis, or Reiter syndrome, also has skin lesions that look similar to psoriasis (although generally they are more extensive and more pustular) and stippling of the nails. However, reactive arthritis is also characterized by urethritis (or cervicitis in women), conjunctivitis, and oral lesions. Thus, inquiring about the presence of these symptoms is useful in evaluating for the presence of an associated systemic process.

Additionally, the sequencing of symptoms is also important in attempting to establish a connection between these various symptoms. For example, the onset of the rash in psoriatic

arthritis typically occurs simultaneously with the onset of the arthralgias; however, it can occur later on in the disease process. And, in Reiter syndrome it is possible for any combination of the symptoms to recur at any time following resolution of the initial disease.

E. Has he recently had strep throat?   NONESSENTIAL

Large papulosquamous plaques like Mr. Queen is describing are not a common dermatologic manifestation of group A β-hemolytic *Streptococcus* or any other common pharyngitis pathogen.

Guttate, or eruptive, psoriasis can occur following streptococcal pharyngitis (or other upper respiratory tract infection). Still, these lesions are not the characteristic scaly, papulosquamous lesions on extensor surfaces as seen in typical psoriasis but rather small (3–10 mm) erythematous lesions on an erythematous base with more extensive body involvement.

2. Physical Examination

A. CAGE alcohol screen   ESSENTIAL

Because Mr. Queen regularly consumes 12 beers per setting, two nights per week, yet describes his alcohol consumption as "occasionally," there is a concern that he might have more of a problem with alcohol abuse than being a binge drinker. Therefore, it is appropriate to perform a brief screen to determine whether further evaluation or treatment is required. This is relevant to his chief complaint because some plaque-type skin lesions can be exacerbated by alcohol intake.

B. Oral examination   NONESSENTIAL

Although there are some conditions characterized by papulosquamous skin lesions and oral lesions, these associated oral lesions tend to by symptomatic. Because Mr. Queen denied any oral complaints, a mouth examination is not indicated.

C. Skin examination   ESSENTIAL

Because Mr. Queen's chief complaint is a rash, a skin examination is indicated. The information that needs to be obtained via the visualization and palpation of the lesions is outlined in Case 5-5.

D. Scalp examination   ESSENTIAL

Because questioning identified that Mr. Queen suffers from chronic dandruff, a scalp examination is indicated to obtain additional information that is going to assist in formulating an appropriate differential diagnosis list for him. The scalp examination should consist not only of inspecting the skin itself for color abnormalities and skin lesions (including their characteristics and distribution if present) but also palpating it for texture changes. Also, the distribution of the hair needs to be evaluated. If an abnormality is identified, it needs to be further defined and characterized. For example, an area of alopecia needs to be evaluated to ensure that it is singular in number, to assess its distribution (e.g., consistent with male-pattern baldness or contact "friction" as seen over the occiput in infants), to examine the underlying skin's appearance and texture, to determine whether hair follicles are present, and/or to look for evidence of broken hair shafts. All of these can provide clues regarding whether the cause is a metabolic, hormonal, dermatologic, or psychological condition because any of these can be responsible for these findings.

E. Nail examination   ESSENTIAL

Additionally, because Mr. Queen admits to chronic nail changes, a nail examination is indicated. A multitude of conditions extending over several specialties (e.g., dermatology, pulmonology, hematology, endocrinology, infectious diseases, and/or psychology) and processes (e.g., traumatic, infectious, inflammatory, malignant, and/or metabolic) can be responsible for nail changes. Therefore, it is essential to examine for changes occurring at the junction of the finger (or toe) and the nail (e.g., clubbing is generally seen in chronic hypoxic states; spooning generally indicates anemia; and erythema, edema, tenderness, and occasionally a purulent discharge are frequently evident with a paronychia), color changes in the nail bed (e.g., bluish discoloration can be seen with hypoxia, acrocyanosis, or Raynaud phenomenon; a bright red discoloration is suspicious for acute carbon monoxide poisoning), thickness of the nail (e.g., atrophy can indicate circulatory abnormalities, neurologic conditions, or trauma), lesions under the nails (e.g., darkened areas can be a hematoma or a melanoma), lesions within the nails (e.g., Beau lines are associated with a recent serious illness or metabolic insult; stippling, ridges, or pitting is most commonly found in psoriasis; gross distortions could represent inflammation or compression of the matrix), color changes in the nails (e.g., yellowing can be secondary to tobacco smoking or carotenemia; generalized hyperpigmentation can result from treatment with chemotherapeutic agents), and the condition of the distal aspect of the nails (e.g., ragged edges can be seen with dermatologic, metabolic, and psychological conditions). Any abnormality identified must be considered in conjunction with the patient's history and other physical examination findings to formulate a clear meaning of its significance.

3. Diagnostic Studies

A. Potassium hydroxide preparation (KOH prep) of skin lesions   NONESSENTIAL

A KOH prep is used to identify the presence of dermatophyte infection. Although fungal infections of the skin can present as papulosquamous lesions, they are generally associated with more erythema, less plaquing, and less scaling lesions than Mr. Queen has. Additionally, they tend to affect the flexure, not extensor, surfaces of the extremities. Because Mr. Queen's condition should be diagnosable based on history and physical examination alone and he lacks the typical symptoms seen with a fungal skin infection, a KOH prep is not indicated at this time.

B. Human immunodeficiency virus (HIV) testing   NONESSENTIAL

An HIV test would be indicated for Mr. Queen if his skin lesions were significantly more extensive, this outbreak represented his initial episode of the lesions, and he was at risk for acquiring HIV because of his lifestyle.

C. Antistreptolysin O titer (ASO)   NONESSENTIAL

An ASO titer is primarily utilized to confirm the suspicion that a recent streptococcal infection is responsible for the

patient's current condition. It is not indicated because Mr. Queen lacks findings suggestive of such.

D. Complete blood count with differential (CBC w/diff) and coagulation studies   NONESSENTIAL

The combination of a CBC w/diff and coagulation studies is generally ordered when there exists suspicion that a bleeding disorder is either responsible for or associated with the patient's chief complaint. Thus, because such a suspicion was not identified through Mr. Queen's history and physical examination, these tests are not indicated.

E. Skin biopsy   NONESSENTIAL

Mr. Queen would require a skin biopsy if his diagnosis could not be established with a high degree of certainty based on his clinical presentation. Furthermore, it would be indicated if he failed to respond to appropriate treatment to ensure the diagnosis was correct. Nevertheless, at this time, a skin biopsy is not necessary because his diagnosis can be made clinically.

4. Diagnosis

A. Guttate (eruptive) psoriasis   INCORRECT

As stated previously, guttate, or eruptive, psoriasis is characterized by an extensive number of small (3–10 mm) erythematous papules that tend to have neither a specific pattern of distribution nor a predilection of body location. It frequently follows a streptococcal pharyngeal infection and is most common in children and young adults. It is rapidly developing, especially in comparison to the typical plaque-type psoriasis. Because this clinical picture is inconsistent with Mr. Queen's, guttate (eruptive) psoriasis can be ruled out as his most likely diagnosis.

B. Plaque-type psoriasis exacerbated by beta-blocker and binge drinking   CORRECT

Scaly, "silverfish" plaques with an erythematous base located on the extensor surfaces of the elbows and knees associated with fine stippling ("pitting") of the nails and seborrheic dermatitis are characteristic of plaque-type psoriasis.

Additionally, several medications, including the beta-blocker propranolol, have been known to worsen or exacerbate this condition. Other medications capable of producing this same type of a reaction include other beta-blockers, lithium, NSAIDs, statins, chloroquine, and other antimalarials.

Comorbid conditions have also been implicated in exacerbating or worsening plaque-type psoriasis; these include binge drinking, infectious processes, immunocompromised status, and emotional stress.

Because Mr. Queen's clinical picture is consistent with plaque-type psoriasis, he was placed on propranolol shortly before his condition exacerbated, and he admits to binge drinking, his most likely diagnosis from the list provided is plaque-type psoriasis exacerbated by beta-blocker and binge drinking.

C. Erythrodermic psoriasis exacerbated by beta-blocker   INCORRECT

Erythrodermic (pustular) psoriasis is very acute in onset and typically accompanied by fever and generalized pustular formation (including the palms of the hands and the soles of the feet) on a severely erythematous background. Medications, infections, irritants, immunocompromising conditions, pregnancy, and glucocorticosteroid withdrawal have been associated with the development of this condition. Although it can be exacerbated by beta-blockers, the discrepancy in the clinical picture prevents erythrodermic psoriasis from being Mr. Queen's most likely diagnosis.

D. Lichen simplex chronicus   INCORRECT

Lichen simplex chronicus is a papulosquamous eruption that occurs on an erythematous base. However, unlike plaque-type psoriasis, its borders are not as well demarcated, it plaques and patches are more rectangular in shape, it is more pinkish than silvery in color, and it is associated with an itch–scratch cycle that often results in a linear appearance to the lichenified areas. Therefore, lichen simplex chronicus can be eliminated as Mr. Queen's most likely diagnosis.

E. Reactive arthritis (Reiter syndrome)   INCORRECT

As previously stated, reactive arthritis (Reiter syndrome) can be associated with papulosquamous skin lesions; however, the hallmark of the disease is the coexistence of arthritis, urethritis (or cervicitis), conjunctivitis, and mucous membrane lesions. Because Mr. Queen lacks the defining symptoms, reactive arthritis (Reiter syndrome) is not his most likely diagnosis.

5. Treatment Plan

A. High-potency corticosteroid ointment twice a day for 2 weeks, then decrease to once a day if responding   CORRECT

The underlying principle in the treatment of psoriasis is the opposite of what is typically done in prescribing medication for most medical conditions. Instead of "starting low and going slow" in an upward taper, the theory is to "hit it hard and fast" and then taper downward. An appropriate combination strategy to achieve this goal is to use a high-potency (or even ultra-high-potency) corticosteroid ointment in addition to another effective agent, and then taper the steroid dose to the minimal effective dose of the lowest potency possible. Therefore, this would be an appropriate treatment option for Mr. Queen.

B. Calcipotriene ointment twice a day for 2 weeks, then decrease to once a day if responding   CORRECT

An excellent adjunct medication, especially in combination with topical corticosteroid therapy, in the treatment of psoriasis is the vitamin D analog calcipotriene ointment. It should also be tapered downward as the patient improves.

C. Clotrimazole ointment twice a day for 2 weeks, then decrease to once a day if responding   INCORRECT

Antifungals, such as clotrimazole, do not have a role in the treatment of psoriasis unless a coexisting fungal infection is present. Because there was no evidence to suggest this was a possibility in Mr. Queen's case, clotrimazole ointment is not indicated as part of his treatment plan.

D. Change propranolol to another antihypertensive outside of the beta-blocker class   CORRECT

Because beta-blockers have been associated with an exacerbation of psoriasis and Mr. Queen's symptoms dramatically worsened shortly after beginning one of these agents (propranolol), it is appropriate to discontinue his propranolol

and institute another antihypertensive outside of the beta-blocker class in hopes of being better able to control his psoriasis. However, it is essential to remember that in addition to monitoring his psoriatic activity, his hypertension is going to likewise need monitoring to ensure that he achieves good control on the new agent and doesn't suffer from unwanted adverse effects because of it.

E. Encourage him to stop, or at least significantly decrease, his alcohol consumption because of the likely effect it is having on his psoriasis and blood pressure   CORRECT

Mr. Queen should be encouraged to stop, or at least significantly decrease, his alcohol consumption because of its known adverse effects on both of his known medical conditions, psoriasis and hypertension. Additionally, he should be made aware of other potential medical, emotional, and social consequences that are potentially possible as a result of his frequent binge drinking despite his negative CAGE screen.

Epidemiologic and Other Data

Psoriasis is one of the most prevalent dermatologic conditions in the world, affecting approximately 1% of the world's population. There appears to be a genetic and immunologic (T-cell–mediated) basis to psoriasis. It occurs most frequently in non-Hispanic whites of northern European descent and much less frequently in African Americans. However, if not treated adequately and promptly, African Americans are more likely to develop keloidlike plaques that tend to be treatment resistant.

CASE 11-5
Rachel Smith
1. History

A. Has Rachel been in contact with a cat or kitten? If yes, could she have been scratched, bitten, or licked by it; where is the animal located; what is its current health; and is it current on its rabies vaccination?   ESSENTIAL

The affected axillary structure (e.g., lymph nodes, skin, muscles, bone, or a subcutaneous mass) is going to provide the most information in guiding the differential diagnoses in the correct direction. A wide array of musculoskeletal, dermatologic, infectious, and malignant causes are possible. A common bacterial infection that has a clinical presentation similar to Rachel's is cat-scratch disease; therefore, it is important to know if Rachel has been scratched, bitten, or even licked by a feline because saliva is the primary mode of transmission of the zoonosis *Bartonella henselae*, which, it is theorized, the cat acquired via an infected flea.

Furthermore because cats are a known reservoir of the rhabdovirus (the virus known to cause rabies), it is essential to know the cat's immunization status, location, and current health because the initial symptoms of rabies in humans can consist of headache, fever, malaise, fatigue, and nausea that can occur anywhere from 10 days to several years after exposure (average is 3–7 weeks).

B. Has Rachel experienced any type of a rash within the past 2 months?   ESSENTIAL

Inquiring about the presence of a rash, its appearance, its course, its location, and its time frame in relationship to her current symptoms is crucial. For example, cat-scratch fever can be responsible for several dermatologic manifestations (i.e., a puncture wound, laceration, or abrasion from the claws and/or teeth of the cat or a maculopapular rash once the patient becomes infected with *Bartonella henselae*). The time from inoculation to symptoms ranges from 3 to 50 days, with an average of 14 to 21 days, before the onset of the lymphadenopathy. Therefore, it is important to ensure that the historical time frame is sufficient to acquire the necessary information.

Other potential causes of a dermatologic manifestation in conjunction with a fever and unilateral axillary lymphadenopathy include viral exanthems; infectious mononucleosis; superficial and deep bacterial infections of the hand, arm, breast, and anterior and posterior chest; and malignancies of these same areas.

C. Has she been complaining of arthralgias or bone pain? ESSENTIAL

Typical and atypical cat-scratch disease; osteomyelitis of the bones of the extremity, scapula, or ribs; bone tumors of these same bones; viral syndromes; and autoimmune conditions can present with arthralgias and/or frank bone pain in a patient with unilateral axillary lymphadenopathy.

Additionally, if she has been experiencing these symptoms, it is important to know if there is true inflammation (erythema, edema, and increased temperature) at the site, indicating an increased likelihood of an autoimmune, inflammatory, or infectious process. The number of bones/joints involved is also important. If the symptoms were confined to a single joint, then trauma unknown to her mother or a septic arthritis must be high on her list of differential diagnoses. A hemarthrosis or a synovitis is also a potential differential diagnosis. However, if multiple joints are affected and exhibit true inflammation, the most likely culprit would be an inflammatory arthritis, of which juvenile rheumatoid arthritis (JRA) would be the most likely. Joint pain without inflammation is most commonly a result of degeneration; however, in Rachel's age group, it more than likely represents a viral process.

Furthermore, knowing which joints are affected is essential in providing clues as to the correct diagnosis because different disease processes have affinity for different diseases. For example, rheumatoid arthritis prefers the proximal interphalangeal (PIP) joints and metacarpophalangeal (MCP) joints, whereas psoriatic arthritis primarily affects the distal interphalangeal (DIP) joints. Finally, if Rachel had joint pain and it seemed to be in a long bone, then unknown trauma, osteomyelitis, and bony tumors must be included on the list of potential diagnoses. However, it is essential to attempt to determine whether the pain is truly skeletal in nature because it can be confused with involvement of the associated structures, especially in children.

D. Has she experienced any eye discharge, conjunctival injection, eye pain, or photophobia?   ESSENTIAL

An eye discharge and conjunctival injection can represent a wide array of viral, bacterial, allergic, and irritative processes. Of particular concern for Rachel would be a viral syndrome or direct inoculation of the *Bartonella henselae* organism. This results in the atypical form of cat-scratch disease

known as Parinaud oculoglandular syndrome, which also causes ipsilateral preauricular lymphadenopathy.

Ocular pain and photophobia are also important symptoms to inquire about in a patient with a fever and unusual lymphadenopathy pattern. They could indicate the presence of an associated central nervous system infection (e.g., meningitis or encephalitis), which incidentally would include rabies or a complication from cat-scratch disease.

E. Which hand is her dominant one?   NONESSENTIAL

Logically, injuries should occur at a greater frequency on the dominant hand; still, this doesn't have any particular significance in regards to Rachel's evaluation and doesn't need to be asked.

2. Physical Examination

A. General appearance   ESSENTIAL

The evaluation of the patient's general appearance is an important component of every medical encounter. This is especially important in patients who present with fever and atypical symptoms, in patients who have difficulty responding appropriately to questions (i.e., children, individuals with subaverage intelligence, or dementia patients), or when nonverbal clues are likely to be exceedingly valuable. In Rachel, one of the most important concerns is whether she is toxic and its severity, if present.

B. Lymph node examination   ESSENTIAL

The axillary lymph nodes are composed of three different sets of lymph nodes: the anterior (or pectoral), the posterior (or subscapular), and the lateral. The anterior group is responsible for draining the lymphatic flow from the anterior chest wall and the majority of the breast. The posterior group is responsible for the drainage of the posterior chest wall and part of the arm. The lateral nodes are responsible for the drainage of the majority of the arm. Infections, carcinomas, and inflammation are the main causes of lymphadenopathy. Therefore, any of these conditions at any of these sites can be responsible for an enlarged (tender or nontender) axillary lymph node. The chain of nodes involved provides additional clues to the exact source of the problem.

Because of the possibility of a systemic problem (despite Rachel only complaining of right axillae discomfort), it is essential to evaluate for the presence of cervical, epitrochlear, and inguinal lymphadenopathy as well.

C. Heart examination   ESSENTIAL

Atypical cat-scratch disease, some autoimmune processes, and a few bacterial infections not only can cause superficial skin problems with an associated lymphadenopathy but also can produce endocarditis. Therefore, it is important to perform a heart examination to identify signs that could indicate the presence of this serious complication.

D. Abdominal examination   ESSENTIAL

An abdominal examination is an important component of Rachel's physical examination to evaluate for the presence of splenomegaly, which can be seen in several febrile conditions with lymphadenopathy (e.g., atypical cat-scratch disease, viral syndromes [including infectious mononucleosis], autoimmune diseases, and malignancies, all of which can have presentations similar to Rachel's). Furthermore, mesenteric adenitis can be a complication of atypical cat-scratch disease. This and other conditions can be suspected by the presence of other abnormalities on the abdominal examination.

E. Bilateral hand/arm/shoulder/axilla examination   ESSENTIAL

The focal point of this examination is Rachel's right axillae to determine which structures are affected. A bilateral examination is essential because it will hopefully provide a "normal" for comparison; however, there is always the potential that an abnormality will be detected on the contralateral side as well.

Additionally, Rachel's upper extremities, shoulders, and axillae need to be examined not only to evaluate the "scratches" she has received from her kitten but also to evaluate for the presence of additional skin lesions, areas of discoloration, temperature changes, edema, and tenderness. Furthermore, this examination should include a musculoskeletal examination to identify any potential abnormalities in structure and function. If not previously conducted, a bilateral lymph node examination would complete this assessment.

3. Diagnostic Studies

A. Abdominal ultrasound   NONESSENTIAL

Because Rachel's only potential gastrointestinal symptoms are nausea and fever and her abdominal examination was unremarkable, an abdominal ultrasound is not indicated.

B. Biopsy with Gram stain, culture and sensitivity of the largest affected lymph node   NONESSENTIAL

A biopsy with Gram stain, culture and sensitivity of an enlarged, tender axillary lymph node is indicated if there are no other nodes involved; a likely diagnosis cannot be established based on the clinical picture; the lymph node is very large, extremely tender, or suppurative; and/or it is unresponsive to a trial of an antibiotic. In the case of a very large, extremely tender, suppurative node, this procedure is therapeutic as well because it often results in significant pain relief.

C. Purified protein derivative (PPD) skin test   NONESSENTIAL

Although tuberculosis (TB) is a potential cause of isolated lymphadenopathy and fever, a PPD test is not indicated because it would be extremely unlikely for Rachel to have acquired a clinically significant TB in the month that has passed since her last nonreactive TB skin test.

Additionally, there exists controversy regarding whether frequent repeat skin testing for TB via PPD, especially at the same site, can produce a false-positive result.

D. Spinal tap for cerebrospinal fluid (CSF) analysis including Gram stain and culture with sensitivity   NONESSENTIAL

A spinal tap for CSF analysis including Gram stain and culture with sensitivity would be indicated if Rachel was exhibiting signs and symptoms that were suspicious for meningitis, encephalitis, or a brain abscess.

E. Serology for *Bartonella henselae* titer   ESSENTIAL

The majority of the time, Rachel's condition can be diagnosed based on history and physical examination alone, especially if the lymphadenopathy has been present for several

weeks. However, because Rachel has only had her lymphadenopathy for a couple of days now, it is best to attempt to confirm her most likely diagnosis by performing a serology test for *Bartonella henselae*.

4. Diagnosis

A. Atypical cat-scratch disease   INCORRECT

Cat-scratch disease is an infectious process caused by *Bartonella henselae* that is characterized by fever and regional lymphadenopathy. Although cat-scratch disease tends to be self-limiting, the associated lymphadenopathy typically remains from weeks to months. The site of inoculation is generally evident as the lesion itself can persist for as long as 3 weeks. Other symptoms tend to be fairly mild and can include anorexia, nausea, vomiting, abdominal pain, headache, myalgias, and malaise.

Atypical cat-scratch disease is the term utilized to describe the approximately 25% of cases of cat-scratch disease that have unusual presentations or complications (e.g., Parinaud oculoglandular syndrome, bacillary angiomatosis, peliosis hepatitis, encephalitis, endocarditis, mesenteric adenitis, osteomyelitis, seizure disorder, or other neurologic abnormalities).

Despite Rachel having an elevated *Bartonella henselae* titer and a clinical picture consistent with the diagnosis of cat-scratch disease, atypical cat-scratch disease is not her most likely diagnosis because she lacks signs and symptoms indicative of an unusual presentation or complicating condition.

B. Infectious mononucleosis   INCORRECT

Infectious mononucleosis (IM), which is discussed in greater detail in Case 11-5, can cause symptoms similar to Rachel's (e.g., fever, sore throat, axillary adenopathy, and vague systemic symptoms); however, infectious mononucleosis is not her most likely diagnosis because she did not have a history of tonsillar enlargement, cervical lymphadenopathy, or splenomegaly, which are characteristic for IM. Additionally, IM is caused by the Epstein-Barr virus not *Bartonella henselae*, which Rachel has a positive (elevated) titer for the latter.

C. Lymphogranuloma venereum   INCORRECT

Lymphogranuloma venereum is a sexually transmitted infection that probably represents a late complication of a chlamydia urethritis or cervicitis (although some believe it is a distinct disease). It is characterized by very painful perineal and perianal ulcerations; proctitis; rectal and/or anal strictures; and severely enlarged, tender, and ulcerated inguinal lymphadenopathy (called buboes). Because Rachel lacked these characteristic symptoms of the disease and has tender, axillary lymphadenopathy and an elevated *Bartonella henselae* titer, lymphogranuloma venereum can be eliminated as her most likely diagnosis.

Furthermore the presence of this condition in a 5-year-old would be considered to result from sexual molestation/assault until proven otherwise and would be reportable to the appropriate authorities.

D. Typical cat-scratch disease   CORRECT

Given the aforementioned description of the disease, Rachel's history of kitten scratches, and her positive titer for

Bartonella henselae, typical cat-scratch disease is her most likely diagnosis.

E. Burkitt lymphoma   INCORRECT

Burkitt lymphoma is a malignancy that is typically associated with abdominal pain, abdominal fullness, and painless lymphadenopathy that generally involves multiple nodes in the inguinal, retroperitoneum, mesenteric, and/or pelvic regions. However, axillary lymphadenopathy is generally not part of the clinical picture. Based on Rachel's clinical picture and elevated *Bartonella henselae* titer, Burkitt lymphoma is not her most likely diagnosis.

5. Treatment Plan

A. Continue acetaminophen   CORRECT

Because acetaminophen is currently controlling her pain and fever and she has no evidence to suspect the presence of a hepatic dysfunction, it should be continued. However, it is important to determine that her mother is using an appropriate formulation for Rachel's age and a correct measuring device, and does not exceed the recommended daily dose.

B. Doxycycline 100 mg with rifampin 300 mg twice a day for 4 to 6 weeks   INCORRECT

Because her disease appears to be mild at present, an antibiotic is not indicated. Furthermore, because of its potential adverse effect on the color of children's teeth, doxycycline is contraindicated in children unless no other suitable antibiotic is available.

C. Ciprofloxacin 500 mg twice a day for 2 weeks   INCORRECT

Again, because her disease is currently mild, she does not require antibiotic therapy. Furthermore, because of ciprofloxacin's potential adverse effect on tendons, it is also contraindicated in children unless there is not another viable antibiotic choice available.

D. Diphtheria, tetanus, acellular pertussis (DTaP)   INCORRECT

Tetanus prophylaxis is typically not discussed as a component of the management of cat-scratch disease, probably because of the delay from inoculation to symptom onset. Additionally, excoriations, superficial lacerations, and abrasions from cat scratch are debatable as to whether they constituted a "dirty" wound, despite there being the potential for them to be contaminated with soil, feces, or saliva. However, once cat-scratch disease is apparent, there is no doubt that the wound contained infected saliva. Still, the time lag from inoculation to symptom development is beyond the time frame where active immunity via vaccine or passive immunity via tetanus immune globulin (TIG) would be a beneficial prevention strategy in patients with an inadequate tetanus immunization status. Nevertheless, it is probably beneficial to provide unimmunized, partially immunized, or inadequately immunized patients with an appropriate vaccination and a schedule to ensure immunity remains active because they will likely have continued exposure to cat scratches, punctures, and bites.

DTaP is the appropriate vaccine for Rachel; however, she does not require one because her history indicated that she received this immunization approximately 1 month ago. Thus, even with a "dirty" wound, she will not need an additional immunization against tetanus for 5 years.

E. Have vet decapitate the cat and send its head to the state health department to be examined for rabies   INCORRECT

The cat is in a confined area where it can be observed for any signs or symptoms of illness, and it will need to remain there for the next 10 to 14 days as a precaution. Additionally, it is current on its rabies vaccination program. Therefore, destroying Rachel's pet is unnecessary at this time.

Epidemiologic and Other Data

Cat-scratch disease is typically a disease of childhood and adolescence, with over 80% of all cases being in individuals younger than the age of 21 years. The annual incidence in the United States is estimated to be approximately 6.5 cases per 100,000 individuals.

It generally takes anywhere from 2 to 6 months for the lymphadenopathy to completely resolve. Obviously, close follow-up is required during this time frame to ensure complications do not develop and resolution is complete.

CASE 11-6
Sabrina Tabatherson
1. History

A. What has been the pattern of her cough since becoming ill? ESSENTIAL

A cough that persists for greater than 2 weeks in a patient who does not appear critically ill (e.g., suffering from untreated pneumonia) can be caused by a variety of conditions. The most common respiratory causes are asthma, chronic bronchitis, pertussis, and chronic postnasal discharge. However, nonrespiratory causes can also be responsible for a chronic cough. The most common one is gastroesophageal reflux disease (GERD).

Furthermore, the pattern of the cough can provide significant clues to the patient's most likely diagnosis. For example, a cough that is most prominent at night is most often associated with GERD or the early onset of pertussis. However, the cough of pertussis eventually becomes diurnal.

B. Does she experience dyspnea between coughing episodes? ESSENTIAL

The lack of dyspnea between the episodes makes an acute infection (e.g., bronchiolitis, acute bronchitis, and pneumonia) much less likely to be causing the patient's symptoms. However, the lack of dyspnea between episodes supports the diagnosis of pertussis, chronic postnasal discharge, and GERD. Asthma could be present in either manner.

C. Are her immunizations up to date, including a recent tetanus toxoid, diphtheria toxoid and acellular pertussis (Tdap) vaccine?   ESSENTIAL

It is essential to inquire regarding Ms. Tabatherson's immunization status, especially her Tdap. If this immunization is current, pertussis is much less likely, but not impossible, to be the cause.

D. What color is her rhinorrhea?   NONESSENTIAL

Knowing the color of Ms. Tabatherson's rhinorrhea does not provide any additional information because recent studies revealed that the color of nasal discharge (and even sputum) does little to assist in differentiating between viral and bacterial infections.

E. Has she ever had pertussis, or "whooping cough"? NONESSENTIAL

A history of pertussis is irrelevant because having the disease does not confer lasting immunity.

2. Physical Examination

A. Ear, nose, and throat (ENT) examination   ESSENTIAL

An ENT examination is indicated to evaluate for residual signs of an infection or other problem because Ms. Tabatherson probably had an upper respiratory infection early in the course of her illness.

B. Bilateral eye examination   ESSENTIAL

A bilateral eye examination is indicated because Ms. Tabatherson is complaining of a painless "red eye." Therefore, an examination is needed to determine whether the cause is benign (e.g., conjunctivitis or subconjunctival hemorrhage) or serious and potentially emergent (e.g., acute uveitis, glaucoma, or trauma).

C. Heart examination   ESSENTIAL

A cardiac examination is indicated because she has been experiencing a new onset of intermittent dyspnea. Arrhythmias, new-onset or advancing valvular abnormalities, and a recently occurring cardiomegaly are among some of the clinical findings that could be associated with a cardiac cause of the dyspnea.

D. Lung examination   ESSENTIAL

A lung examination is indicated because Ms. Tabatherson has a chronic cough and intermittent dyspnea. The location (e.g., generalized, localized to one lobe, unilateral, or bilateral) and type (e.g., absent breath sounds, wheezing, rhonchi, prolonged inspiratory phase, or prolonged expiratory phase) of findings can assist in supporting or eliminating some of the patient's potential differential diagnoses.

E. Abdominal examination   NONESSENTIAL

The most likely GI cause responsible for a chronic cough is GERD; it is generally associated with a normal physical examination, especially in patients without GI symptoms.

3. Diagnostic Studies

A. White blood cell count with differential (WBC w/diff)   ESSENTIAL

A WBC w/diff is indicated in Ms. Tabatherson's case to assist in ruling in or ruling out an infectious process. Furthermore, it will provide clues as to whether an infection, if present, is more than likely viral or bacterial in origin as well as its severity.

B. Nasal swab for culture on Bordet-Gengou agar and a DNA polymerase chain reaction (PCR) assay for *Bordetella pertussis*   ESSENTIAL

A nasal swab for culture on Bordet-Gengou agar and DNA PCR assay for *Bordetella pertussis* are indicated based on

Ms. Tabatherson's description of her cough and her lack of adequate pertussis immunization to rule-out (or -in) pertussis.

Bordet-Gengou agar, or other special media, must be utilized because the gram-negative organism, *Bordetella pertussis* will not grow on regular culture media. Bordet-Gengou is the most commonly utilized agar for this possible organism.

DNA PCR assays are probably the quickest technique to determine the presence of *Bordetella pertussis*. A positive result confirms the diagnosis of pertussis; however, a negative result does not necessarily rule it out. Furthermore, they are not available at all facilities.

C. Enzyme-linked immunosorbent assay (ELISA) IgA and IgG serum antibody titers for pertussis   ESSENTIAL

ELISA IgA and IgG serum antibody titers for pertussis are indicated to assist in ruling in or ruling out the diagnosis of pertussis. A single positive ELISA IgA or IgG antibody is not necessarily confirmation that the patient has pertussis; however, it does indicate that the patient has been exposed to it at some time in the recent past. Therefore, the titers should be repeated in 1 week; a two- to four-fold increase confirms the diagnosis.

A high index of suspicion must be maintained for the disease and the use of empiric antibiotics must be considered as early as possible in the course of the illness. Pertussis should be considered the diagnosis until proven otherwise in patients who have had a cough that has persisted for 14 days or longer, a paroxysmal "whoop" with their respiratory illness, or any signs or symptoms of a respiratory illness if they have been exposed to a confirmed case of pertussis.

D. Chest x-ray (CXR)   NONESSENTIAL

Because of the minimal findings on Ms. Tabatherson's lung examination, a CXR is not indicated.

E. Electroencephalogram (EEG)   NONESSENTIAL

An EEG is not going to provide any useful information unless her clinical course becomes complicated by a seizure or other neurologic disorder.

4. Diagnosis

A. Bronchiolitis   INCORRECT

Bronchiolitis is an acute respiratory illness characterized by bronchial inflammation. It is most commonly caused by the respiratory syncytial virus. It can be eliminated as Ms. Tabatherson's most likely diagnosis because it is rare beyond the age of 2 years, does not have three distinct disease phases, and is associated with dyspnea between coughing episodes. Furthermore, her DNA PCR to *Bordetella pertussis* is positive and the initial ELISA IgA and IgG antibodies to *Bordetella pertussis* are elevated, which is also inconsistent with this diagnosis. Hence, bronchiolitis is not Ms. Tabatherson's most likely diagnosis.

B. Pertussis with subconjunctival hemorrhage probably secondary to cough   CORRECT

Pertussis, or "whooping cough," is a respiratory infection that generally exhibits three distinct phases. The first one, known as the catarrhal stage, lasts approximately 2 weeks. It consists of a nonproductive cough that initially occurs at night but later becomes diurnal as well as symptoms of an upper respiratory tract infection, malaise, and anorexia.

This is followed by the paroxysmal stage, which generally lasts approximately 2 weeks (however, up to 4 weeks' duration is not uncommon). During this stage, all the symptoms improve except the cough. The cough starts occurring in rapid spasms accompanied by high-pitched inspiratory "whoops" and dyspnea. Between paroxysms, the patient is essentially asymptomatic after recovering from the episode. It is not uncommon during the paroxysms for the patient to develop subconjunctival hemorrhages or small petechial hemorrhages anywhere on the body.

This is followed by the final, or convalescent, stage. During this phase, the cough, spasms, and dyspnea gradually subside. Based on the information thus far obtained, Ms. Tabatherson's most likely diagnosis is pertussis with subconjunctival hemorrhage probably secondary to cough.

C. Acute asthma   INCORRECT

The symptoms of acute asthma result from airway hyperresponsiveness and inflammation; and, they include dyspnea, wheezing, and cough. However, these symptoms tend not to be limited to the coughing episodes. Furthermore, patients with acute asthma may or may not have the moderate to severe degree of leukocytosis with lymphocytosis as seen in this patient. Additionally, they are not positive for DNA via PCR and only have elevated ELISA IgA and IgG antibodies to *Bordetella pertussis* if they have recently had the illness, or at least been exposed to it. Therefore, acute asthma is not Ms. Tabatherson's most likely diagnosis.

D. Gastroesophageal reflux disease (GERD)   INCORRECT

GERD has been implicated as a cause of cough. However, it tends to be more gradual in onset and not associated with spasms, as Ms. Tabatherson's is. Additionally, GERD patients generally, but not always, have at least some minimal GI symptoms (e.g., pyrosis, reflux of stomach contents, or dysphagia). Furthermore, it is not associated leukocytosis with lymphocytosis or a positive DNA via PCR test for *Bordetella pertussis*. Hence, GERD is not Ms. Tabatherson's most likely diagnosis.

E. Adenovirus infection   INCORRECT

Adenovirus can cause acute upper respiratory tract infections, conjunctivitis, gastroenteritis, and hemorrhagic cystitis in patients of Ms. Tabatherson's age group. The acute upper respiratory tract infection produced by the adenovirus is self-limiting and rarely persists beyond 1 week. Thus, an adenovirus infection can be eliminated as Ms. Tabatherson's most likely diagnosis because of the length and course of her symptoms and her positive PCR test for *Bordetella pertussis*.

5. Treatment Plan

A. Azithromycin 250 mg two tablets stat, then one tablet a day for 2 to 5 more days   CORRECT

Azithromycin is considered to be one of the first-line drugs of choice for patients with pertussis. However, it generally does not shorten the paroxysmal phase associated with pertussis. Essentially, it must be given during the catarrhal phase to have any effect on the course of the illness. It is

beneficial in eliminating the organism from the upper respiratory tract and hopefully will prevent the spread of the infection to others.

B. Erythromycin estolate 500 mg twice a day for 5 days INCORRECT

Erythromycin estolate 500 mg twice a day for 5 days would not be considered an appropriate treatment plan. Although erythromycin estolate is considered to be another first-line choice for pertussis, the dosage is 500 mg four times a day for 14 days.

Other effective antibiotics include double-strength trimethoprim-sulfamethoxazole twice a day for 14 days, clarithromycin 500 mg twice a day for 7 days, or extended-release clarithromycin 1 g once a day for 7 days.

C. Prophylaxis of household/dormitory contacts   CORRECT

Prophylaxis of household/dormitory contacts is an important public health measure and should be instituted regardless of their pertussis immunization status, because even with appropriate immunizations, there is a 20% infection rate if someone in the household develops pertussis. Among inadequately immunized individuals, the infection rate is between 80 and 100% if a household contact develops the disease.

D. Esomeprazole 20 mg once a day   INCORRECT

Esomeprazole 20 mg once a day is a suitable treatment for GERD, but not for pertussis; therefore, it is not an appropriate component of Ms. Tabatherson's treatment plan.

E. Prednisone tapered over 14 days, starting with 60 mg INCORRECT

Prednisone tapered over 14 days, starting with 60 mg is also not indicated in the treatment of pertussis and therefore should not be given to Ms. Tabatherson.

Epidemiologic and Other Data

Despite immunization, pertussis still has outbreaks that cycle between 3 and 5 years. In the United States, there is a peak in the incidence of cases in the summer and autumn.

The mortality rate of pertussis in female patients is greater than that of male patients. The majority of cases occur in children younger than the age of 5 years. However, rates have been gradually increasing in adolescents and adults in the United States over the past several years.

Recently, a Tdap vaccine was approved for preadolescents. There are two formulations: one is indicated for individuals who are 10 years of age or younger; the other is indicated for individuals who are 11 years of age or older. Its administration is recommended to all children at the age of 11 or 12 years old if they successfully completed their initial series of DTP/DTaP and have not yet had their booster immunization (which generally occurs between the ages of 14 and 16 years, 10 years after the completion of the initial series). If not received in that preadolescent period, it is recommended that it be provided as a "catch-up" immunization somewhere between the ages of 13 and 18 years, especially if the patient plans on attending college or joining the military after high school.

Furthermore, it is recommended that adults from the ages of 19 to 64 years replace one of their Td (tetanus diphtheria)

boosters, which is recommended to be given every 10 years, with Tdap if they are certain they had the initial primary series as a child. Adults with a negative or unknown childhood immunization history should receive the primary series.

CASE 11-7

Tami Upjohn

1. History

A. When was her last menstrual period (LMP) and was it normal?   ESSENTIAL

Inquiring as to when Ms. Upjohn's LMP occurred and whether it was normal is essential because if it was very recent, the nausea and vomiting that she is currently experiencing could be caused by a pregnancy (despite the fact she is reliably using oral contraceptives) that was too early to be detected by a urinary pregnancy test. If that was the case, then a quantitative serum HCG would be indicated.

B. Has she had any constipation, diarrhea, or color change of her stool?   ESSENTIAL

Diarrhea could indicate a viral gastroenteritis, a bacterial gastroenteritis (e.g., *Salmonella choleraesuis* or *Shigella dysenteriae*), a bacterial overgrowth infection as a result of toxin production of normal flora caused by the antibiotic (e.g., *Clostridium difficile* or *Escherichia coli*), or other adverse effect from the antibiotics, to name a few.

A black, tarry-appearing stool could indicate gastrointestinal bleeding, whereas a light-colored stool could indicate a hepatic or pancreatic abnormality.

C. Has she noticed any changes in her skin or yellowing of her sclera?   ESSENTIAL

Inquiring about the presence of jaundice, icterus, and/or any rash is important. Jaundice, icterus, could be an indicator of the presence of a sexually transmitted hepatitis, especially hepatitis B, or a complication of pelvic inflammatory disease (PID), particularly Fitz-Hugh and Curtis syndrome.

A rash could indicate an adverse drug reaction or a complication of PID (e.g., disseminated gonococcal infection [DGI], bacteremia, or endocarditis).

D. Has she had any nasal discharge?   NONESSENTIAL

Because she is only complaining of gastrointestinal symptoms and does not have a fever, it is unlikely that a process associated with rhinorrhea could be producing her symptoms.

E. Has she been drinking any alcohol?   ESSENTIAL

Knowing whether Ms. Upjohn had been drinking any alcohol with her antibiotics is important because the combination of alcohol and metronidazole can cause a disulfiram-like reaction, which consists of nausea, vomiting, flushing, and hypotension (if severe).

2. Physical Examination

A. Ear and nose examination   NONESSENTIAL

Examining these areas is unnecessary because given Ms. Upjohn's symptoms is highly unlikely to yield any clinically relevant information concerning her chief complaint.

B. Sclera and skin examination   ESSENTIAL

Her skin and sclera should be examined for the presence of icterus and jaundice, respectively; either would increase the possibility of an associated hepatitis, perihepatitis, severe hepatic reaction/failure, or significant adverse effects secondary to her medications.

C. Abdominal examination   ESSENTIAL

An abdominal examination is definitely indicated on Ms. Upjohn because she is complaining of two distinct types of pain in two different areas of the abdomen.

D. Pelvic examination   ESSENTIAL

She also needs a repeat pelvic examination to ensure that her PID is continuing to improve and has not developed complications (e.g., abscess formation).

E. Back examination   NONESSENTIAL

Because Ms. Upjohn's symptoms do not appear to be musculoskeletal or renal in nature, a back examination is unlikely to yield any useful clinical information especially since she is not complaining of back pain.

3. Diagnostic Studies

A. Abdominal ultrasound   ESSENTIAL

An abdominal ultrasound is indicated for Ms. Upjohn because of the presence of her right upper quadrant pain associated with nausea and vomiting. This could represent coexisting conditions (e.g., cholelithiasis or hepatitis), complications from her current disease process (e.g., perihepatitis), or effects of the treatment (e.g., adverse effects from the antibiotics). Furthermore, it will provide a superficial scan of the pelvic structures for gross abnormalities that might need to be evaluated further (e.g., ectopic pregnancy, tubo-ovarian abscess, other masses, or organomegaly).

B. Repeat complete blood count with differential (CBC w/diff) and erythrocyte sedimentation rate (ESR)   ESSENTIAL

A repeat CBC w/diff and ESR are indicated to provide confirmation that Ms. Upjohn's PID is indeed improving despite the development of these new symptoms.

C. Repeat testing for gonorrhea and chlamydia   NONESSENTIAL

Repeating the DNA amplification testing for gonorrhea and chlamydia at this time is not going to provide any additional information because they will still be positive. In fact, this testing technique remains positive for several weeks after the infection has been resolved. Therefore, if repeat testing is desired because of concerns of noncompliance, reinfection, or having to utilize a medication that has questionable coverage (e.g., a fluoroquinolone for gonorrhea), it should be performed a minimum of 4 weeks posttreatment.

If there is concern regarding an unresolved infection or a reinfection that must be confirmed within this time frame, a cervical (or other sites if indicated [e.g., pharynx and anal]) culture on appropriate media (e.g., Thayer-Martin ["chocolate auger"] for gonorrhea and cell culture for chlamydia), should be obtained and transported under proper conditions.

D. Liver function tests (LFTs)   ESSENTIAL

LFTs are indicated for Ms. Upjohn because of the location of her pain as well as the possible hepatic conditions in the differential diagnoses.

E. Testing for hepatitis B and C   NONESSENTIAL

Testing for hepatitis B and C is premature at this time. It is very unlikely for acute, symptomatic hepatitis to be present because of her normal LFTs. Therefore, it is best to obtain the LFT results; then, if the results are suspicious for hepatitis, testing can be done with the appropriate antibodies. In acute hepatitis, all the liver enzymes are elevated with the alanine aminotransferase (ALT) > aspartate aminotransferase (AST) > lactate dehydrogenase (LDH) > alkaline phosphatase (ALP).

F. Electrolytes   ESSENTIAL

Because of Ms. Upjohn's frequent vomiting, electrolytes are indicated to evaluate the hydration status and determine the presence of any electrolyte abnormalities that need to be corrected before complications (e.g., cardiac arrhythmias secondary to hypokalemia) occur.

4. Diagnosis

A. Hyperemesis gravidarum   INCORRECT

Hyperemesis gravidarum is severe nausea and vomiting caused by pregnancy. It is generally associated with dehydration, metabolic acidosis, and/or weight loss. From the diagnostic studies obtained, if any alteration of the acid-base balance is present, it would be metabolic alkalosis based on Ms. Upjohn's hypokalemia.

Nevertheless, hyperemesis gravidarum is not Ms. Upjohn's most likely diagnosis because it is uncommon for it to be associated with frank abdominal pain. Additionally, she has a negative pregnancy test and has been using a very effective contraceptive method consistently and correctly.

B. Acute hepatitis B and/or C   INCORRECT

Hepatitis B and C can essentially be eliminated as the most likely diagnosis for Ms. Upjohn because of her normal LFTs; absence of constitutional symptoms before the onset of her right upper quadrant pain; and lack of jaundice, icterus, hepatomegaly, and definite liver tenderness on her physical examination.

C. Fitz-Hugh and Curtis syndrome   INCORRECT

Fitz-Hugh and Curtis syndrome is a perihepatitis that generally occurs as a complication of PID. It can also be ruled out as Ms. Upjohn's most likely diagnosis based on her normal LFTs and lack of physical examination findings suggesting hepatic involvement. Furthermore, her abdominal ultrasound failed to reveal any signs of inflammation of the hepatic capsule, which is one of the hallmark features of the disease.

D. Hepatoma secondary to oral contraceptives   INCORRECT

A hepatoma is a liver tumor that can occur as a rare complication with oral contraceptive usage. Although the majority of cases are asymptomatic, it frequently produces hepatomegaly that is palpable on physical examination. Thus, hepatoma can also be eliminated as her most likely diagnosis for her presenting illness, especially considering one not being visualized on her ultrasound.

E. Gastrointestinal (GI) intolerance of antibiotics causing mild dehydration and hypokalemia   CORRECT

Based on the information available, Ms. Upjohn's most likely diagnosis for her epigastric and right upper quadrant abdominal pain associated with nausea and vomiting is intolerance to her antibiotics with a mild secondary dehydration resulting in the mild hypokalemia. The most likely culprit is the doxycycline, which has a very high rate of discontinuation because of GI intolerability; however, metronidazole has been known to cause GI symptoms as well.

Diagnostic confirmation for this diagnosis consists of a continued improvement of her PID as indicated by an improving CBC w/diff and a decreasing ESR, a normal abdominal ultrasound, and a mild hypokalemia.

5. Treatment Plan

A. Change oral doxycycline and metronidazole to ciprofloxacin 500 mg bid for 14 days and continue treatment as an outpatient   INCORRECT

Stopping the doxycycline and metronidazole should be effective in resolving the nausea and vomiting and correcting her electrolyte disturbance secondary to her vomiting within a few days. However, ciprofloxacin is not recommended for the treatment of PID because of its high incidence of resistance in gonorrhea. Furthermore, it is not an appropriate medication to treat chlamydia either.

B. Add esomeprazole 20 mg once a day to outpatient regimen   INCORRECT

Adding esomeprazole 20 mg once a day to the outpatient regimen is also not an appropriate treatment option for Ms. Upjohn because it may or may not alleviate her nausea and vomiting; therefore, her dehydration and electrolyte abnormality would only worsen. Furthermore, it could potentially interact with her antibiotics, causing a decrease in their serum levels and effectiveness.

C. Hospitalize and provide antibiotics by IV and treat hypokalemia   CORRECT

Ms. Upjohn requires hospitalization for IV antibiotics and to treat her hypokalemia. This decision is based on clinical grounds and supported by the CDC's guidelines recommending hospitalization of patients with PID, because she is unable to tolerate oral medications and has an electrolyte abnormality as a result of her vomiting.

Additional criteria/conditions that the CDC guidelines strongly encourage hospitalization for a patient with PID include the inability to appropriately follow an outpatient regimen, a severe illness, a high fever, pregnancy, a tubo-ovarian abscess, not responding to outpatient treatment, or a surgical emergency (e.g., appendicitis or ectopic pregnancy cannot be excluded during the evaluation).

Remember that these are only guidelines; and, clinical judgment must be utilized on a case-by-case basis.

D. Add potassium chloride orally twice a day   INCORRECT

Adding potassium chloride twice a day to the outpatient regimen might be effective in managing her hypokalemia, if she were able to tolerate anything orally. Because she is vomiting an average of more than once per hour, it is unlikely that she would be able to maintain enough of the medication for it to be effective. Furthermore, potassium chloride is irritating to the stomach and would probably only intensify her GI symptoms.

E. Refer to gastroenterologist for a liver biopsy   INCORRECT

Ms. Upjohn has normal LFTs and a normal abdominal ultrasound; therefore, a hepatic biopsy is not indicated at this time.

Epidemiologic and Other Data

Although PID is considered by most to be a sexually transmitted infection (STI), only approximately 50% of cases are caused by a sexually transmitted infection, either *Neisseria gonorrhea* or *Chlamydia trachomatis*. The other half are caused by organisms found in the normal vaginal flora (e.g., *Haemophilus vaginitis, Gardnerella vaginitis, Mycoplasma hominis, Prevotella* species, *Peptostreptococcus* species, and *Mobiluncus* species) and other miscellaneous organisms (e.g., *Mycoplasma genitalium, Escherichia coli, Haemophilus influenzae,* group A *Streptococcus*, and various anaerobes). Rarely is it caused by some other atypical organism.

In 2005, there were approximately 176,000 cases of PID in the United States in females between the ages of 15 and 44 years old. This incidence rate is less than half of the rate seen in the 1980s despite the "loosening" of the defining criteria.

The fertility rate is estimated to decrease approximately 15 to 25% for each incidence of PID. Hence, if a woman had PID three times, her fertility rate would be anywhere from 45 to 75% lower than an average age-matched woman. Condom usage decreases, but does not totally eliminate, the acquisition of sexually transmitted infections, including PID.

CASE 11-8

Ulisa VanDyke

1. History

A. Have there been any recent changes in soaps, shampoos, lotions, detergents, fabric softeners, or other products that come into contact with Ulisa's body?   NONESSENTIAL

This question is irrelevant because Ulisa's extensive symptoms; the severity of her condition, and the limited location and nature of her rash, make it extremely unlikely that her problem is a contact dermatitis.

B. Has Ulisa been experiencing any myalgias, arthralgias, seizures, lightheadedness, vertigo, presyncope, or syncope?   ESSENTIAL

When presented with a patient with a probable infectious process, it is imperative to distinguish relatively benign, self-limiting infectious illnesses from serious, potentially life-threatening, systemic infectious conditions while concurrently attempting to establish the correct diagnosis. Oftentimes this decision has to be made quickly and based on the limited data to prevent adverse outcomes, significant morbidity, and even mortality.

Critical decisions that must be made during the visit include determining the severity of the infection; interpreting that severity in conjunction with the patient's past medical history; hospitalization; determining frequency of follow-up if managing as an outpatient; deciding to utilize empiric antibiotic therapies immediately, after observation, or not at all, in this age of multidrug resistance; and establishing what constitutes appropriate monitoring and prevention strategies for potential complications.

Although there are some guidelines available to assist in making these decisions for particular conditions (e.g., pneumonia, pelvic inflammatory disease, strep throat, otitis media, and sinusitis), there are no evidence-based guidelines available for the majority of infectious diseases, especially without a firmly established diagnosis; therefore, the HCP must rely on his or her clinical judgment and maintain a high index of suspicion to reach the most appropriate treatment plan in a timely manner.

It can be assumed from the rapid progression of Ulisa's symptoms from being mildly "flulike" early in the day to being toxic appearing, being inconsolable by her mother, developing petechial lesions, becoming confused, and complaining of head and neck pain later in the day that she has a serious infectious process occurring.

Therefore, it is essential to determine whether she is experiencing any other symptoms that could be associated with a severe systemic infectious process, including septic shock.

C. Has Ulisa's rash changed in any manner since it began?   ESSENTIAL

The progression of symptoms is an essential component in the evaluation process. In regards to a rash, it is important to ascertain its initial and current locations, the direction of spread, the initial appearance, type of evolution (if any), and the development of associated symptoms (e.g., pain, paresthesias, or pruritus) in relationship to its onset and progression.

D. What does she mean by "confused"?   ESSENTIAL

When evaluating a patient's complaint, it is essential that the HCP has a clear understanding of exactly what the patient's symptoms are. Thus, it is sometimes necessary to obtain clarification regarding what is meant by certain complaints (e.g., confusion) because different words have different meanings for different individuals. Misinterpreting what a patient/parent means by a symptom can lead to delay in the evaluation, diagnosis, and treatment of a patient's condition, or worse, result in a critical error.

E. Has she noticed any changes in Ulisa's urine's frequency or color?   ESSENTIAL

The hydration status of an individual can be estimated by his or her urine output. If a patient is urinating at least every 6 to 8 hours, then a clinically significant dehydration is unlikely. Furthermore, urinating less frequently and urine that is darker in color (more concentrated) can also suggest the presence of mild dehydration.

Additionally, tears when crying, moist lips, moist oral mucosa, and normal skin turgor on physical examination are gross indicators that a significant dehydration is not present.

2. Physical Examination

A. General appearance   ESSENTIAL

Any time an HCP sees a patient, he or she makes a gross assessment of the patient's general appearance upon entry into the examination room and throughout the encounter. The majority of the time, the patient's appearance is unremarkable and not noteworthy. Therefore, frequently nothing is documented on the chart. However, there are circumstances in which it is essential to pay specific attention to and document these findings.

In children, the major observations include hygiene, appropriateness of dress, signs of abuse, severity of illness, consistency of appearance with given history, overall demeanor and mood, interactions between child and parent, reaction to the HCP, and interfacing with the overall environment. In adults, all of these areas are assessed except for the interaction with parent; however, if accompanied by a significant other, the HCP would notice how they interacted with that individual, their mannerisms, manner of speech, and overall body language.

However, there are times that the history or the initial gross assessment of the patient causes the HCP to really focus on some of these aspects as part of the evaluation. The rapidity of Ulisa's illness, her elevated temperature, her toxic appearance, and not being able to be consoled by her mother are important reasons the HCP needs to take that "extra look."

B. Skin examination   ESSENTIAL

A skin examination is essential for Ulisa because of her rash. It is essential not only to observe the rash but also to evaluate for signs of developing ecchymoses, purpura, or gangrene because these are often signs of a severe, rapidly progressing systemic process.

It should also include an assessment of her skin turgor as a gross assessment of her hydration status because she is young and experiencing a high fever, vomiting, and diarrhea.

C. Eyes, ears, nose, and throat (EENT) examination ESSENTIAL

An EENT examination is essential because Ulisa's illness began with a low-grade fever and rhinorrhea. It should include a comprehensive evaluation of all areas for a focus of infection and the presence of petechiae on her mucous membranes to assist in ruling in or eliminating various infectious processes. Additionally, clues to the patient's hydration status can be determined during the evaluation for presence of tears and a moist appearance to her lips and oral mucosa. (Note: the injection of Ulisa's tympanic membranes in the absence of decreased mobility and middle ear effusion is most likely caused by her crying, not inner ear pathology [e.g., otitis media]).

D. Abdominal examination   ESSENTIAL

An abdominal examination is indicated because of her vomiting and diarrhea to determine whether there are any signs to indicate that a gastrointestinal or peritoneal cause is responsible for, or a component of, Ulisa's illness.

E. Neurologic examination   ESSENTIAL

With the confusion, headache, neck pain and fever, a neurologic examination is indicated to look for signs of a central nervous system infection (the most likely being meningitis). Additionally, it assists in determining whether a lumbar puncture can be relatively safely performed if indicated. Finally, it permits evaluation for any signs (e.g., focal neurologic deficits, seizures, clonuses, myoclonus, or weakness) indicating that another neurologic condition might be present.

3. Diagnostic Studies

A. Blood culture and sensitivity (C&S) with Gram stain ESSENTIAL

With the degree of toxicity exhibited by Ulisa, blood cultures and sensitivities with Gram stains are definitely indicated. If possible, they should be performed before the initiation of an empiric antibiotic to maximize the yield of them producing the causative organism. However, if clinical judgment indicates the antibiotic cannot wait, it should be administered.

The purpose of the Gram stain is to ensure that the specimen is adequate for culture. However, it can supply some useful clinical information (e.g., identification of the type [rods, cocci, or both], configuration [paired, clumped, or linear], and stain uptake [positive or negative]), which can assist in making appropriate empiric antibiotic selections based on the potential pathogens involved in the infection.

The culture and sensitivity, if positive, can identify the exact bacterial pathogen and provide information regarding sensitivity and resistance of tested antibiotics to the organism. Unfortunately, these results are generally not available until 48 to 72 hours postprocedure.

B. Lumbar puncture (LP) with Gram stain, culture and sensitivity (C&S), and routine analysis of the cerebrospinal fluid (CSF)   ESSENTIAL

An LP with Gram stain, culture and sensitivity, and routine analysis of the CSF is also indicated. Again, the Gram stain and C&S will provide the same information as those performed on the blood, if an organism is identified, within the same time frame. Ideally, it should also be performed prior to the administration of antibiotics; however, if that is not possible, performing it within the 2-hour window following the antibiotics does not appear to alter the results.

The CSF analysis can provide confirmatory information of the presence of a central nervous system infection as well as whether it is most likely viral or bacterial in nature. For example, an increased opening pressure can be seen with meningitis; however, it is not specific for this condition. It can also be seen with any condition that can elevate the spinal or intracranial pressure (e.g., intracranial hemorrhage, tumors, hydrocephalus, jugular or superior vena cava obstructions, and other central nervous system infections). An extensive variation between the opening and closing pressure is most often associated with hydrocephalus.

Normally, the CSF is clear and thin in consistency. Infection can make it colored and purulent in appearance. A pinkish appearance or the appearance of gross blood can be caused by an intracranial bleed or a traumatic puncture. If caused by a traumatic puncture, the pinkish color decreases as more fluid is removed. The presence of blood and other metabolic conditions can also be responsible for discolorations of the CSF (e.g., melanoma, hyperbilirubinemia, hypercarotenemia, and protein elevations).

Red blood cells (RBCs) signify the amount of frank blood in the CSF. Normally, there should not be any present. However, an intracranial bleed or a traumatic puncture can elevate the RBC count. WBCs generally do not have any relationship to bleeding except if the spinal needle pierces a blood vessel during the procedure. In that case, more than 1 WBC for 500 RBCs is still considered to be pathologic. A few WBCs can normal be seen in CSF, and the number varies by age. However, if a significant amount is present, the most likely reason is meningitis, but other infections (e.g., cerebral abscesses, viral meningitis, and viral encephalitis) and cancers (e.g., leukemia, primary brain tumors, and metastatic brain lesions) can also cause an elevation in the number of WBCs present in the CSF. Neutrophils predominate in bacterial meningitis and cerebral abscesses. Lymphocytes predominate in viral meningitis, encephalitis, and meningitis secondary to TB.

In general, there is minimal protein in the CSF because it does not easily cross the blood–brain barrier; however, conditions such as meningitis, encephalitis, and myelitis can cause an elevation of total CSF protein.

Other tests of the CSF can provide additional clues to infection and other diseases. The glucose level in CSF decreases with a bacterial infection, inflammation, and/or a malignancy. The LDH elevates with bacterial infections and/or inflammation. Lactic acid (LA) can be seen in bacterial or fungal, but not viral, meningitis. And glutamine elevations are seen with hepatic encephalopathy and coma.

C. Complete blood count with differential (CBC w/diff) ESSENTIAL

A CBC w/diff is essential to perform because it provides additional information regarding the severity of the infection based primarily on the WBC count and provides clues to a bacterial or viral nature by a predominance of neutrophils or lymphocytes, respectively. Additionally, a normal platelet count provides some reassurance that there is currently no evidence of DIC, which is a serious complication of meningococcal disease (the most common organism causing both meningitis and dermal petechiae).

D. Electrolytes, serum glucose, blood urea nitrogen (BUN), creatinine, prothrombin time (PT), and partial thromboplastin time (PTT)   ESSENTIAL

A PT and PTT should also be performed to look for signs of DIC. The PT remains normal in DIC; however, the PTT is elevated in established DIC but is often decreased in early DIC.

Electrolytes are important to perform because they can provide information on Ulisa's hydration status. Vomiting and diarrhea can cause electrolyte disturbances such as hypokalemia, hypochloremia, hypercapnia, elevated carbon dioxide, and hyponatremia. However, true dehydration from the vomiting and diarrhea tends to produce hypokalemia with hyperchloremia. Additionally, serum potassium levels can be increased in acute infections.

The serum BUN and creatinine provide information regarding not only renal functioning but also hydration status. If both are elevated, then a renal problem is the most likely cause; if the BUN is elevated and the creatinine is normal, dehydration could be the culprit. However, there are a multitude of other conditions that could be responsible (e.g., gastrointestinal bleeding, congestive heart failure, myocardial infarction, or shock). That is why it is essential to "treat the patient, not the labs."

Finally, a blood glucose level should be performed to determine whether an undetected diabetes mellitus with or without ketoacidosis is the cause of Ulisa's confusion and/or the severity of her infection.

E. Polymerase chain reaction (PCR) testing of blood and cerebrospinal fluid (CSF) for *Neisseria meningitides*   ESSENTIAL

Based on Ulisa's history, physical examination, Gram stain findings of gram-negative diplococci, and knowledge of the most common pathogens associated with meningitis-like symptoms and petechiae, *Neisseria. meningitides* is the most likely etiologic agent for her infection. Therefore, PCR testing of blood and CSF fluid for *Neisseria meningitides* is appropriate.

On rare occasions, other bacterial infections (e.g., *Staphylococcus* and *Streptococcus*) can produce the combination of a petechial rash and meningitis-like symptoms. However, *Staphylococcus* is a gram-positive coccus that appears in irregular clusters and *Streptococcus* is a gram-positive coccus that appears in pairs or chains of varying lengths.

Viruses (e.g., rickettsia and echovirus) can also produce a similar clinical picture of meningitis-like symptoms associated with a petechial rash.

4. Diagnosis

A. Meningococcemia with meningitis   CORRECT

Meningococcemia with meningitis is caused by the gram-negative diplococci, *Neisseria meningitides*, and is characterized by rapidly progressing symptoms, petechiae, confusion, and meningitis. Based on the information thus far available, this is Ulisa's most likely diagnosis.

Other symptoms and complications can include DIC, seizures, sensorineural hearing loss, cranial nerve palsies, mental retardation, subdural empyemas, subdural effusions, and hydrocephalus.

B. Disseminated gonococcal infection (DGI) with meningitis INCORRECT

DGI is caused by a gram-negative diplococcus, *Neisseria gonorrhoeae*; however, the hallmark of the disease includes the slow development of symptoms, an intermittent fever, and true arthritis with or without tenosynovitis (especially of the knees, ankles, and wrists). Its rash can be maculopapular, pustular, or hemorrhagic; however, it is rarely petechial in nature. Meningitis is rare; and, if it does occur, it develops slowly over time. Thus, DGI with meningitis is not Ulisa's most likely diagnosis.

If DGI was confirmed as Ulisa's diagnosis, then child protective services must be notified to perform an investigation because the transmission of *Neisseria gonorrhoeae* is almost exclusively sexual after the neonatal period; thus, sexual abuse must be considered.

C. *Haemophilus influenzae* meningitis with disseminated intravascular coagulation (DIC)   INCORRECT

H. influenzae meningitis is meningitis caused by *Haemophilus influenzae*, which is a gram-negative bacillus, not a diplococcus. Furthermore, Ulisa's clinical signs and symptoms as well as her platelet count, PT, and PTT do not indicate the presence of DIC at this time. Thus, *Haemophilus influenzae* meningitis with DIC can be eliminated as Ulisa's most likely diagnosis.

D. Pneumococcal meningitis with dehydration   INCORRECT

Pneumococcal meningitis is caused by the gram-positive (not gram-negative) diplococci *Streptococcus pneumoniae*. Thus, pneumococcal meningitis with dehydration can be eliminated as Ulisa's most likely diagnosis.

E. Viral encephalitis   INCORRECT

Viral encephalitis generally has a gradual onset of symptoms. Lymphocytosis (not neutrophilia) tends to be the most common lymphocyte abnormality in both the serum and CSF of a patient with viral encephalitis. Additionally, Ulisa's CSF protein, glucose, LDH, and LA are more consistent with a bacterial, not a viral, process. Thus, this can be eliminated as Ulisa's most likely diagnosis.

5. Treatment Plan

A. Hospitalization   CORRECT

Because of her rapid decline to toxicity, her electrolyte disturbances, and the potential severity of her illness and its consequences, Ulisa needs to be hospitalized for monitoring and treatment.

B. IV dexamethasone with first dose of IV antibiotics   CORRECT

Studies have revealed that a single dose of IV dexamethasone along with, or 15 to 20 minutes prior to, the first dose of IV antibiotics has improved the outcome in children with meningococcal meningitis. However, in the absence of neurologic symptoms, it does not appear to alter the course of meningococcemia.

C. IV ceftriaxone every 12 hours   CORRECT

Ulisa should also receive empiric antibiotic therapy with IV ceftriaxone every 12 hours because it is the drug of choice for meningococcal meningitis. Once her C&S results are back, if there is another more appropriate option, then her antibiotic can be changed at that time.

D. IV vancomycin every 6 hours   INCORRECT

IV vancomycin every 6 hours is not effective in treating meningitis caused by *Neisseria meningitides* or meningococcemia and is therefore not an appropriate component of Ulisa's treatment plan.

E. GI rest and IV fluids to maintain hydration   CORRECT

GI rest and IV fluids are essential in all patients with meningococcemia to maintain hydration.

Epidemiologic and Other Data

In the United States, the age groups that most commonly affected by meningococcemia with meningitis are children younger than 5 years (particularly younger than 2 years) and late adolescence/early adulthood.

Risk factors include being immunocompromised, smoking cigarettes, being exposed to passive smoke, living in close proximity with others (e.g., military barracks and college dormitories), and being in close contact with someone else who has had the disease.

Vaccinations are now available for the prevention of meningococcal disease, including a polysaccharide vaccine (MPSV4) that is indicated for individuals between the ages of 2 and 10 years or older than the age of 55 years and a conjugate vaccine (MCV4) indicated for individuals from 11 to 55 years of age. The CDC's Advisory Committee on Immunization Practices recommends a single dose of the conjugate vaccine for 11- to 12-year-olds (or upon entrance to high school if not previously immunized). Furthermore, it is recommended for college freshmen who are going to live in dormitories if they have not been previously vaccinated. Additionally, they recommend the MPSV4 for children between the ages of 2 and 10 years who are at high risk of acquiring meningococcal disease (e.g., those with complement deficiencies, asplenia, or nonfunctioning spleen).

CASE 11-9
Van Watson
1. History

A. Has he been bothered by pruritus?   ESSENTIAL

Headaches frequently present a diagnostic challenge regardless of the clinical setting and specialty because they can represent a benign to serious headache disorder or they can be a symptom of an illness in virtually every organ system. Therefore, a comprehensive as possible history is essential to evaluate for the many potential causes.

Because Mr. Watson's headaches are associated with erythromelalgia, the possibility of a myeloproliferative disorder should rank high on his list of differential diagnoses. A symptom that is common in myeloproliferative disorders is pruritus following exposure to heat, including hot baths and showers. This phenomenon is presumably caused by the release of histamine from the elevated number of basophilic leukocytes. Thus, this is an essential follow-up question when pruritus is present.

B. Has he experienced any fatigue, night sweats, malaise, unintentional weight loss, fever, or chills?   ESSENTIAL

With the exception of chronic myeloid leukemia, myeloproliferative disorders are generally associated with fatigue but not many other constitutional symptoms; therefore, it is important to inquire about the presence of this and other constitutional symptoms (e.g., night sweats, malaise, unintentional weight loss, fever, or chills) to assist in ruling in or ruling out the various myeloproliferative disorders as the cause of Mr. Watson's headaches. Brain cancer can potentially be associated with any (or all) of these constitutional symptoms.

C. Is he experiencing any insomnia, appetite change, excessive worry, panic attacks, depression, difficulty with memory, anhedonia, or feelings of worthlessness?   ESSENTIAL

Additionally, because Mr. Watson is attributing his headaches to stress, it is important to rule out a stress-related mood disorder as the cause of or being associated with his headaches.

D. Has he experienced any abdominal pain, discomfort, or pressure?   ESSENTIAL

Myeloproliferative disorders are almost always associated with splenomegaly; therefore, it is important to inquire as to whether or not he has any symptoms suggestive of the condition.

E. Has he done any recent traveling or mountain climbing?   ESSENTIAL

A secondary cause of a myeloproliferative disorder, especially polycythemia, is hypoxia as a result high altitudes. Therefore, inquiring about any recent traveling or mountain climbing is important.

2. Physical Examination

A. Oxygen saturation and evaluation for hypoxia   ESSENTIAL

This is an essential component of Mr. Watson's physical examination because they will provide a gross estimate of the patient's oxygenation status. Hypoxia alone can cause headaches. Additionally, hypoxia can cause headaches in conjunction with a primary myeloproliferative disorder or secondary myeloproliferative disorder caused by pulmonary, cardiovascular, and neurologic conditions; high-altitude; and/or smoking.

B. Skin examination   ESSENTIAL

Because of his erythromelalgia, a skin examination is indicated.

C. Heart, lung, and pulse examination   ESSENTIAL

Heart, lung, and pulse examination are also indicated to evaluate for the presence of a primary or secondary pulmonary or cardiovascular condition that could account for his symptoms.

D. Abdominal examination   ESSENTIAL

Although Mr. Watson is not complaining of abdominal pain, an abdominal examination is still indicated because myeloproliferative disorders are included on his list of differential diagnoses. The presence of splenomegaly makes one of these disorders much more likely.

E. Neurologic examination   ESSENTIAL

A neurologic examination is indicated because Mr. Watson is complaining of a headache.

3. Diagnostic Studies

A. Computed tomography (CT) of the head, with and without contrast   ESSENTIAL

Although the primary working diagnosis for Mr. Watson's headaches is either a primary or secondary myeloproliferative disorder, he still requires a CT scan of his head to evaluate for structural problem(s) that might be responsible. This is indicated because he has a new-onset type of headache and is older than the age of 50 years. Furthermore, patients are not limited to a single diagnosis for their complaints.

B. Complete blood count with differential (CBC w/diff) and absolute reticulated platelet count   ESSENTIAL

A CBC w/diff and absolute reticulated platelet count can not only provide confirmation for the diagnosis of a myeloproliferative disorder but also to assist in determining which disorder is present and its severity. A manual platelet count is necessary because of the clumping that normally occurs with automated counts producing a 10 to 15% error in the results; and in Mr. Watson's case, an accurate count is essential.

C. Erythropoietin (EPO)   ESSENTIAL

Decreased oxygenation of one or both kidneys will stimulate the production of EPO. EPO then stimulates the bone marrow to produce more RBCs, which will result in improved renal oxygenation. When the renal hypoxia is decreased, the level of EPO decreases. Therefore, an EPO level is essential in determining which myeloproliferative disease, if any, is present.

D. Carboxyhemoglobin   ESSENTIAL

A carboxyhemoglobin level is indicated for Mr. Watson because one of his differential diagnoses is secondary polycythemia,

which can result from hypoxemia caused by coexisting pulmonary diseases (e.g., chronic bronchitis or lung cancer) or from a chronically elevated carboxyhemoglobin level caused by smoking. Furthermore, chronic low-dose CO_2 toxicity/exposure alone can result in headaches, lightheadedness, fatigue, and possibly even erythromelalgia.

E. Abdominal ultrasound   ESSENTIAL

An abdominal ultrasound is indicated for Mr. Watson because of his palpable spleen. This test will not only supply additional information regarding his spleen but also evaluate for a potential erythropoietin-secreting tumor in his kidneys, liver, pancreas, or gallbladder.

4. Diagnosis

A. Chronic myeloid leukemia   INCORRECT

Chronic myeloid leukemia is a myeloproliferative disorder that could account for Mr. Watson's symptoms; however, it is associated with a significant elevation of WBCs (median 150,000/mm³) and a normal HCT; thus, because of his CBC results, this can be eliminated as his most likely diagnosis.

B. Myelofibrosis   INCORRECT

Fibrosis of the bone marrow frequently occurs in conjunction with a myeloid metaplasis of the spleen and other organs. It is characterized by an abnormal RBC morphology with nucleation. Typically, a leukoerythroblastic anemia and thrombocytopenia are present. The total WBC count can be normal, elevated, or decreased. Because of Mr. Watson's CBC results, myelofibrosis can be eliminated as his most likely diagnosis.

C. Polycythemia vera   CORRECT

Polycythemia vera, or primary polycythemia, is a myeloproliferative disorder of the bone marrow that is characterized by an independent overproduction of erythroid cells that leads to an overproduction of all three of the primary hematopoietic cell lines, especially RBCs.

It can be distinguished from other myeloproliferative disorders by its elevated RBC count of normal morphology, its increased HCT, its normal to slightly elevated WBC count (rarely over 20,000 mm³) with a predominance of basophils and eosinophils, and a normal to elevated platelet count. Additionally, splenomegaly is almost always present. Thus, from the information thus far obtained, Mr. Watson's most likely diagnosis is polycythemia vera.

D. Secondary polycythemia   INCORRECT

Secondary polycythemia, in contrast to primary polycythemia, is caused by another disorder. Unlike polycythemia vera, it is not associated with splenomegaly or an increase in all three cell lines (only the HCT is elevated). Because of Mr. Watson's splenomegaly as well as an increase in all three cell lines being identified on his diagnostic studies, secondary polycythemia can be eliminated as Mr. Watson's most likely diagnosis.

E. Essential thrombocytosis   INCORRECT

Essential thrombocytosis is characterized by a significantly elevated platelet count (in some cases to levels exceeding 2,000,000/mm³) and a normal HCT. Even though the

WBC count can be normal to moderately elevated (rarely over 30,000/mm³), the RBC morphology is normal. Therefore, this can be eliminated as Mr. Watson's most likely diagnosis on the basis of his platelet count and HCT.

5. Treatment Plan

A. Phlebotomy, 1 unit every 7 days until HCT is less than 45%, then as necessary to maintain his HCT at 45% (but no more frequently than once every 7 days)   CORRECT

The treatment of choice for patients with polycythemia vera is phlebotomy consisting of the removal of 1 unit of blood every 7 days until the HCT is less than 45%. Then, the phlebotomies should be continued as necessary to maintain the HCT at 45%; however, maintenance treatment with phlebotomies should not be done more frequently than once every 7 days.

B. Hydroxyurea 500 to 1500 mg/day   INCORRECT

Hydroxyurea is approved by the FDA as a antineoplastic agent. However, it is utilized as a myelosuppressive agent to suppress the platelet count below 500,000/mm³. However, because Mr. Watson's platelet count is only 450,000/mm³, it is unnecessary for him to take this medication currently.

C. Low-dose aspirin 75 to 81 mg/day   CORRECT

Low-dose aspirin 75 to 81 mg/day is indicated for Mr. Watson and should be included in his treatment plan. It has been proven to be effective in reducing the risk of thrombosis without inducing excessive bleeding.

D. Diphenhydramine 25 to 50 mg every 4 to 6 hours as needed up to four times per day   CORRECT

Diphenhydramine 25 to 50 mg every 4 to 6 hours as needed up to four times a day has been shown to be effective in alleviating the pruritus associated with polycythemia vera; therefore, it is also an appropriate component of Mr. Watson's treatment plan. Second-generation antihistamines are not as effective but may be used if drowsiness or other side effects prevent the utilization of first-generation agents.

E. Daily paroxetine if diphenhydramine is ineffective   CORRECT

If the diphenhydramine (or other antihistamines) is ineffective, studies have shown that selective serotonin reuptake inhibitors (SSRIs) offer good benefit in alleviating the pruritus associated with polycythemia vera. However, they do not have FDA approval for this indication.

Epidemiologic and Other Data

The incidence of polycythemia vera is approximately 2 per 100,000 individuals in the United States The prevalence rate increases with age. The average age of presentation is 60 years. It is unusual for this condition to be seen in patients who are younger than 40 years.

It is theorized that this abnormality is caused by a genetic mutation in JAK2 because this signaling molecule has been identified in approximately 95% of all patients who have the condition. Polycythemia affects men at a slightly greater rate than it does women.

CASE 11-10
William Xylophone
1. History

A. How much ibuprofen and which formulation has she been giving him?   ESSENTIAL

Over-the-counter ibuprofen comes in a variety of strengths and dosing formulations. The oral drops provide 40 mg of ibuprofen per milliliter. The oral suspension contains 100 mg of ibuprofen per teaspoon (5 ml). The ibuprofen chewable tablets are available in either a 50- or 100-mg strength. The caplets contain 100 mg of ibuprofen each.

The recommended dosage for children older than the age of 6 months for fever below 102.5°F is 5 mg/kg every 6 to 8 hours as needed. However, for fevers above 102.5°F or pain, the recommended dose is 10 mg/kg divided every 6 to 8 hours as needed. Maximum daily dose is 40 mg/kg/day or 2400 mg.

With all of these options, it is easy for parents to under- or overdose their child. For example, William weighs 13.5 lb, or 6.1 kg (weight in pounds ÷ 2.2 = weight in kilograms), and is having pain; therefore, he should be taking 61 mg per dose (6.1 × 10 [mg/kg/dose] = 61), which is 1.5 ml of the ibuprofen oral drops (61 ÷ 40 [mg in each ml] = 1.5) every 6 to 8 hours as needed. However, his foster mother was only giving him 33% of that recommended dose.

Furthermore, the use of a medication dropper, a plastic syringe without a needle, or a measuring spoon is essential to ensure the patient received the correct dosage.

B. Has he been experiencing any skin lesions or facial edema?   ESSENTIAL

One of the conditions that must be explored when confronted with acute symmetric hand and foot swelling in an allergic process. By the hands and feet being involved as well as the edema being symmetrical, a systemic process is more likely than a contact dermatitis. Nevertheless, it is important to determine whether William is experiencing any other skin lesions or facial edema (e.g., perioral, periorbital, and eyelids) that would be consistent with this potential diagnosis. The prototypical skin lesions indicative of an allergic process are urticaria; however, many other manifestations can occur including macules, papules, plaques, vesicles, scaling, and/or excoriations.

C. Has she noticed any changes in his skin color, sclera, or urine?   ESSENTIAL

Another condition that must be included on William's differential diagnosis list is acute dactylitis caused by vascular occlusion from a sickle cell anemia. This is an especially important consideration because William is of African American descent and his sickle cell status is currently unknown. Because sickle cell disease is almost exclusively found in African Americans, it is important to inquire whether William has been experiencing any other signs or symptoms of the condition.

Because hemolytic anemia is virtually always present in patients with sickle cell syndrome, pallor may be evident, especially of the palpebral conjunctivae. However, it is critical to remember that all dermatologic conditions appear different in individuals of color. Subtle changes, can be easily overlooked, such as pallor in early anemia and jaundice in hepatic diseases. Therefore, it is essential to have a high index of suspicion and evaluate the patient's skin carefully.

Other symptoms/complications that can be associated with sickle cell disease/anemia include hematuria, inability to concentrate urine, renal failure, hyperbilirubinemia, hepatic diseases, and cholelithiasis; any of these could cause a change in the amount, frequency, or color of William's urine.

D. Which immunizations did he receive at his well-child examination?   ESSENTIAL

Fever, fussiness, anorexia, and slight decrease in activity are common immunization reactions. Foot and hand edema are not. Nevertheless, it is worthwhile to know which vaccines he received.

E. Is he being breast- or bottle-fed?   NONESSENTIAL

William is in foster care. Therefore, unless a "wet nurse" is being utilized (which is highly unlikely in the United States), he is not being bottle-fed. This question itself holds little, if any significance, regarding William's symptoms. However, specific questions regarding his diet (e.g., recent introduction of new items or amount of sodium) could be important.

2. Physical Examination

A. General appearance   ESSENTIAL

An assessment of the patient's overall appearance is an essential component of a physical examination regardless of the patient's chief complaint. In William's case the main concerns include how ill he appears, his hydration status, and overall impression of toxicity.

B. Eyes, ears, nose, and throat (EENT) examination   ESSENTIAL

An eye examination is essential to evaluate for the presence of icterus of his sclerae, suggesting an elevated bilirubin level; pallor of his conjunctivae, indicating a diagnosis of anemia; and the presence of lid edema, suggesting an allergic, metabolic, or cardiovascular abnormality.

His ears, nose, and throat should be examined for erythema, paleness, edema, or discharge suggesting an upper respiratory tract infection or allergic process.

C. Abdominal examination   ESSENTIAL

Although William does not seem to be having any abdominal pain, jaundice, vomiting, or bowel changes, an abdominal examination is still indicated because of the association of splenomegaly with sickle cell disease as well as other hereditary anemias and/or hemoglobinopathies.

Additionally, because RBC abnormalities are often associated with these conditions and total bilirubin (and its fractions) is produced from RBCs by the reticuloendothelial system, he also needs evaluation for the hepatomegaly.

D. Hand and foot examination   ESSENTIAL

A bilateral hand and foot examination is essential because this is what prompted William's foster mother to bring him in for evaluation. They need to be closely evaluated for joint swelling/involvement, tenderness, color change, temperature change, rash symmetry, and evidence of trauma.

E. Skin examination   ESSENTIAL

Even though William's foster mother has not noticed any discoloration or rashes, it is important to perform this examination with good exposure of the skin and in very good light. In individuals of color, minimal jaundice, mild erythema, slight pallor, and faint rashes are not always apparent under other light sources and exposure.

3. Diagnostic Testing

A. Complete blood count with differential (CBC w/diff) and manual smear   ESSENTIAL

Because William appears to have some pallor of his conjunctivae, nasal mucosa, and oral mucosa as well as being slightly febrile and underweight (when compared to his height and head circumference), a complete blood count with differential and manual smear to identify potential clues to his final diagnosis is essential.

The RBC indices provide much useful information regarding the various types of anemia. The mean corpuscular volume (MCV), a measurement of the size of the RBCs, and the mean corpuscular hemoglobin (MCH), a measurement of the weight of the RBCs, are correlated to permit the anemias to be divided into three general categories: microcytic, normocytic, and macrocytic. The mean corpuscular hemoglobin concentration (MCHC) is an expression of the hemoglobin concentration of RBCs. It permits further separation of the classification of anemias by determining whether they are hypochromic, normochromic, or hyperchromic. The combination of the volume plus the Hgb concentration assists in determining which diagnostic tests are indicated for the additional evaluation of the anemia, if present.

For example, a microcytic, hypochromic anemia is most commonly due to an established iron deficiency anemia, a thalassemia, or lead poisoning. But a normochromic, normocytic anemia can be caused by an early iron deficiency anemia, an acute blood loss, an aplastic anemia, or an acquired hemolytic anemia. However, if the anemia is macrocytic and normochromic, the most likely culprits are B_{12} and/or folate deficiencies, chemotherapy, or a medication.

The red blood cell distribution width (RDW) is calculated by the autocounter machine and confirmed by manual review of the slide. It determines the degree of anisocytosis, or variation, in the size and morphology of the RBCs. If anisocytosis is present, it can represent an atypical, congenital, or hereditary hematologic abnormality.

Generally, nowadays the indices are automatically determined by the autocounter. However, if not, they are simple to calculate. The MCV is obtained by multiplying the HCT by 10 and dividing the result by the RBC count. The MCH is calculated by multiplying the Hgb by 10 and dividing that amount by the RBC count. The MCHC is derived by multiplying the Hgb by 100 and dividing the result by the HCT.

B. Manual reticulocyte count and level   ESSENTIAL

A manual reticulocyte count and level are indicated because of the possibility of William having some type of anemia. This test and level are useful in determining the type of anemia checking the erythropoietin system's activity, and providing information regarding the functioning of the bone marrow. A manual count is required because RBCs with Howell-Jolly bodies (produced by hyposplenism) are often read by an automated counter as reticulocytes and will falsely elevate the result.

The reticulocyte index is determined by taking the patient's HCT and dividing it by the average, normal HCT for that patient based on age and gender; the result is then multiplied by the reticulocyte count (in %). If the index is then less than one, the bone marrow generally lacks the ability to compensate for anemia and a bone marrow test is indicated.

C. Blood typing and cross-match   ESSENTIAL

Because William appears to be markedly ill and anemias, including sickle-cell, are included in his differential diagnoses, he might require a blood transfusion; therefore, blood typing and cross-match would be appropriate to do at this time so that they are available if required.

D. Hemoglobin electrophoresis   ESSENTIAL

Normally a hemoglobin electrophoresis is not routinely ordered until the results of the CBC w/diff are available. However, because a hemoglobinopathy is strongly suspected in William's differential diagnoses and no prior testing is available, it should also be done at this time. The purpose of this test is to assist in determining which hemoglobinopathy is present based on the percentage of the types of hemoglobin tested—Hgb A_1, Hgb A_2, Hgb C, Hgb F, Hgb H, and Hgb S.

Normal adult hemoglobin is almost completely Hgb A_1, whereas fetal hemoglobin is virtually all Hgb F. In newborns, the majority of hemoglobin is still Hgb F. However, somewhere in the first year of life, most often between 6 and 12 months of age, γ-globin production is replaced by β-globin production and the values become essentially the same as those of adults. If the Hgb F fraction is still greater than 2% by the age of 3 years, a thorough evaluation for the cause must be undertaken. The most likely cause is a chronic hypoxia from a recognized or undiagnosed congenital cardiac defect.

E. Total, conjugated, and unconjugated bilirubin levels ESSENTIAL

Despite the fact that William is not jaundiced, the suspicion of a hemoglobinopathy justifies total, conjugated, and unconjugated bilirubin levels be performed.

With the breakdown of RBCs, heme and globin molecules are formed. From the heme molecules, biliverdin is manufactured by the body, which in turn is transformed into bilirubin. This type of bilirubin is considered to be unconjugated, or indirect, bilirubin. Normally, it makes up 70 to 85% of the total amount of bilirubin; however, in the presence of jaundice (or a slightly elevated total bilirubin level), if the percentage is 80 to 85% or greater, it is considered to be an unconjugated hyperbilirubinemia and dysfunction of the hepatic cells or accelerated RBC destruction is generally responsible; therefore, the diagnostic work-up is directed toward hepatocellular and hematologic abnormalities (e.g., hepatitis, cirrhosis, Gilbert syndrome, sickle cell disease/anemia, hemolytic anemia, and pernicious anemia).

However, unconjugated bilirubin is combined in the liver with a glucuronide to produce conjugated, or direct, bilirubin, which then leaves the liver via the intrahepatic pathway and moves to the hepatic duct and into the small intestines. Obviously, if 70 to 85% of all bilirubin is normally unconjugated, then only 15 to 30% is normally conjugated. However, in the presence of jaundice (or a slightly elevated total bilirubin level), if the percentage is 50% or greater, it is considered to be a conjugated hyperbilirubinemia and extrahepatic obstructions (e.g., cholelithiasis, cholestasis, ductal obstructions anywhere along the pathway, or Dubin-Johnson syndrome) are the most likely cause.

Jaundice is generally not clinically apparent until the total bilirubin level is greater than or equal to 2.5 mg/dl.

4. Diagnosis

A. Acute gastrointestinal blood loss and cholestasis from ibuprofen   INCORRECT

Although ibuprofen can cause GI bleeding, it would be rare for it to occur after only three doses. Furthermore, acute gastrointestinal blood loss should result in a black, tarry-appearing stool or gross blood in the stool, which William did not have. Anemia caused by acute blood loss is generally a normocytic, normochromic anemia, whereas William has a microcytic, normochromic anemia. Ibuprofen is not known to cause cholestasis, which generally produces a conjugated hyperbilirubinemia. However, it has been associated with rare cases of hepatitis, which could cause unconjugated hyperbilirubinemia. Nevertheless, acute gastrointestinal blood loss and cholestasis from ibuprofen is not William's most likely diagnosis.

B. Hand-foot syndrome of sickle cell anemia   CORRECT

The pain of hand-foot syndrome of sickle cell anemia is a result of dactylitis produced by bony infarcts, which are caused by emboli produced by the "sickled cells" seen in sickle cell anemia. This finding is characteristic of infants with sickle cell anemia. This, combined with an atypical anemia pattern combination (microcytic, normochromic), the presence of predominately Hgb S on the hemoglobin electrophoresis, and the mild unconjugated hyperbilirubinemia, essentially establishes this as William's most likely diagnosis.

C. Sickle cell trait arthropathy   INCORRECT

Sickle cell trait rarely produces any symptoms unless the patient is at a high altitude; then, an arthropathy is possible. However, the finding of an anemia and RBC abnormality on William's CBC is inconsistent with this diagnosis. Furthermore, the hemoglobin electrophoresis of a patient with sickle cell trait consists of 60 to 80% of Hgb A_1 and 20 to 40% of Hgb S, plus a maximum of 2% of Hgb F and 2 to 3% of Hgb A_2. Thus, this is not his most likely diagnosis.

D. Thalassemia major   INCORRECT

The anemia from thalassemia major is microcytic and generally normochromic. The hemoglobin electrophoresis of thalassemia major consists of 65 to 100% of Hgb F, 5 to 20% of Hgb A_1, and 2 to 3% of Hgb A_2. Additionally, it is most often found in individuals of Mediterranean descent, not African. Hence, thalassemia major is not William's most likely diagnosis.

E. Viral syndrome and iron deficiency anemia   INCORRECT

Other than a fever, William has very few symptoms that are consistent with a viral syndrome. Additionally, iron deficiency anemia is normocytic, normochromic in its early stages or microcytic, hypochromic in its later stages; William's anemia pattern is consistent with neither. Therefore, viral syndrome and iron deficiency anemia are not his most likely diagnosis.

5. Treatment Plan

A. Increase ibuprofen oral drops to 1.5 ml every 6 to 8 hours as needed for pain/fever up to four times per day and return if still symptomatic in 2 days   INCORRECT

Having William's foster mother increase his ibuprofen oral drops to 1.5 ml every 6 to 8 hours as needed for pain/fever up to four times per day would at least put him at the proper dosage. However, its use in sickle cell disease is controversial. Some experts feel that it is a viable option for mild to minor vaso-occlusive crises. However, others are concerned that with significant anemia, thrombopenia, and a hemoglobinopathy, ibuprofen might put him at a greater risk of internal bleeding despite the fact that ibuprofen does not have any direct platelet effect. Nevertheless, there have been cases where it has been known to interact with warfarin, causing the international normalized ratio (INR) to elevate. Additionally, some experts believe that for a sickle cell anemia vaso-occlusive crisis, narcotic analgesics are justified. Regardless, because he is younger than 1 year of age, has an Hgb less than 6.0 g/dl, and his total platelets are less than 150,000/mm^3, he should not be treated as an outpatient.

B. Hospitalize   CORRECT

Additional criteria for hospitalization include temperature greater than 40°C (or 104°F), WBC count less than 5000/mm^3 or greater than 30,000/mm^3, dyspnea, pulmonary infiltrates, prior episode of sepsis, two or more visits during the same episode, or uncertain/unreliable follow-up.

To convert Fahrenheit temperatures to Celsius, take the temperature in Fahrenheit and subtract 32 from it, multiply this sum by 5, and take the result and divide it by 9. Therefore, William's rectal temperature was 101.1 − 32 = 69.1; 69.1 × 5 = 345.5; 408.5 ÷ 9 = 38.4°C.

To convert Celsius temperatures to Fahrenheit, take the temperature in Celsius and multiply it by 9, divide this result by 5, and add 32 to the result. For example, to determine whether the hospitalization criteria of 40°C is met by William, 40 × 9 = 360; 360 ÷ 5 = 72; 72 + 32 = 104°F.

C. Provide blood transfusion   CORRECT

Blood transfusions are recommended for all sickle cell anemia patients who have an Hgb that is 1.5 g/dl below their average. The goal of these transfusions is to increase the Hgb to 8 to 9 g/dl. Because William's baseline Hgb is unknown, it seems reasonable to transfuse him to these levels.

D. Refer for splenectomy   INCORRECT

Splenectomies are almost always reserved for children who are older than the age of 2 years. Hence, it is not currently indicated for William because he is younger than 2 years old. Studies indicate that patients in this age group do better with blood transfusions compared with surgical solutions.

E. Ensure adequate hydration and pain control   CORRECT

Adequate hydration and pain control are considered to be essential mainstays in the treatment of any type of sickle cell anemia/disease. Most experts recommend replacing IV fluids at 1.5 times the normal rate and not hesitating to use narcotics when indicated. Pain management is difficult when dealing with very small children.

In a child as young as William, it is difficult to determine exactly how much pain he is experiencing. He certainly cannot quantify it on a scale of 1 to 10. Even the face pain scales are too advanced for him to comprehend. They are indicated for children from the age of 5 to 12 years.

Currently, the FLACC scale is the best objective measurement of pain in infants and younger children such as William. FLACC stands for **f**ace, **l**egs, **a**ctivity, **c**ry, and **c**onsolability. Each category is given between 0 and 2 points depending on where they fall on the scale. For example, regarding the leg, 0 points would be provided if the child is lying quietly and moves normally; 1 point is provided if the child appears to be squirming, moves back and forth, and appears tense; and 2 points are assigned if there is rigidity, jerking, or arching of the back. This is repeated for the other four categories, with 0 being essentially asymptomatic and 2 experiencing significant discomfort/frustration/aggravation. Because a maximum of 2 points is provided in each of five categories, the score can easily be related to the adult version of selecting a number from 1 to 10.

Epidemiologic and Other Data

In the United States, sickle cell disease is found almost exclusively in African Americans. It is estimated that approximately 7% of African Americans carry the trait and 0.5% are affected by this genetic disorder. It can also be found in individuals who are descendants from southern Mediterranean countries. Only 50% of patients affected by sickle cell disease live beyond their 45th birthday.

REFERENCES/ADDITIONAL READING

Aghababian RV, ed. *Essentials of Emergency Medicine.* Sudbury, MA: Jones & Bartlett Publishers; 2006.
  Basior JM. Red blood cell disorders. 267–271.
  Murphy P, Bachur R, Manno M, O'Neill, Brent A, Harrison K. Infectious diseases.550–569.
  Nichols CG, Schmidt E. Viral infections. 168–169.
  Singletary EM, Holstege CP. Bites and stings: insects, marine, mammals, and reptiles. 771–782.
  Volturo GA, Griffin J, Germano T, Brunell A, Schmidt J, et al. Bacterial infections. 309–328.
Centers for Disease Control and Prevention (CDC) Advisory Committee on Immunization Practices (ACIP). Recommended adult immunization schedule–United States, 2010. *MMWR Quick Guide.* 2010;59(1):1–4.
Centers for Disease Control and Prevention (CDC) Advisory Committee on Immunization Practices (ACIP). Recommended immunization schedules for persons aged 0 through 18 years–United States, 2010. *MMWR Quick Guide.* 2010;58(51, 52):1–4
Centers for Disease Control and Prevention (CDC) Advisory Committee on Immunization Practices; Healthcare Infection Control Practices Advisory Committee. Preventing tetanus, diphtheria, and pertussis among adults; use of tetanus toxoid, reducing diphtheria toxoid and acellular pertussis vaccines recommendations of the Advisory

Committee on Immunization Practices (ACIP) and recommendations of ACIP, supported by the Healthcare Infection Control Practices Advisory Committee (HICPAC), for use of Tdap among healthcare personnel. *MMWR Recomm Rep*. 2006;55(RR-17):1–37.

Centers for Disease Control and Prevention. Sexually transmitted diseases treatment guidelines, 2006. *MMWR*. 2006;55(RR-11):1–94.

Dienstag JL, McHutchison JG. American Gastroenterological Association technical review on the management of hepatitis C. *Gastroenterology*. 2006;130(1):231–264.

Dworkin RH, Johnson RW, Breuer J, et al. Recommendations for the management of herpes zoster. *Clin Infect Dis*. 2007;44(suppl 1):S1–S26.

Fauci AS, Kasper DL, Longo DL, et al., eds. *Harrison's Principles of Internal Medicine*. 17th ed. New York: McGraw-Hill Medical; 2008.
  Auerbach PS, Norris RL. Disorders caused by reptile bites and marine animal exposures. 2741–2748.
  Dienstag JL. Acute viral hepatitis. 1932–1949.
  Dienstag JL. Toxic and drug-induced hepatitis. 1949–1955.
  Ghany M, Hoofnagle JH. Approaches to the patient with liver disease. 1918–1923.
  Halperin SA. Pertussis and other bordetella infections. 933–936.
  Holmes KK. Sexually transmitted infections: overview and clinical approach. 821–835.
  Langford, CA, Gilliland BC. Arthritis associated with systemic disease, and other arthritides. 2177–2184.
  McCall CO, Lawley TJ. Eczema, psoriasis, cutaneous infections, acne, and other common skin disorders. 312–320.
  Pollack RJ, Maguire JH. Ectoparasite infestations and arthropod bites and stings. 2748–2754.
  Pratt DS, Kaplan MM. Evaluation of liver function. 1923–1926.
  Spach DH, Darby E. Bartonella infections, including cat-scratch disease. 987–990.
  Spivak JL. Polycythemia vera and other myeloproliferative diseases. 671–677.
  Wessels MR. Streptococcal and enterococcal infections. 881–890.
  Wetzler LM. Meningococcal infections. 908–914.
  Whitley RJ. Varicella-zoster virus infections. 1002–1005.

Foucault C, Brouqui P, Raoult D. Bartonella quintana characteristics and clinical management. *Emerg Infect Dis*. 2006;12(2):217–223.

Gershman K. Dermatology. 12.1 Skin problems (benign and malignant). In: Gershman K. (Onion DK, series ed.). *The Little Black Book of Geriatrics*, 3rd ed. Sudbury, MA: Jones and Bartlett; 2006:425–432.

Gilbert ND, Moellering RC Jr, Eliopoulos GM, Sande MA, eds. Clinical approach to the initial choice of antimicrobial therapy. In: Gilbert ND, Moellering RC Jr, Eliopoulos GM, Sande MA, eds. *The Sanford Guide to Antimicrobial Therapy 2008*. 38th ed. Sperryville, VA: Antimicrobial Therapy Inc; 2008:4–58.

Greaves MW. Itch in systemic disease: therapeutic options. *Dermatol Ther*. 2005;18(4):327–327.

Headache Classification Subcommittee of the International Headache Society. The international classification of headache disorders, 2nd ed. *Cephalalgia*. 2004;24(Sept. 1).

Heymann WR. Itch. *J Am Acad Dermatol*. 2006;54(4):705–706.

Kroger AT, Atkinson WL, Marcuse EK, Pickering LK. Advisory Committee on Immunization Practices (AICP), Centers for Disease Control and Prevention (CDC). General recommendations on immunization: recommendations of the Advisory Committee on Immunization Practices (ACIP). *MMWR*. 2006;55(RR-15):1–48.

Lalani A, Schneeweiss S, eds. *The Hospital for Sick Children: Handbook of Pediatric Emergency Medicine*. Sudbury, MA: Jones & Bartlett Publishers; 2008.
  Ansari, K, Pope E. Dermatology. 399–408.
  Jarvis DA, Kirby M. Sickle cell disease. 275–285.
  Schneeweiss S. Meningitis and encephalitis. 259–265.
  Schneeweiss S. Pain management. 503–510.

Luba KM, Stulberg DL. Chronic plaque psoriasis. *Am Fam Physician*. 2006;73(4):636–644.

Merkel SI, Voepel-Lewis T, Shayevitz JR, Malyvia S. The FLACC; a behavioral scale for scoring postoperative pain in young children. *Pediatr Nurs*. 1997;23(2):293–297.

National Center for Infectious Diseases, Centers for Disease Control and Prevention, Advisory Committee on Immunization Practices. Prevention and control of meningococcal disease: recommendations of the Advisory Committee on Immunization Practices (ACIP). *MMWR Recomm Rep*. 2005;54(RR-7):1–21.

Onion DK, series ed. *The Little Black Book of Primary Care*. 5th ed. Sudbury, MA: Jones & Bartlett Publishers; 2006.
  Onion DK, Sahn E. Dermatology. 3.2 Dermatoses. 173–190.
  Onion DK, Sahn E. Dermatology. 3.5 Miscellaneous. 203–220.
  Onion DK. Gastroenterology. 6.4 Hepatic diseases. 352–373.
  Onion DK. Hematology/oncology. 8.3 Hemoglobinopathies. 454–463.
  Onion DK. Hematology/oncology. 8.8 Myeloproliferative disorders. 484–491.
  Onion DK, Sears S. Infectious diseases. 9.2 Gram-positive organisms. 528–543.
  Onion DK, Sears S. Infectious disease. 9.3 Gram-negative organisms. 543–572.
  Onion DK, Sears S. Infectious disease. 9.8 Rickettsia and related organisms. 601–607.
  Onion DK, Sears S. Infectious diseases. 9.21 Viral infections. 666–706.

Pagana KD, Pagana TJ. *Mosby's Diagnostic and Laboratory Test Reference*. 8th ed. St. Louis: Mosby Elsevier; 2007 (multiple pages utilized to provide normal reference values for laboratory tests).

Saucier JR. Arachnoid envenomation. *Emerg Med Clin North Am*. 2004;22(2):405–422.

Singh M, Lingappan K. Whooping cough: the current scene. *Chest*. 2006;130(5):1547–1553.

Smith CH, Barker JNWN. 1. Psoriasis and its management. *BMJ*. 2006;333(7547):380–384.

Stuart MJ, Nagel RL. Sickle-cell disease. *Lancet*. 2004; 364(9442):1343–1360.

Terreri A. Polycythemia vera: a comprehensive review and clinical recommendations. *Mayo Clin Proc*. 2003;78(2):174–194.